Maternal-Newborn Nursing

Care of the Growing Family

THIRD EDITION

Maternal-Newborn Nursing | *Care of the Growing Family*

Adele Pillitteri, R.N., P.N.A., B.S.N., M.S.N.

**Professor of Nursing,
Chairperson, Advanced Department of Nursing**

*Niagara University
Niagara Falls, New York*

Little, Brown and Company

Boston   Toronto

To Joe, with love

Library of Congress Cataloging in Publication Data

Pillitteri, Adele.
  Maternal-newborn nursing.

  Includes bibliographies and index.
    1. Obstetrical nursing.   2. Infants (Newborn)—
Care and hygiene.   3. Infants (Newborn)—Diseases—
Nursing.   I. Title.   [DNLM: 1. Obstetrical Nursing.
2. Pediatric Nursing.   WY 157 P641n]
RG951.P64   1985   610.73'678   84–29738
ISBN 0–316–70794–5

Library of Congress Catalog Card No. 84–29738

ISBN 0–316–70794–5

9 8 7 6 5 4 3 2 1

Published simultaneously in Canada
by Little, Brown & Company (Canada) Limited

Printed in the United States of America

Credits

Table 1–3: From T. H. Holmes and R. H. Rahe, "The Social Readjustment Rating Scale," from *Journal of Psychosomatic Research* 2:214 (1967). Reprinted by permission.

Table 2–6, 2–7: From The Robert Wood Johnson Foundation, Princeton, NJ, *Special Report*, No. 2 (1978). Reprinted by permission of The Robert Wood Johnson Foundation.

Text excerpt and Table 4–2: From E. M. Duvall, *Marriage and Family Development*, Fifth Edition. Reprinted by permission of J. B. Lippincott Company.

Table 8–1: From J. M. Tanner, *Growth at Adolescence*, Second Edition. Reprinted by permission of Blackwell Scientific Publications, Oxford, England.

Table 9–5: Adapted from G. Abraham, "Nutritional Factors in the Etiology of the Premenstrual Tension Syndrome," in *Journal of Reproductive Medicine* 28 (1983). Reprinted by permission.

Table 11–1: From J. G. Dryfoos, "Contraceptive Use, Pregnancy Intentions, and Pregnancy Outcomes Among U.S. Women," in *Family Planning Perspectives* 14 (1982). Reprinted by permission.

Table 11–3: Adapted from A. Torres and J. D. Forrest, "The Costs of Contraception," in *Family Planning Perspectives* 15 (1983). Reprinted by permission.

Table 12–1: From R. W. Kistner, *Gynecology Principles and Practices*, Third Edition. Reprinted by permission of Year Book Medical Publishers, Chicago.

Table 13–1: From J. Rose (Chapter 12) in G. Caplan (Editor) *Preventions of Mental Disorders in Children: Initial Explorations* (1961). Reprinted by permission of Basic Books, Inc.

Table 13–2: From L. McNall and J. T. Galeener (Editors) *Current Practice in Obstetric and Gynecologic Nursing* (Volume 1) (1976). Reprinted by permission of C. V. Mosby Company.

Figure 14–4: From R. S. Snell, *Clinical Embryology for Medical Students*, Second Edition (1975). Reprinted by permission of Little, Brown and Company.

Table 18–12: From C. Mahan and S. McKay, "Let's Reform

(continued on page 1214)

Preface

Consumers' demands for better health care and the expanding limits of practice within the nursing profession pose a dual challenge for both students of nursing and educators. Scientific and technical knowledge that applies to the field of maternal-newborn nursing is increasing faster than ever. Yet this rapid growth in knowledge and information means that less time is available in nursing programs to cover every aspect of care.

Maternal-Newborn Nursing: Care of the Growing Family is written with this challenge in mind. Covering nursing care of the mother and family from planning of pregnancy through the child's first weeks, this third edition, like previous editions, is intended for use in a single course in maternal-newborn nursing or for a curriculum in which concepts of maternal-newborn care are integrated throughout the program. This book will also be useful for graduate nurses who are interested in reviewing or expanding their knowledge on this subject. A companion volume, *Child Health Nursing: Care of the Growing Family*, follows the child and family from the child's birth through adolescence.

Several themes vital in studying maternal-newborn care are emphasized throughout this new edition:

— Childbirth as a family-centered event.
— Pregnancy and childbirth as a time of wellness; the nurse's role in both ambulatory and in-patient settings in emphasizing health maintenance in preference to restoration of health.
— The nursing process as the basis of nursing care.
— The ability to form a nursing diagnosis from assessment data. Nursing diagnoses from the North American Association of Nursing Diagnoses are included where appropriate.
— The importance of nursing research as a method by which nursing progresses.
— Changing areas of practice, such as the increase in alternative birth centers; the increase in the rate of cesarean birth; the effects of pregnancy both on adolescents and on women of more than thirty years of age having their first child; the pregnant handicapped woman; and the frequency with which trauma strikes pregnant women because of the frequency of automobile accidents among young adults.

— Common drugs used in maternal-newborn nursing. A separate drug compendium is provided in Appendix A as a quick reference source.

Each chapter is organized to provide a complete learning experience. Important elements include:

— *Objectives*. These learning objectives are included at the beginning of each chapter to illustrate the most important concepts to be covered and to help the student understand what behavioral outcomes are expected after the material in that chapter is mastered.
— *Procedures*. Techniques of common procedures specific to maternal-newborn care are boxed and presented in list format for easy reference.
— *Nursing Care Highlights*. Material that is necessary for quick reference or for safe practice is boxed for special emphasis.
— *Nursing Research Highlights*. These boxes summarizing research carried out by nurses on topics related to maternal-newborn nursing appear throughout the text.
— *Utilizing Nursing Process* and *Nursing Care Planning*. These sections follow most chapters and serve as summaries and care applications of the nursing process.
— *Questions for Review*. Each chapter has a list of multiple-choice and discussion questions designed to help you review the material covered in the chapter. The answers to the multiple-choice questions appear in Appendix I.
— *Suggested Readings*. At the end of each chapter is a list of up-to-date readings relevant to the topics of that chapter. Reference works have been chosen that are readily available in most nursing school libraries.

Like that of previous editions, the content in this third edition is organized so that the entire cycle of pregnancy, labor, delivery, and newborn care is presented first as a wellness phenomenon; illness associated with pregnancy or the newborn is covered in the last part of the text. In response to feedback from users of the second edition, coverage of complications during the childbearing process has been greatly expanded: nine chapters on specific topics related to the high-risk mother and newborn have been added. The emphasis, however, remains on childbearing as a normal and healthy family process. The psychosocial implications of this process are considered throughout and much attention is given to anticipation of the needs of the childbearing family during one of the most thrilling, yet often stress-producing, events in their lives.

Unit I, Maternal-Newborn Nursing, introduces the book's subject. A framework is presented for practice, and standards and theories of nursing as well as ethical and legal considerations and current trends in practice are discussed.

Unit II, Childbearing in Today's World, places maternal-newborn nursing in the context of the family and community; the effect of culture on childbearing practices and the nurse's role as a genetic counselor are discussed.

Unit III, The Interpartal Period, is a discussion of how important are both developmental and physiological readiness for childbearing, as well as the physiology of reproduction, sexuality, and reproductive life planning. The nurse's role with couples who are infertile is studied, as are also problems of menstruation, such as premenstrual syndrome and toxic shock syndrome.

In Unit IV, The Prepartal Period: Preparing for Parenthood, all aspects of normal pregnancy, including diagnosis of pregnancy, psychological and physiologic changes in the mother during pregnancy, growth and development of the fetus, and the nurse's role in providing high-quality prenatal care, including teaching and counseling of nutrition are discussed.

Unit V, The Period of Parturition, covers both the psychological and physiologic processes of labor. The nurse's role in providing high-quality nursing care in alternative birth settings and with a minimum of analgesia and anesthesia is stressed.

Unit VI, The Postpartal Period: Parenthood, covers both the psychological and physiologic changes in this period, emphasizing the nurses' roles in providing high-quality nursing care to set the stage for both infant and family health.

In Unit VII, The Newborn, both psychological and physiologic development of the newborn and the nurse's role in health assessment and in counseling on nutrition and infant care are discussed.

Unit VIII, High-Risk Pregnancy, introduces the concept of the high-risk mother. In these chapters, both the woman with preexisting illness and the woman who develops a complication in pregnancy, labor and delivery, or the postpartal period are discussed. In separate chapters, the woman at age extremes, the injured woman, trauma and pregnancy, teratogens and fetal health, and specific problems of cesarean birth are covered.

Unit IX, The High-Risk Newborn, introduces the concept of the high-risk newborn. In specific chapters the newborn with a congenital anomaly, the newborn who is ill at birth, and the newborn who is born with an abnormal gestation age or birth weight are discussed.

Appendixes supply quick reference to drugs commonly used in the maternity setting, organizations connected with childbearing, recommendations for family-centered care, rights of the pregnant woman, normal laboratory values, and growth charts. A full glossary defines terms used in maternal-newborn nursing.

To help instructors use the text most effectively, an *Instructor's Manual* prepared by Ann Lyness and Kathy Ammon of the University of Pittsburgh is available. This manual provides a summary, terminology list, suggested classroom and clinical activities, and multiple-choice and discussion questions for each chapter in the text. In addition, several "Teacher's Corner" sections throughout assemble special information on specific teaching matters.

For consistency, the term "patient" is used to describe a person for whom a nurse provides care. The present broad definition indicates a person during health or illness. The reason for this choice (rather than "client") is semantic: care is presented with the belief that people should have input into their care, no matter which term is used to describe them. For readability, nurses are most often referred to as "she," but this does not mean to suggest that men do not also provide maternal-newborn nursing care of high quality. Also for readability, the people significant to a patient are referred to as "support people" or "family" rather than the redundant "significant others."

Contributors

I would like to express a special thanks to the following contributors to this edition of *Maternal-Newborn Nursing*:

Jayson B. Bulmahn, R.P.H., Pharmacist, DeGraff Hospital, North Tonawanda, New York, *Drug Compendium*; Mary Fruscione, R.N., C.P.N.P., M.S. Ed., M.S.N., Assistant Professor, College of Nursing, Niagara University, Niagara Falls, New York, *Research Highlights*; Carol A. Patti, R.N., C.P.N.P., M.S. Ed., M.S.N., Assistant Professor, College of Nursing, Niagara University, Niagara Falls, New York, *Research Highlights*.

Acknowledgments

I would also like to thank the following reviewers who provided many helpful comments and suggestions throughout the revision process: Nedra Caccomo, R.N., M.S., Assistant Professor, Division of Nursing, Saint Joseph College, West Hartford, Connecticut; Verna Carson, B.S., M.S., Assistant Professor, College of Nursing, University of Maryland, Baltimore, Maryland; Susan Leonard, Ph.D., R.N., Assistant Professor, College of Nursing, Tcxas Woman's University, Dallas, Texas; Sharon McGowan, R.N., M.S.N., formerly Instructor of Maternal-Child Nursing/ College of Nursing, University of South Carolina, Columbia, South Carolina; Frances Monahan, Ph.D., R.N., Professor and Chair, Department of Nursing, Rockland Community College, Suffern, New York.

I would also like to express my sincere appreciation to Brian S. Smistek and Timothy R. Palaszewski, Department of Medical Photography, Children's Hospital, Buffalo, New York, for their photographic skill; Eileen Walsh, Graphic Designer, Niagara University, Niagara Falls, New York, for her excellent illustrations; Mary and Mary Lynn Fruscione, JoAnn and Charles Brunetto, Arlene and Paul Dietrick, and Carol Gutt for their willingness to pose for photographs; and Ann West and Sally Stickney, Little, Brown editors, George McLean, designer, and Max Cavitch, editorial assistant, for their assistance and guidance throughout the project.

I hope that this third edition of *Maternal-Newborn Nursing: Care of the Growing Family* not only provides students with the basic knowledge and philosophy needed to meet the challenges offered by nursing practice today, but also that it gives information in a manner that is as interesting and enjoyable as reading and learning about maternal-newborn nursing care should be.

A.P.

Contents

VIII

High-Risk Pregnancy   787

Notice

The indications and dosages of all drugs in this book have been recommended in the medical literature and conform to the practices of the general medical community. The medications described do not necessarily have specific approval by the Food and Drug Administration for use in the diseases and dosages for which they are recommended. The package insert for each drug should be consulted for use and dosage as approved by the FDA. Because standards for usage change, it is advisable to keep abreast of revised recommendations, particularly those concerning new drugs.

I

Maternal-Newborn Nursing

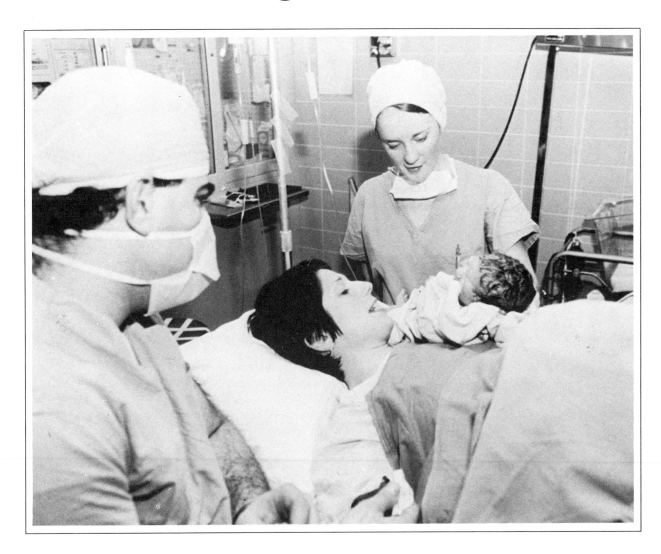

1

A Framework for Maternal-Newborn Nursing

OBJECTIVES

Following mastery of the content of this chapter, you should be able to

1. Describe the evolution and scope of maternal-newborn nursing.
2. Describe the concept of childbearing as a time of crisis in people's lives.
3. Identify the goals of maternal-newborn nursing.
4. Identify generally accepted assumptions or philosophies of maternal-newborn nursing.
5. Analyze the ANA standards for maternal-newborn nursing and their implications for care.
6. Synthesize a framework for maternal-newborn nursing utilizing theoretical, personal, and professional guidelines.

A SPERM AND AN OVUM meet in the velvety softness of a fallopian tube. They fuse. A pregnancy begins.

Subtle changes start in the woman's body. She wakes in the morning with nausea. She looks in a mirror and notices a glow in her face. She finds herself humming while she is doing dishes one morning. She visits a physician, who tells her that what she has suspected is true: She is pregnant. The doctor shows her a calendar and circles a date. On that day, a Monday in March, seven months away, she will give birth. Pregnancy should be uncomplicated. A nurse-midwife will follow her during pregnancy and help her at delivery.

The woman tells no one but her husband about her pregnancy, yet everyone who knows her seems to guess her secret. Her walk, her preoccupation with herself, and finally her growing abdomen betray her.

One afternoon at work she feels a flutter inside her abdomen. She wonders what is happening, then laughs as she realizes this strange new feeling inside her is one she has been longing to experience: the feel of life. She begins to visualize and plan for this new person who is to be by contemplating her life and her readiness to care for another life. She questions her ability to be a mother, her ability to deliver the child, her ability to love a stranger.

She and her husband choose a paint color for the baby's room and buy some stuffed animals. They wait. They rehearse children's names. They wait. They practice breathing for contractions. They wait. And at the end, after she takes a leave from work, she grows impatient and angry with waiting. The months seem to stretch out ahead of her as she grows uncomfortable and angry with her pregnant body.

Finally, when it seems as if she cannot wait any longer, she wakes at night to contractions, announcement of the child's readiness as well as her own. The contractions grow stronger. She goes with her husband to a hospital. The contractions strengthen and change. She pushes. The child is born.

The child cries with a first breath. Both parents laugh with exhilaration. The woman has just participated in an experience that only half the population of the world can ever experience. Both she and her husband have come through a crisis period in their lives with new self-esteem and confidence in themselves and in each other.

Of course not all children are greeted with such joy when they are born, nor will all children be given good care as they grow. It is foolish to believe that all people should be or need to be parents to find personal fulfillment. For the person who chooses this life style, however, the moment of delivery of a child can provide unmatched fulfillment. Being with a couple through a pregnancy and delivery in a nursing role can likewise be unmatched as a source of job satisfaction.

Definition of Maternal-Newborn Nursing

Obstetrics is the branch of medicine that deals with the medical management of pregnancy, parturition (labor and delivery), and the puerperium (the 6-week period following childbirth). The word *obstetrics* is derived from the Latin word *obstetrix*, meaning "midwife," or the person who "stands by" (*obstare*) a woman during childbirth. In light of the range of increased responsibilities and concerns now involved in the care of a woman throughout pregnancy and childbirth, the older term *obstetrical nursing* has been replaced by the more descriptive and broader terms *maternal-newborn nursing* or *perinatal nursing*. Because the father of the new child is always included in planning and care, an even better description of this area of nursing today might be *parental-newborn nursing*. That the father of the child or the woman's important support person is always included in planning and implementing

Nursing Care Highlight

Philosophy of Maternal-Newborn Nursing

1. Pregnancy is a stress circumstance because it is a maturational crisis. It alters family life in both subtle and extensive ways.
2. Not only do adults and children have the right to be healthy; a newborn has a right to be *born* healthy.
3. The maternal-newborn nurse serves as an advocate to protect the rights of the fetus as well as of the woman and family.
4. Pregnancy, labor and delivery, and the puerperium are part of a continuum of a total life cycle. They are meaningful only in the context of a total life.
5. Personal, cultural, and religious attitudes and beliefs influence the meaning of pregnancy for individuals and make each experience unique.
6. Maternal-newborn nursing is family cen-

tered. The father of the child is as important as the mother.
7. Maternal-newborn nursing is research oriented, always trying to achieve optimal health for women and their fetuses/newborns.
8. Maternal-newborn nursing is community centered: The health of individuals is dependent on the health of the community.
9. Maternal-newborn nursing utilizes a high degree of independent nursing functions because teaching and counseling are such frequent implementations.
10. Maternal-newborn nursing is a challenging role for the professional nurse and is a major contribution to promotion of high-level wellness in families.

---

nursing care is implied by this book's subtitle, *Care of the Growing Family.*

All the time stages surrounding pregnancy are equally important in ensuring that the health of the family is maintained. Maternal-newborn nurses should be as directly concerned with the care of women during three trimesters of pregnancy and the puerperium (sometimes termed the fourth trimester) as with their care at parturition; likewise, care of children prenatally, during the neonatal period (the 28 days following birth), as well as intrapartally is also important. Maternal-newborn nursing also deals indirectly with the women before and after pregnancies (interpregnancy health), performing such services as reproductive life planning and teaching concepts of sexuality. These factors influence the optimal health of any woman and child. Because no woman lives without interaction with others, a woman's relationships with her new child, her family, and community are also relevant to planning nursing care and ensuring her sound health at the present and in the future.

Goals and Philosophies of Maternal-Newborn Nursing

The goals of maternal-newborn nursing are broadly stated because the scope of practice itself

is so broad (ranging from health care at birth to women's needs through menopause) and the practice settings so varied (ranging from intensive care nurseries to homes). The overall encompassing goal can be stated simply, however, as *the promotion and maintenance of optimal health for women and their fetuses/newborns.* In other words, to ensure that children are not only physically, mentally, and emotionally well born but also born well. The major philosophical assumptions of maternal-newborn nursing and the role of the maternal-newborn nurse are summarized in the Nursing Care Highlight above.

The Maternal-Newborn Nurse

Roles for maternal-newborn nurses can be found at all levels of nursing preparation. Some people believe that no one can be a good maternal-newborn nurse without the experience of giving birth because with that event comes an understanding of the stress of pregnancy and the force and overwhelming helplessness of labor contractions. Such a criterion would of course restrict the number of persons who could become maternal-newborn nurses.

It is more important that a nurse caring for a pregnant woman and her family be able to empathize with feelings of joy, pain, fear, threat, hope, achievement, disappointment, satisfaction, and terror: All these emotions occur with pregnancy and childbirth. If you can anticipate the feeling that comes with planning and hoping against hope for something, yet constantly being steeled for instant, devastating disappointment, come. You are ready to learn the skills that a nurse in maternal and newborn care must have.

Standards of Maternal-Child Health Nursing Practice

Every nurse is responsible for practicing with a level of care that will provide optimal protection and safety to a woman and her unborn or newborn child. In order to promote consistency of care among nurses, various organizations in nursing have developed standards of nursing practice as guidelines. Individual health care agencies supplement these guidelines with policies for actions and care in that particular setting, based on the specific woman or child or current circumstances.

In 1973, the Executive Committee and the Standards Committee of the Division of Maternal-Child Health Nursing Practice of the American Nurses Association (ANA, 1973) developed 13 process standards for maternal-child health nursing practice. These are summarized in the box on page 7.

Nursing Theory

One of the requirements of a profession (along with other critical determinants, such as members setting their own standards, monitoring the quality of practice, and participating in research) is that the concentration of knowledge flow from a theoretical base. Most current theories of nursing address three separate issues: How is the person who is to be nursed to be viewed; what are the goals of nursing care; and what are the activities of nursing care that will meet these goals.

The first facet, that of characterizing the person to be nursed, seems at first to be an unnecessary question. People who are to be cared for are certainly people who have an illness or are in need of preventive aspects of care in order to remain well. Nursing theorists can help to determine the most helpful ways to view people, however, so that nursing activities can best meet their needs—seeing the patient, for example, not simply as a physical form, but as a dynamic force with important psychosocial needs. In maternal-newborn nursing it is vital to understand people as an extension or active member of a community

as well as a holistic being. Only this wide a focus can bring an appreciation of the degree of change caused by a new family member.

The second issue involves the overall goals of nursing care, which have changed in recent years along with the scope of nursing. At one time the goal of nursing could have been stated as the care and comfort of the injured and ill; today most nurses would perceive this goal as limited: They are equipped to do much more. Nursing theorists help to identify new goals for nursing, which help nurses strive to be all that they can be. Maternal-newborn nursing is, again, an area that has seen extensive change in nurses' scope of concern. Standards of care that were accepted as routine twenty years ago—women being separated from their husbands during delivery, the use of general anesthesia for birth, and all mothers using formula feeding—are viewed today as obsolete.

As nursing goals become broader, so do nursing activities. For example, when the goal of nursing was considered to be care of the ill, nursing actions were mainly bathing, feeding, and providing comfort. Today, with promotion of health as a goal, teaching, counseling, supporting, and advocacy are also common nursing roles. Nurses fill these roles extensively in maternal-newborn nursing.

Nurses need to examine the basis of nursing practice in the context of the three issues discussed above; in this way they can best meet people's health needs and continue to change as people's health needs change. At the present time, no unanimous agreement supports any one theory of nursing as superior to any other. Nursing schools base their curricula on a chosen theorist or integrate a number of theorists' concepts throughout a program. Table 1-1 summarizes the basic tenets of a number of nursing theorists and ways the theories apply to maternal-newborn care for one theoretical patient.

Until one theory of nursing does prove to be superior to others, it is likely that schools of nursing and individual nurses will continue to use diverse theories for care. By examining the third column of Table 1-1, however, you can see that although the theoretical basis of nursing organization differs among theories, the end result of every theory is provision of a high level of nursing care. Differing views of nursing theory are, in the end, not contradictory.

Nursing Process

The amount of knowledge a person must have in order to function as a professional nurse today in a maternal-newborn setting is ten times more

Standards for Maternal-Child Health Nursing Practice

Standard I
Maternal and child health nursing practice is characterized by the continual questioning of the assumptions upon which practice is based, retaining those which are valid and searching for and using new knowledge.

Nurses have a responsibility to be aware of new research findings because these influence their practice, and they should participate in research as needed to evaluate techniques or hypotheses. An example of how nurses have met this standard in maternal-newborn nursing is seen in the increased participation of nurses in helping women to deliver children with a minimum of anesthesia and learn to breast-feed their newborn infants following birth. Twenty years ago, women were taught that anesthesia was the route to painless childbirth. Today it is acknowledged that prepared childbirth can achieve if not a painless birth, one so emotionally satisfying that the pain becomes irrelevant. New mothers were once taught that formula-feeding was the safest and most nutritious choice for newborns. Now, almost all health care personnel accept human milk as the best food for infants. The assumptions have remained the same—childbirth should be a satisfying experience and infants should be fed in the best way possible; but now new methods are used to achieve these goals.

Standard II
Maternal and child health nursing practice is based upon knowledge of the biophysical and psychosocial development of individuals from conception through the childrearing phase of development and upon knowledge of the basic needs for optimum development.

The success of nurses in meeting this standard is reflected in nurses' increased interest and participation in health screening tests as part of routine nursing assessments during the newborn period. In this way, newborns with less than optimal development potential can be identified early and be provided with the special services or care needed. Teaching principles of normal growth and child development to parents helps them to be better caregivers. Helping women learn more about how their body functions at all stages of life, especially during preg-

nancy and parturition, helps to maintain better health practices.

Standard III
The collection of data about the health status of the client/patient is systematic and continuous. The data are accessible, communicated and recorded.

As nurses meet this standard, they become more involved in problem-oriented recording systems. These systems allow data collected during prenatal months to be easily transmitted to the health care personnel who are with a woman at the time of labor and delivery. Participating in problem-oriented recording systems lets nurses share their expertise and their concerns with other health care persons. Thus the nurse can be both a teacher and a learner of better health care practices. A nurse's designing and communicating nursing care plans from prenatal to parturition settings can be instrumental in providing continuity of care.

Standard IV
Nursing diagnoses are derived from data about the health status of the client/patient.

As nurses initiate more independent nursing functions, making nursing diagnoses becomes a more intrinsic part of optimal care and practice. Utilizing scales that identify women as high risk for having a child born with some form of difficulty is an example of an independent nursing action in everyday practice that helps to safeguard women and their unborn children.

Standard V
Maternal and child health nursing practice recognizes deviations from expected patterns of physiologic activity and anatomic and psychosocial development.

Nurses in prenatal, natal, and postnatal areas are in first-line positions to identify deviations from the normal that will affect either a woman or her child. Because many of the problems that occur during pregnancy, such as pregnancy-induced hypertension, begin with subtle symptoms, the continuity of care that nurses offer to women and families enables them to detect small changes before these become irreversible and compromise the pregnancy.

Standard VI
The plan of nursing care includes goals derived from the nursing diagnoses.

The goals that families choose for birth today may range from selecting a hospital, an alternative center, or their own home for birth. Nurses have important roles in all three of these different care settings. Because pregnancy is a time of crisis, pregnant women are easily influenced and are "ripe" for health teaching. Establishing specific goals for each woman allows the most effective and far-reaching results.

Standard VII
The plan of nursing care includes priorities and the prescribed nursing approaches or measures to achieve the goals derived from the nursing diagnoses.

In an area in which health care practices always affect not one but two individuals (and often an entire family), it is easy for secondary concerns (such as worry about a newborn's appearance) to "slip through the cracks" unless nursing care plans detail priorities of action. The nurse is often the person who first recognizes a patient's second concern and is therefore able to initiate the alleviation of the problem.

Standard VIII
Nursing actions provide for client/patient participation in health promotion, maintenance and restoration.

In no other area of nursing are patients allowed to participate more fully in their care than in maternal-newborn nursing. Teaching women to care for their own health during pregnancy and for that of their newborn child, and then to maintain their health following pregnancy, is an intrinsic part of maternal-newborn nursing. Learning to give anticipatory guidance is also a major role of the nurse in this area.

Standard IX
Maternal and child health nursing practice provides for the use and coordination of all services that assist individuals to prepare for responsible sexual roles.

Nurses in maternal-newborn nursing can explain methods of reproductive life planning, thereby helping people assume responsible sexual roles. As a source of information about sexual responses, nurses can help people to view childbearing as an extension of their sexual roles. Young couples look to nurses as models of female or male adult roles.

Standard X
Nursing actions assist the client/patient to maximize individual health capabilities.

This standard reflects the nurse's role in helping a woman with heart disease, diabetes mellitus, or a kidney disorder maintain a long-hoped-for pregnancy; or helping a mother or father touch and accept an ill newborn with an understanding of the child's strengths as well as the extent of the handicap.

Standard XI
The client/patient's progress or lack of progress toward goal achievement is determined by the client/patient and the nurse.

Some women set unrealistic standards for themselves or their children. Couples who are seen for infertility problems may need guidance in setting appropriate goals for themselves and evaluating progress toward their goals. Only by evaluation are people able to assess what is happening at the present time and make plans for the future.

Standard XII
The client/patient's progress or lack of progress toward goal achievement directs reassessment, reordering of priorities, new goal setting and revision of the plan of nursing care.

Because pregnancy is such a major life change, goals that are applicable at the beginning of pregnancy may not be applicable at a later point. If a complication occurs, goals may need to be revised to meet new demands; if a newborn's health is compromised at birth, goals may need to be revised again and again in the first few years of life.

Standard XIII
Maternal and child health nursing practice evidences active participation with others in evaluating the availability, accessibility and acceptability of services for parents and children and cooperating and/or taking leadership in extending and developing needed services in the community.

Maternal-newborn nursing is a rapidly growing area of nursing. At one time nurses interacted only with obstetricians, anesthesiologists, and occasionally dieticians in order to coordinate health care for women and their newborns. They must now interact with perinatologists, geneticists and genetic counselors, respiratory therapists, childbirth educators, neonatologists, pediatric nurse practitioners, clinical nurse specialists, endocrinologists, internists, cardiac surgeons, community health nurses, orthopedists, nurse midwives—members of as many specialties as exist.

In addition to this extended coordination role, nurses are responsible for direct care and often provide many of the educational services needed by women during pregnancy, such as preparation-for-childbirth and childrearing classes. They are active participants in the women's health movement, with the goal of making women more aware of their health during their entire life cycle.

The standards outlined above serve as guidelines for planning quality care. They allow for coordination with other health care providers. They are also important as criteria for assessment of nursing practice in an area of health care delivery that is expanding rapidly.

---

than it was five years ago and as much as one hundred times more than it was twenty years ago. This increasing amount of knowledge, technical innovations, and increased expectations from consumers of health care combine to make nursing a more complex and challenging field every day.

In order for nursing care to be designed and implemented in a thorough manner that ensures quality and consistency in care for patients, it must be done by an organized series of well thought-through steps. Using nursing process as the basis for assessing and planning care is using a form of proven problem-solving, or scientific method, to organize care. That nursing process is applicable to maternal-newborn settings that are largely wellness settings is proof that the system is large enough to serve as the basis for nursing care.

It takes two people to make the nursing process happen: a person who is a nurse (or who is learning to be one) and a person with whom this nurse interacts. The actual interaction may consist of physical ministrations, counseling to improve health, teaching to prevent illness, or even an agreement between the two parties that no intervention is necessary.

A person who enters a purposeful relationship with a nurse has traditionally been called a patient. A *patient* is usually defined as a person under medical care.

Because the modern nurse may give nursing care to people not under medical supervision at that time, the term *patient* is viewed today as old-fashioned by many theorists in nursing. The term *client*, referring to a person who actively participates in a relationship, such as a lawyer-client relationship, may be used instead. *Client*, however, is identified by Webster as a word that stems from a vassal or serf or one who must give service to a master, or whose participation is less than willing, actually forced. This is not the relationship implied or desired in a nursing relationship.

In this text, therefore, persons with whom nurses interact are termed *patients* or, more specifically, *women, newborns, mothers, fathers, parents,* or *families.* This puts the responsibility on nurses to establish and maintain the relationship. Patients who are ill or under stress (the reason they are in need of nursing services) can be free to act ill and under stress and not have to put on a false front to please the nurse who takes care of them.

In most instances, a nurse-patient relationship is a one-to-one relationship. The person involved in the relationship changes during maternal-newborn nursing, depending on the stage of the pregnancy, the health of the newborn, and the circumstances of the individual situation. The relationship is established with a woman alone when she always comes for prenatal care by herself, with a husband singly at such visits if he has concerns he wants to voice separately from those of his wife; sometimes the relationship is established with the husband and wife together when they are interacting as a unit (during labor or at the time a couple is told that their child has been born with a health problem). Sometimes the relationship is established with an entire family (at a time when a family—parents, brothers, and sisters—are told that their new family member is going to die or when they are first getting acquainted with their new family member). Even when the relationship involves a nurse and a single person, it is influenced by other people around that person (family centered), because childbearing and childrearing are influenced strongly by social and cultural factors (Figure 1-1). The interaction between outside influences and the nursing process in maternal-newborn nursing is shown in Figure 1-2.

The NCLEX-RN format for the nursing process including the five steps of assessment, analysis (nursing diagnosis), planning, implementation, and evaluation is used throughout this text; examples of nursing care plans using this format are shown at the ends of chapters to illustrate the process. In addition, Nursing Care Highlights are

Table 1-1 Summary of Common Nursing Theories in Relation to Planning Maternal-Newborn Care

Theorist	Tenets of Theory	Application to Care Example*
Imogene King	Nursing deals with humans as thinking beings. Nursing is a process of action, reaction, interaction, and transaction. Needs are identified based on patient social system, perceptions, interpersonal relationships, and health.	To plan care for Mrs. Baco, discuss with her the way she views herself and her illness. Because she sees herself as being able to return to her previous role of mother and part-time worker, structure care to help her meet these perceptions of herself.
Florence Nightingale	The role of the nurse is viewed as changing or structuring elements of the environment such as ventilation, temperature, odors, noise, and light to assist the patient in recovery.	To plan care for Mrs. Baco, turn her bed so sunlight falls on it; provide adequate covers for warmth; leave her comfortable and resting.
Dorothea Orem	The focus of nursing is on the individual: Patients are assessed in terms of ability for complete self-care. Care given may be wholly compensatory (patient has no role); partly compensatory (patient participates in care); or supportive-educational (patient performs own care).	To plan care for Mrs. Baco, encourage her in self-care within the limitations of bedrest she must maintain. Organize room so she can obtain needed supplies for self-care
Hildegard Peplau	The promotion of health is viewed as the forward movement of the personality. This is accomplished through interpersonal process, including orientation, identification, exploitation, and resolution.	Plan care together with Mrs. Baco. She is unable to assume full responsibility for herself due to bedrest, so encourage her to speak of children and job accomplishments to retain self-esteem.
Martha Rogers	The purpose of nursing is to move persons toward optimal health. The nurse should view people as a whole, constantly changing, and help them to interact in the best way possible with the environment.	Help Mrs. Baco to accept and maintain bedrest so that she returns to optimal health and functioning as soon as possible.
Sister Callistra Roy	The role of the nurse is to aid people in adapting to the change caused by illness. Levels of adaptation depend on the degree of environmental change and state of coping ability. Full adaptation includes physiological factors, self-concept, role function, and interdependence.	Assess Mrs. Baco's physical and psychosocial ability to adapt to continuous bedrest. Direct nursing care toward replacing analyzed deficits with other alternate measures.
Ernestine Wiedenbach	Nursing is nurturing and caring for someone in a motherly fashon. It involves three processes of establishing a central purpose of care, developing a prescription to fulfill the purpose, and consideration of the realities of the immediate situation of the care.	To plan care for Mrs. Baco, establish her need for bedrest, establish a plan of care to accomplish this need, while being aware of her resistance to it.

*Theories are applied to one theoretical patient, Mrs. Angie Baco, who is hospitalized on complete bedrest because of hypertension during pregnancy.

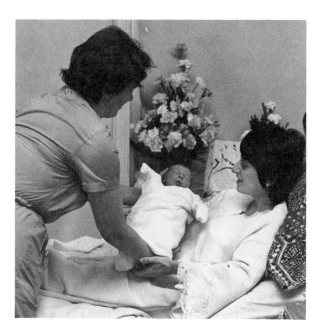

Figure 1-1 *Nurse-patient relationships in maternal-newborn nursing invariably involve more than one patient. (Courtesy of the Department of Medical Photography, Children's Hospital, Buffalo, N.Y.)*

included as additional reminders of safe and well-planned care.

Nursing Research

Research is the controlled investigation of a problem using the scientific method. Bodies of professional knowledge grow and expand to the extent that people in that profession plan and carry out research. *Nursing research* is the controlled investigation of a problem that has implications for nursing practice. It is the method by which the foundation of nursing grows and expands and improves.

The classic example of how the results of nursing research can affect nursing practice is the application of knowledge gained from Rubin's investigation of the mother's approach to her newborn (Rubin, 1963). Prior to this published study, nurses assumed that a woman who did not immediately hold and cuddle her infant at birth was a "cold" or unfeeling mother. Rubin reported that attachment is not a spontaneous procedure, but more commonly begins with only fingertip touching. With this new knowledge available to nurses, women following a normal pattern of attachment are now recognized as not unfeeling, but normal; with normal parameters documented, those women who do not follow a nor-

mal pattern can be isolated and helped with gaining a stronger attachment to their new infant.

Many problems of maternal-newborn nursing still remain unanswered. Problems that warrant more investigation are: What is the best stimulus to encourage women to come for antepartal care? What method is most effective to encourage parent-infant bonding? What are the most effective ways to encourage women to continue breast-feeding after they return home from a health care setting? What are the most appreciated and effective methods to support a woman in labor? Do all fathers want to be included in labor and delivery procedures as much as we currently assume? How much self-care is optimum to encourage in the immediate postpartal period? What is the optimum way to encourage self-esteem in the couple who have had a child born with a birth defect?

In order to assist you to view nursing research as appropriate and practical to your future nursing practice, Nursing Research Highlights have been included in various chapters throughout the text. The intent of these presentations is to expose you to some aspects of maternal-newborn nursing care currently being questioned and/or investigated. It is hoped that these will assist you in developing a questioning attitude regarding current nursing practice and in thinking of ways to incorporate research findings in care.

Pregnancy and Delivery as a Crisis Period

Although they are often planned for and joyfully anticipated, pregnancy and childbirth are always stress-producing times of changing roles. A second, third, or even a ninth pregnancy, although each contains familiar aspects, is no less stressful than the first: Each is the family's first experience with that particular pregnancy. When stress becomes long term and a person fails at efforts in reduction, a crisis situation results.

Life crises may be situational (for example, death of a loved one, ill health, or loss of wealth or love) or developmental (toddlerhood, with its increasing independence; adolescence, with its new body functions and changes; pregnancy; adulthood, with new responsibility). A crisis state will occur with these stresses if the person experiencing the stress does not have or cannot use previously developed coping mechanisms. A period of disorganization or disturbance will occur (crisis) as the person makes various unsuccessful attempts at solution. Eventually, some kind of resolution will be achieved—one that may or may not

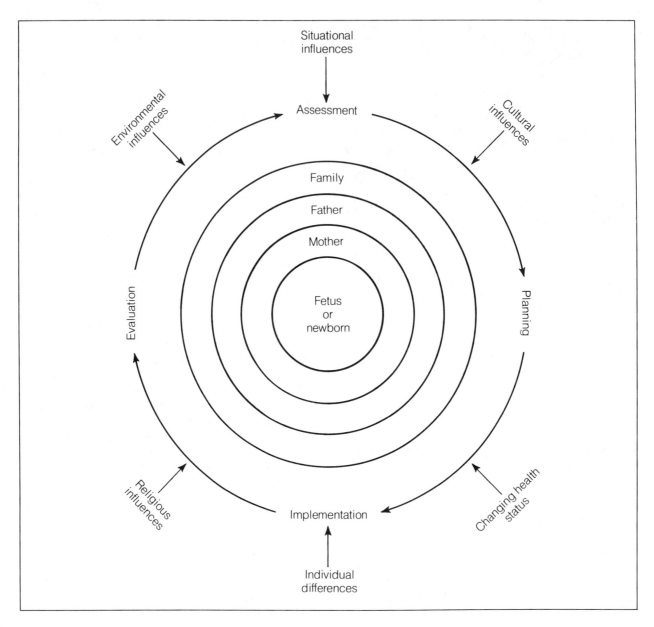

Figure 1-2 *The nursing process and outside influences.*

be in the best interests of that person or the family involved.

If the resolution is reality-oriented, that is, if it indicates acceptance of the inevitable, strengthens interpersonal relationships, and restores equilibrium, it is an *adaptive* resolution. The person has not only resolved a crisis but has also enriched her ability to cope with future crises. If the resolution is not reality-oriented, that is, if it results in lasting interpersonal disturbances or in newly formed neurotic or psychotic syndromes, it is a *maladaptive* resolution (Caplan, 1964). Preventing maladaptive resolutions of crises is essential for the promotion of mental health. This task is a vital nursing role in care of the expanding family and serves as the framework of practice.

Methods you can employ to help an individual deal with stress are outlined in the Nursing Care Highlight on page 13.

People who are reaching a point of exhaustion in their coping strategies begin to evidence typical behaviors, as shown in Table 1-2. Because these responses may be subtle, the better you know a person, or the longer a time period you have given care, the easier it is to recognize them.

Rating Events by Stress Level

Although events are individualized and mean different things to different people, they can be categorized to some extent in terms of their level of stress. Common life events and their stress

════════ *Nursing Care Highlight* ════════

**Methods to Help a Person
Deal with Stress**

1. Help the person to recognize her individual stress level, a level that differs from person to person. Because she works next to someone who is not upset by some condition does not mean that she will not be annoyed or upset. On the other hand, if a situation does not annoy a person, she should not feel that she has to react to it just because a friend does. Help your patients to understand and accept individual differences in stress levels.

2. Help the person to learn to change those things she cannot accept and to learn to accept those things she cannot change. Trial and error is often required to determine the difference between the two categories. Often a total change is not necessary; a modification will make the difference.

3. Help the person to reach out for support. People under stress are often so involved in their problem that they do not realize that people around them want to help. Often the people closest to the person feeling stress are under a similar threat and thus are no longer able to offer support. The person must then call on second- or third-level support persons (family or community people) for help.

4. Help the person to develop a habit of reaching out to give support when others are in threat. Survival is a collaborative function of social groups; a favor offered now can be called in when the person is in need at a later date.

5. Help the person to face the situation as honestly as possible. As a rule, knowing the exact nature of a threat is less stressful than a shadow-haunting, something-is-out-there feeling. On the other hand, people should not be urged to face intense threats, such as a serious complication of pregnancy, until they have had time to mobilize their defenses.

6. Help the person not to rush decisions or final adaptive outcomes to a stress situation. As a rule, major decisions should be delayed at least six weeks after an event; six months is an even better time interval.

7. Help the person anticipate life events and plan for them to the extent possible. Anticipatory guidance will not totally prepare a patient for a coming event but will at least serve notice that distress over the situation is normal.

8. Alert the person to the fact that accidents increase when people are under stress. A person worrying about a complication of pregnancy is more apt to have an automobile accident or burn herself on a hot stove than a person who is stress free.

9. Action feels good during stress. Doing something brings a sense of control over feelings of helplessness and disorganization. Action often is so satisfying that people do things, such as write threatening letters or make hurtful remarks, that they later regret. Help a person to channel this energy into therapeutic action (such as going for a long walk).

10. Encourage the person to verbalize personal reactions. Nothing limits the extent of a threat more than being able to describe it.

───────────────────────────────

values are shown in Table 1-3. If a person's total score from the table is 150 to 199, the person is under mild stress; up to 37 percent of people with this level of stress will become physically ill. A score between 200 and 299 points reflects a medium stress level; up to 51 percent of people in this category will become ill within two weeks. A total score over 300 reflects a high stress level; 79 percent of the people in this group will become physically ill.

Notice that pregnancy is rated as number twelve on the list. If you add the points of common situations that are often present in young adulthood or accompany a pregnancy—such as the wife stopping work (26), a change in financial state (38), a mortgage more than $10,000 (31), ending school (26), a change in living conditions (25), revision of personal habits (24), change in recreation (19), and change in eating habits (15)—to the rating of pregnancy (40), the total is 244. That total places the person within the medium stress range. If any additional situations, such as marital separation (65), change in health of a family member (44), foreclosure of a loan (30), or trouble with

Table 1-2 Evidences of Poor Coping Ability

Behavior	Description	Example
Accentuated use of a particular behavior pattern	Structuring, or repeating an activity over and over, controls stress because it prevents surprises from impinging on a person's thoughts.	A woman, waiting for the results of a pregnancy test, may wash her hands over and over.
Disorganized behavior	Under stress, a woman may be unable to think clearly.	A woman may be unable to organize her day to arrive at a prenatal care appointment on time.
Change in activity from usual pattern	Changing a usual pattern is an effort to avoid facing a stressful situation.	A woman who is usually meticulous may become careless in her personal hygiene during pregnancy.
Decreased sensitivity to the environment	An increased stress level may make a person less aware of her surroundings.	A woman does not notice food burning on the stove the afternoon she learns she is pregnant.
Misinterpretation of reality	A woman may misunderstand what she has been told, only hearing what she wants to hear or reading what she would like into another person's reaction.	A woman being prepared for cesarean birth does not hear you tell her not to drink any fluid before surgery.
Psychosomatic symptoms	Stress is manifested in such symptoms as nausea and vomiting, heartburn, diarrhea, or headache.	A woman experiences a headache on the afternoon she learns she is pregnant. NOTE: A symptom such as stress headache can be very perplexing to assess since headache is one of the danger signs of pregnancy.
Poor memory	Under stress, a person may not even be able to recall such basic information as age and name.	A woman is unable to remember to take a daily iron supplement during pregnancy.
Lessened self-esteem	A woman may feel helpless to act, such helplessness causing a loss of self-confidence.	A woman in labor who had planned on being at her best finds herself frozen, unable to remember even simple breathing exercises.

in-laws (29), is added to this total, the number can easily be raised over 300.

Crisis Intervention

Specifically, whether an individual can manage crisis situations or needs help in handling life events is influenced by three main variables: the individual's perception of the event, the type and availability of support people to call on, and the ways of coping or managing stressful events the person has found to be successful in the past (Aguilera and Messick, 1974). The components of effective crisis resolution are shown in Figure 1-

3A. Figure 1-3B shows ineffective crisis resolution.

Perception of the Event

Families involved in childbearing usually consist of young adults, although a woman may be as young as 11 or 12 or as old as 45 or 50. By young adulthood, most persons have had experience with both success (for example, completion of a school experience) and lack of success (refusal of a loan or a job they especially wanted). They have achieved a degree of responsibility for their own care and possibly that of another if they have cho-

Table 1-3 Social Readjustment Rating Scale for Life Changes

Rank	Life Event	Mean Value
1	Death of spouse	100
2	Divorce	73
3	Marital separation	65
4	Jail term	63
5	Death of close family member	63
6	Personal injury or illness	53
7	Marriage	50
8	Fired at work	47
9	Marital reconciliation	45
10	Retirement	45
11	Change in health of family member	44
12	Pregnancy	40
13	Sex difficulties	39
14	Gain of new family member	39
15	Business readjustment	39
16	Change in financial state	38
17	Death of close friend	37
18	Change to different line of work	36
19	Change in number of arguments with spouse	35
20	Mortgage more than $10,000	31
21	Foreclosure of mortgage or loan	30
22	Change in responsibilities at work	29
23	Son or daughter leaving home	29
24	Trouble with in-laws	29
25	Outstanding personal achievement	28
26	Wife beginning or stopping work	26
27	Begin or end school	26
28	Change in living conditions	25
29	Revision of personal habits	24
30	Trouble with boss	23
31	Change in work hours or conditions	20
32	Change in residence	20
33	Change in schools	20
34	Change in recreation	19
35	Change in church activities	19
36	Change in social activities	18
37	Mortgage or loan less than $10,000	17
38	Change in sleeping habits	16
39	Change in number of family get-togethers	15
40	Change in eating habits	15
41	Vacation	13
42	Christmas	13
43	Minor violations of the law	11

Source: From T. H. Holmes and R. H. Rahe. (1967). The social readjustment rating scale. *Journal of Psychosomatic Research, 2,* 214.

sen to marry. They have had opportunities to make decisions. They are at a time in life when they are ready for children.

The woman who is only an adolescent when she becomes pregnant has had much less experience in decision making. The biggest decision an eighth grader or a high-school freshman may have made is whether to have long or short hair or whether to take English or math in the last period of a school day. Most adolescents have had little experience with real responsibility (occasional baby-sitting is not the same as 24-hour-a-day care of an infant). In the light of her background, a pregnant adolescent may perceive her pregnancy as a tragedy rather than as an anticipated event.

A woman who is past young adulthood when she becomes pregnant has the advantage of being experienced in decision making and responsibility, but she also may cherish the freedom that absence of infant care gives her life style. The stage of life, therefore, of a woman and her family can cause a pregnancy to be viewed as a major crisis, a manageable one, or not a crisis at all.

Whether a woman is married, has other children, has career plans, or has adequate financial resources, are all other factors that influence her perception of pregnancy because they influence how readily a new baby can be incorporated into family life.

Support Persons

Support persons play a significant part in giving counsel or guidance in times of stress. In order to be effective, they must be capable of offering support and must be available when needed. A husband is the traditional support person for a woman, as she is for him, while parents are usually important to adolescents. Pregnancy may turn people in other directions, however: A close friend or a neighbor who has had children may be a stronger support person than a spouse who knows little about children or angry, confused parents. The father of the child of an unmarried pregnant woman may or may not be supportive, depending on what the coming event means to him.

Some persons who ordinarily would be supportive may not be available because of physical distance. Distance is not an absolute barrier, however: Some families separated by great distance maintain close contact by mail or phone and so are very supportive. Husbands who are separated from their wives by work (salesmen, military personnel, truck drivers) may be very supportive throughout a pregnancy—more supportive, perhaps, than a husband who is home every evening

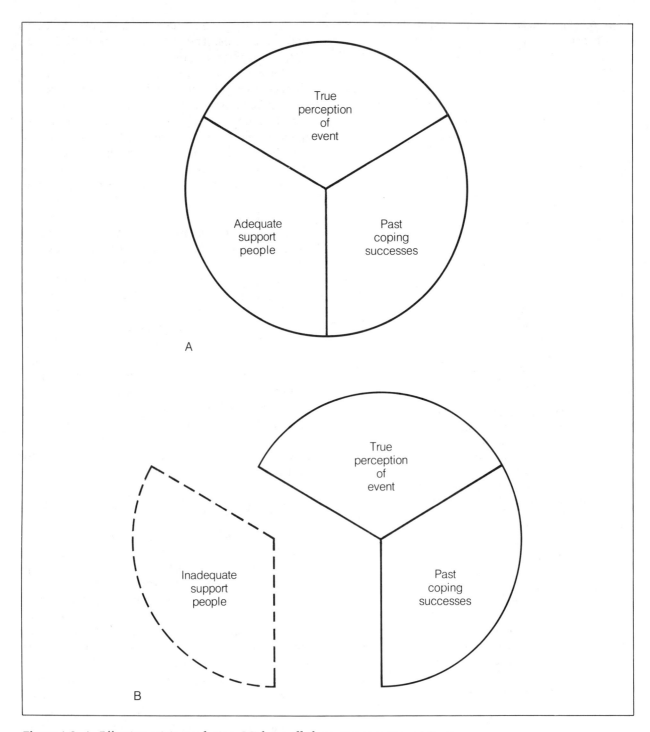

Figure 1-3 *A. Effective crisis resolution. Without all three components, crisis resolution will be ineffective. B. Ineffective crisis resolution. With a missing component, crisis resolution cannot be completed.*

but who does not perceive the coming child in the same way that his wife does.

During labor, the actual physical presence of the support person is important. A husband's absence at this time can be deeply disappointing to a woman. To be kept away from the event by health care personnel (a practice that is fortunately decreasing) can be devastating to both the woman and her support person.

When families were extended—that is, when they contained grandparents, aunts, and uncles in addition to the nuclear family of father, mother, and children—a couple easily received their main support and intervention from the family group during pregnancy. Preparing the family cradle ("four generations of the family have slept in it"), choosing the baby's name ("all male babies in the family are given the middle name John"), and polishing a family baby spoon ("this is the spoon you ate from when you were small") were activities that gave proof that childbirth is a positive, endurable, continuing, generation-to-generation process.

Some of the support a woman used to receive from an extended family was in the form of old wives' tales: "Don't reach up during pregnancy, or you'll twist the baby's cord." "Don't eat strawberries or your child will be born with a birthmark." "Don't sew on Sunday, or the baby's cord will knot." As unfounded as these warnings were, they nonetheless provided a sense of continuity, of security that the women who handed down these tales had successfully passed through the birth process.

Many young couples today do not have the support of an extended family because families today are largely nuclear in structure (parents and children only). Further, more and more unmarried women are having children (single-unit families). Nuclear families, for the most part, live in apartments or suburban communities where they may know their neighbors only well enough to say "hello" on the elevator or across the backyard fence. For support during health crises, they turn to health care personnel. During pregnancy, they rely on health care personnel for reassurance that they are well, that they will be adequate parents, and that their babies will be healthy.

The adaptive resolution the couple achieves in handling the stress and crises of pregnancy and birth—whether they become more able to cope with stress, more aware of their family's support, more attuned to and appreciative of life than before; or become bitter and disappointed and less able to cope with stress—depends a great deal on the amount and kind of support or crisis intervention they receive from the health care personnel who care for them during pregnancy, labor, delivery, and the days following birth. Having a child is never accomplished alone. Interaction with family members and friends and most importantly, the father of the child, helps a woman manage during pregnancy. In turn, how well these individuals cope with crisis may depend on the amount and kind of support they receive from health care personnel (Figure 1-4).

Besides family and health care personnel, individuals have a network of additional support persons, such as from church groups, community organizations, or social clubs. Some people join a specific group for needed support, such as Alcoholics Anonymous; others originate support groups to meet their needs (for example, Parents of Retarded Children or the La Leche League for Breast Feeding Mothers). During a complication of pregnancy, such groups may become primary

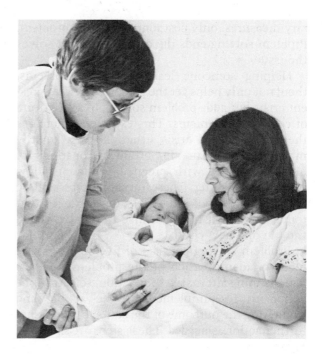

Figure 1-4 *Having a baby is a family affair. If a ready support person such as this father is not available at the time, health care personnel need to fulfill this role. (Courtesy of the Department of Medical Photography, Children's Hospital, Buffalo, N.Y.)*

support sources because of the specific need they serve and help they can offer.

Coping Mechanisms

A person copes with a new stress situation in the same manner used to cope with past situations. Because a coping mechanism worked once, however, is no guarantee that it will work again, even under similar circumstances. A 2-year-old, for example, uses temper tantrums as a coping mechanism. This type of behavior is not likely to be effective for a person trying to resolve a dispute with an insurance company or for a woman who has just learned that she is pregnant.

Another choice, ignoring the situation, is an ineffective coping mechanism for pregnancy: A pregnancy cannot be ignored. Some coping mechanisms, such as crying or aggression, are effective for short-term resolutions. They force other people to change the degree of stress in order to stop the crying or the anger. These methods are ineffective during a long-term crisis—a pregnancy, for example. No one can cry for nine months; no one will listen to someone crying for nine months.

The most effective coping mechanism in any situation is problem solving. Problem solving is superior to such mechanisms as manipulating, ignoring, or fighting because the latter, as temporary measures, only postpone facing the problem. Problem solving ends the crisis because it solves the issue.

Helping someone learn to solve problems, then, not only helps get the person through a present crisis but adds problem solving to a repertoire of coping mechanisms. This experience prepares the person to end crisis situations in a healthy manner in the future. Important implications for nurses working with pregnant women follow from this teaching: These mothers-to-be will be responsible for not only those disturbances that touch their own lives but also those that touch the life of a new child.

Problem solving consists of five steps: assessment or identification of the problem, analysis and planning alternatives for action, selecting one action to try, implementing the action, and evaluating the outcome of the action and whether further action is needed. These steps are shown in Figure 1-5.

Identifying the Problem

Helping someone identify a problem is often more difficult than it appears: Your own values of what is or is not a problem tend to interfere. If you find a woman moaning in labor, for example, you might naturally assume that her labor contractions are beginning to hurt. When you give her

Figure 1-5 *Steps in problem solving.*

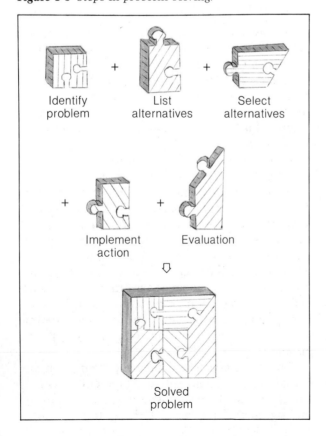

Identify problem + List alternatives + Select alternatives

+ Implement action + Evaluation

Solved problem

something for pain, she does not get better, however. Her problem was not the discomfort of labor contractions but of extreme thirst. You failed to solve her problem by not clearly identifying it.

Another example of imposed values involves a 17-year-old who comes into a prenatal clinic with nausea, wondering if she might be pregnant. The clinic doctor suggests a menstrual extraction to abort a possible pregnancy without asking her if the nausea or the pregnancy is the problem.

No problem can be solved until everyone concerned is certain what the problem is. To identify a problem, ask, "What out of everything wrong concerns or worries you the most?" "If I could do only one thing for you, what would that thing be?" Once a person is sure what the problem is, solutions begin to be possible.

Planning Alternatives

The only alternatives that people can choose in any situation are those they know. For health care personnel a major function in problem solving is letting people know all the available alternatives. A 17-year-old who cannot stand being nauseated every day during early pregnancy, for example, has a number of alternatives: taking medication, eating dry crackers (the time-honored advice for nausea from pregnancy), eating nothing each day until noon, ending the pregnancy, or killing herself. The last solution is extreme; however, some people actually do attempt suicide because they do not know any other way to end their upsetting situation. Better education of the available alternatives could prevent this drastic action.

Choosing from Alternatives

Most people do not have much difficulty choosing from available alternatives once they know what they are. Before they choose, they must think through "what would happen if" they took any given alternative. If the 17-year-old with morning sickness, for instance, chooses to take an over-the-counter medication daily for her nausea, she will cure that symptom. She may also cause fetal malgrowth. If, instead, she is able to view nausea as a normal consequence of pregnancy and eat sparingly during the morning (being certain to eat nutritionally for the remainder of the day), she will also not have nausea. The alternatives people choose to try in situations differ greatly between individuals and according to their values and priorities.

Implementing the Action

Some people are talkers, some are talkers and doers, some are doers. People who can talk their way through problems to the point of selecting an alternative, but then fail to carry it out, do not handle stress well. (In many instances, however, talking about what they should do is so therapeutic that it becomes an action.) Doers who do not plan (for example, solving the problem of not being able to buy a crib for a newborn by getting one on credit) also invariably have trouble handling stress situations. By stabbing in the dark this way, such people waste their energy (and have more problems than originally). Some people need urging to carry out the plan they have decided is most effective. Others need urging to think one more time before they act, to find a balance between planning and implementation in problem solving.

Evaluation

Evaluation—a step often forgotten in problem solving—is necessary because it sets the stage for further problem solving, and for identifying or re-identifying the problem until the person seeking help is at least temporarily crisis-free. Suppose the young girl who has the nausea of early pregnancy is advised to manage it by simple nutritional regulation without medication. Unfortunately, the nausea does not improve. Unless an evaluation is made as to whether the intervention was effective, health care personnel will proceed as if the problem is solved. The girl, frustrated and disappointed, might not return for further care.

Successful Intervention

During crisis periods, people are usually able to devise a first (primary) coping action. In the event that this is unsuccessful, they are usually able to construct a secondary intervention. They often have difficulty, however, initiating a third response (a tertiary coping mechanism). At this point, they need some form of help.

Pregnancy is an extremely vulnerable time in life because it is the announcement of a major life change (not for another 18 years will a couple sleep soundly at night—waking at first to listen for infant breathing or crying, later at the sound of a restless child's nightmares, and still later, unable to sleep until the child is home at night); and of a major accomplishment of an unusual order (building bridges, companies, or computers takes great skill, but they do not smile back at you). As a potentially sustained crisis, it may exhaust a person's usual coping mechanisms before the end of the 9-month course. As you monitor a pregnancy, your offers of support and suggestions for problem solving (tertiary coping mechanisms) can be influential in ensuring an adaptive, fulfilling outcome to a pregnancy. The use of outside intervention to reduce crisis, in contrast to the outcome of unresolved crisis, is depicted in Figures 1-

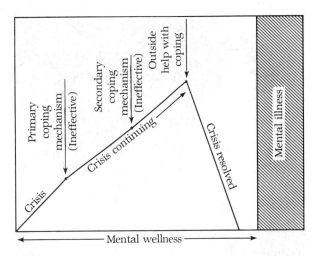

Figure 1-6 *Tertiary coping mechanism. A person's primary and secondary coping mechanisms are both inadequate to effect crisis resolution. Outside implementation is necessary to bring about resolution and keep the person within bounds of mental wellness.*

6 and 1-7. Nurses are health care providers very involved in offering this level of crisis intervention. The use of nursing process as a basis for this is illustrated in further chapters.

Family-Centered Care

Although families vary a great deal in structure, a family can be defined as a group of people who interact with care and concern for each other. A great many children are born into traditional nuclear families with two parents (Figure 1-8). An increasing number of children are being born to a

Figure 1-7 *Unresolved crisis. If a person seeks no help (or is offered no help) after primary and secondary coping mechanisms fail, the crisis situation proceeds unchecked; the outcome will be a continued inability to cope with life situations.*

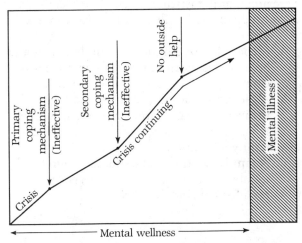

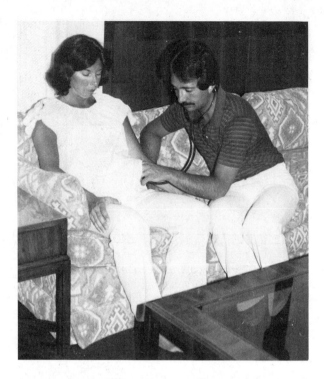

Figure 1-8 *Childbearing is an exciting event for the whole family. Planning nursing care within a framework of crisis awareness allows it to be optimal.*

single parent. Still other children have the luxury of an extended family in which grandparents and other relatives are present. Chapter 4 discusses different types of families and the role of the nurse in interacting with these families. Chapter 5 discusses the effects of culture and religious practices on childbearing: Except for rituals of dying, few events are more culturally influenced than childbirth or childrearing.

No matter what type of family is represented, nursing care must include consideration of the family and the community in which the woman lives. Otherwise, care measures will ultimately be made ineffective because of the strong influence of family and community on a mother and her newborn.

Position Statement

In 1978, the American College of Obstetricians and Gynecologists, the American College of Nurse-Midwives, the Nurses Association of the American College of Obstetricians and Gynecologists, the American Academy of Pediatrics, and the American Nurses Association issued a joint statement endorsing the philosophy of family-

---

Summary Points of the Joint Position Statement on Family-Centered Maternity/ Newborn Care

1. The family is the basic unit of society.
2. The hospital setting provides the maximum opportunity for physical safety and psychological well-being for childbirth if a family-centered philosophy of care is adopted and implemented.
3. The major manner that a family-centered program is instituted is by the accepting attitude of the family by all health care providers.
4. Preparation of families for childbirth should be included as an important component of care.
5. A diagnostic/admitting room should be utilized for examination of women in early labor to avoid unnecessary admission and family separation.
6. A family waiting room should be provided in labor areas so a woman can visit with members during this time.

7. A birthing room with a home-like atmosphere should be available as an alternative to a traditional delivery room.
8. Husbands or a support person should be allowed to visit freely in labor and delivery, recovery, and postpartum rooms.
9. The opportunity to breastfeed should be provided in the delivery room.
10. Rooming-in should be available on a postpartum unit.
11. Family visiting should be available on postpartum units.
12. Early discharge should be available to unite the woman most quickly with her family.

Source: Joint Position on the Development of Family-Centered Maternity/Newborn Care in Hospitals. The Interprofessional Task Force on Health Care of Women and Children, June 1978.

centered maternity/newborn care. Major points of this document are summarized in the box on page 20 and in Appendix C.

Conclusion

Knowing the basis of individual theories of nursing increases your basic knowledge of nursing; using any theorist's basic assumptions as a framework for organization offers increased opportunity for depth and thoroughness as you use nursing process for care. Being aware of the standards of maternal-newborn nursing allows you to nurse with assurance that your care is optimal for developing families. Finally, a framework of crisis intervention allows you to appreciate the impact of pregnancy and so individualize nursing care for a woman and her family.

Questions for Review

Multiple Choice

1. Mrs. Adrian is a 20-year-old woman you meet in a prenatal setting. You plan to base your care for her on Standards of Nursing Practice. Standards of maternal-newborn nursing help to establish
   a. a body of nursing knowledge.
   b. consistency among nurses on ways to practice.
   c. legal criteria for nursing practice.
   d. all of the above.

2. Mrs. Adrian states she is happy to be pregnant. Which action below, however, learned during your assessment, would lead you to believe she is under a high level of stress?
   a. She laughs at a physician's joke even though it is not funny.
   b. She states she is a poor driver.
   c. She has difficulty recalling simple directions you give her.
   d. She tells you she fell yesterday.

3. In planning care, you would decide that the ability of Mrs. Adrian to manage the stress of pregnancy depends *least* on
   a. her perception of the event.
   b. her support people available.
   c. her past experience with coping.
   d. involvement of family members.

4. You attempt to identify Mrs. Adrian's most important support person. From her descriptions below, which person would you rate as being her support person?
   a. her husband, who provides the family income
   b. her physician, who ordered her pregnancy test
   c. her neighbor, who said being pregnant was fun
   d. her mother, who discussed the feeling of being pregnant with her

5. In helping Mrs. Adrian to isolate her problem, which question or statement below would be most helpful?
   a. Tell me exactly what it is you are worried about.
   b. Tell me about everything that is worrying you.
   c. If there would be one thing I could help you with, what would it be?
   d. Why don't you tell me what your problem is?

6. In helping Mrs. Adrian develop a plan of action, which action below would be most important to include?
   a. a solution Mrs. Adrian believes will work
   b. a solution that a textbook on nursing recommends
   c. a solution you know works well because you have tried it
   d. a solution that is family-centered

Discussion

1. What are ways that maternal-newborn nursing has been influenced by nurses beginning to control their own profession?
2. If you were a nurse in a labor and delivery setting in the 1940s, how would your practice differ from that of today?
3. After assessing a pregnant woman you care for using the Stress Rating Scale, what ways could you use to help her reduce her level of stress? What mannerisms did she evidence that she is under any stress?

Suggested Readings

Aguilera, D., & Messick, J. (1974). *Crisis intervention: Theory and methodology.* St. Louis: Mosby.

American Nurses Association. (1973). *Standards of maternal-child health nursing practice.* Kansas City, MO: American Nurses Association.

Beard, M. T. (1982). Life events, method of coping, and interpersonal trust: Implications for nursing actions. *Issues in Mental Health Nursing, 4,* 25.

Berg, M., et al. (1983). Criteria revisited . . . maternal child health. *M.C.N., 8,* 101.

Bradley, C. F., et al. (1983). An evaluation of family centered maternity care. *Women's Health, 8,* 35.

Caplan, G. (1964). *Principles of preventive psychiatry.* New York: Basic Books.

Cousins, E. B., et al. (1981). Maldistribution of primary maternal-child health care: Mandate for nursing. *Issues in Health Care of Women, 3,* 241.

Cronenwett, L., et al. (1983). Models of helping and coping in childbirth. *Nursing Research, 32,* 84.

Field, P. A. (1982). What this country needs now: Nurses prepared to work with today's parents to revolutionize family-newborn care. *Canadian Nurse, 78,* 37.

Free, T. A. (1983). The states' challenge to provide maternal and child care. *Nurse Practitioner 3,* 46.

Gomez, E. A., et al. (1984). Anxiety as a human emotion: Some basic conceptual models. *Nursing Forum, 21,* 38.

Gray, A. (1979). The courts, the government, and the obstetric care consumer: An inventory. *Birth Family Journal, 6,* 227.

Leininger, M. (1981). Woman's role in society in the 1980s. *Issues in Health Care of Women, 3,* 203.

McClure, D. L. (1982). Wellness: A holistic concept. *Health Values, 6,* 23.

Mulligan, J. E. (1983). Some effects of the women's health movement. *Topics in Clinical Nursing, 4,* 1.

Pridham, K. F., et al. (1983). Parental goals and the birthing experience. *J.O.G.N. Nursing 12,* 50.

Raphael-Leff, J. (1984, January 11). Varying needs . . . women vary greatly in their response to birth. *Nursing Mirror, 158,* Midwifery Focus V.

Roskin, M. (1982). Coping with life changes—a preventive social work approach. *American Journal of Community Psychology, 10,* 331.

Rubin, R. (1963). Maternal touch. *Nursing Outlook, II,* 828.

Sandelowski, M. (1983). Perinatal nursing: Whose specialty is it anyway? *M.C.N., 38,* 317.

Sethi, A. S. (1982). Stress coping. *Canadian Journal of Public Health, 73,* 267.

Steer, P. J. (1983). Some impressions of obstetrics and midwifery in the United States. *Midwives Chronicle, 96,* 39.

Tierney, A., & Tierney, I. (1984). Perennial problems of parenthood—adopting a behavioral approach. *Nursing, 2,* 546.

Woolery, L. F. Self-care for the obstetrical patient: A nursing framework. *J.O.G.N. Nursing, 12,* 33.

2

Trends in Maternal-Newborn Nursing

OBJECTIVES

Following mastery of the material in the following chapter, you should be able to

1. Define statistical terms used to monitor maternal-newborn health, such as fetal, neonatal, and perinatal death rates and infant and maternal mortality.
2. Analyze steps to reduce maternal and infant mortality.
3. Describe the concept of comprehensive pregnancy care.
4. Describe innovations in maternal-newborn health practices that have had an influence on nursing care.
5. Synthesize knowledge of trends in health care with nursing process to achieve quality maternal-newborn nursing care.

EACH YEAR in the United States between 3.1 and 3.7 million women give birth (U.S. Dept. H.H.S., 1984). How safe is it for women to have babies today? How safe is it to be born today? Do women still die in childbirth? Do infants die? How many infants die shortly after birth? Before 1 year of age? What can be done to make pregnancy and childbirth safer for both women and infants? More satisfying for women and their families? The answers to these questions, which will be discussed in this chapter, will enrich your background in maternal-newborn nursing.

The Statistics of Maternal-Newborn Health

A number of statistical terms are used internationally in expressing the outcome of pregnancies and deliveries; therefore, statistics reported from different countries can be compared readily. These terms are listed below:

Birth rate: The number of births per 1,000 population.
Divorce rate: The number of divorces per 1,000 population.
Fertility rate: The number of pregnancies per 1,000 women of childbearing age.

Fetal death rate: The number of fetal deaths (over 500 gm) per 1,000 live births.
Infant mortality: The number of deaths per 1,000 live births occurring at birth or in the first 12 months of life.
Maternal mortality: The number of maternal deaths per 100,000 live births that occur as a direct result of the reproductive process.
Neonatal death rate: The number of deaths per 1,000 live births occurring at birth or in the first 28 days of life.
Perinatal death rate: The number of deaths occurring in fetuses over 500 gm and in the first 28 days of life per 1,000 live births.

Birth Rate

The birth rate in the United States started to decline about 1955. It hit a low of 14.8 per 1,000 in 1976, then began to rise again slightly because of the increasing number of women of childbearing age (15 to 44 years of age) to reach a 1982 level of 16.0 (U.S. Dept. H.H.S., 1984). This increasing trend is expected to continue each year until 1990. The overall decrease in birth rate is due to an accelerated willingness to voluntarily reduce family size by reproductive life planning and the use of contraceptives. The variation in the United States birth rate is shown in Figure 2-1.

Boys are born more often than girls, at a rate of 1,053 boys to every 1,000 girls. The peak months for births are August and September. The average size of the completed family in the United States today is 1.5 children. This low birth rate is threatening to some persons involved in maternal or newborn care, who wonder what will happen to their jobs if fewer and fewer children are conceived and born. The answer will be, it is hoped, that all children born in the future will receive the kind of health care that is advocated but not always available today. The decline in birth rate will perhaps allow the reality of maternal-newborn care to approximate the theoretical standards more closely. Using a broad definition, one of every seven pregnancies today is in some way a high-risk pregnancy. One child in every seven, therefore, requires some form of special concern or care at birth.

Fertility Rate

Fertility rates are always higher than birth rates because some pregnancies are spontaneously lost for unexplained reasons. The fertility rate for 1982, for example, was 67.8, while the birth rate was only 16.0 (U.S. Dept. H.H.S., 1983).

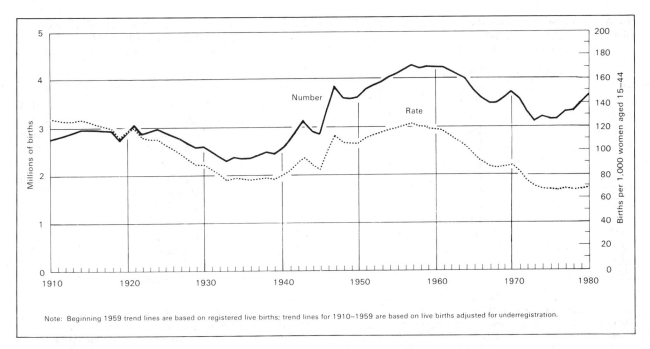

Figure 2-1 *Live births and fertility rates: United States, 1910–80. From U.S. Department of Health and Human Services. (1982, November 30). Advance report of final natality statistics, 1980 (Figure 1),* Monthly Vital Statistics Report, 31, 8, *Supplement. Public Health Service: Hyattsville, MD.*

Fetal Death Rate

Fetal death rate is the number of fetal deaths per 1,000 live births. A fetal death is defined as the death in utero of a child (fetus) weighing 500 gm or more, roughly the weight of a fetus of 20 weeks or more gestation. Fetal deaths may occur because of maternal factors (maternal disease, incompetent cervix, maternal malnutrition) or fetal factors (fetal disease, chromosome abnormality, poor uterine attachment). A large number of fetal deaths still occur for reasons yet unknown. Fetal death rate is important because it reflects the overall quality of maternity care.

Neonatal Death Rate

The first 28 days of life comprise the *neonatal period.* The child during this time is known as a *neonate. Neonatal death rate* is the number of deaths per 1,000 live births occurring at birth or in the first 28 days of life. The neonatal death rate reflects not only the quality of care available to women during pregnancy and childbirth but also the quality of care available to infants during the first month of life.

Immaturity of the infant is the chief cause of these early deaths. Approximately 80 percent of infants who die within 48 hours after birth weigh less than 2,500 gm (5½ lbs).

Perinatal Death Rate

The *perinatal period* is the time beginning when the fetus reaches 500 gm (about the twentieth week of pregnancy) and ending about 4 weeks after birth. The *perinatal death rate* is the sum of the fetal and neonatal rates.

Infant Mortality

Infant mortality is the number of deaths per 1,000 live births occurring at birth or in the first 12 months of life. It includes the neonatal death rate. This rate is the traditional standard that is used to compare one country's overall conditions of health and health care with those of other countries.

Thanks to medical advances and improvements in child care, infant mortality in the United States is falling. The decline since 1960 is shown in Table 2-1 and Figure 2-2.

The steady drop in total infant mortality in the United States is certainly encouraging. Table 2-2 shows the infant mortality in the United States compared to that in other countries. One would expect that the United States, which has the highest gross national product in the world and has great technological resources, would have the lowest infant mortality. In fact, in 1976 (the most recent year for which world statistics are cur-

Table 2-1 Infant Mortality Rates (Per 1,000 Live Births): United States, 1960–1982

Year	Rate Under 1 Year	Under 28 Days	28 Days to 11 Months
1960	26.0	18.7	7.3
1962	25.3	18.3	7.0
1964	24.8	17.9	6.9
1966	23.7	17.2	6.5
1968	21.8	16.1	5.7
1970	20.0	15.1	4.9
1972	18.5	13.6	4.8
1974	16.7	12.3	4.4
1976	15.2	10.9	4.3
1978	13.6	9.4	4.2
1980	12.6	8.5	4.1
1982	11.2	7.6	3.6

Source: National Center for Health Statistics. (1982). Annual summary of births, deaths, marriages, and divorces: United States, 1982, in *Monthly Vital Statistics Report, 31,* 13. Public Health Service: Hyattsville, MD, 1983.

Table 2-2 Infant Mortality Rates (Per 1,000 Live Births) for Selected Countries, 1976

Rank	Country	Rate
1	Sweden	8.3
2	Japan	9.3
3	Denmark	10.3
4	Netherlands	10.6
5	Switzerland	10.7
6	Finland	11.0
7	Norway	11.1
8	England and Wales	14.2
9	France	14.7
10	Scotland	14.8
11	Hong Kong	14.9
12	Canada	15.0
13	United States	15.2

Source: Health in the United States Chartbook. (1978). U.S. Department of Health, Education, and Welfare, Public Health Service, National Center for Health Statistics, Hyattsville, MD.

rently available) our infant mortality was higher than that of 12 other countries.

Why is infant mortality higher in some countries than in others? One factor may be different systems of health care delivery. In Sweden, for example, a comprehensive health care program provides free maternal and child health care to all residents. Women who attend prenatal clinics early in pregnancy receive a monetary award. Sweden's infant mortality is the lowest of any country tabulated.

Methods of delivering infants may also play a part in mortality. In The Netherlands, for instance, cesarean sections are performed in only a small percentage of all deliveries. In the United States the number of cesarean sections being performed is growing yearly. About 5 percent of all infants delivered by cesarean section have some respiratory difficulty for a day or two after birth. One cesarean section often leads to another, so that the number of such procedures performed tends to pyramid, constantly increasing the risk to newborns.

In the United States, infant mortality varies

Figure 2-2 *Infant mortality rate (per 1,000 live births). From U.S. Department of Health and Human Services. (1983). Changing mortality patterns, health services utilization and health care expenditures; United States, 1978–2003, 3, 23. National Center for Health Statistics: Hyattsville, MD.*

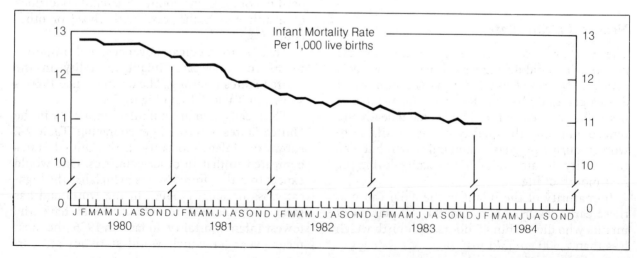

Table 2-3 Infant Mortality Rate (Per 1,000 Live Births) by State, 1982

State	Rate
Wyoming	6.3
Montana	7.4
Wisconsin	7.8
South Dakota	8.4
Idaho	8.6
Vermont	8.6
Hawaii	8.9
Iowa	8.9
Maine	9.2
Pennsylvania	9.3
Minnesota	9.4
Washington	9.5
Kansas	9.7
Arkansas	9.9
California	9.9
New Mexico	9.9
Arizona	10.0
Colorado	10.0
Connecticut	10.1
New Hampshire	10.1
Maryland	10.3
Nebraska	10.4
Ohio	10.5
Massachusetts	10.6
Oregon	10.8
New Jersey	10.9
Rhode Island	11.0
West Virginia	11.0
Texas	11.1
Indiana	11.3
Kentucky	11.4
Oklahoma	11.4
Alaska	11.7
Michigan	11.7
Delaware	11.8
Nevada	11.9
Utah	11.9
Virginia	12.1
Georgia	12.5
Missouri	12.5
New York	12.6
North Dakota	12.7
Florida	12.8
Louisiana	13.0
Illinois	13.3
Tennessee	13.5
North Carolina	13.8
Alabama	14.1
Mississippi	15.2
South Carolina	15.4
District of Columbia	21.9

Source: National Center for Health Statistics. (1983). Annual summary of births, deaths, marriages, and divorces: United States, 1982, in *Monthly Vital Statistics Report,* 31,13. Public Health Service: Hyattsville, MD.

from state to state (Table 2-3). Note that in the District of Columbia, which has the questionable distinction of having higher infant mortality than any state in the country, the rate is more than three times what it is in Wyoming, the state with the lowest infant mortality.

Maternal Mortality

Maternal mortality is the number of maternal deaths per 100,000 live births that occur as the direct result of the reproductive process. As with infant mortality, there has been a consistent decline in maternal mortality since approximately 1940 (Table 2-4 and Figure 2-3). It has declined so much that since 1960 it has been compiled on the basis of 100,000 live births, not on the 1,000 base ordinarily used.

Three causes are responsible for 70 percent of all maternal deaths: hemorrhage, infection, and pregnancy-induced hypertension. Hemorrhage can occur for a number of different reasons, including placenta previa, premature separation of the placenta, and blood dyscrasias, all of which are discussed in detail in later chapters. Infections may occur any time following rupture of the fetal membranes until the uterus returns to its prepregnant state. Infection may be associated with poor technique by health care personnel in caring for the mother in labor, at delivery, or during the days following childbirth when the placental site in the uterus is prone to infection because of its denuded surface. Pregnancy-induced hypertension, a condition peculiar to pregnancy, is manifested by vasoconstriciton, increased blood pressure, proteinuria, edema, and, sometimes, convulsions. The first signs of pregnancy-induced hypertension may occur during pregnancy, labor, delivery, or immediately following birth.

Nurses giving maternal-newborn care should

Table 2-4 Maternal Mortality Rate Per 100,000 Live Births, 1960 to 1982

Year	Rate	Year	Rate
1960	37.1	1972	18.8
1962	35.2	1974	14.6
1964	33.3	1976	12.3
1966	29.1	1978	9.9
1968	24.5	1980	9.2
1970	21.5	1982	8.9

Source: National Center for Health Statistics. (1983). Annual summary of births, deaths, marriages, and divorces: United States, 1982, in *Monthly Vital Statistics Report,* 31,11. Public Health Service: Hyattsville, MD.

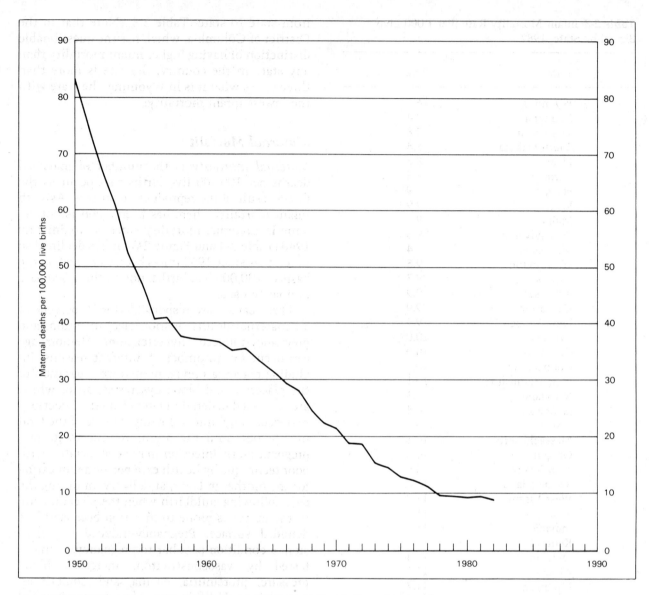

Figure 2-3 *Maternal mortality rates: United States, 1950–82. From National Center for Health Statistics. (1983). Annual summary of births, deaths, marriages, and divorces: United States, 1982, in* Monthly Vital Statistics Report, 31, *13. Public Health Service: Hyattsville, MD.*

impress on their minds the three main causes of maternal mortality so strongly that they flicker like neon signs every time they care for a woman during pregnancy, in childbirth, or during the puerperium. These conditions are for the most part preventable, and nurses who are alert to the signs and symptoms of hemorrhage, infection, and beginning hypertension are invaluable guardians of the health of pregnant and postpartum women.

Divorce Rates

Because maternal mortality is falling, more children than ever before have the chance to be reared in intact families. A high divorce rate, however,

causes this not to be true. The divorce rate for the United States for the years 1960 through 1982 is shown in Table 2-5. The rate in 1982 was 5.1 per 1,000 population, or a total of 1,180,000 divorces a year. Although this rate is reduced from 1980, in many instances, a new mother is single and has had a recent loss of a support person during her pregnancy or postpartum period. Marriage and divorce rates are compared in Figure 2-4.

Steps Toward Reducing Maternal and Infant Mortality

The availability of skilled professional prenatal care and women's recognition of the importance

Table 2-5 Divorce Rate in the United States, 1960 to 1982

Year	Rate	Year	Rate
1960	2.2	1972	4.1
1962	2.2	1974	4.6
1964	2.4	1976	5.0
1966	2.5	1978	5.2
1968	2.9	1980	5.2
1970	3.5	1982	5.1

Source: National Center for Health Statistics. (1983). Annual summary of births, deaths, marriages, and divorces: United States, 1982, in *Monthly Vital Statistics Report*, *31*,13. Public Health Service: Hyattsville, MD.

of such care are important steps in safeguarding the health of women and children. Women today usually either see an obstetrician or a family physician practicing in association with a nurse-midwife or attend a community clinic early in pregnancy. Fewer low-birth-weight babies are born to women who begin prenatal care early in pregnancy than to those who do not (U.S. Dept. H.H.S., 1982). Many health problems of pregnancy are correctable if recognized when they first appear, uncorrectable later. Pregnancy-induced hypertension (the third leading cause of maternal mortality) is an example of a disorder that if recognized early can easily be controlled and will not be detrimental to the woman or her child; if allowed to continue unchecked, it can lead to death of the mother and the infant.

The areas of pregnancy care and perinatal and neonatal care are expanding rapidly today as the overall emphasis of health care in the United States shifts from the treatment of to the prevention of illness, from treating ill newborns to preventing illness in newborns.

Personal Concern for the Patient

Health care consumers are growing more discriminating in what they demand from health personnel. Changes in both private offices and

Figure 2-4 *A. Marriage rate per 1,000 population. B. Divorce rate per 1,000 population. From U.S. Department of Health and Human Services. (1983). Changing mortality patterns, health services utilization and health care expenditures: United States, 1978–2003, 3, 23, National Center for Health Statistics: Hyattsville, MD.*

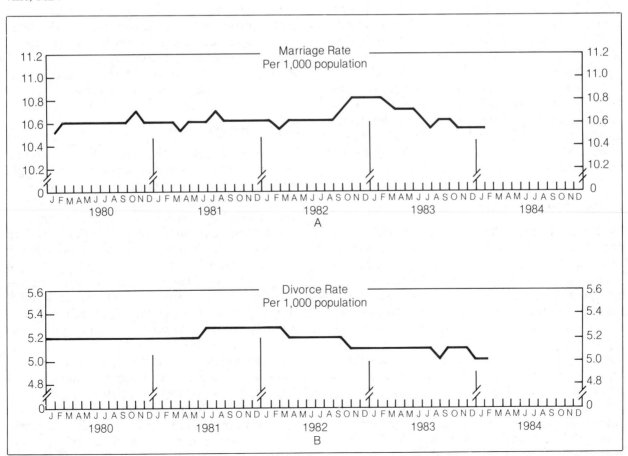

clinics will have to be made if women are to continue to accept prenatal care. Waiting in line, being called by a number, and being treated as a punched data card with little regard for privacy were once accepted fatalistically. Today, women are asking why they must be treated so indifferently and protest such treatment by their poor attendance at health care facilities. Many groups are so distressed by the mechanical way in which women are treated during labor that they are advocating home births.

Personnel in health care facilities may offer excuses for these conditions, claiming, for instance, that no money is allocated to make improvements. The items that women are most concerned with, however, do not cost money. Being addressed by name, being interviewed as if they were important, not just as a repository of wanted facts, having people knock on examining room doors before entering, having examining tables turned so women are not unnecessarily exposed—these courtesies are all free. During and after labor and delivery, being allowed to have a support person with them, being allowed to have their other children visit, being able to care for the newborn in their room rather than having the child taken away to a central nursery—these, too, are free.

Nurses have a great deal to do with creating the atmosphere, conveying the feeling that although a woman is the eighty-sixth patient to be examined in the clinic or seen in the labor unit this week she is still important. She counts. The child inside her counts. Such concern costs nothing.

Nurses are the people who dispense or fail to dispense these amenities. Consequently, nurses bear a great deal of the responsibility for clinic and office attendance and for keeping childbirth in health care surroundings, where safety for the woman and her child can be maintained.

Comprehensive Prenatal Care

During the last two decades maternal and infant care projects have been designed as one way of reducing maternal and infant mortality and morbidity caused by complications of pregnancy and childbirth. These projects provide women of low income with the services of allied health care personnel, such as social workers, nutritionists, and home health aides, as well as nurses and physicians. Great differences have been demonstrated in the outcome of pregnancy in women who make use of the projects, as opposed to nonproject women. In a 1970s project in Chicago, involving women 15 years of age or younger at the time of conception, neonatal mortality was 36.8 for 4,400 nonproject women and 19.0 for those who partici-

pated in the project. In New York City, neonatal mortality was reported as 13 percent lower for infants born to women in the program than for the city as a whole (Pomerance, 1978)

These projects demonstrate what can be accomplished in reducing infant and maternal mortality. Additional comprehensive measures such as these are needed if all the infants delivered to women at the poverty level (about 20 percent of all infants delivered) are to be given good care.

Role of the Community Health Nurse

The home visits of community health nurses can be as important as the monthly visits to a health care facility. A mother who feels too embarrassed to admit at a clinic that she rarely eats may talk about the problem and be receptive to nutrition suggestions in her own home. A mother who feels she will be told she is foolish if she admits to fears while at a busy clinic may feel free to talk about such fears while she is at home. Talking about her fears may put them in a perspective, so that she can start to handle them. Knowing that a person has been concerned enough about her health to visit her home may be motivation enough for her to make the extra effort to get to the clinic or a physician's office and so receive the benefits of prenatal care.

Whether or not the visits of a community health nurse are successful depends on the same factors that determine a woman's acceptance of prenatal care in a health care facility or on whether or not the nurse's attitudes and actions convey a personal, concerned interest.

Improving Nutrition

It is well documented that the nutrition a woman receives before and during a pregnancy strongly influences the course of pregnancy and the health of the baby. The father's nutrition before conception may also have a bearing on the infant's health. According to Antonov (1947), of children born during the siege of Leningrad in 1942 during a period when the little food available was of poor quality, 41.2 percent were premature births. When food was not so scarce, the premature birth rate was only 6.5 percent. In another classic study, Burke (1943) reported that in a study population all stillborn infants, all infants (except one) who died within a few days of birth, all premature infants, all functionally immature infants, and the majority of infants with congenital malformations were born to women on inadequate diets.

Good nutrition is an area of health teaching in which school nurses can be effective, since the nutritional patterns a person learns as a child tend to persist throughout life. Unfortunately, many children are taught nutrition in such a technical way that they are "turned off" by the subject ever afterward. It is a challenge to maternal-newborn nurses to "turn on" women to good health.

Socioeconomic Factors

A number of socioeconomic factors influence infant mortality. The more siblings a mother has, for example, the more likely she is to have a stillborn child. In middle-class women, there is a sharp rise in the number of stillbirths among those who have four or more siblings. Among women whose fathers were unskilled manual laborers, there is a sharp rise in stillbirths between women with no siblings and those with one sibling, and again between women with one sibling and those with two or three. The difference probably occurs at the point at which a scarcity of resources began to have an effect on growth in childhood and thus on the woman's reproductive efficiency.

If stillbirths are related to depletion of resources in the mother's family, reproductive life planning or choosing to have only the number of children who can be economically and emotionally cared for should reduce infant mortality in future generations. Reproductive life planning is an area of health supervision in which the maternal-newborn nurse must develop expertise, since a nurse may be the person with whom the woman feels she can best talk about such subjects.

Child spacing can have a direct influence on perinatal mortality. Data from the Maternity and Infant Care Project in New York City (Pomerance, 1978) show that when deliveries occur a year or less apart, the neonatal death rate is 35 per 1,000. If the interval following delivery is 1 to 2 years, the neonatal death rate drops to 17 per 1,000. After a 2-to-3-year interval, the rate drops to 7 per 1,000.

In infants 2,500 gm or more (normal-birth-weight infants) the morbidity is considered higher during the first year of life for those whose family income is less than $8,000 than for those whose family income is in the middle range ($8,000 to $14,999). This trend is shown in Table 2-6.

Another important factor in planning health care for women in the childbearing age is the number of women in this age range who work in order to bring their family income into the middle range—about 45 percent. This means that many of the old instructions for pregnancy, such as "get lots of rest," have to be modified to "try and get a period of rest each day."

Settings for Childbirth

A factor strongly influencing maternal and infant mortality and related to the current decline in these rates is the trend for women to be hospitalized for childbirth. In 1940 only about 40 percent of live births occurred in hospitals; by 1980, the figure rose to between 96 and 100 percent. Today, although the hospital-born rate is still over 97 percent, a growing number of persons now advocate childbirth at home or in alternative birth settings—in "natural" surroundings, free from the cold, structured hospital environment. They believe that childbirth in these settings is more enjoyable and may be experienced as the truly exciting event that it should be.

In order that childbirth can continue to be safe, nurses have a responsibility to center the operations of labor and delivery units more around concern for the individuality of patients than concern for rules, to make childbirth as enjoyable in a hospital as it is at home. How quickly the laughter

Table 2-6 Infant Morbidity by Family Income

Birth Weight	Family Income	Severe Impairment (%)	Moderate Congenital Anomalies (%)	Significant Other Illness (%)	Brief or No Illness (%)
2,500 gm or less	Less than $8,000	4.0	17.0	21	58
	$8,000–$14,999	5.2	16.3	16	62
	$15,000 and more	5.2	14.8	14	66
Over 2,500 gm	Less than $8,000	2.4	12.6	16	69
	$8,000–$14,999	1.5	11.5	13	74
	$15,000 and more	2.2	14.8	15	68

Source: Special Report, No. 2, 1978. The Robert Wood Johnson Foundation, Princeton, N.J. Based on data compiled by The Johns Hopkins University Health Services Research and Development Center.

stops at home when a mother hemorrhages, 30 minutes away from medical help! How long the heartache lasts when a baby never breathes, 30 minutes away from resuscitation equipment!

The Committee on the Fetus and Newborn of the American Academy of Pediatrics and the American College of Obstetricians and Gynecologists (1979) issued the following joint statement:

> Labor and delivery, while a physiologic process, clearly presents potential hazards to both mother and fetus before and after birth. These hazards require standards of safety which are provided in the hospital setting and cannot be matched in the home situation.
>
> We recognize, however, the legitimacy of the concern of many that the events surrounding birth be an emotionally satisfying experience for the family. We support those actions that improve the experience of the family while continuing to provide the mother and her infant with accepted standards of safety available only in hospitals which conform to standards as outlined by the American Academy of Pediatrics and the American College of Obstetricians and Gynecologists.

Because nurses control the atmosphere of hospitals, making them either friendly or cold places in which to be a patient, they can be instrumental in keeping childbirth in hospitals.

Birthing Rooms

One way of making hospital births more like those at home is the use of birthing rooms in hospitals. A *birthing room* is a room furnished with colorful curtains, a comfortable chair for a support person, and a noninstitutional-looking bed. Supplies for labor and delivery are in readiness but are concealed in wall cabinets, so the room has a comfortable, nonclinical atmosphere.

Following labor, the woman is not moved to a delivery room for the birth of her child; rather the bed is converted into a delivery table or the woman is allowed to deliver in a lateral or squatting position without the use of stirrups (the traditional delivery position with a delivery table). Following birth, the infant is cared for in the same room, remaining with the mother and accompanying her to her postpartum rooming-in suite.

Each birthing room must be a self-contained labor and delivery room (Figure 2-5). Thus if a hospital has six labor rooms and one delivery room, it has to purchase equipment for only one delivery room. If it converts its facilities to six birthing rooms, it must have six complete delivery room setups. Obviously this change entails additional expense.

In order to minimize the duplication of equip-

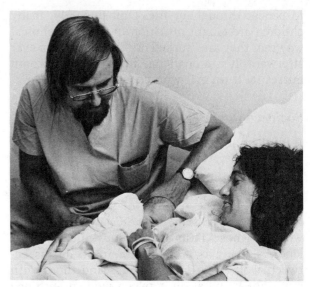

Figure 2-5 *A mother and father share a close moment together in a birthing room. (Courtesy of the Department of Medical Photography, Children's Hospital, Buffalo, N.Y.)*

ment such as radiant heat warmers and anesthetic equipment, many hospitals limit the use of birthing rooms to women who wish to deliver without any anesthetic and who appear to be free from potential delivery difficulties. As satisfaction with such rooms grows, however, even women with complications may use them.

Women appreciate birthing rooms because they do not have to be moved to a cart and transferred to a strange room (possibly away from their support person) at the time labor is becoming hardest for them; husbands are welcome in birthing rooms for the delivery as well as for labor. Husbands do not feel intimidated, as they do by the surgical atmosphere of a delivery room, so they can truly function as support persons.

Use of birthing rooms separates women physically more than traditional labor rooms: Detailed observation by nurses on the women's progress in labor is necessary in order to help physicians coordinate care among so many settings.

Alternative Birth Centers

Another way of making birth more homelike, yet offering the protection of medical or skilled nursing personnel, is the development of alternative birth centers. In such a center, a woman is observed on an ambulatory basis throughout her pregnancy. She delivers at the center in an attractive birthing room, stays only about 24 hours, and then is discharged under well-defined follow-up and supervisory care.

A woman is generally ineligible for care at a

birth center if she has a high-risk factor such as previous cesarean section, is an elderly primipara, or has an accompanying physical illness such as diabetes or a cardiac disease.

Nurse-midwives play a big role in supervising the health and welfare of women who use alternative birth centers and in protecting the health of their newborns.

Observation and Recovery Rooms for Newborns and Mothers

Even though recovery rooms for surgical patients have been available in hospitals for decades, some hospitals still do not utilize a recovery room for women or newborns after childbirth.

A great many mothers still receive some anesthesia during delivery, and they have the same problems of anesthesia recovery as do all surgical patients. All new mothers need careful observation for determination of the amount of bleeding and for signs of postpartum hypertension.

A woman who stays in a birthing room under the watchful eye of a nurse is far safer than one returned immediately to a postpartum unit, where her needs can be overlooked among those of other patients. Mothers who would like a water pitcher filled or ask for medication for suture pain voice their requests strongly and loudly, but hemorrhage, infection, and hypertension are silent killers.

Because of placental transfer, an infant whose mother receives a general anesthetic during delivery also receives some anesthetic. The infant is in just as much need of an anesthesia recovery room as is any postoperative patient. All infants need the protection of a careful watch period following birth because independent respirations are a new experience for them. The change from fetal to extrauterine circulation does not always happen quickly or surely; they may have some mucus or

fluid in the lungs that can lead to obstruction of the airway. Maintaining body temperature at the proper level also poses some difficulty. Heart failure, respiratory obstruction, and hypothermia, like maternal complications, are silent killers. They can be missed in a nursery of crying, hungry infants.

Intensive Care Nurseries

It is generally assumed that newborns with a term birth weight (over 2,500 gm, or 5½ lb) will thrive at birth. In a survey of statistics from high-risk intensive care facilities (Robert Wood Johnson Foundation, 1978), it was discovered that close to 30 percent of infants of normal birth weight experience significant health problems in the first year of life. These findings are summarized in Table 2-7.

Infants who can be categorized as high risk should be transferred to a neonatal intensive care unit or intensive care nursery (ICN). In nine hospitals throughout the United States and Canada, the introduction of neonatal intensive care units resulted in decreased neonatal mortality of up to 42 percent (Robert Wood Johnson Foundation, 1978).

It is sometimes argued that saving small babies from dying at birth is not necessarily good health care, since it is difficult to justify the cost/benefit ratio of such care and since small babies develop such neurologic abnormalities that they cannot function effectively as adults. A team of pediatricians at the University of Southern California in a study of infants born weighing less than 1,500 gm (3 lb, 5 oz) reported that the most striking change in end results—along with an increase in survival (more than 30 percent improvement)—is a decrease in definitely abnormal infants (Teberg, 1977). This study suggests that such care is ethically justified.

Table 2-7 Morbidity in Infants to 1 Year of Age

Birth Weight	Severe Impairment (%)	Moderate to Mild Congenital Anomalies (%)	Significant Other Illness (%)	Brief or No Illness (%)
1,500 gm or less	13.0	29.0	15	43
1,501–2,000 gm	5.3	20.7	17	57
2,001–2,500 gm	3.4	14.6	19	63
Over 2,500 gm	2.0	12.0	15	71

Source: Special Report, No. 2, 1978. The Robert Wood Johnson Foundation, Princeton, N.J. Based on data compiled by The Johns Hopkins University Health Services Research and Development Center.

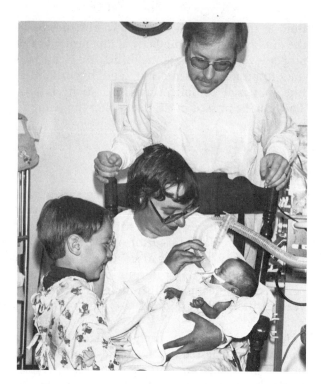

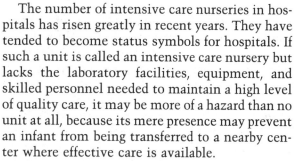

Figure 2-6 *Women should be encouraged to visit with infants who are transported to a high-risk facility for care in order to encourage mother-child bonding. Here a family visits with an ill newborn. The mother holds a source of oxygen near the child's face. (Courtesy of the Department of Medical Photography, Children's Hospital, Buffalo, N.Y.)*

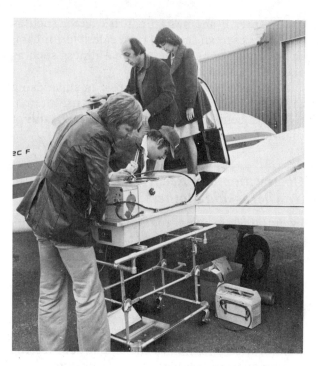

Figure 2-7 *An infant transport unit is moved from the transporting airplane to a transport van. Safe movement of pregnant women and ill newborns to regional centers is an important nursing responsibility. (Courtesy of the Department of Medical Photography, Children's Hospital, Buffalo, N.Y.)*

The number of intensive care nurseries in hospitals has risen greatly in recent years. They have tended to become status symbols for hospitals. If such a unit is called an intensive care nursery but lacks the laboratory facilities, equipment, and skilled personnel needed to maintain a high level of quality care, it may be more of a hazard than no unit at all, because its mere presence may prevent an infant from being transferred to a nearby center where effective care is available.

The cost of keeping an infant in a neonatal intensive care unit is $500 to $1,000 a day. Costs of $20,000 to $50,000 are not rare for care during a high-risk pregnancy and care for a high-risk infant. Almost all states have adopted guidelines for health insurance companies that prevent the companies from excluding coverage of intensive newborn care, so the cost of such high-risk care does not preclude infants from being given it. When infants are hospitalized in regional centers for care (Figure 2-6) the mother who is left behind in a community hospital needs a great deal of support. She has "lost" her infant as surely as the mother whose child dies, unless health care personnel help her maintain contact with the infant through telephone calls or snapshots and encourage her to visit as soon as she is able.

Consolidation of Care

In view of the falling birth rate, no single hospital may be able to afford a corps of highly skilled health care personnel to be available at all times to care for women and newborns (it is impossible to limit births to a 9-to-5 schedule, so it is impossible to limit quality care to only those hours) and the best equipment obtainable to safeguard both mother and child. Thus, concepts of consolidation or regionalization are being explored (Figure 2-7).

When travel was by horse and buggy and roads were rough, small community hospitals at frequently spaced intervals were the answer to health care. With the highways and emergency vehicles now available, the scope of the "community" can be much larger, enabling enough deliveries in one place to justify the cost of the equipment necessary for optimum maternal and infant care.

Transporting High-Risk Patients

When regionalization concepts of newborn care first became accepted, transporting the ill or premature infant was the method chosen. Now, health care providers are looking at the subject in a new light. Instead of transporting the infant, it may be safer to transport the mother, since the uterus has advantages as a transport incubator that far exceed any commercial incubator yet designed.

Unfortunately, transporting mothers has several problems that have yet to be solved. The referring hospital loses a patient and so may lose revenue. Removing a woman from her community places a great deal of stress on her family; it also limits her own doctor's participation in her care. Certainly, women who are transported distances for perinatal care need strong support from nursing personnel or they will feel that they are lost in the system.

It is difficult for many people to relinquish the community concept, to accept a van staffed by a physician and maternal nursing practitioners and traveling from community to community as giving as good prenatal care as that dispensed in a red brick community hospital that has been standing in one spot for 50 years. People find it hard to believe that transporting a woman to a consolidated health care facility for childbirth can be an improvement over the traditional wild dash in the family car to the local community hospital. Nurses, like other people, tend to resist change. On the other hand, nurses have the experience and position to be the prime innovators in changing concepts of maternal-newborn care.

Defining High-Risk Mothers and Infants

Serious attempts to identify a woman who may have difficulty in pregnancy are being made, usually by means of standardized record systems in which point scores are assigned to various criteria such as high blood pressure or previous pregnancy loss. The total risk score can help identify a high-risk woman. Some scoring systems differentiate among more than 150 factors that might affect the woman or the fetus or both, as many as 30 factors that might affect the mother after birth, and an additional 150 items that might affect the newborn infant (Goodwin, 1973).

Some factors that place a woman at risk are (a) age less than 17 years or more than 35 years, (b) hypertension, (c) diabetes, (d) previous premature birth or stillbirth, and (e) abnormal duration of labor or delivery. Some factors that place the newborn at risk are (a) prematurity, (b) difficulty establishing respirations at birth, and (c) congenital anomalies.

Expanding Roles for Nurses

Nurses fulfill important roles in maintaining the quality of maternal-newborn care.

A maternal-newborn practitioner is a nurse able to interview and examine women during pregnancy and so assess their physical and psychological health; obtain pelvic measurements, so that the type of delivery can be predicted; teach women self-care during pregnancy; and prepare them for labor, delivery, and care of the infant. She is able to evaluate the woman in labor, including assessment of her stage of labor and the health of the fetus. Following delivery, she assesses the health of the newborn, teaches self-care to the mother, and helps her with feeding and caring for her infant. She promotes interpregnancy health and provides information for reproductive life planning or child spacing as requested.

The pediatric nurse associate, working with a pediatrician, assesses the health of newborns by examination and advises the mother on the infant's care. She might make a home visit a week after the mother goes home with the infant to be available for the small problems that arise with new babies before the problems become magnified. She is available by telephone for future consultation. She sees the child during his years of growing up for well-child care and preventive health care measures such as immunizations. She offers advice and counsel on the expected crises of childhood and manages minor illness in children in consultation with a pediatrician. Such a role allows physicians or pediatricians to devote more time to ill children and thereby improve the quality of their practice.

A nurse-midwife, in association with an obstetrician, can assume full responsibility for the care and management of women with uncomplicated pregnancies. A nurse who is capable of these functions enables the obstetrician with whom she works to devote the bulk of time to high-risk mothers or to women in whom complications develop during pregnancy or delivery, thereby improving the quality of the practice. In Sweden, a country with a low infant mortality (8.3, versus 15.2 for the United States), nurse-midwives play a much larger role in maternity care than they do in the United States.

All nurses can be instrumental in promoting family-centered care.

Interpregnancy Care

It is becoming more and more evident that the state of the mother's health at the time pregnancy begins is as important as the health she maintains during pregnancy. Women should be urged to have a health assessment prior to conception, so that any existing health problems, including malnutrition, can be corrected before a pregnancy begins. Both women and men should be encouraged to maintain good health practices throughout their childbearing years in preparation for a future child.

Questions for Review

Multiple Choice

1. Mrs. Taylor is a woman you meet in a prenatal setting. She states she wants to have her baby at home. In the United States, statistically the setting where most babies are born today is
   a. in hospital birthing rooms.
   b. at home.
   c. in alternative birth centers.
   d. in hospital delivery rooms.

2. The infant mortality of a country is a gauge of overall health care in that country. The United States' infant mortality
   a. is the lowest in the world.
   b. is steadily decreasing.
   c. has recently been increasing.
   d. is the highest in the world.

3. Infant mortality is defined as
   a. the number of deaths per 1,000 live births occurring at birth or in the first 12 months of life.
   b. the number of deaths compared to live births each month.
   c. the number of deaths per 1,000 pregnancies that occur in the first 12 months of life.
   d. the number of deaths per month of infants under 12 months of age.

3. Nurses in maternal-newborn care are involved in an area of health care that is becoming
   a. overly simplified because of increased technology.
   b. more complex yearly.

   c. no longer in need of nurses as health care providers.
   d. an area with a low-stress environment.

5. Statistically, the number one cause of death in childbirth is
   a. preexisting illness.
   b. infection.
   c. hemorrhage.
   d. hypertension.

6. A concern involving the present intensive care of low-birth-weight infants is that such care will cause
   a. fewer low-birth-weight infants to live than previously.
   b. infants of low birth weight to live but be handicapped.
   c. women to not be as concerned with obtaining pregnancy care.
   d. women to no longer want to carry pregnancies to term.

Discussion

1. How has the declining birth rate in recent years affected maternal-newborn nursing? How will a projected increase in the future affect it?
2. What are ways that nurses are playing a more active role in maternal-newborn care? What caused these trends to develop?
3. The United States has a high infant mortality in comparison to other countries. What are possible reasons for this finding?

Suggested Readings

Antonov, A. N. (1947). Children born during the siege of Leningrad in 1942. *Journal of Pediatrics, 30,* 250.

Bowler, S. (1983). Survival test for babies . . . attitudes to childbirth during the centuries. *Nursing Mirror, 156,* VIII (Midwife Forum 3).

Burke, B. S., et al. (1943). Nutrition studies during pregnancy. *American Journal of Obstetrics and Gynecology, 46,* 38.

Committee on the Fetus and Newborn of the American Academy of Pediatrics and the American College of Obstetrics and Gynecologists. (1979). *Pediatrics, 63,* 166.

de Hann, J., & Smits, F. (1983). Home deliveries in the Netherlands. *Journal of Perinatal Medicine, 11,* 3.

Derby, V. L., et al. (1981). Changing the system to meet the needs of patient and nurse. *M.C.N., 6,* 225.

Fraleigh, D. M. (1984). Combined mother-baby care. *Canadian Nurse, 80,* 25.

Franklin, J. (1978). Home-like deliveries in the hospital. *Birth Family Journal, 5,* 235.

Gillespie, S. A. (1981). Childbirth in the 1980s: What are the options? *Issues in Health Care of Women, 3,* 101.

Gillett, J. (1981). The evolution of thought in obstetrics. *Midwife Health Visitor and Community Nurse, 17,* 458.

Goodwin, J. W., & Hewlett, P. T. (1973). The strategy of fetal risk management. *Canadian Family Physician, 19,* 54.

Gordon, I. T. (1982). The birth controllers: Limitations on out-of-hospital births. *Journal of Nurse-midwifery, 27,* 34.

Haire, D. (1981). Improving the outcome of pregnancy through increased utilization of midwives. *Journal of Nurse Midwifery, 26,* 5.

Jennings, B. (1982). Childbirth choices: Are there safe options? *Nurse Practitioner, 7,* 26.

Joint statement of practice relationships between obstetricians and gynecologists and certified nurse-midwives. (1983). *Journal of Nurse Midwifery, 28,* 10.

Jorgenson, A. J. (1982). Home births. *Journal of Nursing Care, 15,* 14.

Kesby, O. (1982). A case for the birthing chair. *Nursing Mirror, 155,* 37.

May, K. A., et al. (1984). In-hospital alternative birth centers. *M.C.N., 9,* 48.

McGlaughlin, A. (1982). Changing trends in child rearing. *Midwife Health Visitor and Community Nurse, 18,* 48.

Osborne, N. G., et al. (1984). Sexually transmitted diseases and pregnancy. *J.O.G.N. Nursing, 13,* 9.

Pomerance, J. J., et al. (1978). Cost of living for infants weighing 1000 grams or less at birth. *Pediatrics, 61,* 908.

Post, S. (1982). Family-related care is a must . . . maternity and pediatric services. *Hospital Trustee, 6,* 14.

Rising, S. S., et al. (1982). The childbearing childrearing center: A nursing model. *Nursing Clinics of North America, 17,* 11.

Robert Wood Johnson Foundation. (1978). *Special report.* Princeton, N.J.: The Robert Wood Johnson Foundation.

Searles, C. (1981). The impetus toward home birth. *Journal of Nurse Midwifery, 26,* 51.

Sharp, E. S. (1983). Nurse-midwifery education: Its successes, failures, and future. *Journal of Nurse Midwifery, 28,* 17.

Sniderman, S. (1980). Modifying practices to promote family-centered care in the neonatal intensive care nursery. *Birth Family Journal, 7,* 255.

Teberg, A., et al. (1977). Recent improvements in outcomes for the small premature infant. *Clinical Pediatrics, 16,* 307.

Thorne, L. J., et al. (1981). Midwifery laws in the United States, *Women's Health, 6,* 7.

U.S. Department of Health and Human Services. (1983). *Changing mortality patterns, health services utilization and health care expenditures: United States, 1978–2003.* Hyattsville, MD.: National Center for Health Statistics. Series 3, Number 23.

U.S. Department of Health and Human Services. (1984). *Midwife and out of hospital deliveries.* Hyattsville, MD.: National Center for Health Statistics. Series 21, Number 40.

U.S. Department of Health and Human Services. (1984). *Patterns of ambulatory care in obstetrics and gynecology: The national ambulatory medical care survey, United States, January, 1980–December, 1981.* Hyattsville, MD., National Center for Health Statistics.

U.S. Department of Health and Human Services. (1982). *Reproductive impairments among married couples: United States.* Hyattsville, Md.: National Center for Health Statistics. Series 23, Number 11.

3

Ethical and Legal Aspects of Maternal-Newborn Nursing Practice

OBJECTIVES

Following completion of mastery of the material in this chapter, you should be able to

1. Describe the application of the American Nurses Association Code of Ethics to nursing practice.
2. Analyze ways in which ethical considerations arising in maternal-newborn practice have the potential to interfere with care.
3. Describe the sources and types of United States law.
4. Describe the special characteristics of a patient-nurse relationship.
5. Differentiate between the terms *negligence* and *malpractice* and give examples related to maternal-newborn nursing.
6. Describe the reason for Good Samaritan acts.
7. Describe the nurse's role in obtaining informed consent for maternal-newborn procedures of care.
8. Describe the characteristics of a suit-prone nurse and patient.
9. Synthesize personal and professional ethical beliefs with legal considerations to form a foundation for maternal-newborn nursing care.

NURSING PRACTICE in maternal-newborn areas of care, as in all areas of nursing, is affected by both ethical and legal considerations. In this chapter we will look at some of the various ethical and legal issues that can arise in this field of the nursing profession and discuss how you can learn to recognize and deal with potential problems that could have ethical and legal implications.

Ethical Considerations in Maternal-Newborn Nursing

Laws are a society's formal rules of conduct or action, which society members recognize as enforceable by a controlling authority. Ethics are a set of moral principles or values that informally govern individuals in a society. The word *ethics* is derived from the Greek *ethos*, meaning "guided belief" or "custom." Everyone has personal values or a personal set of ethics; all professions establish ethical codes of conduct for their members. Just as people strive to abide by their personal values, nurses agree not only to subscribe to these rules for governing their own conduct but to monitor other members of the profession as well.

Personal Values Clarification

Without clear values people often act with uncertainty or inconsistency. They may flounder, not knowing where to put their best efforts or what actions to take. Their achievements, no matter how strong the effort, may then bring them little satisfaction. Because pregnancy involves a life change, it is often a time when women review their beliefs and values.

Values clarification is the process whereby people examine and determine the things they value (believe in or desire) most. Clarifying values should be done step-by-step, just as is any controlled investigation. The seven commonly accepted steps of values clarification are summarized in Table 3-1. Notice that, depending on the beliefs valued, two separate, different conclusions can be reached for the same problem. It is important to remember that when you are helping patients with value clarification, it is your role to help them determine *what* they value; it is never your role to tell them what *to* value—that is a personal choice. In order to help people clarify their values, you need to help them think about what is important or not important to them. This task is best completed by asking patients how they feel about their actions or decisions (Figure 3-1).

Values are chosen from a range of alternatives. A major role of a nurse in any situation is to be certain that people are aware of all their alternatives and that they have spent time thinking about them. Questions you could ask include "Are there any other things you are considering?" and "What do you think you'll gain by doing that?" Helping a person to explore the freedom of choice can be begun by questions such as "Did that just happen or did you have a choice?" and "Did you have any say in that decision?"

Sometimes people are reluctant to think about how they feel about a choice. Realizing they felt bad would mean knowing they had made a poor choice, which can be a demeaning feeling. You can make this an easier process by phrasing your questions sensitively, such as "How do you feel about that now?" or "Some people feel good when

Table 3-1 Steps in Values Clarification

Problem: Do I want to have a child?

Step	Example A	Example B
List values	Caring and nurturing are values for me. I also value neatness and the self-esteem and money I receive from work.	Caring and nurturing are high values for me.
Examine possible consequences	Pursuing a career will result in greater financial reward for me. Having a baby will leave me with less free time for my career. I do not think of children as being neat.	Having a baby would make me feel fulfilled. Not having a baby would make me feel as if I am not contributing anything to life.
Choose freely	I am healthy so I could either use a contraceptive to prevent pregnancy or have a baby without any harm to me.	I am healthy so I could either use a contraceptive to prevent pregnancy or have a child without harm to me.
Feel good about the choice	I feel most constructive when I am solving a problem at work or organizing a more efficient way to do something.	I have never been so happy as I am thinking about being pregnant for the first time.
Affirm the choice	I have told three separate people that not having children appeals to me.	I tell everyone that I would enjoy being pregnant.
Act on choice	I have started taking an oral contraceptive. I have applied for a promotion at work.	I have stopped using a diaphragm to prevent conception.
Act with a pattern	I have organized my home and social life to be as efficient as possible.	I am "mothering" two dogs while waiting to get pregnant.
	Conclusion: Maintaining a life style without children is a value for me.	**Conclusion: Having a child is a value for me.**

they make a decision, some feel bad; how do you feel?"

To determine if a person is ready to act on a decision verbally or physically, a question such as "Will it be difficult to tell your family about this?" or "Have you done anything to show that you really feel this way?" would probably be effective. To help a person determine if she consistently acts in a pattern, a question such as "Would you do that again?" or "How many times have you done that?" would be helpful.

Notice that in all of these examples your question is phrased to assist a person in thinking through a subject or in clarifying a question. You should never judge a person's response by voicing your opinion ("I don't think that is the right thing to do"), a disapproving remark ("That's not right"), or a teaching point ("It would be better if

you did it this way"). All these responses may have merit at other times (when the person asks you for your personal opinion or when you must prevent the person from harming herself or others); however, they are not effective in clarifying the values of another person, who may be confused by the imposition of your values on the decision process.

What a person values affects and guides how she acts. Any time you are puzzled by what action you should take, take the time to ask yourself, "What are my values in this situation? What do I really want to gain from this situation?" Any time you see a patient acting in a way that seems incongruent with the way you assumed she would act, ask, "Did I read her values wrongly? What is the value that is influencing her to act this way?"

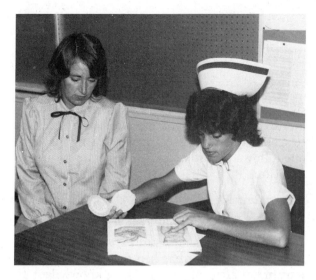

Figure 3-1 *Helping patients with value clarification is a nursing role. Here a nurse helps a woman explore reproductive life planning measures.*

Help people to clarify their values so that they can better understand what motivates them to action. Know your own values so that you can act decisively in those situations in which value judgments must be made while ensuring that your personal ethics do not conflict with your professional ones.

Professional Ethics

All true professions have codes of ethics. These guidelines are intended to demonstrate levels of optimal practice and to maintain standards of conduct within the profession. They also allow people outside the profession to be assured that a member of that profession will consistently act in a certain way.

It is important for you to think through how the Code of Ethics for nursing affects your actions in a clinical area. As a nurse you are expected to adjust your conduct to these statutes. The American Nurses Association Code of Ethics (ANA, 1976) is applied to maternal-newborn nursing in the box on page 42.

Ethical Problems in Nursing

Ethical problems in nursing tend to arise from three principal types of conflict: between what an individual nurse believes and the behavior that the Code of Nursing Ethics advocates; between a nurse's beliefs or the Code of Nursing Ethics and the behavior that is accepted by the agency where she works; and between the Code and a patient's beliefs.

Conflicts Between a Nurse's Values and the Code of Ethics

Various situations arise in nursing that may bring personal and professional ethics into conflict. Suppose, for example, that you do not believe that having an abortion is a woman's individual choice and right. If you are assigned to care for a woman who is scheduled for an induced abortion, what should you do? Refuse the assignment? Take the assignment but give poor care? Take the assignment but tell the patient that you do not approve of her action? Take the assignment and proceed to give the same level of care as you would if she were undergoing a type of surgery that you approve of? Look for yet another option?

This is not an easy question to answer: Each option compromises you in some way. The first three suggested solutions compromise the first professional ethical standard (see the box on page 42). The fourth option compromises your personal values. Is there a fifth option?

Fortunately, as nurses are concerned with respect for human dignity, so is the average health care agency that supplies nursing care. Before you accept a nursing position, you should discuss with the employing agency areas in which your values may conflict with professional ethics. Ask not to be assigned to patients whose care causes these conflicts; this course is more responsible than refusing an assignment later. The health care agency then has the opportunity to choose whether they want to hire you, based on your criteria for employment.

If, after accepting you on these conditions, the health care agency insists that you care for a category of patient discussed in your early interview, you should consider finding another place to work. An agency that does not respect your personal ethics probably has little concern for patients' values either; your experience, rather than being an isolated example, may reflect a philosophical stand of the agency. You would probably be happier in an agency with more respect for you as an individual.

Ethical and legal aspects of care are often interconnected. Legally, once you begin care for a patient (establish a nurse-patient relationship), you are committed to continue care for that patient unless appropriately relieved. This is the reason that you should make clear in advance that you do not choose to care for a patient. Once you begin care, you are legally committed and your per-

Code of Ethics for Maternal-Newborn Nursing Practice

Standard I

The nurse provides services with respect for human dignity and the uniqueness of the client unrestricted by considerations of social or economic status, personal attributes, or the nature of health problems.

Because every woman is unique, women and their support people prepare for labor by different methods. Respecting this individuality and the various types of preparedness reflects this standard.

Standard II

The nurse safeguards the client's right to privacy by judiciously protecting information of a confidential nature.

Much information obtained in a maternal-newborn area is of a very confidential nature. Be careful that lunchtime conversations do not involve information of this type, and guard the patient's identity on written or oral reports that you submit for class assignments by using only the woman's initials. Women have a legal right not to have this type of information spread about indiscriminately: Such information could interfere with obtaining employment or insurance or with personal relationships. When confidentiality is, in addition, stated as an ethical standard, women are twice assured that it will be maintained.

Standard III

The nurse acts to safeguard the client and the public when health care and safety are affected by the incompetent, unethical, or illegal practice of any person.

This standard puts responsibility on you not only to maintain a high standard of care for yourself but to monitor the standards of care of those people around you as well. If everyone performed this task conscientiously, overall care would be improved.

Standard IV

The nurse assumes responsibility and accountability for individual nursing judgments and actions.

This standard puts responsibility on you not to undertake actions that are beyond your ability and not to perform care with inadequate knowledge of individual circumstances and re-quirements. Accountability is also a legal responsibility. You have a strong obligation to be aware of procedures you are not able to do, and to seek help or consultation with them. If everyone follows this standard, patients are assured safe care.

Standard V

The nurse maintains competence in nursing.

This fifth standard assures a patient that the nurse caring for her has kept her knowledge current in her areas of care. Keeping knowledge current is especially important on labor and delivery services and in high-risk nurseries where a great deal of monitoring or high technology equipment is currently used.

Standard VI

The nurse exercises informed judgment and uses individual competence and qualifications as criteria in seeking consultation, accepting responsibilities, and delegating nursing activities to others.

This standard reinforces your responsibility for personal accountability. You must be certain, for example, that when you assign a task to a nurse's aide, the aide knows how to do the task well and will do it at the same level of care that you would have used. Delegating authority in this way has legal implications as well: You are legally accountable to oversee the aide's actions if you assigned her part of a patient's care. This stipulation ensures quality care no matter which member of a health care team actually carries it out. When you are seeking consultation, such as for a medication order, for a pregnant woman, remember that the fetus must be kept safe as well as the mother. In no other area of nursing are you apt to seek consultation for a patient you have not visibly assessed first.

Standard VII

The nurse participates in activities that contribute to the ongoing development of the profession's body of knowledge.

Standard VII places responsibility on you to participate in the nursing research projects of others and to initiate nursing research of your own. It exhorts you to share your areas of expertise with others through writing journal articles or by participating in in-service programs.

Learning to do research begins with being a critical consumer of it.

Standard VIII
The nurse participates in the profession's efforts to implement and improve standards of nursing.

This standard urges nurses to participate in nursing education by serving as preceptors or instructors to students, serving as role models, and, as prescribed by the previous standard, publishing suggestions for improvements in nursing care. It also places responsibility on you to join a nursing professional organization whose interests include improving standards of nursing care. Organizations concerned with maternal-newborn nursing or health care of women are listed in Appendix C.

Standard IX
The nurse participates in the profession's efforts to establish and maintain conditions of employment conducive to high-quality nursing care.

This standard was written to ensure not only a high quality of health care but also a safe environment for that care. It would be unethical for you to ignore conditions that you felt were unsafe from a fire, safety, mental health, or sanitary standpoint.

Standard X
The nurse participates in the profession's effort to protect the public from misinformation and misrepresentation and to maintain the integrity of nursing.

This standard prevents a nurse from advertising or endorsing products. To do so might be misleading, since some people might assume that a nurse would have special knowledge about the product and that it was therefore better than competing brands. Your ethical duty is to help patients interpret advertising claims. You should also monitor newspaper articles or television programs, noting the image they project of nurses or nursing.

Standard XI
The nurse collaborates with members of the health professions and other citizens in promoting community and national efforts to meet the health needs of the public.

This last statement encourages nurses to look beyond their immediate work situation to the surrounding community. They look for unmet needs that they could help meet—for example, a nurse who finds there are no classes for prepared childbirth available could begin to teach some. If every nurse did this conscientiously, the resulting comprehensiveness of care and concern would improve total health care.

---

sonal values may have to be compromised to avoid legal entanglements.

For the same reason, it is important that you as a student make this type of personal value clear to the instructor who will be choosing your patient assignments before these assignments are made. If, after you have explained the conflict of your personal values with the care of a particular type of patient, an instructor insists that you take such an assignment, you need to discuss the problem with her and then, if necessary, your instructor's immediate superior. As a last resort, you might consider transfer to another school of nursing, unless the instructor makes a valid argument—for example, that you can meet a required objective only by taking care of that type of patient. The problem is similar to that of a nurse working in a health care agency that shows little respect for personal values. Check your student manual or college bulletin for statements about this situation. A school of nursing is legally bound by the language in these publications.

This type of values conflict might also arise

with a teaching assignment. As an example, if you are asked to teach a group of women about reproductive life planning and have moral reservations about this area, what should you do? Teach the class and compromise your values? Refuse to teach and therefore receive a failing grade? Teach but state that you do not believe in what you are saying? Search for a fourth alternative?

Again, on most issues where your personal values conflict with professional role expectations, the problem can be solved in a way that maintains and respects your values and yet allows you to function professionally. The objective of such an assignment is probably not to teach reproductive life planning as such but to demonstrate that you are knowledgeable about methods of planning and that you can teach effectively. Make your values known and suggest alternatives, such as writing a paper covering the required material and teaching another subject (bathing a baby, breast-feeding techniques, or stimulation techniques for infants).

If the problem arises as part of a work assignment (someone on the nursing staff must teach this information), the course is part of your contract obligation and a matter you should have discussed before being hired for the position. However, you can usually solve such problems by trading off an equal-time task with someone who has no objection to the assignment. So long as the task is done well, the agency will not care which person does it.

Adopt a philosophy that whenever personal values and professional ethics conflict, you will be firm in refusing to compromise either your personal values or the quality care of your patients.

Conflicts Between a Nurse's Personal Beliefs and Agency Policy

Suppose you believe that a woman whose newborn is dying should be told the truth if she asks and agency policy states that only a physician can answer questions about this subject. Unfortunately, this administrative directive is difficult to carry out when a woman asks, "Is my baby dying?" and you are the only person standing at the side of the bed.

In most instances this type of situation can be solved without compromising either position by a close examination of what you actually believe. Do you feel that you yourself have to inform a person, or just that she should know the exact state of health of her child? You can answer the question she poses by saying, "The rules here don't allow me to answer that question for you; only Dr. Jones can. When she makes rounds this morning, I'll tell her you asked me that so she can talk to you about it." Follow through by telling Dr. Jones of the direct request. Most physicians do not enjoy talking about death; Dr. Jones cannot help but feel that in some way she has failed when one of her patients is dying. She may avoid the subject until a need to discuss it is drawn to her attention. Most physicians appreciate your presence when they discuss painful subjects, such as a poor surgery outcome or death, with patients.

A policy such as the one in question probably should be reviewed by an agency policy committee. Most likely a relic of a former time, this limitation should be replaced by a standard that recognizes a nurse's expertise in discussing this type of information with patients.

Another example of this nature is your discovery that a physician supervising a woman in labor is obviously inebriated. You question the physician's ability to deliver a child safely. Your personal values tell you that it is not nice to be a tattletale; your common sense tells you that the patient's life may be at stake; your professional ethics tell you that you have an obligation to safeguard the patient against incompetent practice. You are also aware that the physician is the sister of the personnel manager, who can block any chance you have for promotion or even retention at the agency. What should you do?

In this instance, because a person's life is at stake, your common sense and your professional ethics make it imperative that you report what you have seen to a supervisor. This is also a legal responsibility. It is not always easy to stand up and be counted when a personal value is at stake; likewise, it is not always easy to be counted when a professional ethic is involved.

Nurse Conflicts with Patients' Beliefs

Patients' beliefs may at times conflict with those of nurses. Parents of children born with birth defects, for example, must make decisions at birth about the child's care and future. In some instances, the decisions to be made are harsh ones; what two parents arrive at may not be the choice you would have liked to see them make. Infants born, for example, with Down's syndrome, a mental retardation syndrome, are also frequently born with heart defects and *atresias* (complete blockage) of the duodenum. At one time parents were told by their physicians that the best therapy for the infant would be immediate surgery for the duodenal obstruction in order to prevent starvation, and they were not asked for input. Surgery was performed so the child would live.

Today, it is a recognized constitutional right of parents to participate in making this type of decision, and they may decide that they do not want the surgery performed. Issues concerning this right have been grouped together in the category "Baby Doe," which refers to an actual decision by parents not to allow surgery and thus to allow a newborn to starve to death. The incident was the catalyst for a bill in Congress that would have made it mandatory for all newborn infants to be fed regardless of their condition at birth. The issue of whether it is a medical or a congressional judgment if a baby with serious birth defects should be fed at birth is still unresolved.

If a decision by parents is in opposition to your personal values—if you believe, for example, that mentally retarded persons have the right to live and develop their potential (as does the average nurse)—it is difficult to stand by and let a decision for a contrary course go unchallenged. Such a decision is also in opposition to nursing's professional ethics, since it does not respect human dignity or uniqueness.

Fortunately, in most instances in which parents make decisions not in a newborn's best interests, the decision is made based on inadequate information about available alternatives. People who make this type of decision are really making the decision not to raise the child; invariably they do not know about their other alternatives, such as signing the responsibility for the child's rearing over to the state.

The state will authorize the surgery to correct the physical defects and arrange for the infant to be initially cared for in an institutional setting or foster home. In many instances an informed, caring adoptive family can be found and formal adoption proceedings accomplished. Informing patients of all their alternatives protects the child and solves the ethical problems of a conflict of beliefs.

Principles of Ethical Decision Making

Ethical decision making is made difficult because there are no black and white solutions, no right and wrong answers. In practice, you will be faced

with situations complicated by many more inter-related factors than those posed in the examples given in this chapter (Figure 3-2).

A model for ethical decision making is shown in Figure 3-3. Using this model (Curtin, 1978), you would first obtain the facts or background information of the situation, then identify the ethical components or problems (truth vs. withholding the truth, etc.). Identifying ethical agents (the third step) refers to locating those people who will have a significant impact on the decision such as the patient, the family, the family's clergyman, and even the court. The fourth step (identification of options) includes not only isolating the options available but thinking through what would be the result if each option were taken (an infant would live but be handicapped; an infant would die, etc.). Application of principles includes applying not only professional ethical principles (a nurse does not discriminate among patients) but personal values (you hold all people to be equal). These steps are basic to problem solving and should result in a resolution and,

Figure 3-2 *Designing care for ill newborn infants requires consideration for ethical decision making. (Courtesy of the Department of Medical Photography, Children's Hospital, Buffalo, N.Y.)*

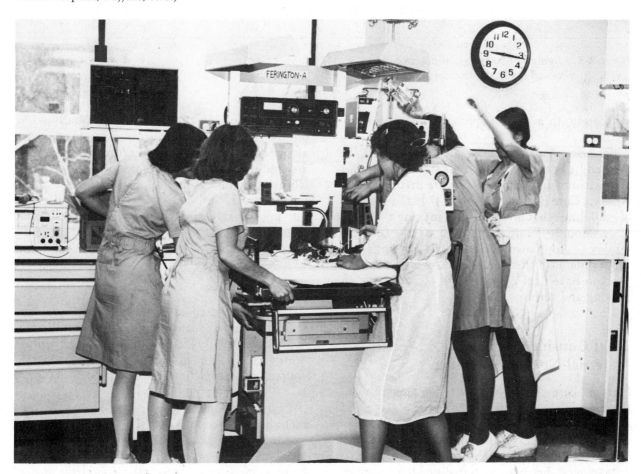

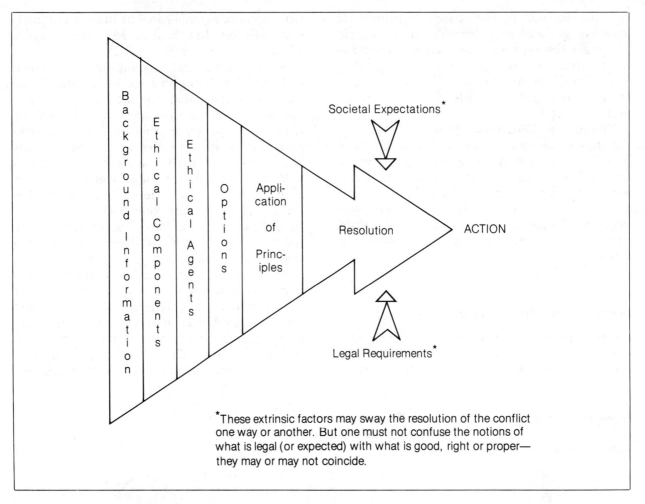

Figure 3-3 *Schematic of a proposed decision making model (From Curtin, L. L. (1978). A proposed model for critical ethical analysis. Nursing Forum, 17:17.).*

ultimately, in a way to approach the ethical dilemma.

Because these instances are so emotionally charged, it is easy for people to argue more than they reason when ethical issues are involved. The Nursing Care Highlight on page 47 lists a number of guidelines that are helpful in making this type of decision. It is important to be aware of the interplay of your own personal value system and the standards of the nursing code of ethics so that you can have firm guidelines for ethical decision making and action.

Legal Considerations in Maternal-Newborn Nursing

Nursing care should always be directed toward the optimal well-being of the patient. It should always be carried out thoroughly and with deliberate thought. Legally, nurses are required to offer a level of care that is reasonable under the circumstances. Because maternal-newborn care is

an area of nursing that is changing rapidly—and often deals with patients with multiple concerns along with a "hidden" patient, the fetus—it is an area of nursing that has specific legal responsibilities involved in care. Reviewing sources of United States law as well as its application to nursing helps to establish the basis for the special responsibility involved in maternal-newborn nursing.

Sources of Law

A law can be defined as a *man-made rule* that regulates human social conduct in a formally prescribed and legally binding manner. In the United States, laws are derived from two separate sources: statutory (legislative) law and common law.

Legislative law is law originated by a government body. Since the supervision and licensing of nursing is delegated to the state level, the state legislative body is the influential and controlling body on nursing for each state. State legislatures,

Nursing Care Highlight

Helpful Guidelines for Ethical Decision Making

1. *Know your values.* Take some time and use values clarification to determine what you value highly enough to defend. This step ensures that you do not compromise an important value by not realizing its significance to you; at the same time it prevents you from spending time fighting for a value that in the end is not important to you (winning battles but losing wars).

2. *Do not allow your values to be compromised.* Giving in to a situation may temporarily solve a problem, but in the end it can breed disrespect for yourself and the agency or person asking you to compromise. You cannot continue to function well if you do not feel good about yourself or the people around you. This type of compromise is often destructive and negatively affects the nursing care you give.

3. *Know professional nursing ethics.* Knowing what is expected of you ethically as a nurse is as important as knowing what is expected of you in any other area. Acting within ethical guidelines is what makes you a professional nurse—one who is dependable and consistently gives quality care.

4. *Do not allow your nursing ethics to be compromised.* Allowing your personal ethics to be violated leads to disrespect; similarly, violation of professional ethical standards lessens your professional reputation.

5. *Do not be disappointed when some people fail to meet your standards.* Values differ among people. Feeling disappointed with someone because he does not value something as highly as you do is destructive to your relationship. Such a person may have a higher value in another area, and in the end you may wish that you were not so quick to feel superior.

6. *Do not force your personal values on others.* Personal values are just that: personal. What works for you may not work at all for another; trying to remake others in your image is not often workable.

7. *Remember that fetal safety is your ethical responsibility as much as is the parent's safety.* Maternal-newborn nursing is a unique area of care because of your responsibility to a "hidden" patient. Medicine administration is of particular concern: Almost all medications cross the placenta to the fetus.

---

for example, originate nursing practice acts (the written statement of what a nurse is allowed and forbidden to do in that state).

Common law, sometimes referred to as the law of *precedent* or judicial law, is necessary because state, federal, and local legislatures cannot anticipate every crime that people will commit or every civil law violation that will require a judicial remedy. Common law decisions often serve as an interim measure until new legislation on the subject can be passed. Because many legal questions of nursing involve new procedures or new roles for which the legislature has not established statutes, common law decisions, which are just as binding as legislative law, have important relevancy to nursing.

Types of Law

In the United States, in addition to two sources of law, there are two major divisions, or types, of law: criminal and civil.

Criminal law is designed to protect the physical safety and property of people at large. If a person is found guilty of criminal law, he pays a penalty to the governing body that originated the law (imprisonment or a fine or both).

Civil law controls most offenses against individuals. If a person is found legally liable for a civil law violation, he pays a sum of money to the offended individual. Most legal controversies in which nurses are involved are civil actions. Violations of civil law causing injury or serious inconvenience to individuals are sometimes described as *torts*.

A Nurse's Responsibility or Legal Accountability for Care

Nurses must take their responsibility for patient care seriously and conscientiously: That responsibility or relationship to a patient's need is recognized, legally speaking, as being on a higher level than an everyday person-to-person relationship. A patient-nurse relationship may be established by the simple introduction, "Hello, I'm Miss

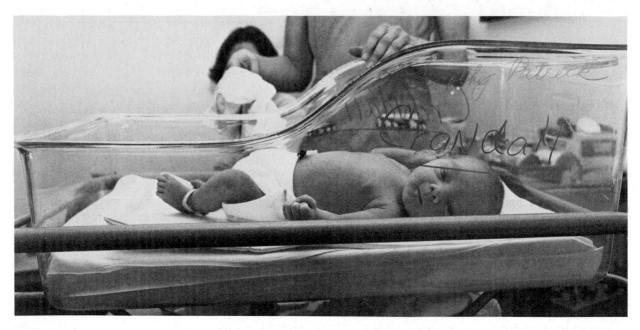

Figure 3-4 *A nurse owes a special duty of care to all patients, especially those such as newborns who are not able to voice their concerns. (Courtesy of the Department of Medical Photography, Children's Hospital, Buffalo, N.Y.)*

Jones (or Mary Jones); I'm going to be caring for you today," or by beginning care. The fact that the legal beginning may lie in giving care—in other words, not only in an oral or written commitment—means that your relationship with an unconscious patient or a newborn is just as binding as your relationship with a patient where an oral contract is made. Once a nurse-patient relationship is established, you are required to render quality care to that individual until such time as you are relieved by another health care provider (Figure 3-4).

Abandonment

Part of the legal nursing-patient relationship involves your providing or supervising the care of the patient until properly relieved. If you should leave the person without care and harm should come to him during that time, your departure and absence might be labeled as *abandonment*. This legal pitfall emphasizes the importance of notifying someone before you leave a patient unit to run an errand, eat lunch, or leave for the day. Someone should be observing your patients while you are absent, after being made aware of any special problems or worries of yours concerning them. Otherwise you may be liable for neglecting their care.

Remember that a nurse-patient relationship is established by the act of *beginning* care. If you should agree to assist a physician with a procedure in an operating room, for example, but after

arriving in the room and beginning care discover that the procedure is a distasteful one to you (or, in the instance of abortion, one immoral to you), you cannot merely announce at that time that you will not assist and leave. If harm should result from your absence, your action could be interpreted as abandonment or irresponsibility. Abandonment could result in a lawsuit and suspension or loss of a nursing license.

The time to announce that you do not wish to assist with a type of procedure because of personal, religious, or ethical beliefs is when you are hired or as soon as you become aware that you may be called on to assist in one. Putting your health care agency on early notice gives it sufficient time to contact persons who can competently assist and follow through with the care of such patients. The nurse-patient relationship is a special bond respected by law: It must not be initiated lightly or irresponsibly.

Respondeat Superior

Respondeat superior is a Latin phrase that means "let the master answer." It implies that employers are responsible for the work of their employees. If you take your watch to a repair shop, for example, and speak with the owner of the shop about having it repaired, you expect that the repair will be of the quality that you have agreed on, no matter who actually does the repair—the shop owner or someone to whom he delegates the work.

People being seen for health care have the same right to know that no matter who gives them care—a nurse, an aide, a student nurse—the employer involved will be legally liable for any negligence involved in its rendering. Nurses, as the representatives of the employer, are responsible for the actions of auxiliary clinical personnel who work with them. If, for example, a nurse asks an aide to take some medicine to Mrs. Smith in Room 312 (a duty far beyond an aide's job description for that agency) and the aide administers it to Mrs. Smith's roommate, who sustains harm, the nurse is just as responsible for the error as if she had given the wrong medicine herself. When you ask an auxiliary worker to help you with patient care, you must be certain that it is a type of care that the worker is qualified to do, as well as is authorized to do by law and by that worker's job description.

This doctrine of *respondeat superior* extends upward as well as downward in lines of authority. Student nurses are legally accountable for their own actions. A nursing instructor might also be found liable, however, if the action of a student resulted in injury to a patient and if it could be shown that the student was not properly instructed or supervised. A health care agency is responsible for the actions of its nurses. If you, as a nurse employee, should negligently cause harm to a patient, both the agency and you can be sued. If you were acting within the scope of your employment and following agency policy, the entire out-of-court settlement or court judgment for money damages would probably be paid by the health care agency because of the *respondeat superior* doctrine.

All nurse graduates or students are ultimately responsible for their own actions, however. If by your not following agency policy, a patient is injured and sues your agency, the agency may settle the law suit and pay a money settlement—and then sue you to recover damages. Nurses working on private duty are always regarded as independent contractors, thus without the insurance protection usually provided by the hospital or health agency for its employees. A nurse who comes into a hospital specifically to act as a childbirth coach is also viewed as an independent contractor. Nurses working in these roles should investigate carrying personal malpractice insurance.

A Nurse's Responsibility for Personal Actions

As mentioned, most legal controversies of nursing involve areas of civil law (torts) or a violation of a duty owed to a patient by the provider of care.

Such instances usually involve the areas of negligence and malpractice.

Negligence

Negligence laws apply to all citizens. Negligence is the omission (not doing) or the commission (doing) of an act that the average prudent (sensible) person would or would not do. Carelessness in some nursing paperwork duties, such as preparing laboratory forms, that leads to improper treatment might fall under the category of negligence because these duties are outside direct patient care.

Malpractice

Malpractice is negligence while performing nursing care. It consists of the omission or commission of an act that the average prudent nurse would or would not do. Negligent actions of nurses (aside from some paperwork, as mentioned above, or actions outside nursing time) are described as acts of malpractice rather than of common negligence. Taking vital signs frequently for the first hour following childbirth, for example, is an activity that the average nurse appreciates is important and does conscientiously. Not taking vital signs during that time could be interpreted as malpractice if injury happened to the patient during that time.

Elements of Malpractice. In order for malpractice to be established, three criteria must be present: a patient injury, a nursing error, and an association between the two (proximate cause). For example, Mrs. *K* develops a urinary tract infection following delivery of her infant, and you are asked to administer 250 mg of ampicillin to her. You make an error in calculating the dose and administer 500 mg of ampicillin instead. You have made an error; the first criterion is present. Because safe ampicillin doses vary widely, however, no harm occurs to the patient; the second criterion does not exist, so grounds for malpractice are scant.

In another instance a physician orders ampicillin to be given to a woman in her sixth month of pregnancy to treat a urinary tract infection. You ask her whether she is allergic to penicillin and you check her records to see that she has no previous allergy to penicillin. A few minutes after you inject the medication, however, the woman becomes extremely short of breath and undergoes an anaphylactic reaction. This leads to a spontaneous abortion. The woman brings suit against you for administering an unsafe drug to her. Although there is patient injury (abortion) and the administration of the drug led directly to the injury, because you did what the average nurse does before administering penicillin (asked about allergies, checked the chart for allergies) one of the criteria necessary for malpractice is absent. It is very unlikely these circumstances would result in a successful legal action.

In a third example, you make an error and give an injection of ampicillin meant for Mrs. *A* to Mrs. *B*. Although there was no medical reason for Mrs. *B* to receive the ampicillin, the drug is not contraindicated during pregnancy (so no harm from the medicine error results). A month later, following childbirth, the woman develops a thrombophlebitis. She brings suit against you for the medication error. Two criteria for malpractice are present: an error on your part (wrong medicine administered) and an injury (the thrombophlebitis). Since there is no proximal cause between an injection of ampicillin and the development of a thrombophlebitis, however, the third criterion for malpractice is still not present.

It is important to remember the components that are essential for malpractice to be proven (and it is the patient's responsibility to prove it exists) in charting nursing actions. Always chart the precautions that you took to make a procedure safe as well as the type of procedure and its outcome.

The Importance of Practice Standards.

In order that lawyers for plaintiffs (persons bringing legal action) can prove that nurses being accused of malpractice did not act in a reasonable and prudent manner, a number of practice standards are used.

NURSE PRACTICE ACTS. Every nurse is responsible for practicing nursing within the limitations and the full scope of the nurse practice act in the state where he or she is employed. Contrary to what many people assume, nurse practice acts are not detailed lists of actions that nurses may or may not do. Such a listing would have to be updated at least every six months as new equipment is designed or new procedures originated. Instead, practice acts specify broad categories of duties (case finding, health teaching, or executing medical regimes) that are within the scope of practice and equally broad categories that are excluded. For example, a nurse may not vary a medical regime; such an action by a nurse would be interpreted as the practice of medicine. A nurse is allowed to evaluate patient response to illness but not to diagnose disease, which is the realm of a doctor, not a nurse.

All nurses work under the provisions of the nurse practice act of the state in which they are licensed. A nurse failing to meet this standard of practice would be legally liable for the deviation.

STANDARDS OF NURSING CARE. The American Nurses Association has published Standards of Nursing Care for the profession. The Standards for maternal-newborn nursing are discussed in Chapter 1. A nurse acting outside the stipulations of these standards could be found liable for not practicing in the normal manner.

HEALTH AGENCY POLICIES AND PROCEDURES. All health care agencies have written policies and procedures that specify how actions should be carried out. You should be familiar with the policies and procedures of the health agency with which you work because being in compliance with them is normal behavior.

JOB DESCRIPTIONS. The average nurse works under the job description of her nursing position. If a job description is too limiting or "just not you," you are best advised to bend your efforts toward having the job description changed or obtaining a different position. It is difficult to justify performing functions outside your job description in the eyes of the law.

PATIENT BILLS OF RIGHTS. The American Hospital Association has devised a Bill of Rights for the Hospitalized Patient. Specialty groups have listed rights for the pregnant woman, the handicapped person, the child, the aged, the mentally ill, and the mentally retarded. The Bill of Rights for the Pregnant Patient is shown in Appendix D. Such lists have implications for the determination of average practice standards because the average nurse protects patient's rights and arranges her care in accordance with them.

LEVEL OF NURSING KNOWLEDGE. The more background and experience a nurse has, the higher the standard of care she is expected to provide. This places a responsibility on nurses to use all their knowledge every time they give patient care. For example, a new graduate would be expected to detect changes on a fetal heart monitor printout at the point they first become specific. A nurse who has had experience caring for patients with fetal heart monitors in place or who has taken an advanced course in fetal heart monitoring would be expected to pick up subtle changes even before they become truly definite on the printed monitor strip. This philosophy—that nurses must perform at the highest level they have attained—ensures patients the best care possible.

NURSES AS EXPERT WITNESSES. Nurses with a broad range of professional expertise are occasionally called on to serve as expert witnesses. A nurse expert witness may be asked to testify in court as to whether she considers the action of a nurse defendant to be consistent with what the average nurse, under those same circumstances, with the same background, education, and experience, would have done. Although nurse expert witnesses are generally nursing instructors or care coordinators, many nurses are considered experts at general nursing care by reason of years of experience. They too might be asked to be an expert witness in court.

USE OF PERIODICALS AND TEXTBOOKS. Nursing periodicals and textbooks set out commonly accepted standards of care. If most textbooks state, for example, that a woman in labor should be asked to void every 4 hours, this becomes a standard for care in labor against which nursing actions and safe practice can be measured.

A Nurse's Responsibility for Patient Safety

Nurses have a high degree of responsibility for keeping patients in their care safe, both physically and psychologically. A number of legal concerns center directly on patient safety; an example of this is the use of restraints.

Using restraints to hold a body part secure or to confine a person to a bed is a form of imprisonment and therefore cannot usually be instituted without a physician's order. A nurse can always apply as much restraint as necessary, however, to prevent a patient from hurting himself or someone else, even in the absence of a medical order.

At one time, all women in delivery rooms had their hands restrained to prevent them from touching the sterile delivery field. Today it is difficult to justify this form of restraint: Educating the women achieves the same purpose. Many modern women interpret the use of stirrups or a lithotomy position for delivery as a form of restraint. For this reason, insistence that women be placed in a lithotomy position for childbirth is becoming obsolete. If the lithotomy position is used, the woman should be placed in it with care, and the length of time she remains in this position must be thoughtfully assessed.

A Nurse's Responsibility for Emergency Care

Because childbirth may occur suddenly or because a complication, such as hemorrhaging, during pregnancy can happen, emergency situations are not uncommon in maternal-newborn nursing. The circumstances of health care vary from emergency to nonemergency settings, but even in the former, a high standard of care must still be provided. A woman has the right to expect that additional complications will not result from someone's carelessness in an emergency situation. For this reason, *Good Samaritan laws* were originated.

At one time, because of the existing laws, nurses took great risks by giving care at accident scenes. For example, suppose you stopped at the site of an automobile accident where you found a pregnant woman bleeding heavily from a neck vein. You tore off the bottom of your shirt to make a compress to apply pressure to the wound. Later, after the woman was removed to the hospital, the wound site became infected and the woman developed septicemia. As a result, she began premature labor and delivered an immature child who died. In the past, the woman could have sued you for placing a clean, not sterile, compress on an open cut and causing the infection (even though you saved her life): As a nurse you should know never to place anything less than a sterile compress on an open wound. Consequently, nurses and physicians were reluctant to stop at accident scenes to administer emergency care.

Good Samaritan laws were passed to ensure that as long as health care providers followed the best procedure *under the circumstances* they could not be held responsible for the nature of their response. Using a clean handkerchief for a compression in the above example was a sensible solution under roadside conditions; using a greasy rag from the car trunk, on the other hand, would not have been a sensible alternative for care. Emergency care to pregnant women includes the responsibility to guard the health both of the woman and of the fetus, if at all possible.

A Nurse's Responsibility for Informed Consent

A woman has the right to choose whether she desires medical care and to sign a consent form detailing what care she desires before it is begun. This consent, to be legal, must be *informed*. Before she signs, the patient must be told what the treatment consists of, what the relevant risks are (to both herself and the fetus), and what alternatives to the therapy could be considered.

Nurses are frequently asked to witness a patient's signature. Before you serve as a witness, you must listen to the physician's explanation of the procedure so that you are certain that what you are witnessing is *informed* consent. Consent is not informed if the explanation of the procedure was given when the person was too sleepy or otherwise too distraught to process the information; if a sedative or preoperative medication had been given; if the explanation was so technical that it could not be comprehended by the person; or if it was incomplete (no risks were mentioned).

People on admission to a health care facility sign a general health care consent form, while for a specific procedure that involves risk (surgery, research, amniocentesis, for example), additional consent must be obtained. Consent is not necessary for lifesaving procedures such as tracheotomy, intubation, or cardiopulmonary resuscitation when the time involved in giving the explanation would interfere with the emergency measure. It is assumed that the average person would consent to lifesaving measures such as these.

Do not witness a consent that you recognize as not an informed one. Ask the physician to repeat the explanation if you did not hear it or explain why in your opinion it is not an informed situation. Some patients may interrupt a physician's explanation of risks by a comment, such as "I don't want to hear any bad news." You may need to inform them that knowing risks as well as benefits of a procedure is their right and for their protection.

Emancipated minors are adolescents who provide the bulk of their own financial support or are the mother or father of a child. Even though such adolescents are not of legal age, they may sign for their own medical care or for the care of their children.

High-Risk Areas of Practice

All of maternal-newborn care is a high-risk area: with a pregnant woman, you are caring for two persons; with newborn infants, you are caring for individuals unable to protest or guide you into safe practice; with a woman in labor or during a complication of pregnancy, you are caring for a person under a high level of stress. Within this area some situations have higher risk for potential legal entanglements than others.

Medicine Administration

Medicine administration is a high-risk area because error may readily occur and the number of drugs for which a nurse is responsible is constantly increasing. You have an added responsibility in maternal-newborn nursing not to administer a drug that has teratogenic (capable of causing fetal injury) properties to pregnant women.

Application of Heat or Cold

Whenever you work with equipment that has the potential to heat or cool, you are working with equipment that has the potential to burn and, if an electrical apparatus is involved, to cause electrical injury. Never use electrical equipment that is not well grounded (has a three-prong plug) or that has a frayed or damaged cord. Do not use electrical equipment around water.

Postpartum women often have sitz baths, K-pads, or heat lamp treatments ordered for them to encourage perineal healing. Infants of low birth weight are often placed in Isolettes or under radiant heat sources or phototherapy light. You must be aware of proper use of such equipment. Be meticulous about temperature settings, time limits, distance required from the heat source, and specific precautions such as shielding the baby's eyes from phototherapy lights. If a woman has received a sedative or analgesic or has a condition that interferes with her perception of heat, your responsibility for keeping her safe increases in proportion to the degree of the loss of sensation.

New Equipment

Any time you are dealing with new equipment or equipment with which you are unfamiliar, you must be certain that you thoroughly understand the purpose of the equipment and how to operate it (Figure 3-5). Ignorance of operational instructions is no defense if patient injury should occur. Get proper instructions before beginning care.

Transfers and Ambulation

Helping patients ambulate or transfer to a wheelchair or stretcher is always a high-risk area because of the possibility that the person will fall. Not using adequate siderails and leaving beds in high positions are also situations that invite patient injury. Pregnant women are particularly prone to falls because their sense of balance is distorted by the increased size of their abdomen. Women following cesarean birth are often dizzy on standing because of the loss of blood (up to 1,000 ml) involved in this procedure.

Teaching

In order for a woman to make decisions regarding her health care, she needs to be well informed of medications or treatments that she is receiving. Not being informed of alternatives could re-

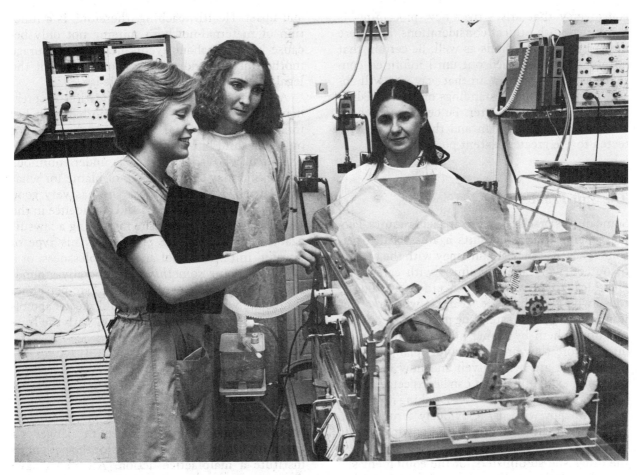

Figure 3-5 *For both legal and safety measures, be certain you are familiar with all equipment you use in patient care. (Courtesy of the Department of Medical Photography, Children's Hospital, Buffalo, N.Y.)*

sult in less than optimal decision making and outcome. You must be certain that the information you are supplying to patients is accurate.

If you do not know the answer to a patient's question, simply answer, "I don't know—but I'll find out for you," rather than trying to guess what the answer would be. If you neglect to tell a woman that drowsiness is a common side effect of an analgesic, for example, she might injure herself trying to ambulate. Teaching is not a nicety of nursing; like almost all aspects of nursing care, it has legal implications.

Poor Communication

Some instances of legal liability occur not because of an action a nurse took but because she neglected to communicate her action or her assessment findings to the patient's physician or the care coordinator. Because of that omission, the responsible party was unaware of the necessity to initiate further measures of care. Be certain that you know precisely what assessments you are expected to make on patients (not "Watch her," but "Take her pulse every 15 minutes and report if it rises above 100 beats per minute") or what procedures you are expected to do (not "Give her a lot of fluid," but "Give her a minimum of 100 ml every hour for the next 4 hours"). This type of instruction not only clarifies your actions but alerts you to an expected point of communication.

Controversial Areas

In previous generations, childbearing was regarded as a process so unique that few interventions were attempted to interfere or even assist. Today, pregnancy may be initiated by artificial insemination or embryo transfer; it may be ended by abortion or cesarean birth. The fetus may be viewed by a fetoscope and even have a blood transfusion administered in utero. Infants may be born in a hospital or home setting. Most of the controversy that arises over new procedures is concerned with ethical considerations, but there may be legal dimensions as well. Be certain that no procedure is carried out until informed consent has been obtained; in that way you will ensure that no misunderstandings of the procedure will be brought forth later. Be certain that both the safety of the woman and the fetus are protected to the greatest extent possible.

The Suit-Prone Nurse

Some nurses practice as if to attract lawsuits. People generally bring lawsuits against health personnel because they are unhappy with the quality or outcome of care. Happiness with care has a great deal to do with the concern or attitude of those who give that care. A nurse who practices impersonally—not extending people the courtesy of calling them by name, not explaining procedures before they are done, not explaining what medications are being given and how they will work, not explaining what can be expected from a treatment or laboratory test—is asking for people to be unhappy with her. Obviously, a nurse who practices on the edge of safety, knowing a little but not a lot about the danger signs of pregnancy, the drugs she administers, or the equipment she uses, is suit-prone. She is not practicing with a high level of care and concern.

The Suit-Prone Patient

Pregnancy, labor and delivery, and the first days of the postpartum period are stressful. People under stress may not "hear" instructions given to them or may interpret them wrongly. During all phases of maternal-newborn nursing, therefore, instructions should be given with the understanding that they are being offered to people under stress, which means they may have to be repeated. People under stress need support persons around them. If they do not have them, they turn to health care personnel. If they do not receive support from health care personnel, they may turn to lawyers.

A major role of a nurse in maternal-newborn care, then, is to help women locate support people or to serve as a supportive, concerned person for anyone who needs this type of interaction during a particularly important time in her life. A patient who understands what is going to happen to her because she had adequate health teaching about pregnancy will not be surprised. That knowledge also makes her less likely to be angry and upset. Health teaching, therefore, is a function of maternal-newborn nursing not only because knowing about events helps to encourage mother-infant bonding but also because of the legal implications of that knowledge.

A woman who has a complication of pregnancy that results in death or morbidity of her infant loses a great deal. Sometimes she loses not only her child but future childbearing potential. A woman who is feeling loss is under enormous stress. She may seek a source of blame for what has happened to her. Unless she has very good explanations and feels trust and confidence in the people who care for her, she may bring a lawsuit against her health care providers. This type of lawsuit, initiated out of anger, helplessness, or a feeling of doing *something*, is generally groundless. It can be prevented if health care personnel appreciate what the loss of a child means and offer more constructive ways to deal with the frustration that these families face.

Legal Responsibility and Nurses

If you commit an error in nursing practice today, you will not feel completely free of the danger of a suit until it is no longer possible for the patient to institute a malpractice action. All states have *statutes of limitations*, or time spans, in which people can bring suit. After that period of time has passed, the threat of lawsuit is over. In most states the time span is 3 to 5 years, though the maternal–child health area of nursing has been given an exception. When parents have chosen not to bring a lawsuit against health personnel concerning a child's injury, there have been instances in which the child was allowed to bring the suit himself after reaching legal age. The time periods involved have implications for detailed charting. No one can remember what she did or what she was thinking 3 or 5 years past, much less 20 years past. You must rely on your chart notes to be so complete that they will still adequately explain the situation 20 years in the future.

Nursing grows more complex daily. The responsibilities undertaken by nurses today were not even imagined by nurses 10 years ago. As nursing grows more complex, it must continue to remain safe or technical advances will in the end not be therapeutic. Functioning at a safe level within the standards of practice with patients who are well informed about the actions and procedures you are taking is your best assurance that you are working within the legal dimensions of quality patient care.

Questions for Review

Multiple Choice

1. The manufacturer of a new brand of prenatal vitamins asks you to appear in uniform in a commercial. Your ethical response to this should be:
   a. It is all right as long as she does not pay you.
   b. Nurses cannot ethically advertise products.
   c. You must have conclusive proof that it is a good product first.
   d. It is illegal for nurses to advertise medicine.

2. You are assigned to care for Mrs. Smith, a patient who is ill because she attempted a self-abortion. When you begin to care for her, you realize that she is a neighbor. At dinnertime, your mother asks you what person you cared for at the hospital. Which of the following answers is best ethically?
   a. a patient named Mary Smith who had an illegal abortion
   b. Mary Smith, a patient who did something illegal
   c. a person from the neighborhood who attempted an abortion
   d. a patient who was ill from an abortion

3. You are working as a staff nurse and the agency you work for has bought a new type of fetal monitor. You have difficulty getting it to work correctly, and your nursing supervisor chides you because you did not read the article in a current nursing journal on such a monitor. She says your action is unethical. On what statement from the American Nurses Association Code of Ethics does she base this accusation?
   a. Nurses should subscribe to nursing journals.
   b. Nurses have particular responsibility in regard to monitors.
   c. Nurses have an obligation to maintain competence in nursing.
   d. Nurses have a particular responsibility in regard to electrical equipment.

4. Mrs. Burrows is a difficult patient to care for because she uses abusive language. Which decision about her care reflects your most ethical course of action?
   a. Refuse to care for Mrs. Burrows and ask to have her moved to another unit.
   b. Give less than quality care so Mrs. Burrows asks to be transferred.
   c. Maintain quality care despite the difficulty.
   d. Agree to give quality care only if Mrs. Burrows changes her behavior.

5. You are using a new resuscitator with Mrs. Smith's newborn infant. You realize after a few minutes that it is causing damage to the baby's lungs because you are using it improperly. Legally,
   a. you cannot be held liable for damage to the baby because use of new equipment exempts you from blame.
   b. the hospital, not you, is liable, because it is their equipment.

   c. you are liable for your own actions as a nurse.
   d. you are liable only if you have used the equipment before.

6. You begin care for Mrs. Smith at 3:00 P.M.; at 3:30 P.M., your nursing shift is over but no evening nurse has yet arrived. If you leave without providing adequate supervision for Mrs. Smith's care,
   a. you might be held guilty of abandonment if injury happened to Mrs. Smith in your absence.
   b. you owe Mrs. Smith no obligation after the time your usual nursing shift ends.
   c. you owe no legal obligation because you did not care for her 1 full hour.
   d. you would not be held liable for abandonment as long as you stated in your notes that you were leaving.

7. Your patient-nurse relationship with Mrs. Smith is established legally when you
   a. chart your first nursing note.
   b. begin care.
   c. have given care for 1 hour.
   d. have given care for 8 hours.

8. If you suspect the dosage of a medication order for Mrs. Smith is too high, your *best* action in regard to this would be
   a. to delay giving it until an adequate explanation is given to you about the dosage.
   b. to give it one time; do not repeat the medication until the dosage is confirmed.
   c. to give it if the medication is oral; delay if it is an injection.
   d. to give the dose you know is appropriate.

9. The statute of limitations refers to
   a. the time limit you have to file an incident report after a patient care error.
   b. the limit of the amount of money for which a nurse can be sued.
   c. the time an injured patient has to bring legal suit against you.
   d. the limit to the number of times you can be sued in a lifetime.

10. Three criteria necessary to prove malpractice are
    a. injury, error, and accusation.
    b. error, proximal cause, and lack of consent.
    c. proximal cause, negligence, and nurse error.
    d. error, injury, and proximal cause.

Discussion

1. Ethical concerns about health care are often reported in the newspaper. Evaluate a currently reported situation as to how you would react. What would be your ethical and legal responsibilities?

2. Suppose a hospital where you practice originates a new policy that is against a personal value of yours. How would you resolve the conflict of practicing in such a setting?

3. Suppose a nursing instructor asks you to care for a patient who has a continuous fetal heart monitor in place and you are not familiar with the particular brand. What are your legal responsibilities in this situation?

Suggested Readings

American Nurses Association (1976). *Code for Nurses.* Kansas City: American Nurses Association.

Annas, G. J. (1981). Invasion of privacy in the hospital. *Nursing Law Ethics, 2*(3).

Bayles, M. D. (1980). The value of life—by what standard? *American Journal of Nursing, 80,* 2226.

Beyrer, M. K., et al. (1980). Ethics for the eighties. *Health Education, 11,* 9.

Carper, B. A. (1979). The ethics of caring. *Advances in Nursing Science, 1,* 11.

Creighton, H. (1983). Law for the nurse manager. Should nurses report negligence in medical treatment? *Nursing Management, 14,* 47.

Creighton, H. (1980). Withdrawal of life support systems. *Supervisor Nurse, 11,* 52.

Crisham, P. (1981). Measuring moral judgment in nursing dilemmas. *Nursing Research, 30,* 104.

Curtin, L. (1978). A proposed model for critical ethical analysis. *Nursing Forum, 17,* 17.

Curtin, L., & Flaherty, M. J. (1982). *Nursing Ethics.* Bowie, MD: Robert J. Brady.

Cushing, M. (1981). "No code" orders: Current developments and the nursing director's role. *Journal of Nursing Administration, 11,* 22.

Davies, B. L. (1983). Decision-making in prenatal genetic diagnosis. *Issues in Health Care of Women, 4,* 69.

Davis, A. J. (1980). When parents disagree on treatment. *American Journal of Nursing, 80,* 2080.

Dean, K. A. (1983). The nurse as witness: Deposition. *Focus on Critical Care, 10,* 20.

Dolan, M. B. (1984). Where do we stand on the coding question? *Nursing 84, 14,* 42.

Doll, A. (1980). What to do after an incident. *Nursing 80, 10,* 73.

Eldridge, T. M. (1979). Adolescent health care: The legal and ethical implications. *Pediatric Nurse, 5,* 51.

Feliu, A. G. (1983). The risks of blowing the whistle. *American Journal of Nursing, 83,* 1387.

Finch, J. (1983). Reasonable standard in determining negligence and avoiding dangers. *Nursing Mirror, 156,* 38.

Fromer, J. J. (1982). Solving ethical dilemmas in nursing. *Topics in Clinical Nursing, 4,* 15.

Harris, E., et al. (1983). Nothing but the truth? . . . How much information to give a patient. *American Journal of Nursing, 83*(1), 121.

Hemelt, M. D. (1984). Steering clear of legal hazards. *Nursing 84, 14,* 81.

Horsley, J. E. (1980). Think twice before you give advice. *R.N., 43,* 95.

Horsley, J. E. (1981). You can't escape the Good Samaritan role—or its risks. *R.N., 44,* 87.

McNally, J. M. (1980). Values. *Supervisor Nurse, 11,* 27.

Nardecchia, M. A., et al. (1980). The policy manual: A basis for legal protection. *Nursing Administration Quarterly, 5,* 57.

Northrup, C. E. (1980). Responding to the malpractice crisis. *American Journal of Nursing, 80,* 2245.

O'Sullivan, A. L. (1980). Privileged communication. *American Journal of Nursing, 80,* 947.

Prato, S. J. (1981). Ethical decisions in daily practice. *Supervisor Nurse, 12,* 18.

Regan W. A. (1981). You don't have to tolerate substandard hospital practices. *R.N., 44,* 99.

Robbins, D. (1982). Developing your ethical perspective. *Journal of Emergency Nursing, 8,* 100.

Salladay, S. A., et al. (1980). Moral authority in OGN nursing. *J.O.G.N. Nursing, 11,* 387.

Scott, D. W. (1982). Ethical issues in nursing research: Access to human subjects. *Topics in Clinical Nursing, 4,* 74.

Smith, S. J., et al. (1980). Ethical dilemmas: Conflicts among rights, duties and obligations. *American Journal of Nursing, 80,* 1462.

Steele, S. M., & Harmon, V. M. (1979). *Values Clarification in Nursing.* New York: Appleton-Century-Crofts.

Strong, C. (1983). Defective infants and the impact on families: Ethical and legal considerations. *Law Medicine and Health Care, 11,* 168.

Thompson, H. O., et al. (1980). Ethical decision-making in nursing. *M.C.N., 6,* 21.

Uustal, D. (1978). Values clarification: Application to practice. *American Journal of Nursing, 78,* 2058.

Wiemerslage, D. (1982). Informed consents. *Critical Care Update, 9,* 39.

II

Childbearing in Today's World

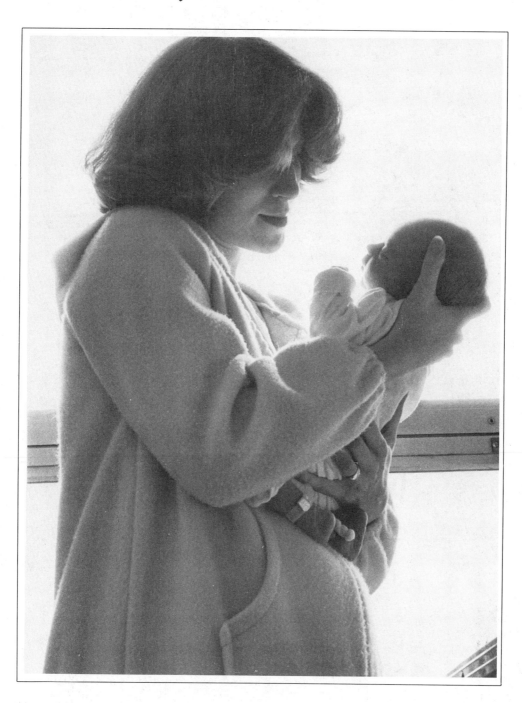

4

Individual, Family, and Community Dynamics

OBJECTIVES

Following mastery of the material in this chapter, you should be able to

1. Define individuality.
2. Describe characteristics or influences that make individuals unique.
3. List basic principles of ensuring that you respect individual differences in people.
4. Describe the role of the family in maternal-newborn nursing.
5. Describe different family structures and life stages.
6. Describe important facets of a family to assess.
7. Define the term *community*.
8. Analyze the important facets of community assessment.
9. Describe the concept of community as a source of third-ring support people.
10. Analyze ways that individual, family, and community characteristics affect maternal-newborn nursing care.
11. Synthesize respect for individual, family, and community characteristics into nursing process to plan and implement maternal-newborn nursing care.

CHILDBEARING DOES NOT occur in a vacuum; it is a phenomenon highly influenced by family, community, and a woman's own individual characteristics. These influences affect such important considerations as whether a woman finds monitoring her own health care a comfortable process and whether she accepts pregnancy as a healthful or as an illness-oriented time. It is, therefore, very important to assess each woman's individual characteristics as well as how she is influenced by her family and community.

Individuality

Individuality refers to those characteristics that make a person unique or not exactly like any other person (Figure 4-1).

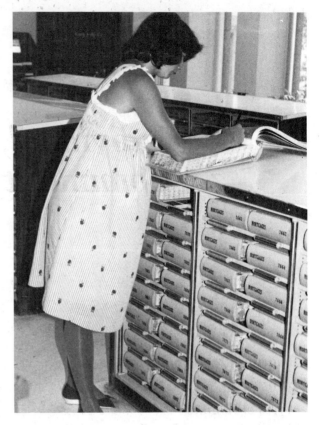

Figure 4-1 *Pregnancy is perceived differently by different women because of individual characteristics. Here a woman perceives no difficulty in continuing to work during pregnancy.*

Characteristics of Individuality

Some characteristics that differentiate people are maturity, intelligence, education level, ordinal position in the family, temperament, state of health, sex roles, past experiences, environment, life style, locus of control, and wellness-illness concepts.

Maturity

Maturity refers to a person's development in terms of judgment and reasoning ability. Maturity is associated but not synonymous with age level; some people reach old age without maturing, while some children are very mature even before legal adulthood.

A mature person is one who is able to delay immediate satisfaction for better or larger rewards at a later date, to view two sides of an argument, and to use progressive steps of problem solving to reach answers to questions. Chapter 7 discusses maturation in terms of the development necessary for successful childrearing.

Intelligence

The higher a person's intelligence, the more easily he or she will grasp principles for self care.

In addition, a more intelligent person will probably learn self-care techniques faster and more thoroughly than a less intelligent person. Under stress any person may lose the ability to solve problems, however: As a result, an intelligent person may become frustrated because of a seeming inability to learn and change as easily as expected during a crisis period such as pregnancy.

Education Level

A person's education level does not necessarily correlate with intelligence level, but theoretically the more education a person has, the more broad-minded and tolerant she will be, and the better is her problem-solving ability. In practice, this correlation does not always hold, because these abilities are influenced by factors other than education.

Ordinal Position in the Family

No two children in a family are exactly alike; and one factor responsible for these individual differences is their birth order. First children are generally asked to assume responsibility for care of young children, while the youngest child in the family has no opportunity to assume such responsibility. Consequently, a first child may strive for a more responsible position as an adult than does a subsequent child.

First-born children also usually have more restrictions on their behavior, such as having to go to bed earlier or not being able to date until later, than do middle or younger children: As parents become more skilled at caring for their children, they relax their controlling measures. This balance increases the older child's ability to follow rules and promotes the younger child's problem-solving ability. Middle children, on the other hand, may grow up feeling insecure because they do not feel "special" (by being the oldest or the youngest); they may also learn diplomacy by being the "middleman," or the peacemaker, in the children's arguments.

Of equal importance in creating differences in children is the period in the family life cycle at which a child is born. If a child is born at a time when her parents are ready for childrearing, they generally view her as a "good" child: When she brushes an expensive vase off the coffee table the first time she pulls herself up to stand, the parent sees the action as "creative, exploring behavior."

If a child arrives at a less than perfect time in a family's life (for example, when the father has no work, the marriage is failing, or the mother was planning to return to school), her knocking over a vase in the same way may be viewed as "troublemaking" or "bad" behavior. These emotions are subconscious; parents are not usually aware that they treat different children in different ways. A child who is told that he is bad and always starting trouble, however, may as an adolescent view himself as only being capable of this role and enter adulthood in opposition to rather than in concordance with most of society's rules. Thus, a person's ordinal position in a family may affect ability to accept or follow health care regimens insofar as it has influenced her sense of responsibility and attitude toward authority.

Temperament

Temperament can be defined as a person's characteristic reaction pattern to situations. The pattern is not developed during childhood or in adult life but is rather an in-born trait. Manifestations of temperament become apparent when a child is about 3 months of age. Temperament determines whether a person is passive or intense, quick or slow to react or adapt to situations, persistent or easily distracted.

Thomas et al. (1971) have identified nine different reactivity patterns by which temperament is manifested. These include *activity level, rhythmicity* (or regularity of physiological functioning), *approach* (a person's response to a new situation), *adaptability* (ability to change reaction to a stimulus over a period of time), *intensity of reaction, distractibility* (the ability to shift focus to a new activity), *attention span, threshold of response* (which refers to the intensity of the stimulation necessary to evoke a response), and *mood* (the overall tone of the feeling projected). The ways in which these patterns apply to a newborn infant's development are discussed in Chapter 30.

It is important in maternal-newborn nursing to assess the elements that make up every person's temperament so that you can better understand various reactions to stress situations. A woman who approaches situations readily and adapts quickly to them is more apt to view a pregnancy that brings acute change to her life as an exciting happening. A woman who approaches tentatively and adapts slowly may need the entire 9 months to begin to view her circumstances in a positive light.

State of Health

A person's state of health can influence her ability to adapt or respond to situations. If fatigued, nauseated, or in pain, a person does not have the adaptive resources or tolerance level that she might otherwise have. On admission to a labor and delivery unit, for example, the behavior of women who are uncomfortable from labor contractions is often very different from that seen immediately after delivery when women are not only free of discomfort but feel an immense sense of accomplishment. Women who think of themselves as chronically ill (perhaps someone with kidney disease) may have a great deal of difficulty adjusting to the physical changes that occur with pregnancy. They may view themselves as ill rather than well and not able to withstand the changes that come with this exceptional year in their lives.

Sex Roles

At a time when sex roles were more clearly delineated, men and women used to react to situations presented to them in markedly different ways. Men, for example, were supposedly always assertive and women always restrained. Sex roles in occupations and behavior now overlap: Many men are involved in childrearing, while many women supply the main financial resources of their family. These changes have resulted in men and women reacting to stimuli in ways that are no longer predictable by sex. Perception of sex-role behavior can influence reactions, however, and must be a factor in assessment.

Past Experiences

What people are is closely related to what they have been. It is often important to ask people about their past experiences with health care providers since this interaction may influence the way they will interact with you. If a woman had a poor outcome from a previous pregnancy, for example, she may not be as anxious to participate in measures to protect the outcome of the following pregnancy as you would expect (she foresees that the outcome will be poor, no matter what she does). Alternatively, she may follow your suggestions for preventive care faithfully (she wants to prevent what happened the last time from happening again).

Environment

A person's reaction to situations differs according to the situation. If you were working as a nurse in an industrial setting, for example, you might find a woman who worked there as an executive rarely demonstrating any quality but stern control. If as a community health nurse you visited her in her home, however, you might find that she would be very willing—even anxious—to discuss how overwhelmed and out of control she feels at times. If you cared for her in a hospital setting close to the time of a frightening event, such as a complication of pregnancy, you might find her sitting by her bed crying. If an employee visited, however, she might quickly regain her composure. Her behavior would vary according to her environment and perception of appropriate actions.

Life Style

Life style is the manner in which a person conducts daily activities and responses, which in turn is influenced by other behavioral characteristics. Some people have a rigid life style: Each day is more or less like the one before it. Others operate with a free-flowing life style that invites constant change and stimulation. For some a life style in which they are constantly surrounded by people is best; others prefer one in which they are more or less alone. Life style also includes such factors as smoking or not smoking; using alcohol not at all, socially, or heavily; and whether a person chooses marriage and children, a nontraditional cohabitation pattern, remaining single, or communal living.

Pregnancy may cause a woman to have to change her life style—to discontinue traveling or participating in formal sports activities, for example. With the forced changes in life style may come more difficulty in accepting a pregnancy than would be caused by a life style with no necessary modifications.

Locus of Control

Many people believe that rewards or circumstances that happen to them result from their own actions; others believe that external forces determine these things. People in the latter group are said to have an *external* locus of control; those in the former have an *internal* locus of control.

Whether a woman believes fate or her own self governs what happens has a great deal to do with how she responds to pregnancy. Women with an internal locus of control are more apt to plan pregnancies, attend preparation for childbirth classes, and be generally more active consumers of health care (Figure 4-2).

Wellness-Illness Concepts

Pregnancy is a well state for the average woman. Women who think of themselves as well during pregnancy (in other words, manifest wellness behaviors) are more apt to cope with the stress of pregnancy and to view health teaching more favorably than are women who view themselves as ill (an ill person has less control of a situation, is more helpless, less able to make decisions than one who is well). Whether women view pregnancy as a time of illness or a time of wellness is culturally and educationally determined. It is important to assess a woman's concept of herself as a well or an ill person in order to best plan care for her.

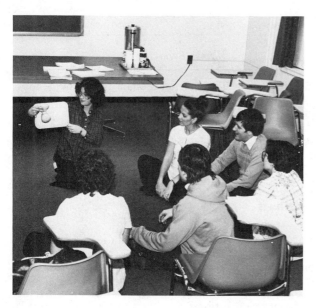

Figure 4-2 *This is a class for prepared childbirth. Women with an internal locus of control may be more apt to actively prepare themselves for labor than others. (Courtesy of the Department of Medical Photography, Children's Hospital, Buffalo, N.Y.)*

behavior may be demonstrating a cultural variation (she believes that illness behavior during pregnancy will improve the outcome of the pregnancy), but she also may be a woman who is overwhelmed by the changes in her life caused by pregnancy. Women in the latter situation need crisis intervention in order to complete their pregnancies in optimum wellness.

Assessment factors related to the characteristics of individuality just discussed are listed in the box below.

Individuality and Nursing Care

Because no two people ever react exactly alike to situations or live identical lives, appropriate nursing care for any two women during pregnancy may be vastly different. A current tendency among some health care agencies is to write standard nursing care plans for the care of people with common conditions, such as pregnancy, postpartal recovery, or adjustment during the newborn period. In practice, there is no such thing as a standard care plan; such plans may actually impede good nursing practice, as they do not focus on individualizing care.

This determination can be made by analyzing whether she consistently evidences more wellness than illness behaviors. Table 4-1 contrasts typical wellness and illness behaviors as a basis for comparison in assessment. It is often helpful to assess a woman for these characteristics as she first enters pregnancy and again about midway in pregnancy to see if she has maintained the same level of wellness actions.

A woman who does not maintain this level of

Take the following example: Angie Baco is a woman who has developed gestational diabetes, and you must teach her about daily insulin injections during pregnancy. You also plan to teach her husband this skill so that he can give the injections on any day that Angie does not feel well. Her husband tends to approach new situations reluctantly; he finds the thought of daily injections difficult to accept. Angie, on the other hand,

---

Assessment Factors Related to Individuality

1. What are the woman's needs based on her level of maturity or development?
2. What are her special needs based on her intelligence or level of education?
3. What are her special needs based on her state of health or comfort?
4. What are her special needs based on her past experiences?
5. What are her special needs based on her coping ability and locus of control?
6. What are her special needs based on her temperament and wellness-illness concepts?
7. What are her special needs based on her life style?
8. What are her special needs based on her perception of her sex role?
9. What are her special needs based on her environment?
10. What are her special needs based on the fact that she is unlike any other individual you have ever cared for before?

Table 4-1 Assessment of Wellness and Illness Behavior

Area of Assessment	Wellness Behavior	Illness Behavior
Family life	Is an active, contributing member of a family. Takes measures to protect against fire and hazards in home (has a fire alarm; uses proper size fuses; has a fire extinguisher in kitchen). Arranges a set time daily for members to "touch base" with each other. Shares feelings with family members and encourages time to share feelings with them.	Depends on the family to provide for her needs or is in opposition to family. Maintains unsafe living quarters. Operates as a "loner" in respect to other family members.
Self-responsibility	Is able to say no without feeling guilty. Can problem solve on daily problems. Can delay immediate rewards for future greater rewards. Does not spend time worrying about problems that are out of her realm to solve. Rarely takes medication other than vitamins or oral iron. Maintains weight within 15% of ideal weight for age and height. Drives defensively and with the use of a seat belt.	Is afraid to say no for fear of being disliked. Is unable to solve problems without extensive aid from others. Is unable to delay immediate satisfaction. Becomes frustrated over problems that are out of her realm to solve. Depends on medication for stimulant or depressant effects. Is over- or underweight by more than 15%. Expects other drivers to respect her; avoids use of seat belts and car seats for children.
Mood	Finds it easy to laugh Has more "good" moments than "bad" moments. Expresses anger, fear, sadness, and happiness easily and in constructive ways. Has no nervous habits such as biting fingernails.	Exhibits a sad, angry, or inconsistent mood quality most of the time. Allows outbursts of emotion to interfere with daily interactions or contains emotions. Exhibits nervous mechanisms.
Sexual role	Finds fulfillment in sexual role. Takes responsibility for reproductive life planning.	Finds her sexual role unfulfilling. Unwilling to consider the consequences of sexual relationships.
Life style	Maintains a life style that is fulfilling to herself and those important to her.	Maintains a life style that is detrimental to herself or caring others.
Self-esteem	Views herself as a worthwhile contributing person Tries to role model measures of good citizenship.	Feels she is less than others; that her suggestions would not be well received by others.
Future outlook	Able to make future plans and set realistic goals for herself.	Makes few future plans; goals are unrealistic for situation or capabilities. Talks or plans about ending life.
Personal care	Is responsible for self-care. Does not smoke. Limits alcohol consumption to none or during social interaction. Does monthly self breast examinations, and has a Pap test done every 3 years. (If a man, does monthly testicular self-examinations; if over age 45, has a yearly prostate gland exam.) Avoids or uses protection to guard against loud noise levels to prevent hearing damage. Keeps immunization level up-to-date.	Depends on others for self-care or neglects self-care. Smokes over a pack of cigarettes a day. Drinks excessively or alone. Does not carry out self-examination techniques or does them only sporadically. Exposes herself to excess noise levels. Neglects suggested immunizations. Brushes teeth infrequently, does not use dental floss, eats many sweetened foods, neglects a yearly examination. Neglects to eat one or more of 5 basic food groups.

Table 4-1 (continued)

Area of Assessment	Wellness Behavior	Illness Behavior
	Is aware of incidence of dental disease, uses good techniques of oral hygiene, and has a yearly examination. Uses little salt in foods; eats a diet high in uncooked fruits and vegetables. Includes basic 5 food groups in meal pattern every week. Plans for and achieves adequate rest and sleep.	Maintains an inconsistent or inadequate pattern of rest and sleep.
Work or school practices	Achieves at work or school setting. Has few absences. Usually enjoys the work she does. Feels financially secure (or has an active plan for achieving security). Is able to accept constructive criticism. Rarely feels tired or fatigued.	Totally involves herself in school or work to the detriment of other life facets or finds work or school requires more concentration or effort than she can expend. Is absent frequently. Lives "beyond her means" and does not see a route for improving this. Reacts defensively to criticism. Feels chronic fatigue and lack of energy.
Social contacts	Has at least 1 person she can identify as a loyal, dependable friend. Plans social contacts for both how much she enjoys the association and the importance of the contact to the other person. Can occupy herself during a time span when she is alone. Enjoys touching and being touched by other people.	Has few friends or no friends. Tends to make social contacts for business or because of "obligations," not enjoyment. Resists being alone or is bored if others are not around. Resents others touching her; rarely spontaneously touches (although this is culturally influenced).
Recreation	Maintains a consistent program of moderate physical effort recognizing age and capabilities. Regularly walks or bicycles instead of taking car for short errands. Does anaerobic or muscle toning exercises at least 2 times weekly. Climbs stairs of 1 flight rather than uses elevator.	Maintains a recreation program that is too intense or not consistent. Rarely walks or exercises. Never uses stairway even to walk down.
Community awareness	Is an active, contributing member of neighborhood and community; works at one or more community improvement projects a year, and belongs to at least one community organization such as church or political group. Votes regularly; is well informed of local, national, and world events. Knows neighbors and is considerate of their property and needs. Recycles articles to limit environmental pollution; supports programs that encourage clean air and water. Prevents crime by supporting police authority.	Is poorly informed and does not participate in community or national issues or concerns.

Nursing Care Highlight

Principles of Respect for Individual Differences

1. No behavior is right or wrong; behavior in any situation is "right" for that individual or moment in time.
2. Do not expect people to react to situations as you do; if their temperament or basic life style is different from yours, their reactions will be different.
3. Assume that people are doing the best they can for that particular circumstance; if their behavior is less than what you would like it to be, it is probably due to the intensity of the circumstances.

4. Changing basic individual characteristics is difficult—and exceedingly difficult when a person is under stress, such as during a pregnancy.
5. The more people you become acquainted with, the easier you can accept and appreciate their individual differences. Make a point of meeting as many people as possible and discussing their life styles and values with them: By doing so you are preparing yourself to individualize your nursing care according to specific patient characteristics.

---

prides herself on quickly taking command of new situations and immediately initiating action.

Your teaching plan for her husband, therefore, would probably include a day or two of quiet nonthreatening exploration of his knowledge of his wife's illness and how a daily insulin regimen could fit into her daily schedule. You might even not produce a syringe and needle until the third or fourth day. For Angie, on the other hand, you might demonstrate the use of a syringe and needle on the first day after only a preliminary introduction.

Individuality dictates learning styles, and different learning styles require different teaching strategies. The Nursing Care Highlight above presents some principles to follow to ensure that you are respecting individual differences.

Family

A family can be defined as a group of individuals living together for the mutual benefit of each other. Individuals typically turn to family members when they are in need of advice or are physically dependent for care. A person's family is his first ring or level of support people. Various functions that almost all families undertake are the care and rearing of children, the socialization of family members into the community, and the transmitting of family and cultural values to the next generation (Figure 4-3).

If a person has difficulty carrying out her own care or accepting a health problem, her family is also probably experiencing difficulty with the ad-

justment. To change a person's nutritional state, for example, you often have to talk not just to the person who is going to eat a new diet, but to the person who is going to prepare it as well. In order to ensure an infant's health, you have to consider the health of his caregivers and often the physical condition of his home. Family assessment is invariably important in maternal-newborn nursing because with a pregnancy and a newborn infant, the family will never be exactly the same again. Whether the family is able to adjust to the change the infant brings will influence the woman's perception of the pregnancy and the environment and acceptance of the infant.

Just as individuals manifest wellness behavior, so do families. The box on page 67 lists the characteristics of a "well" or functioning family. Assessing families for these characteristics is helpful in establishing the wellness or illness behavior of a family.

Types of Families

The support that people receive from their family depends a great deal on the type of family. People come from different types of families, and families change in structure as they mature or are affected by such happenings as divorce or death of a marriage partner. Assessing a woman's family type at a health care visit helps you appreciate her home circumstances and locate support people who will help her through the life change of pregnancy and the postpartum period. Common types of families today include nuclear, extended, single-parent, and communal.

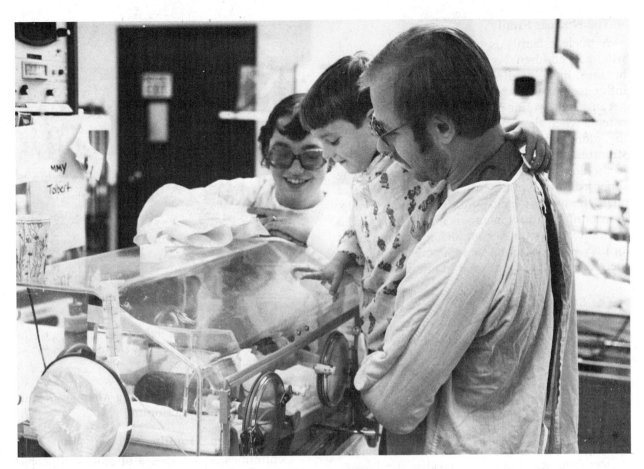

Figure 4-3 *Families provide a supportive environment in which people can grow. Here a family visits with their new family member even though the newborn is ill at birth. (Courtesy of the Department of Medical Photography, Children's Hospital, Buffalo, N.Y.)*

Behaviors Reflecting a Well Family

1. The ability to provide for the physical, emotional, and spiritual needs of family members.
2. The ability to be sensitive to the needs of family members.
3. The ability to communicate thoughts and feelings effectively.
4. The ability to provide support, security, and encouragement.
5. The ability to initiate and maintain growth-producing relationships.
6. The capacity to maintain and create constructive and responsible community relationships.
7. The ability to grow with and through children.
8. The ability to perform family roles flexibly.
9. The ability to help oneself and to accept help when appropriate.
10. The capacity for mutual respect for the individuality of family members.
11. The ability to use a crisis experience as a means of growth.
12. A concern for family unity, loyalty, and interfamily cooperation.

Source: Otto, H. (1963). Criteria for assessing family strengths. *Family Process, 2,* 329.

The Nuclear Family

A nuclear family is composed of a husband, wife, and children. As a rule, a woman receives her most meaningful support and is most strongly influenced by the values of her nuclear family. Because most young people move away from their parents when they marry or establish housekeeping, more and more families today are nuclear in structure (no grandparents, aunts, or uncles live in the home). Although a person receives strong support from such a family structure, in time of crisis the nuclear family may offer limited help. For example, family members may be as worried or frightened as the person undergoing the crisis (or may be undergoing the same crisis), and they therefore cannot be effective in offering support.

The Extended Family

An extended family is one that includes not only the nuclear family but also other family members, such as grandmothers, grandfathers, aunts, uncles, cousins, and grandchildren. Extended families offer more people to serve as resources in times of crisis and more role models for behavior and learning values. In an extended family, a person's strongest support person or a child's primary caregiver may not be the obvious choice: The grandmother may give the largest amount of child care, even though the child's mother is also present every day.

The Single-Parent Family

In as many as 50 percent of families with school-age children today, only one parent lives in the home (Figure 4-4). This trend has resulted from the high divorce rate and the increasingly common practice of women raising children outside marriage. A health problem in a single-parent family is almost always compounded: If the parent is ill, no backup person is available to handle child care. If a child is ill, there is no close support person to reassure the mother or give a second opinion on whether the child is becoming better again.

Low income is often an additional problem encountered by single-parent families. This parent is most often a woman, and, nationally, women's incomes are lower than men's. In addition, single parents often have difficulty with role modeling or identifying their own role in the family: A woman wants to "mother" but must also be the breadwinner. Trying to fulfill two parental roles is not only time consuming but mentally and physically fatiguing—and, in many instances, not satisfying. Such a woman may feel low self-esteem if her husband left her or if the father of her child refuses to marry her; low self-esteem

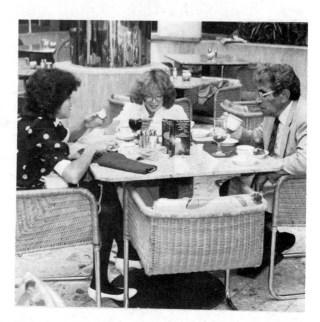

Figure 4-4 *Many families today are headed by single parents. Here a father treats his two daughters to Sunday lunch.*

interferes with decision making, thereby impeding effective daily functioning.

The Communal Family

Communes are composed of groups of people who have chosen to live together as an extended family group; their relationship to each other is social-value or interest motivated rather than kinship based. The values of commune members are often more free choice oriented than those of a traditional family structure: Members may have fewer set roles. People with such philosophies may have difficulty conforming with health care regimes; health care itself may be seen as an established system that they are rejecting. On the other hand, people who reject traditional values may be the most creative people in a community and most interested in participating in their own care. They may have the best outcomes from therapy.

Cohabitation Families

Cohabitation families are couples who are raising children but remain unmarried by choice. Such people can offer as much support to each other as do married couples. Although the relationship may be temporary in some instances, in others it is as long-lasting and as meaningful as more traditional alliances. Common-law marriages fit this category of family.

Homosexual Unions

Homosexual unions involve persons of the same sex living together as married partners for both companionship and sexual fulfillment. Although such marriages currently contradict most people's value systems, they offer firm support in times of crisis comparable to that offered by a traditional nuclear family. Children reared in this type of household need exposure to traditional male-female roles, however, so that they have the opportunity to make a more traditional life-style decision for themselves if they choose.

Family Tasks and Functions

Duvall (1977) has described eight tasks that are essential for a family to perform in order to survive as a unit. These tasks differ in degree from family to family; they also vary according to the stage of the family.

1. *Physical maintenance.* A family must provide food, shelter, clothing, and health care for its members. Being certain that a family has ample resources to provide for a new member is important in maternal-newborn nursing.
2. *Socialization of family members.* This task prepares children to live in the community and interact with people outside the family. A family that is located in a community with a culture or values different from its own may find this a very difficult task.
3. *Allocation of resources.* Determining which family needs will be met and their order of priority is called allocation of resources. Resources include not only financial wealth but material goods, affection, and space.
4. *Maintenance of order.* This task includes opening an effective means of communication between family members, establishing family values, and enforcing common regulations for all family members. Determining the place of a new infant and what rules she will need to follow may be an important task for a developing family.
5. *Division of labor.* The issue here is who will be the family provider and the children's caregiver, and who will be the home manager. Pregnancy may change this familial arrangement and cause the family to have to rethink this task.
6. *Reproduction, recruitment, and release of family members.* Often not a great deal of thought is given to this task: Who lives in a family often happens more by changing circumstances than by true choice. Having to accept a new infant into an already crowded household may make a pregnancy a less-than-welcomed event.
7. *Placement of members into the larger society.* This task consists of selecting community activities, such as school, religious affiliation, or a political group, that correlates with the family's beliefs and values. Selecting a birth setting is part of this task.
8. *Maintenance of motivation and morale.* A sense of pride in the family group, when created, helps members serve as support people to other members in times of crisis.

Types of Family Styles

Families are organized on any of a number of common structures. Recognizing such structures helps you to plan care for families because of your assessment of the difficulties with health care that may arise with differing family patterns.

The Autocratic Family

In an autocratic family, one member is in charge and all other members are subordinate. The dominant member controls not only decision making but the economic purse strings as well. This member is usually a male, although the changing role of women is causing a rise in women undertaking the role.

A woman who is a subordinate in a family might have difficulty coming for health care if the dominant member does not accept its importance. She might be pregnant from sexual relations that she felt she had to submit to rather than as a result of a planned pregnancy. The woman may have little experience in decision making, which may result in difficulty with the daily decisions of newborn care. Fortunately, the number of truly autocratic families is on the wane.

The Patriarchal Family

In a patriarchal family a male member is the dominant person. Such a cultural pattern arises when fathers work close by the home and therefore are available to make childrearing or financial decisions. This family pattern is typical of northern European families: Many fathers are shopkeepers and therefore readily accessible to the family, who live in the rear or upstairs of the store. Because early settlers in the United States were predominantly northern Europeans, this pattern has also come to be regarded as typical in the United States.

The Matriarchal Family

In a matriarchal family, the woman is the dominant or decision-making member. This family pattern arose in cultures where the male member was a hunter or sailor, which meant he was not readily accessible for decision making or childrearing during the day. Because the pattern is not dominant in the United States, saying that a family or culture is matriarchal is often viewed as derogatory. The arrangement is merely a reflection of a cultural pattern, however, and many women find it actually enlightened.

The Democratic Family

In a democratic family, male and female roles are equal and decisions are made based on mutual consultation. Infants have a voice in family life and, as they grow older, are expected to participate in decision making.

A woman from a democratic family may have difficulty asking for health care if the cost will mean a sacrifice of some activity the remainder of the family would have enjoyed. She should be experienced in the kind of decision making necessary for newborn care, but she may be reluctant to make these decisions without consultation with other family members.

Roles of Family Members

People typically assume a unique role within a family; that role depends on each individual's personality characteristics and the changing structure or stage of the family. Identifying a woman's role can help you individualize nursing care for her.

The Nurturer

The nurturer in a family is not only in charge of childrearing but also assumes responsibility for making all family members feel cherished and loved. Such a role is often, though not always, undertaken by a woman. If the nurturer is removed from the family due to hospitalization or illness, she is generally missed by other family members: She is the one who brings joy to the family. Your own day will be brightened by making contact with such a person, for she conveys the same feelings of loving to you. A complication of pregnancy may be felt very strongly by such a person: She can adjust quickly to loving a new family member and feels the threatened loss of this new person very strongly.

The Provider

A provider furnishes financial resources for the family and so influences the availability of food, shelter, warmth, clothing, and health care for the family. This role is typically filled by a male although the woman in a family may actually have more earning power. Removing such a person from a family puts a strain on the entire group because of its loss of financial support. Pregnancy may mean an important change of finances for the family if the provider is the one who is pregnant. In any instance, a pregnancy forces the pro-

vider to make some new allotments for financial resources in order to provide for a new family member.

Some providers spend so much time bringing money into the family (working two jobs or a job that takes them away from the family for extended periods) that they are unable to offer support to the family in other ways than supplying financial resources. In a time of crisis, this family member may discover that she is more alone than she anticipated: Family members are used to sharing only financial information with her.

The Decision Maker

The decision maker is often the same person who is the provider because many family decisions are based on the financial level of the family. This correlation is not necessarily true, however; and many women who are not providers influence their family's goals and decisions so strongly that they are the true decision makers. Even if women do not make the decisions concerning major family goals, they often make household and childrearing decisions. Most women, therefore, are capable decision makers for the problems that arise during pregnancy. Some women need to be reminded of their ability, however, as they are unaware of their role in the family.

The Problem Solver

A problem solver is the most creative family member and the first one to match a solution with a presented problem. This person may also be the decision maker, but again these roles do not necessarily overlap. In many families, the decision maker decides *what* will happen; the problem solver decides *how* it will happen. Being able to problem solve has a great deal to do with the person's exposure to this technique as a child and the family philosophy of solving problems.

A problem solver typically adjusts better to pregnancy than others. If removed from a family, her presence is greatly missed, for the family depends on her to keep its various functions and tasks coordinated and to prevent problems from becoming acute or stressful. Such a woman may be very distressed by being removed from her family if she recognizes the extent of her role in these areas.

The Tradition Setter

One member of every family generally assumes responsibility for seeing that family values continue to be transmitted from generation to generation. This person reminds other members when it is time to begin baking for holidays, and she has a large say in culturally influenced happenings such as childbirth (this person's influence causes a young woman to think of the family cradle either as a "treasure" that she wants to refinish or only as something "old-fashioned" that she will discard).

If such a member is removed from the family near an important family happening, family members will notice the difference in the happening without her presence. A woman in this role may resent or be distressed at being absent: She enjoys maintaining traditions.

The Value Setter

This member influences whether the family accepts or rejects traditional cultural, community, and religious values, as well as whether a happening such as pregnancy out of wedlock or a life style without children is accepted and valued by the family.

The Health Supervisor

A family's health supervisor makes health care decisions for family members. This person is often the nurturer, who will first recognize illness in a family member. Because health care involves financial expenses, the provider may also fill the role.

Health care in the United States would improve remarkably if family health supervisors all became interested in preventive health practices rather than in restorative practices, which are most often requested today. Nurses must make family health supervisors aware of the preventive care available for women during pregnancy and the newborn period.

Family Life Cycles

Families, like individuals, pass through predictable developmental stages. Recognizing the stage of a family is as important in assessment as knowing an individual's developmental stage. Currently accepted developmental stages of families, as identified by Duvall (1977), are summarized in Table 4-2. Table 4-3 lists areas of family assessment and questions to ask to elicit family information.

Community

Community is a term that can be defined in many ways, but generally it refers to a limited geographic area in which the residents relate to and interact among themselves. A community serves as a third ring of support in a time of stress such as pregnancy.

Care of patients should be community oriented because people are never totally separate from

Table 4-2 Family Life Cycles

Stage	Characteristics
Stage I: Marriage	Two partners learning to manage finances, leisure time, decision making, and life style.
Stage II: Early childbearing	Two partners with one or more infant children accepting the responsibility for child care.
Stage III: Families with preschool children	Parents are maturing; childrearing has become a way of life.
Stage IV: Families with school-age children	Parents reach middle age and begin to reach peak of earning power.
Stage V: Families with teenagers	Family changes goals to loosen, not strengthen, family ties so children can be independent.
Stage VI: Launching center families	Partners become a two-member family again as children leave home. Must readjust to new life style.
Stage VII: Families of middle years	Return to two-member family is complete.
Stage VIII: Families in retirement or old age	Family may become a single-member family if one partner dies. A final "rounding out" phase of life.

Source: Duvall, E. M. (1977). *Marriage and Family Development* (5th ed.). Philadelphia: Lippincott.

Table 4-3 Family Assessment Techniques

Area of Assessment	Questions to Ask
Type of family	Is the family nuclear, extended, communal, etc.?
Family characteristics	What is the socioeconomic level? The ethnic background? The religious affiliation?
Decision maker	Who makes decisions, particularly in the areas of finances and leisure time?
Nurturing figure	Who is the primary caregiver to children or any handicapped member?
Tradition setter	Who remembers birthdays? Reminds others of holiday preparations or family values?
Value setter	Who determines whether members maintain a religious affiliation? Who determines "right" from "wrong"?

Table 4-3 (continued)

Area of Assessment	Questions to Ask
Problem solver	Who would a family member go to with a problem? Can the family cope with problems adequately?
Provider	Who furnishes family finances? Are finances adequate? If more than one person earns money, is it fairly divided?
Health supervisor	Who is the person who monitors family health? Does the family eat a nutritious diet? Do they get adequate sleep? Are immunizations current? Is there a balance between work and recreation? Is the home safe from fire or accidents? Does a family member know the technique of CPR?
Level of support	Do family members eat together or spend an equal amount of time with each other daily? Do they band together to defend each other from outsiders?
Outside support	Is the family active in community organizations or activities? Do they visit (or are they visited by) friends and relatives? Can the family name one outside person they can always rely on for help in a time of crisis?

Table 4-4 Community Assessment

Area of Assessment	Questions to Ask
Age span	Is the person within the usual age span of the community and thereby assured of third-ring support people?
Education	If the person is school age, is there provision for her schooling? Is there a library for self-education? Is there easy access to such places if the person is handicapped? If a special program such as nutrition counseling is needed, does it exist?
Environment	Are there environmental risks present, such as air pollution? Busy highways? Train yards? Pools of water where frequent drownings occur?

Table 4-4 (continued)

Area of Assessment	Questions to Ask
	Will hypothermia be a problem from cold weather?
Finances, occupation	Is there a high rate of unemployment in the community? What is the average occupation? Will this person have adequate finances to manage comfortably? Are there supplemental aid programs available?
Health care delivery	Is there a health care agency the person can attend for comprehensive care? Is it convenient in terms of finances and transportation?
Housing	Are houses mainly privately owned or apartments? Are homes close enough together to afford easy contact? Are they in good repair? Is upkeep such as constant repair or extensive lawn mowing a problem?
Politics	Is the community active politically? Can the person reach a local polling place to vote or does she know how to apply for an absentee ballot?
Recreation	Are there recreational activities available of interest to the person? Are they economically feasible for her?
Religion	Is there a facility where the person can worship as she chooses? Is there easy transportation to it?
Safety, protection	Is there adequate protection so that the person can feel safe to leave her home or remain home alone? Does she know about "hot lines" available to her? Local and fire department numbers? Is her home safe from fire?
Sociocultural issues	What is the dominant culture in the community? Does the person fit into this environment? Are foods that are culturally significant to her available?
Transportation	Is there public transportation? Will the person have access to it if she is handicapped?

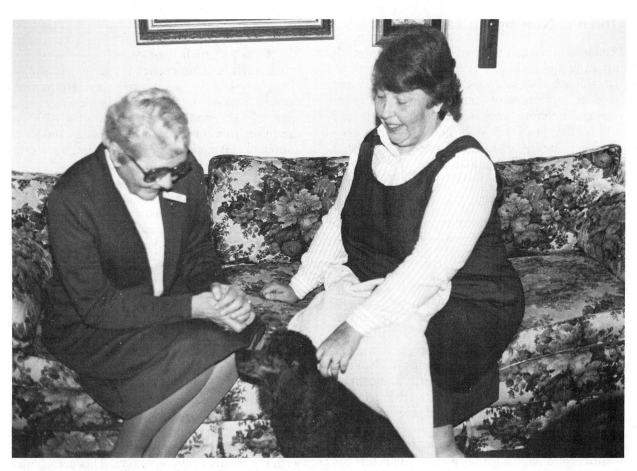

Figure 4-5 *Community health nurses are actively involved in community assessment. Here a nurse makes a home visit to assess a woman's health and environment.*

their families and community. Childbirth adds to the community population and, as the population increases, may eventually place a strain on community functions and resources. Removing a person from the community, such as by hospitalization during a high-risk pregnancy or complications following childbearing, can pose a threat to the integrity both of the person and of the community. When asked what community they are from, people may mention an entire city, a school district, a geographic district ("the east side"), a street name ("Pine Street area"), or a natural marking ("the lower creek area").

Because the health of individuals is influenced by the health of their community, it is important to become acquainted with the communities where you practice. If you are caring for a patient from a community unknown to you, assess her community to see what aspects of it will influence her health during pregnancy or the newborn period (and therefore might need to be corrected) and to determine whether living in that community is beneficial for your patient without extra help and counseling from you.

Community Assessment

Community assessment consists of examining the various systems that are present in almost all communities to see if they are functioning adequately.

Knowing the components of a community allows you to understand why certain diseases occur in some communities more frequently than in others. It helps you plan health care (Figure 4-5). You can better teach women to prepare formula for newborns, for example, if you know whether the Pine Street area has well or city water before you give instructions. You can give better exercise instructions for pregnancy if you know how many flights of stairs someone from the Stevens Plaza area walks to reach her apartment. Finally, you must know the availability of public transportation before telling a woman to return frequently to a clinic for prenatal care from the Creek area. Table 4-4 summarizes areas of community assessment to use in planning care and questions to ask to elicit this type of information.

Utilizing Nursing Process

People do not exist without family and community influences, because even if they are currently living alone, they were socialized by a family and lived in some type of community. In many instances, therefore, you must identify family and community problems and state a nursing diagnosis as a family or community problem rather than as an individual problem.

Assessment

In assessing a family, identify its members and such determinants as the type, stage, and functions of the family. Assess the roles of family members and the amount of wellness-illness behavior displayed by the family.

If a patient you are caring for will need continued care after she returns home, for example, you may want to identify and contact the nurturing member of the family: This person will probably supervise or give the needed care at home. If a pregnancy will cause a major change in life style for a family, you may want to identify and contact the person in the family who is the decision maker or the person who is the problem solver (not necessarily the same). Because pregnancy involves increased expense, you may want to identify and contact the wage earner for the family.

Analysis

The Fourth Annual Conference on Nursing diagnoses approved three diagnoses specifically related to the family: "Coping, ineffective family: compromised," "Coping, ineffective family: disabling," and "Coping, family: potential for growth." The first two diagnoses indicate that a family is not functioning at an optimum level; the third diagnosis is used for a well family or one that is exhibiting enhanced growth in regard to a specific event. These diagnoses can be enlarged to apply to communities.

Locus of Decision Making. The locus of decision making in families and communities is the same as with individuals (the family, the nurse, and shared). Most families and communities are capable of making their own decisions; at a time of crisis, such as a pregnancy, some outside input about available opportunities and alternatives may be needed or the level then changes to a shared level. Families or communities with unusual functions or behavior patterns are unable to complete this task for themselves and need decisions made for them (nurse centered).

Goal Setting. Goal setting for a family or community must be as realistic as for an individual. In helping a family set goals you must be certain that the goal chosen is desired by the majority of family members. It should reflect more than the desires of the family member with whom you have the most contact or who is dominant. If the goal is not respected by all family members, even if it is attained, the family will neither be happy with the outcome nor grow as an intact family unit.

Planning

Planning, like goal setting, must include a design that is appropriate and desired by the majority of family members and fits the community life style. In many families, planning needs to be done with the family decision maker: This person ultimately determines whether or not a plan will be carried out.

Implementation

Implementation of a plan can be accomplished easily if the family agreed on the plan out of support for each other. It may be necessary in some instances to encourage family members to abide by a chosen plan; otherwise they might spend excess energy carrying out an activity that is counterproductive to the major family goal.

Evaluation

Evaluation should reveal not only that the goal of the family was achieved but that the family feels more cohesive than formerly because of working together. If evaluation does not reveal these two factors, reassessment should determine what further steps or new analysis needs to be done.

Nursing Care Planning

Christine McFadden is a 15-year-old you first meet in a prenatal setting. The following is a list of her wellness-illness behaviors.

Assessment

Area of Concern	Prepregnancy Behavior	Pregnancy Behavior
Family life	Enjoys being with family. Shares experiences with older brother.	Barely describes actions to family members. Has not discussed pregnancy with family.
Self-responsibility	Feels pride in cleaning own room and washing own clothes.	Is always angry about having to take care of own clothes because is constantly tired.
Mood	Laughs readily.	Appears angry. Fingernails are chewed.
Sexual role	Pleased to be a woman	Is pregnant because of not using reproductive life planning.
Life style	Full-time high-school student on varsity swimming team.	Discussing quitting school. No outside activities.
Self-esteem	Proud of her accomplishments.	Worried that people are staring at her, because of pigment on face.
Future outlook	Planning on becoming a nurse.	Has no future plans. Will "take whatever happens."
Personal care	Balances activities, sleep, and rest. Takes pride in choosing clothes to	Smokes one package of cigarettes daily. Little interest in clothing.

Area of Concern	Prepregnancy Behavior	Pregnancy Behavior
	wear each day.	States, "no matter what, I look terrible."
Social contacts	Enjoys both male and female friendships.	Says, "Friends don't like me any more. I look like a painted clown."
Recreation	Active in school sports program.	No recreation program.
Community awareness	Recycled bottles, mowed lawn for neighbor.	No participation in community activities.

The following is an assessment you might make of Christine's family.

Family members: father, 50 years old; mother, 48 years old; maternal grandmother, 79 years old; sister, 22 years old; sister's husband, 23 years old; sister's child (Christine's niece), 15 months old; brother, 17 years old; Christine, 15 years old; sister, 5 years old.
Type of family: Extended
Stage of family: Launching center

Area of Concern	Patient's Response
Ability to provide for physical, emotional, and spiritual needs	Family described as "middle-class." Patient wishes family was "kinder" and "more religious." Except for brother, no one is "really kind."
Ability to be sensitive to needs of members	Patient states, "No one understands my needs. Everyone has to be quiet for the baby or grandmother. My sister always gets her way over me."
Ability to communicate thoughts and feelings effectively	Patient states, "No one talks to anyone; everyone shouts."

Area of Concern	Patient's Response
Ability to provide support, security, and encouragement	Patient says, "The family encourages me at swimming. That's nice. And I know we own the house. That's nice."
Ability to initiate growth-producing relationships	Patient explains, "I used to feel good about going home. Now I hate it. When my sister had a baby everyone thought it was great; they think it's terrible for me."
Capacity to maintain community relationships	Patient states, "My father bowls. Otherwise we don't belong to any organizations."
Ability to grow with and through children	Patient says, "My mother lets me share happenings with her. My sister is too busy with her baby."
Ability to perform family roles flexibly	Patient feels, "Anyone could do anyone's job."
Ability to accept help when appropriate	Patient states, "We don't take help from anyone. That's why my sister lives with us. They can't afford a house on their own."
Capacity for mutual respect for individuality	Patient explains, "No one lets me be *me*. I'm supposed to be like my sister."
Ability to use a crisis as a means of growth	Patient comments, "No matter what happens, nothing changes. Life just goes on. My being pregnant isn't going to change anything."
Concern for unity, loyalty, and cooperation	Patient states, "My mother likes us to do things together. Everybody tries to cooperate."

The following is an assessment of Christine's community:

Housing: Patient lives in three-bedroom ranch home with 8 other family members. Has adequate heat, hot water, and furnishings; indoor plumbing.
Support people: Patient lives with moderately supportive family and has a telephone in working order. Has neighbors she states the family can call on for emergencies.
Occupation: Patient is a high-school student and works part-time at a fast-food restaurant. States family is financially "comfortable" although she was unable to buy the winter coat she wanted until it went on sale this spring.
Transportation: Patient does not drive; family does not always have a car available because the father uses it for work. Can ask a neighbor to drive her to any location not accessible by a bus line.
Recreation: Plans to return to an active swimming program at school following pregnancy.
Safety: States she feels safe in her home and on streets near home.
Religion: Attends church once a week. States she can consult with priest if she feels the need for advice or support at any time.
Health care: Has a pediatrician as her primary health care provider. Is aware of emergency rooms in community she could use for emergency care.

Analysis
Coping, ineffective family, compromised.

Locus of Decision Making, Shared.

Goal. Family to provide increased support in six month's time.

Criteria. Christine will tell of any additional support she receives from family.

Nursing Orders
1. Meet with Christine to explore what specific support she needs or expects from family.
2. Meet with mother (nurturer and decision-maker) to discuss Christine's voiced needs and needs viewed by mother (with Christine's permission).
3. Encourage Christine to express her needs so the family can meet those needs.
4. Encourage Christine to participate in family activities so as to feel more like a part of the group.
5. Explore Christine's relationship with older sister; this relationship appears more competitive than cooperative.
6. Promote relationship with brother as this relationship appears to be the "richest" and could be Christine's way back into the family.

Questions for Review

Multiple Choice

1. Barbara White is a woman you meet in a prenatal setting. Which statement below would lead you to believe that Mrs. White's locus of control is *internal*?
   a. "I hate never knowing if I'm having a boy or a girl."
   b. "I leave everything to fate; I feel better that way."
   c. "I like to think what I don't know can't hurt me."
   d. "I hope my baby decides to have an easy entrance into this world."

2. Barbara states she lives with her husband and 2-year-old son. What type of family does this pattern represent?
   a. single unit
   b. extended
   c. nuclear
   d. dyphasic

3. Barbara states that she is a lawyer; her husband is a free-lance photographer. They could not afford to keep their house if she quit work. In assessing the family situation, you would analyze their situation as which family pattern?
   a. She is the provider and her husband is the nurturer.
   b. Her household is patriarchal.
   c. She is the decision maker.
   d. She is the provider.

4. You ask Barbara what effect her being pregnant will have on the family. She answers, "I'll work everything out. I always do." This statement suggests that Barbara's role in the family is also
   a. the comforter.
   b. the problem solver.
   c. the value setter.
   d. the tradition setter.

5. When planning care with Barbara, she states that one of her biggest problems is trying to give equal attention to both her son and her husband. They both want to talk to her the minute she comes in the house. Her ability to keep rivalry down suggests that her role in the family is also
   a. the peace maker.
   b. authoritarian.
   c. matriarchal.
   d. at a line level.

6. In evaluating your goal criteria for the family, you discover the following happenings. Which one suggests that Barbara's family is a "well" family?
   a. Barbara's husband keeps his worries to himself in order not to worry Barbara.
   b. Their son has started having temper tantrums.
   c. Barbara is angry that her husband never helps with dishes.
   d. They both wish they attended church more.

7. The couple's son is struck by a car and brought to the emergency room. Which happening you observe would suggest that the family is *not* functioning optimally?
   a. Barbara's husband comforts the crying child.
   b. Barbara states, "I'll be all right. I'll work this out."
   c. Barbara's husband pays cash for his son's care.
   d. Barbara's husband states, "Emergencies can make a family pull together."

8. Ms. Brown is a 16-year-old patient you meet in a prenatal setting. She lives with her grandmother in a trailer park in a retirement village. In her immediate community, which nursing service might you find infrequently?
   a. a community health nurse
   b. preparation for childbirth classes
   c. a hypertension screening program
   d. a nutrition counseling program

9. What is a community system that might not be adequate for Ms. Brown's needs in her immediate community?
   a. safety
   b. education
   c. religion
   d. politics

10. What would be a factor you would want to assess in her community before you began to organize a teaching plan of formula preparation with Ms. Brown?
    a. the water supply
    b. political system
    c. transportation system
    d. whether horses are present

11. What is a system that would be important to assess in order to ensure safe newborn care?
    a. recreation system
    b. housing system
    c. age-span system
    d. religious system

12. Ms. Brown and her grandmother are of a different ethnic group than most of the people in their community. In which area of their lives will this probably affect them the most?
    a. transportation
    b. recreation
    c. politics
    d. nutrition

Discussion

1. How would the introduction of a newborn into a family affect the family roles of provider, nurturer, problem-solver?
2. Many communities have a rapidly increasing birth rate. What are ways that an increasing birth rate affects a community? A decreasing birth rate?
3. After assessing a pregnant woman for individual characteristics, analyze if she is a woman who will adjust with ease or difficulty to a new role as mother. What would be ways you could help this adaptation?

Suggested Readings

Allor, M. T. (1983). The "community profile" . . . To better understand the community, its strengths and areas of potential or actual need. *Journal of Nursing Education, 22*(1), 12.

Anderson, E. T. (1983). Community focus in public health nursing: Whose responsibility? *Nursing Outlook, 31,* 44.

Balik, B., et al. (1981). Developing a community-based parent education support group. *J.O.G.N. Nursing, 10,* 197.

Ball, J. (1984). Adaptation to motherhood. *Nursing, 2,* 623.

Bartlett, K., et al. (1983). Family nursing: A theory that works. *Canadian Nurse, 79,* 46.

Brandt, M. A. (1984). Consider the patient part of a family. *Nursing Forum, 21,* 19.

Broadman, V., et al. (1982). The development of a family competence instrument related to health. *Nursing Papers, 14,* 11.

Burke, P. J. (1983). A community health model for pregnant teens. *M.C.N., 8,* 340.

Callen, W. B. (1981). The community health advocate. *Journal of Allied Health, 10,* 267.

Collier, P. (1982). Health behaviors of women. *Nursing Clinics of North America, 17,* 121.

Connolly, P. (1983). The family and health. *Midwife Health Visitor and Community Nurse, 19,* 283.

Cromwell, R. E., et al. (1983). Multisystem-multimethod family assessment in clinical contexts. *Family Process, 22,* 147.

Cross, J., et al. (1983). How community health nurses spend their time. *Nursing and Health Care, 43,* 14.

Deuschle, K. W. (1982). Community-oriented primary care: Lessons learned in three decades. *Journal of Community Health, 8,* 13.

Dickson, M. (1982). Community hospital-based obstetrical primary nursing. *J.O.G.N. Nursing, 11,* 292.

Duffy, M. E. (1982). When a woman heads the household. *Nursing Outlook, 30,* 468.

Duvall, E. M. (1977). *Marriage and Family Development* (5th ed.). Philadelphia: Lippincott.

Eigsti, D. V., et al. (1982) The community as client in planning for continuity of care. *Nursing Health Care, 3,* 251.

Erickson, J., et al. (1983). A framework for family nursing. *Nursing Papers, 15,* 34.

Ford, F. R. (1983). Rules: The invisible family. *Family Process, 22,* 135.

Friedman, M. (1981). *Family Nursing.* New York: Appleton-Century-Crofts.

Getty, C., & Humphreys, W. (1981). *Understanding the Family.* New York: Appleton-Century-Crofts.

Goeppinger, J., et al. (1982). Community health is community competence. *Nursing Outlook, 30,* 464.

Green, C. P., et al. (1982). The myth of individuality . . . the impact of illness on the family. *Canadian Nurse, 78,* 49.

Hamilton, P. (1983). Community nursing diagnosis. *Advances in Nursing Science, 5,* 21.

Jacobson, S. E. (1982). Psychosocial stresses of working women. *Nursing Clinics of North America, 17,* 137.

Jerrett, M. D., et al. (1982). Learning to nurse: The family as the unit of care. *Journal of Advanced Nursing, 7*(5), 461.

Kjervik, D. K. (1982). The contemporary American family: Romanticism vs reality. *Journal of Psychosocial Nursing, 20,* 9.

Kutnik, M. L. (1983). Assessing the family of the special-care infant. *Perinatology/Neonatology, 7,* 33.

Leininger, M. (1981). Woman's role in society in the 1980s. *Issues in Health Care of Women, 3,* 203.

Mahan, C. K. (1983). The family of the critically ill neonate. *Critical Care Update, 10,* 24.

McPhee, A. T. (1983). Sharing: Let the family in. *Nursing (Horsham), 13*(1), 120.

Nicholson, J., et al. (1983). Outcomes of father involvement in pregnancy and birth. *Birth, 10,* 5.

Ray, D. W., et al. (1980). Competition vs cooperation in community health nursing. *Nursing Outlook, 28,* 626.

Robbins, M., et al. (1982). Family hierarchies. *American Journal of Nursing, 82,* 284.

Schank, M. J., et al. (1981). Health care practices, problems and needs of young adult women. *Issues in Health Care of Women, 3,* 231.

Shamansky, S. L., et al. (1981). A community is. . . . *Nursing Outlook, 29,* 182.

Sheahan, S. L., et al. (1983). Community assessment: An essential component of practice. *Health Values, 7,* 12.

Siegel, R. (1982). A family-centered program of neonatal intensive care. *Health Social Work, 7,* 50.

Smith, V. (1982). Community neonatal nursing. *Nursing Mirror, 155,* 62.

Stewart, M. J. (1982). Community health assessment: A systematic approach. *Nursing Papers, 14,* 30.

Swanson, A. R., et al. (1983). Family systems: Values and value conflicts. *Journal of Psychosocial Nursing and Mental Health Services, 21,* 24.

Thomas, A., et al. (1971). *Behavioral individuality in early childhood.* New York: New York University Press.

Weissbourd, B., et al. (1981). Family focus: Supporting families in the community. *Children Today, 10,* 6.

Weil, S. G. (1981). The unspoken needs of families during high-risk pregnancies. *American Journal of Nursing, 81,* 2047.

Weltner, J. S. (1982). A structured approach to the single parent family. *Family Process, 21,* 203.

5

The Culture of Childbearing

OBJECTIVES

Following mastery of the contents of this chapter, you should be able to

1. Define *culture* and *transcultural nursing.*
2. Describe ways that cultural variations affect childbirth practices.
3. List basic rules to use to ensure that you respect cultural variations in nursing practice.
4. Analyze ways of improving health care of people from different cultures.
5. Synthesize respect for cultural variations with the nursing process in order to achieve quality maternal-newborn nursing care.

BOTH INNATE characteristics and cultural influences are very strong determinants of human behavior. These factors operate in such a subtle way, however, that a person is usually unaware that they are serving as a basis for action.

Of all the events in life, with the exception of death, few circumstances have more rituals or cultural customs than pregnancy and childbirth. It is important for nurses to be aware of individual and cultural preferences regarding health care practices: These differences influence not only a healthy pregnancy outcome but also the manner in which people accept or reject health care.

Nurses' individual and cultural perceptions may affect how they expect people to act in health care situations. If your own culture places the male in the authority position, for example, you may expect a husband to answer questions about his wife's health at a first pregnancy visit; otherwise, you might find it annoying to have the husband controlling the interview. A nurse whose upbringing places great value on stoic behavior as the "proper" response to pain may be disdainful of a woman who feels that expressing distress in labor is not only proper but expected behavior.

The United States is a country of many varied cultural groups, and any circumstance, medical or otherwise, draws forth a wide range of behaviors. Because of individual response to circumstances combined with disparate cultural mores, there can be no fixed concept of "proper" behavior for an individual at any given time or place.

Culture

Culture may be defined as a view of the world and a set of traditions that a specific social group uses and transmits to the next generation. People's cultures influence their views of themselves and their expectations as well as their approach or lack of approach to health care. Table 5-1 lists a number of commonly accepted facts concerning culture. Basic rules for respecting cultural differences are listed in the Nursing Care Highlight on page 82.

A person's *ethnicity* is the race or cultural group into which he was born. Ethnicity is sometimes used in a narrower context to mean only race. The term *minority* is used in the United States to refer to ethnic or cultural groups other than white. Blacks and those of Oriental heritage comprise about 20 percent of the American population. Minority groups tend to suffer a higher incidence of poverty than do whites, which exacerbates the ethnic discrimination many of these groups face.

All people who move into a new community trade some of their traditions for those of the dominant culture: They become assimilated or *acculturized.* The more different or the more closely knit the two cultures are, the less likely is a high degree of assimilation or acculturation. *Mutual* culture assimilation took place when Italians moved into American communities: The average Italian family coming to the United States learned to speak English; the average American family learned to cook spaghetti with Italian sauce.

Ethnocentrism is the belief that one culture is

Table 5-1 Commonly Accepted Facts Concerning Culture

1. Culture is an organized structure that guides behavior into "acceptable" ways for that group.
2. Each culture differs at least to some degree from every other.
3. Culture is transmitted by formal and informal ways from generation to generation.
4. Although cultural ideas adapt from time to time, they tend to remain constant.
5. Cultural practices arise from environmental conditions: For example, in a country where the men are hunters and away from home, families tend to be matriarchal.
6. Wide variation in values and actions occurs within a culture; its members are individuals who express their own interpretation of their cultural heritage.

— *Nursing Care Highlight* —

Basic Rules for Respecting Cultural Differences in Care

1. Learn as much about different cultures as you can through reading or talking to people from different groups.
2. Examine your own cultural beliefs; you may unconsciously believe they are better than other people's (ethnocentrism).
3. Do not force your cultural values on others.
4. Appreciate that cultural values are ingrained or very difficult to change (in yourself or in others).
5. Do not stereotype. Cultural behavior is learned not inborn. A person's physical char-

acteristics may tell you what her ancestry is, but she may have more "American" cultural values than you do.
6. Remember that poverty is a problem of many minority culture groups as well as whites. Many characteristic responses that are described as cultural limitations are actually the consequence of poverty (seeking medical care late, for example). Solving these problems may be a question of locating adequate financial sources rather than overcoming cultural influences.

---

superior to all others. Ethnocentrism in the United States stems from the 1800s, when the American way (which was actually the northern European way) was thought to be the "best" way. Such a feeling of superiority still affects the American world view. You cannot begin to understand how other people feel about situations or appreciate why they think the way they do unless you accept that the world is large enough to accommodate a diversity of ideas and behaviors.

Caring for people from all cultures with a concerned manner is termed "transcultural nursing" (Leininger, 1979). Some health care facilities maintain an ethnocentric attitude about their care, maintaining that their way is the best way. Maternal-newborn nursing is particularly subject to this limitation: Hospitals often acquire an attitude of their way—no sibling visitation, no fathers in the delivery room, no babies to stay in mother's rooms—as the only way. This attitude on the part of health care providers makes it difficult to change aspects of care to accommodate a person who does not enjoy or want to participate in these set practices.

Stereotyping is expecting people to act in a certain, usually derogatory, way without regard for individual characteristics. A statement such as "Men never diaper babies well" is an example of stereotyping. Stereotyping results from lack of extensive exposure to a particular group and consequently a lack of understanding of its members as individuals rather than as a type. You might believe, for example, that all men cannot diaper babies because you have seen only three men try—and they all did poorly. To avoid stereotyp-

ing, get to know as many people from cultures different from your own as you can. Assess each person you meet as an individual, not as part of a group.

Describing a characteristic of a group that the group is proud of and enjoys supporting, however, is not stereotyping. Stating that Mexican-American women tend to be very loving toward their children, for example, is not stereotyping as much as it is supporting a to-be-envied cultural characteristic. Do not be so worried about stereotyping that you neglect to reinforce positive characteristics of people. Ignoring cultural characteristics is a form of stereotyping. In other words, you are implying that you do not notice someone behaving differently than you would in the same circumstances (or that you expect everyone to mold to your habits and customs).

Health Care Implications of Cultural Differences

When assessing whether cultural influences make special considerations of care necessary, you need to assess at least nine categories of information (see the box on page 83).

Major Cultural Groups in the United States

The United States has a large intermix of cultures because of the constant influx of people into the country. A number of these cultural groups are

Cultural Categories to Assess

Category	*Example of a Potential Problem*
Male-female roles	In a male dominant culture, a woman may be pregnant not from a mutually planned pregnancy but from sexual relations she felt she could not refuse.
Communication ability	Even if a woman is able to converse well at work or in stores, she may not be able to recall the English words for symptoms such as nausea or vaginal discharge.
Time orientation	Mothers who do not have a strict time orientation may view the hospital compulsion of feeding infants at staged times (10 A.M., 2 P.M. etc.) as strange.
Work orientation	In a culture without a strong work orientation, a woman may perceive having to take a job that will pay less but offer more free time as a benefit rather than a drawback of a condition such as pregnancy.
Past, present, and future orientation	If a woman's time orientation is to the present or the past, she may have difficulty accepting a future oriented care plan (resting every day will make a good pregnancy outcome in 9 months).
Family orientation	A woman from an extended family may feel that she has to sacrifice a personal gain in order to maintain the family's welfare; in some instances, such a choice could interfere with her maintaining health following pregnancy. She might decide not to follow through with care in order to save the family money or give care to an ill family member.
Perception of illness	Whether a woman perceives pregnancy as a wellness or illness state guides her activity and nutrition level during pregnancy.
Nutrition practices	In counseling for good nutrition during pregnancy, remember that respect for culturally preferred food is important. People who cannot secure the food you recommend in their own neighborhood may not eat well because of the inconvenience of shopping elsewhere.
Pregnancy and childbirth customs	Many American women visit physicians early in pregnancy, follow all the rules, and at delivery allow the physician to be in charge. In other cultures, pregnancy and childbearing are considered such natural processes that a physician is not necessary (a midwife is sufficient). The woman knows the special rules and restrictions that she must follow in order to ensure a safe birth and healthy child, and she is an active participant in labor and delivery. She may plan to breast-feed until the next child is born, perhaps for 1 to 5 years.

discussed below, though the generalizations made here do not apply to all members of any group.

White Americans

White Americans are the descendants of immigrants who came to the country from a predominantly northern European background. They are usually Anglo-Saxon Protestants (WASPs).

Cultural Orientations

Lisa is a middle-class white woman you meet in a prenatal setting. Her family is nuclear (just her husband and herself). In her household, her husband is the dominant authority figure; she is the homemaker (although in many instances these roles are played more in public than they actually exist at home). She holds a part-time job outside her home. Her husband has finished four years of college; she has finished two. Both she and her husband are conservative in terms of accepting new programs or actions; they take a middle-of-the-road approach to everything from car buying to food preferences to health care. They have a strong motivation to provide a better life for their children and place a good deal of importance on higher education and increased financial security for their children.

The Protestant work ethic is a strong influence. They both believe that people ought to work to support their family and consider a person who accepts handouts to be a failure. They admit to being materialistic, measuring people's worth more by the make of car parked in the driveway than by the number of books read.

They describe themselves as future oriented. They have a personal faith in God although neither attends church regularly.

Health Problems

Neither Lisa nor her husband think about problems associated with illness, although they both carry health insurance. They admit they do not participate in health maintenance programs because incapacitating illness seems so remote from them. They both smoke although they know cigarettes are a major cause of respiratory and cardiovascular disease.

Maternal-Newborn Customs

Both Lisa and her husband are planning to attend a preparation-for-childbirth class during her first pregnancy but admit they will be going for the social interaction more than to learn about labor and delivery (she believes very strongly that what she does not know cannot hurt her). Both believe that it is not manly to cry or complain in the face of pain, but it is all right for women to cry—although not to a point that it is disruptive. Both state that they are not superstitious about happenings during pregnancy, except that saying you want a boy will probably cause the new child to be a girl.

Lisa has visited a physician early in pregnancy; she wants to deliver in a hospital setting. She has no fear or dislike for the use of an analgesic or anesthetic during delivery and would actually prefer one if that would make her most comfortable. She intends to breast-feed her new infant for the first 3 months, as she knows that breast milk is best for newborns. She is aware that nurses will encourage her to ambulate immediately in the postpartal period and accepts this as healthy for her.

Improving Maternal-Newborn Health Care Delivery

A number of attitudes or actions, if accepted by health care providers, could improve health care for the average American:

1. Teach that preventive health care is its own reward (the prize is good health) so that preventive practices will be used more extensively.
2. Respect the cost of health care. People who are materially oriented are cost conscious; they weigh the cost of following your instructions against that of not following them.
3. Respect a future orientation. Making plans for future happenings may be as important as present circumstances.
4. Teach that people should be active consumers of health care and contribute to policies of health care.
5. Teach that preparation for childbirth, which can reduce the amount of analgesia and anesthesia used in labor, is not only healthier for the newborn but can result in a more rewarding experience for the parents.

Hispanic Americans

The term *Hispanic* refers to people with Spanish as a primary language. There are about 12 million documented (legally entered) persons of Mexican, Puerto Rican, Cuban, or other Spanish-speaking origin in the United States; that number, when undocumented or illegal residents are added, grows close to 19 million, or about 9 percent of the total population. Spanish-speaking Americans are the second largest minority population in the United States (blacks comprise about 12 percent of the total population). By 1990, it is estimated that the Hispanic population will be the largest minority (Anthony-Tkach, 1981).

Cultural Orientations

Tina is a Mexican-American you meet as she is being admitted to a labor unit. She has only 8 years of formal schooling, all in Mexico. Her family is extended (her husband, herself, three children, a cousin, and a grandmother). In the family, her husband is the strong dominant force (a characteristic described as *macho*). He takes pride in his ability to support the family and works long hours at several jobs. Tina has never worked outside the home because her husband sees that as his place. She has a warm and nurturing manner, patterning her life style after the warm mothering she received herself.

Both Tina and her husband are Roman Catholic and feel strong bonds to the church. Tina is concerned because it is Sunday and she did not attend Mass this morning. She perceives not being able to attend Mass or speak with a priest as a serious problem. Being out of favor with God, according to an old Spanish belief, is the cause of illness. She describes her family as present, not future oriented.

Health Problems

Tina states that the biggest problems of her family in seeking health care are cost and communication. She does not speak English well enough to describe illness without the use of an interpreter. She often asks her 7-year-old daughter to fill this role, but this reliance has created problems during her pregnancy. Her daughter has had to be absent from school a number of times to help her mother, and Tina feels the subject matter is not appropriate for someone her age.

Although Tina is aware that the majority of diseases are caused by events such as bacteria invasion, she also believes that infant illness can be caused by *mal ojo*, or someone who is envious of her looking at the child with an evil eye. Such an illness is difficult to treat because it has been caused by an unnatural force.

She tells you that delivery of health care in Mexico is less structured than in the United States. There are too few physicians and many drugs are available without prescriptions. A local pharmacist rather than a physician serves as the main health care provider for many Mexicans.

Members of Tina's family first seek help from a respected older member, termed *el que sabe* (he that knows). During an illness this person's approval of therapy is crucial; until it is given, the ill person cannot comply with therapy. Outside the family structure are *yerbero* (herbalists), who grow herbs and instruct people in their use and cures; and healers known as *curandero* help people by the use of herbs or diet. *Espiritualistos* are believed to treat supernaturally caused illnesses, and *brujos* not only revoke evil spells but turn them onto others. Many people turn to a *yerbero* or *curandero* rather than professional health care because these people, instead of charging a fee, accept donations or an exchange of goods or services. Relating health problems to them is also not hindered by a language barrier.

Maternal-Newborn Customs

Tina delivered her first child in Mexico with a *partera*, or midwife. She was encouraged to walk about while in labor, sip an herbal tea for nourishment, use only abdominal massage to control pain, and was delivered from a side-lying position. She is concerned now because she does not like men to examine her and is afraid the physician who will come to care for her will be male (she believes that viewing her genitals is only proper for her husband). She wears a cloth belt she has worn all during pregnancy that she wants to leave in place (she could tell by the loosening of it in the last week that she was at term); she has a *faja*, or cloth binding, in her suitcase she wants to be able to wear after birth to prevent cold from entering her reproductive tract (a condition she has heard will result in sterility). She states she does not want to take a shower following childbirth for at least 14 days, also in order to avoid chilling (a condition called *pasmo*).

If she has a boy she does not want him circumcised; if it is a girl she would like her pediatrician to pierce the earlobes and put baby earrings in place. She has warm socks and a belly band for the infant to keep the baby from becoming cold. Her husband wants to be with her in the labor room; he does not want to follow her to the delivery room, however. Tina's sister will take that role for him. Tina will rest at home for the next 15 days while her mother performs her household work and child care. The couple intends to avoid sexual relations for 40 days following the birth because Tina believes this abstinence will maintain her fertility.

She is most concerned that hospital personnel will insist that she cannot keep the clothing she brought with her for herself and the new baby. She fears they will think these articles are old-fashioned or covered with germs.

Improving Maternal-Newborn Health Care Delivery

A number of attitudes or actions, if accepted by health care providers, would improve health care for Mexican-Americans.

1. Respect the role of *yerberos* and *curanderos*. Disparaging remarks about such people do not strengthen a person's acceptance of professional health care; rather, such a practice demonstrates how different your culture is from that of the person you are trying to help.
2. Respect the role of family. Since Mexican-Americans are family oriented, a woman may have difficulty making a decision about health care, such as whether she should have a diagnostic test, without first consulting the family. Allow time for this exchange of information to take place (call the next day to set up the appointment rather than making it on the spot)—unless, of course, the person's health

would be jeopardized by a delay. It may be very difficult for an individual in the family to change diets or increase daily exercise (especially for women). Try to incorporate the entire family in care so that all members agree to any decision.

3. Overcome language barriers. If a person does not speak your language, take time to record a good health history; the use of an interpreter increases the normal time by at least half. Do not shout to try to make a person understand you. This common habit does not solve the problem; it only allows the confused message to reach him in a louder tone of voice.

Native Americans

Native American beliefs and values are difficult to categorize: They vary from tribe to tribe and between sections of the country. In all there are over 600,000 Native Americans in the United States. The bulk of this population lives in the Southwest.

Land on which Native Americans now live was granted to them by the United States in various treaties as settlers moved further and further west. Unfortunately much of it is waste land, of little value to settlers and unsuitable for farming. In the 1800s, under a major government project to redistribute the land of Native Americans (Dawes Act), each Native American adult was granted an individual portion of land with permission to sell it only after 25 years. Many Native Americans did sell their land at the end of the time period, which then left them with neither property nor a source of income. An unresolved ethical issue is that the United States "granted" Native Americans land they originally owned. Also during the 1800s, an educational project (educating Native American children in government boarding schools) tried to assimilate Native Americans into white culture. Unfortunately all this 10 year project taught Native American children was a culture not applicable to their own way of living; it also left many younger Native Americans with a poor estimation of themselves and little respect for their own cultural traditions.

Cultural Orientations

Mary is a Native American from a New Mexico Pueblo tribe you meet in a labor and delivery unit. She describes her family as matriarchal: her grandmother, the oldest woman in the family, is the person who must be consulted for family problems. Kinship ties are strong and extended. Mary calls many cousins "brothers" and "sisters" because they were all raised in the same house.

The time orientation of the family is the present. Mary describes a typical day as one almost devoid of punctuality or spaced tasks. All the while she answers your interview questions, she speaks gently and does not make eye contact with you. Although she is in active labor on admission to the hospital, she rarely reveals by even a motion that she is uncomfortable.

Health Problems

Poverty is a problem of the Native Americans living on Mary's reservation; measures to promote health, such as care during pregnancy or immunizations for children, are lacking. Frequent health problems include tuberculosis, diabetes, alcoholism, and high infant mortality.

Mary's husband wears a small leather pouch on a cord around his neck. Although it has a pungent odor, he tells you he must retain this item during labor and delivery. It was given to the couple by the tribe's medicine man to safeguard the health of the newborn.

Maternal-Newborn Customs

Mary attended the prenatal clinic at the Indian Health Services hospital. She also visited the tribe's medicine man at the beginning of her pregnancy and again for a special blessing when she realized that she was in labor. She is concerned about her baby's appearance because she was told that eating raisins in pregnancy causes brown marks on a baby, and she ate some early in pregnancy before she was told this. Mary wants to bury the placenta herself rather than have it destroyed by the hospital: She believes this ritual will keep the baby safe from future illness.

Mary's husband prepared a cradle board for their new child. He plans to bring it to the hospital tomorrow to use to carry the infant home.

Improving Maternal-Newborn Health Care Delivery

A number of attitudes or actions, if accepted by health care providers, would improve health care for Native Americans.

1. Native Americans are concerned with the harmonious relationship of man and nature. They respect and preserve life around them and expect their privacy and life style to be respected in return. They will return loyalty to health care providers who show respect for their needs but may give little cooperation to someone who does not make an effort to understand what is important to them and why.

2. Health care for Native Americans is provided free in Native American Health Service facili-

ties. The extreme poverty of Native Americans limits their ability to attend other facilities. Even though care at these facilities is excellent, people may resent the little choice of care available to them.

3. Emotional problems of Native Americans are increasing in incidence (both the suicide and homicide rate for Native Americans is higher than average). Do not assume that an apparently unconcerned patient is a truly unconcerned one.

4. Native Americans may believe very strongly in home remedies or herbal cures. Knowing what remedies the person is taking may prevent medication toxicity, which could be caused by prescribing the same herb in medicine form.

5. Native Americans tend to use touch less than some other cultures. Assess whether a patient wants this type of support or would prefer a close but not touching presence.

Black Americans

The black culture in the United States has arisen primarily from African heritage. A smaller number of the 12 million blacks are immigrants from Caribbean islands such as Haiti, Bermuda, or Nassau. Due to problems of education and discrimination, as many as 40 percent of all black families have low incomes; a great many of the problems that black families encounter, therefore, are those associated with extreme poverty.

Cultural Orientations

Clarissa is a black American you meet in a physician's office. She is an executive secretary; her husband is in college, studying to be an engineer.

Clarissa's family is nuclear (just her husband and herself). She describes her family as patriarchal although her own family was not; she was raised in a three generation–extended, single-parent home (her grandmother, her mother, and two sisters).

Both she and her husband are active in their church, which serves as a center for recreation and social contacts as well as religious activities. Clarissa is aware that her own family orientation was the present; she views that of her husband and herself as the future: She is determined that her children will have a better life not only materially but in terms of freedom from prejudice.

Health Problems

Black Americans are more prone to develop tuberculosis and hypertension than other groups. Infant mortality for blacks is higher than the average rate (probably due to influences of poverty). If the family lives in poor housing, lead poisoning, caused by children eating chips of lead-based paint from walls and windowsills, is also high.

Sickle cell anemia (distortion of the red blood cell structure that governs oxygen transport) occurs in approximately 1 out of every 400 black Americans. About 1 out of every 8 carry the trait of sickle cell anemia, which means they have no symptoms but carry a recessive gene for the disease that their children may inherit. Sickle cell anemia reaches a crisis state if an affected person develops a low blood oxygen level or becomes dehydrated. Any person with the disease is particularly threatened by a fever with profuse sweating or a respiratory illness. These cause clumping of the distorted cells due to loss of fluid or low oxygen blood tension. If a crisis should occur during a pregnancy, the supply of oxygen to the fetus could be seriously impaired.

Clarissa tends to eat small meat portions in comparison with those preferred by northern Europeans. One of her typical foods consists of pork boiled with greens (collards). This diet tends to be high in sodium and low in iron; and it may be deficient in vitamin C due to the loss of this vitamin during boiling. She does not drink milk because she has lactase deficiency, which is an inability to digest milk due to low levels of the enzyme lactase. Drinking milk leads to diarrhea and nausea.

Both Clarissa and her husband perceive illness as an unwanted but acceptable phase of life. They welcome health care for the treatment of physical illness; like most Americans, they may be less receptive to preventive health practices such as immunization programs.

Maternal-Newborn Customs

Clarissa is interested in participating in prenatal care because, although she knows her mother never went for care until the eighth or ninth month of pregnancy, she understands the danger involved. She is interested in diet counseling for pregnancy. She asks about practices of putting a belly band on the baby and giving newborns oil baths for the first week of life.

Clarissa states she does not believe that babies can be "marked" by happenings during pregnancy, yet she knows that her mother believes a birthmark on her sister was caused by eating strawberries. She believes it is bad luck to see a deformed child or view a dead body while pregnant. She is interested in active participation in labor but does not want to breast-feed her new baby.

Improving Maternal-Newborn Health Care Delivery

A number of attitudes or actions, if accepted by health care providers, would improve health care for black Americans.

1. Many mothers of lower-economic-level black families may be young and therefore lack experience in judging illness. Provide educational opportunities based on a philosophy of "Let me help you learn how to do this better next time," not, "You didn't do a good job this time." No one wants to come for health care and be criticized for shortcomings.
2. If poverty is a problem, the cost of health care must be carefully considered. Poor families may not have reliable transportation and returning for follow-up visits may be very difficult if the health care facility is not located close to community transportation systems.
3. The black population is intensely proud of their heritage and of being black. This is evidenced by the popular slogan "Black is beautiful." Be certain in giving instructions that you do not ask a person to violate a value important to her as a black American. Not only will your advice not be followed, but you will lose her respect.
4. Inner-city black Americans often speak a dialect unique to their particular area. Learn the cadence and common words, but do not attempt to imitate it. Black Americans are proud to be different from other people. Trying to speak as they do may be misinterpreted as mockery.
5. Encourage greater problem solving and participation in health decisions.

Chinese-Americans

The largest numbers of Chinese-Americans are concentrated on the West Coast, while large cities on the East Coast have smaller populations. Because Chinese-Americans cluster in cities, they may be less culturally assimilated than are members of other immigrant groups.

Cultural Orientations

Lin Sim is a Chinese-American. She describes her family as extended. Both sets of grandparents live with her family. Obedience and respect for elders are strongly stressed.

Health Problems

Lin Sim's family believes herbal medicine is as important as formal therapy. They try to balance opposing energy forces (yin and yang) in many aspects of their lives, particularly in the foods they eat. Lin Sim describes the majority of health problems in her community as related to poverty (malnutrition and dental caries) and crowded living conditions (tuberculosis and diarrhea).

Maternal-Newborn Customs

Lin Sim is receptive to prenatal care. She would prefer to deliver her baby in a birthing center rather than a hospital because she would like to have her child with a minimum of anesthesia or analgesia. She intends to breast-feed. Except in legal records, she intends to count the age of her child from the date of conception rather than birthdate, as family tradition dictates.

Improving Maternal-Newborn Health Care Delivery

A number of attitudes or actions, if accepted by health care providers, would improve health care for Chinese-Americans.

1. Chinese-Americans rely strongly on the advice of senior family members. They may need time to consult with such members before making a health care decision such as choosing between two alternatives for therapy.
2. Chinese-Americans may not make eye contact during an interview, a social custom that shows respect for the position of the health care professional. They are complimenting you, not avoiding the issues.
3. People who spend the majority of their time in a close-knit community structure may learn little English. In order not to offend you by showing they do not understand what you are saying, they may nod and appear to agree with you. Ask a family member to help you assess the degree of understanding. Make a note in the nursing care plan that the person's nod may be a respectful "I'm listening," not "I'm understanding."
4. Chinese-Americans may have had a bad experience with a health care provider who disregarded their need for family contact or some aspect of their diet. In order to gain their cooperation, you may have to demonstrate by a consistent caring attitude that you are going to respect their needs.

Appalachian Americans

The Appalachian region of the United States is the region from western New York to northeastern Mississippi; the core of this area is West Virginia, eastern Kentucky, and eastern Tennessee. Although many people in this region enjoy middle-class status, at least 20 percent live at a poverty level.

Cultural Orientations

Linda is a woman from eastern Kentucky in your care following the birth of her third child. She lives with her husband, their three children, and her parents on a 20-acre farm that stretches up a hill into very poor soil. Both Linda and her husband have only eighth-grade educations; he works in a coal mine daily to supplement the income they derive from farming.

Linda describes her family as extended; her father is the head of the household, which creates a problem for her husband. Although her nearest neighbor is only a mile away, Linda describes very little family interaction with them: Her family prefers to "make it on their own." Her time orientation is the present; she is much more concerned with what will happen with this year's crop and possible extra income than making long-term plans for future crops.

Health Problems

Linda states her biggest problem with health care is that she has no transportation to the local health clinic. Her husband has the family car away from home most of the day. Paying for care is also a problem; and no member of Linda's family has ever accepted government assistance for income or health care. She would prefer to go without than to accept "charity."

Linda worries that her husband's chronic exposure to coal dust will eventually lead to sarcoidosis (chronic lung disease). She is aware that at times their diet is inadequate, especially in fruit and meat; grocery money is a problem, particularly during the winter when they have no garden.

Maternal-Newborn Customs

The problems Linda experienced during her pregnancy centered on getting to the health clinic for care and money to buy new clothes for the baby. She does not intend to breast-feed as "only really poor people have to do that." She does not want to attend a group class on infant resuscitation; she prefers to learn by herself rather than participate in a group.

Improving Maternal-Newborn Health Care Delivery

A number of attitudes or actions, if accepted by health care providers, would improve health care for Appalachian Americans.

1. People living in Appalachia do not, as a group, accept outsiders well. Be sure you are accepted before you begin to make changes; otherwise you may confront a poor or nonexistent compliance level.
2. Arrange health care services to fit the times of the day when men are home from work. Otherwise women may have no transportation available for health care visits.
3. Appalachian people are often not enthusiastic in affect (facial expression). Although they give warm loving care to infants, they may not make physical contact with other family members as readily as do people from other cultures. This reserve does not imply a lack of caring; in this culture touch is not viewed as necessary to convey affection.
4. Appalachian people often demonstrate a firm sense of pride in their ability to be independent; unable to provide for health care, they may barter with crops. If an exchange arrangement is refused, they may not return for future care. Their resistance to available government supplements may result in a poverty level lower than that of other cultural groups around them who accept these forms of help. Respect the pride that this form of living offers them, even if you disagree with it.
5. These women need to be taught that breastfeeding is the most healthful form of infant feeding. They should not perceive it as associated with poverty, but rather with good mothering ability.

Southeast Asian Americans

During 1980, as many as 14,000 people from Southeast Asia arrived in the United States each month. They came primarily from Indochina, Vietnam, Cambodia, and Laos, often beginning their journey by crossing 900 miles of the South China Sea in rickety, unseaworthy boats. They may have spent time in a refugee camp before being relocated in the community where they now live.

Cultural Orientations

Min Ling is a woman from Vietnam in your care following the birth of her first child. She states that men are the decision makers in her country. Education levels are generally extremely low for both men and women. It is difficult for most of her community to learn English: The dialects and language structures of these nations are so different that transpositions are almost impossible. Time orientation is the present. Time, as a whole, is not regarded as an important entity; Laotians in particular may arrive an hour late for appointments as a form of respect for the person setting the appointment.

Min Ling is Buddhist. She does not believe in using any medicine if not absolutely necessary.

Health Problems

People from Southeast Asia have the problems of people from all poor nations: malnutrition, tuberculosis, and dental caries. They often have few immunizations, and eye and ear disease may have left them with vision and hearing handicaps. There is a high incidence of parasitic and hepatitis B infection. Many are lactase deficient and have difficulty digesting milk, which can give them chronic diarrhea and dehydration.

Hospitals in Southeast Asia are informal; when a person is hospitalized, his family stays at the hospital with him. Therefore, the concept of limited hospital visiting hours in the United States is poorly understood. Vietnamese names are often written backwards from Western custom (the last name is always written first).

Maternal-Newborn Customs

Min Ling expects to have pain with childbirth but to endure it stoically without analgesia or anesthesia. Her husband will not accompany her to the delivery room: The father of a child should not see it until it is cleaned and presentable for him to view. Min Ling has brought worn baby clothes to the hospital with her because she believes that clothing may retain the health or luck of the person who wore them. These clothes are from a neighbor's healthy baby; therefore they are preferable for her newborn to the hospital's clothing.

Min Ling believes that rumpling a person's hair is intrusive and destructive: The head is the home of spirits, who can be disturbed. She dislikes having anyone wipe perspiration from her forehead. She watches the nurse in the newborn nursery wash her baby very carefully every morning. In Vietnam, people do not use diapers on infants. Min Ling states she will use them in this country but worries about the diaper rash that will result.

Improving Maternal-Newborn Health Care Delivery

A number of attitudes or actions, if accepted by health care providers, would improve health care for Americans from Southeast Asia.

1. Respect the vast differences in culture between the Western and Eastern worlds, and between the poverty level of countries that are often involved in war and the relative economic security of the United States.
2. Be aware of the many different religions practiced in Southeast Asian countries. Respect these religious practices in regard to health care.

Changing Cultural Concepts

In the 1800s, when there were a large number of immigrants from many different countries coming into the United States, the United States was viewed as a giant cultural melting pot, where all new arrivals gave up their native country's traditions and values and became Americans as quickly as possible. Any behavior that conflicted with middle-class American views was termed strange and inferior—a mark of a new immigrant or low socioeconomic status.

Today the idea that America ever was a melting pot is being questioned; in addition, it is being stressed that retaining cultural values and traditions is not only acceptable but preferred. Retaining ethnic traditions strengthens and enriches family life; it provides security to younger family members by placing them in a continuing line of people with both a past and a future.

Utilizing Nursing Process

It is important not only to respect people's cultural differences but to help them share their cultural beliefs with you and other health care providers so that you can honor their needs. As a nurse you will meet many people who hold cultural values different from your own. Respecting these differences is as important in giving holistic care as respecting individual traits or characteristics.

Assessment

Assessing for cultural preferences involves observing how people respond to usual health care policies or patterns; it also involves asking them if there is any special action they would like you to implement in any area. Table 5-2 lists areas you should be certain to include in a thorough assessment of cultural variations.

Analysis

The fourth Annual Conference of Nursing Diagnosis accepted no diagnosis that speaks specifically to cultural variations. A diagnosis you might use that would reflect your concern for this area might be, "Communication impairment related to the use of Spanish as the primary language" or, "Anxiety related to a cultural preference for not bathing newborn infants."

Planning

Planning designed to respect cultural preferences may begin with in-service education for health care providers who are unfamiliar with a kind of cultural practice and its importance to the people involved. It may include arranging for variations in policy, such as the length of visiting hours, the types of food served, or the kind of newborn care. Such planning is beneficial not only if it makes health care more acceptable to a patient, but if it causes health care providers to examine policies and question the rationale behind them.

Implementation

Implementation related to cultural diversity may include establishing a network of interpreters from the health care agency personnel or from a nearby university or foreign importing firm; educating a person or community as to the reason for a hospital practice (do not feel that you and the health care agency are always the ones that must adapt; a particular situation may call for both sides to adjust); and carrying out a procedure according to the preference of a person from a different culture.

Evaluation

Evaluation should encompass not only whether a modification of a procedure is still within the safe limits of care but whether the person who asked for the variation is pleased with the result. If a procedure cannot be modified due to the need for asepsis or some other consideration, it may be possible to modify another closely related procedure in order to achieve the same purpose. Eating laundry starch, for example, is a cultural preference of many southern black women as a way to reduce heartburn and ensure a healthy baby. You may not be able to halt this practice in a particular community. The danger of eating laundry starch during pregnancy (why you want to modify it) is that the alkaline medium created by the starch prevents optimal absorption of iron, which is absorbed best from an acid medium. Being certain that a woman is eating an iron-rich diet, taking an iron supplement, and drinking orange juice (an acid beverage) following the starch ingestion may allow the practice to continue and still ensure a high hemoglobin level and storage of iron during pregnancy.

Table 5-2 Important Areas of Cultural Assessment

Area of Assessment	Assessment Factor
Health practices	Does the couple believe in a source of healing other than professional health care? Do they participate in self-monitoring of their health?
Pregnancy	Does the family view pregnancy as a wellness or illness state? What does having a child mean to the couple? Is there any food the woman believes is especially good or harmful for fetal development? Is there any action that, if done during pregnancy, will harm the fetus (killing an animal, tying a knot)? Does the couple believe sexual relations will harm the fetus?
Birth	Does the woman view birth as a private or social process? Is birth viewed as an ill or well time? Do they believe in any practice that will be helpful or harmful to successful birth?
Postpartal period	Is there any special action the woman needs to take during the period to maintain fertility or health? How long does she believe sexual abstinance should be practiced? Does she see a need to rest? Are there special foods she should eat? Are there any activities she should not do?
Role of father	Does the father view his role as a participant in labor and delivery? Is there any action during pregnancy or labor that would harm the fetus?
Child care	What method of infant feeding will the woman use? What actions does she feel are important for keeping the newborn safe?

Nursing Care Planning

Mary Jack is a Native American. She asks you if you can assure her that three tribal customs she believes in strongly can be honored by your hospital while she is in labor. A nursing care plan regarding these considerations is shown below. Notice that this plan is reality oriented in that it requires some compromises from both parties (the hospital allows the knife, and the patient lets it be sterilized).

Assessment

Patient states she wants music played during labor and delivery to welcome the child into the world (otherwise labor will be difficult because the child does not want to enter); a ceremonial knife to be kept under her bed to "cut" labor pains; and her husband to be allowed to cut the umbilical cord with the ceremonial knife (to infuse his strength into the new child).

Analysis

Anxiety related to fear of disregard of cultural preferences during labor.

Locus of Decision Making. Patient

Goal. Patient to feel that cultural preferences were respected in labor by end of birth process.

Criteria. Patient to voice satisfaction with health care during labor and delivery.

Nursing Orders

1. Discuss importance of customs to patient with labor and delivery personnel and gain cooperation.
2. Arrange with hospital in-service personnel to borrow record player to use on labor unit.
3. Delegate responsibility for choosing and providing music of choice to patient and husband.
4. Discuss importance of ceremonial knife being sterilized and obtain patient permission.
5. Wrap and gas sterilize ceremonial knife at next clinic visit so it is sterile for labor.
6. Discuss the advantage of the couple using a birthing room for labor and delivery rather than a delivery room in order to enhance a relaxed birth atmosphere.

Questions for Review

Multiple Choice

1. Mrs. Houston is a Native American. She tells you that she comes from a large family you analyze as extended in structure. Before beginning newborn care teaching with Mrs. Houston, which action below would you want to initiate?
    a. Restrict visitors to reduce the noise level.
    b. Ask the hospital visitor program to see her to prevent loneliness.
    c. Help her contact someone to help her with child care.
    d. Determine who will be the child's primary caregiver at home.

2. You view Mrs. Houston as poor because she describes her home as a "dirt floor" house. In the light of her family structure, in which way might she view you as poor?
    a. You do not practice her religion.
    b. You own only one student nurse's uniform.
    c. You are unmarried and live alone.
    d. You stated that you value honesty.

3. In labor, Mrs. Houston insists on turning her bed so she faces the north star: She believes this will keep the baby in a good delivery position. Your best response to this practice would be to
    a. allow the change as long as you can still view her from the room doorway.

    b. discourage her by saying the hospital disapproves of moving beds.
    c. ask her physician to explain that bed position makes no difference.
    d. explain that fetal position and bed position are unrelated.

4. Miss Crawford is a black American you visit in her home. You are concerned that she does not eat enough vegetables for good pregnancy nutrition. She states that she is preparing "makings" for dinner. You are unfamiliar with this term. In light of this, your best response to the situation would be?
    a. "I hope you eat that with a vegetable."
    b. "I wish you'd eat more spinach and corn."
    c. "Black cooking always sounds exciting; can I have your recipe?"
    d. "I don't know what 'makings' means."

5. Miss Crawford says that before she goes to her physician for prenatal care, she wants to visit a "folk healer" for a special blessing. Your best response to this would be to
    a. encourage her to make both appointments for care promptly.
    b. state that visiting a folk healer will be a waste of her time.

c. explain that prenatal care is very important for the health of her child.

d. state that folk healers are not licensed physicians.

6. Mrs. Wojoynsiak is of Polish heritage. She is angry on hospital admission because so many people have asked her how to pronounce her name. Your best response to her would be,

a. "Polish names *are* pronounced strangely."

b. "No one ever says my name correctly either."

c. "I'll mark in the nursing care plan how to say it correctly."

d. "Why don't I call you Mrs. Wojo? Then I can't say it wrong."

Discussion

1. Suppose a mother tells you she thinks it is important that her own mother bathe the new baby for the first three days following birth or the infant will become ill. A hospital policy states that no one but the mother is allowed to bathe the newborn. How would you go about helping this woman meet her cultural needs?

2. Childbearing is culturally influenced. What are three customs of childbearing that reflect Anglo-Saxon influences in a hospital where you have worked?

3. Women are often referred to as "keepers of culture." How has women's health or women's liberation movements affected childbearing customs?

Suggested Readings

Anthony-Tkach, C. (1981). Care of the Mexican American patient. *Nursing and Health Care, 11,* 424.

Bash, D. M. (1980). Jewish religious practices related to childbearing. *Journal of Nurse Midwifery, 25,* 39.

Beare, J. (1984). Parenthood in other cultures. *Nursing, 2,* 563.

Becerra, R. M. (1981). Knowledge and use of child health services by Chinese Americans. *Health and Social Work, 6,* 29.

Bhanunathi, P. P. (1977). Nurses' conception of "sick role" and "good patient behavior": A cross cultural comparison. *International Nursing Review, 24,* 20.

Bullough, V., & Bullough, B. (1982). *Health care for the other Americans.* New York: Appleton-Century-Crofts.

Carpio, B. (1981). The adolescent immigrant. *Canadian Nurse, 77,* 27.

Clark, A. (1979). *Culture/childbearing/health professionals.* Philadelphia: Davis.

Davis, M., et al. (1981). A model for cultural assessment of the new immigrant. *Canadian Nurse, 77,* 22.

Delgado, M. (1983). Hispanic natural support systems: Implications for mental health services. *Journal of Psychosocial Nursing and Mental Health Services, 21,* 19.

Dempsy, P. A., et al. (1983). The childbearing Haitian refugee—cultural applications to clinical nursing. *Public Health Reports, 98,* 261.

Dobson, S. (1983). Bringing culture into care. *Nursing Times, 79,* 53.

Ellis, D., et al. (1982). Attitudes of Chinese women towards sexuality and birth control. *Canadian Nurse, 78,* 28.

Fanning, J. A. (1980). Culture. In C. C. Hanes & D. H. Joseph (Eds.). *Basic concepts of helping.* New York: Appleton-Century-Crofts.

Gagnon, A. J. (1983). Transcultural nursing, *Nursing and Health Care, 4,* 127.

Grosso, C., et al. (1981). The Vietnamese American family . . . and grandma makes three. *M.C.N., 6,* 177.

Guerra, F. A. (1980). Hispanic child health issues. *Children Today, 9,* 18.

Higgins, P. G. (1983). Pueblo women of New Mexico: Their background, culture and childbearing practices. *Topics in Clinical Nursing, 4,* 69.

Hogan, R. M. (1982). Influences of culture on sexuality. *Nursing Clinics of North America, 17,* 365.

Kalisch, B. J., et al. (1981). Minority nurses in the news. *Nursing Outlook, 29,* 49.

Kegley, C. F., et al. (1983). Working with others who are not like me. *Journal of School Health, 53,* 81.

King, L. S. (1982). Multicultural health beliefs in action. *Health Education, 13,* 198.

Leininger, M. (1979). *Transcultural nursing.* St. Paul, MI: Masson Publications.

Mandelbaum, J. L. (1983). The foodsquare: Helping people of different cultures understand balanced diets. *Pediatric Nursing, 9,* 20.

Martiniz, R. (1978). *Hispanic culture and health care.* St. Louis: Mosby.

Meleis, A. (1981). The Arab American in the health care system. *American Journal of Nursing, 81,* 1180.

Mitchell, A. C. (1978). Barriers to therapeutic communication with black clients. *Nursing Outlook, 26,* 109.

Muecke, M. A. (1983). Caring for Southeast Asian refugee patients in the USA. *American Journal of Public Health, 73,* 431.

Pickwell, S. M. (1982). Primary health care for Indochinese refugee children. *Pediatric Nursing, 8,* 104.

Primeaux, M. (1977). Caring for the American Indian patient. *American Journal of Nursing, 77,* 91.

Rocereto, L. V. (1981). Selected health beliefs of Vietnamese refugees. *Journal of School Health, 51,* 63.

Rodriguez, J. (1983). Mexican-Americans: Factors influencing health practices. *Journal of School Health, 53,* 136.

Satz, K. J. (1982). Integrating Navajo tradition into maternal-child nursing. *Image, 14,* 89.

Schafft, G. (1980). Health care for racial and ethnic minorities and handicapped persons. *Journal of Long-term Care Administration, 8,* 37.

Shutin, S. (1980). Nursing patients from different cultures. *Nursing 80, 10,* 78.

Slevin, K. F. (1982). Motherhood, culture and change. *Pediatric Nursing 8*, 403.

Spector, R. (1979). *Cultural diversity in health and illness.* New York: Appleton-Century-Crofts.

Thomas, R. G., et al. (1982). Maternity care for Vietnamese in America. *Birth, 9*, 187.

Tripp-Reimer, T. (1983). Retention of a folk-healing practice (matiasma) among four generations of Greek immigrants. *Nursing Research, 32*, 97.

Wadd, L. (1983). Vietnamese postpartum practices: Implications for nursing in the hospital setting. *J.O.G.N. Nursing, 12*, 252.

White, E. H. (1977). Giving health care to minority patients. *Nursing Clinics of North America, 12*, 37.

Williamson, D., et al. (1982). American childbirth educators in China: A transcultural exchange. *Journal of Nurse Midwifery, 27*, 15.

Zepeda, M. (1982). Selected maternal-infant care practices of Spanish-speaking women. *J.O.G.N. Nursing, 11*, 371.

6

Genetic Assessment and Counseling

OBJECTIVES

Following mastery of the content of this chapter, you should be able to

1. Describe the nature of inheritance.
2. Describe patterns of recessive and dominant Mendelian inheritance.
3. Describe the reasons for common chromosomal aberrations such as nondisjunction syndromes.
4. Describe common inborn errors of metabolism.
5. Describe the components of genetic assessment in relation to maternal-newborn care.
6. Analyze the role of the nurse as a genetic counselor in maintaining reproductive health.
7. Synthesize knowledge of genetic inheritance with nursing process to achieve quality maternal-newborn nursing care.

THE GENETIC COMPOSITION that a couple brings into the formation of a fertilized ovum has implications for both the successful completion of a pregnancy and the future of the new child. More and more couples are asking about their chances of having a child with a genetic defect or for anticipatory counseling concerning known genetic problems in their family. Being a member of a genetic screening and counseling team is a role for nurses in maternal-newborn care.

The Nature of Inheritance

The material of heredity (deoxyribonucleic acid, or DNA) is woven into strands, called *chromosomes*, in the nucleus of all body cells. *Genes* are designated points along the chromosomes that are responsible for specific body characteristics, traits, or illnesses. In order that cell formation be kept constant, DNA always remains in the cell nucleus. RNA (ribonucleic acid) is a separate protein component that passes out of the nucleus into the cell cytoplasm to guide cell function and reproduction. A wrong communication by an RNA molecule can lead to severe chromosomal abnormalities in the formation of a new cell.

Chromosomes and Their Effects

Chromosomal abnormalities occur in the moment of fusion of the ovum and spermatozoon, or, even earlier in the meiosis division phase of the formation of the gametes (reproductive cells) of the parent. As many as 50 percent of early spontaneous abortions are due to malformations caused by these abnormalities, which are so severe that life is impossible. Sometimes the defect does not affect life in utero; only after birth will the abnormality become apparent. The risk of a chromosomal aberration is so great in human reproduction that as many as 1 in every 150 infants is born with some kind of chromosomal abnormality (Barnett, 1977).

Chromosomes are "like" structures in that they are all composed of four "arms" joined at a point termed the *centromere*. A chromosome is said to be *metrocentric* if the centromere joins so that all four arms are equal length. It is *submetrocentric* if the location of this point results in two long upper arms, *acrocentric* if it results in two short upper arms.

In humans, the spermatozoa and ova each carry 23 chromosomes. For each chromosome in the sperm cell, there is a like chromosome in the ovum of similar size and shape and the same type of gene content (*autosomes* or homologous chromosomes). The exception of this pattern is the chromosome that determines sex. The female sex chromosome is medium-sized, with arms of equal length (metrocentric); the male sex chromosome is small and has an off-center midpoint (acrocentric).

The individual formed from the union of a sperm and ovum has 46 chromosomes in every body cell (44 autosomes and 2 sex chromosomes). If the sex chromosomes are both X (the medium-sized, metrocentric type), the individual is female (Figure 6-1A); if one sex chromosome is an X and one a Y (the small, acrocentric type), the individual is a male (Figure 6-1B).

A person's *phenotype* refers to his outward appearance or the expression of the genes. A person's *genotype* refers to his actual gene composition as shown on karyotyping.

A *karyotype* is a visual presentation of the chromosome pattern of an individual. For karyotyping, a sample of peripheral venous blood is drawn. White blood cells (lymphocytes) are spun off and allowed to grow until they reach a stage of metaphase, which is their most easily observed phase. They are then placed under a microscope, stained, and photographed through the microscope. Chromosomes are identified by banding (stained markings) according to their size and

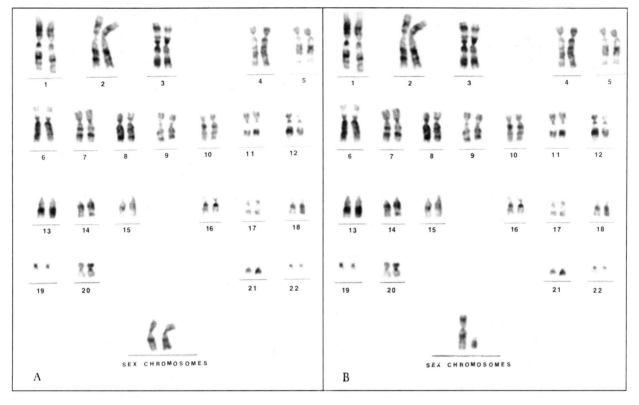

Figure 6-1 *Photomicrographs of human chromosomes (karyotypes). If a blood sample is taken from a newborn and the white cells are examined at the mitotic division phase of reproduction, transferred to slides, and photographed under high-power magnification, then the individual chromosomes can be cut from the photograph and arranged according to size and shape. A. Normal female karyotype. B. Normal male karyotype. (Courtesy of Dr. Judith Brown, Medical College of Virginia, Richmond, and the Department of Medical Photography, Children's Hospital, Buffalo, N.Y.)*

structure, cut from the photograph, and arranged as in Figure 6-1. Visualization of individual genes is now becoming possible: This will allow for even more single-gene-carried diseases to be identified.

A normal karyotype is abbreviated as 46XX or 46XY (designation of the total number of chromosomes plus a graphic description of the sex chromosomes present). If a chromosomal aberration exists, it will be listed after the sex chromosome pattern. In such abbreviations, the letter p stands for short-arm defects, q for the long arm. The abbreviation 46XX5p−, for example, is the abbreviation for a female's karyotype with 46 total chromosomes but missing the short arm of the fifth chromosome (5 p−). This defect is called cri du chat syndrome. Down's syndrome karyotype, in which a person has an extra twenty-one chromosome, is abbreviated 47XX21+ or 47XY21+.

Genetic disorders can be categorized as three types: those that are carried by individual gene abnormalities and inherited according to Mendelian laws, those that are multifactorial (polygenic, or involving many genes), and those that result from either too much or too little chromosomal material. Environmental influences may play a role in all gene and chromosome aberrations.

Mendelian Laws: Patterns of Single-Gene Inheritance

The genetic inheritance of disease follows certain laws, the same laws that govern genetic inheritance of other body characteristics such as eye or hair color. These laws were formulated in the 1800s by Gregor Mendel, an Austrian naturalist, and are known as *Mendelian laws.*

A person who has two like genes for a trait—one for blue eyes from the mother for example, as well as from the father—on two homologous chromosomes is said to be *homozygous* for that trait. If the genes differ (a gene for blue eyes from the mother and a gene for brown eyes from the father, or vice versa), the person is said to be *heterozygous* for that trait. Many genes are *dominant* in their action over others; when paired with

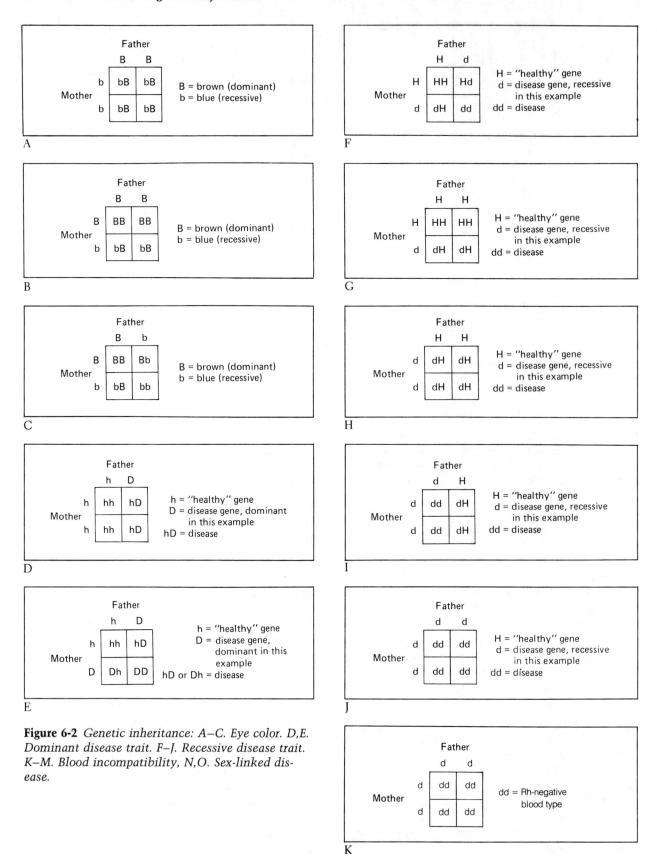

Figure 6-2 *Genetic inheritance: A–C. Eye color. D,E. Dominant disease trait. F–J. Recessive disease trait. K–M. Blood incompatibility, N,O. Sex-linked disease.*

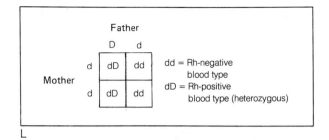

L

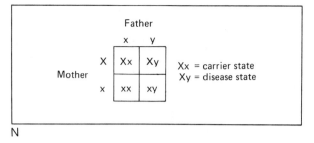

N

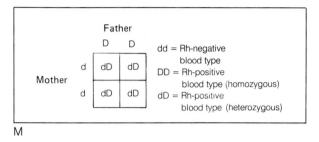

M

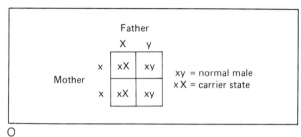

O

other genes, they will always be expressed in preference to the other genes. For eye color, brown is dominant over blue, so a person with a heterozygous pattern of brown and blue would appear to have brown eyes. That individual would be said to be a carrier for blue eyes, however, because of the hidden gene. A person with two homozygous genes for a dominant trait such as brown eyes is said to be *homozygous dominant*; similarly, two genes for a recessive trait such as blue eyes makes a person *homozygous recessive*.

The Mendelian laws permit prediction of inheritance of traits such as illness or eye color in terms of the proportion of children who will be born to parents of a certain genotype. For example, when a person who is homozygous dominant chooses as a sexual partner a person who is homozygous recessive for that trait, 100 percent of their children can be predicted to be heterozygous for the trait (Figure 6-2A); they will appear brown eyed (the phenotype), but will carry a recessive gene for blue eyes (the genotype).

Suppose the mother is heterozygous (has genes for both brown and blue eyes) instead of homozygous recessive. As can be seen in Figure 6-2B, the chances are equal that a child will be homozygous dominant (two genes for brown eyes) like the father or heterozygous like the mother. All the children's phenotypes will include brown eyes.

Suppose both parents are heterozygous. As can be seen in Figure 6-2C, 25 percent of their children will be homozygous recessive (appear blue eyed); 50 percent will be heterozygous (appear brown eyed); and 25 percent will be homozygous dominant (appear brown eyed). This pattern explains how two brown-eyed parents can produce a blue-eyed child, or two brunette parents can pro-

duce a blonde child. A person's genotype cannot possibly be predicted from the phenotype or her outward appearance.

Inheritance of Disease

The same principles of inheritance are applicable to diseases that are carried on the chromosomes by single genes. Diseases may be transmitted either as dominant or as recessive traits.

As a Dominant Trait. The dominantly inherited varieties of disease are few in number. A person with a dominant gene for a disease is usually heterozygous—that is, he has a corresponding healthy recessive gene for the trait. Huntington's chorea, a progressive neurologic disorder with onset usually in middle age, is the traditional example of a dominantly inherited disease. One form of muscular dystrophy (facioscapulohumeral) and osteogenesis imperfecta (a disorder in which bones are exceedingly brittle) are other examples.

If a person with a dominant disease trait—say, facioscapulohumeral muscular dystrophy—chose a sexual partner without the trait, the chances are even (50%), as shown in Figure 6-2D, that their offspring would be born with the disease or be disease-free and carrier-free.

Two persons with a dominantly inherited disease are unlikely to choose each other as sexual partners. However, if they do, their chances of having normal children decline (Figure 6-2E). Only 25 percent of their offspring would be disease- and carrier-free; 50 percent would actually have the disease, and the remaining 25 percent would be homozygous dominant. The two dominant disease genes of the last group would result in a condition that would probably be incompatible with life.

In assessing family pedigrees for incidence of inherited disease, the following findings usually point to a dominantly inherited pattern present in the family:

1. One of the parents of a child with a disorder will also be afflicted.
2. The sex of the affected child is unimportant in terms of inheritance.
3. A history of the disease can usually be documented in past family members.

Figure 6-3 shows a pedigree of a family with a dominantly inherited disorder.

As a Recessive Trait. The majority of heritable diseases are inherited as recessive traits. Such diseases do not occur unless two genes for the disease are present (a homozygous recessive pattern). Cystic fibrosis, adrenogenital syndrome, albinism, Tay-Sachs disease, galactosemia, phenylketonuria, sickle cell anemia, and limb girdle muscular dystrophy are commonly seen examples of recessively inherited diseases.

As an example of recessive inheritance, in Figure 6-2F, both parents are disease-free. However, both are heterozygous in genotype and thus carry a recessive gene for cystic fibrosis. As can be seen, 25 percent of their children will be disease- and carrier-free (homozygously dominant for healthy genes); 50 percent will be, like the parents, free of disease, but carrying the unexpressed disease gene (heterozygous); and 25 percent will have the disease (homozygous recessive).

Suppose a woman with the genotype in Figure 6-2F (heterozygous) chooses a sexual partner who has no trait for cystic fibrosis (Figure 6-2G). A child born to them has equal chances of being completely disease- and carrier-free or of being heterozygous like the mother. None of this couple's children will have the disease. The children should be aware, however, that their own children may manifest the disease if they both carry the trait and choose a sexual partner with the trait (see Figure 6-2F).

Formerly, children with cystic fibrosis died in early infancy and never reached childbearing age. Today, with good management, some can live to have children of their own. If a person with cystic fibrosis should choose a sexual partner without the trait, all their children would be free of the disease. They would all be carriers, however, or carry the recessive disease gene, as shown in Figure 6-2H.

If a person with cystic fibrosis paired with a person with an unexpressed gene for the disease,

Figure 6-3 *Family pedigree. Autosomal-dominant inheritance.*

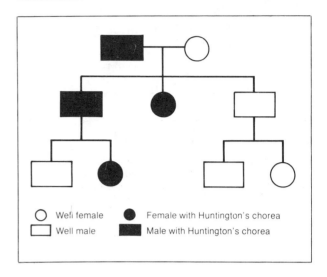

the chances are 50-50 that their children will have the disease or be carriers of the disease (Figure 6-2I). If a person with the disease should choose a person who also has the disease, as shown in Figure 6-2J, all of their children could be expected to have the disease.

When assessing family pedigrees for incidence of inherited disease, a number of common situations which are usually discovered when a recessively inherited disease is present in the family are:

1. Both parents of a child with the disorder will be clinically free of the disorder.
2. The sex of the affected individual is unimportant in terms of inheritance.
3. There is a negative family history for the disorder (no one can identify anyone else who had it).
4. There is often a known common ancestor. This is how both male and female have come to process a like gene for a disorder.

Figure 6-4 shows a pedigree of a family with a recessively inherited disorder.

Inheritance of Blood Type

An important clinical problem that arises during pregnancy is predicting whether a blood incompatibility, such as an Rh and an ABO, between a mother and fetus will occur.

Such a problem occurs when a fetus has a blood type with a protein substance not present in the mother's blood type. The mother's immune system senses a foreign protein invasion and begins to form antibodies against the fetal blood type, just as if the substance were an active disease or

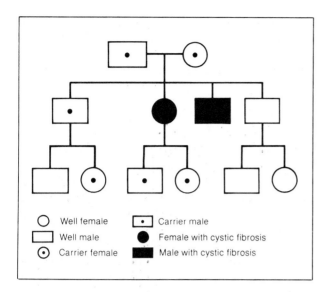

Figure 6-4 *Family pedigree. Autosomal-recessive inheritance.*

viral invader. Maternal antibodies can destroy fetal blood to such an extent that the health of the fetus is severely compromised. (Chapter 47 discusses this problem more thoroughly in reference to overall pregnancy and newborn care).

Rh Incompatibility. The Rh factor is a protein component of red blood cells. Blood incompatibility occurs when a mother whose blood does not contain the Rh factor (i.e., Rh negative) carries a child whose blood does contain the factor (Rh positive). (The Rh factor is also referred to as a D blood antigen.) The Rh factor is recessively inherited: Whether it will occur in a child can be predicted if both parents' blood types are known.

In Figure 6-2K, both the mother and the father have Rh-negative blood or lack a D blood antigen (a dd genotype). As can be seen, all of their children will have Rh-negative blood (dd genotype) and thus there will be no Rh incompatibility.

The father in Figure 6-2L is heterozygous for the Rh factor (a Dd genotype), the mother is Rh-negative (dd genotype). The positive factor (D) is dominant over the negative factor (d), so the heterozygous genotype (Dd) results in Rh-positive blood (the phenotype). In this instance, the chances are equal that a child will have Rh-negative blood (dd) or Rh-positive blood (Dd). The chances that an antigen-antibody reaction could occur during pregnancy are 50 percent. If the father should be homozygous for Rh-positive blood (DD genotype, Figure 6-2M), all the couple's children will have Rh-positive blood. It is extremely doubtful—unless the woman's antibody formation system is not active or she is administered RhoGAM (Rho[D] immune globu-

lin)—that this mother could escape problems of blood incompatibility in her pregnancies.

ABO Incompatibility. Type A and B blood types are dominant over Type O. Both A and B have a protein component lacking in Type O blood. A blood incompatibility in pregnancy will occur if a mother with Type O blood carries a fetus who has either Type A (genotype AO) or type B (genotype BO) blood. Interestingly, neither Type A nor Type B blood is dominant over the other. These types are said to be *codominant* or have a mutual-level expression, which is the reason that Type AB blood occurs.

Sex-Linked (X-Linked). Some genes for disease are located on and therefore transmitted only by the female sex chromosomes (the X chromosomes). This is called *sex-linked*, or X-linked, inheritance. The mother is the carrier for this type of inherited disease; the disease itself is manifested only in her male children.

Hemophilia A, Christmas disease (a blood factor deficiency), color blindness, Duchenne's (pseudohypertrophic) muscular dystrophy, and some forms of gargoylism are examples of this type of inheritance. Such a pattern is shown in Figure 6-2N, in which the mother is the carrier of the disease (the affected gene is on one of her X chromosomes) and the father is disease-free. Half of their male children will manifest the disease, and half of their female children will be carriers like their mother. If the father has the disease and chooses a sexual partner who is not a carrier, all of their daughters will be carriers of the disease—in other words, will have the sex-linked recessive gene. None of their sons will have the disease. This distribution is shown in Figure 6-2O.

In an assessment of family pedigrees, the following findings are usually apparent when a sex-linked inheritance disorder is present:

1. Only males in the family will have the disorder.
2. There is often a history of females dying at birth for unknown reason (These infants had the affected gene on both X chromosomes, a condition incompatible with life).
3. Sons of an affected male are unaffected.
4. The parents of affected children do not have the disorder.

Figure 6-5 shows a family pedigree with a sex-linked inheritance pattern.

Multifactorial (Polygenic) Inheritance

Many congenital disorders such as heart disease, pyloric stenosis, and cleft lip and palate tend to

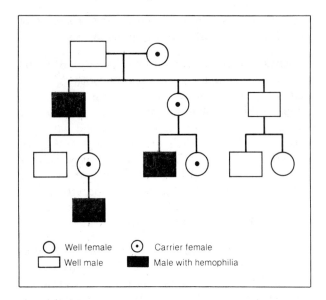

Figure 6-5 *Family pedigree. Sex-linked inheritance.*

"run in families" or have a higher-than-usual incidence in some families. Diabetes, hypertension, and manic/depressive mental illness are other examples of this type.

Multifactorial disorders do not follow the Mendelian laws of inheritance because more than a single gene is involved. Environmental influences may be instrumental in the expression of the disorder. It is difficult to counsel parents regarding these disorders because their occurrence is so unpredictable.

Taking a family history reveals no set pattern. Certain conditions have a predisposition to occur in one sex or the other (cleft palate, for example, occurs most often in females), but they can occur in either sex.

Chromosomal Division Defects

In some instances of chromosomal disease, the abnormality occurs not because of dominant or recessive patterns of genes but because of a fault in division of the reproductive cells: One sperm or ovum receives additional or insufficient amounts of chromosomal material during a cell division.

Nondisjunction Abnormalities

These disorders are the most common chromosome disorders. All sperm and ova initially undergo a meiosis cell division in order to reduce the number of chromosomes in the cell to the haploid number for reproduction (23 rather than 46). In meiosis, half of the chromosomes are normally attracted to one pole of the cell and half to the other pole. The cell then divides cleanly, with 23 chromosomes contained in each new cell (Figure 6-6A). Chromosomal abnormalities occur when the division is uneven (nondisjunction). The result may be one new sperm cell or ovum formed with 24 chromosomes and the other with only 22 (Figure 6-6B). If one of these defective spermatozoa or ova fuses with a normal ovum or spermatozoon, the *zygote* (sperm and ova combined) will have 47 or 45 chromosomes, not the normal 46. The presence of 45 chromosomes does not appear to be compatible with life, and the embryo or fetus will probably be aborted.

Down's Syndrome. Down's syndrome (trisomy 21) (47XX21 + or 47XY21 +) is an example of a disease in which the individual has 47 chromosomes. With Down's syndrome there is an extra number 21 chromosome (three rather than two) (Figure 6-7). Down's syndrome, the most frequently found chromosomal abnormality, was formerly called mongolism because the apparent slant of the eyes (Figure 6-8) makes the child look oriental.

The incidence of Down's syndrome is highest in the children of very young women and of older women (over 35). Thus, both immaturity and aging seem to present an obstacle to clean cell divi-

Figure 6-6 *A. Normal meiosis division. B. Nondisjunction division.*

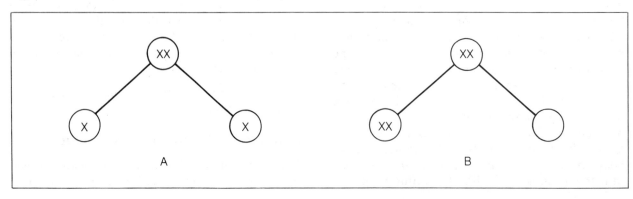

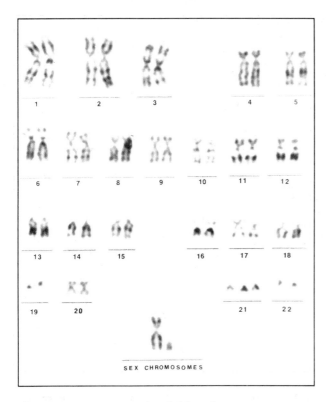

Figure 6-7 *Karyotype of a child with trisomy 21.*

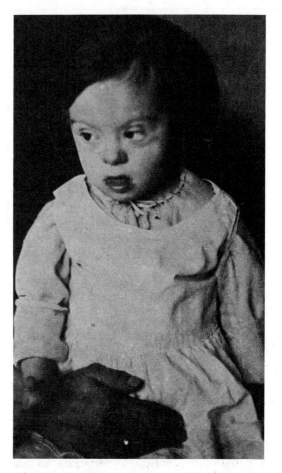

Figure 6-8 *A child with Down's syndrome. From Barnett, H. (1977).* Pediatrics *(15th ed.), p. 899. New York: Appleton-Century-Crofts.*

Table 6-1 Incidence of Down's Syndrome at Birth and at Amniocentesis by Mother's Age

Maternal Age	Incidence at Birth* (per 1,000)	Incidence at Amniocentesis† (per 1,000)
35	2.7	7.5
36	3.0	9.8
37	4.2	13.4
38	5.1	14.6
39	6.4	18.6
40	9.5	23.3
41	11.9	30.6
42	14.3	61.0
43	22.7	40.6
44	27.1	76.9
45	30.3	50.3
46	38.0	135.1

*Nevin, N. C. (1982). Genetic disorders. *Clinics in Obstetrics and Gynaecology, 9*(1), 3.

†Ferguson-Smith, M. A. (1980). Maternal age–specific incidence of chromosome aberrations at amniocentesis. In J. D. Murken, S. Stengel-Rutkowski, & E. Schwinger (Eds.), *Prenatal diagnosis* (pp. 1–14). Stuttgart: Enke.

sion. The actual incidence of Down's syndrome both in live births and by amniocentesis reports is shown in Table 6-1. Note how much higher the actual incidence of the syndrome is by amniocentesis report than by live births. As with other chromosomal disorders, many of these pregnancies end in early spontaneous abortion.

The appearance of the child at birth makes the diagnosis possible. The nose is broad and flat, the eyelids have an extra fold of tissue at the inner canthus (an epicanthal fold) and the palpebral fissure (opening between the eyelids) tends to slant laterally upward. The iris of the eye may have white specks in it (Brushfield's spots).

Even in the newborn, the tongue may protrude from the mouth because of a smaller-than-normal oral cavity. The back of the head is flat; the neck is short, and an extra pad of fat at the base of the head causes the skin there to be so loose it can be lifted up (like a puppy's neck). Ears may be low-set; muscle tone is poor (hypotonia), giving the baby a rag-doll appearance. You are able to touch his toe against his nose, something you cannot accomplish with other mature infants. The palm of the hand shows a peculiar crease (a simian line) or a horizontal palm crease rather than the normal three creases (Figure 6-9).

Children with Down's syndrome are mentally retarded, but the retardation can range from that of an educable child (50 to 70 IQ) to that of a child

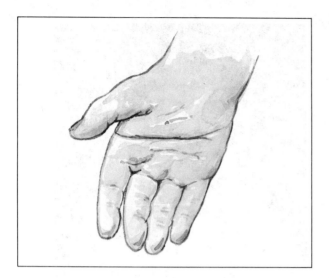

Figure 6-9 *A simian line, a horizontal palm crease seen in children with Down's syndrome. (Courtesy of the Department of Medical Illustration, State University of New York, Buffalo N.Y.)*

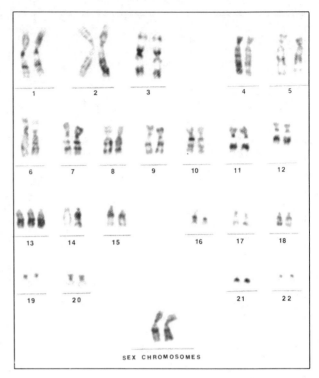

SEX CHROMOSOMES

Figure 6-10 *Karyotype of trisomy 13. Note the extra chromosome 13.*

requiring full care (under 20 IQ). The extent of the retardation will not be evident at birth. Those children with a near normal IQ may manifest mosaic chromosomal patterns (see page 105).

Trisomy 13 and 18. Other common examples of cell nondisjunction are trisomy 13 and trisomy 18 (mental retardation syndromes). Children with trisomy 13, or Patau's syndrome, are severely mentally retarded. The incidence is fortunately low, about 0.45 per 1,000 live births. Midline body defects are present. Microcephaly with abnormalities of the forebrain and forehead; smaller-than-normal eyes (microphthalmia) or no eyes at all; cleft lip and palate; low-set ears; heart defects, particularly ventral septal defects; and abnormal genitalia are common findings. Most of these children do not survive past early childhood (Figures 6-10 and 6-11).

Children with trisomy 18 are severely mentally retarded. The incidence is about 0.23 per 1,000 live births. These children tend to be small for gestational age at birth. They have markedly low-set ears, a small jaw, congenital heart defects, and misshapen fingers and toes (the index finger tends to deviate or cross over other fingers). Also, the soles of their feet are often rounded instead of flat (rocker-bottom feet). Most of these children do not survive beyond early infancy.

Turner's (Gonadal Dysgenesis) and Klinefelter's Syndromes. When nondisjunction occurs in the sex chromosomes, as opposed to in the autosomes, other types of abnormalities occur. Turner's and Klinefelter's syndromes are the most

common of this type of chromosomal abnormality.

In Turner's syndrome (marked by webbed neck, low-set hairline, short stature, sterility, and possible mental retardation) the individual, although female, either has only one X chromosome or has two X chromosomes with one defective. She appears to be female (female phenotype) because of the one X chromosome. The genotype is XO.

In the newborn, there may be appreciable edema of the hands and feet and a number of congenital anomalies, most frequently coarctation of the aorta and kidney defects. The child has only streak gonads, so secondary sex characteristics with the exception of pubic hair do not develop at puberty. Lack of ovarian function results in sterility. The incidence is about 0.33 per 1,000 live births.

In Klinefelter's syndrome (marked by sterility and possibly by mental retardation) the individual has male genitals but his sex chromosomal pattern is XXY. Individuals with Klinefelter's syndrome tend to have poorly developed male secondary sex characteristics, small testes producing ineffective sperm, and gynecomastia (enlarged breast tissue). The syndrome is difficult to recognize in the newborn. Failure of secondary sex characteristics to develop at puberty may be the first clue that an XXY genotype exists. The inci-

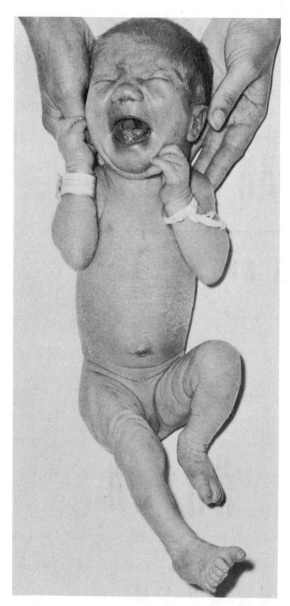

Figure 6-11 *An infant with trisomy 13. Note the cleft palate and polydactyly (7 toes). From Barnett, H. (1977). Pediatrics (15th ed.), p. 901. New York: Appleton-Century-Crofts. Courtesy of Drs. J. Lindsten and P. Zetterquist.*

dence of occurrence is about 1 per 1,000 live births.

Mosaicism. Normally a nondisjunction abnormality occurs during the meiosis stage of cell division when sperm and ova halve their number of chromosomes. Mosaicism is an abnormal condition that is present when the nondisjunction defect occurs following fertilization of the ovum when the structure begins mitotic (daughter cell) division. When this occurs, different cells in a person's body will have different chromosome counts. The extent of the disorder will depend on the proportion of tissue with abnormal chromosome constitution. Children with Down's syndrome who have near normal intelligence may have this type of pattern. That such a phenomenon occurred at this stage of development suggests that a teratogenic (harmful to the fetus) condition, such as x-ray or drug exposure, disturbed normal cell division at that point. This genetic pattern in a female would be abbreviated as 46XX/47XX21 + .

Deletion Abnormalities. Deletion abnormalities are yet another form of chromosome nondisfunction. With deletion, part of a chromosome breaks during cell division. An affected person can either have the normal chromosome count plus an extra portion of a chromosome or only 45¾ chromosomes.

In *cri du chat* (cat's cry) syndrome, a mental retardation syndrome that is marked by the child's peculiar cat-like cry, one portion of the number 5 chromosome is missing. These children have small heads, wide-set eyes, and a downward slant to the palpebral fissure of the eye. Deletion of the long arm of the 18 chromosome (46XX 18q −) results in a syndrome marked by hypotonus, mental retardation, seizures, heart defects, and hyperplastic genitalia.

Translocation Abnormalities

Translocation abnormalities are perplexing situations in which a person has an adequate chromosome count but the structure is arranged differently than normally. A form of Down's syndrome occurs as a translocation abnormality. In these instances, one of the parents has the correct number of chromosomes (46), but one of the 21 chromosomes is misplaced and abnormally attached to a number 14 or 15 chromosome. The parent appears normal and functions normally because the total chromosome count is 46; he is termed a *balanced translocation carrier.* Figure 6-12A)

If during meiosis, however, this abnormal 14 or 15 chromosome plus the one normal 21 chromosome are both included in one sperm or ovum, the resulting child will have a total of 47 chromosomes, including one extra number 21 (Figure 6-12B). Such a child has what is termed an *unbalanced translocation syndrome.* The phenotype (appearance) of the child will be indistinguishable from the form of Down's syndrome that occurs from nondisjunction.

About 2 to 5 percent of children with Down's syndrome have this type of chromosome pattern. It is important that parents who are translocation carriers are identified: Their chance of bearing

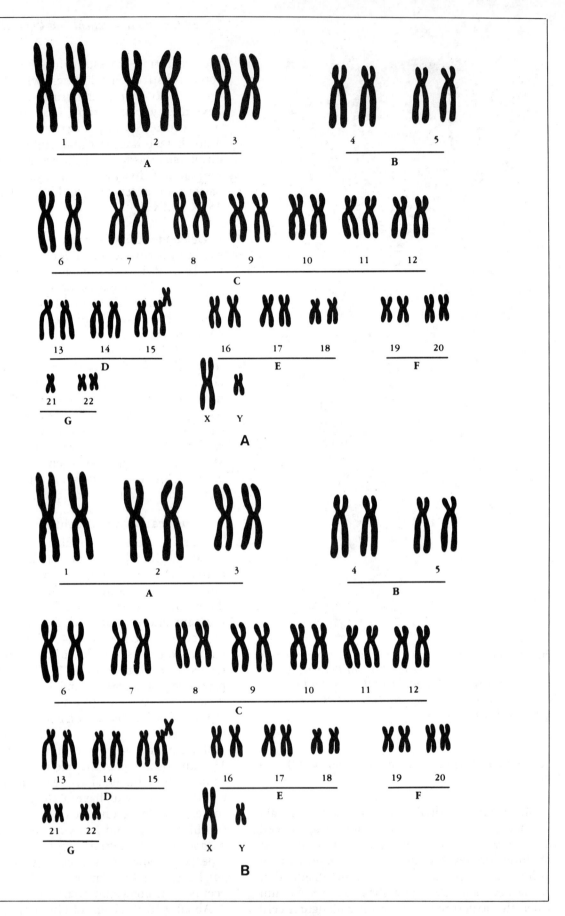

Figure 6-12 *A. Balanced translocation. Notice the 21 chromosome displaced to the 15th pair. B. Unbalanced translocation. Three 21 chromosomes are present because of the additional one attached to the 15th chromosome. Modified from Snell, R. S. (1984).* Clinical Histology for Medical Students. *Boston: Little, Brown.*

only children with Down's syndrome is very high (about 1 in 3). As many as 10 percent of couples who have frequent early spontaneous abortions may have this type of chromosomal aberration (Fitzsimmons, 1981).

Isochromosomes

If a chromosome accidentally divides not by a vertical separation but by a horizontal one, a new chromosome with mismatched long and short arms can result. This is an *isochromosome*. It causes much the same defect as a translocation abnormality where an extra chromosome exists. Some instances of Turner's syndrome (45XO) may occur because of isochromosome formation.

Multiple X, Multiple Y Syndromes

Very rarely, a female is born with more than two X chromosomes (XXX) or a male with more than one Y chromosome (XYY). Such individuals are generally indistinguishable from others at birth. At one time it was believed that men with multiple Y chromosomes were more aggressive or criminally inclined than others, but this finding is no longer accepted as true.

Inborn Errors of Metabolism

Inborn errors of metabolism are inherited disorders in which some body enzyme or metabolic process is absent or inadequate. They are most often representative of Mendelian recessive disorders. A number of them are particularly important to maternal-newborn nursing because of their implications for immediate assessment and planning in the newborn period.

Phenylketonuria

Phenylketonuria (PKU) is an autosomal recessive metabolic disease caused by an inborn error of metabolism. Affected infants lack the liver enzyme phenylalanine hydroxylase and therefore cannot convert phenylalanine, an essential amino acid, into tyrosine. Unconverted, the excessive phenylalanine builds up in the bloodstream and tissues, causing permanent damage to brain tissue and severe mental retardation. The metabolite phenylpyruvic acid (a breakdown product of phenylalanine) spills into the urine to give the disorder its name. It gives urine a typical musty or "mousey" odor.

Tyrosine is necessary for building body pigment and thyroxin; without this important metabolite present, body pigment fades and the child becomes very fair skinned, blonde, and blue

eyed. The skin is very prone to eczema (atopic dermatitis). Conversely, all infants with atopic dermatitis need to be rescreened for PKU because of the association between these two disorders. Affected children fail to meet average growth standards due to the lack of thyroxin production. Many of them develop an accompanying seizure disorder.

Phenylketonuria is found in about 1 in 10,000 births in the United States. It occurs rarely in people of black or Jewish ancestry. That PKU is present cannot be detected by amniocentesis or cord blood because the phenylalanine level does not rise in utero while the infant is still under the control of the mother's enzyme system.

On the third day of life, after two full days of feedings (at least 120 ml of formula at a concentration of 20 calories per ounce or the equivalent amount obtained by breast-feeding), the infant is screened for the disorder by having his heel pricked with a blood lancet. A single drop of blood is allowed to fall on each designated circle of a specially prepared filter paper. The filter paper is then analyzed by a bacterial inhibition process for the amount of phenylalanine contained in the infant's blood (the Guthrie test).

Infants in whom this disease is detected in the first few days of life can be placed on an extremely low phenylalanine formula (Lofenalac is an example). If the diet is begun immediately this way, mental retardation can be totally prevented. For this reason, it is extremely important that every infant with the disease be identified. If an infant is born at home or discharged from a hospital or birthing center before formula feeding is begun, or if the infant is being breast-fed and there is a question as to whether he took in breast milk or only colostrum (the thin fluid expressed before breast milk forms), or is on total parenteral nutrition, the American Academy of Pediatrics recommends that a blood specimen be obtained by the third week of life for a repeat Guthrie test (AAP, 1982).

In order that the child receives *some* phenylalanine (an essential amino acid for growth and repair of body cells), a dietician may include a small amount of milk in the infant's diet every day. This inclusion allows a mother who wants to breast-feed to do so on a limited basis.

The length of time that a child must remain on a restricted low-phenylalanine diet is controversial. The time span should at least be beyond 5 years of age, at which time 90 percent of brain growth is complete. A woman who has PKU must anticipate when she wants to have children and return to a low-phenylalanine diet for about a month before conception. She must remain on the diet during pregnancy; otherwise, her fetus will be exposed to high levels of phenylalanine and be born mentally retarded. Men and women with PKU need genetic counseling to help them realize that, although none of their children will have the disorder like themselves (assuming their sexual partner is disease- and carrier-free), all their offspring will carry the recessive gene for the disease.

Parents need a great deal of support when their child is diagnosed as having PKU. They may appreciate some suggestions on how to "reward" a child in other ways than giving food. The very limited food selection available to PKU children makes such creativity important.

Maple Syrup Urine Disease

Maple syrup urine disease is a rare amino acid metabolism disorder, inherited as an autosomal recessive trait in which a defect in amino acid metabolism leads to cerebral degeneration similar to that of phenylketonuria. The infant appears well at birth but quickly begins to evidence signs of feeding difficulty, loss of the Moro reflex, and irregular respirations. The symptoms progress rapidly to opisthotonos (rigid arching of the back), generalized muscular rigidity, and convulsions. The child may die of the disease as early as 2 to 4 weeks of age.

Although the disorder is rare, it is mentioned here because as early as the first or second day of life the urine of the child develops the characteristic odor of maple syrup; hence the name of the disease. The odor is due to the presence of ketoacids, the same phenomenon that makes the breath of diabetic children in severe acidosis smell sweet.

Theoretically, if maple syrup urine disease could be diagnosed in the first day or two of life and the child placed on a well-controlled diet low in the amino acids leucine, isoleucine, and valine, the cerebral degeneration could be prevented, just as it can be prevented in phenylketonuria. Nurses are the people most likely to detect the characteristic urine odor in the first few days of life. You should be aware of the severity as well as the symptoms of this disorder so that you do not discount the pleasant urine odor as an innocent finding.

Galactosemia

Galactosemia is evidenced by abnormal amounts of galactose in the blood (galactosemia) and in the urine (galactosuria). The commonest form of this disorder is an inborn error of metabolism, in which the child is deficient in the liver enzyme galactose 1-phosphate uridyl transferase enzyme. This is inherited as an autosomal recessive trait.

When lactose (the sugar of milk) is ingested, it is broken down into galactose and glucose. Galactose is then further broken down into additional glucose. Without the enzyme, this second step, or the conversion of galactose into glucose, cannot take place: Galactose builds up in the blood stream destroying body cells and spills into the urine.

Symptoms begin abruptly and grow worse rapidly when the child is begun on formula or breast-feedings: lethargy, hypotonia, and perhaps diarrhea and vomiting. The liver enlarges and cirrhosis develops. Jaundice is often present and persistent; bilateral cataracts develop. Untreated, the child may die by 3 days of age. Untreated children who do survive beyond this time may have mental retardation and bilateral cataracts.

A screening test (the Beutler test) similar to the Guthrie test for phenylketonuria is available. Cord blood can be analyzed for diagnosis. Carriers can be detected by the fact they have a lower level than normal of the effected enzyme.

The treatment of galactosemia consists of placing the infant on a diet free of galactose or a formula made with casein hydrolysates (Nutramingen is an example). Once the child is regulated on this diet, symptoms of the disease do not progress; however, any neurologic or cataract findings already present will persist. Length of time the child should remain on the restricted diet is controversial, but from 6 to 8 years is usually recommended.

Cystic Fibrosis

Cystic fibrosis of the pancreas is a disease in which there is generalized dysfunction of the exocrine glands. Mucous secretions of the body, particularly in the pancreas and the lungs, have difficulty flowing through body gland ducts. There is also a marked electrolyte change in the secretions of the sweat glands (chloride concentration of sweat is two to five times above normal).

The cause of the disorder is unknown, but apparently some compound or enzyme that keeps body fluids free-flowing cannot be manufactured by the affected children. Pancreatic enzymes are unable to flow out of the pancreas into the duodenum, so the children are unable to digest fat, protein, and some sugars. The plugging of the respiratory tree by thickened secretions causes chronic respiratory infection.

The disorder is inherited as an autosomal recessive trait, occurring in about 1 in 2,000 live births. The newborn with cystic fibrosis loses the normal amount of weight at birth (5 to 10% of birth weight) but then does not gain it back at the usual time of 7 to 10 days—perhaps not until 4 to 6 weeks of age. Failure to regain birth weight as a newborn is a significant sign that nurses, who weigh babies, must evaluate.

At birth, meconium may be so tenacious that the baby has intestinal obstruction (meconium ileus) and is unable to pass stool. All babies with meconium ileus should be tested for cystic fibrosis; this testing may be delayed until 6 to 8 weeks of age because newborns do not sweat a great deal and interpretation of the test may not be accurate until then. With newer testing procedures using pilocarpine described below, sweat testing may be done earlier than ever before.

For a sweat test with an infant, pilocarpine (a cholinergic drug that stimulates sweat gland activity) is dropped onto a gauze square. This is placed on the child's forearm, and copper electrodes are connected to it. A small electrical current is applied to carry the pilocarpine into the skin. Because the electrical current is of such low intensity, it should be painless. Following the application of the electrical current, the area on the arm is washed with water and dried, and a filter paper is applied to collect the sweat that forms. The filter paper must be lifted by forceps rather than touched so that sweat from your skin is not transferred to the paper, which would, of course, make the resulting test analysis inaccurate.

A normal concentration of chloride in sweat is 20 mEq per liter. A level of more than 60 mEq of chloride per liter in children is diagnostic of cystic fibrosis.

These children may be seen in a physician's office or clinic at about 1 month of age because of a feeding problem. They eat ravenously because, as a result of poor digestive function, their bodies use only about 50 percent of their intake. The tendency to swallow air, which is associated with this rapid feeding pattern, may be manifested as colic or abdominal distention and vomiting. Stools are large and bulky and perhaps loose and frequent. They feel or look greasy because of undigested fat. The appearance of the stools is an important finding: Children with simple colic do not have this type of stool consistency changes.

These children may also be seen by health care providers between 4 and 6 months of age because of frequent respiratory infections and a chronic cough. On auscultation, wheezing and rhonchi may be heard in the lungs. When weight is plotted on a standard growth chart, they are generally found to be behind.

Therapy for children with cystic fibrosis is a high-calorie, high-protein, moderate-fat diet. Infants are not generally breast-fed because there is not enough protein in breast milk; they need large amounts because they cannot make use of all the protein they ingest. Some of these children are unfortunately initially diagnosed as having a milk allergy and are treated by being placed on a soybean formula. These preparations do not contain enough protein either, and children's malnutrition will increase greatly while they are taking this formula. Probana, a high-protein formula, is generally the milk recommended for them.

Respiratory therapy such as postural drainage and aerosol nebulization will be begun early in life to avoid respiratory tract blocking and infection.

Parents need a great deal of support when they are told their child has cystic fibrosis. Although the prognosis for the disorder is improving with more vigorous treatment, the life expectancy for the average child is not over 12 to 16 years of age. Some children appear to have lighter-than-normal involvement, and these children do reach adulthood. Male adults with cystic fibrosis may not be able to reproduce because of tenacious plugging of the vas deferens from seminal fluid, which tends to cause blockage. Women have such thick cervical secretions that sperm penetration is limited.

Adrenogenital Syndrome

Adrenogenital syndrome is inherited as an autosomal recessive trait. The primary defect is an inability to synthesize hydrocortisone from its precursors. This fault ordinarily occurs at the 21-hydroxylase level. When the adrenal gland is unable to produce hydrocortisone, the pituitary adrenotropic hormone increases, stimulating the adrenal glands to improve function. The adrenals become hyperplastic (enlarged), but, still unable to produce hydrocortisone, overproduce androgen. The effect of androgen is masculinization of the female child or increased size of genital organs in males. This process begins during fetal life: Females are born with an enlarged clitoris that appears more like a penis than a clitoris. As the labia are often fused, the total picture resembles a male infant with undescended testes and hypospadias (displaced urinary meatus). Internal female organs are normal, although a sinus between the urethra and vagina may be present.

When there is a complete block of the formation of hydrocortisone (salt-dumping adrenogenital syndrome), the production of aldosterone will be deficient also. Without adequate aldosterone, salt is not retained by the body; thus fluid is not retained. Within the first month of life, infants begin to have vomiting, diarrhea, anorexia, loss of weight, and extreme dehydration. If they are untreated, the extreme loss of salt and fluid will lead to collapse and death, as early as 48 to 72 hours following birth. This syndrome is one reason newborn babies in hospital nurseries are weighed daily. In males, the inability to gain back their birth weight may be the first sign that the syndrome is present.

These infants must be placed on daily hydrocortisone. If they have the salt-losing form of the syndrome, they must be placed on hydrocortisone and a high salt intake. Desoxycorticosterone acetate (Doca), a synthetic aldosterone, helps to maintain a balance of fluid and electrolytes.

When children were born at home and no close scrutiny was given them at birth by a health care professional, many with adrenogenital syndrome were wrongly identified at birth as males when they were chromosomally female. Some of these people, as adults, have had "sex change" operations that have actually restored their phenotypes (outward appearance) to correspond with their genotypes (actual chromosomal structure)—not very dramatic operations after all. It was formerly recommended that a girl's clitoris be reduced by plastic surgery early in life to give the girl a better cosmetic appearance. This is an ethical concern, however, because clitoral reduction causes a loss of sensation to stimulation. It is now generally recommended that this decision wait until the girl reaches an age to choose for herself whether she desires a more normal vulvar appearance or wants full clitoral sensation.

Parents of females with adrenogenital syndrome need a great deal of support during the first few days of their child's life; their child is imperfect and in an embarrassing, hard-to-explain way. When a *Barr body test* (discussed on page 113) reveals an extra Barr body present, which means the child has two X chromosomes, parents may react with grief for the loss of the son they thought was born to them. They may be embarrassed to call friends and tell them the sex of the child is different from what they first reported. Neighbors may view the child suspiciously as if there were something perverted or provocative about her. Parents need support to accept the child as perfect with the exception of an incompletely formed hormone. In supporting them, health care personnel must recognize the difficulty of this adjustment.

Glucose 6-Phosphate Dehydrogenase (G-6-PD) Deficiency

G-6-PD is transmitted as a sex-linked recessive trait. As the name implies, the children lack the enzyme glucose 6-phosphate dehydrogenase, an enzyme important for red blood cell formation. The disorder occurs most frequently in children of black, oriental, Sephardic Jewish, and Mediterranean descent. As many as 10 percent of American blacks are affected.

In the most frequently occurring form of this illness, children with the disorder are born with normal blood patterns, which are maintained until they are exposed to fava beans or drugs such as acetylsalicylic acid (aspirin) or phenacetin. About two days after the ingestion of such drugs a child begins to show evidence of hemolysis (rapid destruction of red blood cells). Occasionally a newborn with the defect is seen with marked hemolysis because the mother ingested an initiating drug during pregnancy.

Tay-Sachs Disease

Tay-Sachs disease is an autosomal recessive inherited disease in which infants lack the enzyme *hexosaminidase A*. Hexosaminidase A is necessary for lipid metabolism. Without it, lipid deposits accumulate on nerve cells, which causes mental retardation when brain cells are involved or blindness if optic nerve cells are involved.

The disorder is found primarily in the Ashkenazic Jewish population (Eastern European Jewish ancestry: *Ashkenazi* means "German"). A child generally appears normal in the first few months of life except for an extreme Moro reflex and mild hypotonia. At about 6 months of age, the child begins to lose head control and is unable to sit up or roll over without support. On ophthalmoscopic examination, a cherry-red macula is noticeable (caused by lipid deposits).

By 1 year of age, the child has symptoms of spasticity and is unable to perform even simple motor tasks. By 2 years of age, generalized convulsions and blindness occur. Most children die of cachexia (malnutrition) and pneumonia by 3 to 5 years of age. There is no cure for Tay-Sachs disease. The disorder may be detected in utero by amniocentesis. Carriers for the disease trait may be identified by hexosaminidase A assay.

Parents of children with Tay-Sachs disease need a great deal of support when they are told the diagnosis. There is an old saying that children with Tay-Sachs disease die twice: once when the disease is diagnosed, and again when they actually die.

The Impact of Genetic Disease

Many people view inherited disease as a different type of disease from that occurring by bacterial

══════════ *Nursing Care Highlight* ══════════
Genetic Counseling

People who have children with genetic disorders may suffer a severe loss of self-esteem that limits their ability to make decisions or to advocate for their child. Be certain you do not intimidate parents by making decisions for them; instead, strengthen their ability to speak for their child's welfare.

invasion or trauma. The former, it is thought, could have been prevented: Someone is at "fault." If parents of children with inherited disease hold this view, this may leave them with too little self-esteem to parent effectively. Part of the stigmatism arises from early sociologists, who traced inherited diseases through families in order to demonstrate the impact of inherited disease. They often dealt with families who had a syndrome associated with a form of mental retardation, which formed a connection between inherited disease and people too ignorant to care for themselves.

When a child is born imperfect, parents cannot help but ask themselves, Why did this happen? And secondarily, Why did this happen to *me*? It is natural for them to want to blame the occurrence on something. Unless they are counseled otherwise, the parents may begin to feel that the imperfection really is their fault or payment for some past sin. Guilt is a negative emotion that destroys self-esteem and, again, interferes with parenting ability.

Parents need time for a frank discussion of how they feel about themselves, as well as how they feel about their child. They may need counseling to improve their self-esteem before they are ready to parent a very ill child. It is common practice in some health care centers to diagnose children with chromosomal abnormalities as "funny looking kids" before their chromosomal analysis and the specific chromosome problem have been established. This label is unfair and very unprofessional for a nurse interested in improving parents' self-esteem. A parent cannot relate to health care providers who are so callous to their situation that they are not only not sympathetic to their feelings but appear to find amusement in their situation as well.

Genetic Counseling

Any person who is concerned about the possibility of transmitting a disease to his or her children should have access to genetic counseling (see the Nursing Care Highlight above on genetic counseling. The confidentiality, timing, and impact of this counseling is discussed below.

Confidentiality

Genetic screening may reveal information that is dangerous to a person's reputation or could affect a future career or relationship. A woman with a history of mental illness, for example, might seek genetic counseling to find out the chances of the disease occurring in her children. The information would be very helpful if used in this way; it could be detrimental to her if used by a political adversary or given to an employer. Often an entire family should be advised of a member's condition that affects them so that each member can make equally informed, responsible choices. Confidentiality, however, prevents you from alerting them to a problem unless they personally ask for the information. In some instances, confidential information such as a child's adoption, conception by artificial insemination, or having a father not the present husband is involved. The one member of the couple who knows this information has to decide if he or she wants this information imparted to the other member or not.

Timing

The timing of genetic counseling is important: Counseling given "after the fact" is useless; counseling given before a couple is ready to accept the information will not be used. The ideal time for genetic counseling, therefore, is before a first pregnancy. Some couples take the step of genetic counseling before committing themselves to marriage, working out the problem of children who could be subject to an inherited disorder before making a marriage commitment. For other couples, the birth of a child with some disorder signals the need for genetic counseling. Such couples need help before a second pregnancy occurs. They will not be ready for counseling, however, until the initial shock of their child's condition and the accompanying grief reaction has run its course. Only then will they be ready for information and future decision making.

A couple may decide not to have any more children; they should still be aware that genetic counseling is available, as they may change their minds at a future date. They also need to know about the services available to them for their children's information, who may want advice after reaching reproductive age.

Impact

Genetic counseling serves at least four purposes.

1. Reassuring people who are concerned that their children will inherit a noninheritable disorder that their fears are groundless.
2. Allowing people who are affected by inherited disorders to make informed choices about future reproduction.
3. Educating people about inherited disorders and the process of inheritance.
4. Offering support of skilled health care professionals to people who are affected by genetic illness.

In many instances, couples are not aware that genetic counseling is available or even that their first child's condition is inherited. Couples who might benefit from a referral for genetic counseling are:

1. Couples who have a previous child born with a congenital abnormality or an inborn error of metabolism. Many congenital abnormalities occur because of teratogenic invasion during pregnancy (often unknown). More important perhaps for the couple is learning that the abnormality occurred by chance rather than inheritance; then they do not have to spend the remainder of their childbearing years with the fear that other children may be born malformed (although a chance circumstance could occur again). If a definite teratogenic agent, such as a drug the woman took during pregnancy, can be identified, the couple can be advised to avoid this agent in a future pregnancy.
2. Couples whose close relatives have a child with a congenital abnormality or inborn error of metabolism. It is difficult to predict the expected occurrence of "familial" or multifactorial disorders because they are caused by multiple gene defects. Counseling should be aimed

Table 6-2 Common Diseases in Which Carriers Can Be Detected

Disorder	Method of Carrier Detection
Cystic fibrosis	No test available at present, but isoelectrofocusing of protein is encouraging as a future test
Duchenne's muscular dystrophy	Serum creatinekinase, muscle biopsy
Glucose-6-phosphate dehydrogenase	Enzyme assay
Hemophilia A	Factor VIII assays
Phenylketonuria	Phenylalanine loading test
Sickle cell disease	Hemoglobin electrophoresis
Tay-Sachs disease	Hexosaminidase A assay
Thalassemia	Red cell abnormalities; hemoglobin electrophoresis

at helping a couple learn as much as possible about the disorder, what treatment is available for it, and the ultimate prognosis or outcome. Illnesses in which carriers can be detected are shown in Table 6-2. This information allows couples to make an informed reproductive choice.

3. Individuals who are known balanced translocation carriers. Balanced translocation carriers need to understand their own chromosome structure and the process by which their children could be affected. Based on this information, an individual can make a choice to not reproduce or to have an amniocentesis for karyotyping performed during any future pregnancy.
4. Individuals who have an inborn error of metabolism or chromosomal defect. Persons with a disease should know the inheritance pattern of their disease; like balanced translocation carriers, they should be alerted to the wisdom of prenatal diagnosis, if possible, for their particular disorder.
5. Couples who are consanguineous (closely related). The closer related two people are, the more genes they share in common, so the more likely a recessive inherited disease will be expressed. A brother and sister for example, have about 50 percent of their genes in common; first cousins have about 12 percent.
6. Women over 35 years of age. This precaution is directly related to the association between ad-

vanced maternal age and the occurrence of Down's syndrome.

Genetic counseling may result in making an individual feel "well" or free of guilt for the first time—if the disorder they were worried about is not inheritable but occurred by uncontrollable chance. In other instances, individuals learn how they can carry a trait or, through no fault of their own, be responsible for a child's condition. Couples may blame each other so extensively for a child's condition that they can no longer remain together. A person may blame herself so much that she loses all self-esteem.

Anticipating that these actions may occur and laying some foundation to help a couple live with the results of a pregnancy is important. A couple with harsh decisions to make about genetics must, before making them, work out their priorities about children and being life partners.

Laboratory Analysis of Disorders

In order for genetic counseling to be effective, the exact type of involvement the child has must be identified as accurately as possible. Although the term *muscular dystrophy* is used to denote a number of musculoneurologic disorders, for example, the inheritance pattern widely varies. Diagnosis of disorders is made from patient health history, physical examination, and suitable laboratory testing. Helpful techniques of laboratory analysis for genetic screening include karyotyping, Barr body identification, amniocentesis, sonography, fetoscopy, and chorionic villi sampling.

Karyotyping

On the basis of the karyotype (see page 96) and the rules of inheritance, a prediction is made about the chances of children of a couple seeking counseling having an inherited disease. Remember that disease inherited by single or multiple genetic defects is not revealed by karyotyping; only total or partial chromosomal aberrations are revealed by this technique.

Barr Body Determination

To determine whether an individual has two X chromosomes, a simpler test than karyotyping may be performed. Cells are scraped from the buccal membrane of the inner surface of the child's cheek; then they are stained and magnified. Only one X chromosome is functional in females; the nondominant one appears to not be involved in cell metabolism. This second X chromosome, if present, will appear as a black dot on the edge of the cell. This is called a *Barr body*, the test a *Barr*

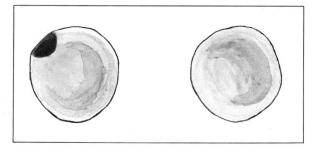

Figure 6-13 *A Barr body determination. The dark spot on the side of the nucleus indicates a second X chromosome.*

body determination (Figure 6-13). It is often performed on newborns to ascertain sex if a child has ambiguous genitalia. The child will then need further chromosomal investigation, including a complete karyotype, to reveal the chromosomal pattern. In order that the laboratory technician carrying out the Barr body test can be certain the cells adequately absorbed the stain, a female's buccal membrane scraping is also examined. Technicians often ask the nurse who is helping them to restrain the child during the buccal membrane scraping for a scraping from her cheek to use as the test control.

Amniocentesis

If a couple chooses to begin a pregnancy, amniocentesis at the fourteenth to sixteenth week of a pregnancy may reveal whether or not the fetus has an inherited disease. Following a sonogram to locate the placenta and establish that there is only one fetus present, the standard amniocentesis technique is used (abdominal skin is anesthetized; then a thin needle is inserted abdominally into the uterus, and 15–20 ml of amniotic fluid is withdrawn). Fetal skin cells, or amnion cells that have flaked off in the fluid, can be used to determine the fetal karyotype. If a twin or multiple pregnancy is present, where two or more separate divisions of amniotic fluid exist, it is important that fluid be removed separately from each compartment. As fraternal twins are derived from separate ova, one twin could have a chromosomal abnormality and the other be normal.

Amniocentesis for chromosomal abnormality is recommended in women over 35 years of age because the incidence of Down's syndrome greatly increases in infants of mothers past this age. It is also recommended if a previous conception in which either parent was a partner resulted in a child with a diagnosable chromosomal defect, if either partner is a known balanced translocation carrier, if both parents are carriers of a metabolic defect, if the woman is a carrier of a sex-

Table 6-3 Common Chromosomal Abnormalities That Can Be Diagnosed Before Birth by Amniocentesis

Disorder	Genetic Defect	Effect on Child
Down's syndrome	Trisomy 21	Mental retardation; protruding tongue, epicanthal folds; hypotonia
Translocation Down's syndrome	Translocation of a chromosome, perhaps 15/21	Same clinical signs as trisomy 21
Trisomy 18	Trisomy 18	Mental retardation, congenital malformations
Trisomy 13	Trisomy 13	Mental retardation; multiple congenital malformations: cleft palate, eye agenesis
Cri du chat syndrome	Deletion of short arm of chromosome 5	Mental retardation, facial structure anomalies, peculiar cat-like cry
Philadelphia chromosome	Deletion of one arm of chromosome 21	Chronic granulocytic leukemia
Turner's syndrome (gonadal dysgenesis)	XO	Short stature, streak gonads; infertility; webbing of neck
Klinefelter's syndrome	XXY	Small testes; gynecomastia; infertility

linked disorder, or if there is a family history of spinal cord defects.

Parents should understand that not all inherited diseases can be detected by amniocentesis. Table 6-3 shows various chromosomal disorders that can be diagnosed prenatally by amniocentesis through karyotyping. Table 6-4 lists common inborn errors of metabolism that can be identified by amniocentesis. These diagnoses are based on the levels of certain enzymes, not on the karyotype. Spinal cord defects can be diagnosed on the presence of extra alpha-fetoprotein in amniotic fluid (see Chapter 15).

Whether to have an amniocentesis done to determine chromosomal normality is a major decision for a couple. As a rule, they are not seeking the information simply out of curiosity: If the amniocentesis reveals that their child is abnormal, aborting the pregnancy seems to most partners to be the next sensible step.

Unfortunately, amniocentesis cannot be done until the fourteenth to sixteenth week of pregnancy when there is a sufficient quantity of amniotic fluid present. By that time the woman is beginning to accept her pregnancy and perhaps to "nest build." Making an abortion decision at this point will be difficult for her—much more difficult than it seemed before or early in the pregnancy when she first agreed to amniocentesis. She needs a great deal of support to carry through with her decision; she will also need support during the remainder of her pregnancy and in the

days following birth if she changes her mind about abortion. It may be hard for her to believe that what the test showed is real. Only when she looks at the baby and sees that the test was accurate—that her child has Down's syndrome, for example—does the realization hit home. The result may be a long-lasting postpartal depression.

Many physicians are reluctant to do amniocentesis, which carries some risk, unless the couple agrees that, if the chromosomal analysis does reveal an abnormality, they will consent to an abortion. Parents do not need to feel bound to this prior agreement, however; any paper they sign previous to an amniocentesis is not informed consent and therefore not binding.

Sonography

Sonography (ultrasound) is a diagnostic tool helpful in assessing general size and structural defects of the spine and limbs of a fetus. It may be used concurrently with amniocentesis because it involves no apparent risk to the fetus and aids in location of the placenta.

Fetoscopy

Fetoscopy is the insertion of a fibrooptic fibroscope through a small incision in the mother's abdomen to inspect the fetus for gross abnormalities, such as spinal cord defects or *anencephaly* (underdeveloped head). This type of examination can be videotaped or Polaroid photos can be taken so the couple can be given extra

Table 6-4 Prenatal Diagnosis of Hereditary Metabolic Diseases

Disorder	Effect on Child
Lipid metabolism	
GM$_2$ gangliosidosis (Tay-Sachs disease)	Degenerative neurologic disorder. Child has cherry red spot within macula. Results in extreme hypotonia, psychomotor retardation, and death
Niemann-Pick disease	Hepatosplenomegaly; skeletal and neurologic involvement
Gaucher's disease	Renal failure; cardiac and ocular involvement
Amino acid metabolism	
Cystinosis	Failure to thrive, rickets, glycosuria, cystine deposition in tissue and aminoaciduria
Homocystinuria	Dislocated lens of the eye; skeletal abnormalities, mental retardation, vascular thrombosis
Maple syrup urine disease	Ketoacidosis, neurologic abnormality, mental retardation, early death
Carbohydrate metabolism	
Glycogen storage disease	Failure to thrive, hepatomegaly, cardiomegaly
Galactosemia	Cataracts, mental retardation, failure to thrive
Glucose 6-phosphate dehydrogenase deficiency	Hemolytic anemia
Mucopolysaccharidoses	
Hurler's syndrome	Gargoyle-like facies, early psychomotor retardation, dwarfism, joint stiffness
Hunter's syndrome	Gargoyle-like facies, psychomotor retardation
Miscellaneous disorders	
Adrenogenital syndrome	Virilization or masculinization of female fetus; adrenal insufficiency with salt loss
Cystic fibrosis	Tenacious body fluids, chronic pulmonary infections, failure to thrive, early death

reassurance that their child does not have the type of defect they were concerned about. This procedure may be important in initiating bonding or attachment to the fetus—a process that may have frozen in development if parents are worried that their child may be abnormal. A photo may, on the other hand, help parents realize that a structural defect does exist so they can make a truly informed choice among alternative next steps.

Chorionic Villi Sampling (CVS)

Karyotyping may also be done by a new technique (chorionic villi sampling) that allows for first trimester pregnancy analysis (as early as the eighth to tenth week). For the procedure, a thin cannula is threaded vaginally and a small sample of chorionic villi is obtained by aspiration. These cells are stained and examined to reveal the chromosomal structure (chorionic villi—cells that will form the placenta—result from the same

basic cells as the fetus so have the same chromosomal structure as the fetus). CVS unfortunately carries a risk that the pregnancy will be interrupted (about 3 to 10 percent). This is in contrast to a risk of only 1.5 percent for amniocentesis and 3 to 5 percent for fetoscopy (Ward, 1984).

Reproductive Alternatives

Some people are afraid to come for genetic counseling because they fear they will be told that it would be unwise to have children (an ignorance-is-bliss philosophy). Helping them to realize that alternatives to childbearing are available for them allows them to seek the help they need.

Artificial insemination by donor (AID) is an attractive option if the genetic problem is one inherited by the male partner or if both partners carry a recessively inherited disorder. AID is available in all major communities and allows the

Guidelines for Genetic Screening and Counseling

Participation in genetic screening programs must be elective, not mandatory.

People desiring genetic screening should sign an informed consent for the procedure.

Results must be interpreted carefully and relayed to individuals as promptly as possible.

The results of the screening must not be withheld from individuals.

The results of genetic screening must not be given to other persons than the individuals directly involved.

Following genetic counseling, persons must not be coerced to undergo abortion or sterilization. This should be a free, individually dictated choice.

---

couple the satisfaction and enjoyment of experiencing a normal pregnancy once fertilization is achieved. If the inherited problem is one caused by the female partner, use of a surrogate mother (a woman who agrees to be artificially inseminated by the male partner's sperm and bear a child for the couple) is a possibility. Donor embryo transfer (an ova is taken from a donor, fertilized in the laboratory by the husband's sperm and then implanted in his wife's uterus) is a procedure that is just becoming possible; like donor artificial insemination, it offers the couple a chance to experience a normal pregnancy.

Choosing to remain childless should not be discounted as a viable option. Many couples who have every reason to believe they would have normal children are choosing this alternative because they find their existence full and rewarding without children. Adoption is a possible alternative certainly; but because of the scarcity of available children, adoption is becoming less and less realistic as an option. It is very unlikely that a couple with an ill child would qualify for adoptive parenthood: Agencies have many childless couples waiting for infants. Theoretically these couples, without the burden of an ill child, would have more time and resources available to parent an adopted child. A couple who has a genetically inherited problem might be able to adopt a "difficult to adopt" child, such as a racially mixed or handicapped child. Such children are usually available through agencies.

Pregnancy interruption or induced abortion of any pregnancy that reveals a chromosomal or metabolic abnormality is yet another option. Early diagnosis and treatment to minimize the prognosis and outcome of any disorder is yet another choice.

Couples need support from health care personnel to decide on the best alternative for them. Be certain that when a couple selects options, they end up with one right for them, not one that they assume you feel would be best. Ultimately, the solution, to be good for a couple, will probably have to coincide with the ethical philosophy or beliefs of other family members.

Legal Aspects of Genetic Screening and Counseling

When participating in genetic screening or counseling, you must keep a number of legal responsibilities in mind, as shown in the box above. Failure to heed these guidelines could result in charges of invasion of privacy, breach of confidentiality, or psychological injury due to a patient's claims of being "labeled" or her fears about the significance of a disease or carrier state.

Ethical Considerations

Many ethical considerations surround genetic screening and counseling—in particular when a couple chooses to abort a pregnancy because of amniocentesis findings. Many people argue that a decision to abort a child because of a mental handicap is unethical, because it is a choice that denies any legal right to handicapped individuals.

The problem becomes even more controversial as men with genetic disorders such as hemophilia A (an X-linked disorder) reach reproductive age. Such a man and his sexual partner might choose to abort all female fetuses so the disorder could not be passed on to another generation (all male children would be unaffected). Another problem occurs if a twin pregnancy is found to include one normal and one affected child. Is it ethical to abort the diseased child, which also might result in the loss of the normal child?

People on a genetic counseling team need to resolve these ethical problems in their own minds, and in a manner consistent with their personal and professional ethics. They may need to help a couple to use values clarification to find an answer for themselves.

Utilizing Nursing Process

Genetic screening and counseling is an area of health care that is changing daily because the number of diseases that can be detected during pregnancy or treated immediately at birth is increasing yearly. Assisting with genetic screening and counseling is both a rewarding and challenging role.

Assessment

Genetic counseling begins with careful assessment of the pattern of inheritance in the family, physical examination of family members, and laboratory analysis such as karyotyping so the extent of the problem and the chance of inheritance can be defined.

A detailed family history is necessary to assess if a disorder occurred by chance or is carried by family members. It is important to trace physical and mental conditions as far back in the family as members can remember. Ask the couple seeking counseling to talk to senior family members about grandparents, aunts, uncles, and other relatives before they come for an interview. Ask specifically for instances of children in the family who died at birth. In many instances these children died of unknown chromosomal disorders or were spontaneously aborted because of chromosomal abnormalities inconsistent with life.

An extensive prenatal history of any affected person helps determine if environmental conditions could account for the condition. Drawing a family pedigree is part of diagnosing the trend of inheritance. Such a diagram not only identifies the possibility of a chromosomal disorder occurring in a couple's children but also helps point out other family members who would benefit from genetic counseling. In drawing a family pedigree, the international symbol for males is a square, for females a circle.

Taking a health history for a genetic pedigree determination is often difficult: You are making people detail facts about themselves that raise accompanying emotions of sorrow or guilt, inadequacy, worthlessness, carelessness, and even the presence of ignorance that no one in the family realized that a disorder was heritable. Many people have inadequate information about their families except for statements such as, "The baby had some kind of nervous disease" or "Her heart didn't work right." You may obtain more helpful information by asking the couple to describe the appearance or activities of the affected individual.

If a child is born dead, parents are usually advised to have a chromosomal analysis and autopsy performed on the infant. If at some future date they want genetic counseling, these procedures ensure the availability of accurate medical information.

Physical Assessment. A careful physical assessment of any family member with a disorder, other children, and the couple seeking counseling needs to be made. Genetic disorders often occur in various degrees of expression. It might be possible for a child to have a minimal expression of a disorder and have gone undiagnosed. *Dermatoglyphics* (the study of palmar hand creases) is often helpful in identifying chromosomal abnormalities because special patterns appear with some disorders.

Careful inspection of newborns is often sufficient to suggest a chromosomal disorder. Infants with multiple congenital anomalies, those born at less than 35 weeks' gestation, and those whose parents have had previous children with chromosomal disorders need extremely critical assessment for chromosomal disorders.

In assessing, special areas to consider are, What is the child's overall appearance? Are the proportions normal? Are congenital defects present? Inspect the level of the ears and the pattern of palm creases. Test muscle strength. Test neurologic function. Are newborn reflexes intact?

Analysis

The Fourth Annual Conference on Nursing Diagnoses did not accept a specific nursing diagnosis for genetic screening or counseling. A typical nursing diagnosis that you might use in this area could be "Fear of outcome of tests related to genetic screening," "Guilt related to identified chromosomal abnormality," or "Lack of knowledge related to inheritance pattern of Down's syndrome." Setting realistic goals that are consistent with the individual's or couple's life style is important.

Planning

Making plans for genetic counseling or further actions must be done with the individual's or couple's input: These plans must be based on very personal decisions. One woman may strongly differentiate, for example, between using a contraceptive to prevent conception (very acceptable) and ending a pregnancy by abortion (totally unacceptable). Other couples do not draw this distinction between the procedures; they may be able to accept either action (or neither). Careful planning must include those options that the couple finds acceptable to them.

Implementation

Nurses play important roles in the assessment of genetic disorders and in offering counsel and support. Be certain when offering advice that you do not impose your opinion on others. Be certain that people are aware of all the options that are available, which is the only way they can choose freely. Otherwise they may reject an option such as artificial insemination because they mistakenly think it involves pain or is an experimental or manipulative procedure.

Genetic counseling is a role for nurses, however, only if they are adequately prepared in genetics. Genetic counseling can be as dangerous and destructive as parlor psychology if it is given "off the cuff"; never state general theories to a couple rather than basing your statements on the specific situation under discussion.

Most people listen to the statistics of their situation ("Your child has a 25 percent chance of having this disease") and misinterpret what they hear. They construe a "25 percent chance" to mean that, if they have one child with the disease, they can then have three normal children without any worry. However, a 25 percent chance means that with each pregnancy, there is a 25 percent chance that the child will have the disease (chance has no memory as to what happened the last time). It is as if the couple had four cards, the aces of spades, hearts, clubs, and diamonds, and the ace of spades represents the disease. When a card is drawn from the set of four, the chances of its being the ace of spades are 1 in 4 (25 percent). That represents the first pregnancy. When the couple is ready to have a second child, it is as if the card drawn the first round is returned to the set. The chances of drawing the ace of spades in the second draw are exactly the same as in the first. Similarly, the couple's chances of having a child with the disease remain 1 in 4.

Nurses can play important roles as members of a genetic counseling team. They can be instrumental in alerting a couple about procedures they can expect to see carried out, offering support during the wait for test results, and aiding in the planning and decision making based on those results. A great deal of time may need to be spent offering support to a grieving couple who realize for the first time how tragically the laws of inheritance affect their lives.

Evaluation

Plans for genetic counseling or decision making are long-term: They can easily change over time. A decision made to not have children, for example, may be made easily at age 20; it may be more difficult to maintain when the couple reaches 30 and begins to feel a time clock of reproduction running out for them. Be certain that people who have asked for genetic counseling have a number to telephone and that they periodically call to update their information on new advances in genetic screening or disease treatment. That way they can benefit from a new screening test or therapy for their particular disorder as soon as it becomes available.

Nursing Care Planning

Mary Kraft is 23-year-old woman whose twin sister has Down's syndrome. She is concerned that she might be a translocation carrier because she had a spontaneous abortion a year ago followed by a period of infertility. A nursing care plan you might design for her genetic counseling is shown below.

Assessment

Patient states' "My twin sister has Down's syndrome. She is severely mentally retarded. My family has always been so ashamed that such a thing could happen in our family. I grew up filled with guilt that it happened to my twin and not to me." (She didn't go to her senior prom in high school because she felt guilty going and having a good time when her twin could not enjoy that type of activity.) She states she wants an amniocentesis during all pregnancies because she will do anything to prevent a child of hers being born that way. She also wants to save her husband the embarrassment of having a retarded child.

The medical chart obtained from her home hospital reveals the patient's sister is karyotype

47XX21 +. Characteristic features include mental retardation, epicanthal folds, bilateral simian palm creases, an endocushion heart defect (repaired), and hypertelorism (wide spaced eyes).

Patient's karyotype is normal (46XX), as is her husband's (46XY). Patient's mother is also normal (46XX). Patient's father refused to have a karyotype done, stating he would rather not know if he was the "fault" of his daughter's retardation.

Analysis

Fear related to possibility of genetic abnormality in children.

Locus of Decision Making. Patient and genetic counseling team.

Goal. Patient to evidence increased understanding of nature of chromosomal disorder in family by 1 week.

Criteria. Patient to voice confidence that she will not have genetically abnormal children except by chance.

Nursing Orders

1. Schedule appointment with couple for report of karyotyping.
   a. Discuss the pattern of nondisjunction as the possible inheritance pattern involved here.
   b. Discuss the cause of twinning and the inability of anyone to control the circumstances of his own birth.
   c. Discuss the attitude of shame in relation to mental retardation as one established before the cause of many disorders were known, but one that, in the light of present-day knowledge, should be obsolete.
   d. Discuss the role of guilt as a deterrent to high self-esteem.
2. Discuss the risk-benefit of having an amniocentesis performed during a pregnancy when chromosomal abnormality is unlikely to occur except by chance.

Questions for Review

Multiple Choice

1. Mrs. Green is a 20-year-old woman who is aware that she carries a recessive gene for sickle cell anemia (Ss). If her sexual partner also has such a recessive gene (Ss), the proportion of their children who can be predicted to develop sickle cell anemia is
   a. 100 percent (all).
   b. 75 percent.
   c. 50 percent.
   d. 25 percent.

2. If Mrs. Green's first child is born with sickle cell anemia, the chances of her second child developing this disease are
   a. 1 in 4.
   b. 2 in 4.
   c. 3 in 4.
   d. 0 in 4.

3. A number of diseases can be detected in utero by amniocentesis. Which disease below can be detected by this method?
   a. diabetes mellitus
   b. spinal cord defects
   c. phenylketonuria
   d. impetigo

4. For what week in pregnancy is amniocentesis for chromosomal analysis usually scheduled?
   a. fourth to sixth week
   b. tenth to twelfth week
   c. fourteenth to sixteenth week
   d. twentieth to twenty-fourth week

5. Mrs. Henry has a child with Down's syndrome. This is an example of which type of inheritance?
   a. Mendelian recessive
   b. Mendelian dominant
   c. chromosome nondisjunction
   d. gene dislocation

6. The ethics of genetic screening encourage you
   a. not to tell a person a finding that would be detrimental to self-esteem.
   b. to spread the findings to all family members as soon as possible.
   c. to promote mandatory screening for high-risk persons.
   d. to relay findings to individuals as soon as possible.

7. Mary has Turner's syndrome. She is 12 years old but has not menstruated yet. You would advise her mother that
   a. Turner's syndrome means that Mary is really a male.
   b. Mary has no uterus so will not menstruate.
   c. Mary's chromosomal structure is XXY.
   d. Mary probably has nonfunctioning ovaries.

8. Mrs. White knows that she is the carrier of a sex-linked disease (hemophilia A); her husband is free of the disease. Which of the following is the incidence of this disease she could expect to see in her children?
   a. All male children would inherit it.
   b. All female children will be carriers like herself.

c. Half of her male children would inherit the disease.
d. Half of her female children would inherit the disease.

9. Mrs. White asks you about reproductive alternatives that would assure she could not have a child with the disease. Which of the following would be an applicable alternative for the Whites?
   a. embryo transfer
   b. artificial insemination by the husband
   c. artificial insemination by donor
   d. contraception use on alternate months

Discussion

1. Parents who have a child with a chromosomal abnormality often develop a severe loss of self-esteem. What are ways you could reinforce a sense of high self-esteem in a woman following childbirth?
2. Deciding to have chorionic villi sampling done is difficult for parents because this procedure may result in the loss of a normal fetus. What would be your role in helping parents make this decision?
3. A patient asks you to tell her what proportion of her children are apt to have a disease you recognize as being autosomally recessively inherited. How would you explain this to her?

Suggested Readings

American Academy of Pediatrics. (1982). Screening guidelines. *Pediatrics, 69,* 104.

Alper J. C. (1982). Genetic counseling: Extending your help beyond treatment. *Consultant, 22,* 159.

Barnett, H. (1977). *Pediatrics* (15th ed.). New York: Appleton-Century-Crofts.

Baskin, J. (1983). Prenatal testing for Tay-Sachs disease in the light of Jewish views regarding abortion. *Issues in Health Care of Women, 4,* 41.

Berry, A. C. (1981). Sexual and genetic counselling. *Nursing (Oxford), 1,* 1067.

Cowie, V. (1982). Genetic causes of retardation. *Nursing Mirror, 15,* 155.

Davies, B. L. (1983). Decision-making in prenatal genetic diagnosis. *Issues in Health Care of Women, 4,* 69.

Ferguson, M. J. (1983). Genetics and genetic counseling. *American Medical Technology, 45,* 18.

Fibison, W. J. (1983). The nursing role in the delivery of genetic services. *Issues in Health Care of Women, 4,* 1.

Fitzsimmons, E. (1981). Genetic counseling: Learning to keep counsel. *Nursing Mirror, 153,* 48.

Golbus, M. S. (1982). The current scope of antenatal diagnosis. *Hospital Practice, 17,* 179.

Goodwin, J., et al. (1976). *Perinatal medicine.* Baltimore: Williams & Wilkins.

Harisiades, J. P. (1983). Maternal serum AFP screening: A programmatic overview. *Issues in Health Care of Women, 4,* 17.

Hopper, W. C., Jr. (1983). A review of genetics in orthopaedics. *Orthopaedic Nursing, 2,* 37.

Jones, O. W. (1981). Genetic counseling: General concepts and principles. *Perinatology/Neonatology, 5,* 32.

Kaback, M. (1979). Genetic screening for better outcomes. *Contemporary OB/GYN, 13,* 123.

LaRochelle, D. (1983). Prenatal genetic counseling: Ethical and legal interfaces with the nurse's role. *Issues in Health Care of Women, 4,* 77.

Lowie, A. F., & Mennie, M. E. (1984). Parenthood—a question of inheritance. *Nursing, 2,* 555.

Nyhan, W. L. (1980). Understanding inherited metabolic disease. *Clinical Symptomology, 32,* 2.

Schimke, R. N., et al. (1983). Genetic counseling. *Hospital Practice, 18,* 35.

Seller, M. J. (1982). Genetic counselling and reproductive patterns. *Midwife Health Visitor and Community Nurse, 18,* 135.

Summer, G. K., et al. (1982). Developments in genetic and metabolic screening. *Family and Community Health, 4,* 13.

Tichler, C. L. (1981). The psychological aspects of genetic counseling. *American Journal of Nursing, 81,* 732.

Tiller, M. J. (1982). A baby with trisomy 13 and necrotizing enterocolitis. *Nursing Times, 78,* 444.

Temple, M. J. (1983). Chromosomal syndromes. *Hospital Practice, 18,* 124a.

Ward, H. (1984). Chorionic villi sampling: Its promise and its problems. *Contemporary OB/GYN, 22,* 31.

III

The Interpartal Period

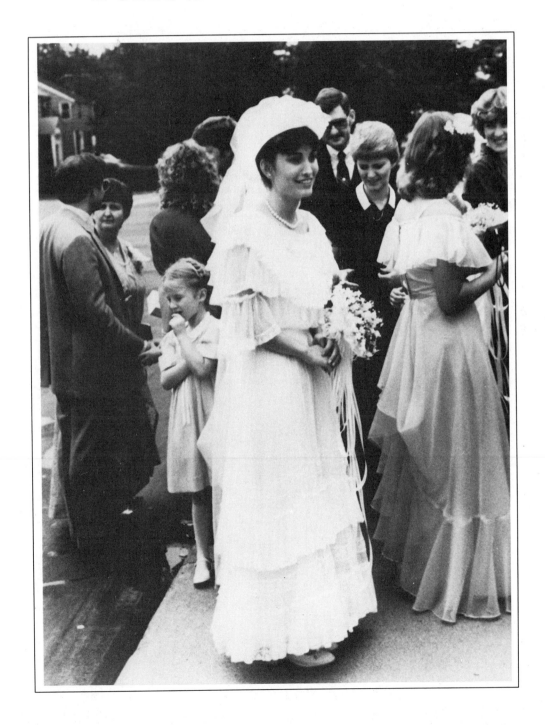

7

Developmental Readiness for Childbearing

OBJECTIVES

Following mastery of the content of this chapter, you should be able to

1. Define the term *developmental task* or *crisis.*
2. Describe the developmental crisis for each age group, as outlined by Erik Erikson.
3. Analyze ways that the achievement of developmental tasks is important for parenting.
5. Synthesize knowledge of developmental tasks with nursing process to achieve quality maternal-newborn nursing care.

BEING READY to be a parent is more than being physically capable of conceiving and producing children. It involves being mature enough emotionally to have another individual dependent on you and being able to sacrifice your own needs when they conflict with those of a child. It means having the maturity to maintain some form of employment so that financial resources are available for childrearing.

Erikson (Erikson, 1950) has described eight stages of life and the psychosocial or developmental steps toward maturity that people take at each stage (Table 7-1). People pass from one developmental stage in life to another, depending not so much on chronological age but on whether they have completed the developmental task of the earlier stage. In order to be effective parents, men and women need to have completed at least the developmental tasks (sometimes called developmental crises) up through adolescence.

Infancy: A Sense of Trust

The developmental task of infancy (birth to 1 year) is that of learning to trust or learning to love. The infant whose needs are met when they arise, whose discomforts are quickly removed, who is cuddled, fondled, played with, and talked to, learns to accept the world as a safe place and people as helpful and dependable.

If infant care is inconsistent, inadequate, or rejecting, however, the opposite of a sense of trust (mistrust) develops in the child. He can become fearful and suspicious of people and the world around him.

People give love to others most freely when they are assured that they will receive love in return. An infant will offer to love the adults who care for him, but if his love is rejected time and again, as happens to a child who is moved from one foster home to another foster home, he will stop trying. After a while he loses the ability to reach out and offer love. Like the burnt child who

Table 7-1 Periods of Developmental Crises

Age Period	Developmental Task	Developmental Outcome
Infancy (1 to 12 months)	Trust	Learns to love
Toddlerhood (1 to 3 years)	Autonomy	Learns to make decisions, to be independent
Preschool age (3 to 5 years)	Initiative	Learns to solve problems, to do things
School age (5 to 12 years)	Industry	Learns to do things well
Adolescence (13 to 18 years)	Identity	Learns who she is and what she wants to do in life; is independent from parents
Young adulthood (19 to 30 years)	Intimacy	Learns to relate effectively on deeper planes
Middle age (30 to 60 years)	Generativity	Learns to look beyond herself at community and world needs
Older age (over 60 years)	Integrity	Learns to be content with what she has achieved, to feel fulfilled in life

Source: Adapted from *Childhood and Society* (2nd ed.). Revised, by Erik H. Erikson, with the permission of W. W. Norton & Company, Inc. Copyright 1950, © 1963 by W. W. Norton & Company, Inc.

avoids fire, the emotionally burnt child avoids the pain of emotional attachment.

Although he continues to grow and learn new motor skills and, on the surface, appears to be progressing normally, emotionally he becomes "stuck" at the infant stage. He may live his life as a "loner," making few close friends. He may have difficulty establishing heterosexual relationships (it is too great a risk to reach out to a partner, to offer love, because he may be rejected again and he has been hurt enough). He will not leave himself that vulnerable again—better to keep to himself and be lonely than be hurt.

Having a sense of trust is vital to being a good parent. It is the cornerstone on which parenthood is built. A parent is asked to give a great deal of time and attention in the early weeks of a newborn's life without getting a great deal of interaction in return. People who have a sense of trust view the early weeks of a newborn's life as enjoyable because giving care is an activity that is enjoyable. People without a sense of trust may interpret the child's inability to follow their finger well, not yet smiling back at their smile, falling asleep instead of listening to them (typical newborn behavior) as rejection. They withdraw into themselves and initiate their protective mechanism—not reaching out to the child any more—and begin another cycle of what happened to them, creating another child who has difficulty loving because he is not loved.

The infant's sense of trust is learned through consistent mother-child interaction. When an infant is hungry, his mother feeds him and takes away his discomfort. When he is wet, his mother changes him and again takes away his discomfort. When he is lonely, his mother comes and holds and talks to him and takes away his discomfort. By this process he learns to trust that when he has a need, someone will come and care for him.

Following some schedule of care goes a long way toward helping an infant form a sense of trust. This does not mean that mothers should plan a rigid schedule of care; but some order to a day (breakfast, then bath, then playtime, then nap) offers direction as to what is coming next. That infants thrive on a routine is shown by their love of nursery rhymes. Even though a rhyme makes no sense, the sound of the same thing said over and over (patty-cake, patty-cake, baker's man . . .) is reassuring.

The mother who works needs to make plans so that her child has consistency when she is not with him. She needs to discuss with the babysitter or day-care center the routine she wants the child to follow so that whether she is present or not consistency will still be there. She needs to choose a day-care center where the child will have as few different caregivers as possible.

Fortunately, although developmental tasks are mastered easiest at that stage of life in which the person seems "ripe" for the task, if the person does not master the task at that age it can be achieved later in life. A child who reaches school age without a firm sense of trust can have it strengthened at school by a teacher who is worthy of trust. A person may enter adulthood without a firm sense of trust but be lucky to find a marriage partner who is so trustworthy and caring he is able to help his partner develop a sense of trust.

At the same time, a child who has developed a strong sense of trust may have it destroyed by the separation or death of a parent or a disastrous marriage relationship. Battered wives, because they are treated so badly by someone they trusted, may have this happen to them.

The Toddler Period: A Sense of Autonomy

The developmental task of the toddler years (12 months to 3 years) is that of gaining a sense of autonomy or independence. It is shown clearly in toddler actions—temper tantrums, foot stomping, shouting "no"—actions that show the child has just glimpsed himself as a person independent of parents, able to do things alone.

Just as people do not learn to do many new tasks without practice, toddlers cannot learn to be independent without practice or making some mistakes. They insist on putting on their own clothes and get their shoes on the wrong feet. They insist on winding a toy themselves and break it. They insist they do not need a nap and fall asleep at the dinner table with their food half eaten.

It takes patience to be the parent of a toddler, but a child, given opportunities to try new things, will learn to be comfortable in going and doing. A child constantly stopped from doing learns, instead of autonomy, a feeling of doubt, or little confidence in personal ability to do things.

A sense of autonomy is necessary for a person to parent; rearing children calls for making many decisions every day. Being able to make a decision is part of being independent; being able to stand by a decision is part of being independent. Standing by decisions leads to consistency and helping children to learn trust in the infant period.

Taking care of a new baby means doing tasks never attempted before. A sense of autonomy allows a mother to try things she has never done before. Without it, she can become overwhelmed by new responsibility.

During a child's growing years, parents may find that they have to change their place of employment. A sense of autonomy allows them to take on new jobs, even in a new city or country, without being overwhelmed.

Children learn a sense of autonomy by being permitted to make decisions. A sense of autonomy is strengthened at any point in life by exposure to decision making. Many new parents need help with decision making about their baby's care in the first few days of the child's life or help strengthening a sense of autonomy at this critical point.

The Preschool Period: A Sense of Initiative

The developmental task of the preschool period (3 to 5 years) is that of developing a sense of initiative or of learning how to do things. The child requires ample opportunity to try new things. He needs play materials that can be arranged or molded into many different shapes and forms. Just as decision making is learned as part of learning independence, problem solving is learned as part of a sense of initiative. At no other time in a child's life is the imagination at a higher peak than during these years. At no other time in life is he able to suggest so many ways of completing a task.

The ability to solve problems is an excellent prerequisite for parenthood. It allows a parent to adapt to changes in the child as she grows from an infant who likes to be held and rocked to a toddler who would much rather be down and doing things alone, from a preschooler who enjoys new experiences to a school-age child who likes to follow rules.

A parent with a poor sense of initiative may be upset by the number of problems any one day of child rearing poses. The newborn period, when everything is new and different from what she is used to, may be extremely difficult if she does not have a strong sense of initiative or an ability to discover alternative routes or solutions to problems.

Pregnancy, because it involves so many changes, may be very difficult for the parent who cannot solve problems.

School Age: A Sense of Industry

A sense of industry or accomplishment is the developmental goal of the school-age period. Learning a sense of initiative is learning how to do things; learning a sense of industry is learning how to do things well.

A 3- or 4-year-old tackles a project energetically and enthusiastically, but the finished product may look little like what the child said in the beginning he was going to make. The edges are raw and unfinished. He does not care. He has created. A school-age child is much more concerned that his project look as he projected. He asks, "Is it all right?" and often adds despairingly, "I do sloppy work."

Achieving a sense of industry is also the ability to learn how to stick with a task until it is done. A parent needs a sense of industry because what he has undertaken—child rearing—is not a transient task but one of the longest he will ever assume, one that lasts 18 to 21 years. That takes a lot of "sticking-to-it."

Having a strong sense of industry is what allows parents to achieve in the working world. Achieving at an occupation gives the parent a strong financial base, and at least some financial base is necessary for child rearing.

Parents without a strong sense of industry may be unable to hold steady jobs and so may move frequently during the child's growing years, creating a potential source of insecurity in the child. They may be ineffective parents in teaching responsibility to a child, enthusiastic about their child's making a hockey team, for example, but not willing to follow through with driving the child to practice. Many of the things a child learns during his growing years are learned by watching the people who are important to him and imitating and adopting what they think is important. It takes an independent person to teach independence, a creative one to teach creativity, a steady, dependable person to teach how to stay with a job until it is finished. Role modeling on how to complete jobs (a sense of industry) is significant in preparing children for their own adult roles in life.

Adolescence: A Sense of Identity

The developmental task of the adolescent period is that of learning a sense of identity (Fig. 7-1) or of knowing who you are. This is a particularly difficult task to achieve because the adolescent's body is changing rapidly. She literally is not the same person one week that she was the week before.

An adolescent is able to list the many people she is—a daughter, a student, a scout, a papergirl, a grandchild, a club member—and she has to learn how to integrate all these roles into one person.

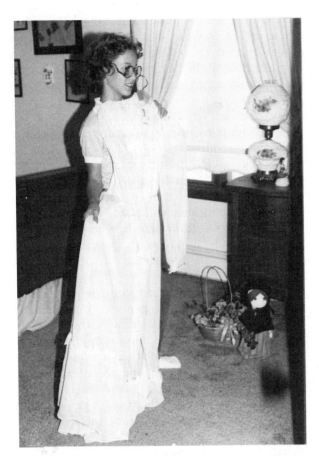

Figure 7-1 *Readiness for childbearing means thinking of oneself as a woman and no longer as a child.*

She begins a day thinking that she is quite pretty, only to look in a mirror and discover that her face is covered with red papules. A boy thinks of himself as short, only to find when he lines up in gym class that his rapid growth over the summer has made him one of the tallest students in the class. A girl thinks of herself as almost mature, but her parents insist on making her decisions, such as whether she should go on vacation with the family or not. How, out of all the contradictions around her, can she find out who she is?

There are four main areas in which an adolescent must make gains in order to achieve a sense of identity: accepting a changed body image, establishing what kind of person to be, making a career decision, and gaining emancipation from parents.

Body Image

The child who has a strong sense of trust, autonomy, initiative, and industry (is able to trust people, be independent, solve problems, and concentrate on a task) is best equipped to deal with the change in body image that occurs with puberty.

A sense of trust allows a girl to believe that even if she is "ugly" and ungainly she will still be loved for what is inside her. A sense of autonomy helps her to function without total dependence on what her peers are telling her about herself. Ability to solve problems allows her to select clothing or activities that complement rather than distract from her new growth.

Girls may have difficulty accepting breast development if they have been led to believe that "nice girls don't do conspicuous things" or are self-conscious because of boys' kidding remarks or other girls' envy. They may limit their social contacts or attempt to slouch continually to hide what is happening to them. Their self-esteem is low. Girls who have late development or little breast development have the same low self-esteem. It is hard to trust yourself to say the right things if one part of your body has betrayed you, because other parts may also betray you.

A girl who has trouble living with her new body because it has changed from the way it was in childhood will have an even more difficult time with body image if she becomes pregnant. That accepting the changing body image in pregnancy is a problem for any woman is reflected in pregnant women's frequent questions about the weight they are gaining and their concern in the postpartal period with losing weight and attempting to fit back into prepregnancy clothing.

What Kind of Person?

Deciding who you are or what kind of person you will be (a miser, a philanthropist, a creator, a destroyer, a religious person, a nonreligious person, a caring person, a noncaring person) is an internal development. Adolescents spend a lot of time talking with each other about how people reacted in a situation and how they would have reacted differently to see if the reaction of the person they are describing "fits" them, if they are that kind of person.

A preliminary step to discovering who you are is that of discovering who you are *not*. Adolescent girls and boys typically form cliques—groups who talk alike, think alike, dress alike—and exclude anyone who talks differently, thinks differently, or dresses differently. This action appears cruel, and many adults remember their adolescence as years of nothing but heartbreak because they were always excluded. It is not so much cruel, however, as developmental, part of knowing who you are. You are like your peers who dress like you; you are *not* like those who dress differently.

Some adolescents are forced into joining boys or girls they really would not have chosen to associate with, except that they are excluded from other associations. Some evidence acting-out or delinquent behavior because being known as the terror of the block is better than not being known at all (having no identity).

In order to be a parent and guide a child into deciding who he or she is, a person first needs to know who *he or she* is. Pregnancy is difficult to accept if a girl and boy are still adolescents. Suddenly, on top of trying to decide what kind of persons they are, they are expecting a baby. An identity has been thrust upon them—that of a parent. For an adolescent, this identity often carries suggestions of being a bad person, or at least an immoral one, and on top of their other problems, it creates a role that is very difficult to handle.

Making a Career Decision

Part of deciding what kind of person you are is deciding what type of job you want to do in life. People identify strongly with their occupations. To the question "What are you?" people rarely answer, "A good person, a mother, a conscientious person"; they answer, "A nurse, an accountant, a housewife."

Because career decisions must be made from such a wide range of choices today, career choice becomes more and more difficult. Because most occupations require education, decision making about a career has to be done in the adolescent years. Parents of children are not very helpful about giving guidance in this area. In a world so changed since they were adolescents the advice that was sound then may no longer be relevant.

Before a person becomes a parent, it is helpful if he or she has made a career decision. This lays the foundation for when and how he is going to live and adds stability to a family unit.

Although pregnant adolescents cannot be excluded from school because of their condition, pregnancy is certain to have some influence on their education. Many girls drop out of school once they are pregnant (they are excluded from their group because they are different). With little education, their income potential will be severely limited just at a time when they need more income than the average person their age because they have a child.

Emancipation from Parents

Gaining independence from parents is often difficult from two standpoints: Parents may not be willing to grant independence yet, and the child is not really sure that he wants to be totally independent. Part of adolescent struggle is related not so much to doing adult things but to struggling for the right to do them. An adolescent, for example, may fight for the right to stay out until midnight on school nights, then, having won the privilege, never use it. Winning the battle is more important than what the battle is about.

Adolescents who are pregnant may do the same thing at prenatal visits. They may fight for the right to weigh themselves, then ask to have their weight rechecked.

As a rule, the closer the parent-child relationship, the more intense will be the struggle to gain independence. A child who has no close ties to his parents can merely walk away. The adolescent who loves his parents has difficulty severing the bond between them.

An adolescent may need some help in understanding that being independent from parents does not mean having to stop loving them; it simply means he must stop depending on them to meet all his needs. Relationships formed as equals can be more lasting and deeper than those of daughter and parent or son and parent.

Before people become parents, it helps if they have gained independence from their own parents. One of the mental tasks of pregnancy for a woman is making a mental switch from thinking of herself as a daughter at the beginning of pregnancy to thinking of herself as a mother at the end. If she is still a daughter, living at home, it may take longer than the nine months of pregnancy to complete this task, so she may not be ready for childrearing at the end of the pregnancy.

Young Adulthood: A Sense of Intimacy

With young adulthood comes the developmental task of achieving a sense of intimacy. The ability to form intimate relationships is strongly correlated with the sense of trust built in the infancy period. If an infant is unable to form a sense of trust, he may be unable to interact with others or develop deep enough connections with them to serve as the basis for lasting relationships. The relationship of developmental tasks is shown in Figure 7-2.

Most sexual relationships between adolescents are built not on a sense of intimacy but on sexual attraction. Those built on sexual attraction (puppy love) are searing in their intensity and in the hurt that occurs when the relationship crumbles. It takes adolescents a number of such relationships before they learn that other values, such as kindness, companionship, and common inter-

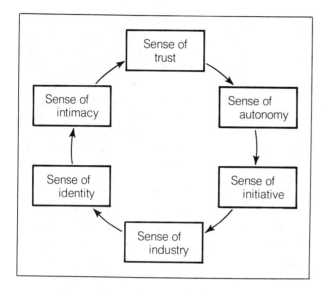

Figure 7-2 *Developmental tasks as the basis for lasting relationships.*

ests, have to be involved in a relationship to make it last.

Acquiring a sense of intimacy means also being able to form lasting relationships with members of the same sex. Anticipating others' needs at a particular time is part of a sense of intimacy. People who have achieved this ability have many close friends or support people. This is important for beginning childrearing, as everything at that point is so new and different that support is necessary.

It is unfortunate when adolescents become parents before a sense of intimacy is achieved. A relationship built on less than that will not be able to stand the rigors of childrearing. A parent needs support people derived from firm relationships at the time of the birth of a child, when a child is ill or hurt, and during many of the expected crises of everyday developmental happenings with children.

The Middle Years: A Sense of Generativity

Although many young couples begin having children while they are adolescents still struggling with a sense of identity, others begin having children while they are struggling to achieve a sense of intimacy in young adulthood. Still others wait until closer to middle adult years to start their families. Many women have their last child as middle-aged adults.

Some people assume that, once they have reached adulthood, the way they are is the way they will always be. They are surprised to see

their bodies change (men become bald; women and men both gain weight); they are unprepared for the developmental task of middle adult life, that of achieving a sense of generativity. *Generativity* means moving away from oneself to become involved with the world or community. The activities of middle-aged adults reflect generativity: being members of committees and clubs, supporting Little League teams, being block parents.

Peck and Berkowitz (1964) have enumerated four subdevelopmental steps that must be taken by the middle-aged adult, not unlike those of the adolescent: increasing self-esteem through self-awareness, separating from parents and children, reviewing his or her value system and changing or reinforcing it, and initiating plans for the future that take into consideration the aging process.

The woman who finds herself pregnant during her middle adult years may have a hard time adjusting to the pregnancy because she has difficulty completing these steps. Her self-esteem may be lowered (she worries that she looks foolish being pregnant "at her age"). She has to face the fact that she will soon be separated from her parents (parents die) but she cannot even begin to consider separating from this child for another 18 years. It is difficult for her to review her value system and change it because it cannot change. She is still a mother, her husband a father. Nothing is changing for them. It is difficult to initiate new plans for the future. The future will go on much like the past in diapers, school plays, high-school proms.

To other women, having a baby at midlife is a joyous event, a last chance to remain young, to have what they thought was over. Each mother's reaction to having a baby during her middle adult years needs to be evaluated individually so that it can be determined whether she accepts the pregnancy as a positive or a negative step in her life.

Older Age: A Sense of Integrity

Few people in the older age category are seen in maternal-newborn settings, as they are past their childbearing years. Many couples have parents or grandparents, however, who are in this age group, so this age group's influence is felt strongly in maternal-newborn settings.

The developmental task of older age is to achieve a sense of satisfaction with what you are. Most people are able to do this by looking back over their lives and realizing that they made some mistakes (they should have bought a house sooner in life; they should have finished college) but overall they have accomplished a great deal (have made a marriage partner happy for forty or more years, have parented children who are responsible adults).

For some older people, having a grandchild or a great-grandchild is the final assurance they need that they have been successful in life. A grandmother's suggestions to a granddaughter (bathe the baby in oil, not water; protect the umbilical cord with a binder) is information a grandmother offers not only to ensure the safety and well-being of the child but also to make the event real to herself, to bring herself to a final life step, or to form a sense of integrity. Rejecting this type of information in the light of this situation is very difficult for granddaughters to do, even after you have pointed out that the advice is old-fashioned and no longer considered appropriate.

The Process of Achieving Maturity

If parents seem to be lacking in a developmental stage of growth, some constructive intervention can be accomplished during pregnancy or the days immediately postpartum.

A Sense of Trust

Helping women to strengthen a sense of trust is important during pregnancy because only by having a sense of trust can one effectively transmit it to others. Being a trustworthy person—that is, being certain that if you tell a woman in labor that you are going to leave her for a few minutes and then coming back after only a few minutes, promising a woman in a prenatal clinic that you will see her at the next visit and then making every effort to be there, telling a woman after delivery that you will review her postpartal instructions with her the next day and making sure that you remember to do it—means acting in ways that demonstrate trustworthiness. Explaining procedures to patients, anticipating events so there are no surprises, taking the time to reassure—all are good examples of trustworthiness.

Rubin (1963) stresses that if a woman is touched in labor and has her needs met the first few days postpartum she is more likely to handle her infant kindly and attempt to meet the baby's needs than if she is left alone in labor and advanced to total independence too quickly after delivery.

A Sense of Autonomy

Some new parents are exceedingly anxious in the newborn period. They worry that their sense of autonomy or their ability to make decisions, in relation to caring for their child, is inadequate. They fear that they will not know whether the child has had enough to eat or whether he is sick. Letting parents make decisions in the first few days after birth (allow some time for just resting and reassurance) helps to strengthen their confidence in their ability to make decisions. Asking "Do you think it's warm enough for the baby to be without a blanket?" is asking for a small decision, but it helps to build practice in making choices about baby care.

Women need to be reassured when they have made a good decision. Many women call prenatal clinics or offices reporting minor discomforts of pregnancy. The statement "That always happens during pregnancy; don't worry about it" is correct, but not as therapeutic as "That is something that often happens in pregnancy; it's nothing to worry about but you were wise to call and check because you weren't certain." The second response reinforces the woman's ability to make decisions even if the decision she made (she was ill) was wrong.

Some women make poor decisions during pregnancy about their own health and in the newborn period about their child because they are not knowledgeable enough about changes in pregnancy or newborns to make good decisions. Providing women with information through classes or one-to-one discussion goes a long way toward making decision making easier.

A Sense of Initiative

People cannot solve problems unless they know the options available to them. Patient education, therefore, is important in helping people to strengthen a sense of initiative.

It is usually helpful to women during pregnancy to review with them some problems you can anticipate they will be facing as pregnancy progresses: How are finances to be reallocated when the woman stops work? Where is a baby going to sleep in a one-bedroom apartment? How is a mother of six children, having her seventh, going to find time for a rest period each day? After the birth of the child, it is advisable to review with women their plans for the first days at home. Does the woman have anyone to help her to keep her from becoming exhausted? If she lives in a two-story house and is not supposed to go up and down stairs more than once a day for the first week, how is she going to manage? In times of stress, thinking through problems is one of the most difficult things to do. Some women find themselves frozen in front of the refrigerator, unable to make even the simplest of choices, such as what meat to defrost for dinner. Having someone to listen to their plans and assure them that the plans sound sensible is always helpful. In many instances, the actual problem solving is not difficult. It is the step before that, getting to a concrete stage of thinking about the problem or realizing that there is one, that poses the obstacle.

A Sense of Industry

It is often hard for women to feel that they are doing things well (sense of industry) during pregnancy because things change so from the beginning to the end of pregnancy that everything is always new; they barely feel comfortable with their body when it changes still more. Parents need reassurance in the newborn period that they are doing things well because, again, everything seems so new and unpracticed. Even women having their second, third, or fourth child have feelings of uncertainty with their newborn because this is their first experience with this child. Everyone, in his eagerness to teach, can easily find himself criticizing the things people are doing wrong and forgetting to comment on the things that are being done right. Being praised for things done right strengthens a sense of industry.

A Sense of Identity

Keeping a firm hold on a sense of identity can be very difficult during pregnancy as a woman evolves from one person at the beginning of pregnancy (a woman with no children or one or two children) to another person at the end of pregnancy (a mother of a child or two or three children).

Knowing what is likely to happen during pregnancy and in labor or delivery, knowing what a newborn will look like beforehand, is information that helps the woman anticipate change and adapt to it more readily. Patient education, again, becomes an important part of yet another developmental crisis.

Some young women develop a sense of identity for the first time during pregnancy. They did not know who they were before; now at least they know they are about to be mothers. Statements such as "I hope I can manage with three under three," or "I can't believe that in just three more weeks I'll be a mother" show that the woman is role playing her new identity. They need to be recognized and discussed so that the sense of identity can be strengthened during pregnancy.

A Sense of Intimacy

Women do not feel instinctive rushes of affection toward newborn babies in many instances. They need assurance that emotions labeled "a strange feeling" or "scared" are much more common in women in the first few days of their child's life.

A great deal of learning how to hold a newborn securely, how to do the "motherly" motions of jiggling, rocking, or stroking is the result of role modeling or watching others. Handling the woman's baby in front of her, therefore, and pointing out positive characteristics of the child (his nose is cute, her hair is curly) help a woman strengthen a sense of intimacy.

A Sense of Generativity

Many women resent a child born to them late in life because they view the child as totally changing their life style or forcing them to continue a life style they were ready to change. Exploring with a woman ways she can continue a career or community service and still be pregnant or care for a newborn can help her to realize that at this time in life she can achieve the best of two worlds, that it might be possible for her to participate actively in her club by addressing envelopes or making phone calls at home as her activity rather than spending days as a volunteer away from home. This type of planning is sensible and will strengthen her sense of generativity or the developmental phase the older woman may be entering as she has her last child.

Utilizing Nursing Process

When civilizations were simpler, physical maturity and developmental maturity occurred close together. Today, when many young people stay in school until they are at least 21 years old and therefore are dependent on parents until that age, they may achieve physical maturity 5 years or more before they have the necessary develop-

mental maturity to use their physical readiness wisely.

Assessment

Just as physical maturity occurs at different ages (some girls have their first menstrual period as early as 9, some as late as 17, yet both groups are normal), so developmental maturity occurs at different ages. Everyone knows a person who, although chronologically mature, still functions as an adolescent. Assessing for developmental maturity is as important as assessing for physical maturity to establish if a person is ready for childbearing and parenting. Table 7-2 lists questions pertinent to use to assess for developmental tasks. The final proof of whether someone has truly achieved a task, however, is whether their behavior reflects that task. Observing actions is important.

Analysis

The Fourth Annual Conference on Nursing Diagnoses accepted no diagnoses specifically related to developmental maturity. Many other diagnoses are applicable to this area, however, because if more developmental maturity were present, the person would probably be able to cope better or experience less anxiety under stress. Anxiety related to fear of being pregnant, fatigue related to poor organization of life style, or anger related to poor coping mechanisms are examples of common diagnoses used in this area.

Be certain when establishing goals in this area that goals are realistic. A person does not become mature overnight and will not change if he does not appreciate the reason for the change.

Planning

It is difficult to plan implementations that are constructive in helping people reach physical milestones more quickly. There *are* implementations to facilitate developmental maturity and readiness to be effective parents. Being certain that people are ready to be parents protects both the physical and the mental health of the next generation. Because each generation lays the groundwork for the next generation, no other nursing implementation may be so far-reaching as that aimed at helping people to be better parents.

Implementation

If parents seem to be lacking in a developmental stage of growth, some constructive implementations can be accomplished during pregnancy or the days immediately postpartum. Such implementations include formal and informal teaching, counseling, and role modeling of mature adult responsible roles.

Evaluation

As with all nursing process, evaluation is an important phase for the determination of the success of implementations. Whether developmental ma-

Table 7-2 Assessment of Developmental Tasks

Developmental Task	Suggested Assessment Questions
Trust	Can you name a close friend you rely on in times of stress? Do you feel loved? Do you find it easy to do things for others? How do you feel about taking care of a newborn? What is your relationship with your mother?
Autonomy	Who makes decisions in your family? Do you have trouble deciding between alternatives? Could you live by yourself if you had to? Do you stand by decisions you make?
Initiative	What do you do when you are faced with a problem? Do you enjoy new situations? Do you find problems challenging?
Industry	Do you usually finish projects you begin? Is your job enjoyable? Do you enjoy hard work?
Identity	What kind of person are you? How do you feel about being pregnant? Do you have future plans for a career? Do you still rely on your parents for decision making?
Intimacy	Do you have a long-term close relationship? Do you have a close friend of your own sex?
Generativity	Do you participate in community activities? Do you listen to world news? Are there things you'd like to see changed in your community?
Integrity	Are there things you would do differently if you had them to do over again? How do you feel about your life? What is your relationship with your children?

turity is present is a question often involving long-term evaluation: A level of maturity may not be readily apparent until a person is under a degree of stress.

Nursing Care Planning

Christine McFadden is a 15-year-old you see in a prenatal clinic (last menstrual period 16 weeks ago). The following is a nursing care plan for her needs with regard to developmental maturity.

Assessment

Patient is a 15-year-old junior in high school. Maintains a B average; swims on girl's varsity team. Has taken responsibility for 5-year-old sister after school since she was 12 (parents own delicatessen and both work). States, "I didn't mean to get pregnant but having a baby will be more fun to take care of than a 5-year-old." Has not told father of child (a high-school senior) or her own parents of possibility of pregnancy as yet. States, "My parents will be wild." No plans for abortion: "I couldn't hurt a baby."

Analysis

Patient with developmental immaturity related to age 15 and current status as a student in school.

Goal. Patient will voice acceptance of pregnancy and birth of child as an individual needing her responsible care by pregnancy term.

Criteria. Patient:

1. Is able to discuss how child will change her life other than being "fun."
2. Will remain in school throughout pregnancy; return to school after delivery.
3. Will establish workable relationship with parents.
4. Will clarify the relationship she wants to have with father of child.

Nursing Orders

1. Discuss how pregnancy may cause changes in friends and family.
2. Discuss how pregnancy may change dietary or social life style.
3. Urge to tell father of child and parents about pregnancy.
4. Later in pregnancy after adaptation has improved, discuss childrearing plans and need for help with baby care.

Mary Kraft is a 23-year-old woman you meet in an obstetrician's office. Her last menstrual period was 9 weeks ago.

Assessment

Patient lives with husband in two-bedroom apartment. Husband has full-time job as high-school English teacher; she works part-time in the public library. Has been planning on being pregnant since spontaneous loss of a pregnancy at 3 months, 2 years ago. Has not mentioned possibility of pregnancy to husband. States, "I can't believe I'm really pregnant." Finances adequate even without her job. Mature mannered.

Analysis

Patient developmentally prepared for childbearing and rearing related to maturity level.

Goal. Patient to maintain developmental preparation for birth of child by end of pregnancy.

Criteria. Patient will make prenatal appointment and realistic plans for new child.

Nursing Orders

1. Give reassurance that pregnancy is real if M.D. confirms.
2. Continue to assure that pregnancy is going well (as appropriate) at continued visits. It may be difficult for her to adapt to pregnancy until time of previous miscarriage has passed.
3. Provide discussion time at visits for worry over loss of last pregnancy to be voiced.
4. Discuss preparation for baby later in pregnancy after she is ready to accept pregnancy as real.

Angie Baco is a 42-year-old woman you meet in a prenatal clinic. Her last menstrual period was 12 weeks ago.

Assessment

Patient lives with husband and four children (19, 17, 15, and 7). Seven-year-old has learning disability; special classroom at school. Husband has full-time job as construction worker. Finances "okay, but not great." Patient was not planning on becoming pregnant (contraception failure). States, "I'm too old for diapers again. My daughter just had a baby." Husband states, "I'll be retiring and this kid will still be in high school." Children's reactions vary from pleasure (the 17 year old) to disbelief (the 15 and 7 year olds) to disapproval (the 19 year old). Religion precludes abortion as an option. States, "I'll just have it, that's all."

Appears tired; nervous mannerisms during interview.

Analysis

Patient with developmental readiness past the optimum for childbearing related to age and life style.

Goal. Patient will voice adaptation to pregnancy and new child by pregnancy's term.

Criteria. Patient:

1. Will discuss with family the reality of pregnancy and how this will affect family members.
2. Will clarify in own mind what pregnancy means to her.
3. Will make prenatal appointments and realistic plans for child.

Nursing Orders

1. Allow discussion time at visits for talk about how life is going to change or is changing.
2. Observe for signs of depression, increased stress due to inappropriateness of childbearing for her now.
3. Later in pregnancy when adaptation is better, discuss plans for baby (physical space and finances may be problems).

Questions for Review

Multiple Choice

1. Mrs. Jones is a woman you care for. She tells you that this marriage is her third. Lack of ability to form a close marriage relationship may reflect lack of which development task?

    a. generativity
    b. trust
    c. autonomy
    d. permeability

2. Mrs. Jones seems unable to decide whether to breast-feed or formula-feed her newborn. Ability to problem solve is learned during which developmental task?

    a. intimacy
    b. trust
    c. initiative
    d. autonomy

3. Which statement by Mrs. Jones suggests that she has a poor sense of autonomy?

    a. "I'll have to ask my husband if he thinks it's all right I'm pregnant."
    b. "I'm not sure if I value children or not."
    c. "I know I don't have any choice but I would love to have a son."
    d. "I'm a very neat person; I like to do things right."

4. Which statement best reflects a sense of industry?

    a. "I don't like to leave a job half done."
    b. "Sometimes I'm not sure I am ready to be a mother."
    c. "I feel confident that I'm having a boy."
    d. "Being loved is a beautiful feeling."

5. A sense of identity is an adolescent developmental task. Which statement below best suggests that Mrs. Jones has a sense of identity?

    a. "I often wonder if God is dead."
    b. "I feel that my school years were happy ones."
    c. "I want to breast-feed my baby."
    d. "I know I will be a good mother."

6. In caring for Mrs. Jones, the best method to strengthen her sense of identity would be to

    a. encourage her to finish tasks she begins.
    b. ask her to tell you about her future plans.
    c. allow her to weigh herself at prenatal visits.
    d. give her a detailed list of foods to eat during pregnancy.

7. Which statement below by Mrs. Jones would best suggest that she has a poorly developed sense of intimacy?

    a. "I'm most comfortable working by myself."
    b. "I'm happy to be pregnant."
    c. "I need advice about baby care."
    d. "I feel awkward holding a new baby."

Discussion

1. After interviewing a pregnant woman, assess her developmental level. What are specific ways you could increase a sense of identity? Of autonomy?
2. Achieving a sense of trust is necessary in order to instill trust in newborns. After assessing a mother for trust, what observations would lead you to believe she had a good sense?
3. A woman over thirty may have difficulty balancing a sense of generativity with one of trust. What are ways in which you could help this woman have the "best of both worlds"?

Suggested Readings

Adams, B. N. (1983). Adolescent health care: Needs, priorities, and services. *Nursing Clinics of North America, 18,* 237.

Baldwin, W., & Cain, V. S. (1980). The children of teenage parents. *Family Planning Perspectives, 12,* 34.

Box, M. (1980). The developing child: Development assessment. *Health Visitor, 53,* 461.

Catrone, C., et al. (1984). A developmental mode for teenage parent education. *Journal of School Health, 54,* 63.

Dominian, J. (1982). Marital stress in the early years. *Health Visitor, 55,* 146.

Erikson, E. (1950). *Childhood and society* (2nd ed.). New York: Norton.

Fleming, R. (1979). Developing a child's self-esteem. *Pediatric Nursing, 5,* 58.

Jarrett, G. E. (1982). Childbearing patterns of young mothers. *M.C.N., 7,* 119.

Johnson-Saylor, M. T. (1980). Seize the moment: Health education for the young adult. *Topics in Clinical Nursing, 2,* 9.

Kraus, M. H., & Kennell, J. H. (1981). *Maternal-infant bonding.* St. Louis: Mosby.

MacCarthy, D. (1980). Psychological influences affecting growth. *Health Visitor, 53,* 461.

Murray, R., & Zentner, J. (1979). *Nursing assessment and health promotion through the life span* (2nd ed.). Englewood Cliffs, NJ: Prentice Hall.

Peck, R. F., & Berkowitz, H. (1964). Personality and adjustment in middle age. In B. L. Neugarten (Ed.), *Personality in middle and late life.* Englewood Cliffs, NJ: Prentice-Hall.

Perry, C. (1982). Enhancing the transition years: The challenge of adolescent health promotion. *Journal of School Health, 52,* 307.

Rubin, R. (1963). Maternal touch. *Nursing Outlook, 11,* 828.

Stranik, M. K., et al. (1979). Transition into parenthood. *American Journal of Nursing, 79,* 90.

Weiss, R. S. (1981). Growing up a little faster: Children in single parent households. *Children Today, 10,* 22.

8

Physiological Readiness for Childbearing

OBJECTIVES

Following mastery of the content of this chapter, you should be able to

1. Describe the embryologic formation of the male and female reproductive systems.
2. Describe normal anatomy and function of both male and female reproductive organs.
3. Describe the measurement of common pelvic diameters and shapes important for childbearing.
4. Analyze anatomic relationships and physiologic functioning to predict physical readiness for childbearing.
5. Synthesize knowledge of readiness for childbearing with nursing process to achieve quality maternal-newborn nursing care.

READINESS FOR CHILDBEARING has both physical and psychosocial aspects; when making this assessment, you need to include both of these areas thoroughly. Anatomy and physiology pertinent to reproductive function is reviewed here as a source of ready information retrieval in this area.

For physical readiness, a woman must have mature endocrine function, ovaries, fallopian tubes and a uterus mature enough to initiate ovulation and sustain a pregnancy, pelvic formation large enough to provide a sufficient-sized canal for birth and additional supporting ligaments, and blood supply and muscles to sustain the pregnant uterus. If she wishes to breast-feed her newborn, she must have mature breast development for milk production.

In order to be fertile, men must have sufficient endocrine and testes maturity to cause formation of spermatozoa; they must have tubal patency and neurologic and circulatory capability for functional ejaculatory ability.

Intrauterine Development

The sex of an individual is determined at the moment of conception by the chromosome formation of the particular ovum and sperm that joined to create the new structure. This distinction cannot be made, however, by appearance early in intrauterine life. A *gonad* is a body organ that produces sex cells (the ovary in females, the testis in males). At about the fifth week of intrauterine life, primitive gonadal tissue appears to be present. Two undifferentiated ducts, the *mesonephric* (Wolffian) and *paramesonephric* (Müllerian) ducts are present. By the seventh or eighth week, in chromosomal males, this early gonadal tissue differentiates into primitive testes and begins formation of testosterone. Under the influence of testosterone, the mesonephric duct begins to develop into the male reproductive organs; the paramesonephric duct regresses. If testosterone is not present by the tenth week, the gonadal tissue differentiates into ovaries and the paramesonephric duct develops into female reproductive organs. All the primordial follicles that will develop throughout the woman's mature years into ova are already formed in this very early structure.

External genitalia develop from a *cloacal* membrane, appearing very similar to inspection by the naked eye until about the twelfth week of intrauterine life. Then, under the influence of testosterone, penal tissue elongates and the urogenital fold on the ventral surface of the penis closes to form the urethra; in females, with no testosterone present, the urogenital fold remains open to form the labia minora. What would become scrotal tissue becomes the labia majora. If, for some reason, testosterone secretion is halted in utero, a chromosomal male will be born with female-appearing genitalia. If a mother should ingest a form of testosterone during pregnancy or, due to a metabolic abnormality, produce a high level of testosterone, a chromosomal female fetus can be born appearing more male than female.

Development at Puberty

Both girls and boys begin dramatic development and maturation of reproductive organs at about 12 to 13 years of age although the initiating mechanism for this is not well understood. The hypothalamus apparently serves as a *gonadostat*, which is set to "turn on" at this age. One theory suggests that a girl must reach a critical weight of about 95 pounds (43 kg) before the hypothalamus is "triggered" to send initial stimulation by releasing a gonadotropin-releasing factor (GN-RF) to the anterior pituitary gland, which then begins gonadotropic hormone (follicle stimulating hormone and luteinizing hormone) formation (Frisch & Reville, 1970). The trigger is even less well understood in boys.

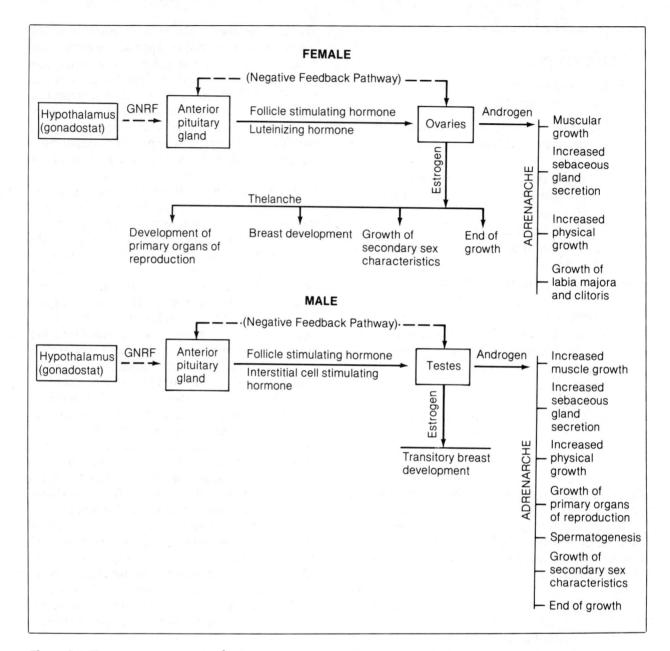

Figure 8-1 *Hormone response at puberty.*

The Role of Androgen

In males, androgenic hormones are produced by both the adrenal cortex and the testes; and in the female, by the adrenal cortex and the ovaries (Figure 8-1).

At puberty, the androgenic hormones are responsible for muscular development, physical growth, and an increase in sebaceous gland secretions, which cause the acne typical in both boys and girls. The level of testosterone is low in males until puberty (about 11 to 13 years of age), when it rises to influence the development of testes, scrotum, penis, prostate, and seminal vesicles; the appearance of male pubic, axillary, and facial hair; laryngeal enlargement and its accompanying voice change; and maturation of spermatozoa.

In girls, testosterone influences enlargement of the labia majora and clitoris and formation of axillary and pubic hair.

The end-products of androgenic hormones are excreted in urine as 17-ketosteroids. Testing for urinary 17-ketosteroids is therefore an often-ordered test as an assessment tool for sexual maturity. Children under 10 years of age usually have little in the urine. Twelve-year-olds excrete about 1 mg of 17-ketosteroids a day; adolescent females, 5–12 mg per day; adolescent males, 8–15 mg per day (Pagano and Pagano, 1982). The development of pubic and axillary hair due to androgen stimulation is termed *adrenarche*.

The Role of Estrogen

At puberty, the hypothalamus stimulates the anterior pituitary gland to begin secreting gonadotropic hormones, the chief of which is follicle-stimulating hormone (FSH). FSH causes maturation of ovarian follicles in females. Ovarian follicles secrete a high level of estrogen, which is actually not one substance but three compounds (estrone [E1], estradiol [E2], and estriol [E3]). It can be considered a single substance, however, in terms of action.

The increase in estrogen level in the female at puberty influences the development of the uterus, fallopian tubes, and vagina; typical female fat distribution and hair patterns; breast development; and an end to growth, as it closes epiphyseal lines of long bones. The beginning of breast development is termed *thelarche*.

In the male, under the influence of FSH, testosterone is secreted by Leydig's cells of the testes and initiates the production of spermatozoa. Estrogen production initiates transient breast enlargement.

Secondary Sex Characteristics

The stages of adolescent sexual development have been categorized by Marshall and Tanner (Marshall and Tanner, 1969 and 1970). These stages are listed in Table 8-1. There is a wide variation in the times that adolescents move through these developmental stages. Any schoolroom reveals a wide difference in the amount of maturity evident in children.

In girls pubertal changes typically occur in the following order: (a) growth spurt, (b) increase in the transverse diameter of the pelvis, (c) breast development, (d) growth of pubic and axillary hair, and (e) vaginal secretions. Menstruation usually begins between the time a girl develops pubic hair and the time she develops axillary hair. *Menarche* (the first menstrual period) may occur as early as age 9 or as late as age 17 and still be within a normal age range. Pubertal changes in girls are shown in Figure 8-2.

Some girls seen at prenatal clinics are afraid they are pregnant because their menstrual periods started regularly for 2 or 3 months, then became irregular or appeared to have stopped. If they are sexually active, they need to have a pregnancy test done to rule out pregnancy, but irregular menstrual periods are the rule rather than the ex-

Table 8-1 Tanner Stages of Secondary Sex Characteristic Development

Boys	
Stage I	Genital size the same as childhood; no distinction between the hair on penis and over the abdomen.
Stage II	Initial enlargement of scrotum and testes; there is reddening and beginning rugae of scrotal skin; there is sparse growth of long, straight, slightly pigmented hair at base of penis.
Stage III	Penis begins to enlarge in length; scrotum becomes more rugated; hair is darker and coarser and curly.
Stage IV	There is increased size of penis; pubic hair is adult in type.
State V	Penis, testes, and scrotum are adult in size and shape; facial and axillary hair as well as pubic hair is present.
Girls	
Stage I	Only slight elevation of the nipple; no distinction between pubic and abdominal hair.
Stage II	Breast bud is present; areola is noticeable; there is sparse growth of long, straight hair at pubic area.
Stage III	The breast nipple and areola further increase in size and pigmentation of the areola is obvious; pubic hair is darker, coarser, and curly.
Stage IV	There is projection of breast areola and nipple to form a secondary mound; pubic hair is adult in type.
Stage V	Breasts and pubic hair are adult in type; axillary and some facial hair is present.

Source: J. M. Tanner (1962). *Growth at Adolescence* (2nd ed.). Oxford, England: Blackwell.

ception for the first year. Menstrual periods do not become regular until ovulation consistently occurs, which does not tend to happen for the first year. This is also one reason that starting estrogen-based oral contraceptives is not recommended until a girl's periods have become stabilized or are ovulatory (so she is not administered a medication to halt ovulation before it is firmly established).

In boys, pubertal changes typically take place in the order of (a) growth spurt, (b) increase in size of genitalia, (c) hypertrophy of breast tissue, (d) growth of pubic, axillary, facial, and chest hair, (e) deepening voice, and (f) production of sper-

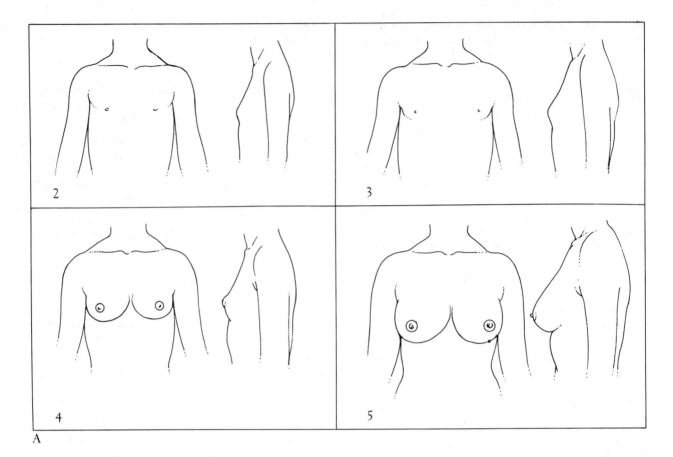

A

matozoa. Puberty changes, as a whole, occur later in boys than in girls, the age range being about 12 to 16 years. Time sequences for developmental changes of boys and girls are shown in Figure 8-3.

Female Internal Reproductive Organs

The study of female reproductive organs and their function is termed *gynecology*. Female internal reproductive organs, as shown in Figure 8-4, are the ovaries, the fallopian tubes, the uterus, and the vagina. Some time when you are observing an abdominal surgical procedure, ask the surgeon if she will show these organs to you. Their appearance is deceptively common compared to their responsibility for the continuity of life generation to generation.

The Ovaries

The function of the ovaries (the female gonads) is to produce, mature, and discharge ova (the egg cells). In the process of performing this function, estrogen and progesterone are produced and menstrual cycles are intiated and regulated. If ovaries are removed prior to puberty (or are nonfunctional), due to lack of estrogen production, breasts will not mature at puberty and pubic hair distribution will assume a more male pattern than normally (normal for females is a triangle shape; for males, a diamond shape). After menopause, or cessation of ovarian function, the uterus and breasts and ovaries themselves undergo atrophy or a reduction in size. Ovarian function, therefore, is necessary for maturation and maintenance of secondary sex characteristics in females. The estrogen secreted by ovaries is also important to prevent *osteoporosis*, or faulty withdrawal of calcium from bones. This frequently happens in women following menopause, making older women prone to major accidents such as vertebrae, hip, and wrist fractures from minor falls. As cholesterol is incorporated in estrogen, the production of estrogen may keep cholesterol levels reduced and so limit the effects of atherosclerosis in women.

The ovaries are about 4 by 2 cm in diameter and about 1.5 cm thick—the size and shape of almonds. They are grayish white in color and appear pitted or with minute indentations on the surface. An unruptured, glistening, clear, fluid-filled *graafian follicle* (an ova about to be discharged) or a miniature yellow *corpus luteum* (the structure left after the ovum has been discharged) may usually be observed on the surface.

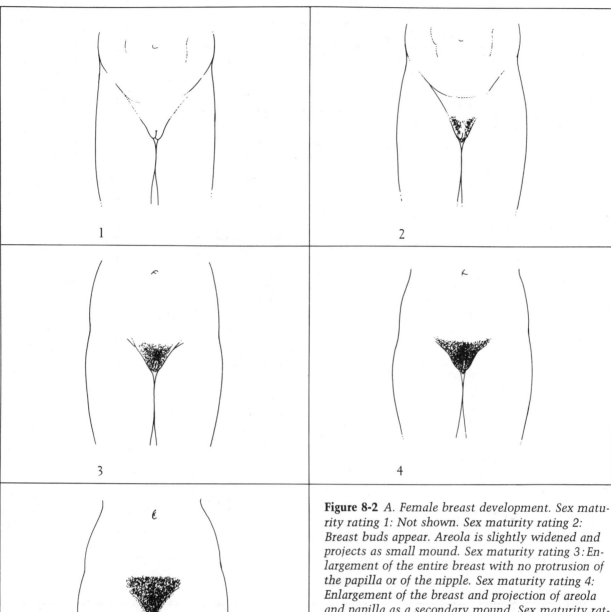

Figure 8-2 *A. Female breast development. Sex maturity rating 1: Not shown. Sex maturity rating 2: Breast buds appear. Areola is slightly widened and projects as small mound. Sex maturity rating 3: Enlargement of the entire breast with no protrusion of the papilla or of the nipple. Sex maturity rating 4: Enlargement of the breast and projection of areola and papilla as a secondary mound. Sex maturity rating 5: Adult configuration of the breast with protrusion of the nipple. Areola no longer projects separately from remainder of breast. B. Female pubic hair development. Sex maturity rating 1: Prepubertal. No pubic hair. Sex maturity rating 2: Straight hair is extending along the labia and between rating 2 and 3 begins on the pubis. Sex maturity rating 3: Pubic hair has increased in quantity, is darker, and is present in the typical female triangle but in smaller quantity. Sex maturity rating 4: Pubic hair is more dense, curled, and adult in distribution but is less abundant. Sex maturity rating 5: Abundant, adult-type pattern. Hair may extend onto the medial aspect of the thighs. From E. Fuller. (1979). A physician's guide to sexual maturity.* Patient Care, 13, *122. Copyright © 1979, Patient Care Publications, Inc., Darien, Ct. All rights reserved.*

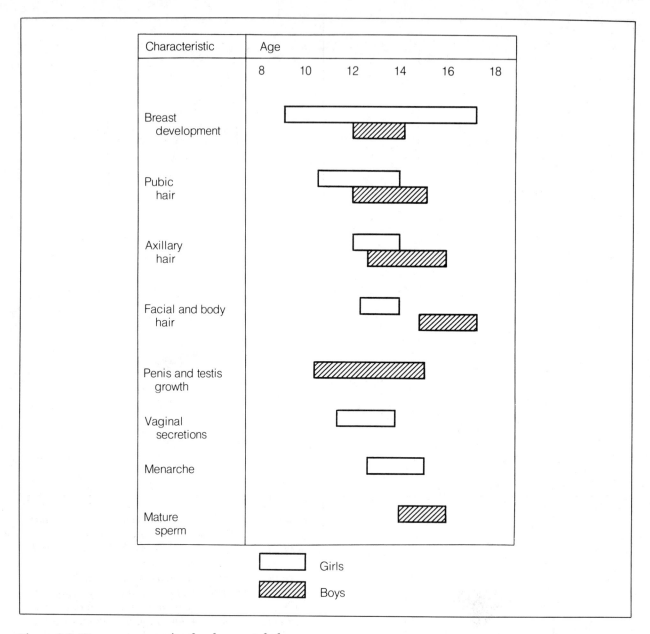

Figure 8-3 *Time sequences for developmental change.*

Ovaries are located close to and on both sides of the uterus in the lower abdomen. It is difficult to locate them by abdominal palpation because they are so low. If an abnormality is present, however,—such as an enlarging ovarian cyst— tenderness of this may be evident on lower left or lower right abdominal palpation.

The ovaries are suspended in the pelvis by two ligaments, the *utero-ovarian* and the *infundibulopelvic* or *suspensory* ligaments. The first of these two ligaments attaches the ovary loosely to the body of the uterus; the second attaches it laterally to the pelvic wall. The ovary is further held in its suspended position and kept in close contact with the fimbriated end of the fallopian tube by attachment to the posterior surface of the pelvic wall by the *broad* ligament.

The ovaries are unique among pelvic structures in that they are not covered by a layer of peritoneum. Because they are not encased this way, ova can escape from them and enter the uterus by way of the fallopian tubes. Because they are suspended in position rather than being firmly fixed in place, an abnormal tumor or cyst growing on them can enlarge to a size easily twice that of the organ before pressure on surrounding organs or the ovarian blood supply leads to symptoms of compression. For this reason, ovarian cancer con-

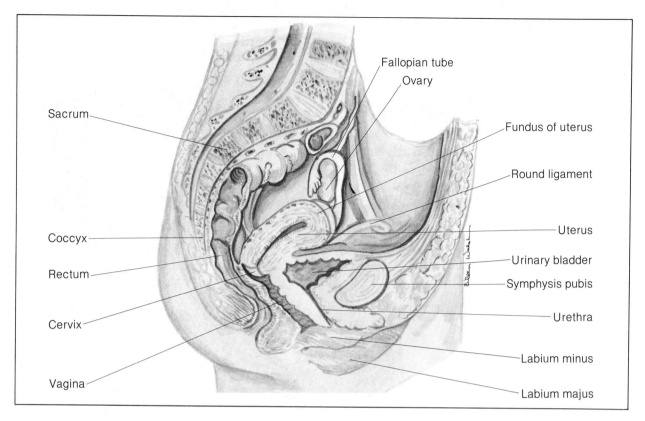

Figure 8-4 *Female internal reproductive organs.*

tinues to be the fourth leading cause of death from cancer in women (the tumor grows symptomlessly for such an extended period of time it has spread before it is noticed). It is also the reason that women should have a yearly pelvic examination during which ovarian pathology is palpated and discovered.

Ovaries are formed with three principal divisions: a layer of surface epithelium, a middle *cortex* area filled with connective tissue, and a still more central area termed the *medulla.* It is in the cortex that immature (primordial) follicles that will mature into ova develop. *Theca* cells, which line these follicles, produce large amounts of estrogen and progesterone important for the physiology of menstrual cycles. This layer of tissue contains a rich supply of nerve fibers and blood vessels to supply the growing cells. The central core contains the blood vessels that lead to the cortex and supporting muscle fibers.

The nerve supply for the ovaries is from both sympathetic and parasympathetic nervous systems. Arterial blood supply is by the ovarian artery, an extension of the aorta; venous return is by the ovarian vein. The lymphatic drainage system is active in the pelvic area, with many large lymph nodes present. A malignancy (cancer) of the ovary is quickly spread to other body sites by this system.

The Fallopian Tubes

A fallopian tube arises from each upper corner of the uterine body and extends outward and backward so that each open distal end lies next to the broad ligament and an ovary. Fallopian tubes are about 10 cm in length in a mature woman. Their function is to convey the ova from the ovaries to the uterus and to provide a place for fertilization of the ova by sperm.

Although a fallopian tube is one smooth hollow tunnel, it can be anatomically divided into four separate parts (Figure 8-5). The *interstitial* portion is that part of the tube that lies within the uterine wall. It is only about 1 cm in length; the lumen of the tube is only about 1 mm in diameter at this point. The *isthmus* is the next distal portion. It is, like the interstitial tube, extremely narrow. The segment is about 2 cm in length. It is the portion of the tube that is cut or sealed in a tubal ligation or tubal sterilization procedure.

The *ampulla* is the next and also the longest portion of the tube. It is about 5 cm in length. It is in this ampulla portion that fertilization of an

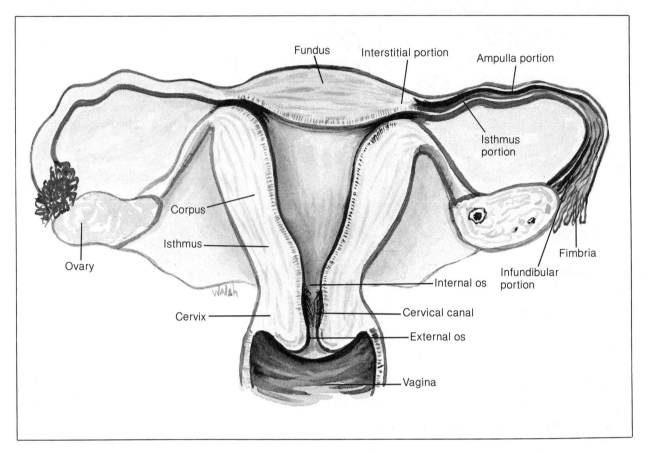

Figure 8-5 *Anterior view of female reproductive organs showing relationship of fallopian tube and body of the uterus.*

ovum usually takes place. The *infundibular* portion is the most distal segment of the tube. It is about 2 cm long and is funnel shaped. The rim of the funnel is covered by fimbriated (hair-covered) cells that help to guide the ova into the fallopian tube.

The lining of the entire fallopian tube is comprised of mucous membrane, which contains both mucus-secreting and ciliated cells. Beneath the mucous lining is connective tissue and a circular muscle layer. Blood supply is by the ovarian artery and vein. The muscle layer of the tube produces peristaltic motions that conduct the ova the length of the tube. This migration of the ova is further aided by the action of the ciliated lining and the mucus, which acts as a lubricant to allow the sperm to migrate easily. The mucus produced, which contains protein, water, and salts, may also act as a source of nourishment for the fertilized egg.

Because the fallopian tubes are open at the distal end, they provide a connection between the outside of the body (vagina to uterus to tube) and the peritoneum. This potential pathway makes childbirth possible. It can, unfortunately, also lead to pelvic inflammatory disease if disease spreads from the external genital organs through the vagina and uterus to the tubes and the peritoneum. Careful, clean technique must be used during pelvic examination or care to prevent this. Vaginal examinations done during labor and delivery are done with sterile technique to ensure that no organisms enter the uterus.

The Uterus

The uterus is a hollow, muscular, pear-shaped organ located in the lower pelvis, posterior to the bladder and anterior to the rectum. During childhood, it is extremely small, about the size of an olive, and its proportions are reversed from what they are later on; the cervix being the largest portion of the organ. At about 8 years of age, an increase in the size of the uterus begins. The maximum increase in size occurs about 17 years of age, a fact that probably helps to account for the low-birth-weight babies typically born to early adolescent women below this age.

With maturity, a uterus is about 5–7 cm long, 5 cm wide, and in its widest upper part 2.5 cm deep. A nonpregnant uterus weighs about 60 gm. The function of the uterus is to receive the ova from the fallopian tube, provide a place for implantation and nourishment during fetal growth, furnish protection to a growing fetus, and, at maturity of the fetus, expel it from the woman's body.

Following a pregnancy, the uterus never returns to quite the small diameters of its nonpregnant size. In the woman who has born a child, uterine dimensions are closer to 9 cm long, 6 cm wide, and 3 cm thick. The organ weighs up to 80 gm.

The uterus consists of three divisions: the body or *corpus*, the *isthmus,* and the *cervix* (see Figure 8-5). The body of the uterus is the uppermost part and forms the bulk of the uterus. The lining of the cavity is continuous with that of the fallopian tubes, which fuse at its upper aspects (the *cornua*). During pregnancy, the body of the uterus is the portion of the structure that expands so greatly to contain the growing fetus. The portion of the uterus between the points of attachment of the fallopian tubes is the *fundus.* The fundus is the portion that can be palpated abdominally to determine the amount of uterine growth during pregnancy, the force of uterine contractions during labor, and the degree to which the uterus is returning to its nonpregnant state following childbirth.

The isthmus is a short segment between the corpus and the cervix. In the nonpregnant uterus it is only 1–2 cm in length. During pregnancy this portion also enlarges greatly to aid in accommodating the growing fetus. It is the portion of the uterus that is cut when a fetus is delivered by a cesarean birth.

The cervix is the lowest portion of the uterus. It represents about one third of the total uterus size and is about 2–5 cm long. About half of it lies above the vagina; half extends into the vagina. Its cavity is termed the *cervical canal.* The junction of the canal at the isthmus is the *internal cervical os;* the distal opening to the vagina is the *external cervical os.* The level of the external os is at the level of the ischial spines (projections of the ischium)—an important relationship in estimating the level of the fetus in the birth canal at delivery.

Uterine and Cervical Coats

The uterine wall is composed of three separate coats or layers of tissue: an inner one of mucous membrane, a middle one of muscle fibers, and an outer one of the perimetrium sheath (Figure 8-6). The mucous membrane lining the cervix is termed the *endocervix;* that lining the uterus is the *endometrium.*

The endometrial layer of the uterus is important in terms of menstrual function and childbearing. It is not a single structure, but composed of two layers of cells. The layer closest to the uterine wall, or the *basal* layer, is not much influenced by hormones. An inner second glandular layer is greatly influenced by both estrogen and progesterone. This is the layer that grows and becomes so thick and responsive each month under the influence of these hormones that it is capable of supporting a pregnancy. If pregnancy does not occur, this layer is shed as the menstrual flow.

The endocervix, continuous with the endometrium, is also affected by hormones, but this is manifested in a more subtle way. The cells of the lining (columnar epithelial cells) secrete mucus to provide a lubricated surface for spermatozoa passing through the cervix; the efficiency of this lubrication increases or wanes depending on hormone stimulation. At the point in the menstrual cycle when estrogen production is at its peak, as much as 700 ml of mucus per day is produced. At the point of low estrogen production, only a few milliliters are produced. Because mucus is alkaline, it decreases the acidity of the upper vagina, aiding sperm survival. During pregnancy, the endocervix becomes plugged with mucus, forming a seal to keep out ascending infections.

The lower surface of the cervix and the lower third of the cervical canal is lined not with columnar epithelium but with stratified squamous epithelium similar to that lining the vagina. Locating this point at which the tissue changes from columnar to squamous epithelium (the transition zone) is important when helping with a *Papanicolaou smear* (a test for cervical cancer). This tissue interface is the most frequent place for cervical cancer to originate.

The *myometrium*, or muscle of the uterus, is composed of three interwoven layers of smooth muscle, the fibers of which are arranged in longitudinal, transverse, and oblique directions, a network that offers extreme strength to the organ. When the uterus contracts at the end of pregnancy to expel the fetus, equal pressure is exerted at all points throughout the cavity because of the unique arrangement of these muscle fibers. Following childbirth, this interlacing network of muscle fibers is able to constrict blood vessels coursing through the layers and so limit loss of blood or hemorrhage in the woman. The middle muscle layer serves an important additional function of constricting the tubal junctions and preventing regurgitation of menstrual blood into the tubes. It also holds the internal cervical os closed during pregnancy to prevent a preterm birth.

The *perimetrium*, or the outer most layer of

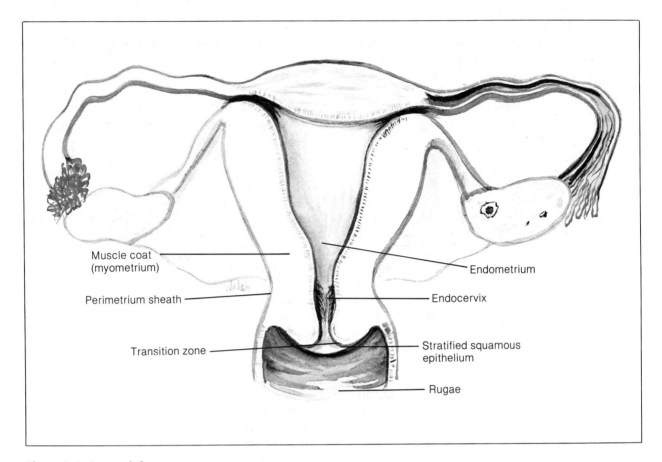

Muscle coat (myometrium)

Perimetrium sheath

Transition zone

Endometrium

Endocervix

Stratified squamous epithelium

Rugae

Figure 8-6 *Coats of the uterus.*

the uterus, is composed of connective tissue and offers added strength and support to the structure.

Uterine Supports

The uterus is suspended in the pelvic cavity by a number of ligaments. A single sheet of fascia (the *anterior* or *pubocervical* ligament) passes from the anterior surface of the cervix to fuse with the fascia covering the symphysis pubis. It supports both the uterus and the anterior bladder. If it becomes overstretched during pregnancy, it may not support the bladder afterward and the bladder may herniate into the anterior vagina, a condition called *cystocele* (Figure 8-7A).

A fold of peritoneum behind the uterus is the *posterior* ligament. The posterior ligament forms a pouch (the cul-de-sac of Douglas) between the rectum and uterus. As the lowest point of the pelvis, it tends to collect any pus or blood in the pelvis. The space can be examined for the presence of pus or blood by insertion of a culdoscope through the posterior vaginal wall (culdoscopy). Damage to the posterior wall of the vagina from childbearing may lead to a pouching of the

rectum into the posterior vaginal wall, called a *rectocele* (Figure 8-7B).

The *broad* ligaments are two folds of peritoneum, one covering the uterus at the front and one at the back, which then extend to the pelvic sides. The lower third of each ligament is composed of dense connective tissue. This is also known as the *cardinal* ligament because it forms the main support for the uterus and, in addition, supports blood vessels and nerves.

The *round* ligaments are two fibrous muscular cords that pass from the body of the uterus near the attachments of the fallopian tubes through the broad ligament into the inguinal canals and insert into the fascia of the vulva. The round ligaments act as "stays" to steady the uterus. If a pregnant woman moves quickly, she may pull one of these ligaments and feel a quick, sharp pain that is frightening in its intensity in one of her lower abdominal quadrants.

The *uterosacral* ligament passes from the upper cervix backward to fuse with the fascia of the sacrum. It counteracts the forward pull of the round ligaments.

That a uterus is a suspended, not a fixed, organ is important in childbearing. Because it is not

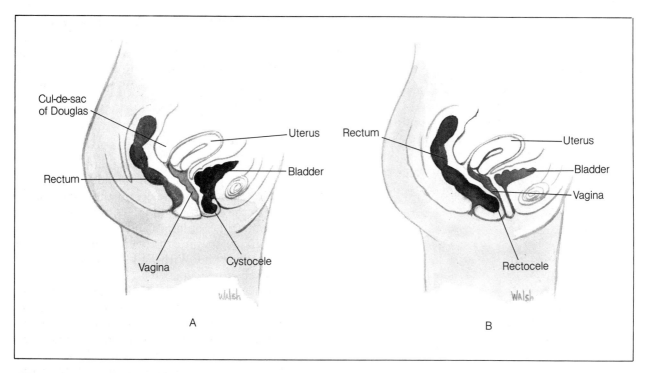

Figure 8-7 *A. Cystocele. The bladder has herniated into the anterior wall of the vagina. B. Rectocele. The posterior wall of the vagina is herniated.*

fixed in one position, the uterus is free to enlarge without discomfort during pregnancy.

Uterine Blood Supply

The large descending abdominal aorta divides to form the two *iliac* arteries; main divisions of the iliac arteries are the *hypogastric* arteries. These further divide to become the *uterine* arteries and supply the uterus. Because of this early division the uterine blood supply is not far removed from the aorta; it is copious and adequate to supply the growing needs of a fetus. In addition, after supplying the ovary with blood, the *ovarian* artery, a direct subdivision of the aorta, joins with the uterine artery; this fail-safe system ensures that the uterus will have an adequate blood supply present. The blood vessels that supply the cells and lining of the uterus are tortuous in appearance against the sides of the uterine body in nonpregnant women. As a uterus enlarges with pregnancy, the vessels unwind, stretching to maintain an adequate blood supply as the organ enlarges. The uterine veins follow the same twisting course as the arteries; they empty into the internal iliac veins.

An important organ relationship is the association of the uterus with the ureters from the kidneys. The ureters pass directly in back of the ovarian vessels near the fallopian tubes; as shown in Figure 8-8, they cross just beneath the uterine vessels before they enter the bladder. This close anatomic relationship has implications in surgery such as tubal ligation and hysterectomy; the ureter may be injured by a clamp if bleeding must be controlled by clamping the uterine or ovarian vessels. This is one reason why observing women for urine output following uterine or fallopian tube surgery is always a critical assessment.

Uterine Nerve Supply

The uterus is affected by both *efferent* (motor) and *afferent* (sensory) nerves. The efferent nerves arise from T5 through T10 spinal ganglia. The afferent (sensory nerves) join the hypogastric plexus and enter the spinal column at T11 and T12. That sensory innervation from the uterus registers lower in the spinal column than does motor control has implications in controlling pain in labor. If an anesthetic solution is injected into the spinal column at a low point (L3 or L4), it will rise and stop the pain of uterine contractions at the T11 and T12 level without stopping motor control or contractions (registered at the T5 to T10 level).

Uterine Deviations

Uterine deviations may interfere with either fertility or pregnancy.

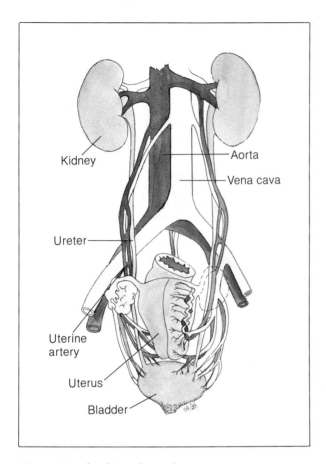

Figure 8-8 *Blood supply to the uterus.*

Uterine Shape

In the fetus, the uterus first forms with a septum or a fibrous division, longitudinally separating it into two portions. As the fetus matures, this septum disappears, so that typically at birth no remnant of the division remains. In some women, the septum never atrophies, and the uterus remains as two smaller compartments. In others, half the septum is still present. Still other women have oddly shaped "horns" at the junction of the fallopian tubes, termed a *bicornuate* uterus, or have yet another remnant of incomplete formation. All these malformations may decrease the ability to conceive or to carry a pregnancy to term. Some variations of uterine formation are shown in Figure 8-9. The specific effects of these deviations on fertility and pregnancy are discussed in later chapters.

Uterine Version and Flexion

Ordinarily, the body of the uterus is tipped slightly forward. *Anteversion* is a condition in which the fundus is tipped very far forward. *Retroversion* means that the fundus is tipped back. *Anteflexion* means that the body of the uterus is bent sharply forward at the junction with the cer-

vix. *Retroflexion* means that the body is bent sharply back. Extreme abnormal flexion or version positions may interfere with fertility by blocking the deposition or migration of sperm. Examples of these abnormal uterine positions are shown in Figure 8-10.

The Vagina

The vagina is a hollow, muscular-membranous canal located posterior to the bladder and anterior to the rectum. It extends from the cervix of the uterus to the external vulva. Its function is to act as the organ of copulation and to convey sperm to the cervix so sperm can meet with the ovum in the fallopian tube. With childbirth, it expands to serve as the birth canal.

When a woman is lying on her back as she does for a pelvic examination, the course of the vagina is backward and downward. Because of this downward slant and the insertion of the uterine cervix into the distal portion, the length of the anterior wall of the vagina is about 6–7 cm long, the posterior wall 8–9 cm long. At the uterine end of the structure, there are recesses on all sides of the cervix termed *fornices*. Behind the cervix is the *posterior fornix*; at the front, the *anterior fornix*; and at the sides, the *lateral fornices*. The posterior fornix serves as a place for the pooling of semen following coitus; this allows a large number of sperm to remain close to the cervix to encourage sperm migration into the cervix.

The vaginal wall is so thin at these points that the bladder can be palpated through the anterior fornix, the ovaries through the lateral ones, and the rectum through the posterior fornix. That these recesses exist has implications whenever a woman is seen in a health care setting for self-induced abortion. An instrument such as a knitting needle, when pushed into the vagina with the intention of inserting it into the cervical os to disrupt a pregnancy, invariably penetrates one of the fornices instead and, rather than induce abortion, introduces pathogenic organisms from the vagina into the peritoneal cavity.

The vagina is lined with stratified squamous epithelium similar to that covering the cervix. It has a middle connective tissue layer and a strong muscular wall. Normally the walls lie in close approximation to each other. They contain many folds or rugae; thus the vagina is very elastic and can expand at the end of pregnancy to allow a full-term baby to pass through without tearing. A circular muscle, the *bulbocavernosus* muscle, at the external opening to the vagina (the introitus), acts as a voluntary sphincter to the vagina.

As one preparation for childbirth, women are

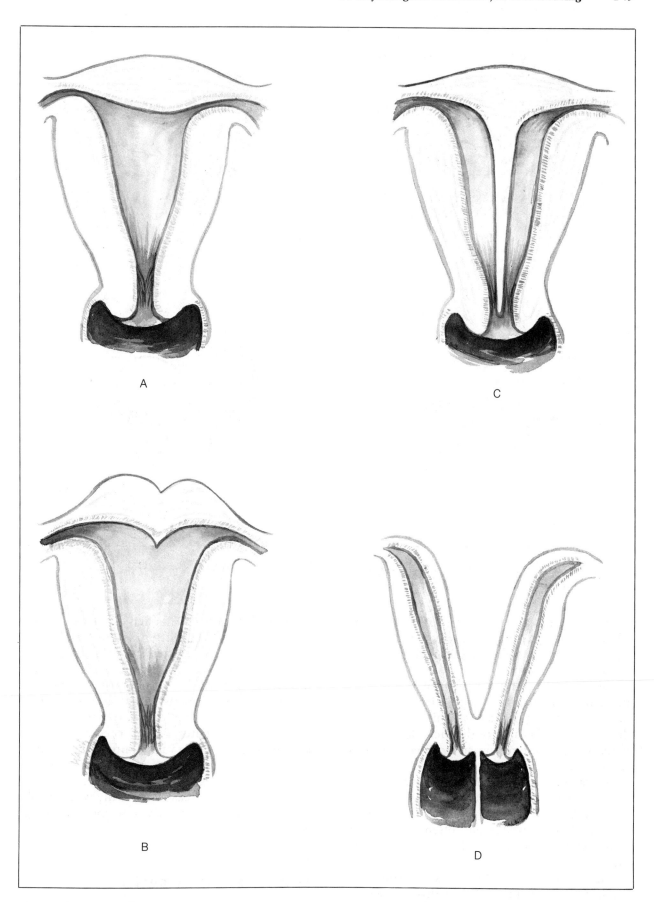

Figure 8-9 *Uterine deviations. A. Normal uterus. B. Bicornuate uterus. C. Septum dividing uterus. D. Double uterus.*

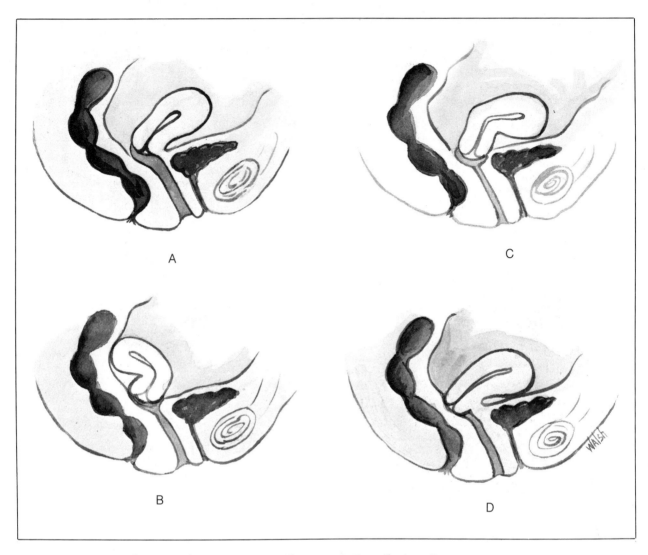

Figure 8-10 *Uterine flexion and version. A. Normal uterus. B. Retroflexion. C. Anteflexion. D. Anteversion.*

advised to relax and tense the external vaginal sphincter muscle periodically to make it more supple for delivery and to help maintain tone after delivery.

The vaginal artery, a branch of the internal iliac artery, provides the vagina with an excellent blood supply. Vaginal tears at childbirth tend to bleed profusely because of this rich blood supply, while for the same reason any vaginal trauma at delivery heals rapidly.

The vagina has both sympathetic and parasympathetic nerve innervations originating at the S1 to S3 level. It is not an extremely sensitive organ, however. Sexual excitement, often attributed to vaginal stimulation, is actually caused mainly by clitoral stimulation.

The mucus produced by the vaginal lining has a rich glycogen content. When this glycogen is broken down by lactose-fermenting bacteria (Döderlein bacillus) that frequent the vagina,

lactic acid is formed. This makes the usual pH of the vagina acid, a condition deterimental to the growth of pathologic bacteria. Even though the vagina connects directly to the external surface, infections are therefore not usually present. Under normal circumstances, use of vaginal douches or sprays should not be a daily hygiene measure: This natural acid medium can be cleaned away, inviting vaginal infections. Following menopause (the end of menstruation cycles), the pH of the vagina becomes closer to 7.5, or slightly alkaline, a reason that vulvovaginitis infections occur so frequently in women in this age group.

Female External Genitalia

The structures that form the female external genitalia are termed the *vulva* (from the Latin

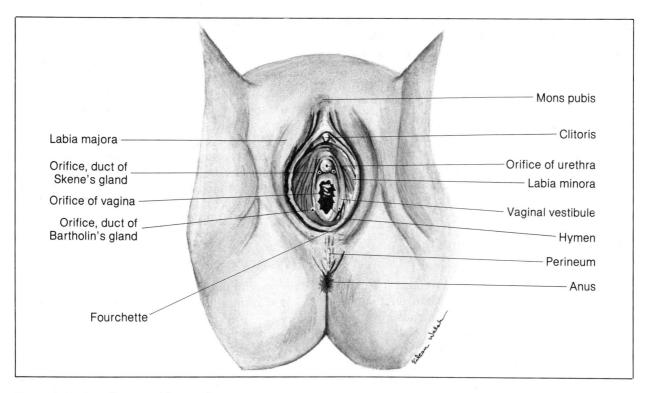

Labia majora

Orifice, duct of
Skene's gland

Orifice of vagina

Orifice, duct of
Bartholin's gland

Fourchette

Mons pubis

Clitoris

Orifice of urethra

Labia minora

Vaginal vestibule

Hymen

Perineum

Anus

Figure 8-11 *Female external genitalia.*

word for covering) and are illustrated in Figure 8-11. An older but still used term for vulva is *pudenda* (from the Latin for "to be ashamed").

Mons Veneris

The mons veneris is a pad of adipose tissue located over the symphysis pubis. It is covered by coarse curly hairs. In females, pubic hair tends to have a triangular distribution (in males, the pubic hair pattern is more diamond shaped). The mons serves to protect the junction of the pubic bone from trauma. Infection of hair follicles or infestation by pubic lice (*Pediculosis pubis*) may occur in the area.

Labia Minora

Just posterior to the mons veneris spread two folds of connective tissue, the labia minora. Prior to menarche (the first menstrual period), the folds of the labia minora are fairly small; by childbearing age they are firm and full. After menopause, they atrophy and again become much smaller. Normally, the folds of the labia minora are pink; the internal surface is covered with mucous membrane, the external surface with skin. The area is abundant with sebaceous glands, which make it a possible site of localized sebaceous cysts.

Labia Majora

The labia majora are two folds of adipose tissue covered by loose connective tissue and epithelium; they are positioned lateral to the labia minora. Covered by pubic hair, the labia majora serve as protection for the external genitalia, the urethra, and the vaginal introitus. They are fused anteriorly, separated posteriorly to form the *posterior commissura.* Trauma to the area such as occurs from childbirth or rape can lead to extensive edema formation in the area because of the looseness of the connective tissue base.

The Vestibule

The vestibule is the flattened, smooth surface inside the labia. The opening to the bladder (the urethra) and the uterus (the vagina) both arise from the vestibule.

The Clitoris

The clitoris is a small (about 1 to 2 cm) rounded organ of erectile tissue at the forward junction of the labia minora. It is covered by a fold of skin, the *prepuce.* The clitoris is sensitive to touch and temperature and is the center of sexual arousal and orgasm in the female (clitoris is Greek for "key"). Arterial blood supply for the clitoris is plentiful. When the ischiocavernous muscle surrounding it contracts with sexual arousal, the venous outflow from the clitoris is blocked. Venous congestion from this blockage is what leads to clitoral erection.

Skene's Glands (Paraurethral Glands)

Skene's glands are located just lateral to the urinary meatus on both sides. Their ducts open into the urethra. Their secretions help lubricate the external genitalia during coitus.

Bartholin's Glands (Vulvovaginal Glands)

Bartholin's glands are located just lateral to the vaginal opening on both sides. Their ducts open into the vaginal introitus. These glands lubricate the external vulva during coitus. The alkaline pH of their secretion helps to improve sperm survival in the vagina. Both Skene's and Bartholin's glands may become infected and produce a discharge and local pain.

The Fourchette

The fourchette is the ridge of tissue formed by the posterior joining of the two labia minora and the labia majora. This is the area cut (episiotomy) prior to delivery of a child to enlarge the vaginal opening.

The Perineal Body

Posterior to the fourchette is the perineal muscle or the perineal body. Because this is a muscular area, it is easily stretched during childbirth to allow for enlargement of the vagina and passage of the fetal head. Many exercises suggested for pregnancy are aimed at making the perineal muscle more relaxed and more expandable so easy expansion during delivery can occur without tearing.

The Hymen

The hymen is a tough but elastic semicircle of tissue that covers the opening to the vagina in childhood. Due to the use of menstrual tampons and active sports participation, even many virginal girls do not have intact hymens at the time of their first pelvic examination. Occasionally, a girl will have an imperforate hymen, or a hymen so complete it does not allow passage of menstrual blood from the vagina or allow for sexual coitus until it is surgically incised.

Vulvar Blood Supply

The blood supply of the external genitalia is mainly from the pudendal artery and a portion of the inferior rectus artery. Venous return is through the pudendal vein. Pressure on this vein by the fetal head may cause extensive back pressure and development of varicosities in the labia majora during pregnancy. Because of the good blood supply, trauma to the area such as occurs from pressure from childbirth can cause the development of large hematomas. This ready blood supply also fortunately contributes to rapid healing of any lesions in the area following childbirth.

Vulvar Nerve Supply

The anterior portion of the vulva derives its nerve supply from the ilioinguinal and genitofemoral nerves (L1 level). The posterior portion of the vulva and vagina is supplied by the pudendal nerve (S3 level). Such a rich nerve supply makes the area extremely sensitive to touch, pressure, pain, and temperature. Much of anesthesia for childbirth is concerned with blocking the pudendal nerve to eliminate pain sensation at the perineum during delivery.

The Pelvic Floor

The pelvic floor is composed of both superficial and deep muscle layers. These muscle layers serve as support for pelvic organs and also to soften the environment of the fetus during intrauterine life and birth. The slope of the pelvic floor is downward and forward due to the muscular attachments. At delivery, when the presenting portion of the fetus touches the pelvic floor, it is pushed forward to be delivered under the pubic arch.

Superficial Muscle Layers

The *bulbocavernous* muscle fibers have their origin in the perineal body. They pass anteriorly, surrounding the vaginal orifice, to insert at the undersurface of the symphysis pubis. It is this muscle that acts as a voluntary vaginal sphincter at the vaginal introitus.

The *transverse perineal* muscle fibers originate at the ischial tuberosities and pass medially to insert at the perineal body. These muscles are so strong, they offer support to both the anal canal during defecation and the lower parts of the vagina during delivery.

The *ischiocavernous* fibers originate at the is-

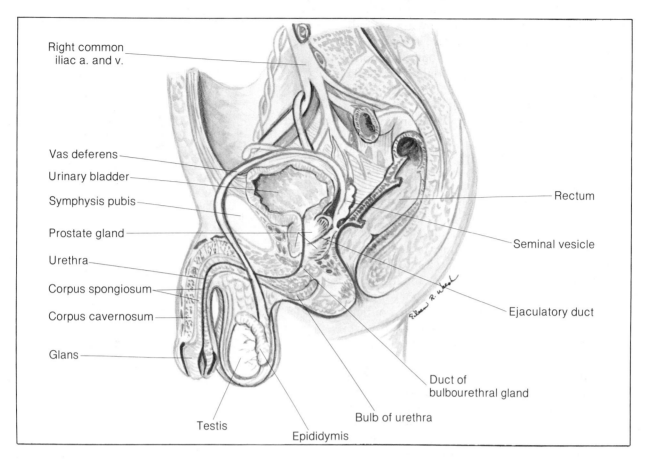

Right common
iliac a. and v.

Vas deferens

Urinary bladder

Symphysis pubis

Prostate gland

Urethra

Corpus spongiosum

Corpus cavernosum

Glans

Testis

Epididymis

Bulb of urethra

Duct of
bulbourethral gland

Ejaculatory duct

Seminal vesicle

Rectum

Figure 8-12 *Male internal and external reproductive organs.*

chial tuberosities and pass obliquely to insert beside the bulbocavernous muscle fibers at the symphysis pubis. By contraction, they cause erection of the clitoris.

The *external anal sphincter* fibers arise from the coccyx and pass on either side of the anus. They fuse and insert into the transverse perineal muscles. As indicated by their name, they allow for voluntary defecation.

Deep Muscle Layers

Although there are three deep muscles of the pelvic floor, they fuse together to form one continuous sheet of muscle, the *levator ani*. Intactness of the levator ani is necessary both for urinary continence and for defecation. This is an important muscle in the second stage of labor: The strength of this muscle allows the fetus to be pushed through the birth canal.

Male External Genitalia

The study of the conditions of male reproductive organs is termed *andrology*. External genital or-

gans of the male are the penis and testes (encased in the scrotum). Male reproductive anatomy showing both internal and external structures is shown in Figure 8-12.

Testes

The testes are ovoid glands that lie in a rugated, skin covered pouch, the scrotum, and are the male analogue of the ovaries. Each testis is encased by a protective white fibrous capsule and is composed of a number of lobules, each lobule containing interstitial cells (*Leydig cells*), a seminiferous tubule and *Sertoli* cells (supporting cells).

Leydig cells are responsible for the production of testosterone, an androgenic hormone, which is in turn responsible for the development of secondary male characteristics such as distribution of pubic hair (a diamond shape in contrast to the triangular shape of a woman's pubic hair), laryngeal and muscle development. When the level of testosterone is at an adult level following puberty, the epiphyseal lines close in long bones, which signals the end of growth in height. During adult life, the level of testosterone in blood influences the production of spermatozoa indirectly: As it increases in amount, it causes decreased production of gonadotropic hormones (follicle stimulating and interstitial cell-stimulating hormones) by the anterior pituitary gland. Under the influence of gonadotropic hormones, spermatozoa are produced by the seminiferous tubules of the testes.

In most males one testis is slightly larger than the other and is suspended slightly lower in the scrotum than the other (usually the left one). Because of this, they tend to slide past each other more readily on sitting or muscular activity and there is less possibility of trauma. Most body structures of importance are more protected than are the testes (the heart, kidneys, and lungs are surrounded by ribs of hard bone, for example). Since spermatozoa do not survive at body temperature, however, the testes are suspended outside the body where the temperature is about 1° lower than body temperature and sperm survival can be ensured.

Production of spermatozoa does not begin in intrauterine life as does the production of ova. Neither are spermatozoa produced in a cyclic pattern as are ova but rather in a continuous process. Sperm production continues throughout a male's lifespan in contrast to female ovarian function. Production of mature ova stops at menopause.

The Scrotum

The scrotum is a rugated skin-covered pouch suspended from the perineum. It contains the testes, epididymis, and the lower portion of the spermatic cord. It is the male homologue of the female labia majora.

The Penis

The penis is the male homologue of the female clitoris. Three cylindrical masses of erectile tissue, two termed *corpus cavernosa* and a third the *corpus spongiosum,* are contained in the shaft. The urethra passes through the corpus cavernosa tissue and serves as the outlet for both the urinary and the reproductive tracts in men. Sexual excitement results in contraction of the ischiocavernous muscle at the penis base. This causes venous congestion in the three sections of erectile tissue, leading to distention and erection of the penis. At the distal end of the organ is a bulging sensitive ridge of tissue, the *glans.* A retractable casing of skin, or *prepuce,* protects the nerve-sensitive glans at birth. In the United States, most male children have the prepuce removed (circumci-

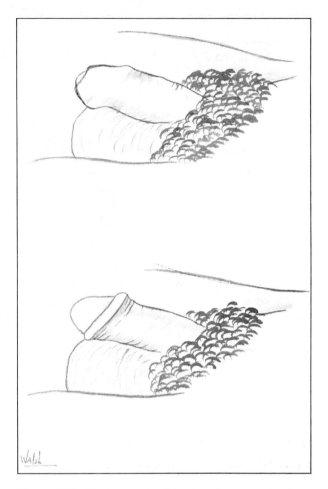

Figure 8-13 *Uncircumcised (top) and circumcised (bottom) penis.*

sion) at birth, although this procedure has little medical necessity or merit (Figure 8-13).

The blood supply for the penis is the penile artery, a branch of the pudendal artery. Penile erection is stimulated by the parasympathetic nerve system; it is inhibited by sympathetic nerve innervation.

Male Internal Reproductive Organs

The male internal reproductive organs are the epididymis, the vas deferens, the seminal vesicles, the ejaculatory ducts, the urethra, the prostate gland, and the bulbourethral glands.

The Epididymis

The seminiferous tubule of each male testes leads to a tightly coiled tube, the epididymis. Because each epididymis is so tightly coiled, its length is extremely deceptive. It actually totals about 20 feet. It is extremely narrow in diameter during its entire length, so infection (epididymitis) can lead to easy scarring of the lumen and prohibit passage of sperm beyond the scarred point.

The epididymis is responsible for conduction of sperm from the testes to the vas deferens, the next step in the passage to the outside. Some sperm are stored in the epididymis. A small part of the fluid that surrounds sperm (*semen*, or seminal fluid) is produced by the cells lining the epididymis. Sperm are immobile and not capable of fertilization as they pass or are stored at the epididymis level. It takes a total of 64 days for sperm to reach maturity and at least 12 to 20 days to travel the length of the epididymis. This is one reason that *aspermia* (absence of sperm) or *oligospermia* (less than 20 million per ml sperm) are problems that do not appear to respond immediately to therapy, taking usually around 2 months to improve.

The Vas Deferens (Ductus Deferens)

The vas deferens carries sperm from the epididymis through the inguinal canal into the abdominal cavity. It is surrounded by arteries and veins and protected by a thick fibrous coating. All together, these structures form the *spermatic cord*. The cord passes over the top of the bladder and at its distal end is joined by the seminal vesicles and the ejaculatory ducts. *Vasectomy*, or severing of the vas deferens, is a popular means of male birth control. Sperm mature in their passage through the vas deferens. They are not very mobile at this point, however, probably due to the fairly acid medium of the semen produced at this level. A *variocele*, or a varicosity of the internal spermatic vein, often contributes to male infertility by causing congestion in the testes.

The Seminal Vesicles

The seminal vesicles are two convoluted pouches that lie along the lower portion of the posterior surface of the bladder and empty into the urethra by way of the ejaculatory ducts. These glands secrete a viscous portion of the semen that has a high content of a basic sugar and protein and is alkaline in pH. Sperm become increasingly motile with this added seminal vesicle fluid as it surrounds them with a favorable pH and nutrients.

Semen (Seminal Fluid)

The content of semen, or the fluid that accompanies spermatozoa, is derived from the prostate gland (60 percent), the seminal vesicles (30 percent), the epididymis (5 percent), and the bulbourethral glands (5 percent). It is alkaline in nature (pH 8.5) and contains a basic sugar and mucin (protein).

The Ejaculatory Ducts

The two ejaculatory ducts pass through the prostate gland. They join the seminal vesicles with the urethra.

The Urethra

The urethra is a hollow tube leading from the base of the bladder that, after passing through the prostate gland, continues to the outside through the shaft and glans of the penis. It is about 8 inches long and lined with mucous membrane, as are other urinary tract structures.

The Prostate Gland

The prostate gland is the homologue of the female Skene's glands and lies just below the bladder. The urethra passes through the center of it, like the hole in a doughnut. The prostate gland secretes a thin, alkaline fluid that, when added to the secretion from the seminal vesicles and that already accompanying sperm from the epididymis, further protects sperm from being immobilized by the naturally low pH level of the urethra (due to the passage of urine through the same lumen).

Bulbourethral Glands

Two bulbourethral, or *Cowper's* glands, the homologue of female Bartholin's glands, lie beside the prostate gland and by short ducts empty into the urethra. Like the prostate gland and seminal vesicles, they secrete an alkaline fluid that helps counteract the acid secretion of the urethra and ensures the safe passage of spermatozoa.

Mammary Glands

The mammary glands or breasts arise from ectodermic tissue early in utero. They remain, however, in a halted stage of development until a rise in estrogen at puberty begins a marked breast maturation in girls and a transient increase in breast size in boys. Increase in male breast size is termed *gynecomastia*. If boys are not prepared for this normal change of puberty, they can be very concerned about abnormal development. Gynecomastia is most evident in obese boys.

The increase in size of breast tissue in both sexes is due to an increase in connective tissue

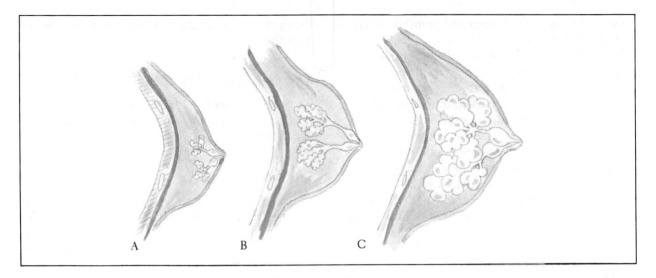

Figure 8-14 *Breast anatomy. A. Nonpregnant. B. Pregnant. C. During lactation.*

and deposition of fat. The glandular tissue of the breasts, necessary for successful breast-feedings, remains undeveloped until a first pregnancy begins.

Breasts are located anterior to the pectoral muscle. In many women, breast tissue extends well into the axilla, a reason that this region must always be included in self breast examination. Milk glands of breasts are divided by connective tissue partitions into about 20 lobes. All the glands in each lobe produce milk by acini cells and deliver it to the nipple by a *lacteriferous* duct. The nipple has about 20 small openings through which milk is secreted. The *ampullar* portion of the duct just posterior to the nipple serves as a reservoir for milk prior to breast-feeding.

A nipple is composed of smooth muscle that is capable of erection on manual or sucking stimulation. On stimulation, it transmits sensations to the posterior pituitary gland to release oxytocin. Oxytocin acts to constrict milk gland cells and push milk forward into the ducts that lead to the nipple. The nipple is surrounded by a darkly pigmented area of epithelium about 4 cm in diameter, termed the *areola*; the areola is rough appearing on the surface due to many sebaceous glands called *Montgomery's tubercles.*

The blood supply to the breasts is profuse, blood being supplied by thoracic branches of the axillary, internal mammary, and intercostal arteries. This effective blood supply is important in bringing nutrients to the milk glands and makes possible a plentiful supply of milk for breast-feeding. It also unfortunately aids in the metastasis of breast cancer if this is not discovered early by self breast examination.

A diagram of breast anatomy is shown in Figure 8-14.

Pelvic Bony Growth

In order for a baby to be delivered vaginally, it must be able to pass through the ring of pelvic bone. Pelvic bone growth must be sufficient, therefore, or the infant will be too large to be born except by cesarean birth. This is not a problem for the average woman; it may be a very real problem for the young adolescent girl who has not yet achieved full pelvic growth (girls under age 14 are most prone to this difficulty) or a woman who has had a pelvic injury.

Structure of the Pelvis

The pelvis serves both to support and to protect the reproductive and the other pelvic organs. It is a bony ring formed by four united bones: the two *innominate* (flaring hip) bones that form the anterior and lateral portion of the ring, and the coccyx and sacrum, which compose the posterior aspect (Figure 8-15).

Each innominate bone is divided into three parts: the ilium, the ischium, and the pubis. The *ilium* forms the upper and lateral portion. The flaring superior border of this bone is what forms the prominence of the hip (the crest of the ilium). The *ischium* is the inferior portion. At the lowest portion of the ischium are two projections, the *ischial tuberosities.* You sit on this portion of the bone. These projections are important markers to use in determining lower pelvic width. The *pubis* is the anterior portion of the innominate bone. The *symphysis pubis* is the junction of the innominate bones at the front of the pelvis.

The *sacrum,* or the upper posterior portion of the pelvic ring, is spoken of as one bone but actually is composed of five bones so tightly fused

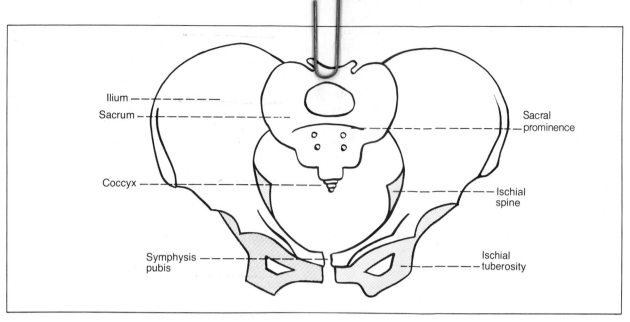

Figure 8-15 *Structure of the pelvis.*

together that they seem as one. There is a marked anterior projection of the sacrum at the point where it touches the lower lumbar vertebrae. This is the *sacral prominence,* a landmark to be identified when securing pelvic measurements.

The *coccyx,* just below the sacrum, is also composed of five very small bones fused together. Although it is stiff, there is a degree of movement possible in the joint between the sacrum and the coccyx (the *sacrococcygeal* joint). This is important because the movement permits the coccyx to be pressed backward, allowing more room for the fetal head as it passes through the bony pelvic ring at delivery.

For obstetrical purposes, the pelvis is further divided into the false pelvis (the superior half of it) and the true pelvis (the inferior half) (Figure 8-16). The *false pelvis* supports the uterus during the late months of pregnancy and aids in directing the fetus into the *true pelvis* for delivery. The false pelvis is divided from the true pelvis only by an imaginary line, the *linea terminalis.* This imaginary line is drawn from the sacral prominence at the back to the superior aspect of the symphysis pubis at the front of the pelvis. Above the line is the false pelvis; below it is the true pelvis.

Other important terms in relation to the pelvis are the inlet, the outlet, and the pelvic cavity. The *inlet* is the entranceway to the true pelvis or the upper ring of bone through which the fetus must first pass to deliver vaginally. It is the level of the linea terminalis or is marked by the sacral prominence in the back, the ilium on the sides, and the superior aspect of the symphysis pubis in the front. A view downward at the pelvic inlet shows that the passageway at this point appears heart-

shaped because of the jutting sacral prominence. It is wider transversely (sideways) than in the anteroposterior dimension.

The *outlet* is the inferior portion of the pelvis, or that portion bounded in the back by the coccyx, on the sides by the ischial tuberosities, and

Figure 8-16 *True and false pelvis. A. Linea terminalis (pelvic inlet). B. True conjugate diameter. C. Pelvic outlet. Portion above linea terminalis is false pelvis; portion below is true pelvis. Arrows show "stovepipe" curve that the fetus must follow to delivery.*

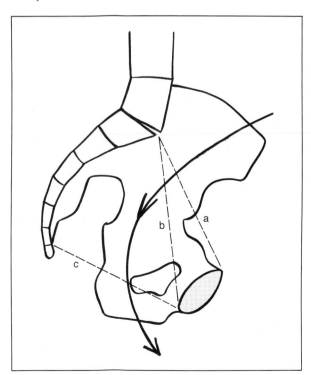

in the front by the inferior aspect of the symphysis pubis. In contrast to the inlet of the pelvis, the greatest diameter of the outlet is its anteroposterior diameter.

The *pelvic cavity* is the space between the inlet and the outlet. This space is not a straight passage but is curved like a stovepipe for an old-fashioned wood stove. The level of the ischial spines marks the *midplane,* or midpoint of the pelvis. This marker is used to assess the level to which the fetus has descended into the birth canal during labor and delivery.

In order to deliver vaginally, a fetus must follow a course of passing through the true pelvis or the inlet, then the pelvic cavity and the outlet of the pelvis. To enter the inlet, the fetus must present the widest head diameter to the transverse diameter of the pelvis, because that is the widest diameter at that level. The fetus must then move through the marked curve of the pelvic cavity. At the outlet, the fetus must turn to present the widest head diameter to the anteroposterior diameter of the pelvis, since that is the widest diameter of the pelvis at that level.

There are physiologic reasons for the design of the pelvis that leads to this much fetal accommodation. The curve slows and controls the speed of birth and therefore reduces sudden pressure changes on the fetal head, which might rupture cerebral arteries. The snugness of the cavity compresses the chest of the fetus while passing through, helping to expel lung fluid and mucus and thereby better prepare the lungs for good aeration at birth.

Pelvic Variations

It is impossible to predict from the outward appearance of a woman whether or not her pelvis is adequate for the passage of a fetus through its center. Some women look as if they have wide pelves but in reality only have wide ilial crests and a normal or even smaller than normal internal ring. Other women appear as if their pelvis will be small because the ilial crests are nonflaring, but the internal pelvis, the part that must be sufficiently large for childbirth, is of average size, and they give birth vaginally without difficulty. Differences in pelvic contour and development occur mainly because of hereditary factors, but disease (e.g., rickets, which may cause contraction of the pelvis), or injury (inadequate repair following an accident) may also play a role.

Types of Pelves

The types of pelves found in women can be categorized into four groups (Figure 8-17):

1. *Gynecoid* pelvis. This is the "normal" female pelvis. The inlet of this type is well rounded forward and back. The pubic arch is wide. This pelvic type is ideal for childbirth.
2. *Anthropoid* pelvis. In this pelvis (an ape-like one), the transverse diameter is narrow and the anteroposterior diameter of the inlet is larger than normal. This does not accommodate a fetal head as well as the gynecoid pelvis.
3. *Platypelloid* pelvis. In this pelvis (a flattened one), the inlet is an oval, smoothly curved, but the anteroposterior diameter is shallow. A fetal head would not be able to rotate to match the curves of the pelvic cavity in this type of pelvis.
4. *Android* pelvis, or "male" pelvis. The pubic arch in this type pelvis forms an acute angle, making the lower dimensions of the pelvis extremely narrow. A fetus has difficulty exiting from this type of pelvis.

Although any of these types of pelves may be adequate for childbearing, the gynecoid pelvis is the one designed for this function. As mentioned, a fetal head might have difficulty fitting into or passing through the other three types, particularly the android pelvis, because of its pointed, rather than rounded, aspects.

Assessment of Pelvic Size

Pelvic measurements are made to determine whether or not the normal vaginal route of delivery will be safe for both the infant and mother. Because an x-ray is not an acceptable technique to use early in pregnancy (it is a potential teratogen, or an agent harmful to the fetus), this information must be obtained manually or by sonogram.

Traditionally, manual pelvic measurements have been made by the physician or a nurse-midwife. There is no reason, however, that they cannot be made, recorded, and interpreted by any nurse who has learned the necessary techniques and appreciates the need for accurate measurements and correct interpretation of the findings.

External Measurements

External measurements of the pelvis, such as the measurement between the femur trochanters, once done routinely, offer so little information as to the size of the internal pelvic ring that they are no longer assessed.

Internal Measurements

Internal measurements give the actual diameters of the inlet and outlet through which the fetus must pass. The following measurements are the ones made most commonly:

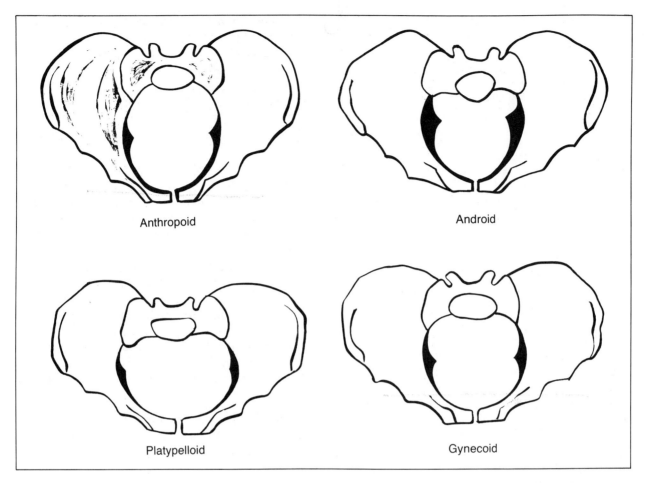

Figure 8-17 *Types of pelves.*

1. The <u>*diagonal conjugate.*</u> This is the distance between the anterior surface of the sacral prominence and the anterior surface of the inferior margin of the symphysis pubis (Figure 8-18). It is the most useful measurement for estimation of pelvic size, as it suggests the anteroposterior diameter of the pelvic inlet (the

Figure 8-18 *Measurement of diagonal conjugate diameter.*

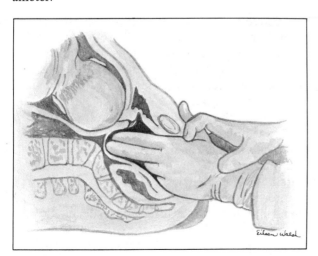

narrower diameter at that level or the one that may cause a misfit with the fetal head).

The diagonal conjugate is measured by asking the woman to lie in a lithotomy position. Introduce two fingers vaginally and press inward and upward until your middle finger touches the sacral prominence. With your other hand, mark the part of your examining hand where it touches the symphysis pubis. Withdraw your examining hand and measure the distance between the tip of your middle finger and the marked point on the glove on that hand by comparing it with a ruler or, for greater accuracy, a *pelvimeter*. If this measurement is more than 12.5 cm, the pelvic inlet is rated as adequate for childbirth (the diameter of the fetal head that must pass that point averages 9 cm in diameter). It is less time consuming for both the woman and health care personnel if the physician or nurse who initially performs the pelvic examination takes this measurement at the same time. Offer a fair warning that the measurement is slightly painful; the woman will feel the pressure of the examining finger as it stretches to touch the sacral prominence. If your hand is small with short

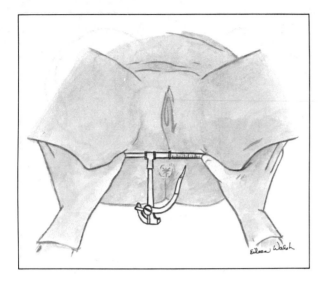

Figure 8-19 *Measurement of intertuberous diameter.*

Table 8-2 Common Pelvic Measurements

Measurement	Diameter (cm)
Diagonal conjugate	12.5
True conjugate	10.5 to 11
Ischial tuberosity	11

fingers, you may not be able to assess pelvic measurements manually because your fingers may not reach the sacral prominence.

2. The *true conjugate, or conjugate vera,* is the measurement between the anterior surface of the sacral prominence and the posterior surface of the inferior margin of the symphysis pubis. This measurement cannot be made directly, but it can be estimated from the measurement you made of the diagonal conjugate. To do this, substract the usual depth of the symphysis pubis (assumed to be 1.2 to 2 cm) from the diagonal conjugate measurement. The distance remaining will be the true conjugate, or the actual diameter of the pelvic inlet through which the fetal head must pass. The average true conjugate diameter is therefore 12.5 cm minus 1.5 or 2 cm, or 10.5 to 11.0 cm.

3. The *ischial tuberosity diameter.* This measurement is the distance between the ischial tuberosities, or the transverse diameter of the outlet (the narrowest diameter at that level or the one most apt to cause a misfit). It is made at the medial and lowermost aspect of the ischial tuberosities at the level of the anus (Figure 8-19). A Williams or Thomas pelvimeter is generally used, although it can be measured by a ruler or by comparing it to a known hand span or clenched fist measurement. A diameter of 11 cm is considered adequate because it will allow the narrowest diameter of the fetal head, or 9 cm, to pass freely through the outlet.

Pelvic measurements ordinarily taken for pelvic capacity assessment and the average diameters of these measurements are shown in Table 8-2.

Pituitary-Hypothalamus Maturity

In order for a person to be able to initiate ova or sperm formation, her or his pituitary-hypothalamic control of gonadotropic hormones must have reached maturity. The initiation and effect of these hormones are discussed in Chapter 9, along with the physiology of menstruation.

Utilizing Nursing Process

Most women and men have little knowledge about their reproductive organs. They speak vaguely about ovaries, "tubes," and "the womb," or "private organs" or "private parts." The fact that people refer to reproductive organs as "private parts" implies that it is more proper for them to know little about the function of these organs than to know a lot about them.

In order to understand why conception occurs, why some pregnancies are lost because of anatomic factors such as an incompetent cervix, why conception cannot occur in the presence of an illness such as endometriosis (abnormal endometrium formation), or what happens during labor

and delivery, women and their male partners need basic knowledge of where organs are located and what organs' primary functions are. In order to understand the therapy or nursing care planned for them, women with gynecologic disorders need the same information.

Women who attend preparation-for-childbirth classes learn about their reproductive anatomy so they can use their bodies effectively in childbirth and not struggle against natural processes. A nursing responsibility is to be an informed source of information about the anatomy and physiology important for childbearing and gynecologic and andrologic health. Such a store of information is necessary as well to allow you to use nursing process to make a thorough assessment of physical readiness for childbearing.

Assessment

Assessment of physical reproductive maturity is done by means of history, physical examination, and possibly sonogram or x-ray. X-ray of pelvic diameters may be performed at a pregnancy's term. As this is only done when a complication of pregnancy is present, this is discussed in Chapter 43.

Analysis

The fourth Annual Conference on Nursing Diagnoses did not accept any diagnoses specifically related to anatomic considerations. This is because nursing diagnoses always deal with problems that a nurse can manage: The nursing diagnosis would always be derived from the effect or secondary problem that arises from the anatomic problem, not the problem itself. Some examples of these might be, dissatisfaction with sexual enjoyment related to anatomic malformation, fear of frequent reproductive loss related to a uterine septum, or lessened self-esteem from inability to conceive related to vaginal anatomic defect.

Planning

Planning with the woman who does not have reproductive maturity or has an anatomic abnormality may involve some very difficult decisions if these problems have led to infertility. The diagnosis of infertility and implementations for problems of infertility are discussed in Chapter 12.

Implementation

If a sister or other family member of a woman had a large baby or another problem during pregnancy that prevented her from delivering vaginally, a woman may worry a great deal during pregnancy about a similar fate. Teach that each woman must be evaluated individually in respect to pelvic structure.

Evaluation

Assessment of pelvic measurements is only done once during a woman's first pregnancy unless the woman is injured in some way that would change her pelvic diameters. These measurements are constants. The fact that she has successfully given vaginal birth once is proof that her pelvis is adequate for childbearing (although fetal position and size may also compromise pelvis adequacy).

Nursing Care Planning

Illustrated below are two individualized nursing care plans related to reproductive readiness.

Christine McFadden
15 years
First prenatal visit; last menstrual period 16 weeks ago

Assessment

Menarche at 12 years; menstrual periods q 28–35 days, 5-day duration, mod. heavy. Cramping enough to keep her home from school 1 day/month.
Good health; no known kidney, heart, diabetes, tuberculosis, sexually transmitted disease; no abdominal surgery; no previous pregnancies (Gravida 1; Para 0).
Pelvic measurements:
Diagonal conjugate: 12 cm.
True conjugate, therefore: 10–10.5 cm.
Ischial tuberosities diameter: 11 cm.

Analysis

Questionable physical readiness for childbearing related to small pelvic measurements (T.D.C. only 10–10.5 cm).

Locus of Decision Making. Patient and mother.

Goal. Patient will accept possibility that vaginal delivery may not be possible due to narrow pelvic measurements.

Criteria. Patient will voice understanding of significance of pelvic diameter determination.

Nursing Orders

1. Mark chart for re-evaluation of pelvic measurements by nurse-midwife.
2. Mark chart for discussion of cesarean birth by twenty-eighth week of pregnancy if nurse-midwife confirms possible need.

Mary Kraft
23 years
First prenatal visit; last menstrual period 9 weeks ago.

Assessment

Menarche at 13 years; menstrual periods now 30–32 days, 6-day duration, heavy; painful cramping. Had infertility work-up during last year. Diagnosis of endometriosis and conservative abdominal surgery for removal of endometriosis implants done 2 months ago. Fully recovered in terms of energy and activity.

Overall health good although she is often "dead tired." No known kidney, heart, diabetes, tuberculosis, sexually transmitted disease. Had surgery for appendicitis (no sequelae) at 12 years. 1 previous pregnancy ending in spont. abortion at 3 months 2 years ago (no known cause). Gravida 2; Para 0.

Pelvic measurements (from old record of previous pregnancy):

Diagonal conjugate: 13.5 cm.

True conjugate, therefore: 11.5–12 cm.

Ischial tuberosities diameter: 11 cm.

Recent abdominal surgical scar appears well healed and strong.

Analysis

Physical readiness for childbearing related to adequate pelvic measurements.

Locus of Decision Making. Patient.

Goal. Patient to complete pregnancy within normal parameters.

Criteria. Patient will deliver vaginally at pregnancy term.

Nursing Orders

1. Inspect recent abdominal incision for stress at prenatal visits.
2. Ask nurse-midwife to stress physical capacity for normal pregnancy because of previous pregnancy loss.
3. Teach preparation for vaginal delivery.

Questions for Review

Multiple Choice

1. Mrs. Andrews is a woman you meet in a prenatal setting. If she has a gynecoid pelvis, this means
   a. the outlet is narrow.
   b. the symphysis pubis does not meet in front.
   c. the pubic arch forms an acute angle.
   d. the inlet is widest in its transverse diameter.

2. Mrs. Andrews is found to have a cystocele. This is
   a. an elongated cervix at the anterior angle.
   b. stenosis of the vagina.
   c. a pouching of the bladder into the vaginal wall.
   d. a cystic growth of the cervix.

3. Mrs. Williams notices a sharp pain in her lower right abdomen when she stands up suddenly. This is proboably a result of tension on which ligament?
   a. broad ligament
   b. round ligament
   c. cardinal ligament
   d. sacral-pubic ligament

4. Following reproductive tract surgery, assessment of urinary status is important. This is because
   a. the ureters pass just behind the uterine arteries.
   b. the ureters pass in front of the uterus.
   c. the bladder is also supplied by the uterine arteries.
   d. the bladder and the cervix surfaces touch.

5. Mrs. Williams asks how the uterine arteries will be able to supply blood to the uterus after the uterus increases to four times its prepregnant size. You would explain that this will happen because
   a. many more arteries form during pregnancy.
   b. the muscle of the uterus decreases during pregnancy.
   c. venous congestion causes stasis of arterial blood.
   d. the uterine vessels are normally twisted and coiled.

6. On pelvic measurements, Mrs. Williams' true conjugate is found to be 10 cm. This is
   a. larger than the average diameter.
   b. an average diameter.
   c. not an important diameter measurement.
   d. less than the average diameter.

7. Mrs. Andrews's daughter is 14 and has not yet menstruated. Which finding would lead you to believe that she is about to menstruate?
   a. She has pubic hair.
   b. She weighs 80 pounds.
   c. Her breast tissue is Tanner Stage I.
   d. She has periodic abdominal pain.

8. At puberty, which of the following statements is true of the action of testosterone in girls?
   a. It has no place in female reproductive development.
   b. It influences growth of axillary and pubic hair.
   c. It causes breast development.
   d. It initiates estrogen production.

9. Mrs. Williams's daughter has a retroverted uterus. This means
   a. the uterus is bent sharply backward at the cervix.
   b. the cervix is located behind the Douglas' cul-de-sac.
   c. the entire uterus is tipped backward.
   d. the uterus is anterior to the bladder.

10. You assess Mrs. Williams for pelvic adequacy by a vaginal exam. In a supine position, the course of the vagina is
    a. almost parallel with the bed surface.
    b. curved sharply downward.
    c. slanted downward and backward.
    d. slanted upward for 2 cm, then downward.

Discussion

1. Male and female reproductive organs are analogues of each other. What are the male analogues of the female organs?
2. What are the advantages of the unique curve and narrow diameters of the birth canal to the fetus? To the woman?
3. How would you explain the function of female reproductive organs to a sixth grade health education class?

Suggested Readings

Austin, J. M., Jr., et al. (1983). The Gravlee method: An alternative to the Pap smear? *American Journal of Nursing, 83,* 1057.

Bernhard, L. A. (1982). Endometriosis. *J.O.G.N. Nursing, 11,* 300.

Brown, M. A. (1982). Primary dysmenorrhea. *Nursing Clinics of North America, 17,* 145.

Dayani, E. (1979). Concepts of wellness. *Nursing Practitioner, 4,* 31.

Edelin, K. C. (1983). Evaluation of female pelvic pain. *Hospital Medicine, 19,* 32W.

Frisch, R. E., & Reville, R. (1970). Height and weight at menarche and a hypothesis of critical body weight and adolescent events. *Science, 169,* 397.

Goplerud, C. P. (1982). Urinary incontinence: An annoying problem in elderly women. *Consultant, 22,* 65.

Gorline, L. L., et al. (1982). What every nurse should know about vaginitis. *American Journal of Nursing, 82,* 1851.

Hammer, S. (1983). Anatomy of a difference: The sexes. *Health, 15,* 18.

Hornick, J. (1982). Evaluating menstrual dysfunction. *Patient Care, 16,* 12.

Marshall, W. A., & Tanner, J. M. (1969). Variations in the pattern of pubertal changes in boys. *Archives of Disease in Childhood, 44,* 291.

Marshall, W. A., & Tanner, J. M. (1970). Variations in the pattern of pubertal changes in boys. *Archives of Disease in Childhood, 45,* 13.

Pauerstein, C. J., & Eddy, C. A. (1983). How the tubes function. *Contemporary OB/GYN, 21,* 121.

Pagano, K. D., & Pagano, T. J. (1982). *Diagnostic testing and nursing implications.* St. Louis: Mosby.

Pritchard, J. A., & MacDonald, P. C. (1980). *Williams Obstetrics* (16th ed.). New York: Appleton-Century-Crofts.

Russo, J. R. (1980). Adolescent menstrual disorders. *Female Patient, 5,* 19.

Waxman, S. (1983). Sexually transmitted disease. *Topics in Emergency Medicine, 5,* 29.

9

The Physiology of Menstruation

The Menstrual Cycle
Menarche
Menopause (the Climacteric)
Menstrual Purpose and Length
Pituitary-Ovarian-Uterine Interplay

Education for Menstruation

Menstruation and Women's Health
Disorders that Cause Discomfort
Frequency Disorders
Infectious Disorders

Utilizing Nursing Process
Nursing Care Planning
Questions for Review
Suggested Readings

OBJECTIVES

Following mastery of the content of this chapter, you should be able to

1. Describe the relationship of the pituitary, ovary, and uterus in the initiation of a menstrual cycle.
2. Describe the phases of the menstrual cycle and the hormones important for their initiation.
3. Describe menstrual cycle disorders such as menorrhagia, dysmenorrhea, and premenstrual syndrome.
4. Analyze the role of menstrual physiology on women's health throughout the life span.
5. Synthesize the role of menstrual physiology with nursing process to achieve quality maternal-newborn nursing care.

IN ORDER TO UNDERSTAND how fertilization and growth of a new human being takes place, it is necessary to understand the physiology of a normal menstrual cycle, or the process that precedes fertilization. There is much misunderstanding among women about the purpose and events of a normal menstrual cycle. Teaching women about what is normal and how to evaluate and judge their menstrual health is a major teaching area in women's health care.

The Menstrual Cycle

A menstrual cycle can be defined as periodic uterine bleeding in response to cyclic hormonal changes. Such a cycle varies greatly in terms of the first and last cycle in a woman's lifetime.

Menarche

The term *menarche* is applied to the first menstruation period in girls. First menstruation occurs as one of a number of maturational changes that are associated with puberty: growth of axillary and pubic hair, broadening of the hips, breast development, and changes in endocrine functions. Although the average age for menarche is 12 to 13 years, it may occur as early as age 9 or as late as age 17 and still be within the range of normal (Barnett, 1977). Because it may occur as early as age 9, school nurses or nurses working in pediatric clinics or pediatricians' offices should routinely include health teaching information on menstruation as part of the care for girls—as early as the fourth-grade level—and for their parents. It is a poor introduction to sexuality and womanhood for a girl to begin menstruation unwarned and unprepared for the important internal function it represents.

Menopause (the Climacteric)

Menopause is the cessation of menstrual cycles. The *postmenopausal* period is the time of life following this change. *Perimenopausal* is a term used to denote the time period during which menopausal changes are taking place. Women have popularly called this time "change of life" because, when childbearing was perceived as their most important role, a cessation of that function did indeed mark a big change in their lives. An important health teaching measure for today is helping women appreciate that loss of uterine function may make almost no change in their lives, and for the woman with *dysmenorrhea* (painful menstruation) may even be a welcome change.

The age range at which menopause occurs is wide, between 40 and 55 years. The age of both menarche and menopause tends to be familial (if menarche occurred early in a mother, it will probably occur early in her daughter; if menopause began early in a mother, it may begin early in her daughter). The earlier the age of menarche, the earlier menopause tends to occur.

Whether women at menopause should be given estrogen supplements to limit or reduce the body changes they experience is controversial: Long-term administration of estrogen has been implicated in the development of uterine cancer. Very low doses of estrogen (administered as Premarin) apparently do not have this effect and may be administered to prevent osteoporosis. The drug is cycled (taken for the first 25 days of each month, then not taken for the remainder of the month) to simulate a premenopausal pattern. Progestin supplementation for the last 10 days of the cycle and daily calcium supplementation may be also advised. This type of supplementation does not increase the risk of breast cancer; however, it has been associated with an increase in risk of endometrial adenocarcinoma and gallbladder disease from gallstone formation (Utian, 1980).

High parity and high socioeconomic status

tend to delay menopause. The climacteric tends to occur early in women who smoke cigarettes.

Menopause is an event marked by ambivalence in most women. Although they may feel fine about being finished with menstrual periods and being free of the concern about unexpected pregnancies, they also may feel "old" because of the loss of a function that so dramatically marked their coming of age.

Menopause occurs as the ovaries become less and less influenced by pituitary hormones. Due to this, the level of estrogen production by the ovaries decreases, as does follicle formation. Since estrogen production by the adrenal glands continues after that of the ovaries decreases, the woman is not without estrogen; she merely has less of it. The type of estrogen produced by the adrenal glands, called *estriol*, is characteristic of postmenopausal women.

Typical symptoms of decreasing estrogen levels are "hot flashes," or sweating and flushing of the face caused by surges of GN-RH. The uterus and vagina reduce in size, and vaginal secretions diminish. The woman may be aware of this change because the resulting vaginal dryness and loss of rugae may make sexual coitus painful. Just as estrogen added to fat deposition at puberty, the loss of estrogen causes fat deposits to be reabsorbed, leading to loss of breast firmness and generally reduced tone. Estrogen at puberty aids bone growth; lowered amounts of estrogen may lead to *osteoporosis*, or bone demineralization. Slender Caucasian women who smoke and have a family history of osteoporosis tend to be at highest risk to develop this disorder (Utian, 1980).

Maintaining an exercise program as well as a high calcium intake is apparently helpful in reducing the process of osteoporosis.

Menstrual Purpose and Length

The purpose of a menstrual cycle is to bring an ovum to maturity and renew a uterine tissue bed that will be responsive to its growth should it be fertilized. The length of menstrual cycles differs from woman to woman, but the accepted average length is 28 days (from the beginning of one menstrual flow to the beginning of the next). However, it is not unusual for cycles to be as short as 20 days or as long as 45.

The length of the average menstrual flow (termed *menses*) is 5 to 7 days, although women may have periods as short as 1 day or as long as 9 days. Because there is such variation in the times that menarche and menopause occur and such variation in length, frequency, and amount of menstrual flow, many women have questions about what is "normal." Contact with health care personnel during a pregnancy or a yearly health examination is often the first opportunity they have to find answers to questions they have had in mind for some time. When you ask a possibly pregnant woman, "When was your last menstrual period?" her answer may be, "I'm awfully irregular," or, "I wish my body did things like the books say," instead of a date. Pregnancy care presents an opportunity for this woman to learn more about her body; ideally, she would also learn to be more comfortable with herself and the way her life is subtly influenced by periodic surges and declines of hormones.

Pituitary-Ovarian-Uterine Interplay

Four body structures are involved in the physiology of the menstrual cycle: the hypothalamus, the pituitary gland, the ovaries, and the uterus. In order for a menstrual cycle to be complete, all four structures must fulfill their roles; if any of these structures is inactive an incomplete or ineffective cycle will result (Figure 9-1).

Hypothalamus

The hypothalamus initiates a menstrual cycle by the release of gonadotropin-releasing hormone. Estrogen represses the release of this hormone. During childhood, the hypothalamus is apparently so sensitive to the small amount of estrogen

Figure 9-1 *The interaction of pituitary-uterine-ovarian functions in a menstrual cycle.*

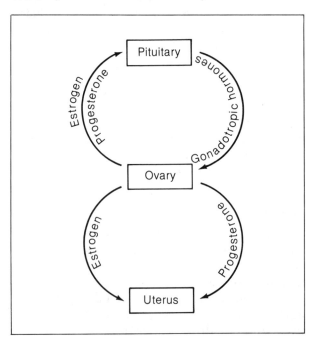

produced by the adrenal gland that this gonadotropic stimulation activity is suppressed. Beginning with puberty—as soon as the hypothalamus has sensed that a sufficient body mass is present—it becomes less sensitive to estrogen feedback; the result is the transmission every month in females of a gonadotropin-releasing hormone (GN-RH)—sometimes abbreviated LH-RH for luteinizing hormone-releasing hormone—from the hypothalamus to the anterior pituitary gland. GN-RH signals the anterior pituitary gland to begin production of gonadotropic hormones.

Diseases of the hypothalamus causing deficiency of this releasing factor result in delayed adolescence. Diseases causing early activation of the releasing factor lead to abnormally early sexual development or precocious puberty. When hormones secreted by the ovary such as estrogen and progesterone rise in amount each month, they create a feedback mechanism that halts production of the releasing factor for the remainder of the month. This inhibition also occurs when high levels of anterior pituitary–based hormones such as prolactin, follicle-stimulating hormone, or luteinizing hormone are present. The cyclic production of gonadotropin-releasing hormone in females is the reason menstrual periods cycle.

One of the most exciting advances in reproductive health today is the ability to produce GN-RH synthetically. Many women who are infertile due to anovulation may be helped with such injections. A contraceptive technique of the future may be the injection of a GN-RH antagonist.

Pituitary Gland

Under the influence of GN-RH, the anterior lobe of the pituitary gland (the *adenohypophysis*) produces two hormones that, by acting on the ovaries, further affect the menstrual cycle. *Follicle-stimulating hormone* (FSH), a hormone that is active early in a cycle, is responsible for maturation of the ovum. *Luteinizing hormone* (LH), which becomes most active at the midpoint of the cycle, is responsible for ovulation or release of the mature egg cell from the ovary and growth of the uterine lining during the second half of the menstrual cycle (Figure 9-2).

Two other hormones produced by the pituitary gland, prolactin and oxytocin, are important for childbearing. *Prolactin* is produced by the anterior pituitary. A feedback effect of prolactin can suppress hypothalamus activity and therefore initiation of GN-RH. This feedback mechanism becomes very active in women who maintain strenuous physical training programs and can totally suppress menstruation in such women. The

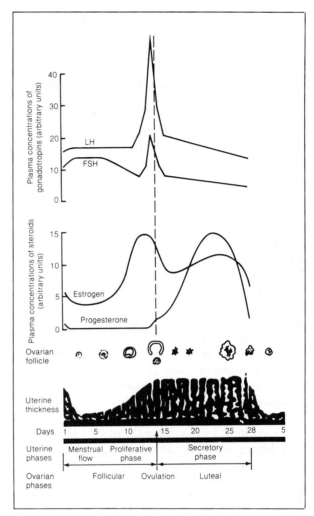

Figure 9-2 *Summary of plasma hormone concentrations, ovarian events, and uterine changes during the menstrual cycle. Reproduced with permission from Arthur J. Vander; James H. Sherman; and Dorothy S. Luciano.* Human Physiology. The Mechanisms of Body Function, *3rd ed. New York: McGraw-Hill, 1980.*

main effect of prolactin, however, is signaled by its name, which means "before milk": prolactin levels increase in response to the drop of estrogen in the blood following childbirth, which initiates milk production in breast glands.

The posterior pituitary (the *neurohypophysis*) produces *oxytocin*, a hormone that is important for the contraction of smooth muscle. Oxytocin levels increase during labor, which helps maintain uterine contractions and achieve a vaginal birth.

Ovaries

Under the influence of FSH and LH—called *gonadotropic* hormones because they cause growth (trophia) in the gonads (ovaries)—each month one ovum matures in one or the other ovary and is discharged.

Division of Reproductive Cells (Gametes).

At birth, each ovary contains about 2 million immature ova (*oocytes*), which were formed during the first 5 months of intrauterine life. Although these cells have the unique ability to produce a new individual, they contain the usual cell components: a cell membrane, an area of clear cytoplasm, and a nucleus containing chromosomes.

They differ from all other body cells in that they contain only half the usual number of chromosomes. They have this lessened number so that when an ovum and spermatozoon combine (fertilization), the new individual formed from them will have the normal number of 46 chromosomes. There is a difference in the way reproductive cells divide that causes the change in chromosome number.

Cells in the body, such as skin cells, undergo cell division by *mitosis*, or daughter cell division. In this type of division, all the chromosomes are reduplicated in each new cell just prior to cell division: Every new cell has the same number of chromosomes as the original parent cell. Oocytes and immature spermatozoa (spermatocytes) divide in intrauterine life by one *mitotic* division. Division activity then appears to halt until at least puberty, when a second type of cell division, *meiosis* (cell reduction division) occurs. In meiosis, the new cells formed contain only half the number of chromosomes as the original parent cell. In the male, this reduction division occurs just before the spermatozoa mature. In the female, it occurs just before ovulation. Following this division, ova have 22 autosomes and an X sex chromosome; a spermatozoon has 22 autosomes and either an X or a Y sex chromosome. A new individual formed from the union of an ovum and an X-carrying spermatozoon will be female (an XX chromosome pattern); an individual formed from the union of an ovum and a Y-carrying spermatozoon will be male (an XY chromosome pattern).

Maturation of Oocytes.

Each oocyte lies in the ovary surrounded by a protective sac, or thin layer of cells, called a *follicle*. The oocyte in this underdeveloped state is called a *primordial follicle*. The maturation of these primitive follicles appears to stop about the fifth month of intrauterine life. The majority never develop beyond the primitive state and actually atrophy. By 7 years of age there are only about 500,000 present in each ovary; by 22 years, there are about 300,000; by

menopause, or the end of the fertile period in females, none are left (all have either matured or atrophied). The point at which no functioning oocytes remain in the ovaries, is one definition of menopause.

Ovulation.

During the fertile period of a woman's life (from menarche to menopause), each month one of the primordial follicles is activated by FSH and begins to grow and mature. Its follicle cells (*theca* cells) produce a clear fluid containing a high content of estrogen (mainly estradiol) and some progesterone. The fluid is termed *follicular liquor* or *follicular fluid*. The structure grows in size, propelling itself toward the surface of the ovary as it develops. It becomes visible on the surface of the ovary as a clear water blister about ¼ to ½ inch across. At this stage of maturation, the small ovum (barely visible to the naked eye, about the size of a printed period), with its surrounding follicle cells and fluid, is termed a *graafian follicle*.

The ovum is at first attached to the edge of the follicle by a thin strand of cells; later, it floats free in the fluid. By the fourteenth day before the end of a menstrual cycle (the midpoint of a typical 28-day cycle), the ovum has divided by a mitotic division into two separate bodies; a primary oocyte, which contains the bulk of the cytoplasm, and a secondary oocyte, which contains so little cytoplasm it is not functional. The structure also has accomplished a meiotic division, or has reduced its number of chromosomes to its haploid number of 23 (haploid means "having only one member of a pair").

Following an upsurge of luteinizing hormone from the pituitary and local production of a prostaglandin, the graafian follicle ruptures. The ovum is set free from the surface of the ovary, a process termed *ovulation*. It is swept into the open end of a fallopian tube. Women should be taught that ovulation occurs on the fourteenth day prior to the onset of the next cycle. Because ovulation happens at the midpoint of a 28-day cycle, many women mistakenly believe that the midpoint of their cycle will be the time of ovulation. If the cycle is only 20 days long, however, their day of ovulation would be the sixth day, not the tenth or middle day. If a cycle was 45 days long, ovulation would occur on the thirty-first day, not the twenty-second or midpoint.

After the ovum and the follicular fluid have been discharged from the ovary, the cells of the follicle still remain in the form of a hollow, empty pit. FSH has done its work at this point and its levels decrease while the second pituitary hormone takes over. Luteinizing hormone acts on the follicle cells of the ovary, causing them to produce, instead of follicular fluid, which was high in estrogen with some progesterone, a bright yellow fluid, *lutein*, which is high in progesterone with some estrogen. This yellow fluid fills the empty follicle, which is then termed a *corpus luteum* (yellow body).

The basal body temperature of a woman drops slightly (1°F) just before the day of ovulation, because of the extremely low level of progesterone present at that time. It rises at least 1°F the day following ovulation, because of the concentration of progesterone (which is thermogenetic) that is present at that time. The woman's temperature remains at this increased level until about the twenty-fourth day of the menstrual cycle, when progesterone level again decreases.

If conception (fertilization by a spermatozoon) occurs as the ovum proceeds down a fallopian tube and the fertilized ovum implants on the endometrium of the uterus, the corpus luteum will remain throughout the major portion of the pregnancy, reaching peak production of progesterone at about the sixteenth to twentieth week. If conception does not occur, the unfertilized ovum atrophies after 4 or 5 days, and the corpus luteum (called a "false" corpus luteum) will then remain for only about 8 to 10 days. As the corpus luteum regresses, it is gradually replaced by white fibrous tissue. The resulting structure is termed a *corpus albicans* (white body).

Uterus

Stimulation from the hormones produced by the ovaries causes specific monthly effects on the uterus.

First Phase of Menstrual Cycle. Immediately following a menstrual flow (the first 4 or 5 days of a cycle), the *endometrium*, or lining of the uterus, is very thin, only about one cell layer in depth. As the ovary begins to form estrogen (in the follicular fluid, under the direction of FSH), the endometrium begins to proliferate, or grow very rapidly, increasing in thickness about eightfold. This increase continues for the first half of the menstrual cycle (from about the fifth to the fourteenth day). This half of a menstrual cycle is termed interchangeably the *proliferative, estrogenic, follicular,* or *postmenstrual* phase.

Second Phase of Menstrual Cycle. Following ovulation, the formation of progesterone in the corpus luteum (under the direction of LH) causes the glands of the uterine endometrium to become corkscrewed or twisted in appearance and

dilated with quantities of glycogen and mucin, an elementary sugar and protein. The capillaries of the endometrium increase in number until the lining takes on the appearance of rich, spongy velvet. This second phase of the menstrual cycle is called the *progestational, luteal, premenstrual,* or *secretory* phase.

Ischemic Phase of Menstrual Cycle. What occurs next in a menstrual cycle depends on whether the released ovum meets and is fertilized by a spermatozoon. As indicated, if fertilization does not take place, the corpus luteum in the ovary begins to regress after 8 to 10 days. As it regresses, the production of progesterone and estrogen decreases. With the withdrawal of progesterone stimulation, the endometrium of the uterus begins to degenerate (at about the twenty-fourth to twenty-fifth day of the cycle). The capillaries rupture, with minute hemorrhages, and the endometrium sloughs off.

The Menses. Blood from the ruptured capillaries—along with mucin from the glands, fragments of endometrial tissue, and the microscopic, atrophied, and unfertilized ovum—is discharged from the uterus as the menstrual flow, or *menses*. This is actually the end of a menstrual cycle, but because it is the only external marker of the cycle, the first day of menstrual flow is used to mark the beginning of a new cycle. A typical 28-day menstrual cycle and the times when hormones are secreted at peak levels are shown diagrammatically in Figure 9-3.

Characteristics of a menstrual flow are reviewed in Table 9-1. Contrary to common belief, a menstrual flow contains only about 25 to 50 ml of blood; it seems more because of the accompanying mucus and endometrial shreds. The blood does not clot, because when the capillaries of the endometrium first ruptured, the blood clotted almost immediately and then liquefied by fibrinolytic activity. Once blood has clotted and liquefied, it will not clot again. The iron loss in a menstrual flow is about 11 mg, enough that many women need to take a daily iron supplement in order to prevent becoming iron depleted during their menstruating years.

In perimenopausal women, menses may typically be a few days of spotting prior to a heavy flow, or heavy flow followed by a few days of spotting as progesterone withdrawal is more sluggish or "staircases" rather than withdraws smoothly.

Cervical Changes. The mucus of the uterine cervix changes each month during the menstrual cycle as does the uterine body lining. During the

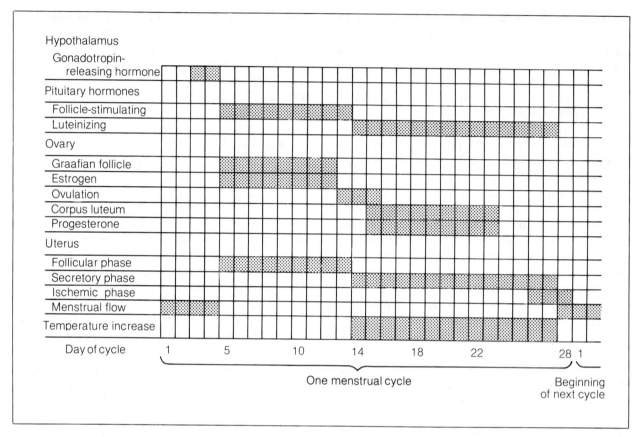

Figure 9-3 *Menstrual cycle of 28 days.*

first half of the cycle, when hormone secretion from the ovary is low, cervical mucus is thick and scant. If you place a drop of it between your finger and thumb and then draw them apart, the mucus will not form a thread but will break at only about a 1-cm distance. If a drop of mucus is placed on a slide, allowed to dry, and then examined under a microscope, it reveals a nondescript pattern. Mucus produced during the first half of the menstrual cycle contains many leukocytes; sperm survival in this type of mucus is poor.

At the time of ovulation, cervical mucus becomes thin and copious, similar in feel to fresh egg white. Its ability to thread or spin is called *spinnbarkeit*, which is so great at this time that the mucus will thread to a distance of 13 to 15 cm before breaking. If this mucus is dried and examined under a microscope, its form resembles miniature fossilized ferns. This pattern is due to sodium and water, which are concentrated in response to high estrogen levels. No leukocytes are present; sperm penetration and survival at the time of ovulation in this thin mucus (termed *type E*) is excellent.

As progesterone becomes the major influencing hormone during the second half of the cycle,

Table 9-1 Characteristics of Normal Menstrual Cycles

Beginning (menarche)	Average age of onset 12 or 13 years; average range of age 9 to 17 years
Interval between cycles	Average 28 days; cycles of 20 to 45 days not unusual
Duration of menstrual flow	Average flow 3 to 7 days; ranges of 1 to 9 days not abnormal
Amount of menstrual flow	Difficult to estimate; average 25 to 50 ml per menstrual period; saturating a pad or tampon in less than an hour is heavy bleeding
Color of menstrual flow	Dark red; a combination of blood, mucus, and endometrial cells
Odor of menstrual flow	Odor of marigolds

Table 9-2 Cervical Changes During the Menstrual Cycle

Assessment Criteria	48 Hours Preovulation	Day of Ovulation	48 Hours Postovulation
Cervical mucus		Type E	Type G
Viscosity	High (thick)	Low (thin)	High (thick)
Quantity	Scant	Copious	Scant
Spinnbarkeit	Little (1 cm)	Extreme (15 cm)	Limited (3 cm)
Leukocytes	Many	None	Moderate
Sperm survival	Little	Excellent	Limited
Fern test	Atypical pattern	Ferning pattern	Negative for ferning
pH	Acid (under 7.0)	Alkaline (7.5)	Acid (under 7.0)

cervical mucus again becomes thick. It loses its property of spinnbarkeit and its ability to fern. Leukocytes are again present; sperm survival is again poor. Mucus at this time is termed *type G.*

The changes in cervical mucus are helpful in establishing fertility. No change in cervical mucus implies that ovulation has not yet occurred. Being aware that such changes take place with ovulation allows women to plan sexual coitus to coincide with ovulation, thus making pregnancy more likely. They will also be able to avoid sexual coitus at the time of ovulation to prevent pregnancy (the natural method of reproductive life planning). Cervical changes are summarized in Table 9-2.

Education for Menstruation

Early preparation for menstruation is important for future childbearing and for a girl's concept of herself as a woman (Figure 9-4). A girl who is told that menstruation is a normal function that occurs every month in all healthy women has a better attitude toward menstruation and toward herself than a girl who wakes one morning to find blood on her pajamas and receives an explanation, "You'd better get used to that. You're going to have to put up with it for the rest of your life." In the first instance, the girl can trust her body; it is doing what every woman's body does. In the second instance, her body is out of control. How can she accept and enjoy growing up if it involves something so unpredictable? In the first instance, menstruation is a mark of pride, of growing up. In the second, it is bothersome and bad; being a woman who menstruates is being second-rate.

Girls who are well prepared for menstruation and view it as a positive happening tend to have fewer episodes of painful cramps and missed school days than those who view it as an ill time. They become better role models of productive women. In defense of some mothers, however, *endometriosis,* a condition that causes menstrual cramping, is familial or occurs at a higher incidence in some families than in others. A mother who has had a history of painful menstruation (dysmenorrhea) may have a difficult time presenting a positive outlook on this life change. Important teaching points regarding menstruation for girls at menarche are shown in Table 9-3. Terms related to menstruation are summarized in Table 9-4.

A woman's overall outlook on menstruation and whether she views it as a healthy function are often reflected by the terms she uses to describe it. "The curse" certainly tends to have a negative connotation. Her inability even to put a name on the happening—"when you-know-what happens. . . "—may indicate a feeling of dirtiness or uncleanliness (something ladies don't talk about any more than they do dust under beds).

Listening to the names used to describe men-

Figure 9-4 *Education about menstruation is an important role for nurses in women's health care. Here a school nurse answers an adolescent's questions on reproduction.*

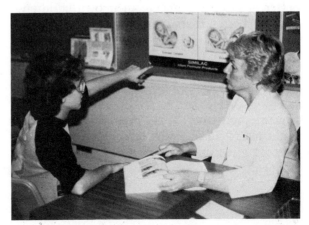

Table 9-3 Teaching Menstrual Health

Area of Concern	Teaching Points
Exercise	Moderate exercise is good to continue during menses. Excess exercise can cause amenorrhea.
Sexual relations	Not contraindicated during menses. Heightened sexual arousal may be noticed during menses. Orgasm may increase menstrual flow.
Activities of daily living	Nothing is contraindicated. (Many people believe washing hair or having a permanent is harmful.)
Pain relief	Any mild analgesic is helpful. Prostaglandin inhibitors are specific for menstrual pain. Applying heat and abdominal breathing are also helpful.
Rest	More rest may be helpful if dysmenorrhea interferes with sleep at night.
Nutrition	Many women need iron supplementation to replace iron lost in menses. Eating pickles or cold food does not cause dysmenorrhea.

Table 9-4 Terms of Menstrual Physiology

Amenorrhea	Absence of menstruation
Catamenia	Menstruation
Hypomenorrhea	Scant amount of menstrual flow
Menopause	Cessation of ovarian function; the last menstrual period
Menorrhagia	Excessively heavy menstrual flow
Menstruation	Periodic discharge of bloody fluid representing the sloughing of the uterine lining from a nonpregnant uterus
Menses	Menstruation
Metrorrhagia	Vaginal bleeding between menstrual flow periods
Mittelschmerz	Lower-quadrant pain in the midmenstrual cycle at the time of ovulation
Oligomenorrhea	Infrequent menstrual flows

These health concerns need time and attention equal to that given other areas by concerned health care providers.

Menstrual problems generally fall into three categories: those resulting in painful or uncomfortable menstruation, those resulting in menses that is either too frequent or too far apart, and infection associated with menses.

Disorders that Cause Discomfort

Mittelschmerz

In some women, abdominal pain results from the release of the ovum from the follicle with ovulation, the release of accompanying prostaglandins, or perhaps irritation caused by a drop or two of follicular fluid or blood in the abdominal cavity. For many women this pain is only a few sharp cramps; other women experience hours of discomfort. The pain is typically one-sided, occurring in one of the lower quadrants of the abdomen (near an ovary). Occasionally it is accompanied by scant vaginal spotting.

Women may need assurance of the innocence of this pain; it may even be advantageous for them, as it clearly marks their day of ovulation. Young girls may be worried that pain in the right lower quadrant is a symptom of appendicitis. However, the lack of associated symptoms (such as nausea, vomiting, and fever), the coincidental timing at the point of ovulation in a menstrual cycle, and the pain's short duration all help to

strual happenings may give you a clue as to how the woman will be able to discuss problems related to a pregnancy: She cannot describe vaginal discharge as a danger sign of pregnancy, for example, if she thinks it is improper to use the term *vaginal*. If she views menstrual flows negatively, how is she going to regard the vaginal discharge she has after a baby is born? Helping women to feel comfortable with their bodies and their physiologic changes each month better prepares them to monitor their own health. They are then in a better position to educate their own children—perhaps better than they were educated themselves.

Menstruation and Women's Health

Because menstruation is a process that is present for at least half of a woman's life, it plays a significant role in the way she thinks about herself. Because a woman's cycle can be a major influence on her daily activities, problems in this area of health are never to be taken lightly: They are not just "something that women have to live with."

differentiate mittelschmerz from other types of abdominal pain.

Dysmenorrhea

Dysmenorrhea is painful menstruation. For generations, dysmenorrhea was thought to be mainly psychological, with no treatment needed other than reassurance of normality. Today it is recognized as the result of prostaglandin (primarily F_2) secretion, which occurs in response to the tissue destruction of the ischemic phase of the menstrual cycle. F_2 causes smooth muscle contraction of organs such as the uterus; the muscle contraction compresses uterine arteries and leads to cell ischemia. Dysmenorrhea can also be a symptom of an underlying illness such as pelvic inflammatory disease, uterine myomas, or endometriosis (abnormal formation of endometrial tissue). Dysmenorrhea is *primary* if no underlying disease condition is present; *secondary* if an accompanying factor such as endometriosis exists.

As many as 80 percent of women have discomfort with menstruation; about 10 percent have enough discomfort to interfere seriously with normal daily plans (Wilson, 1984). Some women notice a bloated feeling and light cramping 24 hours prior to menstrual flow. Pain is mainly noticed, however, with the beginning of the menstral flow. A colicky or sharp cyclic pain is superimposed on a dull, nagging ache across the lower abdomen. Another symptom can be an "aching," or "pulling" sensation of the vulva and inner thighs. Some women have mild diarrhea with the abdominal cramping. Mild breast tenderness, abdominal distention, nausea and vomiting, headache and facial flushing may also be present.

These symptoms can generally be controlled by a common analgesic such as acetosalicylic acid (aspirin). Acetosalicylic acid is a mild prostaglandin inhibitor. Some women are reluctant to take aspirin because they have heard that it interferes with blood coagulation. Fearing an increase in blood loss, they instead take acetaminophen (Tylenol), which does not have a prostaglandin inhibitor effect. A major breakthrough in the relief of menstrual discomfort is the discovery of mefenamic acid (Ponstel), a strong prostaglandin inhibitor. Women with extreme menstrual pain may be treated effectively with this drug. It should be taken with meals because it causes gastrointestinal irritation, and not begun in anticipation of menses but actually with menses as it is potentially teratogenic if pregnancy should be present. Low-dose oral contraceptives to prevent ovulation may also be an effective solution if pregnancy is not desired, though women must

consider the possible negative effects of long-term estrogen administration before using this solution.

Decreasing sodium intake for a few days prior to an expected menstrual flow by omitting salty foods such as potato chips, pretzels, ham and lunch meats, and not adding salt to food at the table may help relieve women who feel "bloated" because of water retention prior to menstruation.

Abdominal breathing (breathing in and out slowly, allowing the abdominal wall to rise with each inhalation) may also be helpful. Applying heat to the abdomen with a heating pad or by taking a hot shower or tub bath may relax muscle tension and relieve pain. Caution young girls to apply heat to their abdomen for abdominal pain only if a menstrual flow is present, not in anticipation of one: Heat applied to an inflamed appendix can cause rupture of the appendix and life-threatening peritonitis. Abdominal massage (effleurage, or very light massage) may feel soothing; resting more than usual tends to relieve vulvar pain. Women who remain sexually active during their menses may discover that orgasm helps relieve pelvic engorgement and therefore lessens cramping.

During the first 1 or 2 years after menarche, dysmenorrhea rarely occurs, probably because early menstrual cycles may be anovulatory. As ovulation begins, so does typical menstrual discomfort, reaching a peak from age 20 to 30. If there is some consolation in dysmenorrhea, then, it is that it usually signifies ovulation.

Menorrhagia

Menorrhagia is an abnormally heavy menstrual flow. It may occur in girls close to puberty and in women nearing menopause because of anovulatory cycles. As ovulation does not occur, progesterone secretion does not occur and therefore estrogen secretion continues to cause extreme proliferation of endometrium. Discharge of this excessive endometrium causes the heavy menses. There is often an unusual amount of flow in women using intrauterine devices (IUDs).

Women who have just discontinued oral contraceptives may misinterpret a normal menstrual flow as excessive when compared to the limited flow they had been experiencing. Heavy flow may indicate endometriosis (abnormal endometrium formation), a systemic disease (anemia), a blood dyscrasia such as a clotting defect, or a uterine abnormality such as the presence of a myoma (fibroid tumor). It can also be a symptom of infection, such as pelvic inflammatory disease (PID), or an indication of early pregnancy loss occurring coincidentally at the time of an expected menstrual flow.

It is difficult to assess what a heavy flow is, but asking a woman to estimate how long it takes her to saturate a sanitary napkin or tampon provides a gross estimate of the amount of flow. A sanitary napkin or tampon holds about 25 ml of fluid. Saturating a pad or tampon in less than an hour is a heavy flow; this should not continue at that rate for more than the first 2 hours.

The causes of menorrhagia should be investigated. Such excessive iron loss can occur that women need to be maintained on iron supplements to achieve sufficient hemoglobin formation. A woman who is losing excessive blood due to anovulatory cycles may be administered progesterone during the luteal phase of her cycle to prevent proliferative growth. Perimenopausal women are in an age bracket with a high risk for the development of uterine carcinoma, which often presents with increased vaginal bleeding: They should be carefully evaluated for causes of menorrhagia.

Metrorrhagia

Metrorrhagia is bleeding between menstrual periods. It can occur as a normal process in some women, who have spotting at the time of ovulation (mittelstaining). It may occur in women for the first 3 or 4 months they take oral contraceptives (breakthrough bleeding). Vaginal irritation from infection might lead to midcycle spotting. Spotting may also represent a temporary low level of progesterone production and endometrial sloughing (dysfunctional uterine bleeding or a luteal phase defect), a condition that tends to occur in women nearing the end of their reproductive years.

If metrorrhagia occurs for more than one menstrual cycle and the woman is not on oral contraceptives, she should be referred to a physician for examination, particularly if she is over 30 years of age. Vaginal bleeding is also an early sign of uterine carcinoma or ovarian cysts.

Endometriosis

Endometriosis is the presence of uterine endometrial cells outside the uterus, often in the cul-de-sac of the peritoneal cavity, on the uterine ligaments, and on the ovaries. This abnormal implantation of tissue is due to excessive endometrial production and a reflux of menstrual blood and tissue through the fallopian tubes at the time of the menstrual flow. As many as 25 percent of women in the United States have endometriosis (Fayez, 1983). The disorder tends to have a familial pattern, with both mothers and daughters affected.

The excessive production of endometrial tissue may be related to a deficient immunologic response. In many women it appears to be related to excessive estrogen production or a failed luteal menstrual phase. Many women with endometriosis do not ovulate or ovulate irregularly, and therefore estrogen secretion continues through the cycle rather than becoming secondary in production to progesterone late in the cycle, as happens in ovulating women. This proliferation of tissue makes it more prone to reflux through the fallopian tubes.

Endometriosis can lead to dysmenorrhea because the abnormal tissue responds to estrogen and progesterone stimulation as if it were intrauterine. At the time of menstruation, it sloughs in the same way as the tissue inside the uterus, which causes inflammation of surrounding tissue and an even greater release of prostaglandins. Tissue present in the pelvic cul-de-sac may cause dyspareunia (painful sexual coitus) because of pressure on the posterior vagina. Infertility can result from fallopian tube blockage by implants or by adhesions that immobilize the tubes and prevent tube peristalsis and ova transport.

Endometriosis then may be either a cause or a symptom of infertility in women. In any event, it is a perplexing disorder. It is always difficult to explain to women why overproduction of uterine tissue leads to infertility; it seems as if overproduction should make them more fertile. The diagnosis, staging, and treatment of this menstrual cycle abnormality and its relation to infertility is discussed in Chapter 12.

Premenstrual Syndrome (PMS)

Premenstrual syndrome refers to a cluster of symptoms that occur just before the menses and disappear with menstrual flow. In order to be diagnostic, identical symptoms should occur in three consecutive cycles; a symptom free stage postmenses should last a minimum of 7 days (Wilson, 1984). As many as 30 percent of women notice some of these symptoms; some women find them incapacitating. They become most acute about age 30 (Dalton 1977). Although the syndrome was described as early as 1931, its official recognition—encouraged by the successful use of PMS as a legal defense for manslaughter in England—has occurred only recently. As many as 80 percent of the violent crimes performed by women are committed just prior to menstruation; PMS is apparently related to this phenomenon (Lauerson, 1983).

PMS may occur due to the withdrawal of progesterone just prior to the menses. Other related causes may be vitamin B complex deficiency leading to estrogen excess, making the ratio of es-

Table 9-5 Premenstrual Tension Syndrome Classification

Classification	Characteristics	Therapies
PMT-A	Premenstrual anxiety, irritability, and nervous tension; behavior patterns detrimental to self, family, and society Elevated blood estrogen and low progesterone Excessive consumption of dairy products Magnesium deficiency	Vitamin B_6 at 200–800 mg/day Progesterone therapy Limit intake of dairy products to two servings per day Increase outdoor exercise
PMT-H	Water and salt retention, abdominal bloating, mastalgia, and weight gain Elevated serum aldosterone May be deficient in vitamin B_6 and magnesium May have elevated prostaglandin E_2	Vitamin B_6 at 200–800 mg/day suppresses aldosterone → diuresis and clinical improvement Vitamin E (600 units) reduces breast symptoms Curtail methylxanthines (coffee, tea, chocolate, and cola) and nicotine Restrict sodium intake to 3 gm/day Limit refined sugar to 5 tbsp/day Prostaglandin inhibitors may provide relief
PMT-C	Premenstrual craving for sweets, increased appetite and food binges followed by palpitation, fatigue, fainting spells, headache, and "the shakes" Altered glucose tolerance Deficiency of prostaglandin E_1 May be deficient in B vitamins, zinc, vitamin C, and magnesium	Restrict refined sugar to 5 tbsp/day Limit alcohol Limit sodium to 3 gm/day ↓ Animal fats to reduce formation of prostaglandin antagonists ↑ Vegetable oils to enhance prostaglandin formation
PMT-D	Depression, withdrawal, insomnia, forgetfulness, and confusion May have altered serum estrogen and serum progesterone May involve deficiencies of B vitamins and magnesium	Therapy should be individualized according to results of serum evaluation

Source: Modified from Abraham, G. (1983). Nutritional factors in the etiology of the premenstrual tension syndrome. *Journal of Reproductive Medicine, 28,*446.

trogen to progesterone abnormal; poor renal clearance, which leads to water retention; an endometrial toxin from ischemic tissue; and hypoglycemia, which can result in a surge of adrenaline.

In order to better classify incidences of premenstrual syndrome, various categories have been established (Abraham, 1983). These classifications are shown in Table 9-5. Women with class A tend to have a high estrogen/progesterone ratio during the luteal phase of a menstrual cycle. Those with class C tend to have a reduced insulin sensitivity or a decrease in carbohydrate tolerance just prior to menses. Those with class H tend to have an elevated aldosterone level during the luteal phase. The course of type D is less well understood but may involve a deficiency of vitamins or minerals.

Therapy is aimed at correcting any identified deficiencies. Increased physical activity and a set exercise program may help to rebuild muscle mass and prevent conversion of fatty tissue into estrogen, which will lower the estrogen/progesterone ratio. A decreased sodium diet may prevent fluid retention. A reduced carbohydrate diet may prevent a rebound hypoglycemia and hopefully prevent an abnormal adrenaline surge. Administration of B_6 (pyridoxine) daily may reduce estrogen excess in women with this specific deficit.

For women with extreme symptoms, progesterone by vaginal suppository 10 to 14 days prior to menses may be necessary. Vaginal suppositories contain a high dosage of medication because of relatively poor absorption due to leakage. Leakage can be reduced if a woman lies down for 15 minutes following insertion. Initially a progesterone suppository may cause a feeling of warmth and flushing. Usage should be stopped at the time of the normal menstrual flow—or if a flow does not occur, because progesterone is potentially teratogenic during pregnancy.

A syndrome similar to PMS may occur in women following tubal ligation. In these women, a decrease in the blood supply to the ovary apparently results in decreased luteal function and resulting low progesterone levels. This complication of tubal ligation has frequently not been discussed with women prior to the decision for ligation.

Women who develop hypertension of pregnancy or postpartal depression are especially prone to developing PMS (Dalton 1977). Women who are concerned that they have premenstrual syndrome should document its occurrence by keeping a diary of what and when symptoms happen. It is important that women recognize whether or not they suffer from premenstrual syndrome; that awareness gives them perspective on other events. They can then remind themselves, for example, that a broken washing machine or missed corporate deadline is just what it is, rather than the total catastrophe it seems when they are about to have their menstrual flow. They could perhaps plan stressful life events so they occur at other times than premenses.

Women need to be aware of public opinion concerning the premenstrual syndrome. One common implication, for example, is that women cannot think rationally once a month. The effects and causes of the syndrome need further study, and affected women should be given individual attention concerning the impact of PMS, both psychologically and physically, on their lives.

Frequency Disorders

Frequency disorders that can occur include amenorrhea, precocious and delayed puberty, dysfunctional uterine bleeding, and postmenopausal bleeding.

Amenorrhea

Absence of a menstrual flow, or *amenorrhea*, suggests, but is by no means diagnostic of, pregnancy. It may result from tension, anxiety, fatigue, or chronic illness; pituitary, ovarian, or uterine disorders; extreme dieting, or strenuous exercise. Many female athletes, such as competitive swimmers, long distance runners (50 to 75 miles per week), and ballet dancers, notice that the more intensely they train the more scant or more irregular their menstrual periods become. A low ratio of body fat to body muscle and an excessive production of prolactin secretion seem to be responsible. With an elevation in prolactin, gonadotropin-releasing factor (GN-RH) from the

hypothalamus decreases and so follicle-stimulating hormone, follicular development, and estrogen secretion declines. What the long term effect of this suppression is is unclear. Menstrual cycles return to normal about 3 months after strenuous training and conditioning is stopped.

Administration of bromocriptine (Parlodel) reduces high prolactin levels by acting on the hypothalamus, thus allowing women training for a sports event to maintain a normal cycle. Bromocriptine should be discontinued if a menstrual flow is delayed: It is potentially teratogenic during pregnancy. Side effects include nausea, headache, and dizziness. If taken with meals, the sensation of nausea can be decreased.

Amenorrhea also occurs when women diet excessively, in part, because the body is trying to conserve fluid. The absence of flow is probably also a defense mechanism to limit ovulation or the chance of a poor pregnancy outcome. Women with anorexia nervosa (excessive dieting to a point of starvation) or bulimia (binge eating followed by induced vomiting) develop amenorrhea after about 3 months due to an increase in prolactin similar to that which occurs in athletes.

Amenorrhea is termed *primary* if a woman has never menstruated, *secondary* if she has had normal menstrual periods. Signs and symptoms of pregnancy and the relationship of amenorrhea to them are discussed in Chapter 16. If no obvious reasons for the amenorrhea such as those mentioned above can be detected, pituitary hormone and skull x-ray examinations and ovarian and uterine studies will be necessary for diagnosis. Therapy would involve hormonal supplementation as necessary.

Precocious Puberty

The development of breasts or pubic hair before the age of 8 or menses before the age of 9 is considered to be precocious sexual development (Balkin, 1983). Most commonly, such development is expressed as isolated breast or pubic hair growth; but it can proceed to complete spermatogenesis and menstrual function.

Precocious puberty is caused by the early production of gonadotropins by the pituitary gland, which stimulate the ovaries or testes to produce sex hormones. Such stimulation can occur because of a pituitary tumor, cyst, or traumatic injury to the third ventricle next to the pituitary gland. It also can occur because of estrogen-secreting cysts or tumors of the ovary or testosterone-secreting cysts of the testes. Rarely, it occurs because of an estrogen- or testosterone-secreting adrenal tumor.

When no physical problem such as a tumor is

present, the phenomenon appears to occur only because the gonadostat of the hypothalamus was triggered several years too early.

In girls, ingestion of their mother's oral contraceptives can initiate menarche-like changes. In all instances, estrogen excess from follicular development will lead to breast development, accelerated skeletal maturation, and vaginal bleeding even though low levels of androgen secretion prevent the stimulation of pubic or axillary hair growth. Girls who develop precociously may tend to be shy and have a poor body image because they appear so different from other members of their group. Their parents worry about them beginning sexual activity and becoming pregnant.

The diagnosis of early puberty is confirmed by the analysis of urine for 17-ketosteroids (the end product of androgen breakdown) and estrogen. These substances may be at adult levels in a child with precocious puberty.

A synthetic analogue to GN-RH manufactured as Factrel (Ayerst) is now available as treatment on a research basis. Administration of this analogue desensitizes the pituitary to the child's own prematurely elevated hypothalamic GN-RH. It is administered subcutaneously daily. The drug is discontinued when the child reaches 12 or 13 years of age, at which point puberty progresses normally.

Parents need reassurance that once the child reaches normal puberty age, she will again be the same as other children; the fact that she started sexual growth early does not mean her genitals will eventually be out of proportion to her body.

Parents must also understand that their child is fully fertile when early puberty occurs—boys are capable of insemination and girls are capable of becoming pregnant. Girls should not be given oral contraceptives at this time: The increased load of estrogen will further hasten the closing of epiphyseal lines of long bones, leading to even shorter stature. Parents may need to be reminded that, although their child appears to be much older, the changes are only in sexual characteristics. Household tasks, responsibility, and expectations must be geared to the child's chronologic age, not to outward appearance.

Delayed Puberty

Delayed puberty in girls is the delay of menstruation until they are past 17 years of age. Often these girls and their parents have experienced years of worry while wondering when a "normal" menarche will occur. Many times a family history reveals a tendency for late maturation. The girls need a thorough physical examination, which usually reveals the presence of some sec-

ondary sex characteristics or the beginning of endocrine stimulation. If pathology has been ruled out, menstrual cycles may be begun by the monthly administration of estrogen. Most girls are willing to wait for normal maturation, however, as long as they receive assurance that they are normal and that their maturation is merely delayed in relation to that of many of their friends.

Dysfunctional Uterine Bleeding (DUB)

Dysfunctional uterine bleeding is a specific type of metrorrhagia, or bleeding between menstrual flows. It can also refer to continuous uterine bleeding and occurs most typically in perimenopausal women. Ninety percent of the time it is caused by lack of ovulation. That ovulation is not occurring can be shown by a persistent ferning mucus pattern during the luteal phase of the menstrual cycle, a flat basal body temperature graph, and lack of secretory endometrium during the luteal phase. Many women have a dilatation and curettage (D&C) done to halt the bleeding. They need to understand that this procedure is only a temporary measure, however; the following month, the problem will probably recur.

Bleeding between menstrual flows is a sign of uterine carcinoma; therefore, caregivers must rule out uterine and cervical carcinoma. As treatment, the woman can be administered estrogen and progesterone to simulate a normal ovulatory cycle (estrogen for 21 days, progesterone during days 15 to 25 of cycle). If the woman wants to ovulate, clomiphene citrate (Clomid) can be administered from days 5 to 9. Dysfunctional uterine bleeding is very frightening to women in this age group because they recognize the tests they are being given, such as an endometrial biopsy, endometrial aspiration, or a Pap test (see Appendix A), as related to uterine carcinoma.

Postmenopausal Bleeding

Any vaginal bleeding in the postmenopausal woman is never normal so needs investigation. At this age the incidence of uterine carcinoma is at its peak.

Infectious Disorders

Because menstrual blood is an excellent growth medium for microorganisms, the chance of infection occurring during menses is always present.

Toxic Shock Syndrome (TSS)

Toxic shock syndrome is an infection by toxin-producing strains of *Staphylococcus aureus* organisms. Organisms typically enter the body

Table 9-6 Symptoms of Toxic Shock Syndrome*

1. Temperature over 38.9°C (102°F).
2. Vomiting and diarrhea.
3. A macular (sunburn-like) rash that desquamates on palms and soles 1 to 2 weeks after illness.
4. Severe hypotension (systolic pressure under 90 mm Hg).
5. Shock, leading to poor organ perfusion.
6. Impaired renal function with elevated blood urea nitrogen or creatinine at least twice the upper limit of normal.
7. Severe muscle pain or creatine phosphokinase at least twice the upper limit of normal.
8. Hyperemia of mucous membrane.
9. Impaired liver function with increased total bilirubin and increased serum glutamic oxaloacetic transaminase (SGOT) at twice the upper limit of normal.
10. Decreased platelet count.
11. Central nervous system symptoms of disorientation or confusion; severe headache.

*Three symptoms must be present for diagnosis.

Source: Centers for Disease Control (1982). Toxic shock syndrome. *U.S. 1970–1982 Morbidity and Mortality Weekly Report 31,* 201.

Table 9-7 Methods to Reduce the Risk of Toxic Shock Syndrome

1. Do not use tampons.
2. Use only tampons with natural materials such as cotton, not synthetics such as cellulose or polyester.
3. Change tampons at least every 4 hours during use.
4. Alternate use of tampons with sanitary pads (use tampons during the day, sanitary pads at night).
5. Avoid handling the portion of the tampon that will be inserted vaginally.
6. Do not use tampons near the end of a menstrual flow when they can cause excessive vaginal dryness from scant flow.
7. Do not insert more than one tampon at a time in order to avoid abrasions and to keep the vaginal walls from becoming too dry.
8. Avoid deodorant tampons, sanitary pads, and feminine hygiene sprays; these products can irritate the vulvar-vaginal lining.
9. If fever, vomiting, and diarrhea occur during a menstrual period, discontinue tampon use and immediately consult a health care provider.
10. Women who have had one episode of TSS are well advised not to use tampons again or at least not until two vaginal cultures for *Staphylococcus aureus* are negative.

through vaginal walls damaged by the insertion of tampons at the time of a menstrual period. As many as 1,660 cases of TSS have been reported; 5 percent of women who have contracted the disease have died (CDC, 1982). As many as 70 percent of U.S. women used tampons in 1980, the year that toxic shock syndrome reached its peak incidence. As women have become wiser about tampon usage, TSS has become less frequent.

The symptoms of TSS are shown in Table 9-6. Any woman who develops fever with diarrhea and vomiting during a menstrual period should be suspected of having TSS. Remember that a number of women have mild diarrhea when dysmenorrhea occurs.

Staphylococcus aureus is generally resistant to penicillin but not to penicillinase-resistant antibiotics (cephalosporins, oxacillins, clindamycins). Women with suspected TSS need a careful vaginal examination with removal of any tampon present and cervical and vaginal cultures for *S. aureus.* Iodine douches may reduce the number of organisms present vaginally. Intravenous fluid therapy to restore circulating fluid volume and increase blood pressure or vasopressors such as dopamine (Intropin) may be necessary to increase the blood pressure. Diuretic therapy to shift fluid back to the intravascular circulation as well as support of renal and cardiac failure may be neces-

sary. Recovery occurs in 7 to 10 days; fatigue and weakness may be present for months afterward.

The risk of developing TSS is higher in young women (20 to 30 years of age) and noncontraceptive users. Bacteria are probably introduced by fingers or the insertion of a tampon (tampons are clean, but not sterile). Once saturated with blood, a tampon presents an optimum growth medium to bacteria, which can enter the body through ulcerations on the vaginal wall made by tampon insertion. Vaginal mucosa may be more likely to be abraded if a mild allergy or irritant reaction to the synthetic material in tampons (cellulose and polyester) or ingredients included to reduce odor has caused inflammation. Superabsorbant tampons made of cellulose may also contribute to the problem: Bacteria can break down cellulose into glycogen, providing an ideal nutrient for growth. Table 9-7 includes teaching points for helping women avoid TSS.

The recurrence rate of TSS is 28 to 64 percent (CDC, 1982). Relapses generally occur within 2 months of the first attack. In these instances the organism was probably not completely eliminated from the body because antibiotics were not fully effective.

Utilizing Nursing Process

Nurses can help women learn more about normal menstruation and therefore act to improve or adapt their self-care in this area.

Assessment

Many women are embarrassed by questions about their menstrual cycles; they are also apprehensive if they are aware that abnormal uterine bleeding is a sign of uterine carcinoma. Assessment of menstrual disorders, therefore, involves careful history taking. Table 9-8 lists specific areas to explore with accompanying questions for eliciting the information.

Analysis

The Fourth Annual Conference on Nursing Diagnoses accepted no diagnosis specifically concerning menstruation, but many diagnoses can be adapted to this health area. Fear related to absence of menstruation, pain related to discomfort from menstruation, or concern related to premenstrual syndrome are examples of commonly used nursing diagnoses.

When helping women to set goals in this area, be certain that the goal is realistic. "Woman will be pain-free by next menstrual cycle" may not be realistic depending on the physical reason for the pain. "Woman will explain reason for pain and take active measures to alleviate it" may be more realistic.

Planning

A major part of planning may be helping a woman to see that she *can* do something about menstrual discomfort or a lack of energy related to excessive blood loss with menstruation. A woman may have to change her primary health care provider if her menstrual pain or premenstrual syndrome has been dismissed as "woman's lot"; a prescription for her individual level of discomfort may be an important aspect of her health care.

Implementation

Implementation in this area of women's health largely involves teaching them what is normal in relation to menstrual function and what is not; role modeling "wellness" behavior regarding menstrual function (males can fill this role through their attitude toward women who are menstruating); and helping them locate health care providers who acknowledge the importance of this area of their lives.

Evaluation

Evaluation is important as a final step in care because problems of menstruation are not necessarily easy ones to solve. If an attitude change is

Table 9-8 Assessment for a Menstrual History

Area	Specific Questions
Menarche	Find out the age at which a woman's first menstrual period began. Document when menstrual periods became stabilized and whether this correlates with the occurrence of any dysmenorrhea. Ask about preparation for menstruation (and teach at the end of the interview that most women have a responsibility to plan better preparation for their daughters than was given to them).
Pattern of menstruation	Document frequency, duration, intensity, description, associated symptoms and actions.
Contraception method	Document if an IUD is used as IUDs may increase bleeding and cramping; also ask about oral contraceptives as these suppress ovulation and therefore dysmenorrhea.
Tampon use	Document use as toxic shock syndrome occurs with constant use, especially of superabsorbant brands.
Reproductive history	Number of past pregnancies, type of deliveries (cervical lacerations may lead to cervical stenosis and increased cramping although dysmenorrhea frequently decreases following a first pregnancy).
Sexual activity	Ask a woman if she has ever contracted a sexually transmitted disease (pelvic inflammatory disease increases dysmenorrhea). Also ask her whether she is sexually active during menstrual flow (orgasm can increase flow).
Menstruation effect	Ask to what extent menstrual flow interferes with activities, and whether she experiences premenstrual syndrome problems.

involved (for example, if the goal is for a woman to change her attitude from one of sickness to wellness regarding menstruation), evaluation is necessary to see that the woman demonstrates a changed attitude (goes to work during her menstrual flow; does not cancel her hair appointment for that week) as well as voices the change ("I know menstruation is a wellness function").

Nursing Care Planning

Below is a nursing care plan for Christine McFadden, a 15-year-old with dysmenorrhea.

Assessment

Patient states that nothing she has tried helps relieve pain. Has diarrhea for most of first day. Misses at least 1 day of school per month. Cringes while describing pain. Began periods at 12 years of age. Normal duration of flow: 5 days; cycle length: 30 days. Sister used to have dysmenorrhea also; improved since birth of a child. No dysmenorrhea in mother.

Analysis

Alteration in discomfort: pain related to dysmenorrhea.

Locus of Decision Making. Shared.

Goal. Patient will maintain normal life pattern during menses.

Criteria. Patient will voice satisfaction with level of comfort and remain in school.

Nursing Orders

1. Discuss physiologic reason for pain with patient.
2. Ask M.D. for prescription for mefenamic acid.
3. Advise to use abdominal breathing as a distraction technique.
4. Stress that menses is a normal phenomena, not an illness.
5. Patient to return to clinic as needed if medication is not effective.

Questions for Review

Multiple Choice

1. Barbara is a 14-year-old you see in an ambulatory setting. Your assessment reveals she has not yet menstruated. In counseling her, you would tell her that in most girls menstruation occurs
   a. before age 12.
   b. between the development of pubic and axillary hair.
   c. before breast development.
   d. following a year of ovulation.

2. You plan to review normal menstruation with Barbara. In doing so you would teach that, during the second half of a typical menstrual cycle, the endometrium of the uterus becomes
   a. thin and transparent, due to progesterone stimulation.
   b. twisted and rugated, due to follicle-stimulating hormone.
   c. thick and purple-hued, due to estrogen stimulation.
   d. corkscrew-like, due to progesterone stimulation.

3. Ovulation is apparently initiated by a surge in
   a. luteinizing hormone.
   b. progesterone.
   c. follicle-stimulating hormone.
   d. estrogen.

4. Mrs. Smith is a 25-year-old who tells you that she always cries for 24 hours preceding her menstrual flow. Based on this information, you would
   a. advise her to see a psychiatrist for depression.
   b. urge her to increase the salt in her diet prior to each menstrual flow.
   c. ask her how much caffeine she takes in daily.
   d. take a complete menstrual history.

5. Mrs. Smith's mother is 50 years old. She is beginning menopause. In planning care with her, which of the following would you teach?
   a. Hot flashes occur only in very emotional women.
   b. Estrogen increases in amount following menopause.
   c. She will notice a decrease in sexual interest.
   d. She needs to maintain a high calcium intake.

Discussion

1. Educating girls about menstruation is one of the roles of a school nurse. How would you present this topic to a class of 12-year-old girls? Would you do it any differently if the class included boys?
2. Teaching prevention for toxic shock syndrome is a major responsibility of nurses. What are the important aspects you would want to teach?
3. Dysmenorrhea is a problem for many women. What measures would you advise a woman seeking relief?

Suggested Readings

Abraham, G. (1983). Nutritional factors in the etiology of the premenstrual tension syndrome. *Journal of Reproductive Medicine, 28,* 446.

Abrams, J. (1982). Menopause: Preventing problems by anticipating them. *Consultant, 22,* 358.

Altchek, A. (1980). Abnormal vaginal bleeding in adolescence. *Consultant, 20,* 103.

Andersch, B., & Milsom, I. (1982). An epidemiologic study of women with dysmenorrhea. *American Journal of Obstetrics and Gynecology, 144,* 655.

Balkin, M. S. (1983). Precocious puberty: Total reversal is now possible. *Female Patient, 8*, 23.

Barber, H. R., et al. (1980). Dysmenorrhea. *Female Patient, 5*, 81.

Barnett, H. (1977). *Pediatrics* (16th ed.). New York: Appleton-Century-Crofts.

Bongiovanni, A. M. (1981). Causes and management of delayed menarche. *Consultant, 21*, 53.

Bongiovanni, A. M. (1983). When girls have delayed puberty. *Contemporary OB/GYN, 21*, 193.

Boyden, T. W., et al. (1983). Sex steroids and endurance running in women. *Infertility and Sterility, 39*, 629.

Brown, M. A. (1982). Primary dysmenorrhea. *Nursing Clinics of North America, 17*, 145.

Carroll, J. S. (1983). Middle age does not mean menopause. *Topics in Clinical Nursing, 4*, 38.

Centers for Disease Control. (1982). Toxic shock syndrome. *U.S. 1970-1982 Morbidity and Mortality Weekly Report, 31*, 201.

Chihal, H. J. (1981). Premenstrual tension: Not "simply in her head." *Consultant, 21*, 99.

Cibublka, N. J. (1983). Toxic shock syndrome and other tampon related risks. *J.O.G.N. Nursing, 12*, 94.

Comerci, G. D. (1983). Diagnosis: Inhibited growth and delayed puberty. *Hospital Medicine, 19*, 138.

Comerci, G. D. (1983). Diagnosis: Excessive growth and precocious sexual development. *Hospital Medicine, 19*, 159.

Cooper, S. L. (1981). Dysmenorrhea: A new approach to an old problem. *Canadian Nurse, 77*, 50.

Dalton, K. (1977). *Premenstrual syndrome and progesterone therapy*. London: Wm. Heineman Medical Books.

Dalton, K. (1981). The importance of diagnosing premenstrual syndrome. *Health Visitor, 55*, 99.

Fayez, J. A., & Taylor, R. B. (1983). Endometriosis: Staging and management. *Female Patient, 8*, 36/1.

Goodmen, S. L. (1982). Toxic shock syndrome. *Topics in Emergency Medicine, 4*, 66.

Gorrie, T. M. (1982). Postmenopausal osteoporosis. *J.O.G.N. Nursing, 11*, 214.

Gough, H. (1982). Premenstrual syndrome. *Nursing Mirror, 154*, 34.

Hammond, C. G. (1983). Estrogen therapy at menopause. *Contemporary OB/GYN, 21*, 25.

Heimburger, D. C. (1981). Toxic shock syndrome. *Critical Care Nurse, 1*, 32.

Hornick, J. (1982). Evaluating menstrual dysfunction. *Patient Care, 16*, 12.

Irwin, C. E., et al. (1982). Emerging patterns of tampon use in the adolescent female. The importance of toxic shock syndrome. *American Journal of Public Health, 72*, 464.

Jennings, B. (1982). Physiology and life stages of the menstrual cycle. In L. Sonstegard (Ed.), *Women's Health*, Vol. 1. New York: Grune & Stratton, 1982.

Kaye, W., & Neff, S. (1983). Could her irregular menses be caused by bulimia? *Contemporary OB/GYN, 21*, 97.

Lauver, D. (1983). Irregular bleeding in women. *American Journal of Nursing, 83*, 393.

Lauerson, N. H., & Graves, Z. R. (1983). Premenstrual syndrome: Court cases and new treatment. *Female Patient, 8*, 41.

Macbicar, M. G., et al. (1982). What do we know about the effects of sports training on the menstrual cycle? *M.C.N., 7*, 55.

Newton, M. (1980). Understanding and managing dysmenorrhea. *Consultant, 20*, 233.

Pearson, L. (1982). Climacteric. *American Journal of Nursing, 82*, 1098.

Premenstrual syndrome . . . test yourself. (1982). *American Journal of Nursing, 82*, 460.

Raisz, L. G., et al. (1984). Osteoporosis: New directions in prevention. *Female Patient, 9*, 38.

Reid, R. L., & Yen, S. S. C. (1981). Premenstrual syndrome. *American Journal of Obstetrics and Gynecology, 139*, 86.

Rosenfield, R. L. (1982). The ovary and female sexual maturation. In S. A. Kaplan (Ed.), *Clinical Pediatric and Adolescent Endrocrinology*. Philadelphia: Saunders.

Skillmen, T. G. (1982). Estrogen replacement: Its benefits and its risks. *Consultant, 22*, 115.

Shahady, E. J. (1982). Gynecology: Common problems in children and adolescents. *Consultant, 22*, 183.

Tudiver, F. J. (1983). Dysfunctional uterine bleeding and previous life stress. *Family Practice, 17*, 999.

Utian, W. H. (1980). *Menopause in modern perspective*. New York: Appleton-Century-Crofts.

Wilson, M. A. (1984). Menstrual disorders: Premenstrual syndrome, dysmenorrhea, amenorrhea. *J.O.G.N. Nursing, 13*, 11s.

Woods, N. F., et al. (1982). Prevalence of perimenstrual syndromes. *American Journal of Public Health, 72*, 1257.

Zarutskie, P. W., Schiff, I. (1984). Corpus luteum dysfunction. *Female Patient, 9*, 38.

10

Sexuality

OBJECTIVES

Following mastery of the contents of this chapter, you should be able to

1. Compare and contrast the terms *sexual gender, sexual identity,* and *sexual role.*
2. Describe the human sexual response.
3. Describe the ways that sexuality affects women's self-esteem.
4. Describe the ways that sexuality affects a woman's attitude toward pregnancy.
5. Analyze methods to promote sexual development and health.
6. Synthesize aspects of sexuality with nursing process to achieve quality maternal-newborn nursing care.

SEXUALITY REFERS to a person's maleness or femaleness, which includes sexual feelings, attitudes, and actions. It is both biologically inherited and culturally learned. It encompasses and gives direction to a person's physical, emotional, social, intellectual, and ethical responses throughout life. Born a sexual being, a child's sexual identity and role behavior evolve from and usually conform to the societal expectations within a given culture.

Sexual gender is the term used to denote chromosomal sexual development: male or female. *Sexual identity* is the sex a person thinks of him- or herself as being (which may be the same as or different from sexual gender). *Sexual role* includes the types of activities a person undertakes (which may or may not seem to be compatible with sexual gender or identity).

Sexual gender is set at the moment of fusion of a female ovum and male sperm. As a male fetus grows in utero and testosterone is secreted by the developing testes, the fetus develops male genitalia and function. If testosterone is not present, female genitalia and function develop. If for some reason testosterone secretion is suppressed, male development may not occur normally. If a chromosomally female fetus should be subjected to a testosterone-like hormone during pregnancy, a female fetus could be born appearing more male than female (such as with the adrenogenital syndrome).

Sexual identity—the feeling of being male or female—appears to be influenced by psychosocial circumstances, although the amount of testosterone secreted in utero may affect this characteristic as well (a process termed sex-typing). How appealing a parent makes a sexual role appear greatly influences how a child envisions him- or herself. If a mother makes being a woman seem second-rate and a father makes being a man appear exciting, a daughter may have difficulty accepting herself as a woman. She may mold herself as much as possible on the characteristics of her more appealing father. Likewise, a son who can relate better to his mother's attitudes and priorities may find himself assuming characteristics often regarded as feminine. In an extreme form, a person may feel trapped in a body of the wrong sex and ask to have a sex change operation to make body and perceived identity correspond.

Sexual role is culturally influenced. Traditionally, women have undertaken supportive and nurturing activities; childrearing and homemaking have been principally their domain. Men were expected to fill roles of responsibility and stability; their duties included providing for and protecting the family. It is difficult for many women today to identify their place in society. The traditional role for women—both during the sexual act, as a passive accepter of the male, and during everyday life—conflicts with a more modern view of women as active, innovative people. It is equally difficult for many men to balance nurturing, caring attitudes with the more traditional male role of dominance and emotional self-control.

The Development of Sexuality

Discussing views on sexuality with patients is made difficult by some people's reticence to discuss sexuality or inability to put their feelings in concrete enough terms for discussion.

In the 1950s, Kinsey and his associates (1953) were the first group of researchers to describe sexual practices and the state of human sexuality. In 1966 (and again in a 1982 revision), Masters and Johnson elaborated on common sexual needs. Their research documented the physiologic responses of both men and women to sexual stimulation. Some of their data-gathering efforts attempted to describe normal female sexual responses and the change in those responses during pregnancy and the postpartal period. They found that concepts about sexuality and related concerns or questions vary with age.

Prenatal Sex Determination

Until about the twelfth week of intrauterine life, it is difficult to tell by gross inspection whether a fetus is male or female. At 12 weeks, either the wolffian duct has become the dominant tract and male external genitalia are apparent, or the müllerian ducts have become dominant and female external genitalia are prominent. Although parents usually respond to the question, "Do you want a boy or a girl?" with the answer, "It doesn't matter as long as it's healthy," most parents actually have a strong preference as to which sex they hope a newborn will be. Many methods for determining whether a fetus will be a boy or girl (whether the fetus is carried high or low, which way a suspended needle spins) do not appear to have a scientific basis or much validity. Their number, however, reveals the interest of couples in determining the sex of their unborn child.

Infants

From the day of birth, there is a tendency for female and male babies to be treated differently by their parents. People are apt to bring girls dainty rattles and dresses with ruffles; on the whole girls are treated more gently by parents and held and rocked more than male babies. People tend to buy boys bigger rattles and sport-related jogging suits. Admonitions given babies may be different. A girl might be told, "Don't cry. You don't look pretty when you cry." A boy might be told, "You've got to learn to be tougher than that if you're ever going to make it in this world."

Because of these subtly different messages babies may get, by the end of the first year, differences in play are usually strongly evident. Girls play for longer periods with quiet, soft toys, checking back with their mother frequently; boys spend more time in gross motor activity, staying away from their mother for longer time periods than do girls (Figure 10-1).

Toddlers and Preschoolers

Children can clearly distinguish between men and women as early as 2 years of age. By age 3 or 4 they know for certain what sex they are, and they have absorbed cultural expectations of that sex role. Watching preschool children at play demonstrates this adaptation. Depending on their role model, children imitate cooking, washing dishes, and cleaning house or pretend to go to work with lunch pails or briefcases. Comments such as "What kind of mommy are you going to be, treating a doll that way?" or "Is that the way a lady

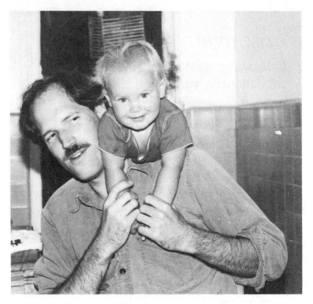

Figure 10-1 *A child's sex role is influenced by "roughhousing" play with a parent.*

sits?" from parents and well-meaning friends help to govern their choice of actions. "Boys will be boys" expresses another attitude representative of the difference expected between the two sexes.

Sex role modeling also comes from watching television. Based on how they see men and women act in these programs, preschool children's actions are strengthened and maintained as right for them or discarded in favor of actions that will bring approval.

If a child lives in a home in which both mother and father are kind, loving people, sex role identification progresses smoothly; it is easy to want to be like someone who treats you well and with whom you feel secure. If one parent does not have a high nurturing capacity, however, it may be hard for a child of the same sex to identify with that person. The identification may occur, but, because the adult is not a good role model, the child may then perpetuate the poor role.

A man who views the masculine role as aggressive, abrupt, and rough may notice in later years that his son is rougher with and less caring about a younger sibling than he likes to see. A man who maintains a passive role in a marriage, relinquishing authority to a more assertive wife, may find that his son finds the female role in this instance, that of the aggressive, decision-making person, more appealing. A girl may view a decision-making male identity as more appealing than a passive female role; or she may be uncomfortable with her mother as an executive because she prefers a quieter, less controlling role.

Although the development of an Oedipus complex may have been overstated by Freud (1962) as a result of sexual bias, many children manifest indications of such a phenomenon. An *Oedipus complex* refers to the strong emotional attachment of a preschool boy to his mother or of a preschool girl to her father. A preschool boy begins to show signs of competing with his father for his mother's love and attention. In what is usually termed an *Electra complex*, a girl begins to compete with her mother for the father's interest. Parents may need reassurance that this phenomenon of competition and romance in preschoolers is normal. They may need help in handling their feelings of jealousy and anger about having to compete with a child for their spouse's attention.

School-Age Children

In the past, the differences between boys and girls used to grow wider during school age. Teachers often contributed to this inflexibility in children's roles by expecting boys to be poorer readers, to write less neatly, and to act rougher in the school hallways.

Today, sex differences are more muted: Girls play in male-dominated activities such as Little League or take shop or auto repair courses, and boys can take homemaking courses. Many activities outside school are now unisex as well. Children this age begin to imitate adult roles and are very interested in what occupations and roles people they admire hold (Figure 10-2).

Adolescents

At puberty, as the adolescent begins the process of establishing a sense of identity—which is a clear understanding of self and personal gains and attitudes—the problem of sex role identification surfaces again. Most early adolescents maintain strong ties to their gender group: boys with boys, girls with girls. Some adolescents choose a teenager of their own sex a few years older than themselves to use as their model of sex role behavior. Parents may worry about this type of attachment and express concerns that the relationship has homosexual connotations. Ordinarily, however, teenagers are just being certain that they understand and feel comfortable with their own sex before they are ready to reach out and interact with members of the opposite sex.

Young Adults

When young adults move away from home to attend college or establish a home, they choose the

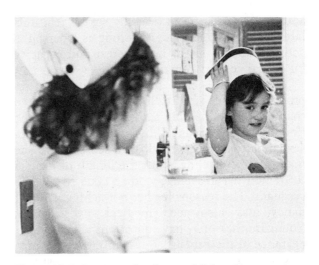

Figure 10-2 *During school age, children begin to imitate adult roles as a part of developing their sexual role.*

way they will express their sexuality along with other life patterns. Many marry with a commitment to one sexual partner. Others establish relationships that are less legally binding but express an equal commitment of long-term concern and support. Many young adults view cohabitation as a means of learning more about a possible marriage partner on a day-to-day basis, in the hope that a future marriage will then be stronger and more lasting. The incidence of sexual behavior outside marriage is increasing yearly. Figures are imprecise, but an estimated 50 to 70 percent of young adults engage in sexual activities outside marriage (Zelnik, 1983).

Homosexuality or bisexuality may be overtly expressed for the first time during this time span. Sexually transmitted disease (STD, or disease spread by coitus) occurs in epidemic proportions in some parts of the country, largely because of the frequent changing of sexual partners in this age group. When young adults are cared for in emergency rooms or admitted to health care facilities for these diseases, they are usually receptive to health teaching information on how better to prevent such diseases as well as about contraceptive choices. They may have questions about sexual practices and want to talk about their feelings about their sex identity or role. The effect of these disorders on pregnancy is discussed in Chapter 36.

Many adolescents and young adult athletes are taught that abstinence from sexual activity will increase their muscle strength and stamina (not true). They may worry that excessive sexual relations early in life will cause them to lose their ability to participate in or enjoy sexual relations later in life (also not true). As long as a person is active sexually, his or her interest and capacity for sexual activity remains.

Young couples often have questions about reproduction and fertility. If a woman anticipated that she would be able to become pregnant the first month she tried and then does not, she or her sexual partner may feel a loss of self-esteem. She may need counseling about the length of time (8 to 10 months) an average woman takes to become pregnant. The reasons for her not achieving pregnancy may also need medical investigation. Young mothers may have questions about the appearance of their infant son's genitals. They may be unaware, for example, that the left testis in most males is slightly larger and lower than the right, which allows the testes to slide past each other more easily and results in less pressure with movement. Most parents are aware that masturbation is normal for preschool boys but are unprepared to see it in preschool girls; they need an explanation that it is normal for both sexes as a part of exploring and growing comfortable with one's own body.

Middle-Aged Adults

For many women and men in midlife, sexuality has achieved a degree of stability. A sense of masculinity or femininity and comfortable patterns of behavior have been established. Although some women may feel financially incapable of leaving a particular life style, the average adult in midlife has resolved earlier conflicts with a mate and has the freedom to satisfy sexual needs, including the freedom to remain with a partner or return to a single state.

In the middlescent woman (woman undergoing menopause), reproductive functioning alters but sexual functioning does not. Menopause is said to have occurred with cessation of menses for at least 1 year. Estrogen levels gradually decrease over a period of about 1 to 7 years, with menopause occurring at about 50 years of age.

A woman's response to the physiologic and emotional components of menopause is, to a degree, culturally determined and includes anticipation of its effects. Generally, a woman engaged in a productive, satisfying life style is more likely to progress through this natural biologic stage with few problems (Figure 10-3).

In the middlescent man, neither reproductive nor sexual functioning alters. Midlife is often reported to be the most difficult period of adjustment in a man's life, however, bringing a need for ego enhancement and reassurance of sexual ade-

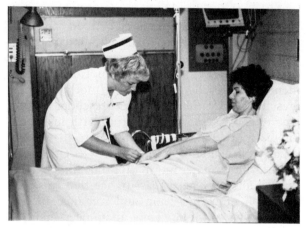

Figure 10-3 *The well older woman maintains her concept of herself as a sexual being and a functioning member of society.*

quacy. He may find he has transitory sexual dysfunction, such as premature ejaculation or impotence, particularly if he has work or family pressure. Men of this age experience an increased incidence of sexual encounters with younger women, which may be their way of reassuring themselves of their attractiveness and virility and of denying the fact of aging. Women who are insecure during this time may encourage the same age-spaced relationships.

A woman who undergoes surgery on her reproductive organs, such as a hysterectomy (removal of the uterus), needs sensitive nurses to listen to her concerns about the meaning of the experience. For some women the loss of their uterus can be synonymous with the loss of femininity. If both ovaries are also removed (oophrectomy), an immediate surgical menopause occurs. The hormonal changes resulting from the removal of both ovaries must be dealt with openly. Limited hormonal replacement is often a means of stimulating the naturally decreasing hormone levels of menopause.

During history taking, be aware that the woman who comments about her need to maintain a reduced activity level at work or a reduced social schedule due to menopausal changes may also be seeking information and direction in other important areas of her life, such as sexual relations.

Older Adults

Both male and female older adults can enjoy active sexual relationships. Some males in this age group experience less erectile firmness or ejaculatory force than when they were younger, but others discover that they are able to maintain an erection longer. Males remain fertile throughout life and so need to continue to be responsible sex partners in terms of birth control.

The older woman has less vaginal secretion because of declining estrogen levels following menopause; therefore she may need to use a lubricant before sexual intercourse for comfort and enjoyment. Women who have been sexually active throughout their lives seem to have fewer problems in this area.

Older women may no longer have a sexual partner, since the average lifespan of women is longer than of men. In many retirement communities, the ratio of women to men is as high as 2:1. These women should be assisted in finding companionship, as well as groups that can provide physical contact, social interaction, and intellectual stimulation. Masturbation can provide sexual gratification for persons of all ages.

Older adults who live with their children may suffer from lack of privacy for fulfilling sexual relationships. Those who are hospitalized or in long-term care facilities should have sexual needs evaluated along with other care needs; because they are older, needs for sexual expression may be ignored or repressed. Nurses need to advocate that couples share a room and provide for privacy. Unfortunately, lifelong partners are sometimes separated. Even in homes for the healthy aged, double-bed facilities are rare.

Handicapped Individuals

Handicapped individuals have sexual desires and needs equal to those of nonhandicapped persons but may have difficulty with sexual identity or enjoyment due to the effects of their handicap. Males with upper spinal cord injury may have difficulty with erection and ejaculation, since these actions are governed at the spinal level. Manual stimulation of the penis achieves erection in most men with spinal cord lesions, which allows the man to have a satisfying sexual relationship with his partner. Women with most spinal cord injuries are not able to experience orgasm but are able to conceive and deliver children (see Chapter 38).

Both males and females with handicaps that are interpreted as disfiguring, such as colostomies, may be reluctant to participate in sexual activities; they fear that the sight of the disfigurement will diminish their partner's satisfaction or enjoyment. Individuals with urinary catheters in place may be concerned about their ability to enjoy coitus. For women, a retention catheter should not interfere with coitus. Males may be taught how to replace their own catheter

so they can remove it for sexual relations. In all instances where one sexual partner is handicapped in some way, the response of a loving partner does much to enhance the body image and feelings of adequacy of the mate.

Sexuality in the handicapped person is a facet of rehabilitation that was not emphasized in the past. If a person could accomplish activities of daily living such as eating, elimination, and mobility, he was considered to be leading a normal or near normal life. Today, establishment of a sexual relationship is included as an activity of daily living and should be considered in rehabilitation programs as well as more technically oriented activities.

Sex Roles and Parenting

People tend to parent as their parents parented. Those who come from intact homes often have rather firmly fixed notions about their roles as parents of children. They may believe, for example, that fathers should play with babies—toss them in the air, play patty-cake with them—but should not be asked to get up at night with them. Fathers may be seen as in charge of physical discipline, while the maternal role encompasses eating habits, manners, and talking to teachers. Conflicts in parenting can occur if parents-to-be do not take time to discuss their views on parenting and come to an agreement about male and female roles and their relationship with their children.

A single parent may have difficulty fulfilling both roles; cultural expectations of proper parental roles may also cause stress to the parent or child. People raised in single-parent homes may have more difficulty with parenting than those who had constant role models; on the other hand, because they are used to an untraditional mixing of parenting roles, they may be more flexible and more able to adapt to the expectations of their marriage partner. As an example of the former response, a man who saw his father only on weekends, with each experience being something special, may have trouble dealing with the day-to-day needs of his children.

Trying to live up to television role models for parenting (the house is always neat, the children are always well behaved, and all problems can be solved by clever one-liners) is also very difficult.

A sad finding that has emerged from studying sex role identification in relation to parenting is that of Kempe and Helfer (1972): Children who are battered by their parents grow up to imitate that role model and become battering parents themselves. They assume the role their parents exemplified for them, even though objectively they can voice the fact that it is not a good role model, that theirs was not a happy childhood, and they would have liked it otherwise.

Conflicts in the role women have chosen for themselves often come to light for the first time during pregnancy as they worry about what type of parent they are going to be or their adequacy as a parent. Being able to talk to health care personnel about the sex role they have adopted in life can be a major step in resolving feelings of inadequacy and preparing these women to parent.

Sexual Responses

Sexual response is another area in which women typically ask questions of health care providers. Since the nineteenth century sex has been viewed in light of male desire, and the average female characterized as a passive recipient. Recent research reveals, however, that women enjoy sexual relations as much as men and that both men and women have typical reaction patterns to sexual stimulation. Recent research suggests there is a sexually responsive spot on the anterior wall of the vagina that may increase sexual response in women.

Stages of Sexual Response

Masters and Johnson (1982), have divided sexual response into four stages: excitement, plateau, orgasm, and resolution.

Excitement

With sexual stimulation either by massage of the glans of the penis or the clitoris or by sights or sounds, parasympathetic nerve stimulation leads to arterial dilatation and venous constriction in the genital area, increasing blood supply to the area, and vasocongestion and increasing muscular tension. In woman, this vasocongestion causes the clitoris to increase in size and mucoid fluid to appear on vaginal walls as lubrication. The vagina widens in diameter and increases in length. The breast nipples become erect. In men, penal erection occurs; there is scrotal thickening and elevation of the testes. In both sexes, there is an increase in heart rate, respiratory rate, and blood pressure.

Plateau

The plateau stage is reached just prior to orgasm. In the woman, the clitoris is drawn forward and retracts under the clitoral prepuce; the lower part of the vagina becomes extremely congested (formation of the orgasmic platform). There is increased nipple engorgement.

In men, the vasocongestion has led to full distention of the penis. Heart rate has increased to 100 to 175 beats per minute, respiratory rate to about 40 breaths per minute.

Orgasm

Orgasm is a vigorous contraction of muscles in the pelvic area. The average woman has 8 to 15 contractions at intervals of one every 0.8 second. This violent contraction expels or dissipates blood and fluid from the area of congestion.

Statistics on whether women achieve a stage of orgasm from coitus with no clitoral stimulation vary from early reports by Freud that women were neurotic if they did not always achieve orgasm through intercourse to findings by Hite (1976) that only 30 percent of women regularly experience orgasm from vaginal intercourse alone. About 90 percent of women are capable of achieving orgasm if manual or direct clitoral stimulation is used in conjunction with coitus.

In men, muscle contractions surrounding the seminal vessels and prostate project semen into the proximal urethra. These are followed immediately by three to seven propulsive ejaculatory contractions, occurring at the same time intervals as in the woman, that force semen from the penis.

Resolution

Resolution is the period during which the external and internal genital organs return to a quiet state. This takes about 30 minutes in both men and women.

Influence of the Menstrual Cycle

During the second half of the menstrual cycle—the luteal phase—there is increased fluid retention and vasocongestion in the woman's lower pelvis. Because some vasocongestion is already present at the beginning of the excitement stage of sexual response, women appear to reach the plateau stage more quickly and achieve orgasm more readily during this time. Women also seem to be more interested in initiating sexual relations at this time.

Influence of Pregnancy

Pregnancy is another time in life when, because of the rapidly growing fetus in the lower pelvic area, vasocongestion of the area already exists. Some women experience their first orgasm during pregnancy due to this phenomenon. Following a pregnancy, many women feel increased sexual interest because the new growth of blood vessels during pregnancy lasts for some time, thus facilitating pelvic vasocongestion. This physiologic response is a good reason to include sexual relationships as a part of health teaching during pregnancy. At a time when a woman may want sexual contact very much she needs to be free of old wives' tales, such as that orgasm will cause a spontaneous abortion. Although the level of oxytocin (a pituitary hormone that strengthens uterine contractions) does appear to rise in women following orgasm, in the average woman without a poor obstetric history this rise should not be enough to cause her any concern about continuing contractions and pregnancy loss.

For some women, the increased breast engorgement that accompanies pregnancy may result in extreme breast sensitivity during coitus. Foreplay that includes gentle sucking or massaging breasts is not contraindicated, however, and actually helps to toughen nipples in preparation for breast-feeding.

Peak Sexual Response

The peak sexual response of men appears to take place in the late teen years. The peak response in women, however, tends to be much more delayed, occurring more frequently during the late 30s. This difference in peak age of response probably stems from the fact that men are taught early in life that sexual activity is expected of them. Girls, on the other hand, are still taught that the proper context of sexual activity is marriage. It may take women until their 30s, therefore, to overcome this inhibition about enjoying or wanting a sexual relationship. The discrepancy in the age of peak sexual response may account for the number of young adult men who find other sexual partners during their mate's pregnancy. Pregnancy, with its restrictions due to awkward body size and possible prohibition of sexual relations (to lessen the possibility of introducing infection if membranes have ruptured) during the last month, occurs for these people at a time in life before the highest point of sexual response in women, at the peak of sexual response in men. The woman who is pregnant after 30 years of age has the opposite situation present, or is most interested in a sexual relationship at a time when her male partner's interest is declining.

Reproductive Life Planning and Sexuality

Because oral contraceptives contain estrogen and excess estrogen can decrease the desire for sexual relations, some women taking oral contraceptives express a lowered interest in coitus. This re-

sponse may be enough to make this method of reproductive planning unacceptable for a woman because of the interference with her relationship with her sexual partner. Other women find that feeling confident about controlling the timing of pregnancy makes sexual relations more pleasurable.

People using barrier methods of reproduction planning (diaphragm, condom, spermaticide foam or sponge) may find insertion of the contraceptive method inconvenient as it inhibits spontaneous expression.

Methods of Sexual Expression

A person expresses sexuality by dress, mannerisms, occupation, way of greeting people, and amount of touching in relationships (see the Nursing Care Highlight on page 190). For example, in social settings, men greet each other with a handshake; women may or may not shake hands. Women typically touch more (patting an arm, adjusting a sleeve on another's dress) than do males. This need for physical contact seems to peak during pregnancy: Women report wanting to be touched more than normally during pregnancy (Ellis, 1980).

Masturbation

Masturbation is self-stimulation for erotic pleasure; it can also be a mutually enjoyable activity for sexual partners. The accompanying sexual release may also serve to relieve overall tension or anxiety. Children between 2 and 3 years of age discover masturbation as an enjoyable activity as they explore their body. A child under a high level of tension may become accustomed to using masturbation as a means of falling asleep at night or at naptime. While doing so they make no attempt at concealment because they have not yet learned that society views such activity as private.

School-age children continue to use masturbation for enjoyment or to relieve tension but limit such activity to private times. In a hospital setting, a school-age child may assume that she has more privacy than she does: If you walk unannounced into her room, you may find her masturbating.

Following reproductive tract surgery or childbirth, women wonder how soon they will be able to resume sexual relations without feeling pain at their incision line. They may masturbate to orgasm to "test" whether everything in their body is still functional, much as the preschooler does. Masters and Johnson (1982) report that women may find masturbation to orgasm the most satis-

Nursing Care Highlight

Health Teaching and Sexuality

Many young adults are interested in knowing what is normal sexual response or expected frequency of sexual relations. A commonly accepted rule of thumb is that any act mutually satisfying to both sexual partners is normal. Frequency and type of activity vary widely within normal parameters.

---

fying sexual expression and use it more commonly than men.

Caution pregnant women that if they have been advised by their physician to avoid coitus in order to avoid orgasm, that orgasm from masturbation is often of a higher intensity than that from coitus and so should be avoided as well. Most restriction of coitus during pregnancy is associated with a danger of introducing penile/vaginal infection due to ruptured membranes, however, not orgasm response; for these women masturbation can serve as a substitute.

Erotic Stimulation

Erotic stimulation is the use of visual materials such as magazines or photographs for sexual arousal. Though usually perceived as a male phenomenon because of the number of girlie magazines on newsstands, centerfold photographs are gaining increasing interest in women's magazines. Some women may need to be assured that pleasure in visual excitement is normal.

Coitus

It is generally assumed that a person admitted to a health care facility is too ill or will be hospitalized for such a short period of time that a desire for sexual relations will not occur. In reality, a woman admitted to a health care facility for something such as a pregnancy complication may not feel ill at all. She may well experience a need for sexual relations or a desire to grant her sexual partner an opportunity to fulfill this need.

Sexuality Problems

Couples seen in ambulatory health care settings for infertility problems may have a sexual problem that is the basis for that infertility. A woman who is seen for pregnancy might comment that she feels lucky to be pregnant because she or her sexual partner has a problem in this area. Asking about satisfaction with sexuality is part of a total database for health assessment. A number of areas lead to sexual dysfunction.

Physical Illness

Following a heart attack, many men forego sexual activity; they are afraid that the stimulation will cause them to have a second attack. Obese men may have difficulty achieving deep penetration because of the bulk of their abdomen. Chronic disease, such as peptic ulcer or severe allergy, that causes frequent pain or discomfort may interfere with a man or woman's overall well-being and interest in sexual activity.

Obese women may have difficulty with sexual relations—again, because of the bulk of their abdomen. Women who have had a mastectomy may feel embarrassed about exposing their bodies. Fortunately, the number of total mastectomies being done now in preference to simple removal of the malignant breast mass is decreasing.

Impotence

Impotence is the inability to achieve or maintain an erection. Some reasons impotence occurs are physical, such as debilitating disease or drug dependence. In many instances, the problem appears to be psychological. Doubts about ability to perform or overall masculinity might be the cause. Excessive stress at home or at work might also be factors. The treatment of impotence depends on the source of the problem. Surgical implants to aid erection are possible, while a psychological block may be helped by sexual counseling.

Premature Ejaculation

Premature ejaculation is ejaculation prior to penile-vaginal contact. The term is often used to mean ejaculation prior to the sexual partner's satisfaction. Premature ejaculation is unsatisfactory for both partners: The woman cannot achieve orgasm because of loss of the man's erection and the man has failed to help her achieve orgasm.

The usual cause of premature ejaculation, like that of impotence, appears to be psychologically based. Masturbating to orgasm (where orgasm is achieved quickly owing to lack of time) may play a role. Other reasons may include doubt about masculinity and fear of impregnating the woman. Sexual counseling to help the female partner put less pressure on the male (and he on himself) may alleviate the problem.

Vaginismus

Vaginismus is involuntary contraction of the muscles at the outlet of the vagina when coitus is attempted. This muscle contraction prohibits penile penetration.

Vaginismus may occur in women who have had negative sexual experiences such as rape. It can also result from early learning patterns in which sexual relations were portrayed as "bad" or "sinful." As with other problems in this area, sexual or psychological counseling may be necessary to reduce this response.

Dyspareunia

Dyspareunia is the pain women may feel during coitus. It can be due to endometriosis, vaginal infection, or hormonal changes such as those that occur with menopause. It can be psychological. Treatment is aimed at the underlying cause.

Failure to Achieve Orgasm

The failure of a woman to achieve orgasm can be due to poor sexual technique, concentrating too hard on orgasm, underlying fear, or negative attitudes toward sexual relationships. Treatment is aimed at relieving the underlying cause, and it includes instruction for both partners in better sexual techniques and counseling about sexual feelings.

Nursing Responsibility and Human Sexuality

Because sexual roles and people's concepts of sexuality influence the ways they think, feel, plan—truly all activities of life—the kind of sexual beings that parents-to-be have become greatly influences the quality of parenting or parents they will become (Figure 10-4).

It is important for health professionals to be well prepared for their clients' questions about sexuality (see the Nursing Research Highlight on page 192). During crisis periods (and pregnancy is a crisis), people often question their life styles and beliefs. For this reason, questions about human

Figure 10-4 *Human sexuality and its effects on childbearing.*

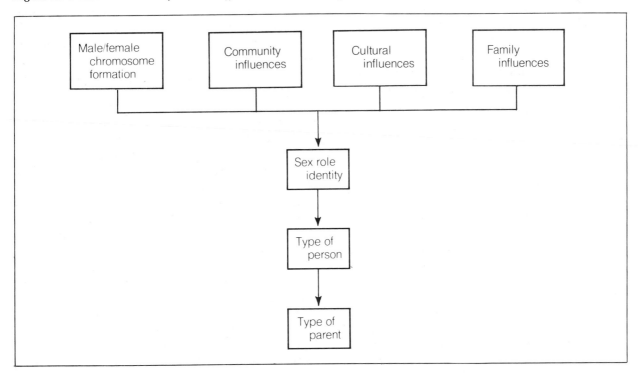

Nursing Research Highlight

Are Nursing and Medical Students Knowledgeable About Human Sexuality?

The literature indicates that student nurses as well as medical students are often inadequately prepared in the area of human sexuality. There are few controlled studies related to this particular area. One study (Kuczynski, 1980) was conducted on 110 voluntary students (55 sophomore medical students and 55 graduate nursing students) drawn from a large, state-supported, urban, midwestern university. It was designed to determine the extent of knowledge about sexuality and to assess attitudes about human sexuality held by graduate nursing students and sophomore medical students. Another purpose was to compare medical, graduate nursing, and nonmedical graduate students' attitudes toward and knowledge of human sexuality.

The findings indicated that medical and nurs-

ing students hold more conservative attitudes in comparison to nonmedical students. It is not enough, this study suggests, to include a course on human sexuality in the medical and nursing curricula: Even if required, such an inclusion will not necessarily change attitudes about sexual needs. Faculty must be made aware that problems in sexuality are as important as physical and psychological problems and in turn impart this attitude to their students. More constructive education in human sexuality must become a planned part of the nursing curricula.

Reference

Kuczynski, J. (1980). Nursing and medical students' sexual attitudes and knowledge. *J.O.G.N. Nursing,* 9(6), 339.

---

sexuality or sex roles may be asked at prenatal health visits. The nurse's largest contribution in this area may be to make it clear that such questions can be discussed. With this attitude, problems of sexuality are brought out of the closet and made as solvable as other health problems.

Utilizing Nursing Process

Problems of sexuality may not be evident on first meeting a patient; she may not be able to voice a problem in this area until she feels more secure with you. Good follow-through and planning is important with this type of problem because a person may find the courage to discuss it once but then will not be able to do so again. If the problem is ignored or forgotten through a change in caregivers, it will be lost.

Assessment

Sexual assessment is not a routine part of every health assessment. Many people are not able or willing to discuss sexual problems or concerns at a first health assessment. Include sexual assessment, therefore, when it is appropriate—such as during pregnancy or following birth of a baby. These are times when most women have concerns in this particular area of care. Any change in physical appearance (such as that caused by pregnancy) can intensify or create a sexual problem. A woman with surgery on reproductive organs, inflammation or infection of reproductive organs,

or the presence of a retention catheter needs to be assessed for problems of sexual function as well as for concerns on other important areas in her life.

Specific questions to ask for a sexual history are included in Chapter 18 along with other aspects of a comprehensive database for women's health. Verbal clues that a person may want more information about a sexual concern or that you need to explore this area in depth are often subtle ("I guess marriage isn't for everybody"; "I'm not the woman I used to be"; "Are there ever funny effects from this medicine I'm taking?"). Telling a seemingly inappropriate sexual joke may be a less subtle indication of need. Nonverbal clues to watch for include extreme modesty, obvious embarrassment at a televised sanitary napkin or douche commercial, or an uncomfortable reaction to a question about voiding or perineal pain or stitches.

Interviewing to obtain a sexual history takes practice and conviction that exploring sexual questions is as important for health as exploring less emotionally involved ones such as dietary intake or activity level. Frank admission that you do not understand words that a person is using helps communication; offering a personal response, such as that you do not always know how to explore this facet of a person's life (if that is true), can also ease any awkwardness. You have let the person know that a difficulty in explaining sexual concerns is a common reaction—and one that you also share.

On physical examination, observe women for normal distribution of body hair (hair on arms, axilla, and triangle-shaped pubic hair). Observe for normal genital and breast development. In adolescents this development is divided into Tanner stages (see Chapter 8) for easy documentation.

Analysis

The Fourth National Conference of Classification of Nursing Diagnoses accepted two diagnoses in reference to sexual functioning: sexual dysfunction and rape trauma syndrome. Another approved nursing diagnosis that could be adapted to a sexual problem is disturbance in self-concept. In addition to these officially approved diagnoses, a nursing diagnosis related to sexuality might express a problem, such as loss of sexual identity related to recent surgery, fear related to loss of sexual partner, or concern related to sexually transmitted disease. Analysis to determine whether a sexual need exists should always be considered in long-term illness and in any illness that results in a change of physical appearance or self-esteem.

Planning

Planning for strengthening a person's sexual identity or sexual role behavior may emphasize interventions that support maleness or femaleness. A woman who perceives her sexual role as assertive needs opportunities for decision making and self-care built into her care plan; a woman who places importance on good grooming and daily hair washing needs time set aside for these activities at the same priority level as other measures of self-care. Planning for these activities must be carefully structured: These needs are easy for a busy health care provider to omit.

Implementation

People who are insecure about their sexual identity may demonstrate acting out or attention-getting behavior—for example, a woman may allow a patient gown to slip, thus exposing her breasts. Adolescents with questions about whether their development is progressing normally are particularly prone to try to reach you in this way. A girl who has one breast slightly larger than the other (a normal development) might want to be certain that you notice this difference so that you will reassure her.

Women recovering from illnesses that have affected their physical capacity such as arthritis, which can make it painful for a woman to lie supine, may ask you about alternative coital positions. They may also wonder about alternative methods of sexual expression, such as oral-genital stimulation or anal intercourse. These questions must be answered in the light of the person's limitation and disability; but be aware that the person is often seeking approval for her interest. When your reply shows that her concern is normal and acceptable, she can then ask her physician about specific physical limitations.

Evaluation

How a person feels about herself has a great deal to do with how quickly she recovers from illness, how quickly she is ready to begin self-care following pregnancy, or even how well motivated she is to do those things necessary to remain well. Evaluating whether goals related to sexuality were achieved is important in being certain that a woman will be able to accomplish activities in all other phases of her life.

Nursing Care Planning

Mary Kraft is a 23-year-old woman you care for in a prenatal setting. Mrs. Kraft had a spontaneous abortion 2 years ago followed by a year of apparent infertility.

Assessment

Patient states that she is concerned because her husband is refusing to have sexual relations with her since she became pregnant (now 12 weeks pregnant) because he is afraid of "hurting the fetus." Prior to pregnancy, the couple mutually enjoyed coitus about two times weekly. She has not discussed the problem with her husband.

Analysis

Anxiety related to lack of sexual interest by husband.

Locus of Decision Making. Patient.

Goal. Patient and husband to achieve satisfactory sexual relationships by 1 month time.

Criteria. Couple to return to prepregnancy relation pattern.

Nursing Orders

1. Discuss reason for husband's concern and that reaction is a positive response to wanting her to complete pregnancy.

2. Patient to ask husband to come for additional health care visit next week to discuss topic of sexual relations during pregnancy.

3. Following childbirth and before discharge, nurse clinician alerted to discuss more positive means of approaching problem solving than she currently uses (withdrawing from situation).

Questions for Review

Multiple Choice

1. Mrs. Jones is a patient in your care. In assessing her sexual gender, which of the following points would you assess?

   a. temperament
   b. hair distribution
   c. occupation
   d. ability to love

2. Mrs. Jones's sexual role refers to

   a. her chromosomal inheritance.
   b. the sex she sees herself as being.
   c. her sexual identity.
   d. her demonstrated sexual behaviors.

3. Mrs. Jones uses masturbation as a tension-release mechanism. Which of the following statements is true concerning masturbation?

   a. It leads to early loss of fertility.
   b. It is practiced by individuals of all ages.
   c. It is less satisfying to women than men.
   d. It is almost exclusively a practice of preschool children.

4. On occasion, Mrs. Jones has difficulty achieving orgasm. Orgasm in females results mainly from

   a. penile penetration.
   b. clitoral stimulation.
   c. uterine stimulation.
   d. sensory arousal.

5. Mrs. Pietrazak tells you her husband likes to continue sexual relations during her menstrual period. She asks you if this will harm her. What would be your best advice?

   a. You don't advise it because orgasm may be painful for her during her menses.

   b. The risk of infection is too great for sexual relations during this time.
   c. She cannot achieve orgasm during the menses.
   d. If this is satisfying for her there is no harm in it.

6. She is also concerned that her husband will want to continue sexual relations during a pregnancy. You might advise her that

   a. sexual relations can safely be continued during a normal pregnancy.
   b. sexual relations are dangerous during pregnancy after 3 months.
   c. this is a problem for her to resolve without outside help.
   d. she will be able to continue relations only if a condom is used.

7. Mrs. Ferdinand is a woman approaching menopause. Which reaction below would you explain to her that she will soon experience?

   a. She can expect to begin experiencing pain with coitus.
   b. She will begin noticing increased sexual interest.
   c. She will experience marked decreased sexual interest.
   d. She can expect to notice no marked change in sexual interest.

Discussion

1. Taking a sexual history may be awkward as a woman may not feel comfortable discussing this aspect of her life. How would you help a woman feel more comfortable responding in this area?

2. A woman's sexual gender may differ from her sexual role. How might differing sexual roles affect a woman's feelings about being pregnant?

Suggested Readings

Aiken, M. M. (1983). When an employee tells you she has been raped. *Occupational Health Nursing, 31,* 42.

Allensworth, D. D., et al. (1982). Sexism in the school: A hindrance to health. *Journal of School Health, 52,* 417.

Bartscher, P. W. (1983). Human sexuality and implications for nursing intervention: A format for teaching. *Journal of Nursing Education, 22,* 123.

Buckwalter, K. (1983). The role of the occupational health nurse in sexual counseling. *Occupational Health Nursing, 31,* 23.

Brodoff, A. S. (1983). Marriage counseling: Helping couples with sexual problems. *Patient Care, 56,* 48.

Cohn, S. D. (1982). Sexuality in pregnancy: A review of the literature. *Nursing Clinics of North America, 17,* 91.

Ellis, D. (1980). Sexual needs and concerns of expectant parents. *J.O.G.N. Nursing, 9,* 306.

Freud, S. (1962). *Three essays on the theory of sexuality.* New York: Hearst Corporation.

Hite, S. (1976). *The Hite Report.* New York: Macmillan.

Hogan, R. M. (1982). Influence of culture on sexuality. *Nursing Clinics of North America, 17,* 365.

Juhasz, M. A. (1983). Sex education: Today's myth . . . tomorrow's reality. *Health Education, 14,* 16.

Kempe, C. H., & Helfer, R. (Eds.). (1972). *Helping the battered child and his family.* Philadelphia: Lippincott.

Kinsey, A., et al. (1953). *Sexual behavior in the human female.* Philadelphia: Saunders.

Krauss, D. J. (1983). The physiologic basis of male sexual dysfunction. *Hospital Practice, 18,* 193.

Masters, W. H., & Johnson, V. E. (1982). *Human sexual response.* Boston: Little, Brown and Company.

McAnulty, E. (1983). The sexuality of childbirth. *Midwives Chronicle, 96,* 236.

McKears, J. (1983). Sex education in schools. *Health Visitor, 56,* 48.

Mead, B. T. (1983). Adolescent homosexuality. *Consultant, 23,* 107.

Mims, F. H. (1982). Sexual stress: Coping and adaptation. *Nursing Clinics of North America, 17,* 395.

Osofsky, H. J., et al. (1984). Gynecologic aspects of sexual dysfunction. *Female Patient, 9,* 150.

Robson, K. M. (1982). Sexual behavior: Falling interest . . . a decline in sexuality during pregnancy. *Nursing Mirror, 15,* 42.

Sapala, S., et al. (1982). Adolescent sexuality: Use of a questionnaire for health teaching and counseling. *Pediatric Nursing, 7,* 33.

Schuster, E. A., et al. (1982). Nursing practice in human sexuality. *Nursing Clinics of North America, 17,* 345.

Sloan, D. (1984). Stress and sex. *Female Patient, 9,* 159.

Tauer, K. M. (1983). Promoting effective decision-making in sexually active adolescents. *Nursing Clinics of North America, 18,* 275.

Taussig, W. C. (1982). Sixth grade children's questions regarding sex. *Journal of School Health, 52,* 412.

Zelnik, M., et al. (1983). First intercourse among young Americans. *Family Planning Perspectives, 15,* 64.

11

Reproductive Life Planning

OBJECTIVES

Following mastery of the contents of this chapter, you should be able to

1. Define *reproductive life planning.*
2. Describe common methods of reproductive life planning.
3. Describe common assessments necessary to assist couples with reproductive life planning.
4. State a nursing diagnosis related to reproductive life planning.
5. Plan specific counseling measures to assist a couple with reproductive life planning.
6. Assist with implementations involved in reproductive life planning.
7. Evaluate goal outcomes regarding reproductive life planning.
8. Analyze the risks and benefits of common reproductive life planning measures.
9. Synthesize knowledge of reproductive life planning with nursing process to achieve quality maternal-newborn nursing care.

REPRODUCTIVE LIFE PLANNING is a broad term that includes active intervention for couples who are having difficulty conceiving children, helping couples space children so they have time to enjoy each child, counseling couples who have the potential for conceiving children with genetic abnormalities as to their best course of action, and helping couples and individuals who do not want to have children to avoid conception. This chapter concentrates on methods of limiting or spacing children. A woman's right to control the size of her family in this way is a fairly recent social innovation. Prior to introduction of "the pill" in the 1950s, available methods of reproductive life planning were so limited that, aside from abstinence, women had difficulty planning and spacing their children.

As women become aware of their ability to change and control all aspects of their lives, preventing unwanted children or delaying children until a more appropriate time in life often becomes both a desire and a concern. As men begin to view having children as a family activity rather than merely "woman's business," they begin to participate more actively in reproductive planning.

As early as 1966, the American Nurses Association issued the following resolution outlining the responsibility of registered nurses (ANA, 1966):

1. To recognize the right of individuals and families to select and use such methods as are consistent with their own creed and mores.
2. To recognize the right of individuals and families to receive information about family [reproductive] planning if they wish.
3. To be responsive to the need for family [reproductive] planning.
4. To be knowledgeable about state laws regarding family [reproductive] planning and the resources available.
5. To assist in informing individuals and families of the existence of approved family [reproductive] planning resources.
6. To assist in directing individuals and families to sources of such aid.

Contraceptive Methods Now in Use

As many as 28 million U.S. women use some form of contraceptive, which is three-fourths of the women of childbearing age (Dryfoos, 1982). Table 11-1 shows the incidence of the use of common methods. Figure 11-1 shows contraceptive users' preferences worldwide.

In order to be ideal as a method of reproductive life planning, a contraceptive should be completely safe and effective, free of side effects, easily obtainable, inexpensive, acceptable to the user, and not have an effect on future pregnancies. Various contraceptive measures are compared on

Table 11-1 Incidence of Use of Contraceptive Measures

Method	Use (%)
Condom	11
Diaphragm	8
IUD	8
Oral contraceptives	32
Rhythm or natural	10
Spermicides	7
Sterilization	24

Source: Dryfoos, J. G. (1982). Contraceptive use, pregnancy intentions and pregnancy outcomes among U.S. women. *Family Planning Perspectives, 14,* 81.

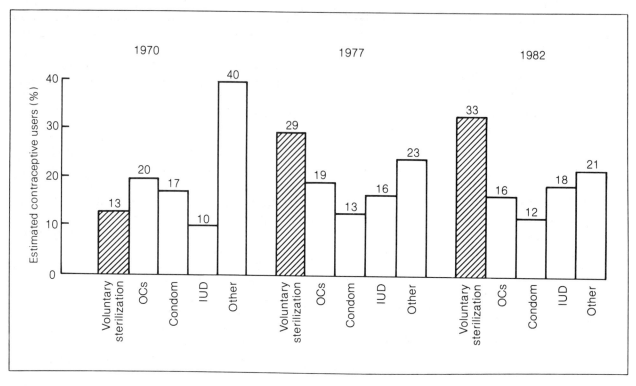

Figure 11-1 *Contraceptive users' preference worldwide. From Huber, D. (1984). Update on techniques for voluntary sterilization.* Contemporary OB/GYN, 23, 130.

the basis of the criteria of effectiveness in Table 11-2, while Table 11-3 lists the current costs of some of these measures. The Nursing Research Highlight on page 200 (top) summarizes some recent studies on contraception preferences. The Nursing Care Highlight on page 200 (bottom) discusses important safety considerations.

Ovulation Suppressants

Oral contraceptives, commonly known as "the pill," are most frequently composed of synthetic estrogen combined with a small amount of synthetic progesterone. The estrogen content acts to suppress follicle-stimulating hormone (FHS) and luteinizing hormone (LH), the gonadotropic hormones of the pituitary, and therefore to halt ovulation. The progesterone action decreases the permeability of cervical mucus, limiting sperm motility and access to ova. Progesterone also interferes with endometrial proliferation to such a degree that implantation is unlikely.

Ovulation suppressants must be prescribed by a physician or a woman's health care nurse practitioner. When used correctly, they are 100 percent effective in preventing conception. Because women occasionally forget to take them, however, their actual effectiveness is between 96 and 100 percent.

Table 11-2 Comparison of Contraceptive Effectiveness

Method	Effectiveness	Ideal Failure Rate (%)	Actual Failure Rate (%)
Tubal ligation	Excellent	0.04	0.04
Vasectomy	Excellent	0.15	0.15
Oral contraceptives	Excellent	0.5	2–3
Minipill	Very good	1–2	5–10
IUD	Excellent	1–3	5–6
Condom and diaphragm	Excellent	1	3–5
Condom and foam	Excellent	1	3–5
Diaphragm and cream or jelly	Good– very good	3	10
Cervical cap	Good	3	18–20
Spermicides	Good	3	18–22
Vaginal sponge	Good	3	18–22
Withdrawal	Fair	9	20–25
Rhythm	Poor to fair	13	20–40
Douching	Poor	Not rated	40+
Breast-feeding	Poor	15	50+

Source: Based on data from R. A. Hatcher, et al. (1980). Contraceptive technology 1980–1981. (10th ed.). New York: Irving. From W. H. Masters, V. E. Johnson, & R. C. Kolodny. (1982). *Human Sexuality.* Boston: Little, Brown and Company.

Table 11-3 First-Year Cost of Common Reproductive Life Planning Measures

Method	Total Cost	Medical Care	Supplies
Prescription			
Pill	$ 172	$ 65	$107
Diaphragm	160	65	95
IUD	131	65	66
Nonprescription			
Foam	50	NA	50
Condom	30	NA	30
Rhythm	NA	NA	NA
Sponge	104	NA	104
Withdrawal	NA	NA	NA
Sterilization			
Tubal ligation	1,180	1,180	NA
Vasectomy	240	240	NA

Source: Modified from Torres, A., & Forrest, J. D. (1983). The costs of contraception. *Family Planning Perspectives,* 15, 71.

Table 11-4 Mortality of Women Associated with Pregnancy and Childbirth Compared to Use of Oral Contraceptives

Age (Years)	Pregnancy and Childbirth[a]	Oral Contraceptives[b]	
		Nonsmokers	Smokers
15–19	11.1	1.2	1.4
20–24	10.0	1.2	1.4
25–29	12.5	1.2	1.4
30–34	24.9	1.8	10.4
35–39	44.0	3.9	12.8
40–44	71.4	6.6	58.4

[a] Per 100,000 live births, U.S.A., 1972–1974.
[b] Per 100,000 users per year.

Source: Tietze, C. (1978). What price fertility control? *Contemporary OB/GYN 12,* 32. Used by permission.

Pills contain estrogen (about 35 µg) and progesterone (0.5 to 1 mg) in a combination form. A former sequential pattern, whereby pills taken during the first part of a cycle contained only estrogen and later pills contained progesterone, is no longer available. The progesterone content of these last pills caused endometrial sloughing to occur and a woman's menstrual period seemed nearly normal. Unfortunately, the sequential forms were suspected of causing an increased rate of endocervical cancer, which is why they were taken off the market. Women who take the combination form now available often report scant menstrual periods; some worry that they are pregnant because their menstrual flow is so atypical.

Although there is a current uneasiness about the safety of chronic pill use (see Table 11-4 for mortality rates of women associated with pregnancy and childbirth compared to use of oral contraceptives), there is no proof of an increase in the rate of breast or cervical cancer with the use of the pill, and the rate of endometrial and ovarian cancer may be reduced by 50 percent in pill users (Mishell, 1983). These women also seem to be less apt to develop benign breast disease, including fibrocystic breast disease. Pelvic inflammatory disease (PID) occurs less often than usual in pill users (Zatuchni, 1984), apparently due to cervical changes. Women who use ovulation suppressants experience little dysmenorrhea because ovulation does not occur; premenstrual syndrome is also lessened due to adequate progesterone levels. The use of ovulation suppressants reduces the amount of menstrual flow so iron deficiency anemia is less likely in pill users. Another benefit is the prevention of salpingitis, or inflammation of the fallopian tubes, from sexually transmitted diseases; due to this, tubal obstruction and infertility may be reduced by ovulation suppressant use (Mishell, 1983).

A pelvic examination and a Pap smear should precede prescription of ovulation suppressants. The instructions for taking pills are roughly similar for all brands. The general method is to take the first pill on a Sunday (the first Sunday following the beginning of a menstrual flow). Following childbirth, a woman should start on the Sunday closest to 2 weeks postdelivery; after an abortion, she should start on the first Sunday following the procedure. The woman takes the pill at the same time every day for 21 days. Pill taking by this regimen will end on a Saturday. No pills are taken for a week; then the woman starts a new month's supply of pills on the Sunday 1 week after she stopped (Figure 11-2). A menstrual flow will occur 4 days after she stops taking pills.

A pattern of this kind helps a woman remember when it is time to start a new dispenser. Sunday may not be a good day for some women to begin new cycles because it is such an atypical day for them so these women should choose another starting day. Another factor to consider is that a woman on the pill has some control over the time of a menstrual period: If she starts taking pills on a Sunday, she will begin her period 4 days after she ends a 3-week cycle, or on a Wednesday; if she starts her 3-week cycle on a Friday, she will begin her menstrual period on a Monday, a pattern that avoids having menstrual periods on weekends.

Nursing Reseach Highlight

Contraception Preferences

Does the Use of Birth Control Pills Depend on a Woman's Perception of her Chances and Ability to Conceive?

Most studies on contraceptive use have not focused on the woman's perception of her chances and ability to conceive but on convenience or cost.

A sample of 32 women seeking abortions was studied (Klein, 1983) to determine if there is a relationship between these factors. Subjects were between the ages of 16 and 29 years, white, unmarried, and gravida 1. Findings from the study indicate that the stronger are a woman's perceptions of her chances and ability to conceive the more effective will be the method of birth control chosen. This correlation has implications for nurses, who are often in contact with women who are at risk or potential risk for unwanted pregnancy. It has particular application to care of adolescents: Educating them that they can become pregnant may be the first step in helping them to choose an effective contraceptive.

The Cervical Cap: Is It Effective?

Use of the cervical cap as a method of contraception has enjoyed a resurgence of interest in recent years. A study by one researcher (Boehm, 1983) to assess the effectiveness of and satisfaction with the cervical cap was conducted on 76 women fitted over a 1-year period. These women were all in their childbearing years and were sexually active. Data indicated that over 80 percent of the women found the cap effective and were satisfied with its use. There was a 51 percent continuation rate over a 1-year period. The use of the cervical cap as a method of contraception is comparable with the user effectiveness of the vaginal diaphragm, and discontinuation rates for this method are not disproportionate to those of other methods of contraception. When women choose to use contraceptives they should have options, and these options should be backed by accurate and complete statistical data.

Is Choice of Contraceptive Related to Age?

The contraceptive methods used by young women were the focus of a study done by Ayvazian (1981) on 78 women, with a mean age of 20 years, who were attending a university contraceptive health education clinic. The study sought to identify whether a relationship existed between age, race, and marital status and choice of contraceptive; whether psychosocial factors affect the decision; and when and why these women change birth control methods. Data indicated a strong relationship between age and choice of contraceptive: The older the woman, the more concerned she was with health risks and choosing a method free from medical side effects. Rated as most important, overall, for contraceptive choice was physical safety and effectiveness, with the most popular method being oral contraceptives (50%) followed by the diaphragm (37%). Health professionals should keep this correlation in mind when counseling and teaching different age groups about contraceptives.

References

Ayvazian, A. (1981). Contraceptive choices of female university students. *J.O.G.N. Nursing, 10*(6), 426.

Boehm, D. (1983). The cervical cap: Effectiveness as a contraceptive. *Journal of Nurse Midwifery, 28*(1), 3.

Klein, P. M. (1983). Contraceptive use and perception of chance and ability of conceiving in women electing abortion. *J.O.G.N. Nursing, 12*(3), 171.

Nursing Care Highlight

Reproductive Life Planning

Be aware of contraindications for certain reproductive life planning methods. IUDs should not be advised for women with multiple sexual partners in order to prevent pelvic inflammatory disease. Ovulation suppressants are contraindicated for women past 35 years of age who smoke, have hypertension, or have a history of thromboembolic disease.

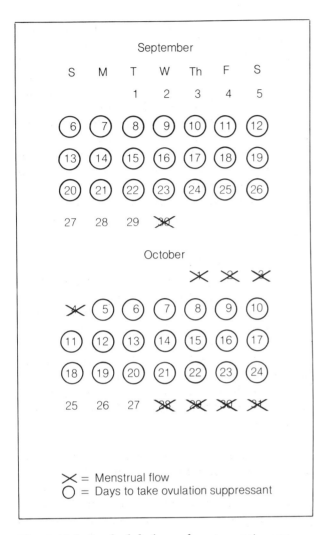

Figure 11-2 *A schedule for oral contraceptive use.*

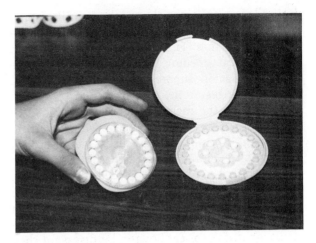

Figure 11-3 *Oral contraceptives are supplied in a circular monthly dispenser.*

Ovulation suppressants are packaged in convenient dispensers (Figure 11-3). In order to help women remember their pattern of pill taking (and to eliminate having to count days between pill cycles), certain brands of oral contraceptives are packaged with 28 pills in a circular dial dispenser. The woman begins to take pills on the first day of her menstrual period. The first five pills are placebos; the next 20 are real. She starts a second dispenser of pills the day after finishing the first dispenser. There is no need to skip days because the placebo tablets do that for her.

In order for birth control pills to be effective, they must be taken consistently and conscientiously. Many women leave them in plain sight on the bathroom or kitchen counter to remind themselves. Women with young children in the house need to be cautioned, however, about child poisoning. Women who have difficulty remembering to take a contraceptive in the morning, because of a busy schedule of getting ready for work or getting children or husband off to school or

work, may find it easier to remember to take a pill at a set evening hour. It makes no difference what time of day the pill is taken; the key word is the same time *daily.* Irregular scheduling can allow FSH levels to rise and ovulation to occur.

If a woman forgets to take one pill, she should take it as soon as she remembers and then continue the following day with her usual schedule. Missing one pill should not initiate ovulation. If the woman misses two consecutive pills, she should take one as soon as she remembers, and then continue the following day with the usual schedule. Missing two pills may be enough to allow ovulation to have occurred, however, so the woman should also use added protection for the remainder of the month such as a vaginal foam. She may experience some breakthrough bleeding and needs to be cautioned not to mistake this bleeding for her menstrual flow.

Side Effects

Some women dislike taking ovulation suppressants because of side effects they experience. Principal side effects include nausea, weight gain, headache, breast tenderness, breakthrough bleeding (spotting in between menstrual periods), acne, monilial vaginal infections, and mild hypertension. Breakthrough bleeding is due to temporary estrogen deficiency that allows the endometrium to begin to slough—a disturbing but not a serious phenomenon. Modern ovulation suppressants contain only one-fifth the amount of estrogen (ethyl estradiol) originally used and only one-eighth the amount of progesterone; these changes have made them more safe and less likely to produce side effects.

Breast-fed infants have lower weight gains when the mother is on ovulation suppressants during lactation, since the mother's milk supply is decreased. Also, as the long term effect of estrogen use in infants is not yet documented, women who are breast-feeding, therefore, should not be taking ovulation suppressants unless they contain only progesterone.

Because of the increased tendency of blood to clot in the presence of estrogen, women with a history of thromboembolic disease or a family history of cerebral or cardiovascular accident should not be routinely placed on the pill. Women who smoke, are over 35 years of age, are obese, or have high blood pressure, high serum cholesterol levels, or pulmonary disease are particularly at risk for cardiovascular disease if they are taking ovulation suppressants (Mishell, 1983).

Estrogen tends to interfere with glucose metabolism due to its liver conjugation. Women with diabetes mellitus or a history of liver disease, including hepatitis, should also be considered individually before being placed on the pill. Other problems that may contraindicate ovulation suppressants are breast or reproductive tract malignancy, undiagnosed vaginal bleeding, migraine headache, epilepsy, or sickle cell disease.

The cost of oral contraceptives and a woman's ability to follow instructions faithfully must both be considered before a prescription is made. A woman on oral contraceptives should return for a follow-up visit in 3 months, 6 months, and 1 year, then yearly for a pelvic examination and breast examination as long as she remains on this form of reproductive life planning.

Mini-Pills and Morning-After Pills

Oral contraceptives may be composed only of progesterone (called *mini-pills*), which allows ovulation but no implantation. This form has advantages for the woman who cannot take an estrogen-based pill and wants high-level contraception assurance; this form can be used while a woman is breast-feeding (Zatuchni, 1984). Mini-pills are taken every day, even through the menstrual flow, which minimalizes necessary planning.

To prevent pregnancy from an unprotected act of sexual coitus, diethylstilbestrol (DES), a synthetic estrogen, may be prescribed by a physician. To be effective, this oral medication, called the *morning-after pill*, must be started no later than 24 hours after the unprotected coitus. The high level of estrogen interferes with the production of progesterone and therefore prohibits good implantation. It is a helpful method for preventing pregnancy in women or girls who have been raped.

DES should always be used cautiously: High levels of estrogen in the body are associated with thromboembolism. If DES is given during early pregnancy, vaginal carcinoma may occur in a female child at puberty; boys may have distorted and infertile testes. Therefore, if DES is ineffective in preventing conception, the child of the pregnancy should be monitored into puberty for vaginal cancer or poor testicular development. Because of the short course of DES that is used (4 days usually), these problems are only possibilities to be watched for, not certainties. Their risk, however, along with the high risk to the woman, prevents DES administration from becoming a routine method of reproductive life planning.

Effect on Sexual Enjoyment

For the most part, not having to worry about pregnancy because the contraceptive being used is reliable makes sexual relations more enjoyable for couples using birth control pills. Some women, however, appear to lose interest in coitus after taking the pill for about 18 months, possibly because of the long-term effect of altered hormones in their body. Sexual interest increases again after they change to another form of contraception.

Women who have been reared to think that coitus is permissible only as a means of producing children may find little enjoyment in the act when they use a birth control method. Other women find the nausea they experience with the pill interferes with sexual enjoyment as well as with other activities. Women taking birth control pills need to be told that there are now many different forms and strengths of pills available. If they are having side effects with one brand, they might be able to take another brand containing a different strength of estrogen without problems.

Effect on Future Pregnancies

If a woman suspects that she has become pregnant, she should stop taking the pill if she intends to continue the pregnancy. High levels of estrogen or progesterone might be teratogenic to a growing fetus—a concern that has, however, lessened now that birth control pills contain very low doses of hormones.

After a woman discontinues an oral contraceptive, she should not expect to become pregnant before 1 to 2 months, and probably 6 to 8 months; the pituitary gland needs a recovery period before beginning cyclic gonadotropin stimulation again. In one study, premature births and infants with congenital anomalies occurred less frequently in women who had been on the pill before conceiving than in women not using oral contraceptives (Peterson, 1969). This correlation may result from the lower neonatal mortality found in children spaced 2 to 3 years apart than in children spaced 1 year apart. If ovulation does not return spontaneously following discontinuation of the pill, it can be stimulated by clomiphene citrate (Clomid) therapy.

Use by Adolescent Girls

Adolescent girls should have a well-established menstrual cycle of at least a 2-year duration before being begun on ovulation suppressants. This caution reduces the chance that the ovulation suppressant will cause permanent suppression of pituitary regulating activity. Estrogen causes epiphyseal lines of long bones to close and growth to halt; therefore, a time delay will also ensure that the preadolescent growth spurt will not be halted. Adolescent girls may not take pills reliably enough to make them effective (adolescent compliance for any form of medicine taking is low). In addition, the cost of a continuing supply of pills may make this a prohibitive method of birth control. On the other hand, oral contraceptives reduce the incidence of facial acne (by increasing estrogen-androgen ratios) and dysmenorrhea, two common adolescent problems, and are therefore very appealing to this age group.

Chemical Protectives

Spermicidal jellies or creams, when inserted into the vagina, cause the death of spermatozoa before they can enter the cervix. These jellies are not only actively spermicidal, but change the vaginal pH to a strong acid level, a condition not conducive to sperm survival.

With an applicator supplied with each product, the woman inserts the jelly or cream into the vagina before coitus (Figure 11-4). She should do this no more than 1 hour prior to coitus for most effective results. She must be certain to insert the product far back in the vagina. She should not douche for 6 hours following coitus to ensure that the cream or jelly has completed its spermicidal action. Since no prescription is necessary for the purchase of such creams or jellies, they offer an independent method of birth control.

A newer form of spermicidal product is the vaginal tablet. The tablet is small and can be inserted into the vagina easily; on contact with vaginal secretions or precoital penile emissions, it dissolves and a carbon dioxide foam forms that protects the cervix against invading spermatozoa. Another new method is a foam-impregnated sponge that is inserted vaginally. Moisture, again, creates an internal foaming action and contraception protection. Also available are cocoa butter–

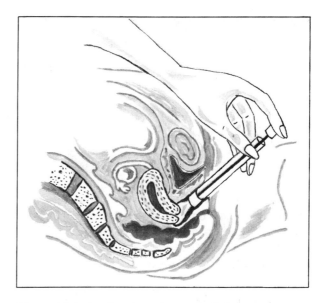

Figure 11-4 *Application of spermicidal preparation.*

and glycerin-based vaginal suppositories. Inserted vaginally, the suppository dissolves and frees spermicidal ingredients. The suppository takes about 15 minutes to dissolve, so coitus should be timed accordingly.

Vaginally inserted spermicidal products are contraindicated in women with acute cervicitis because they may further irritate the cervix. They are generally inappropriate for couples who *must* prevent conception (perhaps the woman is taking a drug that is teratogenic or the couple absolutely does not want the responsibility of children): The effectiveness of all forms of these products is only about 80 percent, compared to the higher 90 to 100 percent effectiveness rate of diaphragms, IUDs, and ovulation suppressants. Women nearing menopause should be advised not to use a type of contraceptive that depends on vaginal moisture to be activated; they may have less at this time of life than they did previously. Some women find the vaginal "leakage" they have after use of these products bothersome. Vaginal suppositories, because of the cocoa butter and glycerin bases, are most bothersome; the sponge is least bothersome. Women who have had toxic shock syndrome should be cautious with using sponges until the method's safety in this regard is more firmly established.

Effect on Sexual Enjoyment

Although spermicidal products must be inserted fairly close to coitus, they also are so easily purchased (no prescription, no physician appointment necessary) that many couples find the inconvenience of insertion only a minor problem. If a couple is concerned that the method does not offer enough protection, worry about becoming pregnant may interfere with sexual enjoyment. Some women and even their partners find the foam or moisture irritating to vaginal and penile tissue during coitus.

Effect on Future Pregnancy

If conception should occur, there is no reason to think that the fetus will be affected. Some women worry that a sperm that survived the cream or foam must have been weakened by migrating through it and will produce a defective child. They can be assured that conception occurred because the product did not completely cover the cervical os; the sperm that reached the uterus was free of the product and unharmed.

Use by Adolescent Girls

Many adolescents use vaginal products as their method of birth control. There is little money involved because a physician appointment is not needed, and no parental permission is required. Adolescents should be cautioned that this method has a high pregnancy rate (20 percent). All women need to be cautioned that preparations labeled "feminine hygiene" products are for vaginal cleanliness and are not spermicidal; they are not birth control products.

Because of the settings in which adolescents engage in coitus (in cars or hurriedly on couches), some girls find having to insert the product awkward and consequently omit using it even though they have purchased it and intended to be more cautious.

Barrier Methods

Barrier methods of birth control work by physically placing a barrier between the cervix and sperm so that sperm cannot enter the uterus and fallopian tubes or by preventing implantation of the fertilized ovum so it will not survive.

Intrauterine Devices (IUDs)

A plastic spiral, S-shape, T-shape, 7-shape, or ring inserted into the uterus can act as a means of contraception. The mechanism of this contraceptive action is not fully understood but possibly a local sterile inflammatory action may result that prevents implantation. If copper wire is added to the IUD, cytotoxins may attack and destroy a blastocyst or destroy the sperm's ability to transverse the uterine space (Kase and Weingold, 1983). Although intrauterine devices have been prescribed for women only in recent years, this ancient method of contraception was used in camels as long ago as 100 B.C. (a stone was inserted into the camel's uterus).

An intrauterine device must be fitted by a physician or a nurse practitioner, who first performs a pelvic examination and does a Pap smear. The device is inserted either during the menstrual flow or before the woman has had coitus following a menstrual flow. The health care provider is thus assured that the woman is not pregnant at the time of insertion, and insertion is easiest while the cervical canal os (entrance to the cervix) is slightly dilated during menses. Insertion may be made immediately following childbirth or before the cervical os closes again. An IUD inserted this soon after childbirth does not affect uterine involution or return to a prepregnant uterine size.

Insertion of an IUD is done in a physician's office or a reproductive life planning clinic. The device is collapsed into a thin inserter; this is introduced into the cervix and uterus by the health care provider. The woman may feel a sharp cramp as the device is passed through the internal cervical os but will not feel the device after it is in place. Although it is inserted in a collapsed position, it takes on its characteristic shape in the uterus when the inserter is withdrawn (Figure 11-5). Properly fitted, the device is contained wholly within the uterus, although an attached string protrudes through the cervix into the vagina.

Progestasert is a special form of IUD (a T-shape of permeable plastic with a drug reservoir in the stem). When progesterone is added to this drug reservoir, it gradually diffuses into the uterus through the plastic and prevents endometrium proliferation. Although most IUDs need to be replaced only every 3 years (copper devices must be replaced within this time frame by FDA regulation), Progestaserts must be changed yearly or the progesterone supply will be depleted.

Intrauterine devices have several advantages over oral ovulation suppressants. Usually only one insertion is necessary, and no further attention is needed except for yearly pelvic examinations. Thus, although the initial insertion involves the cost of a visit to a health care agency, there is no continued expense. The patient may notice some spotting or uterine cramping the first 2 to 3 weeks after insertion; as long as this is present, she should use an additional form of contraception such as a vaginal foam. Some women have a heavier-than-usual menstrual flow for 2 or 3 months with dysmenorrhea. Mefenamic acid (Ponstel), a prostaglandin inhibitor, is helpful in relieving this problem. Occasionally, a woman continues to have cramping and spotting and is likely, in these instances, to expel the device spontaneously. After each menstrual flow, the

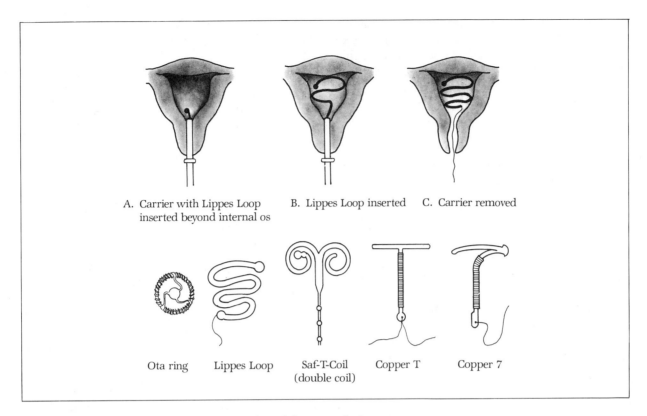

A. Carrier with Lippes Loop inserted beyond internal os   B. Lippes Loop inserted   C. Carrier removed

Ota ring   Lippes Loop   Saf-T-Coil (double coil)   Copper T   Copper 7

Figure 11-5 *Insertion of an IUD and several models currently in use.*

woman should manually check the string attached to the IUD to make certain that the device is still in place.

Some health care providers suggest that the woman not use tampons with an intrauterine device in place to prevent the possibility of the two strings becoming entangled or to prevent trauma to the cervix by pulling on the wrong string in order to remove a tampon. The possibility of staphylococcal infection from the vaginal insertion of tampons traveling by the IUD string into the uterus is being researched as a cause of uterine infections (toxic shock syndrome).

The incidence of pelvic inflammatory disease increases with plain IUDs in place; the copper devices appear to involve a decreased incidence (Young, 1982). Symptoms of pelvic inflammatory disease (PID), most prevalent in women with many sexual partners, include fever, low abdominal tenderness, and dyspareunia. Any woman using an IUD should be familiar with these symptoms. IUDs are contraindicated in women with cervicitis, endometritis, salpingitis, or pelvic inflammatory disease, and in the woman whose uterus is known to be distorted in shape (the IUD might cause increased irritation and spread of infection; it might perforate an abnormally shaped uterus). They are not advised for women with dysmenorrhea, menorrhagia, or a history of ec-

topic pregnancy (their use may increase incidence). Women with valvular heart disease may be advised against the use of IUDs because the possibility of increased pelvic inflammatory disease may lead to accompanying valvular involvement (subacute bacterial endocarditis). As they cause a heavier-than-usual menstrual flow, a woman with anemia is generally not considered to be a good candidate for IUD use.

Effect on Sexual Enjoyment. Women are unable to feel an IUD if it is properly fitted, even during sexual relations, so it does not interfere with sexual enjoyment. The spotting that occurs the first few weeks after insertion is bothersome. Women can be assured that this is a temporary problem. For the occasional woman who continues to have cramping and spotting, another method of contraception is usually recommended.

Effect on Future Pregnancy. If a woman should become pregnant while using an IUD, the device is generally removed vaginally to prevent infection and septic abortion during the pregnancy, although instances of finding the device outside the membranes at the time of delivery, with no damage to the fetus, have been reported. At the time of removal of the device during pregnancy, there is some risk that the intactness of the pregnancy will be disrupted. The use of IUDs is associated with ectopic (tubal) pregnancy due to delay of the zygote in the fallopian tube and an increased incidence of sterility due to pelvic inflammatory disease. They are not recommended for use with the woman who has multiple sexual partners (already at high risk for PID).

Use by Adolescent Girls. It is now possible for nulliparous women (those who have never had children) to be fitted with IUDs (previously these devices were too large for their undeveloped uteruses). A T-shape or 7-shape (copper coated) device is usually chosen. Girls need a review of reproductive anatomy before they have IUDs inserted so that they understand exactly where the device is being positioned; otherwise, they worry that it is somehow free-floating in their abdominal cavity and might become misplaced into the stomach or intestines. If an adolescent has many sexual partners, the increased occurrence of PID must be explained to her and may make the use of an IUD too high a risk.

Diaphragms

A diaphragm is a circular rubber disk that fits over the cervix and forms a barricade against the entrance of spermatozoa. Because it is used with a spermacide jelly, it actually combines a barrier and a chemical method of contraception. A diaphragm is initially prescribed and fitted by a physician or nurse practitioner. Since the shape of the cervix changes with pregnancy, miscarriage, cervical surgery (D&C), or therapeutic abortion, a woman must return for a fitting after any of these occurrences. Gaining or losing more than 15 pounds in weight may change pelvic and vaginal contours to such an extent that having the diaphragm competency checked after the weight gain or loss is also advisable.

Before coitus, the woman coats the rim and the inside of the diaphragm with a contraceptive jelly; in a squatting position, with one leg elevated on a chair, or lying supine, she then inserts the diaphragm into the vagina, sliding it along the posterior wall and pressing it up against the cervix so it is held in place by the vaginal fornices. After insertion, she should always check its position against the cervix by palpating the cervical os through the diaphragm (Figure 11-6). Spermatozoa remain viable in the vagina for 6 hours. Thus, a diaphragm should remain in place for at least 6 hours following coitus, and it may be left in place for as long as 24 hours. If left for longer periods, the stasis of fluid may cause cervical inflammation (erosion). A diaphragm is removed by

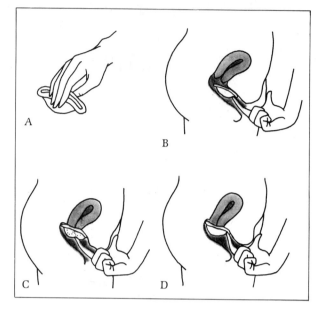

Figure 11-6 *Proper use of a diaphragm. A. After spermicidal jelly or cream is applied, the rim of the diaphragm is pinched between the fingers and the thumb. B. The folded diaphragm is gently inserted into the vagina and pushed downward and backward as far as it will go. C. To check for proper positioning, feel the cervix to be certain it is completely covered by the soft rubber dome of the diaphragm. D. Check that the diaphragm is up under the pubic rim.*

inserting a finger vaginally in order to press against or hook around the anterior rim of the diaphragm, which can then be withdrawn.

If a woman washes the diaphragm in mild soap and water, dries it gently, and stores it in its protective case, it will last for 2 to 3 years. If she inspects the diaphragm periodically to see that the rubber is not deteriorating and checks it with a finger after insertion to be certain it is fitted well up over the cervix, its efficiency as a contraceptive is very high (90%).

Diaphragms may not be competent if the uterus is prolapsed, retroflexed, or anteflexed to such a degree that the cervix is also displaced in relation to the vagina. Intrusion on the vagina by a cystocele or rectocele (walls of the vagina are displaced by bladder or bowel) may make inserting a diaphragm difficult. Diaphragms should not be used in the presence of acute cervicitis, as the close contact of the rubber may cause additional irritation.

Effect on Sexual Enjoyment. Some women dislike using diaphragms because they must insert them prior to coitus (although they may be inserted up to 2 hours beforehand, minimizing this problem). Use of a vibrator as a part of fore-play, frequent penile insertion, or the woman taking the top position during coitus may dislodge the diaphragm, so it may not be the contraceptive of choice for some couples. If coitus is repeated within 6 hours, the diaphragm should not be removed and replaced; instead more spermicidal jelly should be added. Some couples may find this precaution restricting. Use of a diaphragm allows sexual relations during the menstrual flow without menstrual blood interfering with enjoyment.

Effect on Future Pregnancy. If a woman should become pregnant while using a diaphragm, there is no risk to the fetus. People tell bad jokes about babies looking as if they had been strained through diaphragms, and some women may need help separating such jokes from reality.

Use by Adolescent Girls. Adolescents may be fitted for diaphragms, although the device may not remain as effective as with older women because an adolescent's vagina varies in size as she matures and starts sexual relations. Adolescents may need to be reminded that diaphragms must be individually fitted; otherwise, they may borrow a friend's, or a group of girls will pool their money to pay for one. A young girl needs to be shown an anatomic diagram of her cervix. Another option is to use a mirror during a pelvic examination to show a girl her cervix; she can then visualize what she is feeling when she checks for diaphragm placement. Asking the girl to place the diaphragm and then assessing the placement yourself assures you and the girl that she can use the method reliably.

Cervical Caps

A cervical cap is another barrier method of contraception. Caps have been available in Europe for years but are only recently being introduced to any great extent in the United States. A cervical cap is made of soft rubber shaped like a thimble and fits snugly over the uterine cervix in a manner similar to a diaphragm. It is filled just before insertion with a spermicidal jelly that must be used with it—again, like the diaphragm.

Many women are not able to use cervical caps because their cervix is too short for it to fit properly. The caps tend to dislodge more readily than a diaphragm during coitus. One of the few advantages caps have over diaphragms is that they can be left in place longer than diaphragms (weeks if desired) because they do not put pressure on the vaginal walls as diaphragms do, possibly causing interference with vaginal blood supply. Most women notice a vaginal odor if a cervical cap re-mains in place over 24 hours, however, so this difference may be of little practical use to them. Cervical caps, like diaphragms, must be fitted individually by a health care provider.

Condoms

A condom is a rubber or synthetic sheath that is placed over the erect penis prior to coitus. It prevents pregnancy because spermatozoa are deposited not in the vagina but in the tip of the condom. The use of condoms has an efficiency rate of about 85 percent. One of the few "male-responsibility" birth control measures available, condoms do not require a prescription for purchase. As well as having a contraceptive role, these devices lessen the chance of spreading sexually transmitted disease.

There are no contraindications to the use of condoms except for rare rubber sensitivity. Examining the condom following coitus for a tear is an effective method for alerting a couple that conception may occur. As they are not as effective a means of contraception as other forms, they should be used with caution by couples who must for medical reasons delay conception.

Effect on Sexual Enjoyment. In order to be effective, condoms must be applied prior to any penile-vulvar contact because preejaculation fluid may contain some sperm. The condom should be positioned so it is loose enough at the penis tip to collect the ejaculate without undue pressure on the condom. As soon as the penis begins to become flaccid following ejaculation, the penis (with the condom held carefully in place) must be withdrawn. If it is not withdrawn at this time, sperm may leak from the now loosely fitting sheath into the vagina. Some men find that condoms dull their enjoyment of coitus or are unable to achieve erection with one in place; some women resent men having to withdraw promptly following ejaculation.

Many men enjoy the use of condoms because they feel they are taking more of the responsibility for reproductive life planning.

Effect on Future Pregnancy. Children conceived while a condom is being used are not adversely affected.

Use by Adolescents. Adolescents may need to be cautioned that condoms should not be reused: Even a pinpoint hole can allow thousands of sperm to escape. Some adolescent boys have infrequent coitus and therefore use condoms that they have owned and stored for a long time. The efficiency of these old condoms, especially if they are carried in a warm pocket, should be questioned. For many adolescent couples, use of a vaginally inserted preparation by the girl and a condom by her partner is the preferred method of reproductive life planning. Efficiency of these two methods of birth control, used in conjunction, is about 95 percent.

Natural Family Planning

When initial reports on ovulation suppressants were so suggestive of carcinogenicity, many couples turned to natural reproductive life planning choices. These methods involve no expense, nor are any foreign materials used. They are choices approved by the Roman Catholic Church and Orthodox Judaism.

The Rhythm (Calendar) Method

The rhythm method requires a couple to abstain from sexual coitus on the days of a menstrual cycle when the woman is able to conceive (the period surrounding ovulation). Calculating fertile days is based on three assumptions:

1. Ovulation occurs on days 12–16 (14 plus or minus 2) from the end of a cycle.
2. A sperm is capable of fertilization for 48 hours.
3. The life of an ovum is 24 hours. A woman's fertile days are therefore days 11 to 18 (12 to 16 plus 48 hours for sperm life) from the end of a cycle.

In order to have a framework on which to base calculations of safe times, a woman should keep a record of 12 menstrual cycles (a minimum of six). Her *first* fertile day is determined by subtracting 18 from the number of days in the shortest menstrual cycle she has had over the last 12 months. The *last* fertile day is determined by subtracting 11 days from the longest menstrual cycle during the 12-month period. For example, if she had menstrual cycles ranging from 26 to 32 days, her fertile period would be from the eighth day (26 –18) to the twenty-first day (32 – 11). This schedule is shown in Figure 11-7.

In this hypothetical situation, the woman has only 9 days during the first month illustrated that are "safe" for her. In the second month, because her menstrual cycle was fairly short (27 days), there are only 7 safe days available. This short period of safe days is the reason the rhythm method is not an acceptable form of reproductive life planning for some couples.

This method of contraception is about 80 percent effective if the woman has regular menstrual cycles and is motivated to maintain monthly records. In actual practice, irregular cycles and

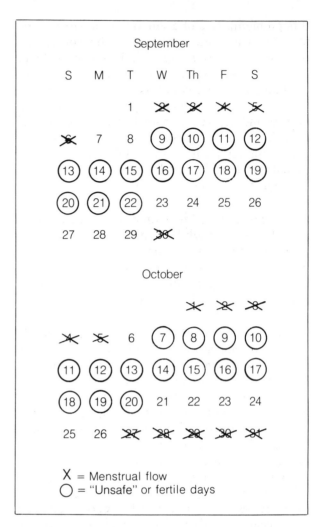

Figure 11-7 *Timetable for using rhythm (calendar) method as a reproductive life planning method.*

failure to keep records over a long period of time make it less effective. The method will not work reliably if the woman's menstrual cycles are irregular or she does not accept the responsibility for calculating fertile days. It is also unreliable both in the postpartal period, until regular periods are reestablished, and in lactating women, who may not have menstrual flows as markers for calculation.

More than do previously mentioned methods of birth control, the rhythm method depends on increased cooperation of the sexual partner. Some women find this a disadvantage; other couples enjoy the feeling family planning has truly become "family" planning.

Effect on Sexual Enjoyment. Because no prescription or medication is involved, no cost is incurred. More spontaneity in sexual relations is possible than with methods that involve vaginal insertion. On the other hand, the required days of abstinence may make the method unsatisfactory and unenjoyable for a couple.

Effect on Future Pregnancy. Since no artificial methods of contraception are involved, no physical harm can be caused to future pregnancies. There is the possibility, however, that a conceived child may be unwanted and that the parents cannot adjust to the conception, pregnancy, and child.

Use by Adolescent Girls. As girls tend to have irregular menstrual cycles for several years after menarche, the rhythm method is often ineffective as a means of reproductive life planning for young adolescents. Girls may also find it difficult to keep a calendar of safe and unsafe days and to be able to say "no" to encounters on unsafe days.

Rhythm and Basal Temperature

Just prior to the day of ovulation, the woman's basal body temperature falls about half a degree. At the time of ovulation, the temperature will rise a full degree. This higher level will be maintained for the rest of the menstrual cycle. Adding basal body temperature taking to a rhythm or calendar method of contraception decreases the number of unsafe days each month.

In practicing this method of contraception, a woman should take and chart her temperature each morning immediately after waking, before she undertakes any activity (a rectal temperature is most accurate but an oral reading will suffice). This is her basal temperature. She should then calculate her first fertile day as in the rhythm method (i.e., shortest menstrual cycle minus 18). This will be her first day of abstinence (as with the rhythm method). As soon as she notices a slight dip in temperature followed by an increase, she knows that she has ovulated. She continues abstinence only until the third day of the sustained high temperature (the life of ova and sperm combined) which usually shortens the period of abstinence by 3 or 4 days (Figure 11-8).

The danger of this method is that a temperature rise may be the result of illness rather than of ovulation. The woman may misinterpret the increase in temperature and think a fertile day is a safe one.

Rhythm and Ovulation Determination

Prior to ovulation each month, cervical mucus is thicker and does not stretch when pulled between the thumb and a finger (the property of spinnbarkeit). With ovulation and for 2 days afterward, the cervical mucus becomes thin and watery and stretches a distance of 11 to 15 cm before

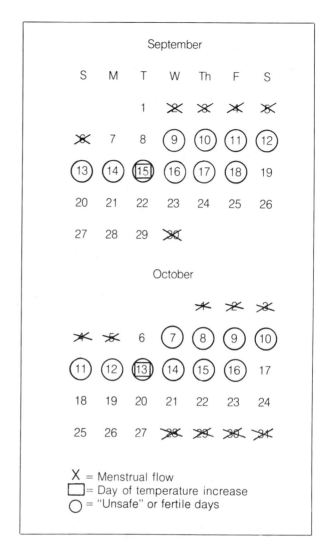

Figure 11-8 *Timetable for using rhythm (calendar method) in conjunction with basal temperature as a reproductive life planning method.*

the strand breaks. With this knowledge, a woman can more accurately predict her day of ovulation than by the rhythm method alone.

To use this method, a woman establishes her first day of sexual abstinence as she would for the basic rhythm method (18 days subtracted from her shortest period). She then tests her vaginal secretions daily for the property of spinnbarkeit. She continues abstinence only 3 days after spinnbarkeit occurs, which, like the basal body temperature modification, allows her to shorten the total period of abstinence each month by 3 or 4 days.

A woman must be conscientious about assessing vaginal secretions daily or she will miss the phenomenon of changing cervical secretions. The feel of vaginal secretions following sexual relations is unreliable: Seminal fluid has a watery, postovulatory consistency and can be confused with ovulatory mucus.

Ovulation Method Alone

Women may rely only on the naturally occurring changes in cervical mucus as a method of natural family planning. Often called the *Billings method* after its originator, the method requires the woman to assess her vaginal secretions daily following her menstrual flow. When the quality of secretions changes, becoming wet and slippery with spinnbarkeit properties, she begins to abstain from sexual relations. She continues abstinence until 3 days after the mucus has become sticky and unstretchable again. For most women, these determinations limit the period of abstinence to a very short time, about 5 to 7 days.

In order to acquaint herself with the feel of vaginal changes during a cycle, a woman should abstain from coitus for a full month. During following months, she should abstain from coitus every other day during the first part of each cycle so she can evaluate cervical mucus free of seminal fluid.

A woman must be highly motivated to use the ovulation method. It may be a good choice for a lactating woman without the menstrual flow markers for the rhythm method or for a woman with such irregular periods that the rhythm method leaves her very few safe days.

Coitus Interruptus

Coitus interruptus is one of the oldest known methods of contraception. The couple proceeds with coitus until ejaculation seems imminent. Then the man withdraws and the emission of spermatozoa takes place outside the vagina. Unfortunately, ejaculation may occur before withdrawal is complete and, despite the care used, some spermatozoa may be deposited in the vagina. Since there are always a few spermatozoa in preejaculation seminal fluid, even though withdrawal seems controlled, fertilization may occur. For these reasons, coitus interruptus offers little protection against conception.

Effect of Sexual Enjoyment. Some couples obtain sexual satisfaction when using this method. Others find that it interferes with satisfaction.

Effect on Future Pregnancy. There are no effects on children conceived when the procedure is used.

Use by Adolescents. Adolescent boys often lack the control or experience to use coitus interruptus.

Permanent Methods

Permanent methods of reproductive life planning involve sterilizing men by vasectomy and women by a tubal procedure. Sterilization should not be undertaken in individuals—male or female—who equate being fertile with being a full person. The self-esteem of these individuals may be lessened after such a change.

Vasectomy

In sterilization of a male, a small incision is made in each side of the scrotum. The vas deferens at that point is then cut and tied, blocking the passage of spermatozoa.

Following vasectomy, some men develop autoimmunity or form antibodies against sperm. Even if reconstruction of the vas deferens is successful, then, the sperm they produce do not have good mobility and are incapable of fertilization. The actual ability to reverse vasectomy procedures is therefore low, about 30 percent (Diebel, 1978). There is currently a concern that vasectomy can lead to coronary artery disease or shorten a man's life span; additional studies on over 10,000 men have shown this fear to be groundless (Zatuchni, 1984). The man should think of the procedure as irreversible, although newer techniques of silicone plugs, stopcocks, and microsurgery can, to a limited extent, give him the chance to change his mind.

Vasectomy can be performed under local anesthesia in a physician's office. The man experiences only a small amount of local pain afterward that can be managed by the administration of a mild analgesic and application of ice. It is 100 percent effective, although spermatozoa that were present in the vas deferens at the time of surgery may remain viable for as long as six months. Although the man can resume sexual coitus within a week, an additional birth control method should be used until two negative sperm reports have been examined.

Some men resist the concept of vasectomy because they are not sufficiently aware of their anatomy to know exactly what the procedure involves. It is important to teach that vasectomy does not interfere with the production of sperm; the testes continue to produce sperm as always. The sperm simply do not pass beyond the severed vas deferens but are absorbed at that point. The man will still have full erection and ejaculation capacity. Because he also continues to form seminal fluid, he will ejaculate that fluid—just without sperm. The incision site for a vasectomy is shown in Figure 11-9.

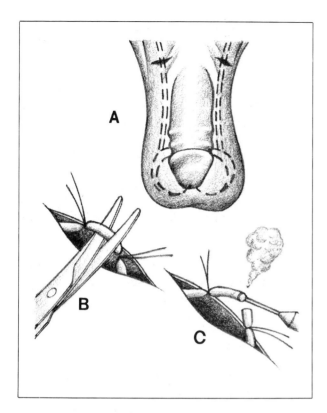

Figure 11-9 *A. Site of a vasectomy incision. B. The vas being cut with surgical scissors. C. Cut ends of the vas being burned with a controlled electric current so that scar tissue forms to block the passage of sperm.*

Tubal Procedures

In some areas of the country, tubal sterilization is a more popular contraceptive choice than even ovulation suppressants. Sterilization of women could involve removal of the uterus (hysterectomy), but it generally refers to a minor surgical procedure, such as tubal ligation, that occludes the fallopian tubes by cauterizing, blocking, crushing, or clamping them. With the tubes no longer patent, sperm are prevented from passing into the tubes to meet the ova. Newer techniques are the instillation of a silicon gel into the tubes as a plug that can be removed at a later date if the woman changes her mind and the use of metal or plastic clips or rubber rings that cause necrosis and scarring of the tubes. "Femcept" is a brand name for a device that can be inserted vaginally into the uterus without anesthesia; a plastic compound is then injected into both tubes to seal them (Zatuchni, 1984). This office procedure can be performed by a nurse or physicians' assistant. A *fimbriectomy*, or removal of the fimbria at the distal end of the tubes, is possible. This procedure prevents the ova from entering the tubes.

Operations Used. The most common operation for female sterilization is *laparoscopy* (Figure 11-10). Following a menstrual flow and before ovulation, under general anesthesia, an incision

Figure 11-10 *Laparoscopy for tubal sterilization. The patency of the tubes is destroyed by application of an electrical current. Two small abdominal incisions are used here. From Richard Wolf Medical Instruments Corporation.*

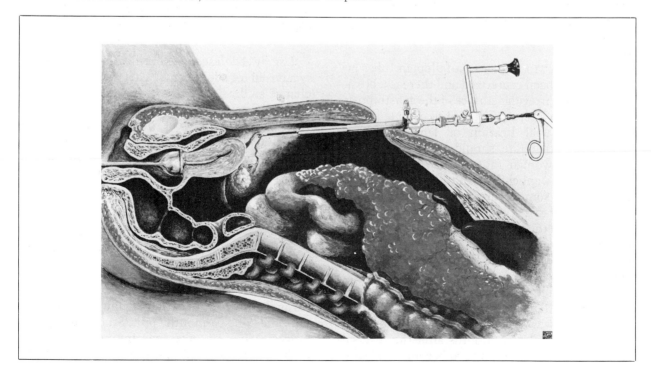

as small as 1 cm is made just under the woman's umbilicus. A lighted laparoscope is inserted through the incision. Carbon dioxide is then pumped into the incision to lift the abdominal wall upward out of the line of vision. The surgeon locates the fallopian tubes by viewing the field through the laparoscope. An electrical current is passed through the instrument for about 3 to 5 seconds, which coagulates the tissue of the tube and seals it. The operation is quick, and the woman is only kept in the hospital overnight or discharged in a few hours. She may notice abdominal bloating following the procedure for the first 24 hours until the carbon dioxide is absorbed. Sharp diaphragmatic or shoulder pain may result if some of the carbon dioxide escapes under the diaphragm. She may resume coitus as soon as 2 to 3 days following the procedure.

Women need to be certain that they have no unprotected coitus before the procedure: A sperm trapped in the tube could fertilize the ova there and cause an ectopic pregnancy. Women need to be informed prior to the procedure that their menstrual cycle will be unaffected by the procedure. Otherwise they may be disappointed or worried that, unlike hysterectomy, the operation does not end their menstrual periods. As with any abdominal surgery, there is a risk of bowel perforation, hemorrhage, and side effects of general anesthesia with the procedure. A contraindication to laparoscopy is an umbilical hernia, which might result in bowel perforation. Extensive obesity probably would require a full laparotomy in order to allow good visualization. If clips were used, the woman may notice a day or two of abdominal discomfort caused by the local necrosis at the clip site.

It is difficult to reconstruct fallopian tubes after they have been cauterized and there is a possibility that the irregular surface of the anastomosis site after such a repair will lead to ectopic (tubal) pregnancy. Tubal ligation or laparoscopy for sterilization, therefore, should not be undertaken lightly: The woman must decide that she not only does not want children now but also will not want them at some future date. After reconstructive surgery of this type (salpingoplasty) to reverse cauterization, the pregnancy rate is only 30 to 60 percent; it may be as high as 80 percent if clamps, not cautery, were used for the ligation (Kase, 1983).

An incision for microsurgical tubal reconstruction is about 10 to 15 cm in length and transverse across the lower abdomen. A woman should be advised to wait 1 or 2 months after the reversal procedure before attempting to become pregnant,

a caution that helps inflammation in the tubes from the surgery to fade; this constriction might lead to ectopic pregnancy.

Women who have been using ovulation suppressants prior to sterilization need to be forewarned that, after discontinuing ovulation suppressants, dysmenorrhea may return if they had been previously affected.

Sterilization can be carried out as soon as 1 day after childbirth. The abdominal distention at this time may make locating the tubes difficult. A *minilaparotomy* is the procedure used during this time or postabortion. Many such procedures are done in the ambulatory surgery department. After a local anesthetic, an incision is made 2 to 3 cm transversely just above the pubic hair. The fallopian tubes are pulled to the surface and lifted out of the incision in order to be visualized. A disadvantage of a minilaparotomy is that it makes it difficult to fully visualize the pelvis.

Culdoscopy (an examining culdoscope inserted through the posterior fornix of the vagina) and *colpotomy* (incision into the vagina) could be the methods of choice, but the incidence of pelvic infection is higher and visualization less.

Metal or plastic clips or rubber rings may be used to seal the tubes.

Effect on Sexual Enjoyment. Sterilization may lead to increased sexual enjoyment by completely eliminating the possibility of pregnancy. If either partner changes his or her mind, however, the surgery may become an issue that interferes not only with sexual enjoyment but with other aspects of their relationship as well.

Use by Adolescents. Sterilization is not usually advised for adolescents. Their future goals may change so drastically that what they want at age 16 or 18 may not be what they want at age 30. Adolescents should be counseled to use more temporary forms of reproductive life planning. Later, if they still feel sterilization is the method of reproductive life planning for them, the option is still open.

Future Reproductive Planning Methods

Since estrogen is responsible for most of the side effects associated with oral contraceptives, studies are being made of extremely low-dose estrogen pills and "once-a-month" pills. Studies using only progesterone are also continuing. In Europe, biphasic and triphasic pills which alter the proportion of estrogen to progesterone during a cycle are being used. It is possible that a progesterone injection once a month, a topical application of progesterone, or a progesterone-impregnated diaphragm will be used in the future. Progesterone or estrogen can perhaps be implanted under the skin once a year in a slowly dissolving plastic capsule. Possibly a woman could be "vaccinated" with antibodies against spermatozoa. A GN-RH antagonist to halt FSH production may soon be available; this could be the first male oral contraceptive. Injection of testosterone-filled microcapsules is another form of male contraception that is being explored. Until some method satisfies all the criteria for an ideal contraceptive—complete safety, no side effects, low cost, easy availability, and user acceptability—research in this field will continue.

Utilizing Nursing Process

Reproductive life planning is a sensitive area of concern because it involves very personal decisions. In order that such planning can be adequate for each individual, it is necessary to use the nursing process in planning care.

Assessment

Due to changing social values and life styles, many more people are able to talk freely about reproductive life planning today than formerly. Remember, however, that many people are still not comfortable with this area of concern and may not voice their interest in the subject comfortably unless they are asked specific questions. Many women in the immediate postpartal period may believe that they cannot conceive immediately (especially if they are breast-feeding). Ask at health assessments if a woman wants more information or any help with planning in this area of her life.

Analysis

The Fourth Annual Conference on Nursing Diagnoses accepted no nursing diagnosis specific to the area of reproductive life planning. Common nursing diagnoses used in this area, however, include these: Knowledge, deficit, related to reproductive life planning; fear, related to use of ovulation suppressant; discomfort, vaginal spotting, related to the side effects of an IUD. When establishing goals for care in this area, be certain that they are realistic for that person. If the person has a history of poor drug compliance, it may not be realistic for her to plan on taking an ovulation suppressant every day. If she has strong religious or cultural beliefs that a system is morally wrong, obviously, this would not be the system to suggest to her.

Planning

Many women are unable to make realistic plans about reproductive life planning because they are uninformed about the many methods available. Planning, therefore, begins with formulating methods of teaching to make the woman a more informed health care consumer.

Implementation

A great deal of the implementation in this area involves informing women and their sexual partners of the variety of measures that are available. Do not discount natural methods of planning, such as ovulation determination. For the woman who intends to maintain planning measures for a long period, this noninvasive, nondrug method may be her best choice.

Evaluation

Evaluation is important in reproductive life planning because the side effects of many methods can cause women to discontinue them and be left without protection. Evaluate early (within 1 to 3 weeks) after a woman begins a system of birth control so that you can assess effectiveness before she might discontinue the system. Evaluation of contraceptive methods is much broader than simply counting unwanted pregnancies; the couple's satisfaction with the system is vital.

Nursing Care Planning

Barbara Harrington is a 17-year-old whom you see in a reproductive life planning clinic. The following is a nursing care plan related to this area of care.

Assessment

17-year-old female seen for advice on contraception. Has been sexually active for 3 months; has not been using any form of birth control. Menarche at 12 years, menstrual cycle 28–35 days duration, moderately heavy flow, dysmenorrhea enough to keep her home from school 1 day/month. Last menstrual flow 1 week ago.

No history of sexually transmitted disease, vaginal infections, pelvic inflammatory disease, uterine malformation. Height: 5'2"; development: Tanner 4.

Analysis

Fear related to unprotected coitus.

Locus of Decision Making. Shared.

Goal. Patient to choose and utilize a method of reproductive life planning by one month's time.

Criteria. Patient:

1. Will voice contraceptive options available and her preference.

2. Can explain how to use the method of her choice correctly.

3. Can explain any follow-up care necessary for method chosen.

Nursing Orders

1. Support choice of IUD suggested by M.D. (at 5'2", growth may not be complete enough for ovulation suppressant; adolescent poor compliance leaves other methods in doubt).

2. Routine VDRL, gonorrhea plate, Pap test with pelvic examination.

3. Discuss ability to say "no" to sexual relationships she does not want.

4. Discuss necessity for yearly pelvic examinations with IUD in place. Possibility of mild cramping and spotting for one week.

5. Discuss symptoms of PID and importance of notifying health care provider if any of these occur.

Questions for Review

Multiple Choice

The following patients are seen at a family planning clinic.

1. Mrs. Green had an intrauterine device (IUD) inserted 2 weeks ago. She calls the clinic and reports that she has had some cramping since insertion and that her present menstrual flow is heavy. You would advise her to
   a. come to the clinic as soon as possible.
   b. consider this normal, as her IUD has been newly inserted.
   c. take her blood pressure for the remainder of the month.
   d. change her method of reproductive life planning.

2. Mrs. Lee visits the clinic to request a prescription for birth control pills. Assessment of which of the following would indicate that an ovulation suppressant would *not* be the method of choice for Mrs. Lee?
   a. She is 30 years of age.
   b. She has irregular menstrual cycles.
   c. She has varicose veins.
   d. She has a history of cervical infections.

3. Mrs. Lee telephones you after taking an ovulation suppressant for 3 months to tell you she has forgotten to take her pill 2 mornings in a row. What would be the best advice to give her?
   a. Start a new cycle of 21 pills immediately, plus additional estrogen for the next three days.
   b. Take 3 pills immediately and avoid coitus for the remainder of the month.
   c. Take a pill now and use a second method of contraception for the remainder of the month.

   d. Take a pill now and return to the clinic to reevaluate whether or not she is best suited for this method.

4. Mrs. Brown uses a diaphragm as a method of reproductive life planning. She should be instructed to return to the clinic to have her diaphragm fit checked following all of the following occurrences *except*
   a. cervical infection.
   b. miscarriage.
   c. weight change of 20 pounds.
   d. childbirth.

5. Mrs. Smith is 40 years old and a heavy smoker. She has very irregular menstrual cycles. She wants a highly reliable contraceptive. Assuming that all the following methods of birth control are acceptable to her, which would you recommend?
   a. an ovulation suppressant
   b. a condom for her partner
   c. the rhythm (calendar) method
   d. an IUD

6. Linda is 14 years old. She hates the thought of an intrauterine device yet wants a method of birth control with high reliability. Which of the following methods would you recommend to her?
   a. an ovulation suppressant
   b. vaginal foam for her; a condom for her partner
   c. postcoital douching
   d. an IUD

7. In helping Mrs. Berg locate her fertile days using the rhythm or calendar method, you would teach her to substract
   a. 14 from 28.
   b. 18 from her shortest period, 11 from her longest.

c. the length of her average period from the ideal of 28.

d. 18 from her longest period, 11 from her shortest.

8. For natural reproduction life planning, at ovulation, cervical mucus can be identified by a woman because it

   a. has a high viscosity and alkalinity.
   b. has properties of acidity and ferning.
   c. is thin and watery.
   d. is filled with increased leukocytes.

9. Tubal ligation is a common sterilization procedure in women. Which of the following concepts should you teach Mrs. Martin about this procedure?

   a. She will have lessened dysmenorrhea following the procedure.
   b. She must think of it as irreversible.
   c. Her menstrual flow will be reduced in amount.
   d. She should schedule it just before a menstrual flow.

10. Mr. Atkins is interested in learning about vasectomy. You would teach him that

    a. it is usually done as an office procedure.
    b. he will no longer have an ejaculate.
    c. he may notice continued scrotal swelling.
    d. his testes will no longer produce sperm.

Discussion

1. Teaching reproductive life planning measures can be a nurse's major role in a health maintenance setting. What are important factors to consider to ensure you will meet a couple's needs?

2. The age of a woman often influences her choice of reproductive life planning methods. How might the choice of a 16-year-old girl differ from that of a 35-year-old woman?

3. Knowing the contraindications of certain reproductive life planning methods is important for ensuring safe practice. What are the contraindications for ovulation suppressants? IUDs?

Suggested Readings

American Nurses Association. (1966). ANA adopts statement on family planning. *American Journal of Nursing, 66,* 2376.

Arthur, C. (1981). Customized cervical cap: Evolution of an ancient idea. *Journal of Nurse Midwifery, 26,* 13.

Atkinson, L., et al. (1980). Prospects for improved contraception. *Family Planning Perspectives, 12,* 173.

Ayvazian, A. (1981). Contraceptive choices of female university students. *J.O.G.N. Nursing, 10,* 426.

Bendett, J. (1980). Current contraceptive research. *Family Planning Perspectives, 12,* 149.

Billings, J. (1975). *Natural family planning: The ovulation method.* (2nd ed.). Collegeville, MN: The Liturgical Press.

Bleden, K. D. (1982). Psychological aspects of family planning. *Midwife Health Visitor and Community Nurse, 18,* 518.

Burbach, C. A. (1980). Contraception and adolescent pregnancy. *J.O.G.N. Nursing, 9,* 319.

Callender-Green, G., et al. (1983). The nurse-midwife in a contraceptive program for adolescents. *Journal of Ambulatory Care Management, 6,* 57.

Capiello, J. D., et al. (1981). The rebirth of the cervical cap. *Journal of Nurse Midwifery, 26,* 13.

Cole, L. P., et al. (1983). Effects of breastfeeding on IUD performance. *American Journal of Public Health, 73,* 384.

Cordero, J. F., & Layde, P. M. (1983). Vaginal spermicides, chromosomal abnormalities and limb reduction defects. *Family Planning Perspectives, 15,* 16.

Cupit, L. G. (1984). Contraception: Helping patients choose. *J.O.G.N. Nursing 13,* 23s.

DeLia, J. E. (1981). Contraception for adolescent girls. *Consultant, 21,* 63.

Diebel, P. (1978). Natural family planning: Different methods. *M.C.N., 3,* 171.

Dryfoos, J. G. (1982). Contraceptive use, pregnancy intentions and pregnancy outcomes among U.S. women. *Family Planning Perspectives, 14,* 81.

Fiscella, K. (1982). Relationship of weight change to required size of vaginal diaphragm. *Nurse Practitioner, 7,* 21.

Gara, E. (1981). Nursing protocol to improve the effectiveness of the contraceptive diaphragm. *M.C.N., 6,* 41.

Gromko, L. (1980). Intrauterine devices. *Nurse Practitioner, 5,* 17.

Hartwell, S. F., & Schlesselman, S. (1983). Risk of uterine perforation among users of intrauterine devices. *Obstetrics/Gynecology, 61,* 31.

Huber, D. (1984). Update on techniques for voluntary sterilization. *Contemporary OB/GYN, 23,* 130.

Kase, N. G., & Weingold, A. B. (Eds.). (1983). *Principles and practice of clinical gynecology.* New York: John Wiley and Sons.

Lane, C., & Kemp. J. (1984). Family planning needs of adolescents. *J.O.G.N. Nursing, 13,* 61s.

Lippes, J. (1981). The mechanism of action of intrauterine contraceptive devices. *Midwife Health Visitor and Community Nurse, 17,* 518.

Maine, D., & Wray, J. (1984). Effects of family planning on maternal and child health. *Consultant, 23,* 122.

Martin, M. C. (1981). Natural family planning and instructor training. *Nursing Health Care, 2,* 554.

Martins, H. (1983). Family planning update. *Health Visitor, 56,* 166.

McCarthy, J. J. (1981). Natural family planning: When other contraceptive methods won't do. *Consultant, 21,* 109.

Mishell, D. R. (1983). Oral contraceptives: The latest facts on their benefits and risks. *Consultant, 23,* 139.

Namerow, P. B., et al. (1983). Follow-up of adolescent family planning clinic users. *Family Planning Perspectives, 15,* 172.

Orr, M. T. (1982). Sex education and contraceptive education in U.S. public high schools. *Family Planning Perspectives, 14,* 304.

Peterson, W. F. (1969). Pregnancy following oral contraceptive therapy. *Obstetrics and Gynecology, 34,* 363.

Quinlivan, W. L. (1983). Postpill amenorrhea: Tests to find the cause. *Female Patient, 8,* 29.

Redmond, M. A. (1982). Couple-directed contraceptive counseling. *Canadian Nurse, 78,* 38.

Skillman, T. G. (1980). Oral contraceptive use: Its risks and benefits. *Hospital Formulary, 15,* 622.

Torres, A., & Forrest, J. D. (1983). The costs of contraception . . . one factor that affects the choice of a birth control method. *Family Planning Perspectives, 15,* 70.

Trimmer, E. (1983). Awkward questions about IUDs. *Midwife Health Visitor and Community Nurse, 19,* 66.

Young, R. L. (1982). Barrier contraception: A trend toward older methods. *Consultant, 22,* 297.

Zatuchni, G. I. (1984). Advances in fertility control. *Female Patient, 9,* 38.

12

The Couple Who Is Infertile

OBJECTIVES

Following mastery of the contents of this chapter, you should be able to

1. Define the terms *infertility* and *sterility*.
2. Describe common reasons for infertility in both men and women.
3. Describe common assessments necessary to detect infertility.
4. State a nursing diagnosis related to infertility.
5. Plan care specific to relieving or coping with a diagnosis of infertility.
6. Assist with implementations involved in a diagnostic fertility study or help a couple achieve fertility.
7. Evaluate goal outcomes regarding infertility management.
8. Analyze alternative reproductive measures that may be undertaken by a couple with a problem of infertility.
9. Synthesize concern for problems of infertility with nursing process to achieve quality maternal-newborn nursing care.

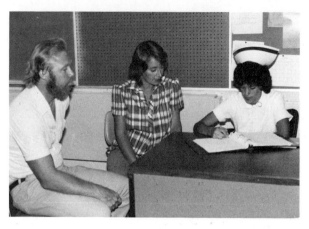

Figure 12-1 *One nursing role in maternal-newborn nursing is helping discover why an infertile couple cannot conceive.*

FROM THE TIME a couple is told that the woman is pregnant until she holds the infant in her arms, both the woman and her sexual partner may worry that she may not be able to carry the child to term. In about 10 percent of American couples, the concern is even greater: They wonder if they will be able to initiate a pregnancy at all. One of them may be infertile or perhaps even sterile.

It is important for the welfare of children, the physical health of women, and the mental health of couples that they have only as many children as they want and can care for. It is equally important that couples who do want children should be able to conceive and bear them, in other words, that conception is considered as important as contraception (Figure 12-1).

Infertility is said to exist when a pregnancy has not occurred after at least 1 year of unprotected coitus. In *primary* infertility, there have been no previous conceptions; in *secondary* infertility, there has been a previous viable pregnancy, but the couple seems unable to conceive again. In *sterility*, some known factor, such as the absence of a uterus, prevents conception. In 30 to 35 percent of couples with an infertility problem, the man is infertile. In 5 to 10 percent of couples, no known cause for the infertility can be discovered despite all the diagnostic tests currently available (Speroff, 1983).

Many couples think they have a problem of infertility because they are unaware of the average length of time it takes to achieve pregnancy. When participating in coitus an average of four times per week, 50 percent of couples take 6 months to conceive; after 12 months, 80 percent of couples will have conceived (Wallach, 1983). These times are longer if sexual relations are less frequent. After 12 months, the 20 percent of couples who have not conceived will begin to have serious doubts about their fertility.

Many young couples today try to organize their lives into time blocks. The first 2 years of marriage, both partners will work and they will furnish their home; or they will both attend school and finish their educations. The third year of their marriage they will have their first child. Couples who program their lives this way grow apprehensive when conception does not occur according to plan. Sometimes simple counseling, with an explanation that conception is not as predictable as a degree after 4 years of college, will alleviate their apprehension. There is a general feeling that infertility tends to occur in couples who desperately want a baby. The woman is said to be "trying too hard." It is difficult to document which is the chicken and which is the egg in such couples.

Nursing Care Highlight

Infertility Testing

A couple having infertility testing done may be asked to make many difficult decisions about their future lives based on how much they value children. Be certain that you do not influence these decisions based on your own values. In the future, the couple, not you, must live with these decisions.

Perhaps they want a child desperately because their plans have been frustrated, and it is not their desperation that is causing the infertility, but their infertility that is causing the desperation.

Women who have been taking ovulation suppressants or using an intrauterine device (IUD) for reproductive life planning may have difficulty becoming pregnant for a number of months after discontinuing the pill or having the IUD removed. Couples should be counseled regarding this possibility. Couples who engage in coitus daily hoping to cause early impregnation may actually have more difficulty with conceiving than those who delay at least every other day: Too frequent coitus can lower a man's spermatozoa count below a point of fertility. In addition, couples who increase their sexual relations to increase sperm-ova exposure may find their lives governed by temperature charts and "good days" and "bad days" to such an extent that their relationship undergoes a great deal of stress. More knowledge about normal conception time intervals helps to relieve these problems.

The responsible nurse's general approach to couples undergoing infertility testing is summarized in the Nursing Care Highlight above.

Fertility Studies

The age of the couple and the degree of apprehension they feel make a difference in determining when they should be referred for evaluation for fertility studies. As a rule of thumb, if the woman is under 30, she should be referred after 1 year of infertility. If she is over 30, she should be referred after 6 months of infertility. The older the woman, the more quickly studies should be undertaken, since adoption, artificial insemination, and embryo transfer—the alternatives to natural childbearing (besides childless living, which must not be discounted)—are limited by age. It would be doubly unfortunate if a couple delayed fertility testing so long that by the time they discovered they were incapable of conception they would also be considered too old to adopt or the woman would have difficulty completing a pregnancy successfully. If a couple is extremely apprehensive over their apparent infertility, no matter what their ages, studies should never be delayed.

Infertility studies are time-consuming; at least 8 to 11 weeks are required for a minimum series. If the first tests reveal abnormalities, further studies may be necessary, extending the time to 3 or 4 months. After all this, the results may reveal no known cause for the apparent infertility. A couple should be prepared for both these eventualities at the first visit, so that they are not unnecessarily alarmed by the time the studies take and do not feel cheated if the results are indeterminate.

Male Infertility

Although infertility is almost automatically assumed to be the woman's problem, fertility studies must involve both partners. The man may be the cause, and the problem is most assuredly the couple's. Also, fertility testing in the male is relatively easier. It is a waste of health personnel time, as well as of the woman's time and money, to conduct extensive fertility studies on her until the man has been demonstrated to be fertile.

Causes

A number of factors may lead to male infertility: a disturbance in spermatogenesis (the production of sperm cells); an obstruction in the seminiferous tubules, ducts, or vessels that prevents movement of spermatozoa; autoimmunity, which immobilizes sperm; qualitative or quantitative changes in the seminal fluid that again prevent motility of spermatozoa; and a problem in ejaculation or deposition that prevents spermatozoa from being placed close enough to the cervix to penetrate it and fertilize the ovum.

Inadequate Sperm Count

The minimum sperm count considered normal is 20 million per milliliter of seminal fluid, or a total of 50 million per ejaculation. At least 60 percent of sperm should be motile, and 60 percent should be normal in shape and form (Speroff, 1983). Spermatozoa must be maintained at a temperature slightly less than body temperature (which is why the testes are suspended in the scrotal sac away from body heat) for the sperm cells to be normal and motile. Inadequate sperm counts may be caused by chronic infection, such as tuberculosis or recurrent sinusitis, because of the slightly elevated temperature accompanying these diseases. Men who work at desk jobs—sitting for long periods increases scrotal heat—are likely to have lower sperm counts than men whose occupations allow them to be ambulatory at least part of each day. Men who drive a great deal each day (salesmen, truck drivers) may be affected the same way. The heat of frequent hot tubs or sauna use may also appreciatively lower a sperm count.

Basic production of spermatozoa may be impaired by a disease such as the orchitis (testicular inflammation and scarring) that follows mumps. This problem cannot be alleviated at present once it has occurred, but it can be prevented by giving children mumps vaccine.

Exposure to excessive x-rays or radioactive substances may impair spermatozoa production by damage to the Leydig cells. Men should have adequate protection from these substances if they are exposed to them in their employment. The testes of boys and men having pelvic x-rays should be covered by a protective lead shield.

Excessive use of alcohol or drugs may affect sperm production by causing general ill health and debilitation or malnutrition. Marijuana use directly inhibits gonadotropin-releasing hormone (GN-RH) and testosterone secretion. It may cause loss of libido as well as a low sperm count, probably due to lessened testosterone (Hembree, 1984). Endocrine imbalance may be responsible for inhibition of spermatogenesis. Thyroid, pancreatic (diabetes mellitus), and pituitary imbalances are the endocrine problems most often at fault.

Low vitamin intake may play a role in male infertility. Although vitamin E apparently aids fertility, the sexual prowess attributed to this vitamin is probably exaggerated.

Surgery on or near the testes (inguinal herniorrhaphy, for example) may impair circulation to the testes, with resultant reduction or absence of spermatogenesis. Trauma to testes such as may occur in a sports accident sometimes causes testicular damage due to fibrous scar formation. The presence of a varicocele, or varicosity of the spermatic vein, may limit sperm formation due to vasocongestion.

Cryptorchidism, or undescended testes, may lead to lowered sperm production if the repair to lower the testes into the scrotal sac was not completed until after puberty or if the spermatic cord was twisted at the time of surgery. Fifty percent of the male children born to women who took diethylstilbestrol (DES) during pregnancy have abnormal sperm or semen (Eisenberg, 1983).

Obstruction of Sperm Motility

Obstruction may occur at any point in the pathway that spermatozoa must travel to reach the outside—the seminiferous tubules, the epididymis, the vas deferens, the ejaculatory duct, and the urethra (see Figure 8-12). Tubal infection, such as occurs with gonorrhea or ascending urethral infection, may result in adhesions and occlusions; congenital stricture of a spermatic duct is sometimes seen. Hypertrophy of the prostate gland occurs in many men beginning about 50 years of age; resulting pressure on the vas deferens may interfere with sperm transport.

It has been shown that men who have vasectomies may develop an autoimmune reaction or may form antibodies that immobilize their own sperm. It is conceivable that men with obstruction in the vas deferens from other causes could also develop such a reaction that immobilizes sperm.

Changes in Seminal Fluid

Infection of the prostate gland through which the seminal fluid passes or infection of the seminal vesicles will change the composition of the seminal fluid to such an extent that sperm motility may be reduced. These infections may be spread from urinary tract infections.

Difficulty with Ejaculation

Too frequent coitus may reduce sperm count. The use of precoital lubricants may inhibit deposition of sperm near the cervix. Anomalies of the penis, such as *hypospadias* (urethral opening on the ventral surface of the penis) or *epispadias* (urethral opening on the dorsal surface) may cause deposition of spermatozoa too far from the cervix to allow for cervical penetration. Extreme obesity may interfere with penetration.

Psychological problems and debilitating diseases may result in an inability to achieve ejaculation (*impotence*). Impotence is *primary* if the man has never been able to achieve erection and ejaculation, *secondary* if at one time it was not a problem. Impotence can be easily solved if it is associated with stress, such as work or home responsibility, and this stress can be relieved. Impotence can also be a manifestation of an underlying psychological problem, however, such as that the man tends to view sex as aggressive, attacking behavior and does not want to treat his partner that way. If the impotence is caused by a deep-seated psychological issue (psychogenic infertility), a solution to the problem will include psychological or sexual counseling and may involve long-term care.

Premature ejaculation (ejaculation before penetration) is another problem usually attributed to psychological causes. It may affect the proper deposition of sperm.

Assessment

As mentioned, it is best to begin fertility testing with the man because these tests are inexpensive and simple in nature and therefore easy to carry out. Occasionally, a man cannot admit that he might be infertile. In such an instance, testing may have to be initiated in the woman. The man can be tested when he has reconciled himself to the need.

History

As with any health investigation, a male fertility study begins with a careful history. The history should cover general health; nutrition; alcohol, drug, or tobacco use; congenital health problems such as hypospadias or cryptorchidism; illnesses such as mumps orchitis, urinary tract infection, or sexually transmitted disease; and operations such as herniorrhaphy, which could have resulted in a blood compromise to the testes. The history should also cover present illnesses, particularly endocrine in nature, and the man's occupation and work habits, both present and past (sitting at a desk all day or exposure to x-rays or other forms of radiation). Other essential facts are the frequency of coitus and masturbation, the occurrence of impotence or premature ejaculation, coital positions used, whether or not lubricants are used, what contraceptive measures have been used, and whether or not the man has ever fathered children by a previous marriage or relationship. Ask if he uses hot tubs or saunas frequently to evaluate whether this increased heat might have decreased his sperm count. Cultural or religious values could be factors. In Orthodox Judaism, for example, coitus is not permitted for 7 days after the last day of the menstrual flow. This long a period of abstinence could interfere with conception if the woman has a relatively short menstrual cycle and ovulates earlier than 7 days following the menstrual flow.

Ask about drug or medication use (include marijuana). Ask if the man knows if his mother took any medications during his pregnancy to detect diethylstilbestrol use.

Physical Assessment

The man needs a thorough physical assessment to rule out present illness. Of particular importance is the observation of secondary sexual characteristics and genital abnormalities, such as the absence of a vas deferens or undescended testes. Assess for the presence of a varicocele, an enlargement of a testicular vein, or a hydrocele (collection of fluid in the tunica vaginalis of the scrotum). Hydrocele is not directly associated with infertility but should be documented if present.

Semen Analysis

For a semen analysis, after 3 or 4 days of sexual abstinence, the man ejaculates by masturbation into a clean, dry specimen jar, and spermatozoa are examined under a microscope within 2 hours. If the man brings in the specimen to the health care facility, he must be certain that it is not exposed to extreme cold or heat in transport, which can destroy sperm mobility. The number of spermatozoa in the specimen are counted, and their appearance and motility are noted. An average ejaculation should produce 2.5 to 5.0 ml of semen. As previously noted, it should contain a minimum of 20 million spermatozoa per milliliter of fluid, or a total of 50 million per ejaculation (the average normal sperm count is 50 to 200 million per milliliter). Two hours after ejaculation, 60 to 70 percent of sperm cells should still be vigorously active; 6 to 8 hours later, 25 to 40 percent should still show good motility. Liquefaction of the sample usually occurs within 10 to 30 minutes.

If the man is unwilling to submit to a semen analysis, a sperm analysis may be made at the same time as the test for female cervical mucus (the Sims-Huhner test) is done, although this is never preferable. If the result of a single sperm and semen analysis is substandard, two or three specimens should be examined for verification: There may be a wide variation of sperm production within even a 24-hour period. A further test of sperm that is available in large centers better measures the ability of sperm to penetrate ova. Hamster ova are prepared on a laboratory dish and then exposed to human sperm (Zacar, 1983). The ability of human sperm to penetrate the ova reveals not only mobile but also penetration capacity of sperm. Testing sperm in bovine cervical mucus may demonstrate their ability to migrate successfully through cervical mucus.

Laboratory Tests

In order to rule out poor health as a causative factor for infertility, the following laboratory tests are also usually included in the male studies: urinalysis; complete blood count; blood typing, including Rh factor; serologic test for syphilis and sometimes a sedimentation rate (increased if inflammation is present); protein-bound iodine test (thyroid function); cholesterol level determination; and assessment of gonadotropin, prolactin, and testosterone levels. A more extensive study is a bioassay of urine for 17-ketosteroids, which are the breakdown product of androgen in urine. Testicular biopsy or x-ray study of the excretory portion of the genital tract using a contrast medium might rarely be indicated.

Psychological Assessment

The man needs an opportunity to discuss with the physician or nurse his overall attitude toward sexual relations, pregnancy, and raising children. It is good to explore with the man how he gained his knowledge of sexual relations—from school classmates or a reliable source? What is his attitude toward coitus? What does he know about sexual technique?

How sexually active was he before this relationship? Some men worry that because they were very active sexually when they were young, they have spent all their viable sperm (and so are unable either to conceive or to have normal children). They need to be assured that normally sperm are continually produced and sperm quality does not deteriorate with aging. Other men may think that not being able to have children is punishment for earlier irresponsibile encounters. They may worry that their masturbation will cause deformed children (a very old wives' tale).

Some men may worry that their wife may die in childbirth and so they really do not want her to be pregnant. Others are afraid that they will not be able to support a family or be a good father: They want things to remain as they are. Some of these men need referral to a psychologist for counseling. Others benefit most from a frank discussion, separating fears from reality, or preparing their minds as well as their bodies for possible fatherhood.

Plans and Implementations

The management of male infertility involves treating, if possible, the underlying cause of the infertility, such as chronic disease or current infection. If the vas deferens is obstructed, the obstruction is usually extensive and difficult or impossible to relieve by surgery. If spermatozoa are present but the total count is low, a man might be advised to abstain from coitus for 7 to 10 days at a time in order to increase the count. If the underlying cause cannot be corrected, which unfortunately often happens (for example, the reason for infertility is a prior infection such as mumps orchitis, which has left extensive scarring), artificial insemination is a possible solution.

If spermatozoa appear to be destroyed by vaginal secretions due to an immunologic factor, the response may be reduced by abstinence or condom use for about 6 months. The administration of corticosteroids to the woman to reduce her immune response may have some effect. Direct insemination of the sperm into the cervix to bypass the vagina may also be a solution.

Artificial Insemination

Artificial insemination is the instillation of sperm into the uterus in order to aid conception. It can either be accomplished by the introduction of the husband's sperm (AIH, or artificial insemination by the husband) or by introduction of donor sperm (AID, or artificial insemination by a donor).

To prepare for artificial insemination, the woman must take her basal body temperatures for a number of months in order to be able to predict the day during her cycle ovulation usually occurs. Just before, on, and 2 days after the day of ovulation, a physician takes the seminal fluid of the husband's or donor's ejaculate and, using a syringe, places it at the opening to the cervix. The woman rests in a supine position for approximately 15 minutes in order to allow the spermatozoa ample opportunity to enter the cervix. A cervical cap may be fitted to ensure that the sperm remain in contact with the cervix.

Donors for artificial insemination are traditionally medical or nursing students who have no history of disease and no family history of possibly heritable disorders. The blood type, or at least the Rh factor, can be matched with the mother's to prevent Rh incompatibility. Sperm banks, supplying frozen spermatozoa, are now available. Sperm from these sources is from screened donors and can be selected according to desired physical characteristics. It has the added advantage of being available any day of the month. Sperm used from sperm banks has been frozen and tends to have slower mobility than nonfrozen specimens; although the rate of conception may be lower from this source, there is no increase in the congenital anomalies in children.

A man who has a low sperm count may pool and freeze ejaculations for a week or more, and then this pooled specimen can be used in the insemination. This technique may not be as effective as hoped, however, as the individual with a low sperm count usually has poor sperm mobility as well. The added insult of freezing can prevent conception under these circumstances.

Artificial insemination may be done with unmarried or married women. There are legal complications in some states that must be considered (the question of inheritance or child support and responsibility are in doubt). Some couples have religious beliefs that deter them from using artificial insemination, especially donor insemination.

Artificial insemination may be a discouraging process to some couples: The method does not speed up the average time of 6 months that an average couple takes to effect conception. These months seem long and filled with the tension of having pregnancy so near and yet so elusive.

Female Infertility

Causes

The factors that cause infertility in women are analogous to those causing infertility in men: anovulation (faulty or inadequate production of ova); problems of ova transport through the fallopian tubes to the uterus; uterine factors such as tumors or poor endometrial development; and cervical and vaginal factors that immobilize spermatozoa. In 30 to 35 percent of instances of female infertility, the fallopian tubes are involved; in 20 percent, the cervix; and in 15 percent, a hormonal factor.

Anovulation

Anovulation is the most serious cause of infertility in women because it is the one most difficult to correct. Anovulation may occur not as a primary ovarian problem but as an imbalance of hypothalamus-pituitary-ovarian interplay; therefore, a condition such as hypothyroidism may contribute to anovulation. Chronic or excessive exposure to x-rays or radioactive substances may be involved. General ill health or poor diet may contribute to poor ovarian function. Ovarian tumors may produce anovulation due to feedback stimulation on the pituitary. There are several tests for ovulation.

Basal Body Temperature. Basal body temperature is a test for the slight temperature increase that normally occurs with the release of progesterone following ovulation. Before getting out of bed each morning, the woman takes her rectal temperature (oral temperature may be used but it

tends to be less accurate). She must be certain to take her temperature before moving around, since activity changes the basal level. She plots the daily temperature on a monthly graph, noticing conditions that might affect her basal temperature (colds, other infections, sleeplessness). At the time of ovulation, the basal temperature dips slightly, then rises a degree higher and stays at that level until 3 or 4 days before the next menstrual flow. The increase in basal body temperature marks the time of ovulation (actually the beginning of the luteal phase of the menstrual cycle that only occurs when ovulation occurs). A temperature rise should last 10 days or there is a luteal phase defect present (progesterone production begins but is not sustained). Graphs of basal body temperature are shown in Figure 12-2.

In Figure 12-2A, the woman's temperature dips slightly at midpoint in her cycle, then rises sharply, an indication of ovulation. Toward the end of the cycle (the twenty-fourth day) her temperature begins to decline, indicating that progesterone levels are falling and that she did not conceive.

In Figure 12-2B, the woman's temperature rises at midpoint in the cycle and remains at that elevated level past the time of her normal menstrual flow, suggesting that pregnancy has occurred.

In Figure 12-2C, there is no preovulatory dip and no rise of temperature anywhere during the cycle. This is the typical pattern of a woman who does not ovulate.

Fern Test. When high levels of estrogen are present in the body, as they are just prior to ovulation, the cervical mucus forms fern-like patterns when it is smeared and dried on a glass slide. This phenomenon is caused by crystallization of sodium chloride on mucus fibers and is known as *arborization*, or ferning. When progesterone is the dominant hormone, as it is just after ovulation when the luteal phase of the menstrual cycle is beginning, a fern pattern is no longer discernible. Fern tests are usually done at midcycle and again before menstruation, so that both patterns can be demonstrated. Women who do not ovulate continue to show the fern pattern throughout the menstrual cycle (progesterone levels never become dominant), or they never demonstrate it because their estrogen levels never rise.

Spinnbarkeit Test. At the height of estrogen secretion, the cervical mucus becomes thin and watery and can be stretched into long strands. This stretchability (to a distance of 13 to 15 cm) contrasts to its state when progesterone is the dominant hormone. Taking spinnbarkeit patterns at a midpoint and a late point in the menstrual

Basal body temperature

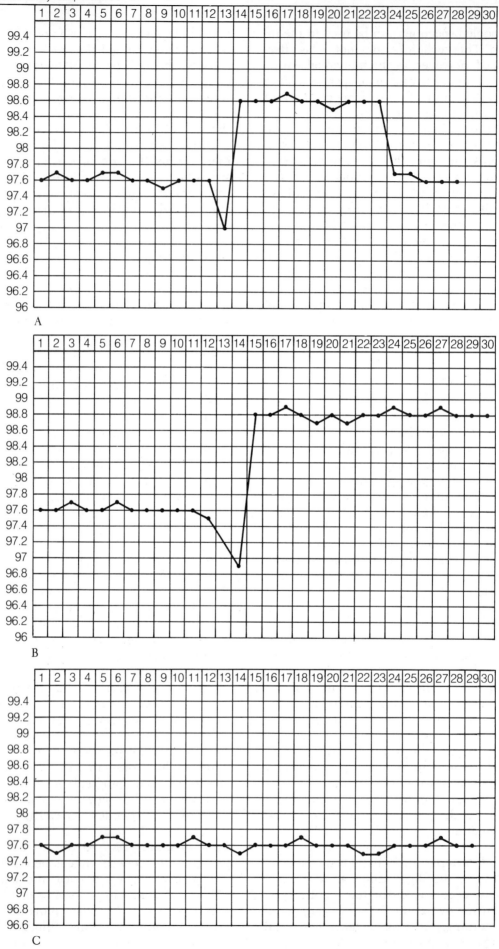

cycle can demonstrate that progesterone is being produced and, by implication, that ovulation has occurred. A woman can do this herself by stretching the sample between thumb and finger; you can test it in an examining room by smearing a cervical mucus specimen on a slide and stretching the mucus between the slide and cover slip.

Uterine Endometrial Biopsy. Uterine endometrial biopsy may be used as a test for ovulation or luteal phase defects. A corkscrew-like appearance of the endometrium (typical if progesterone-dominated) suggests that ovulation has occurred.

Endometrial biopsy is done by introducing a thin probe and biopsy forceps through the cervix after the cervix is washed with iodine. It involves slight discomfort from the maneuvering of the instruments, and there is a moment of sharp pain as the biopsy specimen is taken from the anterior or posterior uterus. The procedure is usually performed 2 to 3 days prior to an expected menstrual flow (the twenty-fourth to twenty-sixth day of a typical menstrual cycle). The date an actual menstrual flow does occur is noted; this day is assigned an arbitrary date of day 28. The findings of the endometrium biopsy are examined, "dated," and compared with what finding should have been present on that day. If the appearance of the endometrium lags behind what appearance it should have achieved by more than 2 days, a luteal phase defect is present. The risks of endometrial biopsy are pain, excessive bleeding, infection, or uterine perforation. It is contraindicated if pregnancy is suspected, although the chance of interference with a pregnancy is probably under 10 percent. It is also contraindicated if an infection such as acute pelvic inflammatory disease (PID) or cervicitis is present. Caution the woman to expect a small amount of spotting following the procedure, but she should call back if she develops a temperature over 101°F, has a large amount of bleeding, or passes clots. Be certain she has instructions to telephone you when her next menstrual flow begins so the biopsy specimen can be histologically dated and analyzed.

Hysteroscopy. Hysteroscopy is visual inspection of the uterine lining by the insertion of a hysteroscope through the cervix. This procedure is helpful if uterine adhesions were discovered on the hysterosalpingogram (x-ray of the uterus and fallopian tubes).

Figure 12-2 *Basal body temperature chart for determining ovulation. A. Ovulation without conception. B. Ovulation with conception. C. An anovulatory cycle.*

Culdoscopy. Culdoscopy is a sterile procedure that permits direct visualization of the organs of reproduction through a culdoscope inserted into the posterior fornix of the vaginal canal. A culdoscope is a thin hollow metal tube with a small light at the distal end. With the culdoscope in place, both ovaries can be inspected grossly for the presence of a graffian follicle, corpus luteum, or corpus albicans, providing evidence of previous ovulation (Figure 12-3). The procedure is little used today because laparoscopy allows better visualization.

Laparoscopy. Laparoscopy is the introduction of a thin, hollow, lighted tube through a small incision in the abdomen just under the umbilicus in order to examine the tubes and ovaries. It is scheduled during the follicular phase and done under general anesthesia to allow for good relaxation and a steep Trendelenburg's position (which brings the reproductive organs up out of the pelvis). Carbon dioxide is introduced into the abdomen to cause the abdominal wall to move outward and allow for better visualization. Caution women that they may feel bloating of their abdomen afterward; if some carbon dioxide escapes under the diaphragm, they feel extremely sharp shoulder pain following the procedure.

Laparoscopy is the same procedure used to enter the abdominal cavity to sterilize fallopian tubes by placing clips or cautery to the tube (see Figure 11-10). Be certain the woman understands that the term simply means "opening into the abdomen," or she may worry that the exact opposite of what she wants (patent tubes) will be the result.

Tubal Factors

Difficulty with tubal transport usually occurs because of chronic salpingitis (inflammation of the tubes), which is most often due to chronic pelvic inflammatory disease, but sometimes results from a ruptured appendix or abdominal surgery in which infection was involved and adhesions formed. Occasionally, congenital webbing or strictures of the fallopian tubes occur.

Pelvic inflammatory disease (PID) is infection of the pelvic organs: the uterus, fallopian tubes, ovaries, and their supporting structures. The infection can extend to cause pelvic peritonitis. Although sexual transmittal accounts for about 75 percent of all PID, infections from causes other than sexually transmitted diseases (STDs), such as *Escherichia coli* and *Streptococcus*, are beginning to occur more frequently and may be as severe. PID tends to occur at a higher incidence in women with IUDs in place than in other women.

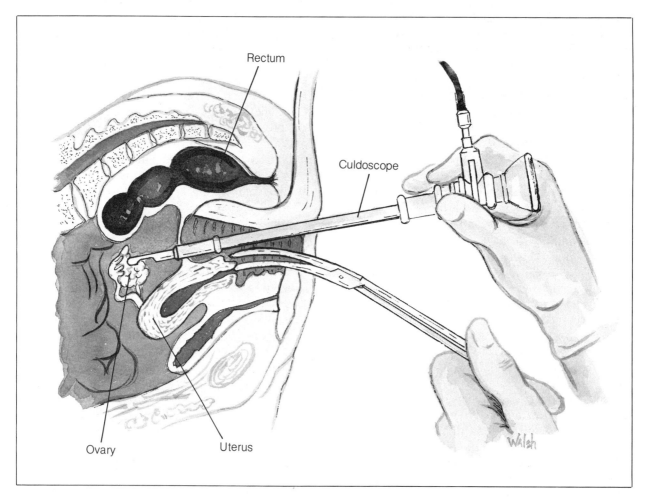

Figure 12-3 *Culdoscopy. A lighted scope is introduced into the posterior vaginal fornix.*

The initial phase of PID begins with a cervical infection that spreads by surface invasion along the endometrium to the tubes and then the ovaries. Spread is most apt to occur at the end of a menstrual period: At that time, menstrual blood provides an excellent growth medium for bacteria and there is loss of the normal cervical mucous barrier.

As tissue becomes inflamed and edematous, a purulent exudate forms. If the process is untreated, the process enters a chronic phase and fibrotic scarring with stricture of the fallopian tubes will result. With acute PID, the woman notices severe pain in the lower abdomen. She may have an accompanying heavy purulent discharge. As the infection progresses she will develop a fever. Leukocytosis and an elevated sedimentation rate will be present on laboratory testing. On a pelvic examination, any manipulation of the cervix causes severe pain. It may be difficult to palpate ovaries because of abdominal guarding resulting from tenderness. If the PID enters a chronic phase, the abdominal pain lessens but dyspareunia or dysmenorrhea may be ex-

treme. If the ovaries are affected, intermenstrual spotting may occur.

Diagnosis can be aided by sonogram and laparoscopy. Therapy involves administration of specific antibiotics and analgesics. Limiting activity aids in pain relief. In some women, a pelvic abscess forms, which must be drained through the cul-de-sac before healing will take place.

Women who have had one PID have an increased chance of having a second occurrence because the immune protection of the tubes and ovaries may be damaged. Such a woman should be certain not to have coitus with an infected partner and to avoid coitus during menstruation, when her protective mechanisms are at their lowest level. She should consider childbearing early in life because fertility may be a problem if extensive tubal scarring is present.

There are several tests of tubal patency.

Laparoscopy. Laparoscopy may be used to view the proximity of the ovaries to the fallopian tubes (if the distance is too great, the discharged ovum cannot enter the tube). Dye can be injected into the uterus by a polyethylene cannula through the cervix and tubal patency assessed by observing if the dye appears in the abdominal cavity (tubal lavage). Inspection of the tube fimbria reveals whether they are present or not; these fringe-like structures are necessary for conduction of the ovum into the tube.

Rubin Test. A Rubin test is a traditional test for patency, but one used less today than formerly as laparoscopy or tubal X-ray is preferred. It is done on the third day following cessation of menstrual flow, before an ovum could have entered the fallopian tube. The woman lies in a lithotomy position. Carbon dioxide under pressure is then instilled into the cervix through a slender tube. The gas passes through the uterus and fallopian tubes into the pelvic cavity if the tubes are patent; with normal patency, carbon dioxide passes through with a pressure of under 100 mm Hg. When pressure over 100 mm Hg is necessary for passage, stricture is suggested. No passage whatsoever with a pressure of 200 mm Hg indicates occlusion.

As the carbon dioxide is diffused into the peritoneum and collects under the diaphragm, the woman experiences sharp, almost excruciating pain in one or both shoulders. She should be warned in advance; otherwise she may worry about a heart attack or torn shoulder ligament. Auscultating the abdomen with a stethoscope while the carbon dioxide is infusing may aid in establishing bilateral patency; the passage of the carbon dioxide can be heard as a faint hissing sound with a stethoscope.

Rubin tests should not be done when uterine bleeding or infection is present. Infective organisms or blood might be forced up the tube into the abdominal cavity.

Hysterosalpingography. Hysterosalpingography (uterosalpingography) is an X-ray study of the fallopian tubes using a radiopaque medium. It is done at the same time of the month as the Rubin test, with similar contraindications. The radiopaque material is introduced into the cervix under pressure (Figure 12-4), where it outlines the uterus and both tubes, provided the latter are patent. Because the medium is thick, it distends the uterus and tubes slightly, causing uterine cramping that is momentarily painful. Following the study, the contrast medium will drain out through the vagina. The instillation of carbon dioxide or of a radiopaque material may be therapeutic as well as diagnostic. The pressure of the gas or solution may actually break up adhesions as it passes through the fallopian tubes, thereby increasing their patency. It is important that

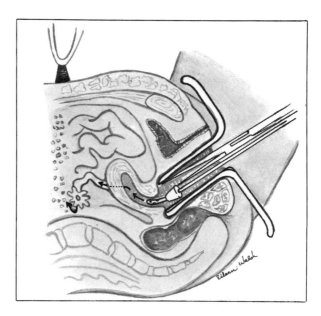

Figure 12-4 *A hysterosalpingogram. A contrast dye is introduced via the cervix to outline the uterus and fallopian tubes.*

tubal X-ray examinations be done just following menstruation so a growing zygote is not irradiated. The procedure carries a degree of risk of infection, allergic reaction to the contrast medium (it is iodine based), and embolism from dye entering a uterine blood vessel.

Uterine Factors

Tumors such as fibromas (leiomyomas) may result in infertility because of their blockage of fallopian tubes or limiting of the space available for effective implantation; many women with huge fibromas, however, become pregnant. A congenitally deformed uterine cavity may also limit implantation sites, but this is a rare occurrence. Inadequate endometrium formation resulting from poor secretion of estrogen or progesterone from the ovary is the main cause of infertility due to a uterine factor (the primary factor here is actually ovarian). Endometrial biopsy will reveal any inadequacies of the endometrium.

Endometriosis. Endometriosis is the implantation of uterine endometrium outside the uterus. The most common sites of endometrium spread are the cul-de-sac of Douglas, the ovaries, the uterine ligaments, and the outer surface of the uterus and bowel (Figure 12-5).

The spread of endometrium is probably due to regurgitation through the fallopian tubes at the time of menstruation. Viable particles of endometrium regurgitated this way begin to proliferate and grow at the new sites. On laparotomy, the implants appear as ragged purplish growths. On the ovaries, cysts filled with old blood are often

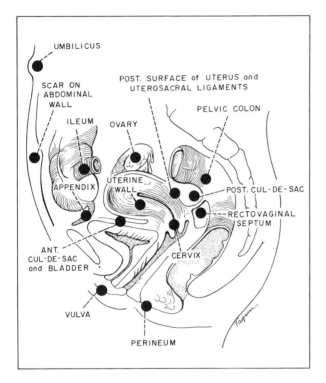

Figure 12-5 *Common sites of endometriosis formation. From Thomas H. Green. (1977). Gynecology: Essentials of Clinical Practice, (3rd ed.), p. 329. Boston: Little, Brown.*

seen (brown or chocolate cysts). Endometriosis acts to cause infertility, perhaps because fallopian tube implants cause fallopian tube obstruction; or the presence of peritoneal macrophages drawn to the abdominal tissue destroy sperm. That endometriosis occurs may reveal an endometrium that has different or more friable qualities than normally (perhaps due to a luteal phase defect) and so does not support implantation as well.

ASSESSMENT. Endometriosis tends to occur most often in white, nulliparous women. Pelvic examination may show that the uterus is displaced by tender, fixed, palpable nodules. Nodules in the cul-de-sac or on an ovary may be palpable as well. If endometriosis is minimal, the woman will not be aware of any related symptoms. If moderate or extensive, the woman may feel painful cramping at the time of menstruation; patches of ectopic endometrium also undergo preflow breakdown and bleeding, and blood is irritating to the peritoneal membrane. The woman may report dyspareunia (pain at penile-vaginal penetration) if the implants are in the cul-de-sac of Douglas.

Endometriosis is staged according to the extent of involvement. A common method of staging is shown in Table 12-1.

ANALYSIS. A common nursing diagnosis related to endometriosis is pain related to dys-

pareunia, or fear related to possibility of infertility. Be certain that goals established are realistic as to time: The problem is not easily corrected.

PLANNING AND IMPLEMENTATION. Treatment for endometriosis can be either medical or surgical and differs according to the stage the process has reached. Use of estrogen/progesterone-based ovulation suppressants may cause regression of the implants, due primarily to the extreme sloughing of tissue following progesterone administration. It is difficult for a woman who wants to have children to understand why she is being asked to take birth control pills. It seems to be the exact opposite treatment from what she needs. Be certain the woman has a good understanding of what is being attempted: She needs a diagram of uterine and tubal anatomy so she can understand what *regurgitation* means, an appreciation of how progesterone acts on endometrial tissue, and support of her patience for a minimum of 6 months during therapy. Danazol, a synthetic androgen, taken orally, may be used to cause shrinkage of the tissue. Laparotomy to excise the implants is often more effective. A laparotomy is major surgery, however, so a course of conservative medical treatment may be undertaken first.

EVALUATION. The best proof that treatment has been effective is that the woman becomes pregnant. Following birth of the child, the woman is usually advised to have a second child (provided she wants more than one child) as soon after the first child as possible. Waiting the traditional 2 or 3 years between children could give endometrial implants a chance to grow again. Be careful in the postpartal period that you do not give traditional advice (spacing children conserves maternal energy, produces healthier children, and encourages infant-parent bonding)—advice that does not apply here. Endometriosis tends to be familial. Daughters of women with the condition may develop symptoms of dysmenorrhea early in life and may need to be advised to have their families fairly early in life before extensive overgrowth of endometrium occurs.

Asherman's Syndrome. Trauma from uterine infection or repeated uterine surgery may lead to such uterine scarring that no implantation sites are available. Infertility results from this condition, called Asherman's syndrome.

Cervical Factors

Infection or inflammation of the cervix (erosion) may cause such changes in the cervical mucus that spermatozoa cannot penetrate easily

Table 12-1 Endometriosis Staged Based on the Degree of Spread

Area	Stage I	Stage II-A	Stage II-B	Stage III	Stage IV
Broad ligaments	No implants more than 5 mm	No implants more than 5 mm	Covered by adherent ovary	May be covered by adherent tube or ovary	May be covered by adherent tube or ovary
Tubes	Avascular adhesions, fimbria free	Avascular adhesions, fimbria free	Adhesions not removable by endoscopy, fimbria free	Fimbria covered by adhesions	Fimbria covered by adhesions
Ovaries	Avascular adhesions, no fixation	Endometrial cysts 5 cm or less (stage A-1), over 5 cm (stage A-2), ruptured (stage A-3)	Fixed to broad ligaments, implants over 5 mm	Adherent with or without implants or endometriosis	Adherent with or without implants or endometriosis
Cul-de-sac	No implants more than 5 mm	No implants more than 5 mm	Multiple implants, no adherent bowel or fixed uterus	Multiple implants, no adherent bowel or fixed uterus	Covered by adherent bowel or fixed retrodisplaced uterus
Bowel	Normal	Normal	Normal	Normal	Adherent to cul-de-sac, uterosacral ligaments, or corpus
Appendix	Normal	Normal	Normal	Normal	May be involved
Bladder	Normal	Normal	Normal	Normal	Implants
Uterus	Normal	Normal	Normal	Normal	May be fixed and adherent posteriorly

Source: Kistner, R. W. (1971). *Gynecology principles and practice* (3rd ed.), p. 464. Chicago: Year Book Medical Publishers.

or survive. A tight cervical os or obstruction of the os by a polyp may compound infertility but is rarely enough of a problem to be the sole cause. The woman who has had several D&Cs or cervical conization should be evaluated in light of the possibility that scar tissue and tightening of the cervical os has occurred. These women as well as those who have had vacuum extractions for abortions performed may develop a cervix that does not close completely. This problem is not so much one of conception, however, as of maintaining a pregnancy: An incompetent cervix is the end result.

At the time of ovulation, cervical mucus becomes thin and watery and can be easily penetrated by spermatozoa for a period of 12 to 72 hours. If ovulation does not occur, or estrogen levels do not increase at the midpoint of the cycle, the cervical mucus does not become receptive in this way to penetration. The Sims-Huhner test is used to determine whether or not this change has occurred.

Sims-Huhner Test (postcoital). In the Sims-Huhner test, the time of ovulation is predicted from the woman's basal body temperature rate. The couple has coitus just prior to the expected ovulation date, using no precoital lubricants. Following coitus, the woman lies on her back for at least 30 minutes to ensure that spermatozoa will reach the cervix. She uses no postcoital douche and reports to the health care facility within 2 to 8 hours following coitus.

With the woman in a lithotomy position, a specimen of cervical mucus is removed and examined microscopically for ferning and cell count, and grossly for its ability to form long strands (spinnbarkeit). It is further examined under the microscope for viable spermatozoa. At the time of ovulation, the amount of cervical mucus present should be moderately large to profuse (up to 700 mg a day is produced at this time). It should appear clear and thin (low viscosity), have few cells (under five leukocytes per high-power field), have an alkaline pH, and form strands 13 to 15 cm in length. If the male partner is fertile and there is little destruction of spermatozoa, spermatozoa will be present in the cervical mucus (over five per high-power field at 2 hours postcoitus), more than 25 percent will be motile, and penetration will be at the rate of 1.5 to 2.0 mm per minute.

A postcoital test may be stressful for some couples because it requires the couple to initiate coitus "on command"; give sensitive support in light of this.

Vaginal Factors

Infection of the vagina may cause the pH of the vaginal secretions to change, limiting or destroying the motility of spermatozoa; the use of feminine hygiene products or frequent douching may also cause this. Some women, particularly those with an ABO blood incompatibility to their sexual partner, appear to have sperm-immobilizing or sperm-agglutinating antibodies in the blood plasma, which act to destroy sperm cells in the vagina. This is actually a systemic response to a local invasion.

Tests for vaginal adequacy usually include a pelvic examination for gross abnormalities and probably a vaginal secretion culture. Abnormal results from a postcoital test may suggest a vaginal sperm agglutination problem.

Assessment

History

To aid assessment, the woman's menstrual history should be obtained, including the age of menarche, the length and frequency of menstrual periods, the amount of flow, and any difficulties she experiences. She should be asked about present or past reproductive tract infections; her overall health, with a stress on endocrine problems; and abdominal or pelvic operations she might have had. How often does she use douches or intravaginal medication or sprays? Is she exposed to occupational hazards such as x-rays or toxic substances? It is also important to obtain a history of previous pregnancies or abortions and to ask questions about her use of contraceptives.

Physical Assessment

A thorough physical assessment is necessary to rule out present illness. Of particular importance is the presence of secondary sex characteristics, since these are an indication of maturity and pituitary function. A complete pelvic examination is needed to rule out gross anatomic defects and infection.

Laboratory Tests

To determine the woman's general state of health, laboratory tests like those done on the man will be ordered: urinalysis, a complete blood count and possibly a sedimentation rate, a serologic test for syphilis, and a T3 and T4 uptake determination for thyroid function. A basal metabolic rate may be taken. If the woman has a history of menstrual irregularities, the urine may be assayed for 17-ketosteroids, follicle-stimulating hormone, estriol, and pregnanediol (the breakdown product of progesterone). If a luteal phase defect is suspected, plasma progesterone levels taken on days 3, 8, and 11 after ovulation may be necessary (a level under 5 ng per milliliter is diagnostic of decreased progesterone levels). A serum midcycle LH peak may also be taken.

Psychological Assessment

As with a man, a woman needs the opportunity to discuss with the physician or a nurse her overall attitudes toward sexual coitus, pregnancy, and raising children. It is good to explore with her how she was introduced to the phenomenon of menstruation. Was she prepared for it or not? Is her present husband her only current sex partner? Did she have premarital coitus?

Some women are afraid of pregnancy because they worry that old sperm from premarital encounters will be activated, and the resulting child will look like their previous sexual partner, not like their present one. Others fear punishment for premarital affairs by the birth of a defective child. Others are so frightened at the thought of labor and delivery that, although they say they want to have a child, they are actually petrified of the undertaking. Some of these women need referral to a psychologist for counseling. Many of them will benefit from a frank discussion that separates old wives' tales from reality preparing their minds as well as their bodies for possible motherhood.

Plans and Implementations

As with men, treatment of infertility in a woman is directed toward the underlying cause. If a vaginal infection is present, the infection will be treated according to the causative organism. Vaginal infections such as trichomonas and monilia are obstinate and tend to recur, requiring close supervision and follow-up. The possibility that the sexual partner is reinfecting the woman also needs to be considered. Many women do not believe that the single act of using an antifungal vaginal suppository daily will have that much effect; despite their strong desire to become pregnant, they may not comply with the medicine regimen. Teach that medicine does not have to be injected or swallowed in order to be effective. Caution women who are prescribed metronidazole (Flagyl) for a trichomonas infection that this substance is teratogenic and should not be continued during a pregnancy. Without this precaution, a woman who notices a vaginal discharge during pregnancy may remember she has some medicine left and use it.

If there are white blood cells in the cervical mucus, an endocervical or endometrial infection may be present. Culturing the specimen will reveal the specific organism and allow for appropriate antibiotic therapy. *Chlamydia trachomatis* infections are becoming more and more common. Culturing for this bacteria involves a complex microimmunofluorescence technique, which is not available in all communities. The treatment for *Chlamydia* infection is oral tetracycline. Caution the woman that if pregnancy should occur, she should not continue the drug: Tetracycline is associated with tooth and long bone defects in the fetus.

If the problem is that spermatozoa do not appear to survive in the vaginal secretions because secretions are too scant or tenacious, the woman may be placed on low-dose estrogen in order to increase mucus production during days 5 to 10 of her cycle. Premarin is a brand of estrogen used this way. Women may develop antibodies to sperm or semen that interfere with sperm mobility or penetration of the mucus or the zona of the ovum. If sperm immobility appears to be an immunologic response, advising abstinence from coitus or condom use for 6 months may reduce this effect. Administration of corticosteroids to the woman during this time may also be effective. Artificial insemination with the sexual partner's sperm may offer a solution because placing the sperm directly into the cervix bypasses cervical mucus.

If the problem appears to be a luteal phase defect, progesterone vaginal suppositories beginning on the third day of the temperature rise and continued for the next 6 weeks if pregnancy occurs or until the menstrual flow may be a solution. Oral progesterone is not used because of possible fetal reproductive tract abnormalities if pregnancy occurs.

If the cause of infertility is a myoma (fibroid tumor), removal of the tumor by surgery may be necessary (a myomectomy). Myomectomy may be done with a hystoscope inserted through the cervix if the growth is small. If the problem of infertility is abnormal uterine formation, such as a septal uterus, surgery is now available. Septal defects, however, are generally a problem of early pregnancy loss, not of infertility. Uterine adhesions may be lysed by hysteroscopy, or insertion of a hystoscope into the uterus. Following this procedure, an IUD may be placed for 3 months and estrogen administered to prevent adhesions from reforming. Women find it difficult to accept the IUD as a means of eventually achieving, not preventing, pregnancy.

If the infertility problem is tubal insufficiency, diathermy or steroid administration may be helpful in reducing adhesions. A Rubin test or hysterosalpingography may be repeated as a therapeutic measure. Plastic surgical repair (microsurgery) is feasible. If peritoneal adhesions are holding the tubes fixed and away from the ovaries, these can be removed by laparotomy or possibly laparoscopy. If the fimbria of the tubes have been destroyed due to a pelvic inflammatory reaction, the chance for normal conception is small: ova seem unable to enter the tubes without fimbrial currents present.

If a disturbance of ovulation exists, endocrine therapy may be necessary. In some instances, therapy with estrogen and progesterone is sufficient. In other women, ovulation must be stimulated by the administration of human menopausal gonadotropins (Pergonal) followed by administration of human chorionic gonadotropin. Human menopausal gonadotropins (derived from postmenopausal urine) are combinations of follicle-stimulating hormone and luteinizing hormone. Clomiphene citrate (Clomid), an estrogen antagonist that stimulates pituitary FSH release, may also be used to stimulate ovulation.

The administration of clomiphene citrate and human menopausal gonadotropins may overstimulate the ovary, and multiple births may result. Women who are administered these compounds should be counseled about this possibility. Clomiphene citrate is administered beginning on the fifth day of the cycle. This allows one follicle to come to maturity. Caution women that if clomiphene is started on day 1, it brings multiple follicles to maturity. The drug is given for 5 days. If prolactin levels are increased, bromocriptin (Parlodel) is added to the medicine regimen, to help reduce these levels and stimulate gonadotropin production.

In Vitro Fertilization (IVF)

In vitro fertilization is fertilization of a mature oocyte recovered from a woman's ovary by laparoscopy; the oocyte is exposed to sperm under laboratory conditions outside the woman's body. Embryo transfer (ET) is insertion of the laboratory-grown embryo into the woman's uterus about 40 hours following fertilization, where it will hopefully implant and grow.

IVF is available for women who have blocked or damaged fallopian tubes that prevent sperm from normally meeting an ovum. It is also useful if a man has oligospermia or a low sperm count. Because of the controlled, concentrated conditions, fewer sperm are necessary—perhaps as few as 50,000, in contrast to the nearly 50 million normally required. The procedure may be advisable for women without enough cervical mucus for sperm to negotiate the cervix or who have sperm antibodies that cause their immobilization. A donor ovum may be the answer for a woman who carries a sex-linked disease she does not want to pass on to her children.

Prior to the procedure, the woman is administered an ovulation induction agent such as clomiphene citrate (Clomid) or human menopausal gonadotropin (Pergonal). These are given early in a cycle so under the influence of these medications, ovaries generally mature more than one oocyte. The chances of aspiration of an oocyte are greater if more than one is present. Beginning about the tenth day of the menstrual cycle, ovaries are examined daily by sonography for follicle development; cervical mucus and serum estriol are also examined daily. When follicles appear to be mature, the woman's LH level is assayed. As soon as a surge of LH begins, ovulation will occur within 24 hours. If the woman does not have a sufficient LH increase to trigger ovulation, she can be administered an injection of HCG (human chorionic gonadotropin) hormone. HCG creates an LH effect and causes ovulation. Encouraging ovulation by this synthetic means allows aspiration of the ripe oocyte to be specifically timed (ovulation occurs about 38 hours past HCG injection).

A laparoscopy under general anesthesia is done to aspirate the oocyte with a needle and sterile tubing from its follicle just prior to ovulation. Such aspiration from the follicle prevents the oocyte from being lost in the peritoneum following ovulation and prevents the oocyte from being exposed to the carbon dioxide used to distend the peritoneal cavity. Such exposure apparently renders the oocyte incapable of cleavage: Even if it is successfully fertilized, it will not grow.

Following aspiration and removal, the oocyte is incubated for at least 8 hours to be certain it is whole; it is then exposed to sperm (obtained by masturbation) in a petri dish. If fertilization oc-

curs, the zygote formed will almost immediately begin to divide and grow. By 40 hours postfertilization, it will have undergone its first cell division. Following this step, it is transferred to the uterine cavity through the cervix by a thin catheter.

A woman may be administered progesterone to support a luteal endometrium phase because corpus luteum formation may have been affected by the aspiration of the follicle. The zygote's implantation can be demonstrated by a serum pregnancy test as early as 11 days after transfer.

The results of IVF and ET are often disappointing; as with in-tube fertilization, implantation is a risky step. The overall pregnancy rate is about 15 to 20 percent. Although IVF programs do not result in an increase in birth defects, about 25 percent of pregnancies will end in spontaneous abortion (Gardner, 1983)

IVF is expensive, not available except at specialized centers, and a psychological strain (waiting to be accepted by a center's program and waiting to obtain the oocyte, let it grow in the laboratory, and be assured of pregnancy success). Once a pregnancy has been successfully implanted, the woman's pregnancy care is as with any other normal pregnancy.

Ethical considerations are involved in interfering with nature to this extent. There is a risk that if bacteria are introduced at any point in the transfer, maternal infection could occur. It is unfortunate that the term *test-tube baby* has come to be used for this process: It implies more manipulation than actually occurs. IVF should not evoke an image of infants growing in the giant test tubes of science fiction books and films; it is instead an alternative method to help a couple achieve pregnancy and produce children.

Adoption

Adoption, once a ready alternative for infertile couples, has been made difficult by the decreasing numbers of children available for adoption. In addition, as with other alternatives, adoption may not be right for every couple. The average parent has 9 months to prepare physically and emotionally for the coming of a baby. Usually it takes that long for the parents to accept the pregnancy and to begin to think of themselves as parents. Although adoptive parents may have been planning on a baby for much longer than 9 months (the waiting time at some adoption agencies may be as long as 5 years and many are no longer even taking applications), the actual appearance of the child occurs quite suddenly. They are called and told "their child" has been born; they go to the hospital or agency 2 days later to bring the infant home. In 2 short days they are asked to make the mental steps toward parenthood that biologic parents make over 9 months.

Because adoptive parents tend to be older than nonadoptive parents at the time of the birth of their first child (the average couple conceives a child within 2 years of marriage; the average adopting couple waits 2 years, then undergoes fertility testing for an additional year, then waits for agency adoption up to 5 years), the parents may be less able to adjust their lives to the presence of a new baby in the home. Adoptive parents may need a great deal of "talk time" at health care visits to explore their feelings about the child and about being parents; they need frequent assurance that they are good parents until they grow accustomed to their new role.

Surrogate Mothers

A surrogate mother is a woman who agrees to be impregnated by a man's sperm and then to carry a fetus to term for him or his sexual partner. A surrogate mother is often a friend or family member who takes the role out of friendship or compassion. She can be a woman who is interested in the arrangement for monetary gain.

An infertile couple can enjoy the pregnancy as they watch it progress by this arrangement. A number of problems may arise with surrogate motherhood. What if the surrogate mother decides at the end of pregnancy that she wants to keep the baby despite the prepregnancy agreement she signed? What if the child is imperfect and the infertile couple no longer wants it? Who should be responsible? Couples and the surrogate mother should be certain they have given adequate thought to the process before attempting it.

Childless Living

Childless living is an alternative life style that an infertile couple may choose. Childless living has the advantage of making it easier for a couple to pursue dual careers. It offers them a more varied life style in terms of travel and allotment of resources, pursuing hobbies, continued education, and lessened responsibility. Childless living can be just as fulfilling as having children by giving a couple more time to help other people and to contribute to society through personal accomplishment. Many couples today who feel that overpopulation is a major concern are choosing childless living even when a problem of infertility is not present.

Utilizing Nursing Process

Since tubal insufficiency is a major cause of infertility (in 30 to 35 percent of instances) and gonorrhea infection is a prime cause of tubal insufficiency, infertility problems can be expected to increase in the future along with the currently rising incidence of gonorrhea. Since the solutions to infertility are also increasing, however, more and more infertile couples will eventually conceive. At one time a woman who was anovulatory could not be helped. Now she not only can be stimulated to ovulate but may find herself the mother of twins, triplets, or even quintuplets.

Caring for couples who have a problem of infertility is a stressful area of care. Proper nursing process must be used to ensure quality care.

Assessment

Couples are in a vulnerable position when they call a health care facility to ask for help with infertility. They are admitting that they need help with one of life's major areas, a concession many people find difficult to make. Social and family pressure may make admitting they cannot conceive a child seem demeaning. The couple may be worried about the future of their marriage or rela-

tionship. Each partner may wonder whether the other will be able to accept marriage with a person who is infertile. Some people would rather not have the infertility investigated on the theory that no news is at least not bad news.

Couples need to discuss at the first visit to the health care facility the reason for their being interested in a fertility series. Those who seriously desire children because they love and want children should be differentiated from those who are attempting to strengthen a weak marriage with a child; from those who want to know for their own peace of mind that they are fertile, but who do not want children; and from those who want to know that they are indeed infertile so that they can discontinue a contraceptive measure.

Not all couples know what motivation lies behind their visit. Encouraging them to examine their motivations helps them to clarify their feelings about children and offers clues about their reactions to the outcome of the studies. Depending on their motivation for undertaking the studies, a couple's reaction to the results may vary from relief to stoic acceptance to grief for children never to be born. They need the support of health care personnel throughout the course of infertility studies; if the news is bad, it should come from people who have stood by them from the first day they steeled themselves to ask, "Exactly why are we childless?"

History taking for the couple should include not only the factual details of their health and reproductive status but their plans and feelings about infertility as well.

Analysis

The Fourth Annual Conference of Nursing Diagnoses accepted no diagnoses directly related to infertility. The diagnosis "Sexuality, alterations in," might be applicable if a specific problem in this area is determined. Other commonly used diagnoses are "Fear related to outcome of infertility studies" and "Grieving, dysfunctional, related to inability to conceive children."

In setting goals with a couple for fertility testing, be certain that they realize that testing will take a period of time; they should not expect results to be instantaneous. They also may change or modify their goals as tests begin to show that what they first wanted—to have a child without medical interventions—is not possible.

Planning

Few health insurance programs provide money for fertility testing although coverage of surgery such as that to relieve endometriosis is available. When helping a couple to make plans, you may have to help them determine the cost of fertility testing and interventions and budget and plan their resources accordingly.

Resolve is a national support group for couples with infertility; it can offer referral sources and support that a couple can use in planning.

Implementation

A couple's anxiety becomes more and more acute as fertility studies proceed. Some physicians give the results of each test as it is done; others prefer to wait until the basic series of tests is completed before the couple is told the outcome.

A woman who has had to seek help for infertil-

ity may have less confidence in her body than one who becomes pregnant with ease. She is likely to worry more during pregnancy than the average woman about whether she will carry the pregnancy to term. Back pain, frequency of urination, heartburn—all normal occurrences of pregnancy—may be interpreted as ominous signs. She needs added support during pregnancy and added reassurance that her difficulty in conceiving is unrelated to the complications of pregnancy.

Couples who are unable to be helped in achieving fertility and conception need time and support to grieve. Until they can accept an alternative method of having children, such as a surrogate mother, artificial insemination, or adoption, many future plans have been crushed for them. It is not unusual to see a couple move through steps of denial, anger, bargaining, and depression before they reach a level of acceptance that they are different in this one area of life from others. Eventually they will have to make some adjustments in their wants or plans in order to feel fulfilled.

Evaluation

Evaluation should be ongoing with a couple who has a problem of infertility. As circumstances around them change, so may their goals and desires. A couple who decided at age 20 that they wanted to choose childless living might change their minds at a later date. A couple who chose artificial insemination might decide after a number of unsuccessful attempts that they are no longer interested in this method of conception. Keeping evaluation an ongoing process allows you to stay up-to-date and modify a current plan if necessary. Couples seen for fertility testing should feel free to telephone or make a reappointment at a later point in life; at these times they can inquire about new discoveries in the field of fertility and any application to their situation. In this way they can be certain that any decision they make is based on the most current information available.

Nursing Care Planning

Mary Kraft is a 23-year-old you see in a health care setting for a fertility evaluation. The following is a nursing care plan designed for her.

Assessment

Patient had a spontaneous abortion 1½ years ago, unable to conceive since. Sexual relations about 2 × week. Keeps temperature chart daily; is aware of concept of fertile and infertile periods. Has temperature increase suggesting ovulation on

17th day of cycle as a rule. Menstrual cycle 30–32 days, 6 days duration, heavy flow with painful cramping. No history of sexually transmitted disease, normal activity level although she has a scanty diet pattern. Had abdominal surgery for appendicitis as 12-year-old. No Gyn surgery. Sometimes has dyspareunia.

Patient became pregnant first time after 3 months of sexual relations. Spontaneous abortion at 2½ months, no known cause, no apparent sequelae, no D&C performed. Has slight vaginal discharge now, some pruritus.

Hemoglobin: 12 mg, normal urinalysis.

Analysis

Fear related to apparent infertility.

Locus of Decision Making. Patient.

Goal. Patient to be cognizant of reason for infertility by 3 months' time.

Criteria. Patient to complete infertility studies and voice conclusions of studies.

Nursing Orders

1. Discuss treatment for vaginal discharge as outlined by M.D.
2. Schedule fertility testing pattern determined by M.D.
3. Discuss husband-wife relationship and coping ability in view of frustration and disappointment of infertility and possible length of testing period.

Questions for Review

Multiple Choice

1. Charles is a 25-year-old male who visits a health care facility because he is worried he has an infertile sperm count. Which circumstance below would you want to be certain to ask about during his health history?
   a. if he works at a desk job
   b. if he eats a low lipid diet
   c. if he jogs frequently
   d. if he takes a vitamin supplement

2. Charles will bring a semen specimen into clinic tomorrow for analysis. Which instruction below would you give him regarding this?
   a. It should be obtained immediately after voiding.
   b. It should be collected immediately after coitus.
   c. It should be protected against chilling.
   d. It should be diluted with saline for transport.

3. Charles is interested in artificial insemination if he is proven to be infertile. He asks you if its use would be appropriate for him and his sexual partner. Which statement below would be your best advice?
   a. "The chance of twins is increased with artificial insemination, so be prepared."
   b. "It is only useful if your sexual partner has an allergy to your sperm, not if you are infertile."
   c. "You need to consider donor artificial insemination if you are found to be infertile."
   d. "You and your sexual partner should consider embryo transfer first, as it is safer."

4. Wanda is a 22-year-old woman you see in an infertility clinic. She and her husband have been trying for a year to become pregnant. In a year, what proportion of couples usually do conceive?
   a. 40 percent
   b. 60 percent
   c. 80 percent
   d. 100 percent

5. You are asked to schedule a uterosalpingogram for Wanda. Which question would be important to ask her before doing this?
   a. When does she expect her next menstrual flow?
   b. Is she allergic to any sedatives?
   c. What is her blood type and Rh factor?
   d. Does she have an allergy to radioactive test material?

6. Wanda is also to have a Sims-Huhner test. Which instruction below would you give her concerning this?
   a. She should douche before coming to the clinic.
   b. It will be scheduled immediately after her menstrual flow.
   c. She can expect no pain from the procedure.
   d. Her sexual partner should use a condom for 3 days afterward.

7. Wanda is discovered to have endometriosis. She asks you to explain why this causes her to be infertile. Your best explanation would be,
   a. "The lining of your uterus appears to have different properties than usual."
   b. "Your uterine cervix fails to close because it is engorged with tissue."
   c. "Menstrual sloughing does not occur, so there is never a new base for embryo growth."
   d. "You do not ovulate because of endometrial implants on the ovaries."

8. Wanda is placed on birth control pills. Which of the following would you explain to her?
   a. how progesterone acts on endometrial tissue
   b. how estrogen reduces inflammation
   c. how estrogen acts on the pituitary
   d. how sperm cannot survive with endometriosis

Discussion

1. Taking a history from an infertile couple often reveals the cause of infertility. What areas are important to ask about in a male history? A female history?
2. A Rubin test and a hysterosalpingogram are tests used to establish tubal patency. How would you prepare a woman for these tests?
3. Most couples do not understand artificial insemination. How would you explain the use of this procedure?

Suggested Readings

Alexander, N. J. (1983). A new test of sperm function: In vitro CMP. *Contemporary OB/GYN, 21,* 203.

American Nurses Association. (1966). ANA adopts statement on family planning. *American Journal of Nursing, 66,* 2376.

Barnett, H. (1977). *Pediatrics.* New York: Appleton-Century-Crofts.

Behrman, S. J. (1979). Artificial insemination. *Clinical Obstetrics and Gynecology, 22,* 245.

Bernstein, J., et al. (1982). An overview of infertility. *J.O.G.N. Nursing, 11,* 309.

Boyden, T. W., et al. (1983). Sex steroids and endurance running in women. *Infertility and Sterility, 39,* 629.

Eisenberg, E. (1983). Fertility problems of DES daughters. *Contemporary OB/GYN, 22,* 197.

Fleming, C., et al. (1983). Microscopic tubal reversal. *Association of Operating Room Nurses Journal, 37,* 199.

Friedmen, B. M. (1981). Infertility workup. *American Journal of Nursing, 81,* 2040.

Gardner, C. H. (1983). In vitro fertilization and embryo transfer. *J.O.G.N. Nursing, 12,* 71.

Gray, M. J. (1980). Sexual problems in infertility. *Female Patient, 5,* 21.

Hakim-Elahi, E. (1982). Infertility: Diagnosis and clinical management. *Family and Community Health, 5,* 61.

Hembree, W. C. (1984). Long-term marijuana use: Can it reduce fertility? *Contemporary OB/GYN, 20,* 67.

Hendershot, G. E., et al. (1982). Infertility and age: An unresolved issue. *Family Planning Perspectives, 14,* 287.

Isaacs, J. H. (1983). Vaginal reconstruction. *Female Patient, 8,* 6.

Kapstrom, A. B. (1981). Does the career woman face infertility? *Supervisor Nurse, 12,* 54.

Kaufman, S. A. (1984). Stress and infertility. *Female Patient, 9,* 107.

Kaye, W., & Neff, S. (1983). Could her irregular menses be caused by bulimia? *Contemporary OB/GYN, 21,* 97.

Lamb, C. (1983). Battling sexually transmitted diseases. *Patient Care, 17,* 19.

McCusker, M. P. (1982). The subfertile couple. *J.O.G.N. Nursing, 11,* 157.

Menning, B. E. (1982). The psychological impact of infertility. *Nursing Clinics of North America, 17,* 155.

Ollivier, S., et al. (1984). Providing infertility care. *J.O.G.N. Nursing, 13,* 85s.

Rebar, R. W. (1983). Premature ovarian failure: A multifactorial disorder. *Contemporary OB/GYN, 21,* 175.

Sawatzky, M. (1981). Tasks of infertile couples . . . four psychological tasks . . . to deal with the childlessness. *J.O.G.N. Nursing, 10,* 132.

Sheinfeld, M. (1983). Helping the infertile orthodox Jewish couple. *Contemporary OB/GYN, 21,* 137.

Siegler, A. M. (1983). HSG to diagnose uterine and tubal anomalies. *Contemporary OB/GYN, 21,* 137.

Speroff, L. (1983). Avoiding the pitfalls of infertility management. *Contemporary OB/GYN, 21,* 127.

Wallach, E. E. (1983). Solving the riddle of unexplained infertility. *Contemporary OB/GYN, 21,* 142.

Weathersbee, P. S., & Werlin, L. B. (1984). Pelvic ultrasound in infertility management. *Female Patient, 9,* 55.

Williamson, J. K. (1983). Reproductive decisions: Adolescents with Down's syndrome. *Pediatric Nursing, 9,* 43.

Zacar, H. A., & Rock, J. (1983). Diagnosis and treatment of infertility. *Female Patient, 8,* 39.

IV

The Prepartal Period: Preparing for Parenthood

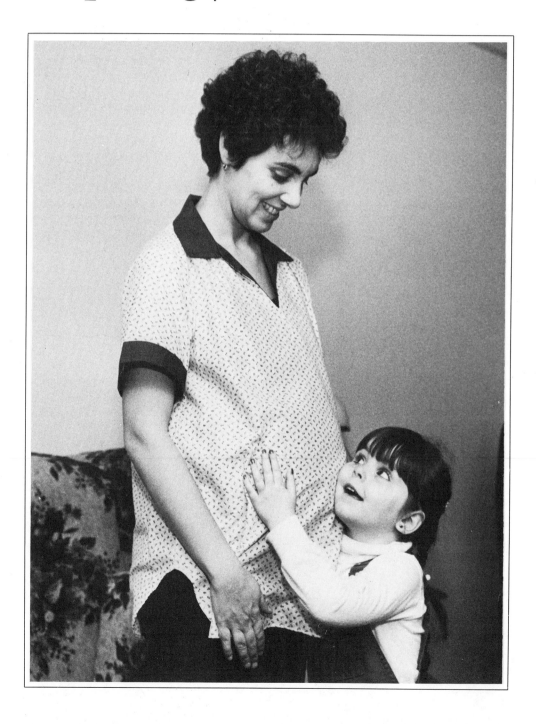

13

Psychological Aspects of Pregnancy

OBJECTIVES

Following mastery of the contents of this chapter, you should be able to:

1. Describe the common initial psychological reactions to pregnancy by both a woman and her sexual partner.
2. Describe the steps of psychological preparation for childbirth.
3. List common assessment areas to detect whether psychological adjustment to pregnancy is occurring.
4. State a nursing diagnosis and establish patient goals related to a psychological aspect of pregnancy.
5. Plan nursing implementations for a woman regarding psychological aspects of pregnancy.
6. Implement nursing care to encourage healthy psychological adaptation to pregnancy.
7. Evaluate goal outcomes regarding psychological adjustment to pregnancy.
8. Analyze the effect of pregnancy and childbirth on a family.
9. Synthesize knowledge of psychosocial aspects of pregnancy with nursing process to achieve quality maternal-newborn nursing care.

THE PSYCHOLOGICAL CHANGES of pregnancy are a direct consequence of the child growing within the woman, the physical changes this pregnancy entails, and the increased responsibility and concern for the new family member resulting from the pregnancy. It is unrealistic to discuss the psychological aspects of pregnancy apart from its physiologic aspects, or the development of the unborn child. In terms of nursing care, the psychological aspects are inseparable from the physiologic. Both must be kept in mind during prenatal visits if a woman is to have an uncomplicated pregnancy and establish a healthy mother-child relationship, and if the family is to adjust adequately to its new member.

The Pregnant Woman

Because the first signs of pregnancy are subtle—nausea in the morning, a feeling of fatigue, the absence of a menstrual flow—the woman is the first to know or suspect that she is pregnant.

Initial Reactions to Pregnancy

A woman may run the gamut of emotions during pregnancy, from the surprise of finding herself pregnant (or wishing she were not), to pleasure and acceptance as she feels the child stir within her, to fear for herself and her child, to boredom with the process and wishing to get it all over so that she can get on with the next step—rearing her child—to surprise again that the process is over and she really has given birth.

From a physiologic standpoint, it is fortunate that a pregnancy is 9 months long. This gives the fetus time to mature and to be prepared for life outside a protective uterine environment. The psychological preparation of the family also hinges on this long waiting time: They must get ready for the coming of the child.

The availability of birth control measures today would seem to prevent pregnancy from being a surprise. In reality, every pregnancy is a surprise (Rubin, 1976). The woman who was not planning on being pregnant will obviously be surprised. The woman who was looking forward to being pregnant is surprised that it has really happened (no woman is absolutely certain in advance that she can conceive whenever she wishes to) and that it happened this month instead of next month or the month before.

If pregnancy announced itself by more reliable signs, women could be more certain how they feel about being pregnant. It is strange that such an important life function is heralded by the absence of a body function rather than by the addition of something.

Along with the first flush of surprise that they are pregnant, as many as 80 percent of women experience a feeling that is less than pleasure and may be disappointment or anxiety (Rubin, 1965). The reasons they give for their displeasure at the news are many: "I don't want a baby." "I don't want a baby *now*." "I want a baby, but I don't want to be pregnant for the next 9 months." "I want a baby and I want to be pregnant, but I don't want any part of labor and delivery." "I can't afford to give up my job." "My husband doesn't want a baby." Fortunately, most of these women change their attitudes toward the pregnancy by the time they feel the child stir inside them.

Cultural Influences

A woman's attitude toward a pregnancy depends a great deal on the culture in which she was raised, the culture in which she lives now, and the individual experiences she had with pregnancy as a child.

Despite efforts to change this focus, childbearing in the United States is still a medically oriented process. The woman goes to a physician or nurse midwife during pregnancy; she is treated for discomforts of pregnancy with a medical prescription; at the time of delivery, she is admitted to a health care facility. Maternal and infant mortality figures attest to the value of this kind of care during pregnancy and delivery, but the emphasis on medical management also conveys a feeling that pregnancy is an illness. Some women therefore view being pregnant as being ill. When a woman perceives herself as ill, she may resist encouragement to get enough exercise or eat sufficient nourishing food: Ill people, after all, typically need to rest and to eat sparingly.

A pregnant woman often visits the physician's office alone—which implies that childbearing is a woman's business. A husband who accepts this attitude will be hard put to understand that his wife needs his emotional support during pregnancy.

In the United States, most women are made to feel that they are responsible for the health of the child growing within them. In many other cultures there is little stress on this responsibility, and the outcome of a pregnancy is felt to depend on some supernatural agency. It is difficult to teach a woman to take extra precautions during pregnancy, such as discontinuing the use of a potentially harmful medication, if she believes that the health of her newborn is ultimately out of her hands.

When planning health instruction you should keep in mind that the material taught must be chosen for its relevance to the patient, not for its relevance to you. If you believe that, ideally, parents should be over 21 before they have children, or that the best home is a shuttered cottage surrounded by a white picket fence, take a deep breath before you begin to talk to a pregnant, unmarried adolescent about nutrition during pregnancy. If you believe strongly that families should be limited to two children for zero population growth, be careful of the tone of your voice when you talk to a woman who is pregnant with her tenth child. These are your beliefs, and they work for you, but they may mean little or nothing to the girl or woman in front of you because of the differences in your backgrounds.

The home in which a woman was raised is as important as the general culture from which she comes. If she was raised in a family where children were loved or viewed as pleasant outcomes of a marriage, she is more likely to have a positive attitude toward a pregnancy than is the woman who was reared in a home where children were felt to be in the way or were blamed for the breakup of a marriage. No matter how often a girl is told that pregnancy is natural and simple, if she has heard horror stories about excruciating pain and endless suffering in labor, she cannot be overjoyed to find herself pregnant. If her mother has constantly reminded her, "If you hadn't come along, I could have gone to college" or "I could have had a career," she is likely to think of pregnancy as a kind of disaster.

That people love as they have been loved is said so often now that it has become a cliché, but it has a great deal of relevance to whether pregnancy and childbirth are viewed positively or negatively. If a woman has difficulty loving, she will have difficulty accepting a fetus growing within her. In order to mother well (being a mother is a second adjustment step, over and above being pregnant) the woman must feel pleasurable anticipation at the prospect of rearing a child. The woman who views mothering as a positive activity because her mother was able to view it as a fulfilling life role is more likely to be pleased when she becomes pregnant than one who devalues mothering.

The Psychological Tasks of Pregnancy

A number of developmental and psychological tasks must be accomplished by the woman during pregnancy. The first of these is accepting the pregnancy.

Accepting the Pregnancy

Nausea and vomiting, frequency of urination, tiredness, perhaps slight tingling in the breasts, and amenorrhea are the first indications of pregnancy; however, they cannot be taken as absolute proof. A visit to a physician or clinic and a diagnosis of pregnancy is a major step in helping a woman to accomplish the task of accepting the pregnancy. The fetus may be only an hour older when the woman leaves the health care facility than when she entered it, but if a diagnosis of pregnancy was the outcome of the visit, she *feels* "more pregnant."

Our culture structures celebrations around important life events. Christenings, bar mitzvahs, marriages, birthdays, deaths—all have a ritual to help those concerned take a step toward or accept the coming change in their lives. A diagnosis of pregnancy is a similar initiation ceremony. Think of a diagnosis visit as having special, hidden meaning, different from an ordinary visit to a health care facility.

A second ceremony of pregnancy is *quickening*, or the moment the woman first feels life. Until this time she tended to think of the life inside her as an integral part of herself. She knew it was there; she ate for it, slept for it, but it was just a part of her body like her arms or legs. With quickening, the child becomes a separate entity, and the mother begins to give the child an identity. She imagines how she will feel in the delivery room when the physician announces, "It's a boy!" or "It's a girl!" She imagines herself picking out baby clothes, selecting toys, mending little blue jeans, teaching her child the alphabet or how to cook. She pictures herself seeing a daughter off to college, watching a son play football. She sees herself as the mother of the bride, or groom, at a wedding. This anticipatory role playing is an important task for the woman: It leads her to a larger concept of her condition. Not only is she pregnant, but she is going to have a child as well!

Most women can name a point during pregnancy when they knew they wanted their child. For some who carefully planned the pregnancy, it is the moment after they recover from the surprise of suspecting they are pregnant. For others it is the day of diagnosis. In one woman it may be a personal moment: her father and mother expressing their joy, or a look of pride on her husband's face. It might be quickening, the moment she realized that the fetus inside her was not passive but active, when she suddenly knew the stranger she had lived with for 5 months. It might be a moment she first shopped for baby clothes and picked up a size 0 shirt. It might be the moment she set up the crib; seeing a crib in *her* house made the pregnancy, the coming baby, real and desired.

Accepting the pregnancy might not come until labor begins, or hours into labor. It might be the moment she first hears the baby cry, or first touches or feeds the baby. The moment may come late, a week, or 3 weeks, after she takes the baby home. But at some point—the usual times tend to cluster around diagnosis and quickening—a woman will know that she and her baby are going to get along, that they will make a go of it.

How close the woman is to achieving acceptance is sometimes evident in her ability to follow prenatal instructions. Until she views the growing structure inside her as something of value, she will have difficulty following a proper diet. If she wants very much to be pregnant but is not yet convinced that she is, she may have difficulty eliminating excessively high carbohydrate foods from her diet. After all, her weight gain may be the most certain proof she has that she is pregnant.

Preparations for a baby's coming imply that acceptance has been achieved. Thus, it is good to ask the woman what she is doing to get ready for her baby. Once she has accepted her pregnancy and that she is having a baby, she begins to "build the nest." Between the fifth and seventh months of pregnancy, most women begin to plan where the infant will sleep, what he will wear, how he will be fed, what his name will be.

It is easy to infer that a woman who uses the term *it* for the fetus inside her has not yet accepted her pregnancy. However, many women, although they have chosen a name for the child and are very sure which sex they want, continue to refer to the baby as *it* during pregnancy. They would deny being superstitious, but nonetheless they are worried that referring to the child as *she* will somehow turn the child into *he*, or vice versa.

Caplan (1959) has documented several abnormal maternal fantasies about a pregnancy or a child. The first of these is a conception of the fetus as an older child. A woman with such a fantasy may feel despondent in the newborn period, when she must care for a helpless, dependent infant rather than the older child she fantasized.

A second fantasy that may reveal nonacceptance of the pregnancy or of the reality that a child is to be born is that the baby is already an adult. "I hope she has her grandmother's tiny feet; she can be a dancer." "I hope she's as athletic as my husband; I want her to get a varsity letter." "I want him to major in international law." These are typical examples of this kind of fantasy. Such a woman may be attempting to fulfill her own ambitions through her child rather than accepting the child as having individual needs and desires.

A third woman who may have difficulty is the one who knows exactly what her child will look or be like. She may not be able to accept her child's actual looks or personality, but will instead expect her fantasy standard to be met. Yet another woman who may have difficulty is the one who insists she can tell that she is having a boy or a girl. She may have a hard time mothering a child of the opposite sex.

Whether or not a woman feels secure in her relationship with the people around her, especially the father of her child, is important in her acceptance of a pregnancy. Pregnancy is easier to accept when a woman has confidence in the solidity of her marriage or, if she is not married, that the father of the child will be there to give her emotional support. She will be less comfortable when she learns she is pregnant if she has an unreliable partner who may shortly disappear, leaving her alone with the responsibility of child-rearing.

A woman's ability to cope with or adapt to stress, to resolve conflict, and to adapt to new life contingencies plays a major role. Part of this ability to adapt (to be able to mother and no longer need mothering, to love a child as well as a husband, to be a mother of four, not just of three) involves the woman's basic temperament, that is, whether she always adapts quickly or slowly, whether she faces new situations with an intense or a low-key approach, and whether or not she has had past experience with change and stress.

Some women view a pregnancy as a threat. A woman who thinks of brides as young but mothers as old may believe that pregnancy will rob her of her youth. If she thinks of children as sticky-fingered and time-consuming, she may view the pregnancy as taking away her freedom. If she has heard that pregnancy will stretch her abdomen and breasts permanently, her concern may focus on losing her looks. She may feel that the pregnancy will rob her financially and ruin her chances for promotion on her job. These are very real feelings, and they must be taken seriously when you are working with pregnant women. They cannot be shrugged off by a cliché ("A door closes, another one opens") or repression ("You shouldn't think that way; you'll love having a baby in the house"). The woman needs an opportunity to express such feelings so she becomes aware of their intensity and can begin to work them through to resolution.

Reworking Developmental Tasks

Women work through previous life experiences during pregnancy as one of the tasks of pregnancy. Needs and wishes they have repressed for years surface to be studied and reworked, to such an extent that if the woman were not pregnant, such behavior might be called pathological.

Primary among those life experiences are the woman's relationship with her parents, particularly with her mother. For the first time she finds she can empathize with her mother's concern when she used to return late from high-school

dates. She herself is already worrying about her child if she feels no movement within her for a few hours, yet she is only 5 months pregnant!

Fear of dying is a common fear of childhood that is revived during pregnancy. Thinking along these lines is not unrealistic; women do die in childbirth.

In order for the woman to work through past fears and conflicts, she needs to think about them when she is alone and to talk about them with others. She "throws out comments" when talking to her husband or to health care personnel, to test their reactions. "I really hated my mother when I was a kid" is a typical opener for a woman during pregnancy. If you respond to that in a therapeutic way ("Would you like to talk about that?"), she will feel free to reveal the intensity of her conflict with her parents, how much she hated them at times, how she cannot bear to think of the child inside her feeling that way about her (it almost makes her dislike her child before birth). If the response to her remark is less than therapeutic ("Oh really? Now where is the urine specimen you said you brought in?") or trite ("Don't worry; everyone feels that same way"), she will usually not repeat the comment at that visit or may try it out on other health care personnel.

Her cues to what she is thinking may be subtle. "Am I ever going to make it through this?" might mean that she is tired of her backache, but it might also be a plea for reassurance that she will survive this event.

A woman needs to have confidence in the health care personnel who care for her during pregnancy, so that she can express some of the thoughts that are bothering her. It is easier and less time-consuming to ignore the comments that pregnant women make about their relationships with their families or husbands or their fears about the baby. However, an aim of maternal-newborn nursing is to ensure the welfare of the baby, and helping a woman to verbalize her thoughts, to straighten out old conflicts or crises, contributes to the establishment of a good mother-child relationship, which is essential for the baby's well-being.

Preparing for Motherhood

Preparing for motherhood is an extension of the phenomenon of accepting the pregnancy and the child. It is necessary, however, that it be completed during pregnancy or during the weeks afterward, or parenting cannot proceed.

Kempe and Helfer (1972) relate the battered-child syndrome to a poor mothering image. Poor mothering ability may also produce children who exhibit the syndrome of failure to thrive because of the parents' lack of attachment and emotional concern.

Rubin (1976) has identified a number of steps through which a woman must pass before she is ready to be a mother. These steps are as important to the woman about to become a mother for the second, third, fourth, or sixth time as they are for the woman about to become a mother for the first time.

Mimicry

The process of mimicry in the pregnant woman is not so different from that of the pre- schooler who mimics parental roles. When a pre- schooler follows after her mother dusting the fur- niture, her parents may express approval. When she mimics the position in which her father stands to use the toilet, her parents may express disapproval. As a result, the child chooses to im- itate her mother.

The pregnant woman begins to spend time with other pregnant women or acquaintances of hers who have young children. She may spend more time talking to her own mother; this may be the first time she has truly talked to her since the conflicts of adolescence set up a barrier. She imitates actions, words, and tasks that exemplify mothering.

Role Playing

The second step in the process is role playing. The woman offers to babysit for a neighbor or relative who has a new baby. She imitates the way the mother deals with the child. She is role playing at "being a mother" (Figure 13-1).

Fantasy

In fantasy, the woman performs much the same work she did in accepting the pregnancy. She fantasizes what it will be like to be the mother of a boy, the mother of a girl. She sees if she can find a "fit" that is comfortable for her. Hopefully, she sees herself as fitting both roles, because she has no way of knowing which she will be called on to assume.

Taking-In

The fourth step is a taking-in. Rubin (1965) re- fers to this step as introjection-projection-rejec- tion. It is a continuation of actively acquiring a mother role "fit." The step begins with a woman becoming aware of her need to learn to mother (introjection). She then finds a role model of a mother among her friends or family (projection).

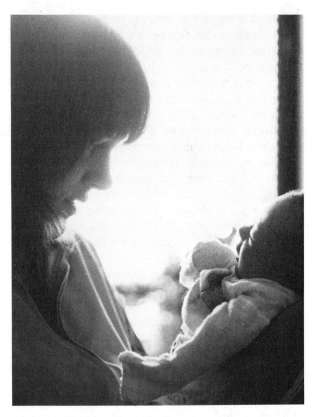

Figure 13-1 *Psychological preparation for childbirth involves caring for babies or role playing what being a mother will be like.*

The behavior of the role model is observed closely. The mother transposes herself into the model person's role. If the other woman's behav- ior seems to fit how the pregnant woman will be able to mother, then this woman adds to her ex- isting knowledge and behavior repertoire. If the behavior does not seem to fit—the role model chosen was too rough with her children or too unconcerned—the woman will cast this model aside (rejection). She will then choose another role model and will continue this process until she finds one that is right for her.

This step is an important one in helping an adolescent girl to become a good mother. If the only role models she has are other girls her own age, who typically are not very interested in the commitment to mothering, or if the role model is her own mother, and the mother is unable to cope with poverty, or too many children, or an ineffec- tual husband, then the young girl will probably assume the same role. She needs exposure to good role models—in mothers' classes, at the clinic, in the physician's office, in a social agency—to be able to find a maternal role that will be worth copying and integrating into her own behavior.

Grief Work

The thought that grief could be associated with such a positive process as childbirth is at first bizarre. But before a woman can firmly take on a mothering role she has to "give up" present roles. She cannot be the mother of three and the mother of four at the same time; the mother-of-three image will have to go. She cannot be a child if she is to be an effective mother. The child in her will have to go. She cannot think of herself equally as a career woman and a mother. Either she will be a career woman who mothers in her spare time or a mother who squeezes in a career; one of the roles will have to be suppressed or perhaps temporarily put aside. This is grief work. The result will be a woman ready to accept a new role as a mother.

There are a number of life contingencies that may interfere with a woman's developing a relationship with her new child (accepting the pregnancy) or becoming a mother. Some of these are listed in Table 13-1. These life situations should be kept in mind when working with pregnant women. All too often, in both prenatal clinics and physicians' offices, considerable time is spent on taking a history on the initial visit, but on subsequent visits very few questions are asked. Thus, life contingencies may be overlooked that could have as great an effect on the newborn child as the physical things that have happened to the woman since she was last in the office.

It is easy to convince yourself that asking questions such as "How does your husband feel about your being pregnant?" or "Has anything changed in your home life since you were in the clinic last time?" is meddling. But such questions are not meddling to one who believes that mental health has as high a priority as physical health. Some nurses are reluctant to ask questions about these kinds of situations because they are aware that they cannot handle all the feelings that will be aroused. It is a fallacy to think that *any* person has the solutions to all the problems that people will pour out to health care personnel if they are given even the slightest opening to talk of things other than the swelling in their ankles or how much weight they have gained. You need the wisdom to recognize what you can handle, together with knowledge of the persons or social agencies who are equipped to deal with problems you cannot solve. This is a much more positive approach to mental health and one that is not very different from the way you handle medical problems. For example, you may or may not be in a position to correct beginning hypertension in a woman during pregnancy, but knowing that pregnancy-induced hypertension is a major cause of maternal mortality, you will not neglect to take a blood pressure simply because you will not be making the decision as to how to correct the problem.

Table 13-1 Life Contingenices Associated with Mothering Breakdown in the Perinatal Period

1. Multiple births
2. Children born within 10 to 12 months of each other
3. Dislocating moves in pregnancy or newborn period involving changing geographical areas and need to find new ties
4. Moving away from a family group or back to the group for economic reasons at a critical period for mother and child
5. Unexpected loss of security by reason of job losses, to husband; to the pregnant woman
6. Marital infidelity discovered in prenatal period
7. Illness in self, husband, or relative who must be cared for at a critical period
8. Loss of husband or of the infant's father close to prenatal period
9. Role reversals if a previously supporting person becomes dependent
10. Conception and course of pregnancy associated with loss of a person with whom there was a deeply significant tie
11. Previous abortions, sterility periods, traumatic past deliveries, loss of previous children
12. Pregnancy health complications
13. Experience with close friends or relatives who have had defective children
14. The juxtaposition of conception with a series of devaluing experiences

Source: Rose, J. (1961). The prevention of mothering breakdown associated with physical abnormalities of the infant. In G. Caplan (Ed.). *Prevention of mental disorders in children: Initial explorations* (Chap. 12). New York: Basic Books.

Emotional Responses to Pregnancy

Pregnancy is an intrusive process. A separate individual has invaded the woman's body and is growing inside it. She cannot ignore its presence any more than she can ignore that of a stranger who walked into her home and sat for 9 months at her dining room table. She might try to pretend no one was there, or forget he was there when out of the house. Sometimes, if he conversed with her or told amusing stories, she might be grateful he was there. But it would be virtually impossible not to have some feeling about his presence.

A great deal of a woman's reaction to pregnancy is similar—that is, *ambivalent.* She wants the pregnancy and yet she does not want it. She enjoys being pregnant and yet she does not enjoy it. Some nurses assume ambivalence means that the positive feelings counteract the negative feelings, the accepting feelings the rejecting feelings, so the woman is left feeling almost nothing toward her pregnancy, making pregnancy a calm, neutral period 9 months long. This is not the case. No matter how neutral she wants to be, sooner or later she will have to walk into the dining room. A stranger will be sitting at the table. She has to experience some emotion at his being there.

Narcissism

A woman's reaction to the intrusion of pregnancy can be manifested in a number of ways. Self-centeredness is generally an early reaction to pregnancy. A woman who previously was barely conscious of her body, who dressed in the morning with little thought about what to put on, who was unconcerned about her posture or her weight, suddenly begins to concentrate on these aspects of her life. She dresses so that her pregnancy will or will not show, and dressing becomes a time-consuming, mirror-studying procedure. She makes a ceremony out of fixing her meals. Remember, there is a stranger in her life, someone coming to dinner, someone who is watching her (the stranger sitting in the dining room).

A woman sometimes manifests narcissism by a change in her activities. She may stop playing tennis, even though her physician tells her it will do no harm in moderation. She criticizes her husband's driving when it never bothered her before. She is unconsciously "protecting" her body and thus her baby. She may be so unaware of what she is doing that she rationalizes her behavior. Tennis becomes "too tiring" or "boring." She describes her husband's driving as "reckless." What she means in both instances is that she feels threatened.

When working with a pregnant woman, it is important to remember that she feels a need to protect her body, that her *self* is important to her. She regards unnecessary nudity as a threat to her body (be sure to drape properly for pelvic and abdominal examinations). She resents casual, thoughtless remarks, such as "Oh, my, you're getting fat!" (a threat to her appearance) or "You don't like milk?" (a threat to her judgment).

There is a tendency to organize health instruction to pregnant women around the baby. "Now be sure to keep this appointment. You want to have a healthy baby." "You really ought to drink more milk for the baby." This approach is particularly inappropriate early in pregnancy, before the fetus stirs and before the woman is convinced not only that she is pregnant but that there is a baby inside her who is going to be born. At this stage

she may be much more interested in doing things for herself, since it is her body, her tiredness, and her well-being that will be affected.

Introversion versus Extroversion

Although introversion, or turning inward to concentrate on oneself and one's body, is common during pregnancy, some women react in an entirely opposite fashion and become more extroverted. They become active, appear healthier than ever before, and are more outgoing. Their faces glow, and they appear to "bloom" more and more with each month. Some women who undergo this change are just extremely happy to be pregnant. It tends to occur in women who are finding unexpected fulfillment in pregnancy, who had seriously doubted that they would be lucky enough or fertile enough to conceive. Such a woman regards her expanding abdomen as proof that she is equal to her sisters. In her eyes her pregnancy is a badge certifying equality. Although such a woman may become more varied in her interests during her pregnancy, she is certain to confuse those around her, who may have regarded her as quiet and self-contained.

Decreased Decision Making

People who were dependent on a woman before pregnancy may feel hurt because now that she is pregnant she seems to have strength only for herself. A pregnant woman may lose interest in her job because the work seems alien to the events taking place in her body, which constantly remind her that a new round of life is beginning. She may have difficulty with decision making because she does not have enough interest to concentrate on a problem. This reaction does not mean that a pregnant woman should not work. Pregnancy is not an illness; the outside interest and stimulation make the time go faster; the social contacts and the work she does are helpful to her and to her employer.

Decrease in responsibility taking is a reaction to the stress of pregnancy, not the pregnancy itself. Nonpregnant women and many men function under just as much stress at work because of marital discord or illness or death of a loved one and have just as much difficulty with decision making in these circumstances. Pregnancy may actually be less stressful than these situations because of its predictable outcome.

Emotional Lability

Mood changes occur frequently in a pregnant woman, partly as a manifestation of narcissism

Nursing Research Highlight

What are the Sexual Needs and Concerns of Expectant Parents?

Pregnancy brings with it changes in the sexually related roles and functions of an expectant couple, which can potentially contribute to marital stress. In many instances couples are reluctant to discuss sexual concerns. A study by one researcher (Ellis, 1980) was conducted to elicit the perceived needs of expectant couples regarding sexuality. Volunteer couples were recruited from urban classes for expectant parents. A questionnaire was completed by 15 couples. Findings indicate that these expectant parents perceived a variety of needs related to sexuality during pregnancy. As a group, women reported

they were satisfied with their woman's role during pregnancy but felt a decrease in the degree of sexual enjoyment. Their desired sources of sexual information were listed as books, prenatal instructors, and, lastly, physicians. This study gave couples an opportunity to state their needs and also offers valuable information to prenatal educators in the development of content for teaching.

Reference

Ellis, D. J. (1980). Sexual needs and concerns of expectant parents. *J.O.G.N. Nursing, 9*(5), 306.

(her feelings are easily hurt by remarks that would have been laughed off before) and partly because of hormonal changes, particularly the sustained increase in estrogen and progesterone. Mood swings are so common they make the woman's reaction to her family and to clinic or office routines unpredictable. What she found acceptable one week she may find intolerable the next. She may cry over her children's bad table manners at one meal and find the situation amusing and even charming at the next. A husband needs to be forewarned of these mood swings before his wife becomes pregnant, or at least very early in pregnancy, so that he will accept them as a part of a normal pregnancy. Otherwise, such changes in mood may cause him concern about his wife's mental health or about their relationship.

Changes in Sexual Desire

Most women report that their sexual desires change, at least to some degree, during a pregnancy. For women who were always worried about becoming pregnant, sex during pregnancy may be truly enjoyed for the first time. Others may feel a loss of desire or may unconsciously view sexual relations as a threat to the body they must protect. Some may be frightened that sexual relations may bring on early labor.

Both wives and husbands should be warned early in pregnancy that such changes may occur, so that they will be interpreted in the correct light, that is, as differences, not as loss of interest in the sexual partner. The physiologic changes

due to the increase in estrogen and progesterone may well serve as a physical basis for these changes. (See the Nursing Research Highlight above.)

Body Image and Boundary

Body image (the way your body appears to yourself) and body boundary (a zone of separation you perceive between yourself and objects or other people) (Fawcett, 1978) both change during pregnancy as the woman begins to envision herself as a mother in addition to a daughter and/or wife. This change in body image is the basis for the woman becoming narcissistic and introverted. Changes in the body boundary concept lead to a firmer distinction between objects and yet, at the same time, the boundary is perceived as very vulnerable as if the body were very delicate and easily harmed (Fawcett, 1978). This change in boundary perception is so striking that pregnant women may walk far away from an object such as a table in order to avoid it and, of course, accounts for the increasing "guarding" of the body as pregnancy progresses.

The Practical Tasks of Pregnancy

In addition to the main tasks of pregnancy, Duvall (1971) has identified a number of practical adjustments that must be made during pregnancy before the woman is ready for her baby. Although some of these are housekeeping adjustments, such as preparing a sleeping space for the infant, some are psychological adjustments, such as those involved in financial changes or changes in attitudes.

Arranging for the Infant's Physical Care

If the parents already have an extra bedroom and the additional equipment needed for a baby will be no financial burden, arranging for the baby's physical care may be a minor task (Figure 13-2). Frequently, however, providing space for a baby means moving to a larger apartment, or changing the older children's sleeping arrangements, or buying a new home. Purchasing a crib on a minimum income may require the sacrifice of some other item the couple very much wants. For these reasons, this task of pregnancy may be one of the most difficult.

Developing New Economic Patterns

At least 50 percent of women work during their first pregnancy. Then, just at a time when the couple's expenses are increasing (medical expenses, clothing, food, more costly living arrangements), the woman takes a leave of absence or resigns, cutting the family income drastically. If the woman's income was counted on to maintain the family's style of living—and it generally is—adjustment to a lesser income will be difficult to make. The woman may also have some strong feelings about not contributing to the family income or may fear that she will have no control over how income is to be spent. This is a devaluing experience that may make accepting her pregnancy difficult for her or may interfere with her relationship with her newborn child.

Reevaluation of Household Assignments

If the woman has intense nausea and vomiting early in pregnancy, or she tires easily in later pregnancy, the husband may, for the first time, find himself assuming chores in the home that he never imagined he would do. If he was raised to believe that household tasks are strictly women's work, he may find the demands too devaluing to endure. Even if he is used to a sharing of chores, he may chafe at suddenly having to do more than was originally agreed on. By envisioning household chores not as sex-related but merely as jobs that must be done in order to ensure the smooth running of the home, he will find them easier to

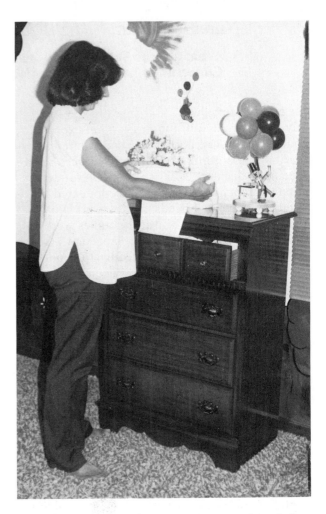

Figure 13-2 *"Nest-building," or preparing for a baby, is a positive sign of pregnancy acceptance.*

perform—because *"We* are having a baby at our house."

Acquisition of Knowledge About Pregnancy, Childbirth, and Parenthood

A woman is more likely to acquire knowledge about pregnancy, childbirth, and childrearing than a man because, as part of her role-playing behavior during pregnancy, she is drawn into a world of talk about babies. It is helpful to most couples to attend education-for-childbirth or -parenthood classes during a pregnancy. Attending such classes helps the couple accept the pregnancy ("I must be going to have a baby, otherwise why would I be here?"), exposes the woman to role models of mothering, and provides information about pregnancy and child care to both parents. The content of such classes is discussed in Chapter 21.

The Expectant Father

The father has traditionally been the forgotten person in the childbearing process. There are still many men who are raised to think of childbearing as a woman's concern. Thus, a man may expect that during pregnancy and at childbirth he will be relegated few tasks other than to "boil water" (with no idea what he is to do with the water once it is boiled!). He suspects that such tasks are merely busywork to keep him out of the mainstream of events. Fortunately, it is beginning to be recognized that men have an important role in childbirth and must take many of the same steps during pregnancy that women take.

Accepting the Pregnancy

For the husband, accepting the pregnancy means not only accepting the certainty of the pregnancy and the reality of the child to come but also accepting his wife in her changed state. As noted before, it is helpful to forewarn the husband of the changes he can expect in his wife. Otherwise, he will interpret her mood swings, change of sexual interest, introversion, or narcissism as loss of interest in him.

A man needs to give his wife emotional support while she is working through accepting a pregnancy, and she should reciprocate when he is going through the process in his turn. A husband may feel jealous of the growing baby, who, although not yet physically apparent, seems to be taking up a great deal of his wife's time and thought. He may feel as if he has been left standing in the wings, waiting to be asked to take part in the event. To compensate for this feeling he may become absorbed in his work, in producing something concrete, feeling that he must demonstrate that he, too, is capable of creativeness. This preoccupation with work may limit the amount of time he spends with his wife, just when she needs his emotional support most.

Whether or not he is able to accept the pregnancy and the coming child depends on the same factors that are crucial in women, namely, his cultural background, past experience, and relationship with family members. If he was raised to believe that men do not show emotion, he may not be able to say easily, "I want this baby; I'm glad," when his wife tells him of the diagnosis. He may not be able to say, "It's great to feel it kick. That's a reassuring feeling." He may be unable to say, "I love you. Looking fat, unhappy with yourself, stomach full of baby or not, I love you."

However, even though he is inarticulate, he may be able to convey such emotions by a touch or a caress—a reason his presence is always desired at a prenatal visit and certainly in a labor and delivery room. His wife will know that his hand on hers is as meaningful an expression of emotion as the spoken word.

Many men experience physical symptoms known as a *couvade syndrome*, such as nausea, vomiting, and backache, the same way as or more intensely than their wives experience them. As their wives' abdomens begin to grow and they begin to take up more body space, men may perceive themselves as taking up more body space as if they, not their wives, were the ones who were pregnant. This change is most noticeable about the eighth month of pregnancy and extends as long as the twelfth postpartum month afterward (Fawcett, 1978). (See the Nursing Research Highlight below.)

Nursing Research Highlight

Which Type of Fathers with Couvade Symptoms Seek Help?

A retrospective review of records of 267 couples was conducted by two researchers (Lamb and Lipkin, 1982) to identify which expectant fathers with couvade symptoms seek help. Couvade symptoms refer to the somatic symptoms the expectant father experiences in response to his mate's pregnancy. Data analysis indicated that there was no relationship between the expectant father's age, socioeconomic position, education, occupation, or ethnicity and seeking care for his couvade symptoms. It was noted that men who sought care for couvade symptoms seemed to be less well educated and less experienced fathers than the men who did not seek care. Awareness of these characteristics should help care providers identify these men and prepare them for a period of change through anticipatory guidance.

Reference

Lamb, G. S., & Lipkin, M., Jr. Somatic symptoms of expectant fathers. *M.C.N.*, 7, 110.

These are healthy happenings and show the interest and the depth with which the man is accepting the pregnancy.

Reworking Developmental Tasks

Men have to do the same reworking of old values and forgotten developmental tasks as do women. Many men obtained their sex education from other boys and so come into manhood believing in many old wives' tales, sometimes not even being certain in what part of the woman's body a fetus grows. A man may believe that breast-feeding will make his wife's breasts pendulous and no longer attractive to him. He may believe that childbirth will stretch his wife's vagina so much that sexual relations will no longer be enjoyable. He needs factual education to update his knowledge.

He has to rethink his relationship with his father and to come to a better understanding of the kind of father he is going to be.

Preparing for Fatherhood

The man has role playing and grief work to do during pregnancy before he can be a father. He has to imagine himself as the father of a boy, the father of a girl. He has to cast aside a father-of-two image to accept a father-of-three image (difficult to do if he keeps concentrating on the cost of baby clothes or tuition or the loss of his wife's income during a maternity leave). If this is the first time he is to be a father, he has to relinquish the image of being "one of the boys" or a "carefree bachelor." These freedoms may not seem so precious if he examines them truthfully, but giving them up is difficult. A man does not seem thirsty until you tell him he cannot have any water; a man does not mind giving up a well-ordered, uncluttered life until a pregnancy compels it.

Concerns of Expectant Fathers

Fathers-to-be may not voice their concerns well because they feel that the things they are concerned about are things they should somehow already know and so should not ask about, or they do not want to compound their wives' anxieties by appearing anxious themselves.

In one study (McNall, 1976), when fathers were asked after delivery of their child what things concerned them most about pregnancy, labor, or delivery, they showed that the matters it is often assumed fathers will worry about (getting to the hospital on time, infant care, and finances, for example) were not great worries. They were more concerned with their wives' physical health during pregnancy, with having sufficient knowledge about what was happening during labor, and with their ability to help their wives during labor. These findings are summarized in Table 13-2.

Although this study utilized a small sample of fathers, it shows the significance to them of a statement such as "Your wife is doing fine" at the end of a prenatal visit. A question such as "Could I review what's going to happen in labor with you?" might be the most important question that the man is asked in 9 months.

The Expectant Family

Most parents today are aware that older children in a family need some warning that a new baby is on the way. However, knowing that such preparation is called for and being able to give it are two different matters. Many couples need suggestions from health care personnel as to how this task should be accomplished.

"How soon should I tell the older children?" is a common question. The answer depends on the ages and personalities of the older children and on the parents' ability to accept the pregnancy. School-age children should probably be told of the coming event when the parents know that it is definite. Parents are bound to discuss the pregnancy, and it is frightening for a child to walk into a room and hear the conversation suddenly halt. It is far more perplexing and worrisome to know that *something* is going on, *something* is happening, than to know *exactly* what is happening: that no matter how much you may dislike the prospect, a new baby is coming.

Preschoolers should be told at the time preparations for the coming infant begin. This is the point at which they become aware that something is happening. They need limits or boundaries put on the happening, so it does not loom so large in their minds that they cannot cope with it. "A baby is coming. Soon our family will be Mommy, Daddy, you, and a new baby. Four of us. That's what is happening."

It is important that parents prepare a preschool child for the initial helplessness of the infant. There is a tendency to say, "Soon you'll have a little brother or sister to play with." The child who is prepared by that explanation will be disappointed when his mother shows him a very small baby who does not respond at all to his favorite toys.

If a toddler is going to be moved from the crib to an adult bed, it is important that the parents make the change at least by the sixth month of

Table 13-2 Concerns of Expectant Fathers

Much Concern

Feelings about being able to help wife in labor.
Preference for a boy or girl.
Concerns about wife's physical health during pregnancy.
Feelings about pain or discomfort that wife experienced during delivery.
Feelings about not being with wife during delivery.
Concerns about having sufficient knowledge or being kept informed about what was going on during the period of labor.

Some Concern

Concerns about the amount of time wife will have to spend with the baby at home.
Feelings about change in wife's figure.
Feelings regarding mood changes in wife.
Concerns about sexual relations during pregnancy.
Feelings about being able to ease wife's discomforts.
Concerns about providing wife with emotional support and understanding.
Concerns about health of unborn child, possibility of mental and physical defects.
Concerns about being a father.
Concerns about discipline of child.
Temporary mood changes experienced by expectant fathers.
Changes in feelings toward wife.
Feelings about love and attention received from wife.
Concerns about environmental effects of war, crime, drugs, and pollution on child's health and development.
Feelings toward babies of friends and neighbors.

No Concern

Physical discomforts experienced by expectant fathers.
Concerns about loss of freedom and less spare time.
Feelings about attention that wife received from friends and neighbors.
Concerns about the kind of mother the wife would be.
Concerns about what to expect during pregnancy.
Concerns about being able to maintain social and leisure-time activities once the baby was born.
Concerns about medical care wife received during pregnancy.
Concerns about providing for child's needs without depriving himself and his wife of their needs.
Concerns about getting wife to hospital in time.
Concerns about holding, feeding, and taking care of newborn.
Concerns about role parents or parents-in-law played during wife's pregnancy.
Concerns about finances.
Difficulties deciding on name for child.

Source: McNall, L. K. (1976). Concerns of expectant fathers. In L. K. McNall & J. T. Galeener (Eds.). *Current practice in obstetric and gynecologic nursing* (vol. I). St. Louis: Mosby.

pregnancy. It is a positive experience to be moved from a crib to a regular bed because "you are a big girl (or a big boy) now." It is a crushing experience that plants seeds of jealousy to be moved because "the new baby needs your bed."

The same principle applies to starting a toddler in nursery school or kindergarten. He should be started, if possible, during the pregnancy, or about 6 months afterward, but not in the period shortly after the new baby's birth. He will feel unloved and rejected if he is sent off to school just when the new baby comes home. Later, he will feel proud that *he* is old enough to go to school while the baby has to stay home.

Children ask many questions about a new baby. Where is she growing? What is she doing? Is she eating now? How does she get out? How did she get in? If these questions are answered one by one during the process of childbearing, easily and naturally as they occur, childbearing becomes once and for all a positive, miraculous aspect of life. Examples of answers to the above questions are: "A baby grows in a special place in Mommy's tummy." (It is important that the preschooler knows it is a special space so he does not envisage the new baby smothering in the food his mother eats.) "A baby doesn't seem to do much in his special place. He just grows and gets ready to be born." "She doesn't have to eat while she's inside Mommy. A special cord gives her food through her belly button. See where your special cord fed you when you were inside me?" "I'll go to the hospital when it's time for the baby to come and the doctor will help the new baby be born. Babies come out of a special opening between the mother's legs." "Babies begin to grow as a seed so tiny you can't even see it. When two people love each other, the father puts his penis inside the place in mother's body where babies are born. A seed from Daddy's penis mixes with a seed from Mommy's body, and that makes a baby start to grow."

These are simple explanations but enough to answer the child's questions truthfully. If the first question is answered responsibly and openly, the child will feel free to ask a second. There is no reason to tell the child any more than is asked. Remember the boy who came home from school and asked, "Where did I come from?" His mother spent a half hour explaining the birds and the bees to him. When she was finished, the child said, "Thanks, I wondered. The kid who sits behind me said he comes from Cleveland."

If parents feel uncomfortable answering questions about childbirth, they might arrange for the child to see a dog or cat in the neighborhood giving birth to a litter. The child will be able to relate these observations to the birth of the new baby. Warn parents to stress, however, that although the puppies and kittens are going to be given away, the new brother or sister will be here to stay.

Children under school age need to be prepared for the separation from their mother that childbirth will entail. Overnight stays with grandparents or at a neighbor's are a good way to accustom both children and mother to being apart briefly.

Both preschool and school-age children need to be reassured periodically during pregnancy that a new baby is *adding* to the family and will not replace anyone in either parent's affection.

The Unwed Pregnant Woman

An increasing number of women are choosing to have children out of wedlock today and to raise their child as single parents. Along with this increase in out-of-wedlock pregnancies, acceptance of such pregnancies has grown—or if not acceptance, at least a recognition that they occur, that they occur frequently, and that health care personnel have the same obligation to meet the needs of these women during pregnancy and childbirth as they do to meet the needs of married women.

Accepting the Pregnancy

Pregnancy comes as a surprise to all women, and it should not necessarily be any more of a surprise to an unmarried woman than to a married one. Any woman who does not use a reliable contraceptive runs the risk of impregnation.

There are many reasons for an unmarried woman to want a baby. She may imagine that it will give her a hold on a boyfriend she does not want to lose (married women sometimes have children to prevent a divorce). She may be lonely and want someone to love or to love her (again, married women have children for the same reason). Some unmarried women deliberately plan to have a child (perhaps by artificial insemination) because they want children.

These are important concepts to keep in mind when mentioning the subject of adoption or abortion to unmarried women. They may have as great an attachment to the baby or as much of a desire to have the child as a married woman.

Facing a Pregnancy Alone

Pregnancy is a crisis situation. Almost automatically, the single woman has more difficulty adjusting to and accepting a pregnancy and a new child because she almost automatically has fewer support people around her than her married counterpart. She may feel acute loneliness during pregnancy. Acute loneliness brings with it depression, and a common symptom of depression is inability to function or make decisions.

Deciding whether to cook green beans or corn for dinner becomes a major problem for a depressed person. Whether to walk outside or not, whether the twinges she feels in her back are beginning labor contractions or just backache, whether she should phone a doctor or not—all are difficult decisions for someone depressed. The single woman needs thorough history taking at prenatal visits so loneliness and depression can be revealed and evaluated.

Some women begin a pregnancy married and then, through trauma (a car accident, a work injury) or illness, separation or divorce, lose their husbands during pregnancy. These women need to be evaluated very carefully, as their loneliness is likely to be extremely acute during this time, when they feel the need stronger than ever before for someone around them to care about them. A loss of this nature during pregnancy also has the potential for interfering with parent child bonding.

Becoming a Mother

Role playing and fantasy may be hard for the young unmarried woman. It may be impossible for her to cast aside the role of daughter in her grief work because she is still so obviously a daughter.

She needs support from the father of the child. If he can talk about the pregnancy, if it seems real to him, then it will seem more real to her. Emotional support from the unwed partner has special significance—it is given absolutely voluntarily. Remember this when debating whether or not an unmarried father should be allowed in the examining room or in the labor or delivery room. If he is there, it is because of emotional ties, not marriage ties. He can be an important person for the woman to have with her in a stress situation.

The major need of unwed women during pregnancy is additional talk time—time to voice their concerns and to begin to think through solutions. If this additional time and attention are not given, because of busy clinic or office schedules or nurses who think of patients as stereotypes rather than as persons with individual needs, the woman with few support people may reach the end of pregnancy with many of its tasks unresolved.

The Unwed Expectant Father

For generations, the unwed father has been dismissed as a person who had no interest in a pregnancy or further concern about the mother's or infant's health. Statements such as "It's always the woman who pays" or "Love 'em and leave 'em" reflect these societal values.

In the past, many men were forced into the role of disinterested observer, whether or not that was truly the role they wanted, for both financial reasons and an unwelcoming attitude of health care providers for them. If they were still in school or were married and had another family to support, the only way they could be free of the expense of doctors and hospital bills was to disappear quietly into the background as soon as the diagnosis became certain.

Today, with health care costs and childbearing costs usually being covered by third-party payers rather than individuals, unmarried fathers are free to have an emotional interest in the pregnancy. They should feel as welcome at prenatal visits or at the time of delivery as their married counterpart. Before, when most children were placed for adoption, it was easier to pretend that nothing had happened, to dismiss the pregnancy as none of their concern. Now, with most women choosing to keep their babies, the situation is less easy to ignore. Those fathers who planned on having children without ever marrying see having children but not marriage as their life style; although their last name is different from the woman's, they are very much fathers and have exactly the same involvement and commitment to the pregnancy and child as their married counterpart. Some men who want to have a child but not marriage arrange for a surrogate mother to have a child for them. They usually show more interest in the pregnancy than even the woman.

Accepting the Pregnancy

An unwed father may have a great deal of difficulty accepting the pregnancy if he has doubt whether the baby belongs to him. He tries to picture what the child will look like; fears that the baby will not look like him appear and dissolve the image. He tries to picture himself as a father, then realizes he will never play a father role to this child; the image disappears again. Because the unwed father can relate to some extent to being a father, however (and sometimes more easily than the woman can see herself as a mother), if the woman decides to have an abortion (and that is her decision, not one he needs to be consulted on) or the baby is born less than perfect, the man may be left with a deep sense of loss and may have few people around him for support who are even aware than he has lost anything.

Reworking Developmental Tasks

The unwed father has to rework developmental tasks the same as the married man—as difficult a problem for him as it is for his unmarried partner. It is hard to review his relationship with his parents if they insist that he handle this problem by ignoring it. It is equally hard to review a sense of identity because his identity is now so unclear. He is a father and yet he is not a father. People may tell him that the woman took advantage of him, that she became pregnant to trap him. He may begin to doubt his ability to evaluate people. He loses self-esteem. He feels in many ways a helpless, second-rate person in this situation.

Grief Work

The unmarried father has very real grief work to do during pregnancy, grieving not only for life the way it was before but possibly for the loss of his child's mother (angry with him because she is pregnant, told by her parents to stay away from him, so introverted by her own pregnancy work that she is unable to meet any of his needs) and for loss of the child (it will be placed for adoption, or the woman will keep it but he doubts that he will be allowed to visit).

Unmarried fathers need time during pregnancy to talk about how it feels to be a father when they have little outward connection with the pregnancy, yet have deep emotional ties with the woman or the growing fetus that are stronger than even they may realize.

Utilizing Nursing Process

Pregnancy is such a unique experience that nursing care during the period must be carefully planned, with nursing process used so that it is comprehensive and goal oriented.

Assessment

Much of assessment in psychological areas is gained through history taking. Be certain early in pregnancy that you establish an in-depth relationship with a woman so she sees your role as a person who is capable of counseling and helping her to problem solve. Otherwise she may interpret a question such as "How does it feel to be pregnant?" as merely a conversational opening and answer it only at a conversational level ("Fine, thank you").

Be certain to use your observational powers to gain insight into unverbalized psychological areas. A woman who says it is fun being pregnant, yet moves slowly as if she is extremely fatigued or has a lot of back pain, surely cannot be having all that much fun.

Analysis

The North American Nursing Diagnosis Association (NANDA) accepted no diagnosis specific for pregnancy. A number of diagnoses easily adapted to this period, however, are "Fear related to diagnosis of pregnancy," "Self-concept, alteration in, related to changing body image," or a well diagnosis of "Sound mental health related to acceptance of pregnancy." Be certain when establishing a goal with a woman or a couple during this time that it is realistic. A 9-month time span only permits limited change to occur.

Planning

Because pregnancy is a family event or at least affects all family members in some way, planning should include not only the woman but her support person (if she has one) and any other children

as well. For most women, telling their family about the pregnancy is a time of happiness; for others, this creates a stress period; for still others, determining how a new child will fit into the family is a major problem.

Implementation

A major amount of implementation time in relation to psychological aspects of pregnancy may be spent in helping the woman to locate a support person whose opinion she values and whom she can relate to during this unusual year in her life. In many instances, health care personnel serve in this role because the woman's sexual partner (her usual support person) is as overwhelmed or as uninformed by the event as she is.

Evaluation

Evaluation of how well a woman is adjusting to pregnancy should be ongoing during pregnancy. Ultimately whether women become good mothers and men become good fathers relates directly to how well they resolved the psychosocial adjustment to pregnancy.

Nursing Care Planning

Mary Kraft
23 years old
First prenatal visit: LMP 9 weeks ago

Assessment

Married 4 years; planned pregnancy after surgery for endometriosis 4 months ago. "Unbelievably happy" is reaction to pregnancy confirmation. Husband attends night school so "some nights are lonely." Family is out of town; she has few close friends, "One at work." Only black family in condominium and sometimes feels "out of place."

Last pregnancy ended in spontaneous abortion at 2½ months. She asked, "How do I know that won't happen again?" Appeared happy at discussing pregnancy; nervous at discussing lack of friends.

Analysis

Sound mental attitude (although limited support people) related to acceptance of pregnancy.

Locus of Decision Making. Shared.

Goal. Patient to continue good adaptation throughout pregnancy.

Criteria. Patient:

1. Establishes a satisfying relationship with at least one neighbor or new acquaintance outside work.
2. Is able to use health care personnel as support people until outside sources are established.
3. Has continued positive adaptation to pregnancy (difficult to maintain due to previous pregnancy loss).
4. Accepts and views herself as a mother by end of pregnancy.

Nursing Orders

1. Urge to communicate with family out of town by letter, telephone.
2. Urge to have husband accompany her for at least 1 prenatal visit.
3. Discuss ways to fill in free time to counteract feelings of loneliness.
4. Discuss ways of meeting more people in order to establish her own network of friends outside husband's acquaintances.
5. Assure that pregnancy is going well (as appropriate) at visits because of previous pregnancy loss to ensure parent-child bonding.
6. Schedule appointments so consistent health care personnel are present for support people.

Mary Kraft
23 years old
Gestation length: 20 weeks

Assessment

Attended prenatal visit with husband. States, "I have never been so happy. I'm past the point when I lost the last one; I feel safe now." Has bought crib and wallpaper for baby's room. Appears happy discussing pregnancy.

Analysis

Sound mental attitude related to good adaptation to pregnancy (nest building beginning).

Goal and Criteria. Unchanged.

Nursing Orders

1. Provide opportunities for discussion at visits so any problems that do arise can be aired.
2. Continue assurance that pregnancy is going well.
3. Continue to include husband in health care.

Questions for Review

Multiple Choice

1. Mrs. Jones is a woman you care for in a prenatal clinic. She tells you that her pregnancy was unplanned and unwanted. At what point in pregnancy does the average woman change her mind about an unwanted pregnancy?
   a. the third month
   b. quickening ✔
   c. lightening
   d. the seventh month

2. Psychological adjustment to pregnancy includes working through developmental tasks. Which statement below would lead you to believe Mrs. Jones is doing this?
   a. "My mother and I are closer than ever before."
   b. "I don't care what sex baby I have as long as it's healthy."
   c. "I'm thinking about everything I eat these days."
   d. "There are a lot of allergies in my husband's family."

3. Which situation during pregnancy is a happening that is most likely to be high-risk for interfering with mother-child bonding?
   a. Mrs. Jones's neighbor is planning an extensive vacation.
   b. Mrs. Jones's father has been very ill during the pregnancy.
   c. Mrs. Jones's husband was awarded a large year-end bonus.
   d. Mrs. Jones's sister recently had a baby.

4. You would like Mrs. Jones to increase the amount of milk she drinks daily. Early in pregnancy, which statement below would probably be most effective as a health teaching measure?
   ✔a. "Milk will strengthen your fingernails as well as be good for the baby."
   b. "The fetus needs milk in order to build strong bones and teeth."
   c. "Milk is a rich source of calcium that is important for fetal growth."
   d. "Your future baby will benefit from a high milk intake."

5. Most mothers fantasize about their newborn child. Which statement below would lead you to believe that Mrs. Jones is not accepting the pregnancy realistically?
   ✔a. "One thing I'm sure of: this child is going to college."
   b. "I want to have my baby at a birthing center."
   c. "I wish I wasn't so sick to my stomach in the morning."
   d. "I'm lucky. I like children and they like me."

6. Mrs. Jones's husband does not voice concerns at prenatal visits. Which of the following concerns might you guess is present (because the average man is highly concerned about it)?
   ✔a. whether the child will be a boy or girl
   b. the level of medical care his wife is receiving
   c. concern about loss of his free time
   d. if he will get his wife to the hospital on time

7. To prepare his son for the new baby, which statement below would you suggest Mr. Jones use?
   a. "The new baby will need your bed so we're buying you a new one."
   b. "It will be fun to have a sister or brother to share your toys."
   ✔c. "A new baby takes time to grow to be big enough to play."
   d. "You'll have to set a good example as a big brother."

Discussion

1. Some women are reluctant to discuss emotional responses to pregnancy in a health care setting. What environment would be most conducive to helping a woman discuss her feelings about pregnancy?
2. The emotional changes that a woman experiences during pregnancy can interfere with a marriage relationship. What changes would you want to be certain to include in anticipatory guidance at a prenatal visit?
3. Nest building is an outward sign that a woman is actively planning on having a child. What activities would you ask about to determine if a woman is engaged in this?

Suggested Readings

Caplan, G. (1959). *Concepts of Mental Health Consultations.* Washington, D.C.: U.S. Children's Bureau.

Cohn, S. D. (1982). Sexuality in pregnancy: A review of the literature. *Nursing Clinics of North America, 17,* 19.

Cranley, M. S. (1981). Development of a tool for the measurement of maternal attachment during pregnancy. *Nursing Research, 30,* 281.

Duvall, E. (1971). *Family development.* Philadelphia: Lippincott.

Fawcett, J. (1978). Body image and the pregnant couple. *M.C.N., 3,* 227.

Grace, J. T. (1984). Does a mother's knowledge of fetal gender affect attachment? *M.C.N., 9,* 42.

Josten, L. (1982). Contrast in prenatal preparation for mothering. *Maternal Child Nursing Journal, 11,* 65.

Keimar, R. (1984). Motherhood and mental illness: The role of the midwife in prevention and treatment. *Midwives Chronicle, 97,* 70.

Kempe, C. H., & Helfer, R. (Eds.) (1972). *Helping the battered child and his family.* Philadelphia: Lippincott.

Lee, G. (1982). Relationship of self-concept during late pregnancy to neonatal perception and parenting profile. *J.O.G.N. Nursing, 11,* 186.

May, K. A. (1982). Three phases of father involvement in pregnancy. *Nursing Research, 31,* 337.

McNall, L. K. (1976). Concerns of expectant fathers. In L. K. McNall and J. T. Galeener (Eds.), *Current Practice in Obstetric and Gynecologic Nursing* (Vol. I). St. Louis: Mosby.

O'Connell, M. L. (1983). Locus of control specific to pregnancy. *J.O.G.N. Nursing, 12,* 161.

Richardson, P. (1983). Women's perceptions of change in relationships shared with their husbands during pregnancy. *Maternal Child Nursing Journal, 12,* 1.

Richardson, P. (1983). Women's perceptions of change in relationships shared with children during pregnancy. *Maternal Child Nursing Journal, 12,* 75.

Rose, J. (1961). The prevention of mothering breakdown associated with physical abnormalities of the infant. In G. Caplan (Ed.), *Prevention of mental disorders in children.* New York: Basic Books.

Rubin, R. (1965). Cognitive style in pregnancy. *American Journal of Nursing, 65,* 97.

Rubin, R. (1976). Maternal tasks in pregnancy. *Journal of Advanced Nursing, 1,* 367.

Sherwen, L. N. (1981). Fantasies during the third trimester of pregnancy. *M.C.N., 6,* 398.

Stichler, J. F., et al. (1979). Pregnancy: A shared emotional experience. *M.C.N., 4,* 153.

Tilden, V. P. (1983). Perception of single vs partnered adult gravidas in the midtrimester. *J.O.G.N. Nursing, 12,* 40.

Valentine, D. (1982). Adaptation to pregnancy: Some implications for individual and family mental health. *Children Today, 11,* 16.

Webster-Stratton, C., & Kogan, K. (1980). Helping parents parent. *American Journal of Nursing, 80,* 240.

Wheeler, L. A. (1979). Sexuality during pregnancy and the postpartum. *Perinatal Press, 3,* 131.

14

Growth and Development of the Fetus

OBJECTIVES

Following mastery of the contents of this chapter, you should be able to

1. Describe the process of fertilization and implantation.
2. Describe the growth and development of the fetus by lunar months.
3. Describe the role of the accessory organs of fetal growth such as the placenta, amniotic membranes, amniotic fluid, and umbilical cord.
4. Analyze the changes in the woman that occur as a result of fetal requirements and growth.
5. Synthesize knowledge of growth and development of the fetus with nursing process to achieve quality maternal-newborn nursing care.

BEFORE THE nineteenth century, people had a variety of concepts and superstitions concerning the fetus. Medieval artists depicted the child in utero completely formed as a miniature man. Leonardo da Vinci, in his notebooks of 1510 to 1512, made several sketches of unborn infants, indicating that he believed the fetus was immobile and essentially a part of the mother, sharing her blood and internal organs. During the seventeenth and eighteenth centuries, two separate theories were explored. According to one theory, the baby was contained fully formed in the mother's ovaries, and when male cells were introduced, the baby expanded to birth size. The second theory suggested the child existed in the head of the sperm cell as a fully formed being, the uterus being used only as an incubator in which the child grew. It was not until 1759 that Kaspar Wolff proposed that both parents contribute equally to the structure of the baby.

Fertilization: The Beginning of Pregnancy

Fertilization is the union of the ovum and a spermatozoon. Other terms used to describe this phenomenon are *conception*, *impregnation*, or *fecundation*.

Following ovulation, as the ovum is extruded from the graafian follicle, it is surrounded by a ring of mucopolysaccharide fluid (the zona pellucida) and a circle of cells (the corona radiata). These structures increase the bulk of the ovum, facilitating its migration to the uterus, and probably also serve as a protection from injury (Figure 14-1). The ovum and surrounding cells are propelled into the near fallopian tube by currents initiated by the fimbriae, the fine hair-like structures that line the openings of the fallopian tubes. The ovum is propelled the length of the tube by peristaltic action of the tube and movement of the tube cilia. Fertilization must occur fairly quickly after release of the ovum because an ovum is capable of fertilization for only 24 hours (48 hours at the most) after ovulation. After that time, it atrophies and becomes nonfunctional.

Although only one ovum reaches maturity each month, a normal ejaculation of semen averages 2.5 ml of fluid that contains 60 to 100 million spermatozoa per milliliter, or an average of 200 million per ejaculation. To promote the possibility of a sperm reaching the ovum, there is a reduction in the viscosity of cervical mucus at ovulation, which makes it easier for spermatozoa to penetrate. Sperm transport is so efficient at this time that spermatozoa deposited in the vagina during sexual coitus generally reach the cervix of the uterus within 90 seconds after deposition and the outer end of a fallopian tube in 5 minutes (this is the reason douching is not an effective contraceptive measure unless it is done within 90 seconds of ejaculation). Spermatozoa move by means of their flagella (tails) and uterine contractions through the cervix, the body of the uterus, and into the fallopian tubes, where one spermatozoon meets the waiting ovum.

Fertilization sometimes occurs because spermatozoa are already present in the fallopian tube at the time of ovulation. The functional life of a spermatozoon is about 48 hours, so sexual coitus as far away as 48 hours before ovulation may result in fertilization. That makes the total critical fertilization time span in which fertilization may occur about 72 hours (48 hours preceding ovulation; 24 hours afterward).

Freshly ejaculated spermatozoa cannot fertilize ova; apparently some sort of change must occur in the head of the spermatozoon (capacitation) before it is capable of fertilization. This change takes place during passage through the uterus. The mechanism whereby spermatozoa are drawn toward an ovum is unknown. It may be a species-specific reaction similar to an antibody-antigen reaction.

Fertilization usually occurs in the outer third of a fallopian tube, the ampullar portion (Figure 14-1). All the spermatozoa that reach the ovum

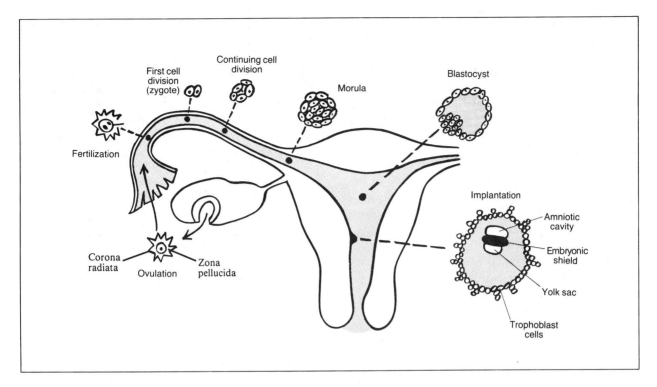

Figure 14-1 *Schema of ovulation, fertilization, and implantation. At the time of implantation, the blastocyst is already differentiated into germ layers (ectoderm, mesoderm, and entoderm). Cells at the periphery of the structure are trophoblast cells that mature into the placenta.*

cluster around its protective layer of corona cells. Hyaluronidase, a proteolytic enzyme, is apparently released by the spermatozoa. This enzyme acts to dissolve the layer of cells protecting the ovum. Once a spermatozoon penetrates the zona pellucida, a reaction sweeps throughout the entire zona that makes it difficult for other spermatozoa to penetrate it. Similarly, only one spermatozoon is able to penetrate the cell membrane of the ovum. After it has done so, the cell membrane apparently becomes impervious to other spermatozoa.

The chromosomal material of the ovum and spermatozoon fuse, and the resulting structure is called a *zygote*. Since the spermatozoon and ovum each carry 23 chromosomes (22 autosomes and 1 sex chromosome), the fertilized ovum has 46 chromosomes. Because it contains some hereditary material from the mother and some from the father, it is exactly like neither of them and also uniquely like no other person.

If an X-carrying spermatozoon enters the ovum, the resulting child will have two X chromosomes and will be female (XX). If a Y-carrying spermatozoon fertilizes the ovum, the resulting child will have an X and a Y chromosome and will be male (XY).

Fertilization is not a certain occurrence be-cause it depends on at least three separate factors being present: maturation of both sperm and ovum, ability of the sperm to reach the ovum, and ability of the sperm to penetrate the zona pellucida and cell membrane and achieve fertilization.

Out of the fertilized ovum (the zygote) will form not only the future child but also the accessory structures needed to support the fetus during intrauterine life: the placenta, the fetal membranes, the amniotic fluid, and the umbilical cord. These accessory structures plus the zygote are referred to as the *conceptus*.

Implantation

Once fertilization is complete, the zygote migrates toward the body of the uterus, aided by the currents initiated by the muscular contractions of the fallopian tubes. It takes 3 or 4 days for the zygote to reach the body of the uterus. During this time, mitotic cell division, or *cleavage*, begins at a rapid rate. The first cleavage occurs at about 24 hours; cleavage divisions continue to occur at a rate of one about every 22 hours. By the time the zygote reaches the body of the uterus, it consists of 16 to 50 cells. At this stage, because of its bumpy outward appearance, it is termed a *morula* (from the Latin word *morus*, meaning "mulberry").

The morula continues to multiply as it floats free in the uterine cavity for 3 or 4 more days. Large cells tend to mass at the periphery of the ball, leaving a fluid space surrounding an inner cell mass at one of the poles. At this stage, the structure is termed a *blastocyst.* The cells in the outer ring are known as *trophoblast cells.* They are the part of the structure that will later form the placenta and membranes. The inner cell mass (*embroblast cells*) is the portion of the structure that will later form the embryo.

After the third or fourth day of free floating (about 8 days from ovulation), the last residues of the corona and zona pellucida are shed by the growing structure. The blastocyst brushes against the rich uterine endometrium (in the second [secretory] phase of the menstrual cycle), a process termed *apposition;* it then attaches to the surface of the endometrium (*adhesion*) and settles down into its soft folds (*invasion*). Stages up to this point are depicted in Figure 14-1.

The blastocyst is able to invade endometrium because, as the trophoblast cells on the outside of the blastocyst touch the endometrium, they produce proteolytic enzymes that dissolve the tissue they touch. This action not only allows the structure to burrow deeply into the endometrium but to receive some basic nourishment of glycogen and mucoprotein from the endometrial glands. As invasion continues, the structure establishes an effective communication network with the blood system of the endometrium. The touching or im-

plantation point is usually high in the uterus and on the posterior surface. If the point of implantation is low in the uterus, the growing placenta may occlude the cervix and make delivery of the child at term difficult (*placenta previa*).

Implantation is an important step in pregnancy; as many as 50 percent of zygotes never achieve it. In these instances, a pregnancy ends as early as 8 to 10 days after conception, often before the woman is even aware it had begun. Occasionally, a small amount of vaginal spotting appears with implantation, since capillaries are ruptured by the implanting trophoblast cells. A woman who normally has particularly scant menstrual flows may mistake implantation bleeding for her menstrual period, and the predicted date of delivery of her baby (based on the time of her last menstrual period) will then be calculated one month late.

The Decidua

When conception has occurred, the corpus luteum in the ovary continues to function rather than to atrophy under the influence of human chorionic gonadotropin hormone secreted by the trophoblast cells. Thus the endometrium of the uterus, instead of sloughing off as in a normal menstrual cycle, continues to grow in thickness and vascularity. The endometrium is now termed *decidua* (the Latin word for "falling off"), since it will be discarded following the birth of the child. The decidua has three separate areas: the *decidua basalis,* or the part of the endometrium lying di-

Figure 14-2 *Division of uterine decidua into three areas.*

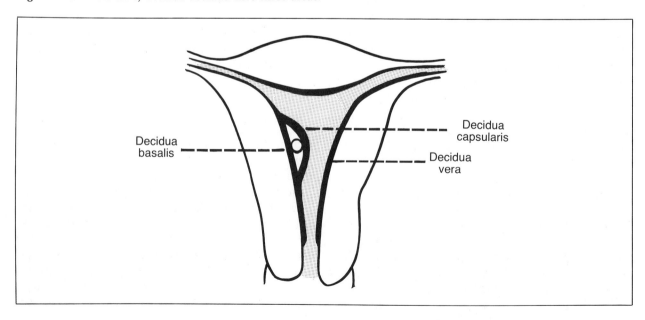

Decidua basalis

Decidua capsularis

Decidua vera

rectly under the embryo (or the portion where the trophoblast cells are establishing communication with maternal blood vessels); the *decidua capsularis*, or the portion of the endometrium that stretches or encapsulates the surface of the trophoblast; and the *decidua vera*, or the remaining portion of the uterine lining (Figure 14-2).

As the zygote grows during pregnancy, it pushes the decidua capsularis before it like a blanket. Eventually, enlargement brings the decidua capsularis into contact with the opposite uterine wall. There, the decidua capsularis fuses with the endometrium of the opposite wall. This is why, at delivery, the entire inner surface of the uterus not just that of the implantation site is stripped away and the organ becomes highly susceptible to hemorrhage and infection.

Chorionic Villi

Once implantation is achieved, the trophoblastic layer of cells of the blastocyst begins to mature rapidly. As early as the eleventh or twelfth day, miniature villi, or probing "fingers," reach out from the single layer of cells into the uterine endometrium; these are termed *chorionic villi*. At term, nearly 200 such villi will have formed.

Chorionic villi have a central core of loose connective tissue surrounded by a double layer of trophoblast cells. The central core of connective tissue contains fetal capillaries. The outer of the two covering layers is termed the *syncytiotrophoblast*, or the *syncytial layer*. This layer of cells is instrumental in the production of various placental hormones, such as human chorionic gonadotropin, somatomammotropin (human placental lactogen), estrogen, and progesterone. The inner layer, known as the *cytotrophoblast* or *Langhans' layer*, is present as early as 12 weeks of gestation, appears to be functional early in pregnancy, but then disappears at about the fourth or fifth month. Apparently this layer protects the growing embryo and fetus from certain infectious organisms such as the spirochetes of syphilis. This is why syphilis is considered to have high potential for fetal damage late in pregnancy, when Langhans' cells are no longer functioning. Unfortunately, Langhans' cells appear to offer little protection against viral invasion.

Placenta Formation

The word *placenta* is Latin for "pancake," which is descriptive of its size and appearance at term.

The placenta arises out of trophoblast tissue and thus is fetal in origin. It serves as the fetal lungs, kidneys, and gastrointestinal tract and as a separate endocrine organ throughout pregnancy. It offers some protection to the fetus against invading microorganisms or chemical substances. Its growth is as phenomenal as that of the fetus, from a few identifiable cells at the beginning to an organ 15 to 20 cm in diameter and 2 to 3 cm in depth at term. It covers about half the surface of the internal uterus.

Circulation

As early as the twelfth day of pregnancy, maternal blood begins to collect in spaces (intervillous spaces) of the uterine endometrium surrounding the chorionic villi. By the third week, oxygen and other nutrients, such as glucose, amino acids, fatty acids, minerals, and vitamins and water, diffuse from the maternal blood through the cell layers of the chorionic villi to the villi capillaries. From there, the nutrients are transported back to the developing embryo.

For practical purposes, there is no direct exchange of blood between the embryo and the mother during pregnancy; the exchange is carried out only by selective osmosis. The osmosis is so effective that all but a few substances cross the placenta into fetal circulation. It is important that a woman take no drugs (including caffeine, alcohol, and nicotine) other than those prescribed for her during pregnancy because almost all drugs cross into the fetal circulation.

Substances cross the placenta by four separate processes: diffusion, facilitated diffusion, active transport, and pinocytosis. These are much the same processes that allow substances to pass from the gastrointestinal tract into the bloodstream in adults. They are summarized in Table 14-1.

As the number of chorionic villi increases, the villi form a network of communication with the maternal blood that becomes more and more complex. A basal plate of support tissue forms along the surface of the endometrium and a chorionic plate forms along the fetal side of the placenta to give structure to the intervillous spaces, which grow larger and larger and become separated by a series of partitions, or septa. On a mature placenta there are as many as 30 separate segments, called *cotyledons*. These compartments make the maternal side of the placenta at term look rough and uneven.

Placental circulation is depicted in Figure 14-3. Maternal blood reaches the intervillous spaces through coiled or spiral endometrial uterine ar-

Table 14-1 Mechanisms by which Nutrients Cross the Placenta

Mechanism	Description
Diffusion	When there is a greater concentration of a substance on one side of a semipermeable membrane than on the other, substances of correct molecular weight cross the membrane from the area of higher concentration to the area of lower concentration. Oxygen and carbon dioxide cross the placenta by simple diffusion.
Facilitated diffusion	In order that the fetus receives enough concentrations of necessary growth substances, some substances cross the placenta more rapidly or more easily than would occur if only simple diffusion were operating. Glucose is an example of a substance that crosses by this process. Fetal plasma maintains a glucose level about 60 to 70 percent that of the maternal concentration.
Active transport	Essential amino acids and water-soluble vitamins cross the placenta against the pressure gradient or from an area of lower molecular concentration to an area of greater molecular concentration. Amino acid concentrations in the fetal plasma are twice what they are in the mother, a situation that must occur to provide building substances for active fetal growth.
Pinocytosis	Pinocytosis is absorption by the cellular membrane of intact microdroplets of plasma and dissolved substances. Globulins, lipoproteins, phospholipids, and other molecular structures that are too large for diffusion and that cannot participate in active transport cross in this manner. Unfortunately, viruses that then infect the fetus may also cross in this manner.

teries, which open directly onto the floor of the intervillous spaces. About 100 maternal arteries supply the mature placenta. In order to provide enough blood for exchange, the rate of uteroplacental blood flow in pregnancy increases from about 50 ml per minute at 10 weeks to 500 to 600 ml per minute at term. No additional maternal arteries appear to be added after the first 3 months of pregnancy; to accommodate the increased blood flow, the arteries increase in size. Systemically, the mother's heart rate, total cardiac output, and blood volume all increase to supply the placenta.

In the intervillous spaces, maternal blood jets from the arteries in streams or spurts. It is propelled from compartment to compartment by the currents initiated and not through definite anatomic channels as it is conducted from the arteries to spaces around the villi. Thus, its movement appears to be controlled physiologically rather than anatomically. As the blood circulates around the villi, and nutrients osmose from it into the villi, the blood gradually loses its momentum and is crowded toward the placental floor. From there, it enters the orifices of maternal veins and is returned to the maternal circulation. Braxton Hicks' contractions, or the barely noticeable uterine contractions that are present from about the twelfth week of pregnancy, aid in maintaining pressure in the intervillous spaces by closing off the uterine veins momentarily with each contraction: this aids nutrient exchange.

Uterine perfusion is most efficient when the mother lies on her left side. This position lifts the uterus away from the inferior vena cava and prevents blood from being trapped in the vena cava, unable to circulate. Placental circulation can be sharply reduced if the mother lies on her back; in this position, maternal blood pressure decreases as surely as would occur with sudden hemorrhage or the administration of a hypotensive drug.

At term, the placental circulatory network is so extensive that a placenta has increased in weight to 400 to 600 gm (1 pound) and is one-sixth of the weight of the baby. If a placenta is smaller than this, circulation to the fetus may have been inadequate. Interestingly, a placenta greater in size may also indicate that circulation to the fetus was threatened. It means the placenta was forced to spread out in an unusual formation in order to organize a sufficient blood supply. A fetus who develops syphilis during pregnancy usually develops a large placenta (for unknown reasons). A fetus of a woman with diabetes may develop a larger-than-usual placenta, probably from excess fluid collected between cells.

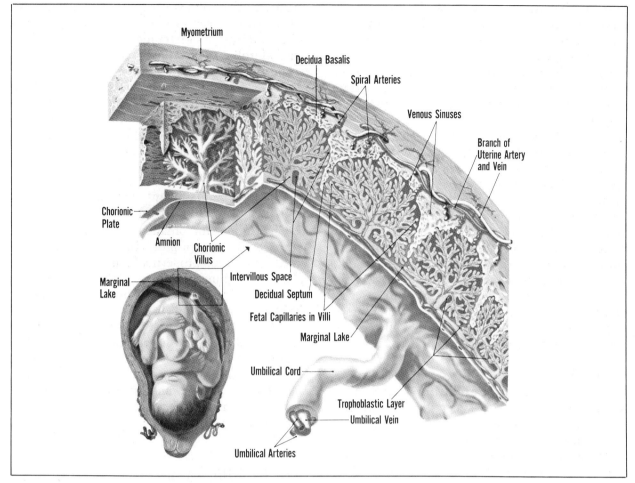

Figure 14-3 *Schema of placental circulation. From Clinical education aid, No. 2, Ross Laboratories, Columbus, Ohio, 1960.*

Endocrine Function

Aside from serving as the source of oxygen and nutrients for the fetus, the placenta develops into a separate, very important hormone-producing organ. These hormones are produced by the syncytial layer of the trophoblast villi.

Human Chorionic Gonadotropin

The first hormone to be produced by the placenta is human chorionic gonadotropin (HCG). It was previously assumed that this hormone was produced by the inner layer of cells, or the Langhans' layer, because their courses closely approximate each other. The presence of HCG can be demonstrated in maternal blood serum as early as before the first missed menstrual period (on the sixth or seventh day after implantation). It reaches a peak level at about the sixtieth day of pregnancy and then recedes so by the twentieth week of pregnancy it is greatly diminished in amount. By the end of pregnancy, levels are barely detectable.

The purpose of HCG is to act as a fail-safe measure to ensure that the corpus luteum of the ovary continues to produce progesterone and estrogen. If the corpus luteum should fail, falling levels of progesterone would cause endometrial sloughing with loss of the pregnancy followed by a rise of pituitary gonadotropins to induce a new menstrual cycle.

Kangaroos and opossums are examples of an animal species (marsupials) that apparently does not have a pregnancy-prolonging factor such as chorionic gonadotropin. This is the reason that pregnancy in one of these animals ends while the fetus is still grossly immature; the offspring must complete maturation by being sheltered in the mother's abdominal pouch, where they are at greater risk than in utero. HCG may also play a role in suppressing the maternal immunologic response so placental invasion is not rejected. Because the structure of HCG is similar to luteinizing hormone of the pituitary gland, it exerts an effect on the male fetal testes to begin to produce testosterone. Testosterone's presence causes the maturation of the male reproductive tract, rather than the female reproductive tract in the fetus.

At about the second month of pregnancy in the

human, the syncytial cells of the developing placenta begin to produce progesterone so the corpus luteum is no longer needed. At this time, production of HCG decreases.

Chorionic gonadotropin is an important hormone in pregnancy, not only because its action guarantees the production of progesterone by the corpus luteum but also because its presence in the mother's blood and urine serves as the basis for pregnancy testing. By the seventh day of pregnancy it rises to a level great enough to be detected on blood serum analysis. It is present in urine in significant titer for these purposes from about a week after the first missed menstrual period (the thirty-fifth day) through the one-hundredth day of pregnancy. Before or after these times, a false-negative result from a pregnancy test may be reported. The mother's urine will be completely negative for HCG within 1 to 2 weeks after delivery. Testing for HCG hormone following delivery can be used as proof that all the placental tissue has been delivered.

Estrogen

Estrogen (primarily estriol) is produced as a second product of the syncytial cells of the placenta. Estrogen contributes to the mother's mammary gland development in preparation for lactation and stimulates the uterus to grow to accommodate the developing fetus. It is excreted by the mother in urine as estriol. Assessing the amount of estriol excreted serves as a test of fetal welfare because the immediate precursor of estrogen synthesis by the placenta is a compound produced by the fetal adrenal gland and liver. When a fetus is in difficulty, the production of this fetal compound is decreased, estrogen cannot be synthesized, and estriol excretion in maternal urine will then be decreased. After the thirty-second week of pregnancy, a level below 12 mg suggests that the fetus is in difficulty.

Progesterone

Estrogen is often referred to as the "hormone of women"; progesterone as the "hormone of mothers." Its presence is indisputably necessary to maintain the endometrial lining of the uterus during pregnancy. Progesterone is increased as early as the fourth week of pregnancy due to the continuation of the corpus luteum. When placental synthesis begins during the third month of pregnancy, this causes the level to rise progressively during the remainder of the pregnancy. A second function of this hormone appears to be induction of quiescence of the uterine musculature during pregnancy, which prevents premature labor. Such quiescence is probably produced by a

change in electrolytes (notably potassium and calcium), which decreases the contraction potential of the uterus. Progesterone is synthesized from cholesterol; it is excreted in the maternal urine as pregnanediol. Assay of this compound can be used as a measure of placental, and therefore indirectly of fetal, well-being. Because the analysis of the compound is more difficult than that of estrogen, however, it is used infrequently. A normal urine level of pregnanediol is 180 to 560 mg per 24 hours.

Chorionic Somatomammotropin (Human Placental Lactogen)

Chorionic somatomammotropin is a hormone with both growth-promoting and lactogenic (milk-producing) properties. It is produced by the placenta beginning as early as the sixth week of pregnancy. It then increases in amount to a peak level at term. It can be assayed in both maternal blood and urine. It functions to promote mammary gland (breast) growth in preparation for lactation in the mother (accounting for its name). It also serves the important role of regulating maternal glucose, protein, and fat levels so that adequate amounts of these are always available to the fetus.

The Umbilical Cord

As chorionic villi form and begin to function, initiating circulatory communication with the maternal blood pools, they join together into larger and larger veins and arteries until they become the umbilical cord. Also called the *funis* (Latin for "cord"), the umbilical cord is about 53 cm (21 inches) in length at term. It is about 2 cm (¾ inch) in thickness. It contains one vein (carrying blood from the placental villi to the fetus) and two arteries (carrying blood from the fetus back to the placental villi). It arises from the center of the fetal surface of the placenta. The remnant of the yolk sac (see page 266) may be found in the fetal end of the cord as a white fibrous streak at term. The bulk of the cord is a gelatinous mucopolysaccharide termed *Wharton's jelly*, which gives the cord body and prevents pressure on the vein and arteries. The outer surface is covered with amniotic membrane. The function of the cord is to transport oxygen and nutrients to the fetus from the placenta and to return waste products from the fetus to the placenta.

The number of veins and arteries in the cord is always assessed at birth because about 1 percent of all infants are born with a cord that contains only a single artery. About 15 percent of these

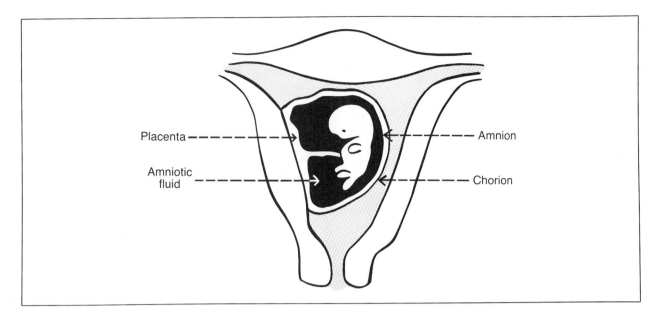

Figure 14-4 *Membranes, with embryo lying within amniotic sac.*

infants are found to have accompanying congenital anomalies, particularly kidney and heart anomalies (Barnett, 1977).

The rate of blood flow through an umbilical cord is rapid (350 ml per minute at term). This rapid flow makes it unlikely that a cord will twist or knot enough to interfere with the fetal oxygen supply. In 20 percent of all deliveries, a loose loop of cord is found around the fetal neck. If this loop of cord is removed before the shoulders are extruded, so that there is no traction on it, it is not constricted, and nutrition supply to the fetus remains unimpaired. Smooth muscle is abundant in the arteries of the cord; the constriction of these circular muscles after birth contributes to the hemostasis and helps prevent hemorrhage of the newborn through the cord. Since the umbilical cord contains no nerve supply, it can be cut at birth without discomfort to the child or mother.

The Membranes and Amniotic Fluid

The chorionic villi on the medial surface of the trophoblast (those that are not involved in implantation because they do not touch the endometrium) gradually thin and leave the medial surface of the structure smooth (the *chorion laeve,* or smooth chorion). The smooth chorion eventually becomes the *chorionic membrane,* the outermost fetal membrane. Once it smooths, its purpose for the remainder of pregnancy is to offer support to the sac that contains the amniotic fluid. A second membrane lining the chorionic membrane, the

amniotic membrane or amnion, forms beneath the chorion (Figure 14-4). Early in pregnancy, these membranes become so adherent that they seem as one at term. They cover the fetal surface of the placenta and give it its typical shiny appearance. Like the umbilical cord, they have no nerve supply. Thus, when they rupture at term, neither mother nor child experiences any sensation.

The purpose of the amnion membrane is not only to offer support to amniotic fluid but to actually produce the fluid. It also produces a phospholipid that initiates the formation of prostaglandins. Prostaglandins are proven to cause uterine contractions and may be the "trigger" that initiates labor.

Within the amnion and chorionic membrane forms the clear albuminous fluid (*liquor amnii,* or amniotic fluid), in which the embryo (later the fetus) floats. This fluid is constantly being newly formed and reabsorbed, so it is never stagnant. It is apparently produced from the cells of the amniotic membrane although a portion may be formed from a transexudate from maternal serum. It is formed at a rate of about 500 ml per 24 hours. At term, the average amount of fluid present is 1,000 ml. The fetus swallows the fluid rapidly, and it is absorbed across the fetal intestine into the fetal bloodstream; from there the umbilical arteries exchange it across the placenta. Some fluid is probably absorbed in direct contact with the fetal surface of the placenta. If for any reason the fetus is unable to swallow (esophageal atresia or anencephaly are the two most common reasons), *hydramnios,* or excessive amniotic fluid (over 2,000 ml), will result. Early in fetal life, as soon as the fetal kidneys become active, fetal urine adds to the quantity of the amniotic fluid. A disturbance of kidney function may cause *oligo-hydramnios*, or a reduction in the amount of amniotic fluid (under 300 ml).

Amniotic fluid is an important protective mechanism for the fetus. It shields against pressure or a blow to the mother's abdomen, and it protects the fetus from changes in temperature, since liquid changes temperature more slowly than air. Because it allows the fetus freedom to move, it probably aids muscular development.

Even if the membrane ruptures prior to birth and the bulk of the amniotic fluid is lost, some will always surround the fetus in utero because of the constant formation of amniotic fluid. Amniotic fluid is slightly alkaline, with a pH of about 7.2. This might be important at the time of rupture, in differentiating it from urine, which is acidic (pH 5.0 to 5.5). The specific gravity of amniotic fluid is only slightly heavier than that of water—1.005 to 1.025.

Origin and Development of Organ Systems

The fertilized ovum is a zygote until implantation. From implantation to the end of the fifth to eighth week, it is an *embryo*. From the fifth to eighth week until the end of pregnancy, it is a *fetus*. The terms used to describe fetal growth are summarized in Table 14-2.

From the beginning, development of the fetus proceeds in a cephalocaudal (head to tail) direction; head development occurs first, then development of middle and finally lower body parts. A baby is born with cephalocaudal development still incomplete—that is, the newborn has the ability to lift up his head but not to walk, to control sucking and swallowing functions but not urinary or bowel function.

Fetal development follows the principle of *induction*, or of one tissue transmitting a stimulus to an adjoining tissue to begin development. If at any point the stimulus is inadequate for some reason, the adjoining tissue cannot respond and so growth or development of body parts will not proceed beyond that point. Thalidomide, a drug that caused infants to be born without arms or legs if taken by the mother during early pregnancy, is an example of a substance that interferes with induction. In some instances, interference with induction leads to the double formation of structures, such as double ureters.

Table 14-2 Terms Used to Denote Fetal Growth

Common Name	Time Period
Ovum	From ovulation to fertilization
Zygote	From fertilization to implantation
Embryo	From implantation to 5 to 8 weeks
Fetus	From 5 to 8 weeks until term
Conceptus	Developing embryo or fetus and placental structures throughout pregnancy
Low-birth-weight infant (previously termed a *premature infant*)	Infant born after the twentieth week but before the thirty-seventh week of intrauterine growth
Abortion	Loss of conception before twentieth week of pregnancy

Primary Germ Layers

At the time of implantation, the blastocyst has already differentiated to a point at which two separate cavities appear in the inner structure: a large one, the *amniotic cavity*, and a smaller one, the *yolk sac*. These are illustrated in Figure 14-1.

The walls of the amniotic cavity are lined with the cells of a primary germ layer, the *ectoderm*; the cavity is filled with amniotic fluid. The yolk sac is lined by another distinctive layer of cells, the *entoderm*. In chicks the yolk sac serves as a supply of nourishment for the embryo throughout its development. In human reproduction, the yolk sac appears to supply nourishment only until implantation. It then provides a source of red blood cells until the embryo's hematopoietic system is mature enough to perform this function (at about the third month of intrauterine life). In addition it forms a portion of the epithelium of the gastrointestinal tract and the ovaries and testes. It atrophies after the hematopoietic function is complete and remains only as a thin white streak discernable in the cord at birth.

Between the amniotic cavity and the yolk sac forms a third layer of primary cells, the *mesoderm*. The embryo will begin to develop at the

Table 14-3 Origin of Body Systems by Tissue Layer

Tissue Layer	Body Portions Formed
Mesoderm	Supporting structures of the body (connective tissue, bones, cartilage, muscle, and tendons), the upper portion of the urinary system (the kidneys and ureters), the reproductive system, the heart, the circulatory system, and the blood cells.
Entoderm	Lining of the gastrointestinal tract, the respiratory tract, the tonsils, the parathyroid, thyroid, and thymus glands, and the lower urinary system (bladder and urethra).
Ectoderm	The nervous system, the skin, hair, and nails, the sense organs, and the mucous membranes of the anus and the mouth.

point where these three cell layers meet: the *embryonic shield.*

Each germ layer of primary tissue develops into distinctive body systems, shown in Table 14-3. It is helpful to know which structures rise from each germ layer because coexisting congenital defects found in newborns usually arise from the same layer. For example, a tracheoesophageal fistula (both organs arising from the entoderm) is a common birth anomaly. Heart and kidney defects (both organs arising from the mesoderm) are often found together. It is rare, however, to see a newborn with a heart malformation (arises from the mesoderm) and a lower urinary malformation (bladder and urethra arise from the entoderm). Rubella is always serious in pregnancy because it is capable of affecting all the germ layers and thereby causing congenital anomalies in a myriad of body systems, irrespective of their origin.

Knowing the origins of body structures helps you to understand why certain screening procedures are ordered for newborns with congenital malformations. A kidney x-ray examination, for example, may be ordered for a child born with a heart defect. A child with a malformation of the urinary tract is often investigated for reproductive abnormalities as well.

Major Body Systems

All organ systems are complete, at least in a rudimentary form, at 8 weeks' gestation (the end of the embryonic period). It is during this early time of organogenesis (organ formation) that the growing structure is most susceptible to invasion by teratogens—in other words, any factor that adversely affects the fertilized ovum, embryo, or fetus.

Cardiovascular System

The cardiovascular system is one of the first systems to become functional in intrauterine life. The circulatory system progresses from simple blood cells joined to the walls of the yolk sac, to a network of blood vessels, to a single heart tube, which begins to form as early as the sixteenth day of life and to beat as early as the twenty-fourth day. The heart beat is governed by the sinoatrial (SA) node and spreads to the ventricles by the atrioventricular (AV) node, the same as in adults. The septum that divides the heart into chambers develops during the sixth or seventh week, and the heart valves begin to develop in the seventh week. Using a Doppler system, the heart beat may be heard as early as the tenth week of pregnancy. An electrocardiogram may be recorded on a fetus as early as the eleventh week, although the accuracy of such ECGs is in doubt until about the twentieth week of pregnancy.

The heart rate of a fetus is affected by fetal oxygen level, body activity, and circulating blood volume, as in adults. After the twenty-eighth week of pregnancy, the sympathetic nervous system has matured to such an extent that the heart rate will begin to show a baseline variability, or a baseline variation, of about 5 beats per minute on a fetal monitor.

Fetal Circulation. As early as the third week of intrauterine life, fetal blood has begun to accept nutrients by the chorionic villi from the maternal circulation. Fetal circulation (Figure 14-5) differs from extrauterine circulation in several respects. During intrauterine life the fetus derives oxygen not from oxygen exchange in the lungs but at the placenta. The excretion of carbon dioxide also occurs at the placenta. Blood does enter lung vessels while the child is in utero, but this blood flow is to supply the cells of the lungs themselves, not for oxygenation. The major difference, then, between circulation in utero and after birth is that in the fetus the blood largely bypasses the lungs and primarily serves to carry nutrients to and from the placenta.

Blood arriving from the placenta (with a high oxygen content) enters the fetus through the umbilical vein (called a vein even though it carries oxygenated blood, because the direction of the blood is toward the fetal heart) and into an acces-

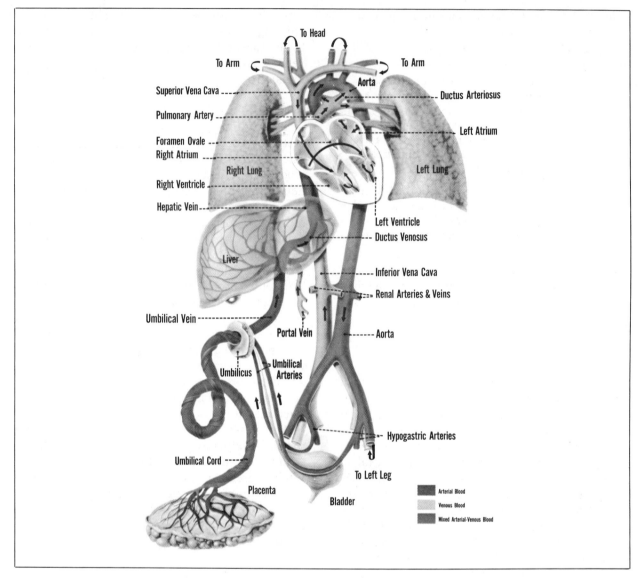

Figure 14-5 *Fetal circulation. From Clinical education aid, No. 1, Ross Laboratories, Columbus, Ohio, 1963.*

sory vein, the *ductus venosus.* The ductus venosus supplies blood to the fetal liver and empties into the inferior vena cava, through which blood flows to the right side of the heart. As the blood enters the right atrium, the bulk of it is shunted into the left atrium through an opening in the atrial septum, the *foramen ovale.* From the left atrium it follows the course of normal circulation into the left ventricle and into the aorta.

Some of the blood that enters the right atrium leaves it by the normal circulatory route, that is, through the tricuspid valve into the right ventricle. This blood leaves the right ventricle through the pulmonary artery in the normal manner. A small portion of this blood flow services the lung tissue; the larger portion is shunted away from the lungs, through an additional vessel, the *ductus arteriosus,* directly into the aorta.

Two umbilical arteries (called arteries because they carry blood away from the fetal heart, even though they are now transporting unoxygenated blood) transport most of the blood flow from the descending aorta back through the umbilical cord to the placental villi, where new oxygen exchange takes place.

The shunts of fetal circulation are necessary to supply the most important organs of the fetus: the brain, liver, heart, and kidneys. The ductus venosus supplies the liver and the foremen ovale allows oxygenated blood to move directly to the left side of the heart and the aorta, the vessel from which the arteries arise that supply the brain, heart, and kidneys.

The fetus exists at a blood oxygen saturation level about 80 percent that of a newborn. The rapid rate of the fetal heartbeat during pregnancy

(120 to 160 beats per minute) is necessary to supply oxygen to cells when blood cells are never fully saturated. Fortunately, fetal hemoglobin has a higher dissociation level than adult hemoglobin so that, again, the movement and release of oxygen are facilitated. Despite this low blood oxygen level, carbon dioxide does not accumulate in the fetal system because of its rapid diffusion into maternal blood across a favorable pressure gradient.

Fetal Hemoglobin. Fetal hemoglobin differs from adult hemoglobin in several ways. As mentioned, it has greater oxygen affinity, which makes it more efficient. It has a different composition (two alpha and two gamma chains as compared with two alpha and two beta chains of adult hemoglobin). It is more concentrated (at birth, hemoglobin is about 17.1 gm per 100 ml compared to an adult normal of 11 gm per 100 ml, and hematocrit is about 53 percent compared to an adult normal of 45 percent). These same changes occur in people who live at high altitudes, where the atmosphere has a reduced oxygen content. The change from fetal to adult hemoglobin begins before birth and accelerates following birth. The major blood dyscrasias such as sickle cell anemia are defects of the beta hemoglobin chain, so clinical symptoms do not become apparent until the bulk of fetal hemoglobin has matured to adult hemoglobin composition at about 6 months of age.

Respiratory System

At the third week of life, the respiratory and digestive tracts exist as a single tube. This is the reason that tracheoesophageal fistulas are a common newborn anomaly. By the end of the fourth week, a septum begins to divide the two systems. At the same time, lung buds appear on the trachea.

Until the seventh week of life the diaphragm does not completely divide the thoracic cavity from the abdomen. During the sixth week of life, lung buds may extend down into the abdomen, reentering the chest only as the chest's longitudinal dimension increases and the diaphragm becomes complete (the end of the seventh week). If the diaphragm fails to close completely, the stomach, spleen, liver, or intestines may enter the thoracic cavity. The child will then be born with a diaphragmatic hernia, compromising the lungs and perhaps displacing the heart.

Alveoli begin to form between the twenty-fourth and twenty-eighth weeks. The alveoli are supplied by capillaries as they develop. Both capillaries and alveoli must be developed before gas exchange can occur in the fetal lungs. This is why 28 weeks is a practical lower limit of prematurity, or the earliest gestation age at which a fetus can survive in an extrauterine environment without a great deal of assistance.

As early as during the first three months of pregnancy, the fetus begins to make spontaneous respiratory movements. Although these movements continue throughout pregnancy and babies are born with fluid in their lungs, it is not amniotic fluid but a specific fluid that has a low surface tension and low viscosity and is capable of being rapidly absorbed after birth. The presence of this fluid aids in the expansion of the alveoli at birth.

At about the twenty-fourth week of pregnancy, alveolar cells begin to excrete *surfactant,* a phospholipid substance that decreases alveolar surface tension on expiration. This prevents alveoli from collapsing on expiration and so greatly adds to the infant's ability to maintain respirations in the outside environment. Surfactant has two components: lecithin and sphingomyelin. Early in the formation of surfactant, sphingomyelin is the chief component; at about 35 weeks there is a surge in the production of lecithin, which becomes the chief component in a ratio of 2:1. As surfactant is mixed with amniotic fluid due to lung movements, it becomes present in amniotic fluid. Analysis of the lecithin/sphingomyelin (L/S) ratio by an amniocentesis technique is one of the primary tests of fetal maturity. Lack of surfactant, or a reversed L/S ratio, is a factor in the development of respiratory distress syndrome (RDS), formerly called hyaline membrane disease.

Nervous System

Like the circulatory system, the nervous system begins to develop extremely early in pregnancy. During the third and fourth weeks of life, at a time when the woman may not even realize that she is pregnant, active formation of the nervous system has already begun, and the sense organs are developing along with it.

By the third week of gestation, a *neural plate* (a thickened portion of the ectoderm) is apparent in the developing embryo. The top portion of the neural plate differentiates into the neural tube, which will form the central nervous system (brain and spinal cord), and the neural crest, which will develop into the peripheral nervous system.

Although all parts of the brain (the cerebrum, the cerebellum, the pons, and the medulla oblongata) form in utero, the brain is not yet mature at birth. It continues rapid growth during the first year; growth continues at high levels until 5 or 6 years of age. Thus the newborn infant still has many findings of neurologic immaturity such as a positive Babinski's sign (toes flare on stroking of the bottom of the foot).

The neurologic system seems particularly prone to insult during the early weeks of the embryonic period. All during pregnancy and at birth it is vulnerable to damage from anoxia.

Endocrine System

The fetal adrenal glands play a direct role in placental estrogen production, as they supply a precursor of estrogen synthesis. One of the theories of why labor begins is that the uterus receives a message from the fetal adrenals that the fetus is mature and ready to be born. The fetal pancreas produces the insulin needed by the fetus (insulin is one of the few known compounds that does not cross the placenta from the mother to the fetus).

Digestive System

Once the digestive tract is separated from the respiratory tract (at about the fourth week), the intestinal tract grows very rapidly. During the sixth week of intrauterine life the abdomen becomes too small to contain the intestine, and a portion of the intestine enters the base of the umbilical cord. Intestine remains in the base of the cord until about the tenth week, until the fetal trunk has extended and enlarged the abdominal cavity so it can accommodate all the intestinal mass. If intestinal coils remain outside the abdomen, in the base of the cord, a congenital anomaly, called *omphalocele*, develops.

Meconium forms in the intestines as early as the sixteenth week. It is the end product of fetal metabolism, consisting of cellular wastes, bile, fats, mucoproteins, mucopolysaccharides, and portions of the *vernix caseosa*, the lubricating substance that forms on the infant's skin at the fifth month of intrauterine life. Meconium is black or dark green and it is sticky in texture. It derives its dark color from bile pigments. White meconium is a sign of biliary obstruction. Children with cystic fibrosis have such thick, tenacious meconium that they may have bowel obstruction and intestinal perforation and die in utero. Meconium is apparently excreted early in intrauterine life; excretion late in intrauterine life suggests the infant has suffered anoxia and a vagal reflex has occurred.

The gastrointestinal tract is sterile at birth. Because vitamin K is synthesized by the action of bacteria in the intestines, vitamin K levels may be low in the newborn infant.

Sucking and swallowing reflexes are not mature until the fetus is about 32 weeks or weighs 1,500 gm. The development of these functions, so necessary for survival outside the uterus, so late in pregnancy has implications for nursing care of the fetus born before this time.

The ability of the gastrointestinal tract to secrete enzymes essential to the digestion of carbohydrate and protein is mature at 36 weeks. Amylase, an enzyme found in saliva and necessary for digestion of complex starches, is not mature until 3 months after birth. Lipase, an enzyme needed for fat digestion, is not available in many newborns. This fact has implications for newborn nutrition.

The liver is active throughout intrauterine life, functioning as a screen between the incoming blood and the fetal cells. It is still immature at birth, however. Two of the biggest problems of infants in the first 24 hours of life are hypoglycemia and hyperbilirubinemia, both related to immature liver function.

Skeletal System

In the first two weeks of fetal life, cartilage prototypes provide position and support. Ossification of bone tissue begins in the third month. The ossification process continues all through fetal life and until adulthood. A fetus cannot be detected by X-ray until a degree of ossification has taken place. A fetal X-ray film has been demonstrated as early as the fourteenth week of gestation, but on the average it is not accurate until the fifth lunar month (and contraindicated during pregnancy because X-ray is potentially harmful to the fetus). Carpals, tarsals, and sternal bones do not generally ossify until birth is imminent.

Reproductive System

Whether the child will be male or female is determined at the moment of conception by a spermatozoon carrying an X or a Y chromosome. At about the sixth week of life, the gonads (ovaries or testes) form. When testes form, the secretion of testosterone apparently influences the sexually neuter genital duct to form other male organs (maturity of the wolffian, or mesonephric duct). In the absence of testosterone secretion, female organs form (maturation of the müllerian, or paramesonephric, duct). This is an important phenomenon: If the mother ingests androgen or an androgen-like substance during this stage of pregnancy, the child, although chromosomally female, may look more male than female at birth because of clitoral growth. This characteristic has sometimes been seen in children whose mothers were given synthetic progesterone to prevent spontaneous abortion.

Masculinization may also occur in female infants with *adrenogenital syndrome,* a genetic disease in which there is deficient production of cortisol and excess production of androgen by the adrenal gland. These female infants are born with a clitoris that resembles a penis, and if close inspection is not carried out at birth, they may be assumed to be males with cryptorchidism (undescended testes). Males with this syndrome are born with abnormally enlarged genitalia.

Testes in a normal male tend to descend from the pelvic cavity, where they first form into the scrotal sac late in intrauterine life, in the seventh to ninth month. Thus many male low-birth-weight infants are born with undescended testes. These children should be followed closely to see that the testes descend when the child reaches the seventh to ninth month of gestational age, since testicular descent does not always occur as readily in extrauterine life as it does during intrauterine existence.

Urinary System

Although rudimentary kidneys are present as early as the end of the fourth week, kidneys do not appear to be essential for life before birth. Urine is formed by the twelfth week and is excreted into the amniotic fluid by the sixteenth week of pregnancy. The complex structure of the kidneys is gradually developed during pregnancy and for months afterward. The loop of Henle, for example, is not fully differentiated until the child is born. Glomerular filtration and concentration of urine in the newborn are not efficient, since the kidney is not fully mature at birth. At term, fetal urine is excreted at a rate of 500 ml per day.

Early in the embryonic stage of urinary system development, the bladder extends to the umbilical region. On rare occasions, an open lumen between the urinary bladder and the umbilicus fails to close. This is a *patent urachus* and is discovered at birth by the persistent drainage of a clear, acid-pH fluid (urine) from the umbilicus.

Immunologic System

Maternal antibodies cross the placenta during the third trimester of pregnancy to give a fetus passive immunity against diseases for which the mother has antibodies. These usually include poliomyelitis, rubella (German measles), rubeola (regular measles), diphtheria and tetanus, infectious parotitis (mumps), and pertussis (whooping cough). The antibodies are of the IgG class of immunoglobulins.

Little or no immunity to varicella (chickenpox) or to the herpesvirus (the virus of cold sores and genital herpes) is transferred to the fetus, and thus the newborn is always potentially susceptible to these diseases. It is important to screen a woman in labor for herpes infections, both type I and II, so that the newborn can be isolated from contact with this potentially hazardous virus. Herpesvirus causes a systemic disease in the newborn that may be fatal.

Since the passive immunity passed placentally from mother to fetus lasts about 2 months for diphtheria, tetanus, and pertussis, "baby shots" against these illnesses are typically begun at 2 months' extrauterine age. Passive antibodies to measles have been demonstrated to last over a year; consequently, the immunization for measles is not given until 15 months' extrauterine age.

A fetus is capable of antibody production late in pregnancy. The average fetus is not called upon to use this function, however, because the need for making these antibodies is only stimulated by an invading antigen and no antigen usually invades the intrauterine space. Babies whose mothers have an infection such as rubella during pregnancy typically have IgA or IgM antibodies in their blood serum at birth. Because these antibodies do not cross the placenta, their presence in a newborn is proof that the fetus has been challenged by disease invasion and has actively produced antibodies.

One largely unsolved mystery of fetal and placental growth is why a mother does not reject the placenta as she would any other foreign protein. This phenomenon is probably due to the increase of corticosteroids in the circulation, which depresses her immunologic response. It may be due to a special ability of trophoblast cells or HCG to suppress the immunologic response. Knowing more about this phenomenon would help with understanding the acceptance of any organ transplant.

Monthly Estimates of Fetal Growth and Development

During pregnancy, women often ask, "What is my baby like now?" "Does it have arms or legs yet?" "When can you tell if it is a girl or boy?" "What day will it be born?" In order to answer these questions effectively and to plan care to safeguard the growth of the new child, you should be able to describe the developmental milestones of intrauterine life.

Discussing intrauterine life is sometimes confusing because the life of the fetus is generally measured from the time of ovulation or fertilization, while the length of the pregnancy is generally measured from the first day of the last menstrual period. Because ovulation and fertilization

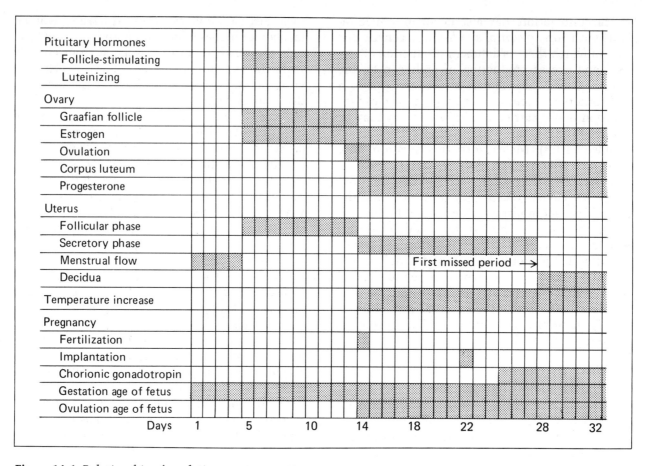

Figure 14-6 *Relationship of ovulation age to gestation age.*

take place about 2 weeks after the last menstrual period, the ovulation age of the fetus is always 2 weeks less than the length of the pregnancy or the gestation age of the fetus.

Both the length of the pregnancy and the life of a fetus are measured in lunar months (4-week periods) or in trimesters (3-month periods) rather than in calendar months. In lunar months a pregnancy is 10 months long; a fetus grows in utero 9½ lunar months. Three trimesters are necessary for full growth. The relationship of ovulation age to gestation age is shown in Figure 14-6.

Methods of Estimation

Haase's Rule

Using Haase's rule, the expected size of a fetus can be approximated. This rule states that the length of the embryo in centimeters can be calculated during the first 5 months of gestation by squaring the number of the month of the pregnancy, and in the sixth to tenth month, by multiplying the number of the month by 5. For example, a 4-month-old fetus is approximately 16 cm long; an 8-month-old fetus is 40 cm long. This rule has little clinical implication because the

length of the fetus cannot be measured except by sonogram in order to tell if it is reaching this length or not. If sonography becomes a more common procedure, more and more fetuses will be actually measured for length in utero.

McDonald's Rule

Mcdonald's rule is based on the measurement of fundal height. This measurement is made from the notch of the symphysis pubis to over the top of the uterus fundus as the woman lies supine (Figure 14-7). To calculate the length of pregnancy in lunar months, multiply the fundal height (in cms) by 2/7. By this rule a fundal height of 14 cm indicates a pregnancy of 4 lunar months.

To calculate the duration of the pregnancy in weeks, multiply the height of the fundus times 8/7. By this rule, a fundal height of 14 cm indicates a pregnancy of 16 weeks (4 lunar months). After 25 weeks, the height of the uterus in cm approximates the length of the pregnancy in weeks (28 cm = 28 weeks).

Expected Date of Confinement

It is impossible to predict the date of confinement (the day of birth of a child) with a high

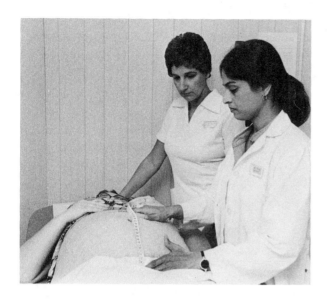

Figure 14-7 *Measuring fundal height. Height is measured from the superior aspect of the pubis to the fundal crest. (Courtesy of the Department of Medical Photography, Children's Hospital, Buffalo, N.Y.)*

degree of accuracy. As mentioned, the average length of a pregnancy from ovulation is 9½ lunar months, or 38 weeks, or 266 days; from the last menstrual period, a pregnancy is 10 lunar months, or 40 weeks, or 280 days. In actuality, fewer than 5 percent of pregnancies end exactly 280 days from the last menstrual period; fewer than half end within one week of day 280.

Nägele's Rule

Nägele's rule is the standard method used to predict the length of a pregnancy. To calculate the expected date of confinement (EDC) by this rule, count backward 3 calendar months from the first day of the last menstrual period and add 7 days. For example, if the last menstrual period began May 15, you would count back 3 months (April 15, March 15, February 15), add 7 days, and the EDC would be February 22.

If fertilization occurred early in the menstrual cycle, the pregnancy will probably end "early"; if ovulation and fertilization occurred later in the cycle, the pregnancy will end "late". Because of these normal variations, a pregnancy ending 2 weeks before or 2 weeks after the calculated EDC is considered well within the normal limit (a pregnancy 38 to 42 weeks in length).

Fetal Developmental Milestones

Fetal developmental milestones are listed in Table 14-4. The following discussion of fetal developmental milestones is based on gestation weeks because it is helpful when talking to expectant parents to correlate fetal development to the way they measure pregnancy, which is gestation weeks (dated from the first day of the last menstrual period).

End of First Lunar Month (4 Gestation Weeks)

At the end of the first month the human embryo is a rapidly growing formation of cells, but not yet resembling a human being. Very shortly, the head will become prominent, comprising about a third of the entire structure. The back is bent so that the head almost touches the tip of the tail (yes, a human embryo does have a tail at this point). The heart (still rudimentary) appears as a prominent bulge on the anterior surface. The arms and legs are bud-like structures. Rudimentary eyes, ears, and nose are discernible. Length crown to rump is 4.0 to 4.5 mm. Weight is 400 mg.

End of Second Lunar Month (8 Gestation Weeks)

Length, crown to rump, is 1.3 cm (0.5 inch); weight is 1 gm (1/30 ounce). Organogenesis is complete at the end of 8 weeks. With organogenesis, the structure is termed a *fetus* for the remainder of the pregnancy (fetus is Latin meaning "offspring"). The heart has a septum and valves and is beating rhythmically. The facial features are definitely discernible. Legs, arms, fingers, toes, elbows, and knees have developed. Although the external genitalia are present, sex is not distinguishable by simple observation. The primitive tail is undergoing retrogression. The abdomen appears large as fetal intestine is growing rapidly. A sonogram taken at this time demonstrates a gestational sac and is diagnostic of pregnancy (Figure 14-8).

End of Third Lunar Month (12 Gestation Weeks)

Length, crown to rump, is 6.5 inches; weight is 20 gm (1¾ ounces). For ease of discussion, pregnancy is generally divided into three segments (trimesters), each of 3 months' duration. At the end of the third month the fetus is at the end of the first trimester of pregnancy. Nail beds are forming on fingers and toes. The fetus is capable of spontaneous movements, although they are usually too faint to be felt by the mother. Some reflexes are present, notably Babinski's reflex. Ossification centers are forming in bones, and tooth buds are present. (The latter point is important because if tetracycline is taken by the mother after this point in pregnancy the child may have tetracycline-stained, or brown, teeth.) Male and female fetuses are distinguishable by outward appearance. Kidney secretion has begun, although urine may not yet be evident in amni-

Table 14-4 Timetable of Normal Fetal Development

Age (weeks)	Gross Appearance	Cardiovascular	Digestive	Respiratory	Urogenital	Nervous System	Sense Organs	Musculo-skeletal
1st	Fertilization. Cleavage of zygote. Blastocyst enters uterine cavity.							
2nd	Blastocyst enlarges. Implantation							
3rd	Head and tail folds.	Primitive vascular system established. Heart tube.	Buccopharyngeal membrane breaks down. Foregut. Midgut. Hindgut.			Neural plate. Neural folds. Partial fusion of neural folds.		Somites appear.
4th	Body narrow and tubular; C-shaped. Limb buds appear. Placenta begins to form.	Heart is enlarged and beating. Partitioning of atrium begins. Hemopoiesis in yolk sac.	Esophagus, stomach, liver, and pancreatic buds.	Laryngotracheal tube, trachea, lung buds.	Mesonephros rapidly forming.	Neural tube. Three primary vesicles of brain.	Optic placode and auditory vesicle present.	Most somites formed. Myotome, sclerotome, and dermatome.
5th	Head increases greatly in size. Face is forming. Limb buds show limb, forelimb, hand or foot.	Cardiac septa developing. Atrioventricular cushions fusing.	Stomach starts to rotate. Midgut forms loop. Urorectal septum.	Lobes of lung formed.	Genital ridges. External genitalia.	Cerebral hemisphere.	Lens vesicle. Auditory vesicle.	Condensation of mesenchyme to form cartilage and muscle.
6th	Head dominant. Oral and nasal cavities confluent. Curvature of embryo diminished. Fingers and toes recognizable.	Heart now has definitive form. Foramen primum closes. Aorticopulmonary septation. Hematopoiesis in liver.	Upper lip forming. Dental lamina. Palatal processes. Pleuroperitoneal canals close. Midgut loop herniates. Cecum and appendix. Vitello-intestinal duct atrophies.	Bronchi dividing.	Paramesonephric ducts. Sex cords start to develop in testis. Cloaca divided.	Flexures of brain obvious.	Nasolacrimal duct.	Chondrification. Intramembranous ossification.
8th	Head nearly as large as rest of body. Facial features more distinct. Eyes directed more anteriorly. Neck established. Limbs more developed. Digits of hands and feet separated. Fetus covered with epitrichium. Retrogression of tail.	Ventricular septum completed in week 7.	Enamel organs. Small intestine rotating in umbilical cord. Cloacal membrane has broken down.	Bronchioles dividing.	Genital tubercle and genital swellings further developed. Still sexless. Mesonephros fully developed. Metanephric duct branching to form collecting tubules. Testes and ovaries recognizable.	Rapid growth of CNS. Expansion of forebrain vesicle.	Eyes converging. Eyelids developing. External nares plugged. Auricle of external ear forming.	Fetal muscular movement commences. Endochondral ossification. Smooth muscle.

Table 14-4 (continued)

Age (weeks)	Gross Appearance	Cardiovascular	Digestive	Respiratory	Urogenital	Nervous System	Sense Organs	Musculo-skeletal
12th	Rapid growth in fetal length. Head still relatively large. Eyes look anteriorly. External ears on side of head. Eyelids fused. Nails. Sex recognition possible.	Hematopoiesis in liver and spleen.	Nasal septum and palate fusion complete. Midgut loop returns to abdominal cavity.	Lungs are of definitive shape.	Kidneys have started to secrete urine. External genitalia sufficiently developed to identify sex. Testes close to future deep inguinal ring.	Brain and spinal cord well developed. Cauda equina.	Eyelids fuse. Nasal septum fuses with palate.	Ossification centers forming. Tooth buds present.
16th	Further rapid growth in fetal length. Head still relatively large. Eyes widely separated but eyelids fused. Lanugo present. Auricles of ear high up on side of head. Fetus looks human.	Hematopoiesis in bone marrow commences.	Ascending and descending colon retroperitoneal. Meconium starts to accumulate. Fetus swallowing amniotic fluid.		Mesonephros involuted. Definitive lobulated kidney present. External genitalia well developed.	Cerebellum prominent. Myelination begins in spinal cord.	Eyes, ears, and nose in final positions.	Joint cavities.
20th	Lanugo covers entire body. Hair present on head. Mother detects quickening.	Fetal heartbeat heard with stethoscope.	Meconium reaches rectum.					Distinct movements of limbs felt by mother (quickening).
24th	Skin wrinkled and red. Vernix caseosa present. Head still relatively large. Face childlike. Eyebrows and eyelashes present. Eyelids open.			Pulmonary alveoli appear.		Myelination begins in brain.	Eyelids reopen.	Movements stronger.
28th	Skin wrinkled. Fetal contours more rounded. Hair on head longer.				Testes in inguinal canal.			
32nd	Fetus looks wrinkled and scraggy. Subcutaneous fat appearing. Lanugo hair has disappeared from face. Vernix caseosa thick. Nails reach end of fingers.							
36th	Fetus looks plumper and rounder.				Left testis in scrotum.	Cerebral fissures and convolutions rapidly developing.		Movements much stronger.
40th	Fetus fully developed. More subcutaneous fat present. Lanugo hair disappears. Nails project beyond ends of fingers and toes.	Fetal hemoglobin begins conversion to adult hemoglobin.		Bronchioles and alveoli still developing.	Both testes in scrotum. Kidneys lie opposite L2.	Lower end of spinal cord at L3.	Paranasal sinuses are rudimentary.	Bones of skull are firm. Circumference of skull larger than rest of body.

Source: Adapted from Snell, R. S. (1975). *Clinical embryology for medical students.* (2nd ed.). Boston: Little, Brown.

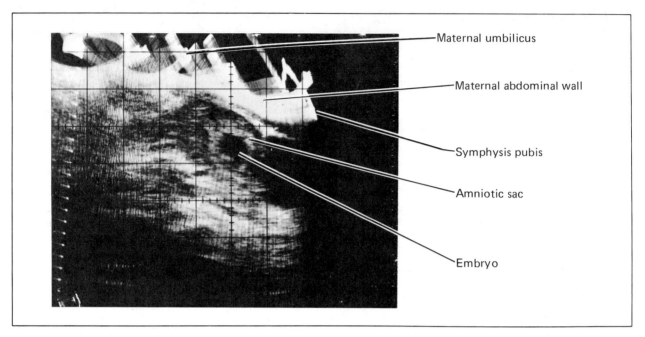

Figure 14-8 *A sonogram showing implantation, or the characteristic circular ring present at 6 weeks' gestation.*

otic fluid. The heart beat is audible by a Doppler instrument, allowing the mother to hear the beat.

End of the Fourth Lunar Month (16 Gestation Weeks)

Length, crown to rump, is 11 cm (4.4 inches); weight is 124 gm (4 ounces). It may be possible to hear fetal heart sounds through an ordinary stethoscope at the end of the fourth lunar month. (The fetal heart rate is between 120 and 160 beats per minute throughout pregnancy.) The formation of *lanugo* (the fine, downy hair on the back and arms of newborns, apparently serving as a source of insulation for body heat) is well formed by this month. The liver and pancreas are functioning. At this time the fetus actively swallows amniotic fluid, demonstrating an intact swallowing reflex. Ossification of bones is complete enough to allow the fetal skeleton to show on x-ray film.

End of Fifth Lunar Month (20 Gestation Weeks)

Length, crown to rump, is 15 cm (6 inches); weight is 300 gm (10 ounces). During the fifth month of intrauterine life the spontaneous movements of the fetus become strong enough for the mother to feel. The sensation is like the fluttering of wings or fluid moving rapidly through the bowels. This event is termed *quickening*. It is a major milestone in pregnancy. For many women it is the first time the pregnancy seems real to them. It

is such an exciting event in a first pregnancy that most mothers can remember for the rest of their lives not only at what month in pregnancy quickening occurred but exactly where they were when it happened.

A 20-week-old fetus is capable of antibody production but apparently produces few antibodies until challenged by antigens at the time of birth. Hair formation extends to include eyebrows and hair on the head. Meconium is present in the intestine. Brown fat, a special fat that aides in temperature regulation, begins to be formed behind the kidneys, sternum, and posterior neck. The fetal heart beat is strong enough to be readily heard through the abdomen with an ordinary stethoscope.

Twenty weeks is sometimes spoken of as the age of "viability," since a few infants born at this age have survived. The designation is mainly academic, however, because the average fetus born at this time does not have enough lung surfactant (necessary to keep the lungs from collapsing on exhalation) for respiration. Definite sleeping and activity patterns are distinguishable: Already at this point in pregnancy, the fetus has developed biorhythms that will guide later life.

End of Sixth Lunar Month (24 Gestation Weeks)

Length, crown to rump, is 20 cm (8 inches); weight is 600 gm (1⅓ pounds). Passive antibody transfer from mother to fetus probably begins as early as the fifth lunar month, certainly by the sixth lunar month.

Infants born before antibody transfer has taken place have no natural immunity and need more than the usual protection against infectious disease in the newborn period.

Vernix caseosa, a cream cheese-like substance produced by the sebaceous glands that serves as a protective skin covering during intrauterine life, begins to form during the sixth lunar month. Meconium is present as far as the rectum. Active production of lung surfactant begins, and features as detailed as eyebrows and eyelashes are well defined.

At 24 weeks, or 600 gm, the fetus has reached a practical lower age of viability if a modern intensive care facility is available when the infant is born.

End of the Seventh Lunar Month
(28 Gestation Weeks)

Length, crown to heel, is 37 cm (14.4 inches); weight is 1,100 gm (2½ pounds). The lung alveoli begin to mature, and surfactant can be demonstrated in amniotic fluid. The eyelids of the fetus have been fused since the third lunar month. Now the membrane that had fused them dissolves, the eyes can open, and the pupils are capable of reacting to light. In the male fetus, descent of the testes into the scrotal sac from the lower abdominal cavity begins.

Many women believe that a fetus born in this month of development has a better chance of surviving than one born in the eighth month. This belief is probably associated in part with the belief that 7 is a lucky number and in part with a superstition handed down from ancient Greek times, when physicians thought that a fetus always attempted to escape the uterus during the seventh month. The fetus who was strong succeeded. If he failed, he again attempted escape at the eighth month. However, the fetus that succeeded on this try was so weak from the two attempts that he died. The theory is doubly fallacious. The fetus appears to be a passive, not an active, passenger during delivery (although the initial signal for labor may come from the fetus or the membranes), and the more months available for maturation in utero, the more capable the fetus is of surviving.

The blood vessels of the retina are susceptible to damage from high oxygen concentrations at 7 months (an important point to be aware of when caring for low-birth-weight infants who need oxygen).

End of the Eighth Lunar Month
(32 Gestation Weeks)

Length, crown to heel, is 43 cm (17 inches); weight is 1,800 to 2,000 gm (3½ to 4 pounds). Subcutaneous fat begins to be deposited in the fetus during this month; the former stringy, "little-old-man" appearance is lost. The fetus is aware of sounds outside the mother's body; an active Moro reflex has been demonstrated, and some have assumed delivery position (vertex or breech). Iron stores to provide iron for the time during which the infant will ingest mainly milk following birth begin to be laid. Fingernails grow to reach the end of fingertips.

End of Ninth Lunar Month
(36 Gestation Weeks)

Length, crown to heel, is 46 cm (18 inches); weight is 2,200 to 2,700 gm (5 to 6 pounds). In the last 2 months of intrauterine life, body stores of glycogen, iron, carbohydrate, and calcium are augmented; additional amounts of subcutaneous fat are deposited. At this time the sole of the foot has only one or two crisscross creases. A full crisscross pattern will be evident at term. The amount of lanugo present begins to diminish.

Many babies turn in utero during this month into a vertex or head-first presentation.

End of Tenth Lunar Month
(40 Gestation Weeks)

Length, crown to heel, is 50 cm (20 inches); weight is 3,100 to 3,400 gm (7 to 7½ pounds).

The fetus kicks actively during this month, hard enough to cause the mother considerable discomfort. Fetal hemoglobin begins its conversion to adult hemoglobin. The conversion is so rapid that at birth about 20 percent of hemoglobin will be adult in character.

Vernix caseosa is fully formed. Fingernails extend over the tips of fingers. Creases on the soles of the feet cover at least two thirds of their surface.

In primiparas (women having their first babies), the fetus often sinks into the birth canal during these last 2 weeks, giving the mother a feeling that her load is being lightened. This event is termed *lightening*. It is a fetal announcement that the third trimester of pregnancy has ended and birth is at hand.

Figures 14-9 and 14-10 illustrate the comparative size and appearance of human embryos and fetuses at different stages.

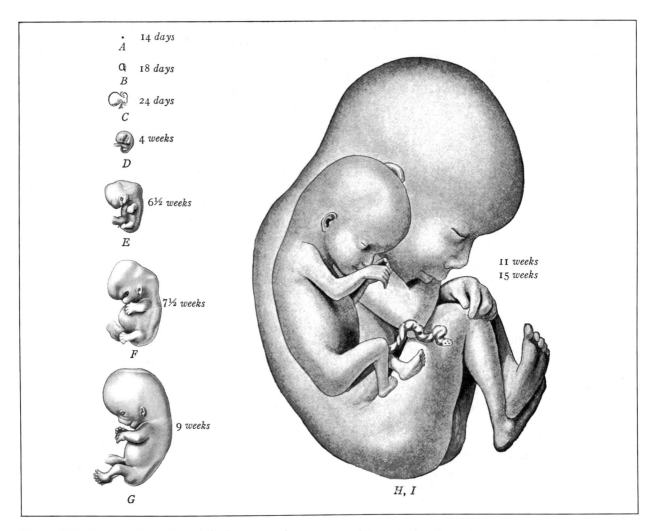

14 *days*
A

18 *days*
B

24 *days*
C

4 *weeks*
D

6½ *weeks*
E

7½ *weeks*
F

9 *weeks*
G

11 *weeks*
15 *weeks*
H, I

Figure 14-9 *Comparative sizes of the human embryo at nine different ages. From Arey, L. (1965).* Developmental anatomy. *(7th ed.). Philadelphia: Saunders.*

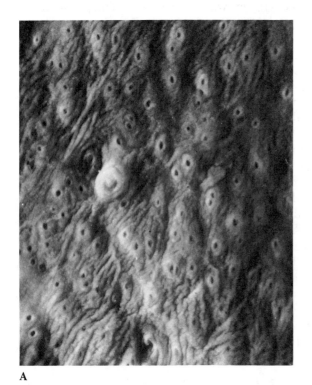

A

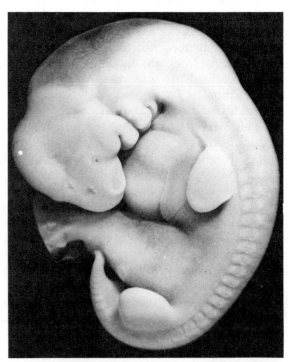

B

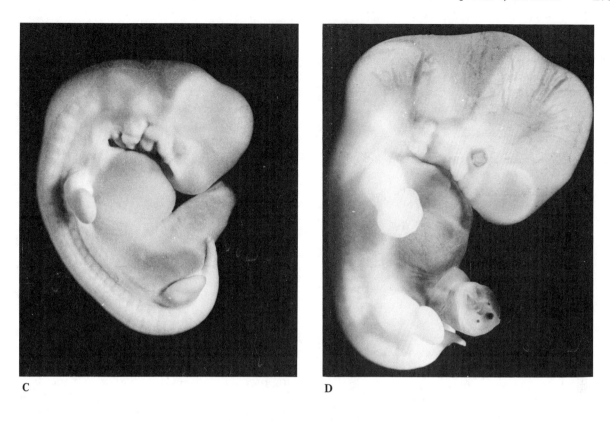

C   D

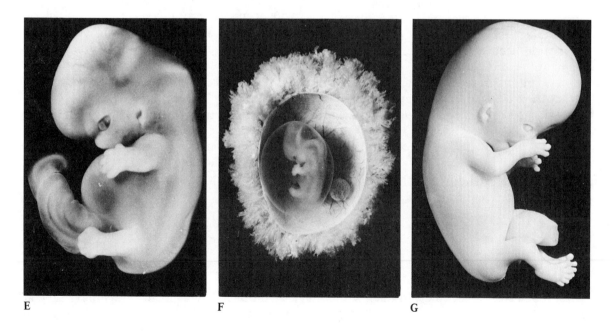

E   F   G

Figure 14-10 *Human embryo at different stages of development. A. Surface view of a human implantation on the uterus 7 to 8 days after conception. The openings of uterine glands of the epithelium appear as dark spots surrounded by light circles. B. Embryo at 32 days. Notice the primitive tail. The heart fills a large portion of the upper torso. C. Embryo at 37 days. The abdominal contents are beginning rapid growth. D. Embryo at 41 days. Arms and legs are becoming clearly defined. The tail is retrogressing. E. Embryo at 48 days. Fingers and toes are formed. The bulk of the fetal intestine is protruded into the umbilical cord. F. Embryo at 48 days, surrounded by amniotic membrane and fluid, the opened chorion, and the projecting chorionic villi. G. Embryo at 57 days (8 weeks). Organogenesis is complete. (Courtesy of Carnegie Institution of Washington, Department of Embryology, Davis Division.)*

Utilizing Nursing Process

Designing safe care for a fetus in utero is just as important as planning care for a more visible patient. To ensure that care is safe and optimal, it must be done using nursing process.

Assessment

Measures used to assess the growth and development of the fetus are fundal height, fetal movement, fetal heart rate, amniocentesis, sonography, and maternal blood serum and urine analysis. These techniques of assessment are discussed in Chapter 15.

Analysis

It is difficult to establish a nursing diagnosis that is fetus-centered as it is impossible to know the desires of a fetus; the problem raises an ethical question concerning the point at which a fetus has desires. It can be assumed, however, that if a fetus has the rights of all individuals, the primary needs of safety and well-being should be safeguarded as well as those of any patient. Typical nursing diagnoses used are "Impairment in fetal growth related to inadequate nutritional intake," "Fear of mother related to lack of fetal movement," or a wellness-oriented diagnosis of "Health promotion need related to fetal growth and development."

Goals of care are instituted with the mother. Be certain that they are realistic as they include actions that must be carried out for 9 months' time.

Planning

Planning in regard to safeguarding fetal health involves planning for maternal education for a life style that includes adequate nutrition and activities that are safe for fetal growth. Remember that without a reward, people do not continue health maintenance measures over a long period of time. Because a fetus does not give a reward early in pregnancy (late in pregnancy, fetal activity can be viewed as a reward or response), it is difficult for a woman to maintain health care measures. Build in rewards in the form of praise from health care providers until the fetus can take over this phase. Teratogens, or factors that are detrimental to fetal health, are discussed and illustrated in Chapter 40.

Implementation

Women are interested in the appearance and size of the fetus inside them at each month of gestation. Teaching women fetal growth and development and helping them to visualize the fetus helps them to maintain the necessary activities during pregnancy to ensure fetal well-being. It is easier for a woman to eat liver once a week, for example, because she views the fetus as a person she is caring for than if she thinks she is carrying a vague accumulation of cells. Table 16-6 which correlates fetal growth with the physiologic changes of pregnancy, is a good teaching aid for helping mothers to understand fetal growth.

Evaluation

Evaluation of fetal health involves the assessment measures discussed in Chapter 15. Ultimately evaluation is completed at birth when a well or ill child is born.

Nursing Care Planning

Christine McFadden is a 15-year-old you meet at a prenatal clinic.

Assessment

Unsure of date of LMP (about 16 weeks). Has been diving on school swimming team from high board with two "wrong dives" hitting abdomen hard against water. Now no longer diving. Nonsmoker; no alcohol consumption. Evasive about usual use of marijuana. None since she thought she might be pregnant. Nutrition: eats two meals at home daily, one at school; "Mom watches her diet." Uterine height 4 cm above symphysis. Fetal heart tones by Doppler at 150.

Analysis

Health promotion need related to fetal growth and development.

Locus of Decision Making. Shared.

Goal. Patient will safeguard fetal health for pregnancy duration.

Criteria. Patient:

1. Will take no nonprescribed drugs during pregnancy.
2. Will keep sports activities to sensible levels.
3. Will carry pregnancy to term.

Nursing Orders

1. Schedule for sonogram per M.D. order for estimation of pregnancy length (LMP not known).
2. Educate about medication, drug, and alcohol use during pregnancy.
3. Caution her to phone clinic for advice if in doubt about what is appropriate sports activity during pregnancy.

Questions for Review

Multiple Choice

1. Mrs. Murphy is a woman having her first pregnancy. She asks you at what day during pregnancy the embryo implants on the uterine surface. Your best answer would be
   a. the 14th day of a "typical" menstrual cycle.
   b. ten days after ovulation.
   c. ten days after the menstrual flow.
   d. four days after ovulation.

2. Implantation generally occurs at which place on the uterus?
   a. the lower anterior surface
   b. the upper posterior surface
   c. directly over the cervical os
   d. directly over an opening to a fallopian tube

3. Mrs. Murphy tends to go a long time between meals because of a busy work schedule. What process safeguards glucose transfer to the fetus during this long period of low glucose intake?
   a. Glucose crosses the placenta by diffusion.
   b. Glucose crosses by facilitated diffusion.
   c. Pinocytosis is necessary for glucose transport.
   d. Active transport allows glucose to transfer freely.

4. Human chorionic gonadotropin hormone is the hormone tested for in urine as a pregnancy test. The purpose of this hormone is to
   a. ensure chorionic somatomammotropin hormone production.
   b. permit the uterus to increase in size.
   c. prolong the life of the corpus luteum.
   d. ensure oxygen transport across the placenta.

5. Mrs. Murphy asks why the amniotic fluid does not grow stagnant. The theory for this is that
   a. amniotic fluid is constantly formed by the amnion.
   b. amniotic fluid is constantly absorbed by the chorion.
   c. the fetal urine increases the bulk of amniotic fluid.
   d. amniotic fluid circulates through the chorionic villi.

6. A fetus is able to maintain blood circulation in utero by the presence of circulatory shunts. The ductus arteriosus in utero shunts blood from
   a. the left to right heart atria.
   b. the aorta to the pulmonary veins.
   c. the right ventricle to the aorta.
   d. the pulmonary artery to the aorta.

7. Omphalocele is a developmental abnormality in which an infant is born with intestines outside the abdomen. This occurs because
   a. the fetus suffered a bowel obstruction at an early point in life.
   b. the fetal abdomen formed with a smaller internal cavity than normal.
   c. the intestines formed without sufficient nerve innervation for contraction.
   d. the intestines normally leave the abdomen during intrauterine life.

8. Assessment for surfactant level is a primary estimation of fetal maturity. Surfactant acts to
   a. prevent alveoli from collapsing on expiration.
   b. increase lung resistance on inspiration.
   c. encourage immunologic competence of lung tissue.
   d. promote maturation of lung alveoli.

9. A fetus is capable of producing antibodies. The finding of IgM antibodies in an infant at birth implies that
   a. antibodies were transferred to the fetus during pregnancy.
   b. the fetus contracted an infection during intrauterine life.
   c. the fetus's liver has reached developmental maturity.
   d. the mother contracted an infection during pregnancy.

Discussion

1. The placenta is indispensible to fetal life. What are the body organs that it takes the function of?
2. It is difficult for women to envision fetal appearance during pregnancy. What are teaching aides you could use to help with this?
3. The ability of low-birth-weight infants to survive depends on their level of development at birth. What would be the differences in a 20-week and a 26-week fetus?

Suggested Readings

Afriat, C. (1983). The nurse's role in fetal heart rate monitoring. *Perinatology/Neonatology, 7*, 29.

Andrews, C. M. (1981). Nursing intervention to change a malpositioned fetus. *Advances in Nursing Science, 3*, 53.

Barnett, H. (1977). *Pediatrics,* New York: Appleton-Century-Crofts.

Burkart-Jayez, S. F. (1982). The effects of congenital rubella on the neonate. *Journal of Neurosurgical Nursing, 14*, 173.

Crelin, E. S. (1981). Development of the musculoskeletal system. *Clinical Symposia, 33*, 2.

Didolkar S. M., et al. (1981). Tracing the heart's action before birth. *Journal of Cardiovascular and Pulmonary Technology, 9*, 55.

Donovan, P. (1983). When does personhood begin? *Family Planning Perspectives, 15*, 40.

Finch, J. (1983). Law: Protection of the unborn child. *Nursing Mirror, 156*, 33.

Hadlock, F. P., et al. (1982). Fetal head circumference: Accuracy of real-time ultrasound measurements at term. *Perinatology/Neonatology, 6*, 97.

Hazinski, M. F. (1983). Congenital heart disease in the neonate: Epidemiology, cardiac development and fetal circulation. *Neonatal Network, 1*, 29.

Ho, E. (1983). Fetal well being . . . the role of preconceptual care and the early and accurate detection of the fetus at risk. *Nursing Mirror, 12*, 156.

Levine, A. H., et al. (1982). Intrauterine treatment of fetal hydronephrosis. *Association of Operating Room Nurses Journal, 35*, 655.

Loper-Hunter, D. (1982). The beginning of the respiratory system . . . embryologic development. *Neonatal Network, 1*, 19.

Malnory, M. E. (1982). A prenatal assessment tool for mothers and fathers. *Journal of Nurse Midwifery, 27*, 26.

Naeye, R. L. (1983). Effects of maternal nutrition on fetal and neonatal survival. *Birth, 10*, 109.

Patterson, P. (1982). Fetal therapy: Issues we face. *Association of Operating Room Nurses Journal, 35*, 663.

Sabbagha, R. E. (1984). Diagnosis and management of fetal growth retardation. *Female Patient, 9*, 128.

Weaver, R. H., et al. (1983). An exploration of paternal-fetal attachment behavior. *Nursing Research, 32*, 68.

Wharton, B., et al. (1982). Organogenesis, fetal growth and food. *Birth, 9*, 111.

Woodward, S. L. (1981). How does strenuous maternal exercise affect the fetus? *Birth and the Family Journal, 8*, 17.

Wynn, M., et al. (1982). The importance of maternal nutrition in the weeks before and after conception. *Birth, 9*, 39.

15

Fetal Assessment

OBJECTIVES

Following mastery of the contents of this chapter, you should be able to

1. Describe common maternal assay tests for fetal well-being.
2. Describe the common fetal monitoring tests based on fetal activity or heart rate.
3. Describe the technique of amniocentesis and its role in fetal assessment.
4. Describe care necessary before, during, and after fetal assessment procedures in reference to both fetal and maternal well-being.
5. Analyze the importance of fetal assessment to the family.
6. Synthesize knowledge of fetal assessment tests with nursing process to achieve quality maternal-newborn nursing care.

TOWARD THE END of pregnancy most women wish they could have a glimpse of their unborn child to see whether it is a boy or girl and to assure themselves that the child is doing well and is ready for extrauterine life. Often, those caring for the woman during pregnancy would also find this information helpful. Although not yet available to satisfy the mere curiosity of parents or health care personnel, various techniques now available make it possible to learn a great deal about the health of an unborn child when this information is essential for care.

Responsibility for Procedures

Nursing responsibility for fetal assessment procedures includes obtaining consent as needed, explaining the procedure to the woman and her support person, scheduling the procedure, preparing the woman physically and psychologically, accompanying her to the hospital department where the procedure will actually be done, providing support during the procedure, assessing both fetal and maternal response to it, and providing aftercare of equipment, of specimens, and to the woman herself.

Obtaining Consent

Consent to perform a procedure must be obtained if the procedure carries any risk that would not be present if it were not performed. In order for a woman to sign a consent form, she must be informed what the procedure consists of and what risk (to both herself or the fetus) is present by having or not having the procedure performed. In order to be certain that you can explain procedures clearly to women and answer their questions concerning them, make every effort to see as many procedures done as you can. Ask a woman following a procedure what sensations she experienced, not only to increase your own knowledge of fetal assessment procedures but to help her work through a possibly frightening situation.

Explaining Procedures

In order not to be unduly frightened by a diagnostic procedure, a woman needs an understanding of the reason for the procedure and a description of it ("you will lie on a table; a physician will clean your abdomen, you will feel a small pinprick as anesthesia is injected . . ."); where the procedure will be done (the X-ray department, a treatment room); any unusual sensations to be expected during the study (alcohol for skin cleaning will feel cold); a fair description of any pain involved (the needle will sting); any strange equipment used (a sonogram scanning transducer); the approximate time the study takes; and any special care following the study (she will need to lie quietly for 15 minutes afterward).

Be careful not to use terms that might be confusing such as trimester, gestation, transducer, or electrode during your explanation unless you define them as part of the explanation. Most women are anxious about undergoing fetal assessment studies and so have difficulty understanding even very simple explanations. To estimate her level of knowledge, ask about a woman's previous experience with similar procedures. A woman may have had a sonogram done for a gynecologic scan, for example, and so is not worried at all about the procedure because it is "old hat" for her.

Be prepared to repeat a description of the procedure immediately before the study to counteract a natural blocking out of information that occurs under stress. If you are unfamiliar with what a procedure entails, do not guess: Nothing is more confusing than receiving two different versions of a procedure. Most technical personnel will take the time to give you a description over the telephone of the specific points the woman should know about the study; having a well-informed woman makes her better able to cooperate and so simplifies their job. Be certain that a support person receives an explanation of the procedure as well. A woman cannot relax if her husband is still anxious because he does not understand what is going to happen. A support person can usually accompany the woman for all fetal assessment tests as they do not involve X-ray (except for pelvimetry at a pregnancy's term), and a meaningful support person can be extremely helpful in reducing the threat of the procedure.

Scheduling Fetal Assessment Procedures

If women are going to have a fetal assessment procedure done on an ambulatory basis, they can be given the responsibility of reporting to the designated department at the scheduled time themselves. Remember that women "guard" their bodies during pregnancy. They are reluctant to allow strangers to perform procedures on them. Always take some time to get acquainted with a woman before attempting any procedure such as blood drawing or a sonogram scan so the woman can grasp that you are not an "attacker" but a helper.

Accompanying the Woman

If a woman is hospitalized because of pregnancy complications, going to the health care facility was probably extremely difficult for her. Once she has become comfortable there and is familiar with the personnel on that unit, *leaving* the unit to go to another department for fetal assessment becomes hard. Always accompany women to other departments to decrease this reluctance and remain with them for the procedure or at least until they have met a primary person who will be with them during the assessment procedure. If the woman is in labor, remain with her during the entire procedure (but not in the X-ray room for pelvimetry) in case labor should suddenly progress rapidly or a complication such as cord prolapse should occur.

Before leaving the patient unit, check that the woman's ID band is securely in place and readily visible despite any intravenous equipment. There may be a considerable wait in another department. Ask the woman if she would like some activity to occupy her, such as reading material. Hallways may be cool. Provide adequate blankets on the stretcher for comfort. Always use cart straps and siderails for safety. A stretcher is very narrow for a pregnant woman and she could fall easily. Always transport pregnant women on

their side, not lying on their back, to prevent supine hypotension syndrome.

Before leaving the patient unit have the woman void for comfort (a sonogram when she needs a full bladder for best transmission is the exception to this rule). Check for a medication or some assessment procedure such as a blood pressure recording that should be given or done before leaving the unit for another department in case the woman is out of the unit for a long time.

Fetal Measurements

Estimation of Fundal Height

Fundal height should be measured at each prenatal visit as a means of assessing fetal growth and well-being. It is a helpful determination, since the increase in the size of the uterus directly reflects the increase in the size of the fetus. Establishing fundal height and length of pregnancy by McDonald's rule is explained on page 272. If the fundal height is more than it should be, multiple pregnancy, miscalculated due date, hydramnios (increased amniotic fluid volume), or hydatidiform mole (see Chapter 39) may be the cause. A fundal measurement much less than it should be suggests that the fetus is failing to thrive or that an anomaly such as anencephaly is developing.

Recording that the fundus reaches milestone measurements, such as over the symphysis pubis at 12 weeks, at the umbilicus at 20 weeks, and at the xyphoid process at 36 weeks, is also a helpful determination.

Fetal Movement

Quickening is much less reliable as a sign of well-being. A woman who wants to have a baby very badly can be deceived by her own desire into "feeling" quickening when in reality there is no child inside her. A woman who has previously felt movement and reports that she no longer feels it needs to be seen immediately; she may be reporting fetal death.

Fetal movement that can be felt by the mother begins at 18 to 20 weeks and reaches a peak at 29 to 38 weeks. Because a healthy fetus moves with a degree of consistency and a fetus affected by placental insufficiency will greatly decrease in movement, asking the mother to observe and record how many movements the fetus makes daily can give a gross assessment of fetal well-being.

One popular method for this counting is the "Count-to-Ten" chart. Beginning at 30 weeks of pregnancy, the mother counts the number of fetal movements beginning at 8 or 9 A.M. daily. As soon as she has counted 10 movements, she marks a chart as to the time of day. If at the end of 12 hours, 10 movements have not occurred, she marks the number that did occur. Such a chart shows a typical pattern for that fetus (10 movements always occur before 1 P.M.). If this pattern changes, or if 2 days pass without 10 movements, the woman calls her health care provider to report this change of activity.

Before being asked to be responsible for this type of observation, mothers must be given good orientation that fetal movements do vary, especially in relation to her activity and proximity to meals during the observation time; periods as long as 75 minutes may pass without fetal activity (Patrick, 1982). Otherwise the strain of waiting for the tenth movement may increase her anxiety level so severely that, although the fetus may be doing well with the pregnancy, the pregnancy becomes an unbearable stress for her.

Fetal Heart Tones

The presence and rate of fetal heart sounds and the response of fetal heart rate to stress are all good indications of fetal well-being.

Fetal Heart Presence

Typically, the sound of the fetal heart is first heard with a stethoscope between the sixteenth and twentieth weeks, so that auscultation at this time is an assessment of well-being as well as a means of establishing or confirming the expected date of confinement (due date) of the pregnancy (Figure 15-1). Fetal heart rates can be heard as early as the eleventh week by the use of an ultrasonic Doppler technique (Figure 15-2). Fetal heart rate should be 120 to 160 beats per minute throughout pregnancy.

Electrocardiography

Fetal electrocardiograms (ECGs) may be recorded as early as the eleventh week of pregnancy. The ECG is inaccurate before the fifth month, however, because until this time the fetal cardiac electrical signal is so weak that it may be masked by the mother's. It may be a helpful tool in differentiating between an intrauterine tumor and a viable pregnancy, however.

All fetal hearts should be monitored by an ECG technique or Doppler technique during labor, when the fetus is under a high degree of stress. Techniques of fetal heart rate monitoring during labor are discussed in Chapter 24 with other important aspects of care during labor.

Nonstress Test (NST)

A nonstress test measures the response of the fetal heart rate to fetal movement. For the test, following a good explanation of the procedure, the mother is placed in a semi-Fowler's position (either in a comfortable lounge chair or an examining table with an elevated back rest) to prevent supine hypotension syndrome (Figure 15-3). An external fetal heart rate monitor is attached abdominally. The woman is asked to report any fetal movement while fetal heart sounds are recorded on a rhythm strip; she can do this by pressing a button to enter a notation on the rhythm strip. When the fetus moves, the fetal heart rate should increase, just as anyone's heart rate increases with exercise. It should decrease again as the fetus quiets. No variability in heart rate to fetal movement suggests poor placental perfusion or that the fetus is at risk in utero.

The woman is monitored until two fetal movements have occurred. The test is *reactive* if two accelerations of fetal heart rate (an increase of 15 beats or higher) lasting for 15 seconds' time occur within any 10-minute time period. The fetal heart rate variability should be six beats per minute or greater. It can be predicted that for 7 days following a reactive test an infant will do well in utero or will be healthy at birth. The test is *nonreactive* if no accelerations occur within 40 minutes or if there is low fetal heart rate variability (under 6 beats per minute) throughout the testing period.

If a 10-minute time period passes without any fetal movement, the mother may be given an oral carbohydrate snack. This increases her blood glucose level and usually causes fetal movement in a well fetus. If a nonstress test is nonreactive, additional fetal assessment, such as an oxytocin challenge test (OCT), must be undertaken to further assess fetal well-being. A delivery decision to remove the fetus from the intrauterine environment may also be made.

Contraction Stress Testing (CST)

Stress testing involves using the response of the fetal heart rate to uterine contractions to assess whether the fetus is receiving adequate oxygen in utero and to assess whether the fetus will be able to do well during labor.

Rhythm Strip Testing

Normally, a fetal heart rate slows with the beginning of a uterine contraction as the oxygen supply to the fetus is compromised and slight fetal myocardial hypoxia occurs. If the placenta is functioning well, however, as the uterine contrac-

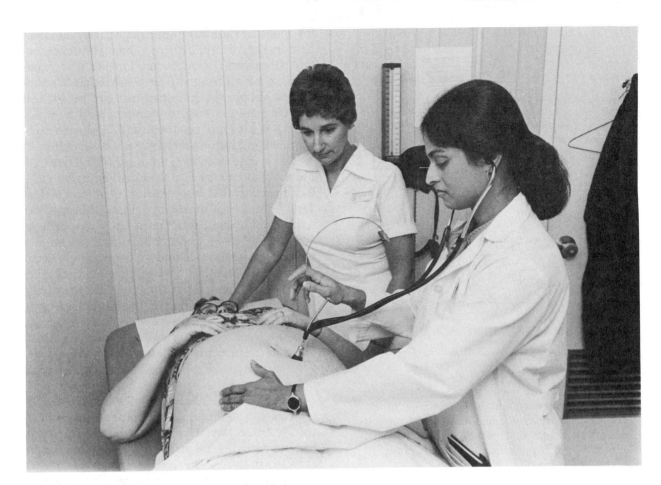

Figure 15-1 *Auscultation of fetal heart sounds by use of a stethoscope.*

Figure 15-2 *A Doppler instrument detects and broadcasts the fetal heart rate so the parents-to-be as well as you can hear and count it.*

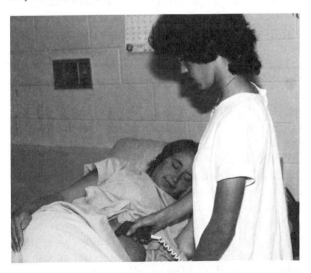

tion ends, the fetal heart rate rises immediately to its precontraction level.

A fetal heart rate that dips late into the contraction and stays down past the end of the contraction (termed *late deceleration*) is a sign that the placenta is not functioning adequately.

Although they are not noticeable by the mother until late in pregnancy, Braxton Hicks, or very light, uterine contractions are present as early as the twelfth week of pregnancy. The fetal heart rate may be assessed in connection with these. Braxton Hicks contractions can be increased in frequency and strength if the woman gently rolls her breast nipples between her fingers for about 5 minutes. This action releases oxytocin, which strengthens the contractions.

A stress test is considered negative if there is no late deceleration with three contractions during any 10-minute time "window." A *negative* test denotes that the placenta is adequate and probably will be adequate for at least 1 more week. A test is *positive* if late decelerations occur with over 50 percent of contractions. Tests may also be interpreted as *suspicious* (there was some

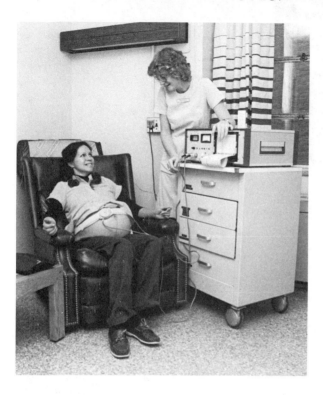

Figure 15-3 *A nonstress test is the recording of the fetal heart rate in association with fetal movements. Here the test is being done on an ambulatory basis. (Courtesy of the Department of Medical Photography, Children's Hospital, Buffalo, N.Y.)*

late deceleration, but the pattern was not persistent), *hyperstimulation* (contractions were so close together than even a fetus with a well-functioning placenta would have late decelerations), or *unsatisfactory* (for some reason, the monitor recording was not adequate for interpretation). Remember that these tests are interpreted based on medical criteria—a "positive" result denotes the finding of pathology not the finding of encouraging wellness—which means the results will have to be carefully interpreted for the mother.

Oxytocin Challenge Testing (OCT)

Women are asked to eat a full meal before they come for an OCT because a full stomach quiets a fetus along with bowel sounds. A woman is placed in a semi-Fowler's position (not flat, so hypotension is avoided). A baseline blood pressure and pulse rate are obtained.

OCT tests may be done in pregnancy as early as the twenty-eighth week of gestation. External fetal and uterine monitors are placed on the woman's abdomen, and a baseline recording is made

for about 10 minutes of uterine activity and fetal baseline heart rate. If there is enough uterine activity (Braxton Hicks contractions) so that a contraction is occurring at a rate of three per 10 minutes, a simple rhythm strip test can be done. If contractions are fewer in number, a dilute intravenous solution of oxytocin will be started until uterine contractions are three per 10 minutes.

The woman's blood pressure and pulse rate must be taken every 10 minutes during an OCT to be certain that hypotension is not occurring. The woman can be assured that, although she will have uterine contractions, they will be light enough not to be extremely painful (more of a feeling of pressure). If tetanic contractions occur (contractions coming so close together that there is no room for placenta filling between them), the oxytocin infusion should be turned off immediately, the woman turned on her left side (to free the vena cava and cause a large return of blood to the placenta for better oxygenation), oxygen administered by mask, and a physician notified.

Oxytocin challenge tests offer a great deal of information about fetal well-being. A test is *positive* if three late decelerations occur in a 10-minute period. Fetal stress caused by this simple exercise indicates the fetus will not be able to remain safely in utero much longer; plans for delivery must be undertaken. This fetus would be compromised to a point of injury during labor, however, when contractions are much longer and much more frequent than those created in the test. Some infants will be delivered by cesarean birth so as not to be stressed by labor; in other instances, a woman may be able to deliver vaginally as long as she lies in a lateral position during labor (the position that increases blood flow to the placenta) and has oxygen administered by mask during labor. OCTs are contraindicated for women who have a placenta previa (a placenta covering the cervical os), multiple pregnancy, premature rupture of the membranes, incompetent cervix, or a previous classical cesarean birth. In these women, the possibility of initiating labor by beginning even a dilute solution of oxytocin is too great a risk. The woman should plan on the test taking about 2 hours. Uterine and fetal monitors are left in place until uterine contractions have quieted again to three or fewer contractions per 10 minutes so there is no danger that continuing contractions will lead to labor and delivery after the woman returns home.

Uterine contractions are strong enough during an OCT to cause discomfort. Teach the woman abdominal breathing or encourage her to use another prepared childbirth method before the procedure. This can make the experience a positive "rehearsal" for real labor. Because an OCT carries so much more risk to the fetus than a rhythm strip or a nonstress test, these methods are usually given preference today.

X-Ray Films

X-rays must always be used with caution during pregnancy because of their known teratogenic effects. Aside from being contraindicated unless they can supply information that cannot be established in any other way, fetal X-ray films are grossly unreliable for estimating fetal age or assessing fetal health. Fetal X-ray examination at term may be helpful in determining maturity. If the distal femoral and proximal tibial epiphyses are both present, the fetus is undoubtedly mature.

X-ray may be used to establish fetal death. Between 48 and 72 hours after death, fetal skull bones override, and the spine becomes extremely curved. If a radiopaque substance is introduced into the amniotic fluid and none of it appears in the fetal intestinal tract within 12 to 24 hours, the fetus either has an obstructing esophageal atresia that prevents swallowing or may be presumed to be dead.

Amniography, an injection of a contrast medium into the amniotic fluid followed by X-ray examination, may be done to localize the placenta. A medium such as Ethiodan coats the fetal skin and so will show soft tissue abnormalities such as meningocele on the film.

Nuclear Magnetic Resonance (NMR)

Although NMR scanning equipment is not yet available in all cities, it is predicted that by 1990 NMR will be a common scanning method for soft-tissue abnormalities (Barber, 1984). NMR uses a computerized axial tomographic (CAT) scanner with a magnetic field substituted for the X-ray tube. The technique has the potential to offer a much more striking gray matter-white matter contrast than even the very best CAT scanners. The pelvis is particularly well imaged by NMR. As the technique apparently causes no harmful effects to the fetus (although extensive testing has not yet been done), NMR has the potential to replace or complement sonography as a fetal assessment technique.

Sonography

In a sonogram technique, intermittent sound waves of high frequency (above the audible range) are projected toward the mother's uterus by a transducer. The sound frequencies that bounce back can be displayed on an oscilloscope screen as a visual image; those from tissues of various thicknesses and properties will have different appearances. A permanent record can be made by timed Polaroid photography.

The intricacy of the image obtained depends on the type or mode of process used. *A*-mode scanning measures simple distances or thicknesses only. The monitor reveals a graph showing vertical spikes or waves to illustrate these differences. *B*-mode scanning is shown on the screen as light spots that merge to form a picture of internal organs or the fetus (called *gray-scale imaging*). *B*-mode scanning is the process most frequently used and generally what is meant by a sonogram. *Real-time* mode involves the use of multiple waves, which allows the screen picture to be two dimensional or actually move. This technique is termed *echocardiography* when it is used to study heart movements. On this type of sonogram, you can actually view the fetal heart moving—and even the movement of extremities, such as the fetus bringing a hand up to suck a thumb. A parent who is in doubt that her fetus is well or whole cannot help but be assured by viewing a real-time sonogram.

Sonography may be used early in pregnancy to diagnose the pregnancy (as early as 6 weeks' gestation age). Later in pregnancy it can be used to confirm the presence, size, and location of the placenta and to establish that the fetus is increasing in size. It may be used at term to predict maturity by measurement of the biparietal fetal head or fetal abdominal circumference diameters.

A placenta changes in the amount and contour of basal and chorionic plate substance as it ages; based on these changes it is possible to grade a placenta from 0 to 3 or document its maturity by sonogram (Grannum, 1979). When a placenta is mature (grade 3), fetal pulmonary function is also likely to be mature, so placental grading can be an additional method for predicting fetal lung maturity. This art is too imprecise at present, however, to replace analysis of L/S ratio for fetal lung maturity (Quinlan, 1982).

Sonography diagnoses the pregnancy by demonstrating the presence of a gestational sac (Figure 15-4). At almost the same time (8 to 9 weeks of pregnancy), movement of the fetal heart can be demonstrated by real-time mode. Sonography can be used to assess fetal well-being by identifying the fetal heartbeat at any point in pregnancy although this will not be common practice until sonography is proven to have no effect on the fetus. Various growth anomalies, such as hydrocephalus, anencephaly, and spinal cord defects,

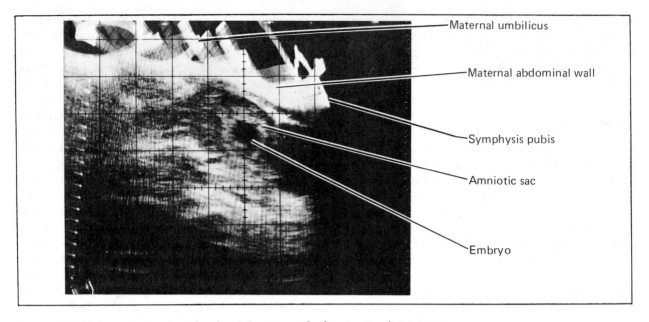

Figure 15-4 *Sonogram showing the characteristic circle diagnostic of pregnancy.*

can be detected on sonogram. Complications of pregnancy, such as the presence of an IUD, hydramnios or oligohydramnios, ectopic pregnancy, missed abortion, abdominal pregnancy, placental previa, premature separation of the placenta, coexisting uterine tumors, and multiple pregnancy, can all be revealed by this method. Fetal death is manifested by the lack of heart beat and respiratory movement on a real-time scan. Just prior to delivery, a sonogram may be used to establish the presentation and position of the fetus. Following birth, sonogram may be used to detect a retained placenta or poor uterine involution.

Sonography allows a health care provider to predict the maturity of the fetus by measuring the biparietal diameter (side to side measurement) of the fetal head on the permanent record. This may be determined as early as the thirteenth week of pregnancy. Thompson et al. (1965) have determined that when the biparietal diameter of the fetal head is 8.5 cm or more, in 90 percent of pregnancies the infant will weigh more than 2,500 gm (5½ pounds). A biparietal diameter of 9.8 cm is accepted as a fetus at mature growth. Serial sonograms which demonstrate a fetal head is growing at 3 mm/week before the thirty-second week of pregnancy and 1.8 mm/week thereafter demonstrate healthy intrauterine growth (O'Sullivan, 1976).

An additional method for estimating fetal weight is to measure the fetal abdominal circumference at the level of the umbilical vein and liver on the sonogram (Campbell & Wilkin, 1975). Table 15-1 shows birthweights that can be pre-

dicted from such a measurement. Until the long-term effects of sonography are known, this will not be a routine measurement of fetal well-being, but it is helpful if fetal growth retardation is suspected or a decision for delivery must be made.

Table 15-1 Birthweight from Abdominal Circumference Scans

AC (cm)	Estimated Birthweight (g)
21	900
22	1,030
23	1,180
24	1,340
25	1,510
26	1,690
27	1,880
28	2,090
29	2,280
30	2,490
31	2,690
32	2,900
33	3,100
34	3,290
35	3,470
36	3,640
37	3,700
38	3,920
39	4,020
40	4,100

Source: Campbell, S., & Wilkin, D. (1975). Ultrasound measurement of fetal abdominal circumference in estimation of fetal weight. *Br. J. OB/GYN, 82,* 689.

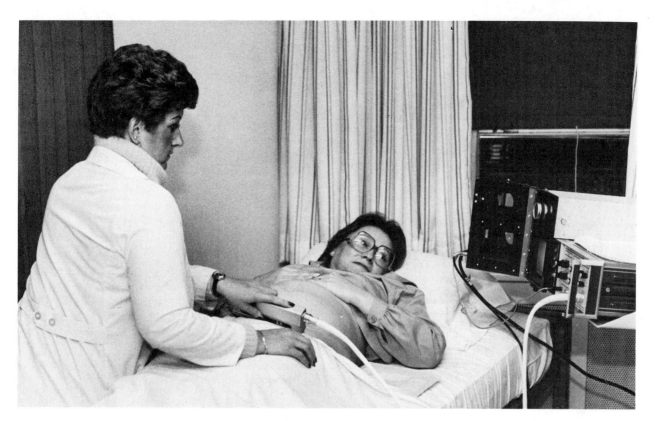

Figure 15-5 *A sonogram being recorded. The mother is watching the screen display of uterine contents. (Courtesy of the Department of Medical Photography, Children's Hospital, Buffalo, N.Y.)*

For a sonogram study, the mother needs to be given a good explanation of what will happen and that this process does not involve X-ray. Comparing it to the same process by which radar detects submarines may be helpful (it is the same process). It is safe for the father of the child to remain in the room during the test, as opposed to an X-ray examination. In order for the sound waves to reflect best, the mother needs a full bladder at the time of the procedure. To ensure this, she should drink a full glass of water every 15 minutes beginning an hour and a half before the procedure and then be certain not to void preprocedure. For the actual procedure, the mother lies on an examining table and is draped for privacy, but with her abdomen exposed (place a folded towel under her right buttock to tip her body slightly, which rolls the uterus away from the vena cava and prevents supine hypotension syndrome). A medium such as mineral oil is applied to her abdomen to improve the contact of the transducer (be certain this is at room temperature or even slightly warmer or you can cause uncomfortable uterine cramping). The transducer is then placed on her

abdomen and moved both horizontally and vertically until the uterus and its contents are fully scanned (Figure 15-5).

Although sonography appears to be safe for both mother and fetus, few long-term effects are yet known. A recent study of these long-term effects reports that children who had a sonogram done while they were in utero have a higher incidence of dyslexia (a learning disability) and an increased number of hospitalizations by the time they are 12 years old than children who did not have an intrauterine sonogram (Stark, 1984). Researchers in this study were unable to document the reason for the intrauterine sonograms so the fact that these children's mothers may have had high-risk status (the reason for the sonogram) may be the cause of the neurologic difficulties, not the sonogram. The procedure is done with caution, and only when necessary, until the long-term effects of sonograms are fully known. It appears to involve no discomfort for the fetus, and the only discomfort for the mother is that the contact lubricant must be applied to her abdomen at the beginning of the scan (she may interpret

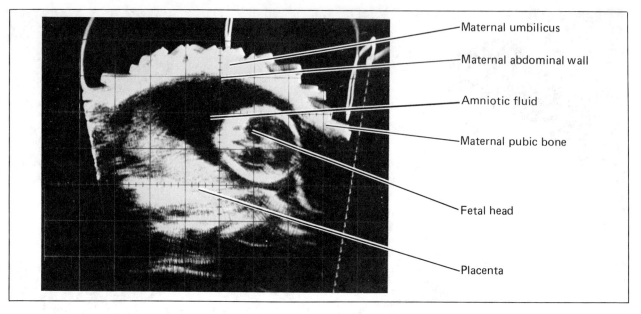

Figure 15-6 *A sonogram at 39 weeks' gestation. The biparietal diameter of the fetus measures only 7.7 cm. There is more amniotic fluid present than normal (hydramnios). The abdominal wall appears shaggy because of the scanning technique. (Courtesy of Richard W. Munschauer, M.D., Children's Hospital, Buffalo, N.Y.)*

this as messy) and she may experience a strong desire to void before the scan is completed.

If Polaroid photographs are taken of the sonogram image, ask if the mother can have one for her baby book. Bonding may be hazardous in any pregnancy where the fetal outcome is in doubt. As shown in the Nursing Research Highlight below, bonding may be strengthened by the mother's ability to view her baby with a sonogram photo. Having a photo can be sure proof to show a support person, if he was not present for the test, that the pregnancy exists and for the moment, at least, the fetus appears well. Figure 15-6 is a sonogram of a fetus near term.

Nursing Research Highlight

Does Ultrasound Have an Effect on Gravida's Image of Her Fetus?

There is a growing emphasis on encouraging maternal-infant bonding. A woman's mental image of her fetus might be an important component of this interaction; if so, making her perceptions of the fetus visual through a real-time sonogram might have profound effects on the mother-infant relationship. A study conducted by researchers (Kohn, Nelson, and Weiner, 1980) on 100 women referred for ultrasound during pregnancy supported the expectation that visualization of the real-time image affects a woman's perception of her fetus. The effects of the visual experience stabilized impressions of the fetus for most women and gave them a greater sense of attachment; for some this attachment also gave a greater sense of vulnerability with regards to outcome of the pregnancy. The potential effects of real-time ultrasound on maternal-infant bonding could be far-reaching and serve as a powerful new facilitator to the attachment process.

Reference

Kohn, C. L., Nelson, A., & Weiner, S. (1980). Gravida's responses to realtime ultrasound fetal image. *J.O.G.N. Nursing, 9*(2), 77.

Fetoscopy

Actually visualizing the fetus by inspecting it through a fetoscope (an extremely narrow, hollow fiberoptic scope inserted by amniocentesis technique) is helpful in assessing fetal well-being in some instances. Intactness of the spinal column can be confirmed by this method. Biopsies of fetal tissue and fetal blood samples can be removed through a fetoscope for analysis. Elemental surgery such as inserting a polyethylene shunt into the fetal ventricles to relieve hydrocephalus or anteriorly into the fetal bladder to relieve a stenosed urethra can be accomplished. A Polaroid photograph can be taken through the fetoscope as assurance for the parents that their infant is well and perfectly formed.

The sixteenth or seventeenth week of pregnancy is the earliest point in pregnancy that fetoscopy can be performed. For a fetoscopy procedure, the mother is prepared and draped as for amniocentesis (see page 296). A local anesthetic is injected into the abdominal skin. The fetoscope is then inserted following a minor scalpel incision in the skin. If the fetus is very active, to avoid injury by the scope or to provide for better observation, the mother may be administered meperidine (Demerol). This crosses the placenta and sedates the fetus.

Fetoscopy carries a small risk of premature labor (5 to 10 percent). Amnionitis (infection of the amniotic fluid) may occur. As a precaution, the mother may be placed on 10 days of antibiotic therapy following the procedure.

Chorion Vaginal Sampling (CVS)

Chorion vaginal sampling is a method whereby chromosome analysis may be done as early as the fifth week of the pregnancy by cervical aspiration of chorionic cells. This is discussed in Chapter 6.

Amnioscopy

Amnioscopy is visual inspection of the amniotic fluid through the cervix and membranes with an amnioscope (a small fetoscope). This may be done to detect meconium staining. It carries some risk of membrane rupture and initiating premature labor.

Maternal Assessments

Maternal History

The history of the current pregnancy, the woman's general health, the outcome of previous pregnancies, and her health during those pregnancies are good indexes to predict the outcome of a current pregnancy. It is time-consuming to take a thorough initial history, but the potential dangers of, for example, a prediabetic condition or a blood incompatibility make it important to discover such conditions early in pregnancy.

Obtaining thorough initial and interval histories is a task a nurse skilled in interviewing can perform. The benefits of extensive interviewing are always surprising, both in terms of the amount of information that can be gained and in terms of the rapport that being listened to (*really* listened to) establishes with women.

Assay of Urine

Whether or not maternal urine can be assayed depends on the reliability with which it is collected. You often want to instruct a woman how to make the collection correctly and then allow her to collect her own 24-hour urine specimen at home. Other women may be hospitalized for 24 hours for a supervised collection. Either way, the responsibility for giving accurate instructions falls to you.

A 24-hour urine collection begins with a "discard" urine. If a urine is not discarded to begin a collection, you are actually measuring not only all urine the woman produced from 8:00 one morning to 8:00 the next, but also the urine that was in her bladder when you started. If the urine collection begins in the morning, it would include urine that has been in her bladder from the time she went to bed the night before, 8 hours earlier or longer. At the end, therefore, you have a 32-, not a 24-, hour urine. Low estriol levels can be masked by these extra hours of collection time. A fetus in distress would go unrecognized.

Women are often reluctant to discard this first urine and need to be given an explanation of the importance of doing it. Otherwise, they may think that every little bit will help in the analysis and not realize that they are interfering with the analysis by saving this urine.

The beginning of the 24-hour period is timed from the discard urine. If the woman does not remember this step, but times from the first urine she is to save, she will again be compromising the analysis of the specimen. Suppose, for instance, she does not void again for 6 hours following the discard urine. If she times the 24-hour specimen from the first voiding, she is again adding too many hours (24 plus the 6 extra hours since the discard). Following the discard urine, the woman saves all urine for the next 24 hours. She should

Table 15-2 Twenty-Four-Hour Urine Collection

Day 1, 8:00 A.M.	*Day 2, 8:00 A.M.*
Void and *discard* urine, but *time* the beginning of collection from this point. Save all urine passed until 8:00 A.M. of Day 2.	Void at this time (24 hours after beginning) to end collection. Add this specimen as final specimen to collection. If a second 24-hour urine collection is to begin, consider the last specimen from the first collection period the discard specimen for the second collection.

void as closely as possible to the time of the end of the collection (24 hours after the time of the discard specimen). This procedure is summarized in Table 15-2.

Urine should be saved in a clean container furnished by the health care facility laboratory or clean quart jars the woman can supply herself. Be certain to ask the laboratory whether a preservative should be added. Refrigerating urine keeps the bacteria count low and aids analysis. When women move their bowels, they invariably also void. Caution them to always void *before* moving their bowels to avoid loss of urine.

A number of constituents of maternal urine can be assayed to help determine fetal well-being and maturity.

Estriol

Estrogen is produced by the placenta from precursors produced largely from the fetal adrenal glands. Measuring estriol, the breakdown product of estrogen, in urine is a measure of both placental function and fetal well-being.

Estriol secretion rises about a thousand-fold during pregnancy. At the seventh week of gestation, the excretion rate is about 0.4 mg per day; by the twentieth week it is between 1 and 3 mg per day. From the twentieth week to the termination of pregnancy the rate increases even more rapidly, reaching 12 to 50 mg per day at term. Estriol levels fall rapidly when the fetus is in jeopardy or dies. Late in pregnancy (after the thirty-fourth week), a level under 1 mg is usually evidence of a dead fetus; levels between 1 and 4 mg suggest that the fetus is in serious danger. Levels between 4 and 12 mg suggest retarded fetal development.

Since estriol levels in urine are influenced by the efficiency of maternal kidney function, they vary widely from woman to woman. For this reason it is important that a woman who will be depending on assay of estriol levels late in pregnancy have a number of 24-hour urines collected at about the thirtieth week of pregnancy. These will serve as her individual baseline level. Urines being assayed for estriol are often analyzed for creatinine also. Creatinine is the end product of muscle action, and is excreted in uniform rates by the kidneys. If the level of creatinine in the urine specimen is low, either the woman's kidney function is impaired (the fetus and placenta are both fine; the fault is with her kidneys) or part of the 24-hour specimen has been lost. This double check on the intactness of the specimen prevents overreading of the seriousness of low estriol levels.

Estriol levels in maternal urine are typically low in pregnancies in which the fetus is anencephalic (little head and brain development) because the fetus's pituitary does not produce ACTH to stimulate adrenal function so the precursor of estrogen is not produced. Estriol levels may be low in women with pregnancy-induced hypertension or diabetes, demonstrating the poor placenta-blood interchange that is occurring. Estriol levels are not a helpful determination in a fetus who has damage due to Rh incompatibility; with this complication, although the fetus's blood is threatened, the adrenal gland is not impaired. Estrogen production remains high (until, of course, the fetus is so severely compromised that no maintenance of any body function is possible).

Ampicillin causes low excretion of estriol. Women being treated with ampicillin must have estriol levels analyzed with this in mind; the fact that they are currently being treated with ampicillin must be marked clearly on the laboratory slip.

Estriol determinations are helpful in assessing placental health in the fetus who is overdue—that is, has remained in utero more than 2 weeks beyond the calculated due date. As long as estriol secretions remain at a high level, 12 to 50 mg per day, the likelihood is that the birth day was calculated incorrectly and the pregnancy is not truly overdue (or at least, placental function is remaining adequate).

Pregnanediol

The chemical determination of urinary pregnanediol is sometimes of use in determining the efficiency of placental function. Pregnanediol is the breakdown product of progesterone; indirectly, it measures the ability of the placenta to produce progesterone.

A woman with a history of repeated spontaneous premature labor might have this determination made weekly or every 2 weeks during pregnancy. If serial determinations of urinary pregnanediol are consistently lower than normal, progesterone suppository therapy may be indicated. It is inadvisable to give progesterone in large doses in early pregnancy until urinary human chorionic gonadotropin levels are also assayed. If these levels are low, placental growth may be faulty; hence, progesterone therapy to keep the decidua from sloughing off and ending a faulty pregnancy might be ill advised.

Bacteriuria

The urine of women should be screened for asymptomatic bacteriuria during pregnancy by a clean catch sample as a further test of fetal well-being, since there is a higher-than-usual incidence of low-birth-weight infants (27% vs 7–10%) in women with bacteriuria.

Assay of Serum

Determinations of the levels of various hormones in maternal blood are being made more and more frequently as assessments of fetal well-being.

Diamine Oxidase

Diamine oxidase (DAO) is an enzyme that is typically found in high levels in maternal blood during pregnancy. The origin of diamine oxidase is the maternal decidua beneath the placenta. Large amounts of histamine are present in fetal tissue (the same quantity as is present in any rapidly growing tissue such as a tumor or a healing wound). Diamine oxidase is formed from histamine. The level of the enzyme is two or three times above nonpregnancy level by the sixth week of gestation. It reaches 100 units by 11 weeks, 500 units at 21 weeks. If levels of DAO are within the normal range for pregnancy during the first and second trimesters, the fetus is probably actively growing (which is why high levels of histamine are present) and a normal outcome of the pregnancy can be predicted. A level that does not rise suggests improper or retarded fetal growth. Unfortunately, levels of DAO do not fall rapidly enough after fetal distress occurs to be used as a marker of distress in a previously healthy fetus.

Oxytocinase

Oxytocinase is an aminopeptide enzyme apparently produced by the syncytiotrophoblast layer of the placenta. It seems to inactivate maternal oxytocin so that the uterus remains quiet during pregnancy. Assay of maternal levels of oxytoci-nase is an indirect assay of placental function. Levels increase steadily from about the eleventh week of pregnancy until term. They are typically low after a pregnancy becomes postterm.

Alkaline Phosphatase

Alkaline phosphatase is an enzyme originating in the placenta. It is released from placental tissue following injury to the placenta the way heart enzymes are released after heart damage. Assay of maternal plasma for alkaline phosphatase might be helpful if placental infarcts or trauma is suspected.

Human Placental Lactogen

Human placental lactogen (HPL) (also called *chroinoic somatomammotropin hormone*) is an enzyme formed by the syncytiotrophoblast layer of the placenta. Levels of HPL can be detected in maternal plasma as early as the sixth week of gestation. They increase throughout pregnancy until the thirty-sixth week, after which they stay the same until term.

Since the half-life of HPL is short (about 20 minutes) the level decreases rapidly following delivery. It may be used to monitor placental function during pregnancy. A level of under 4 μg per milliliter after 30 weeks' gestation suggests that the placenta is not functioning adequately to support a growing fetus.

Plasma Estriol

Plasma estriol levels rather than urinary estriol levels may be monitored to determine the adequacy of the fetal-placental unit because serum analysis requires only a single puncture and withdrawal of blood, rather than a long 24-hour collection. If kidney function in the woman is impaired, the plasma estriol level (because estriol is not being excreted) will be falsely high.

Electrophoretic Bands

A characteristic electrophoretic protein band appears to be present in over 80 percent of pregnant women during the third trimester of pregnancy. Its function is not well understood, but its absence in some women who deliver congenitally deformed infants is suggestive of its importance to a healthy pregnancy.

Alpha Fetoprotein (AFP)

Alpha fetoprotein (a substance produced by the fetal liver) will be present in the maternal serum if the fetus has an open spinal cord defect. Alpha fetoprotein reaches a peak level at 15 weeks' gestation, then steadily decreases until term. In the future, a screening test for alpha fetoprotein may

Table 15-3 Timing of Amniocentesis Procedures

Reason for Procedure	Timing (weeks)
Chromosome determination	14–16
Rh isoimmunization	20–28
Maturity determination	34–42
Assessment of fetal well-being	34–42
Amniography	20–42

be done routinely on all women during pregnancy.

Amniocentesis

Amniocentesis (from the Latin *amnion* for "sac" and *kentesis* for "puncture") is aspiration of amniotic fluid from the pregnant uterus for examination. It can be done in a physician's office or an ambulatory clinic as early as the fourteenth to sixteenth week of pregnancy. The time during pregnancy at which amniocentesis is done depends on the reason it is being done. These times are shown in Table 15-3.

It is a technically easy procedure, with a failure rate of only about 5 percent. However, it may be very frightening to a woman and not totally without risk to the fetus because it involves penetrating the integrity of the amniotic sac. It can lead to complications in rare instances (under 1% of procedures) such as hemorrhage from penetration of the placenta, infection of the amniotic fluid, puncture of the fetus, and irritation of the uterus, which can initiate labor prematurely.

To prepare for amniocentesis, a woman is asked to void (to reduce the size of the bladder, so that it is out of the field). She lies in a supine position on the examining table and is draped for privacy, but with her abdomen exposed (place a folded towel under her right buttock to tip her body slightly to the left, which moves the uterus off the vena cava to prevent supine hypotension syndrome). Take maternal blood pressure and the fetal heart rate for baseline levels. The position of the fetus, a pocket of amniotic fluid, and the placenta are all located by sonogram. The woman's abdomen is then washed with an antiseptic solution, and the skin is infiltrated with a local anesthetic, causing momentary pain, since abdominal skin is tender. This is the extent of the pain the woman will experience; she may feel a sensation of pressure as the needle for the actual aspiration is introduced. Do not suggest that the woman take a deep breath and hold it as a distraction against pressure; this lowers the dia-

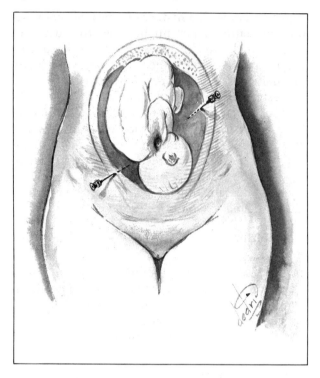

Figure 15-7 *Technique of amniocentesis. The needle is inserted by the back of the fetal neck or by the small body parts after the placenta has been located by a sonogram. (Courtesy of the Department of Medical Illustration, S.U.N.Y. at Buffalo, N.Y.)*

phragm against the uterus and shifts intrauterine contents.

The needle used is a 3 or 4 inch 20 to 22 gauge spinal needle. This is inserted into the abdomen and into the amniotic cavity over the pool of amniotic fluid, carefully avoiding the fetus and placenta (Figure 15-7). A syringe is attached to the needle, and 10 to 20 ml of fluid is withdrawn. The needle is then removed, and the woman rests quietly for a short period. The fetal heart sounds are assessed, and the woman is assured that they are still of good quality. The amniotic fluid is immediately placed in an opaque container so that if bilirubin pigment is present it will not change composition with light. The fluid is then centrifuged to remove blood particles. If the woman has Rh negative blood, RhoGam (Rho[D]immune globulin) may be administered following the procedure. This precaution ensures that maternal antibodies will not form against any placental red blood cells that accidentally were released by puncture of placental villi.

Amniocentesis can reveal information in a number of areas.

Significance of Color

Normal amniotic fluid is as clear as tap water. A yellow tinge to it suggests a blood incompatibility (the yellow resulting from the presence of bilirubin released from the hemolysis of red blood cells). A green color suggests meconium staining or that fetal distress has occurred. Meconium staining in amniotic fluid does not always signal fetal distress but is certainly ominous if in addition the fetal heart rate is below 100 or over 170 beats per minute.

Estriol

The level of estriol in amniotic fluid increases steadily from early pregnancy to term. Late in pregnancy an amniotic fluid level under 100 μg per liter suggests fetal distress.

pH

Acid-base measurements of amniotic fluid provide reliable indications of fetal welfare. Fetal distress from hypoxia results in fetal acidosis due to the rising level of PCO_2 (partial pressure of carbon dioxide). The pH of amniotic fluid is greatly reduced (acidotic) following a fetal death.

Creatinine

Creatinine in amniotic fluid is probably contributed by fetal urine. The amount of creatinine increases progressively as pregnancy advances. A value of 2 mg per 100 ml of fluid is a significant indicator of fetal maturity.

Lecithin/Sphingomyelin (L/S) Ratio

Lecithin and sphingomyelin are the protein components of the lung enzyme surfactant that the alveoli begin to form about the twenty-second to twenty-fourth weeks of pregnancy. When lecithin exceeds sphingomyelin by a 2:1 ratio, fetal lung tissue is mature. Following amniocentesis, the ratio of lecithin to sphingomyelin may be determined quickly by a shake or bubble test, or the specimen may be sent for laboratory analysis.

The Shake Test. To do a shake test, amniotic fluid is placed in a test tube and then diluted with saline; ethanol alcohol is then added and the mixture is shaken. If stable bubbles appear, the L/S ratio is greater than 2:1. If the bubbles are unstable, the L/S ratio is below 2:1—that is, not enough lecithin is present to ensure lung function if the fetus should be delivered at this point.

Laboratory Analysis. More accurate information on lecithin production may be accomplished by laboratory analysis. Lecithin is produced by two pathways. In the early weeks of pregnancy, the route of production (the methyltransferase reaction) is easily interfered with by anoxia or acidosis. The second pathway for lecithin production (the phosphocholine transferase reaction) begins to operate only at about 35 weeks. Usually when the second pathway is fully operative, the fetus is truly ready to be born in terms of lung maturity, as this second pathway is much more stable. Infants of severely involved diabetic mothers may have false mature readings of lecithin because the stress to the infant in utero tends to mature lecithin pathways early. Fetal values must be considered in light of the presence of maternal diabetes, or these infants may be delivered with mature lung function but be immature overall (fragile giants) and so not do well in postnatal life. Some laboratories only interpret an L/S ratio of 2.5:1 or 3:1 as a mature indicator in these infants.

Phosphatidyl Glycerol (PTG)

Phosphatidyl glycerol is an additional phospholipid found in fetal alveoli. Pathways for this compound mature at 36 weeks. When phosphatidyl glycerol is present in amniotic fluid, respiratory distress syndrome will not occur.

Bilirubin Determination

Determining the presence of bilirubin is important when a blood incompatibility is suspected. If the fetal red blood cells are being destroyed by maternal antibodies (as happens with a blood incompatibility), the massive breakdown of red blood cells will release a great deal of indirect bilirubin into the fetal bloodstream. Indirect bilirubin crosses the placenta and is converted by the maternal liver into direct bilirubin, which is then converted into bile and excreted in maternal stool and urine (see Chapter 47 for a full description of blood incompatibility physiology). If the fetus has a high level of indirect bilirubin due to abnormal cell breakdown, the fetus itself begins to convert some indirect bilirubin to direct bilirubin and excretes a portion of it as urobilinogen in urine. As urobilinogen-tainted urine is added to the amniotic fluid, the amniotic fluid becomes yellow in color.

The amount of bilirubin present in amniotic fluid can be analyzed by spectrophotometric analysis. When a monochromatic light is shown on amniotic fluid, the amount of light absorbed depends on the differing amounts of products (bilirubin, protein, uric acid, meconium, etc.) in the fluid. The presence of bilirubin shows a great deal of absorption at a 450 mμ wavelength. If the amounts of light absorbed at wavelengths between 350 and 650 mμ are graphed, this dramatic increase in absorption in bilirubin at 450 mμ is seen as a bulge or lump on the graph.

In the pregnancy without blood incompatibility, bilirubin levels reach a peak at about 24 weeks of pregnancy, and then decline in amount. When none is present any longer, the fetus is assumed to be mature. Specimens of amniotic fluid for bilirubin analysis must be blood-free or the oxyhemoglobin of the blood will show a deceptive 450 mμ bulge (a false positive).

Cell Analysis

A number of epithelial cells are generally obtained by the amniotic fluid sample. When these cells are stained, the proportion of cornified and lipid cells present is revealed. Early in fetal life, basal cells are the major type of cell present. After 32 weeks, precornified cells become apparent; after 36 weeks, cornified cells are present. This form of cell predominates after 38 weeks. At 34 weeks of age, fewer than 1 percent of cells are lipid cells; by 40 weeks, 10 to 50 percent are lipid cells. Over 50 percent lipid cells suggests that the pregnancy is past 40 weeks.

Chromosomes

The study of amniotic fluid for chromosome analysis is done early in pregnancy so that if a significant chromosomal abnormality is detected the woman may choose to abort the fetus. The earliest that there is enough amniotic fluid present to ensure a successful tap is 14 weeks, however. A few fetal skin cells are always present in amniotic fluid. These are the cells to be cultured and stained for chromosomal analysis. It is important that a specimen for chromosome analysis be blood-free, as cells will not grow in bloody fluid. When the cells have grown and are in a mitotic division stage—the stage at which chromosomal contents are best visualized—the cells are stained and examined microscopically. They can be photographed through the microscope, the various chromosome pictures cut out, and the individual chromosomes aligned into a karyotype or chromosome analysis format. The chromosomal diseases that can be detected by prenatal amniocentesis and their significance to health are discussed in Chapter 6.

Inborn Errors of Metabolism

Some inherited diseases that are caused by inborn errors of metabolism can be detected by amniocentesis. In order for a condition to be identified this way, the enzyme defect must be known and must be present in the amniotic fluid as early as 14 to 16 weeks' gestation. Phenylketonuria, for example, a defect that causes serious mental retardation unless the child's diet is carefully controlled, cannot be detected this early in pregnancy because phenylalanine hydroxylase, the defective enzyme, is not present in amniotic fluid this early. Enzyme defects that can be detected in amniotic fluid and their significance to health are also discussed in Chapter 6.

Alpha Fetoprotein

If the fetus has an open spinal cord defect, such as anencephaly or myelomeningocele, alpha fetoprotein will be present in the amniotic fluid because of leakage of cerebrospinal fluid containing the protein into the amniotic fluid. If the defect in the spinal column is fully covered by skin, no alpha fetoprotein may be present in amniotic fluid.

Other Measurements

Amniotic fluid may be tested for protein levels (there is a decrease in protein values as pregnancy advances), and osmolality (osmolar concentration decreases as pregnancy progresses).

In spite of the slight risk associated with amniocentesis, it appears to be the most accurate method available for predicting the maturity of the fetus and certain aspects of fetal well-being, such as the presence or absence of a chromosome abnormality.

Women need support during the procedure, since it is intrusive, there are slight risks involved, and the procedure is a very real "test situation" for them as to whether they are going to have a well newborn or not.

Utilizing Nursing Process

Fetal assessment procedures always carry a level of stress for the woman because no matter how often you explain the situation is not a graded test, the importance of the results to her belies your assurances. In order that assessment procedures can be carried out with the least degree of anxiety, they must be planned and accomplished with the use of nursing process.

Assessment

Assess the level of a woman's knowledge concerning a procedure before it begins: The better informed she is about the procedure, the better she can cooperate and, hopefully, the lower will be her anxiety. Assess anxiety not only by spoken words but by facial tension and other body postures such as clenched fists.

Analysis

The Fourth Conference on Nursing Diagnoses accepted no nursing diagnosis specific for fetal assessment procedures. A number of diagnoses can be easily adapted to the area, however. "Fear related to amniocentesis outcome," "Potential for hypotension syndrome related to lengthy procedure," or "Knowledge deficit, related to 24-hour urine collection" are common diagnoses used. When establishing goals, be certain they are realistic for the circumstances. Fetal assessment is always a stress-related procedure so you can never totally reduce fear or anxiety.

Planning

Some fetal assessment procedures such as nonstress tests may be ordered without a lot of lead time so you need to plan on how to orient a woman to a procedure quickly and yet be certain that you have included all the necessary information in the explanation. Much of planning involves determination of the best time to schedule a procedure (when the woman can take time off from work or her support person can be free to be there). Encourage a woman's support person to be present for testing not only as a support person but also as an active participant in decision making. His presence also allows him to share the news of an assessment finding.

Implementation

During a fetal assessment procedure, you need to function in a trifold role: as a support person for the woman, as an observer of the woman's reactions, and as an assistant to the person performing the procedure. As a rule, the person performing the procedure will inform the woman of the steps of the test and what she can expect before they are performed. If the person neglects to do so because of concentration on a step of the procedure, you should undertake informing the woman as part of your support role.

Do not distract with casual conversation. A woman's having to answer casual questions is more annoying than it is therapeutic (and unnecessary, because your presence is supportive in itself). A hand on her shoulder is comforting. Make space if possible for the support person to come closer to the examining table. Helping the woman concentrate on breathing while a needle is inserted may be effective distraction against pain in that this fulfills the principle of gating for pain relief. Use of gating for pain relief during labor is discussed in Chapter 21.

In your second role, you need to observe the woman carefully for signs of discomfort such as increased pulse, pallor, or dizziness and report these to the person performing the procedure. You may be asked to maintain a flowsheet of vital sign levels for a procedure such as amniocentesis.

In your third role as assistant, you will be asked to hand the person performing the procedure any necessary equipment not contained in a prepared tray. If a specimen was obtained from the procedure, be certain that it is handled correctly and forwarded to the correct department, correctly labeled and accompanied by the correct requisition. Specimens should be transported to the correct department as soon as possible; this keeps them from drying and distorting the analysis. Following a procedure such as amniocentesis, the fluid removed is often hand-carried to the proper laboratory to prevent spilling of a specimen that was removed at some degree of risk to the fetus.

Most women want to know the results of procedures immediately. If a technician performed the procedure, no findings may be available until the results are interpreted by a physician. Let the woman know the reason for any delay so she does not interpret reluctance to give her information as knowledge that there is only bad information to give.

Be certain that fetal assessment procedures are recorded in the woman's record. You may need to mention special considerations in the patient's care plan—such as the fact that although she did not appear nervous, she admitted to being more scared than ever before in her life; thus, other nurses will know her facial expression can mask her emotions. They will then not assume she needs less reassurance than she actually does if another procedure is scheduled.

Evaluation

Evaluation of the test outcome should include not only the test results but whether the woman remains in optimum health and whether the fetal health was found to be compromised by the procedure.

Nursing Care Planning

Angie Baco is a 42-year-old woman you meet at a prenatal clinic.
Gestation length: 12 weeks.

Problem Area. Fetal well-being.

Assessment

No medication except aspirin, 10 gm, 2 days ago, for headache. No spotting, falls, radiation since LMP. Nonsmoker. Alcohol consumption, 2 beers/month.

Advised to have an amniocentesis done for genetic studies (aware that she is high-risk for Down's syndrome). States she will have it done to be informed, but will not abort in any event.

Had gestational diabetes with last pregnancy; no symptoms present here yet. Last child weighed 9 lb, 3 oz at birth. Urine negative, negative this pregnancy.

Uterine height, barely palpable above symphysis. Heart tones by Doppler at 130.

Analysis

Potential for chromosomal abnormality related to maternal age and gestational diabetes.

Locus of Decision Making. Shared.

Goal. Patient to be informed about fetal chromosomal structure.

Criteria. Patient to consent to amniocentesis for chromosomal analysis.

Nursing Orders

1. Schedule amniocentesis for 2 weeks (14th week of pregnancy).
2. Give instructions for out-patient procedure (empty bladder).
3. Schedule for glucose tolerance test next week to assess possibility of gestational diabetes with this pregnancy.
4. Mark chart as high-risk for genetic interference (mother 42 years of age), possible large size (last pregnancy 9 lb, 3 oz).
5. Mark chart to instruct in 24-hour urine for estriol collection for baseline at 20–24 weeks of pregnancy.

Questions for Review

Multiple Choice

1. Mrs. Gray is a woman who is asked to submit urine for estriol determination during pregnancy. You would teach her concerning this test:
   a. estriol determinations are based on 24-hour samples.
   b. not to ingest any coffee during the collection period.
   c. to use a clean catch specimen technique.
   d. the specific gravity of the urine should be over 1.010.

2. Which finding in her history would make you question whether she is a good candidate for an accurate estriol determination?
   a. She is being treated with ampicillin for a sore throat.
   b. She had a urinary tract infection last month.
   c. She takes acetylsalicylic acid for occasional headaches.
   d. She has constipation from her iron supplementation.

3. In early pregnancy. Mrs. Gray is scheduled for a sonogram for detection of the gestational sac. As part of your instructions prior to this study, you would tell her
   a. not to drink any fluid 1 hour prior to the study.
   b. to be prepared for a catheter to be inserted prior to the study.
   c. to empty her bladder just prior to the study.
   d. to drink a large amount of fluid prior to the study.

4. Mrs. Gray is scheduled for an amniocentesis. She asks you how the physician can be certain the placenta is not punctured. You would explain:
   a. "Placentas always form on the posterior uterine wall."
   b. "It would not be harmful even if it were punctured."

   c. "The placenta is located first by sonogram."
   d. "It's possible to locate the placenta by auscultation."

5. Which precaution would you take with Mrs. Gray following an amniocentesis?
   a. remind her not to raise her head for 4 hours
   b. assess fetal heart rate and maternal blood pressure
   c. perform a vaginal exam for a ferning pattern
   d. assess for increased abdominal distention

6. Mrs. Gray is asked to observe fetal movements as a fetal assessment technique. You would instruct her regarding this:
   a. to report if she feels no movement for any ½-hour period.
   b. to count only movements that are strong enough to hurt.
   c. to not eat during the 12 hours she counts fetal movements.
   d. fetal movement is influenced by her level of activity.

7. A nonstress test is an assessment test based on what phenomenon?
   a. Braxton-Hicks contractions cause fetal heart rate alterations
   b. fetal heart rate slows in response to a uterine contraction
   c. fetal movement causes an increase in maternal heart rate
   d. fetal heart sounds increase in connection with fetal movement

8. The fetal assessment technique of a rhythm strip refers to
   a. a fetal EKG, as it is affected by glucose stimulation.
   b. a tracing of fetal heart rate in response to uterine contractions.

c. the rhythm of the fetal heart rate compared to maternal pulse.

d. the response of fetal heart rate to oxytocin-stimulated contractions.

Discussion

1. To parents, fetal assessment procedures are always potentially frightening. What would be meaningful support measures you could use to alleviate anxiety during a procedure?

2. Sonography is a fetal assessment technique commonly used. How would you explain this procedure to an expectant couple?

3. Amniocentesis is also a commonly used assessment procedure. What are nursing responsibilities during such a procedure?

Suggested Readings

Afriat, C. (1983). The nurse's role in fetal heart rate monitoring. *Perinatology/Neonatology, 7,* 29.

Barber, H. (1984). Nuclear magnetic resonance (NMR). *Female Patient, 9,* 113.

Beck, C. T. (1980). Patient acceptance of fetal monitoring as a helpful tool. *J.O.G.N. Nursing, 9,* 350.

Bennett, M. (1981). What do we know in advance? Antenatal diagnosis. *Nursing (Oxford), 1,* 907.

Burkart-Jayez, S. F. (1982). The effects of congenital rubella on the neonate. *Journal of Neurosurgical Nursing, 14,* 173.

Campbell, S., & Wilkin, D. (1975). Ultrasound measurement of fetal abdominal circumference in estimation of fetal weight. *British Journal of Obstetrics and Gynecology, 82,* 689.

Coleman, C. A. (1981). Fetal movement counts: An assessment tool. *Journal of Nurse Midwifery, 26,* 15.

Davies, B. L., et al. (1982). Factors in a woman's decision to undergo genetic amniocentesis for advanced maternal age. *Nursing Research, 31,* 56.

Didolkar, S. M., et al. (1981). Tracing the heart's action before birth. *Journal of Cardiovascular and Pulmonary Technology, 9,* 55.

Grannum, P. A., et al. (1979). The ultrasonic changes in the maturing placenta and their relation to fetal pulmonic maturity. *American Journal of Obstetrics and Gynecology, 133,* 916.

Hadlock, F. P., et al. (1982). Fetal head circumference: Accuracy of real-time ultrasound measurements at term. *Perinatology/Neonatology, 6,* 97.

Harisiades, J. P. (1983). Maternal serum AFP screening: A programmatic overview. *Issues in Health Care of Women, 4,* 17.

Hazinski, M. F. (1983). Congenital heart disease in the neonate: Epidemiology, cardiac development and fetal circulation. *Neonatal Network, 1,* 29.

Hibbard, B. M. (1982). Screening for neural tube defects; Results in practice. *Midwife Health Visitor and Community Nurse, 18,* 460.

Ho, E. (1983). Fetal well being . . . the role of preconceptual care and the early and accurate detection of the fetus at risk. *Nursing Mirror, 12,* 156.

Kleinman, C. S., et al. (1980). Prenatal echocardiography. *Hospital Practice, 15,* 81.

McDonough, M., et al. (1981). Parent's response to fetal monitoring. *M.C.N., 6,* 32.

Milne, L. S., et al. (1981). Cognitive and affective aspects of the response of pregnant women to sonography. *Maternal Child Nursing Journal, 10,* 15.

O'Sullivan, M. J. (1976). Acute and chronic fetal distress. *Journal of Reproductive Medicine, 17,* 320.

Patrick, J., et al. (1982). Patterns of gross fetal body movements over 24-hour observation intervals during the last 10 weeks of pregnancy. *American Journal of Obstetrics and Gynecology, 142,* 369.

Pearce, J. M. (1983). The use of ultrasound in the diagnosis of congenital anomalies. *Midwife Health Visitor and Community Nurse, 19,* 82.

Poundstone, W. (1982). Fetal-neonatal monitoring: A new dimension in care. *Perinatology/Neonatology, 6,* 25.

Powell, J. J. (1981). The tragedy of fetal alcohol syndrome. *R.N., 44,* 33.

Quinlan, R. W., & Cruz, A. C. (1982). Ultrasonic placental grading and fetal pulmonary maturity. *American Journal of Obstetrics and Gynecology, 142,* 111.

Rice, N., et al. (1982). Reflections on prenatal diagnosis: The consumer's view. *Social Work in Health Care, 8,* 47.

Sabbagha, R. E., et al. (1982). Obstetric ultrasonography in perspective. *Perinatology/Neonatology, 6,* 53.

Sabbagha, R. E. (1984). Diagnosis and management of fetal growth retardation. *Female Patient, 9,* 128.

Stark, C. R., et al. (1984). Short- and long-term risks after exposure to diagnostic ultrasound in utero. *Obstetrics and Gynecology, 63,* 194.

Thompson, H. W. et al. (1965). Fetal development as determined by ultrasound pulse echo techniques. *American Journal of Obstetrics and Gynecology, 92,* 44.

16

Physiologic Changes in Pregnancy

Following mastery of the contents of this chapter you should be able to:

1. Describe the physiologic changes that occur with pregnancy.
2. Describe the underlying principles for the physiologic changes of pregnancy.
3. Analyze the systemic effects of the physiologic changes of pregnancy.
4. Synthesize knowledge of physiologic changes in pregnancy with nursing process to achieve quality maternal-newborn nursing care.

THE PHYSIOLOGIC CHANGES of pregnancy are healthy extensions of normal biological functions that occur gradually but eventually affect all organ systems of the woman's body. Although such changes are extensive, they are also temporary, for the duration of the pregnancy, and because they are wellness-oriented changes, at the end of pregnancy the woman's body returns virtually to her prepregnant state. These changes enable her to provide oxygen and nutrients for the growing fetus and extra nutrients for her own increased metabolism during the pregnancy. They ready her body for labor and delivery, and for lactation if she chooses to breast-feed her baby at the end of pregnancy. Because they are only extensions of normal physiology, and despite the large number of bodily changes, pregnancy is not an ill state but a wellness one.

Changes that occur in the woman can be categorized as *local*, confined to the reproductive organs, or *systemic*, affecting the entire body.

Local Changes

Local changes are those involving the reproductive tract, skin, and breasts.

Reproductive Tract Changes

Uterus

The most obvious alteration in the woman's body during pregnancy is the increase in the size of the uterus that occurs in order to accommodate the growing fetus. Over the 10 lunar months of pregnancy, the uterus increases in length from ap-

proximately 6.5 cm to 32 cm; in depth, from 2.5 cm to 22 cm; and in width, from 4 cm to 24 cm. Its weight increases from 50 to 1,000 gm. At the beginning of pregnancy the uterine wall is about 1 cm thick, and its cavity is barely large enough to hold a 2 ml bulk. As pregnancy begins, the wall first hypertrophies and thickens to about 2 cm. Then it begins to thin, so that by the end of pregnancy it is very supple and about 0.5 cm thick—so thin the presence of a fetus can be palpated easily through it. At term, the increase in size is so extensive that the uterus can hold a 7-pound (3,175 gm) fetus plus 1,000 ml of amniotic fluid, or a total of about 4,000 gm.

This great uterine growth is due to development of the decidua and formation of a few new muscle fibers in the myometrium but the increase in capacity is principally due to the stretching of existing muscle fibers (by the end of pregnancy, muscle fibers in the uterus are two to seven times longer than they were pregestationally). The uterus is able to withstand this stretching of its muscle fibers because of the formation of extra fibroelastic tissue between fibers, which binds them closely together. Because uterine fibers only stretch during pregnancy, and are not built new, the uterus returns to a prepregnant state at the end of the pregnancy with very little difficulty and almost no destruction of tissue (which is why the postpartal period is also a wellness, not an illness time).

The woman becomes aware of the growing uterus by the end of the twelfth week of pregnancy, when it is large enough to be palpated as a firm spheroid under the abdominal wall above the symphysis pubis. An important factor to assess in uterine growth is its *constant, steady, predictable* increase in size. By the twentieth or twenty-second week of pregnancy it reaches the level of the umbilicus. By the thirty-sixth week it touches the xyphoid process and makes breathing difficult. About 2 weeks before term in a primigravida (a woman in her first pregnancy), the fetal head settles into the pelvis preparatory to delivery, and the uterus returns to its height at 32 weeks. This settling is termed *lightening*, because the lung expansion and easier breathing pattern seem to lighten the woman's load. When lightening will occur is not predictable in women during an additional pregnancy. In these women it may not be felt until the morning of delivery.

The fundus of the uterus usually remains in the midline during pregnancy, although it may be pushed slightly to the right side because of the larger bulk of the sigmoid colon on the left. The changes in fundus height during pregnancy are shown in Figure 16-1.

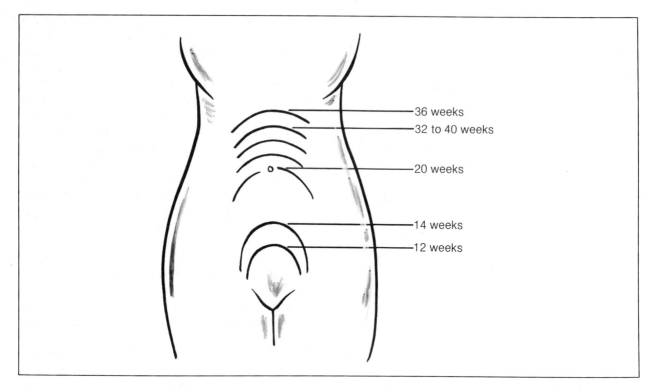

Figure 16-1 *Fundus height at various times during pregnancy.*

As the uterus increases in size, it pushes intestine to the sides of the abdomen and elevates the diaphragm at term. A slender woman may worry that there is not enough room inside her abdomen for the uterus to increase in size as it should and her baby will feel crowded. She can be assured that abdominal contents can be shifted readily to accommodate the size of the uterus (Figure 16-2).

Uterine blood flow increases during pregnancy as the placenta grows and requires more and more blood volume for perfusion. Before pregnancy, uterine blood flow is at the rate of 15 to 20 ml per minute. By the end of pregnancy, it is as much as 500 to 750 ml per minute with 75 percent of that volume going to the placenta. One sixth of the total body blood supply is circulating through the uterus (which is why vaginal bleeding in pregnancy is always potentially serious: one sixth of the blood supply could be lost if uterine bleeding is occurring).

Cervix

During pregnancy, in response to the increased level of circulating estrogen, the cervix of the uterus becomes more vascular and edematous. The increased fluid between cells causes it to soften in consistency. The increased vascularity causes it to darken in color from a pale pink to a violet hue. The glands of the endocervix undergo

both hypertrophy and hyperplasia as they increase in number and distend with mucus. A tenacious mucus plugs or obliterates the cervical canal. This mucous plug, the *operculum*, seals out bacteria during pregnancy and helps prevent infection in the fetus and membranes.

Softening of the cervix is so extensive that the consistency of a nonpregnant cervix may be compared to that of the nose; the consistency of a pregnant cervix more closely resembles that of an earlobe. This softening is so marked it is one of the diagnostic signs of pregnancy (Goodell's sign). Just prior to beginning labor the cervix can be described as having the consistency of butter; it is "ripe" for delivery.

Vagina

An increase in the vascularity of the vagina, beginning early in pregnancy, parallels the vascular changes in the uterus. The resulting increase in circulation changes the color of the vagina from its normal light pink to a deep violet. Under the influence of estrogen the vaginal epithelium and underlying tissue become hypertrophic and enriched with glycogen; they loosen from their connective tissue attachment in preparation for great distention at birth. This increase in the activity of the epithelial cells results in a white vaginal discharge throughout pregnancy.

The secretions of the vagina during pregnancy

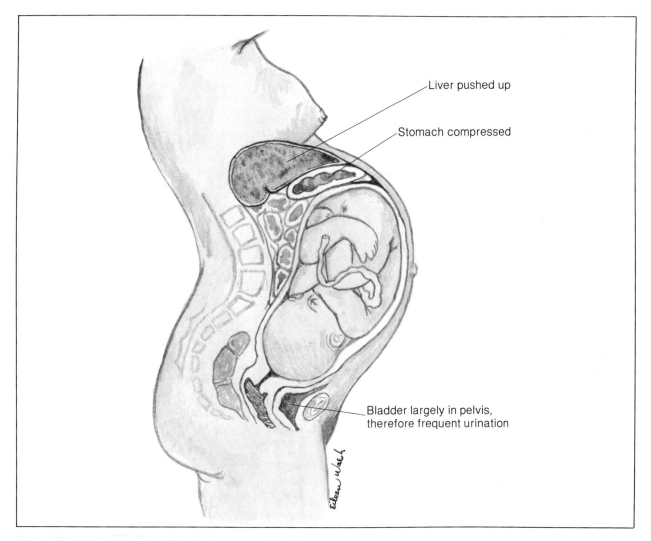

Liver pushed up

Stomach compressed

Bladder largely in pelvis, therefore frequent urination

Figure 16-2 *Crowding of abdominal contents late in pregnancy.*

fall to a pH of 4 or 5 (due to an increased lactic acid content caused by the *Lactobacillus acidophilus*, which grows freely in the increased glycogen environment) and therefore are resistant to bacterial invasion. This change in pH unfortunately favors the growth of *Candida albicans*, a species of yeast-like fungi. A candidal infection is manifested by an itching, burning sensation in addition to a cream cheese-like discharge. A nonpregnant woman needs medication for such an infection to relieve discomfort. A pregnant woman needs medication not only to relieve discomfort but to prevent transmission of the infection to an infant passing through the birth canal at term. Candidal infection is manifested as *thrush* (oral *Monilia*) in the infant.

Many women are reluctant to mention that they have an infection in this part of their body or mistake the excessive discharge of a monilial infection for the normal increase of mucus of preg-

nancy. Make it a nursing responsibility to inquire whether any symptoms of this nature exist at all prenatal health assessments.

Ovaries

Ovulation stops with pregnancy, as does menstruation, because of lack of activity of follicle-stimulating hormone; this is due to the active feedback mechanism of estrogen-progesterone being produced by the corpus luteum early in pregnancy, the placenta late in pregnancy. A small number of women (about 20%) may notice some vaginal spotting at the point that progesterone-estrogen secretion shifts to the placenta (9 to 12 weeks of pregnancy).

On the surface of the ovary the corpus luteum continues to increase in size until about the twelfth week of pregnancy, when the placenta has taken over as the chief provider of progesterone and estrogen. At this point, the corpus luteum, no

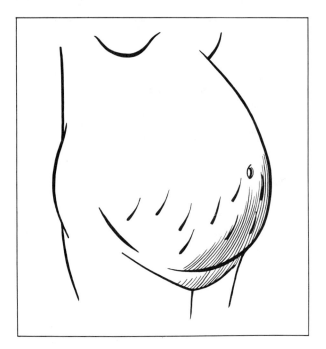

Figure 16-3 *Striae gravidarum. In the later months of pregnancy, reddish, slightly depressed streaks often develop in the skin of the abdomen and sometimes of the breasts and thighs. Following pregnancy, these fade to glistening silvery lines.*

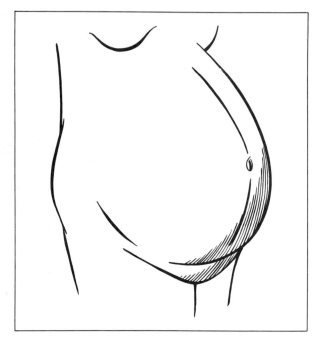

Figure 16-4 *Linea nigra. In many pregnancies, the abdominal skin at the midline becomes markedly pigmented, assuming a brownish-black color.*

longer essential for the continuation of the pregnancy, begins to regress in size.

Skin Changes

As the uterus increases in size, the abdominal wall must stretch to accommodate it. This stretching (and possibly increased adrenal cortex activity) causes rupture and atrophy of small segments of the connective layer of the skin, and pink or reddish streaks (*striae gravidarum*) usually appear on the sides of the abdominal wall and sometimes on the thighs (Figure 16-3). In the weeks following delivery, the striae gravidarum lighten to a silvery-white color (lineae albicantes or striae atrophicae) and are barely noticeable.

Occasionally, the abdominal wall cannot stretch enough, and the rectus muscles actually separate, a condition known as *diastasis*, which will be manifested after pregnancy as a bluish groove at the site of separation.

The umbilicus is stretched by pregnancy to the extent that by the twenty-eighth week it is usually pushed so far outward that its depression becomes obliterated and smooth. In some women it tends to appear as if it has turned inside out and protrudes as a round bump at the center of the abdominal wall.

Extra pigmentation generally appears on the

abdominal wall. A brown or black line (*linea nigra*) may be present, running from the umbilicus to the symphysis pubis and separating the abdomen into a right and left hemisphere (Figure 16-4). Darkened brown areas may appear on the face, particularly on the cheeks and across the nose. This is known as *melasma* (chloasma), or the "mask of pregnancy." The increases in pigmentation are due to melanocyte-stimulating hormone (MSH) secreted by the hypophysis (pituitary). With the fall in the level of the hormone after pregnancy, the areas lighten and disappear.

Vascular spiders (small, fiery-red branching spots) are sometimes seen on the skin of pregnant women, particularly on the thighs. These probably result from the increased level of estrogen in the body. They fade but do not necessarily disappear completely following pregnancy.

There is an increase in the activity of sweat glands throughout the body. This may be manifested as an increase in perspiration that can become annoying by the end of pregnancy.

Breast Changes

Subtle changes in the breasts that occur due to the effect of estrogen-progesterone may be some of the first physiologic changes of pregnancy the women notices. She may experience a feeling of fullness or tingling, due to the increased stimulation of breast tissue by the high estrogen level in the body. As pregnancy progresses, the breast size increases because of hyperplasia of the mammary alveoli and fat deposits. The areola of the nipple darkens in color and its diameter increases from about 3.5 to 5 or 7.5 cm (1½ to 2 or 3 inches). There is additional darkening of the skin surrounding the areola in some woman, forming a secondary areola. As vascularity of the breasts increases, blue veins may become prominent over the surface. The sebaceous glands of the areola (Montgomery's tubercles) enlarge and become protuberant.

Early in pregnancy the breasts begin readying themselves for the secretion of milk. By the sixteenth week, *colostrum,* a thin, watery, high-protein fluid and the precursor of breast milk, may be expelled from the nipples.

Systemic Changes

Although the physiologic changes a woman notices first and is apt to find most interesting are those of the reproductive system and breasts, changes do occur in almost all body systems.

Respiratory System

The increased level of progesterone during pregnancy appears to set a new level in the hypothalamus for acceptable blood carbon dioxide levels (PCO_2), as during pregnancy a woman's body tends to maintain a partial pressure of CO_2 at closer to 32 mm Hg than the normal 40 mm Hg.

This low PCO_2 level in the mother causes a favorable CO_2 gradient at the placenta (the total CO_2 level in the fetus is higher than that in the mother), so CO_2 crosses readily from the fetus to the mother.

To keep the mother's pH level from becoming acidotic from the load of CO_2 shifted to her by the fetus, increased ventilation (mild hyperventilation) to blow off carbon dioxide begins early in pregnancy. Ventilation capacity rises by as much as 40 percent by term. The increased ventilation may be so extreme that the woman develops a respiratory alkalosis. In compensation, plasma bicarbonate is excreted by the kidneys in larger than normal amounts. With greater urine output, additional sodium is lost and therefore additional water. The effect is *polyuria,* an early sign of pregnancy.

The change in CO_2 level and the compensating mechanisms can be described as a chronic respiratory alkalosis fully compensated by a chronic metabolic acidosis.

As the uterus enlarges during pregnancy, a great deal of pressure is put on the diaphragm and ultimately on the lungs. The diaphragm may be displaced by as much as 1 inch upward. This crowding of the chest cavity causes an acute sensation of shortness of breath late in pregnancy, until lightening relieves the pressure.

Even with all the other respiratory changes happening, *vital capacity* (the maximum volume exhaled following a maximum inspiration) of the woman does not change during pregnancy. Although lungs are crowded in the vertical dimension, they can expand horizontally, and the woman expands her rib cage further with each inspiration. *Residual volume* (the amount of air remaining in the lungs following expiration) is decreased by the pressure of the diaphragm up to 20 percent. *Tidal volume* (the volume of air inspired) is increased up to 40 percent as the woman draws in extra volume to increase the effectiveness of air exchange. Total oxygen consumption increases up to 20 percent.

The net effect of these respiratory changes is often felt by the woman as a chronic shortness of breath. She needs to take a deep breath periodically or sit down to "catch her breath." She waits for her breathing rate to slow in a sitting position and is concerned that it does not. Women need a clear explanation that a breathing rate more rapid than normal (18 to 20 breaths per minute) is physiologic for pregnancy. When you are taking vital signs on a pregnant woman, you should also remember that the respiratory rate is normally elevated.

The slight increase in pH due to the increased expiratory effort slightly increases the binding capacity of maternal hemoglobin and so the oxygen content of maternal blood (the level of PO_2) rises from a normal level of about 92 mm Hg to a level of 106 mm Hg early in pregnancy.

Another change that often occurs in the respiratory system is marked congestion or "stuffiness" of the nasopharynx, a response to increased estrogen levels. Women may worry that this stuffiness indicates an allergy or a cold. Some women take over-the-counter cold medications or antihistamines to try to relieve the congestion before they realize that they are pregnant. Some continue to take the medication, not mentioning it to their physician because they think it is a separate problem and not pregnancy-related. Asking a woman at prenatal visits if she is taking any kind of medicine or if she has noticed or been bothered by nasal stuffiness is a nursing responsibility.

Changes in respiratory function during pregnancy are summarized in Table 16-1.

Table 16-1 Respiratory Changes During Pregnancy

Vital capacity	No change
Tidal volume	Increased
Respiratory rate	Increased
Residual volume	Decreased
Plasma PCO$_2$	Decreased
Plasma pH	Increased
Plasma PO$_2$	Increased
Respiratory minute volume	Increased
Expiratory reserve	Decreased

Temperature Regulating System

Early in pregnancy there is a slight increase in temperature, because of the progesterone activity of the corpus luteum (the temperature elevation that marked ovulation is sustained). As placental function is substituted for that of the corpus luteum at about 16 weeks, the temperature generally decreases to normal.

Some women associate this slight rise in temperature (99.6°F [37.6 C] orally) together with the nasal congestion of pregnancy as a sure sign that they have a cold and need medication.

Circulatory System

Changes in the cardiovascular system are extremely significant to the health of the fetus: They are important for adequate placental and fetal circulation.

Blood Volume

To provide for an adequate exchange of nutrients at the placenta and for fluid to compensate for blood loss at delivery, the circulatory blood volume of the woman's body increases at least 30 percent (possibly as much as 50 percent) during pregnancy. Blood loss for a normal vaginal delivery is about 300 to 400 ml. Blood loss from a cesarean birth is higher, between 800 to 1,000 ml. The increase in blood volume is gradual, beginning by the end of the first trimester. It reaches its peak at about the twentieth to the twenty-fourth week and continues at this high level through the last trimester. As the plasma volume first increases, the concentration of hemoglobin and erythrocytes may decline, giving the woman a pseudoanemia. Her body compensates for this change by producing more red blood cells, so that the concentration of red blood cells reaches normal levels again by the second trimester.

Almost all women need some iron supplementation during pregnancy due to a variety of fac-

tors. They usually have comparatively low iron stores (less than 500 mg) because of their monthly menstrual loss. The fetus requires about 350 to 400 mg of iron in order to grow. The increases in the circulatory maternal red cell mass require an additional 400 mg of iron. This is a total increased need of about 800 mg. As the average woman's store of iron is less than this (about 500 mg), and iron absorption may be impaired during pregnancy due to decreased gastric acidity (iron is absorbed best from an acid medium), she should take in additional iron during pregnancy or she will develop a true anemia.

A hemoglobin concentration less than 10.5 gm per 100 ml, or a hematocrit value below 30 percent, is generally considered a true anemia for which iron therapy above normal supplementation is advocated. Folic acid requirement also increases during pregnancy, and a lack can cause megalohemoglobinemia (large, nonfunctioning red blood cells).

In order to handle the increase in blood volume in the circulating system, a woman's cardiac output increases significantly, by 25 to 50 percent, an increase in heart rate of 10 beats per minute. Like the circulating volume increase, the bulk of the cardiac work increase occurs during the second trimester, a small amount occurring in the last trimester. This rise in circulating load has implications for the woman with cardiac disease. A heart that has difficulty moving a woman's normal circulating load may be overwhelmed by the requirements placed on it by pregnancy. The average woman's heart has great ability to adjust to these changes, however. Although significant changes are occurring inside her related to her circulatory system, she is not even aware that they are happening.

Because the diaphragm is elevated by the growing uterus late in pregnancy, the heart is shifted to a more transverse position in the chest cavity. The heart may then appear enlarged on X-ray examination. Some women have audible functional (innocent) heart mumurs during pregnancy, probably because of the altered heart position.

During the last trimester of pregnancy, blood flow to the lower extremities is impaired by the pressure of the expanding uterus on veins and arteries, which slows circulation. This decrease in blood flow in the venous system leads to edema and varicosities of the vulva, rectum, and legs.

Palpitations

Palpitations of the heart are not uncommon, particularly on quick motion, during pregnancy. A woman should be warned that palpitations may

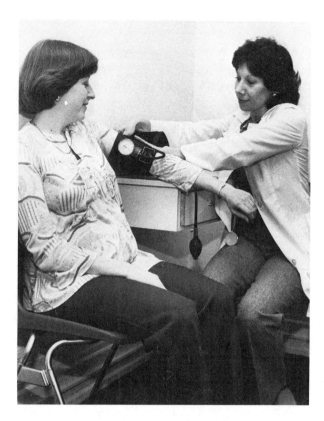

Figure 16-5. *Blood pressure determination is an important assessment during pregnancy.*

Table 16-2 Average Blood Pressures in American Females

	Age	White Women Average (mm Hg)	S.D.	Black Women Average (mm Hg)	S.D.
Systolic	Under 20	111.0	13.7	112.7	13.2
	20–29	116.9	13.8	119.1	14.7
	30–39	121.4	16.3	128.1	20.2
	40–49	129.3	19.6	138.3	22.8
Diastolic	Under 20	69.3	9.8	70.0	10.1
	20–29	73.7	7.2	75.4	9.7
	30–39	76.9	10.7	82.0	13.0
	40–49	80.6	11.6	86.9	13.9

S.D. = standard deviation.

Source: Adapted from Stamler, J. J., et al. (1976). Hypertension screening of one million Americans. *Journal of the American Medical Association, 235,* 2299. Copyright 1976, American Medical Association.

occur, so that she will not be frightened when they do. Palpitations in the early months of pregnancy are probably due to sympathetic nervous system stimulation; in later months, they may result from increased thoracic pressure caused by pressure of the uterus against the diaphragm.

Blood Pressure

Despite the hypervolemia of pregnancy, the blood pressure does not normally rise, as the increased heart action takes care of the greater amount of circulating blood.

In many women blood pressure decreases slightly during the second trimester because of the lowered peripheral resistance in the woman's circulation, which is due to the rapidly expanding placenta. During the third trimester, blood pressure rises again to first-trimester levels.

Determining normal blood pressure in pregnant women is as difficult as it is in the population at large (Figure 16-5). Average blood pressures for adult women are shown in Table 16-2. During pregnancy, blood pressure is often reported as mean arterial pressure rather than a more common systolic/diastolic figure. A mean arterial pressure of 90 mm Hg or more in the midtrimester is an ominous sign. A mean arterial pressure above 105 mm Hg in the third trimester is generally regarded as hypertension.

To determine a mean arterial pressure, subtract the woman's diastolic reading from the systolic reading. This difference is the *pulse pressure.* Divide the pulse pressure by one third and add that number to the diastolic pressure. If a woman's blood pressure is 120 over 70, for example, her pulse pressure is 50 (120 − 70). One third of 50 is 16.6. Adding 16.6 to the diastolic reading (70) gives a mean arterial pressure of 86.6, which is a normal mean arterial pressure for a pregnant woman.

If a woman's blood pressure is 140 over 80, her pulse pressure is 60 (140 − 80). One third of 60 is 20. Adding 20 to the diastolic reading (80) gives a mean arterial pressure of 100, which is ominously high for a pregnant woman in the second trimester.

Supine Hypotension Syndrome

When a pregnant woman lies supine, the weight of the growing uterus presses the vena cava against the vertebrae, obstructing blood flow from the lower extremities (Figure 16-6). This causes a decrease in blood return to the heart and consequent immediate hypotension from decreased cardiac output. The woman experiences this as light-headedness, faintness, and heart palpitations. Supine hypotension syndrome can be easily corrected by the woman turning (or you

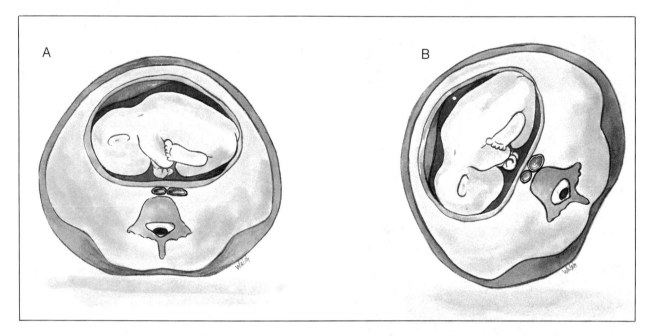

Figure 16-6 *A. During pregnancy, the weight of the uterus can press on the vena cava if a woman lies on her back, limiting the return flow of blood to the heart (hypotensive syndrome). B. If the woman turns to her side, pressure of the uterus is lifted off the vena cava.*

turning her) onto her side to free blood flow through the vena cava. Teach women to always rest on their side rather than their back; even with additional collateral circulation that forms in an effort to lessen the development of the phenomenon, a supine position tends to lead to hypotension.

The Roll-Over Test

Normally, when a woman turns from a prone to a supine position, her blood pressure falls. Interestingly, if a woman is about to develop hypertension of pregnancy (a serious complication of pregnancy), her diastolic blood pressure will show an increase of at least 20 mm Hg when she turns from a side-lying to a supine position. Many physicians include roll-over tests as part of routine health surveillance during pregnancy. This simple test can be done by you as an independent nursing action (directions are given in Chapter 19). It can be helpful in isolating women who will develop hypertension of pregnancy (one of the three most common causes of maternal mortality in pregnancy) before clinical symptoms become apparent. Preventive measures to stop the blood pressure from rising can then be instituted.

Blood Constitution

The level of circulating fibrinogen, a constituent of the blood necessary for clotting, in-creases as much as 50 percent during pregnancy; the clotting factors VII, VIII, IX, and X and the platelet count also rise. All of these changes, which probably result from the increased level of estrogen, form a safeguard against major bleeding should the placenta be dislodged and the uterine arteries or veins open. Total white cell count rises slightly, probably as both a protective mechanism and a reflection of the woman's total blood volume (up to about 15,000 per mm^3). The total protein level of blood decreases, perhaps reflecting the amount of protein needed by the fetus. Because the circulating system has a lowered total protein load with hypervolemia, fluid will readily leave the intravascular spaces to equalize osmotic and hydrostatic pressure. This leads to the very common ankle and foot edema of pregnancy (not to be confused with nondependent edema, which is a symptom of pregnancy-induced hypertension).

Overall, blood lipids increase by a third; cholesterol blood level increases 90 to 100 percent. This latter change provides a ready supply of available energy for the fetus; but, because of its incorporation in bile, a woman who is prone to gallbladder stone formation may form more stones during pregnancy than normally (cholelithiasis).

Changes in the cardiovascular system during pregnancy are summarized in Table 16-3.

Table 16-3 Changes in the Cardiovascular System During Pregnancy

	Prepregnancy	*Pregnancy*
Cardiac output		25–50% increase
Heart rate		10 beats/min increase
Plasma volume (ml)	2,600	3,600
Blood volume (ml)	4,000	5,250
Red cell mass (cu mm)	4,200,000	4,650,000
Leukocytes (cu mm)	7,000	10,500
Total protein (gm %)	7.0	5.5–6.0
Fibrinogen (mg %)	300	450
Blood pressure		Decreases in second trimester; at prepregnancy level in third trimester

Gastrointestinal System

As the uterus increases in size, it tends to displace the stomach and intestines toward the back and sides of the abdomen. At about the midpoint of pregnancy, the pressure may be sufficient to slow intestinal peristalsis and the emptying time of the stomach, leading to heartburn, constipation, and flatulence. Relaxin, a hormone produced by the ovary, may contribute to decreased gastric motility; so may the decrease in blood supply to the gastrointestinal tract (blood is drawn to the uterus). Progesterone also has an effect on smooth muscle, making it less active.

Nausea is one of the first sensations the woman may experience with pregnancy (sometimes before the first missed menstrual period). This is most apparent early in the morning, on rising, or when she becomes fatigued during the day. Known as *morning sickness*, it is probably a systemic reaction to decreased glucose levels, glucose being used in great quantities by the growing fetus, and to increased estrogen levels.

The nausea subsides after the first 3 months, and the woman may acquire a voracious appetite. Although the acidity of the stomach secretions decreases during pregnancy, heartburn may result from the reflux of stomach content into the esophagus, because of the displaced position of the stomach and the relaxed cardioesophageal sphincter.

Decreased emptying of bile from the gallbladder may result in reabsorption of bilirubin into the maternal bloodstream, giving rise to symptoms of generalized itching (subclinical jaundice). A woman with previous gallstone formation may have an increased tendency to stone formation during pregnancy due to an increased cholesterol level and additional cholesterol incorporation into bile. Women with peptic ulcer generally find their condition improved during pregnancy because the acidity of the stomach is decreased.

Some women notice hypertrophy at their gumlines and bleeding of gingival tissue when they brush their teeth. There may be increased saliva formation (hypertyalism). This is probably a local response to increased levels of estrogen—an annoying but not a serious problem. A lower pH of saliva than normal may lead to increased tooth decay if toothbrushing is not continued at the usual pattern. Constructive health teaching reminds women who "expect to be expecting" to keep regular dental checkups so they enter pregnancy with their teeth in good repair.

Our grandmothers expected to lose a tooth a pregnancy, as a growing fetus requires so much calcium to make bones. If a woman ingests a good diet during pregnancy, including a quart of milk a day or a calcium supplement if she cannot drink milk, and continues daily toothbrushing this becomes an old wives' tale. Some women do not go to the dentist during pregnancy because they are afraid that possible X-rays of their teeth will harm their growing baby. Lack of dental care from this practice can be very damaging to their teeth. Women can have dental X-ray examinations during pregnancy, provided their abdomen is protected with a lead apron. Dental care should be continued during pregnancy as it is during other times in life. Before extensive dental work involving a local anesthetic or nitrous oxide inhalation, however, the woman should consult her obstetrician or nurse-midwife.

Urinary System

During pregnancy, the kidneys must excrete not only the waste products of the woman's body but those of the growing fetus as well. Thus, urinary output gradually increases (about 60–80%) and specific gravity decreases during pregnancy. Creatinine clearance is used as a test of renal function; it increases in relation to glomerular filtration rate (GFR). A normal pregnancy value, measured by a 24-hour urine sample, is 90 to 180 ml per minute.

Total body water increases to 7.5 liters; this requires an increased sodium reabsorption in the tubules to maintain osmolarity. Under the influence of progesterone, there is an increased response of the angiotensin-renin system in the kidney. This change leads to an increase in aldosterone, which aids sodium reabsorption. Progesterone also appears to be potassium-sparing; even with diuresis, potassium levels remain adequate.

Occasionally, a trace of albumin will be present in urine, due to congestion in renal capillaries. Glomerular filtration rate (GFR) and renal plasma flow are both most effective, increased up to 50 percent, when a person lies in a lateral recumbent position (on the side). Women should be advised to rest and sleep in this position during pregnancy not only to prevent cardiovascular problems but in order to assist the kidneys to function most efficiently.

Both the glomerular filtration rate and the renal plasma flow increase 30 to 50 percent. The rise is consistent with that of the circulatory system increase, peaking at about 24 weeks. This efficient GFR level leads to a lowered blood urea nitrogen (BUN) and low creatinine levels in maternal plasma. A BUN of 15 mg per 100 ml or higher and a creatinine over 1 mg per 100 ml are considered abnormal and reflect kidney difficulty in handling the increased blood load. High GFR leads to increased filtration of glucose into the renal tubules. Because reabsorption of glucose by the tubal cells occurs at a fixed rate, some accidental spilling of glucose may occur into urine during pregnancy. Lactose, the sugar of breast milk, which is being produced by the mammary glands but is not used during pregnancy, will also be spilled into the urine.

Although some spilling of glucose may occur, the finding of glucose in a routine sample of urine from a pregnant woman is considered abnormal until proved otherwise: It can be an indication of gestational diabetes (see Chapter 36).

To differentiate what sugar is spilling into the urine, a test material for urine analysis specific for glucose (Tes-Tape) must be used. A urine test method that is positive for all sugars (Benedict's solution) will give false-positive results by reporting the presence of harmless lactose.

The ureters increase in diameter in response to increased progesterone in order to accommodate the greater urine flow. Bladder capacity increases to about 1,500 ml. The uterus tends to rise in the right side of the abdomen, since it is pushed slightly in that direction by the greater bulk of the sigmoid colon. The consequent pressure on the right ureter may result in urine stasis and pyelonephritis if it is not relieved.

A woman may notice urinary frequency the

Table 16-4 Urinary Tract Changes During Pregnancy

Glomerular filtration rate	Increased
Renal plasma flow	Increased
Blood urea nitrogen	Decreased
Plasma creatinine level	Decreased
Renal threshold for sugar	Decreased
Bladder capacity	Increased
Diameter of ureters	Increased
Frequency of urination	Present first trimester, last 2 weeks of pregnancy

first 3 months of pregnancy until the uterus rises out of the pelvis and relieves pressure on the bladder. Frequency of urination may return at the end of pregnancy as lightening occurs and the fetal head exerts pressure on the bladder once more.

Changes in the urinary tract during pregnancy are summarized in Table 16-4.

Skeletal System

Calcium and phosphorus needs are increased during pregnancy for the building of the fetal skeleton. As pregnancy advances, there is a gradual softening of the pelvic ligaments and joints to allow for pliability and to facilitate passage of the baby through the pelvis at the time of delivery. The ovarian hormone *relaxin* probably initiates these changes. Excessive mobility of the joints may cause discomfort, and a wide separation of the symphysis pubis may occur.

In order to change her center of gravity and make ambulation easier, a woman tends to stand straighter and taller than usual during pregnancy. This stance is frequently referred to as the "pride of pregnancy." Standing this way with the shoulders back and the abdomen forward creates a *lordosis* (forward curve of the lumbar spine), which may lead to backache.

Endocrine System

The most striking change in the endocrine system during pregnancy is the addition of the placenta as an endocrine organ, which produces large amounts of both estrogen and progesterone. Many women experience palmar erythema during early pregnancy as a response to the high circulating estrogen levels.

The pituitary gland is affected by pregnancy in that, under the influence of high estrogen and progesterone levels, the production of follicle-stimulating hormone and luteinizing hormone is halted. There is increased production of growth hormone and melanocyte-stimulating hormone (the reason skin pigment changes occur in pregnancy). Late in pregnancy, the posterior pituitary begins to produce the oxytocin that will be needed to aid in initiation of labor. Prolactin production is also begun late in pregnancy to aid in lactation at birth.

The thyroid gland is significantly altered. The gland enlarges in early pregnancy. Levels of protein-bound iodine (PBI), butanol extractable iodine (BEI), and thyroxine (T_4) are all elevated. The result is an elevation of basal metabolic rate by about 20 percent.

These thyroid changes, along with emotional lability, tachycardia, heart palpitations, and increased perspiration, may lead to a mistaken diagnosis of hyperthyroidism if the woman has not yet been found to be pregnant. If a sufficient supply of iodine is not present during pregnancy, goiter (thyroid hypertrophy) can occur as the gland intensifies its productive effort.

The parathyroid glands, which are necessary for the metabolism of calcium, also increase in size during pregnancy. Since calcium is an important ingredient of fetal growth, the hypertrophy is probably necessary to satisfy the increased need for calcium.

Glucocorticoid levels increase in pregnancy, perhaps because of increased plasma binding rather than increased production by the adrenals. Although the pancreas increases production of insulin in response to the higher glucocorticoid levels, estrogen, progesterone, and human chorionic somatomammotropin all tend to make insulin less effective. Thus a woman who is diabetic and taking insulin before pregnancy will need more insulin during pregnancy. A woman who is prediabetic may develop overt diabetes for the first time during pregnancy.

Carbohydrate Metabolism

A fetus exists at a glucose level about 30 mg per 100 ml below that of the maternal glucose level. In order to prevent hypoglycemia in the fetus with resultant cell destruction or lack of fetal growth, a maternal glucose level must be maintained at a normal level during pregnancy. Even though a number of "fail-safe" measures are present to help achieve this goal, a fasting blood sugar level is generally slightly low early in pregnancy (80–85 mg/100 ml).

Although the pancreas secretes an increased level of insulin throughout pregnancy, it appears not to be as effective due to the presence of human chorionic somatomammotropin hormone secreted by the placenta and cortisol secreted by the adrenal gland. The high levels of estrogen and progesterone may also be influential in reducing insulin effectiveness. With this decreased effectiveness, fat stores of the woman are used as well as available glucose, which holds maternal glucose levels fairly steady despite long time intervals between meals or days of increased activity. In order to ensure against hypoglycemia, a pregnant woman should be conscientious that her diet is high in calories and she should try never to go longer than 12 hours between meals.

Water Metabolism

Water is retained during pregnancy to aid the increase in blood volume and to be present as a ready supply of fluid to the fetus in interstitial tissue. As nutrients can only pass to the fetus when dissolved in or carried by fluid, this ready fluid supply is a fetal safeguard. Water is retained because of the influence of estrogen/progesterone (steroid hormones) and the increased level of aldosterone secreted by the adrenal gland, which causes increased sodium reabsorption in the tubules.

At one time pregnant women were administered diuretics to help clear this excess fluid from their systems. Today it is recognized that this practice is potentially harmful: This fluid has physiologic benefits for the fetus; if hemorrhage in the mother should occur, the fluid could serve to replenish her own blood volume.

Adrenal Glands

Adrenal gland activity increases in pregnancy as an elevated level of corticosteroids and aldosterone is produced. The function of corticosteroids is generally unknown, but it is assumed that this increased level aids in suppressing an inflammatory reaction or helps to reduce the possibility of the woman's body rejecting the foreign protein of the fetus, just as she would automatically reject a foreign tissue transplant. It also helps to regulate glucose metabolism in the woman. The increased level of aldosterone aids in promoting sodium reabsorption and maintaining osmolarity in the amount of fluid retained. This effect indirectly helps safeguard the blood volume and provide adequate perfusion pressure across the placenta.

Immunologic System

Immunologic competency during pregnancy is apparently decreased, a mechanism that probably prevents the woman's body from rejecting the fetus as she would reject transplanted organs. IgG production is particularly decreased, which may make the woman more prone to infection during pregnancy. The increased white blood count that

Table 16-5 Average Weight Gain in Pregnancy

System	Pounds	Kilograms
Fetus	7.0	3.1
Placenta	1.5	0.6
Amniotic fluid	2.0	0.9
Uterus	2.5	1.1
Blood volume	3.5	1.5
Breasts	1.5–3.0	0.6–1.3
Body fluid	8.0	3.6
Total	26.0–27.5	11.4–12.1

is present may help to counteract the decrease in IgG response.

Weight Gain

All the physiologic changes of pregnancy and the growth of the fetus tend to result in a weight increase of about 25 to 30 pounds (11.3–13.1 kg). A portion of the weight gain can be easily accounted for and is shown in Table 16-5. The remainder of the weight gain comes from the greater-than-normal accumulation of fat and fluid characteristic of pregnancy.

During the first 3 months of pregnancy, weight gain is usually slight (about 3 pounds). If the woman has a great deal of nausea, she may actually lose a small amount of weight. During the second and third trimesters she generally gains about a pound a week (a 3-12-12 pattern). A typical graph of weight gain is shown in Figure 16-7. Whether a woman is taking in a diet sufficiently high in protein and whether her vital signs, particularly blood pressure, remain normal for her are equally as important as the fact she is gaining weight at this rate.

Women who are underweight coming into pregnancy may easily gain (and should gain) more weight than the average woman during pregnancy. An obese woman may gain less. As a rule, women should not diet to lose weight during pregnancy lest nourishment to the fetus be decreased.

Weight gain should be higher for a multiple pregnancy than for a single pregnancy. Adequate weight gain in pregnancy is strongly correlated to adequate birth weight and well-being of newborns. Nurses in the past have been overly conscientious about trying to force women to limit the amount of weight gained during pregnancy. It is true that a rapid increase in weight is a danger sign, since it may herald the onset of pregnancy-induced hypertension. However, weight gain during pregnancy can be kept in a better perspective if you remember that it is the pregnancy-induced hypertension that causes the increase in weight, not the increase in weight that causes the hypertension.

Effects of Physiologic Changes

The physiologic changes of pregnancy may appear insignificant if taken one by one, but together they add up to a major change. Every woman of childbearing age has a mental picture of herself. She has a good idea how she will look in a dress before she tries it on in a store. She chooses a certain style of furniture for her house or takes a vacation in a certain place because it says "this is me."

Then in 9 months, she gains 25 to 30 pounds, and her figure changes so drastically that none of her prepregnancy clothes fit. Toward the end of pregnancy, the extra weight and the strain of waiting make her feel tired and short of breath. Endocrine changes make her moody and perhaps quick to cry. She may never have been concerned with her health before, and now, every month (toward the end of pregnancy, every week), she must think about it as she reports for a prenatal checkup. She may worry that she will never lose all the weight she has gained, that the stretch marks on her abdomen will remain forever, and that she will always be as tired or as nauseated as she is now. Table 16-6 correlates the physiologic changes of the mother with the growth of the fetus.

At prenatal visits, women need help in voicing their concerns over the physiologic changes of pregnancy. The worry these changes may cause, if the woman is not forewarned that they are a normal and necessary but transitory part of pregnancy, compound an already stressful situation. (See the Nursing Research Highlight on page 316 for more information on this topic.)

Utilizing Nursing Process

Although many of the physiologic changes of pregnancy occur subtly and are usually welcome changes because they are a woman's surest proof that pregnancy exists, in order that the woman is

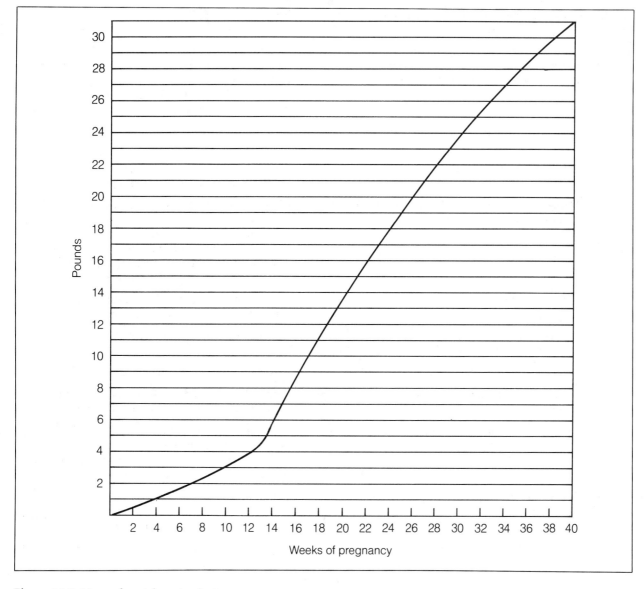

Figure 16-7 *Normal weight gain during pregnancy.*

prepared for them and not concerned by them, nursing care planning is necessary.

Assessment

Women are interested in the physiologic changes of pregnancy because they mark the progress and assess the reality of their pregnancy by the presence of the signs. Physical examination reveals many of these findings. Remember that a pulse rate is usually 10 beats increased during pregnancy; respiratory rate is also on the upper side of normal (18–20 breaths/minute).

Analysis

As a nursing diagnosis does not deal with a physical finding but with the result or concern of that finding, a typical nursing diagnosis involving

physical changes of pregnancy might be "Concern over increased skin pigmentation related to a physiologic change of pregnancy," or "Shortness of breath related to a physiologic change of pregnancy."

Planning

Planning in connection with physiologic changes of pregnancy should involve not only a plan to review concerns but ways to prevent concerns that could arise from other physical changes. Plan a way that education regarding physical changes can be built into a prenatal health teaching program ("a white vaginal discharge is normal; clear secretions from nipples is normal; breast tenderness is normal . . .").

Table 16-6 Correlation of Fetal Growth and Maternal Changes During Pregnancy

Month	Fetal Growth	Maternal Changes
1	Heart is beating; limb buds are present.	Fatigue, breast changes present. Internal vaginal and cervical changes are present. Amenorrhea is present.
2	Fingers are present; head is dominant.	Frequency of urination is present. Morning sickness is present.
3	Sex recognition possible.	Fetal heart rate present by doppler. Uterus palpable over symphysis pubis.
4	Hematopoiesis begins in bone marrow. Meconium starting to accumulate.	Morning sickness fading. Pregnancy is obvious by abdominal contour. Striae gravidarum begin to appear. Colostrum secretion begins. Blood volume beginning marked expansion. Begins to gain a pound of weight a week.
5	Lanugo covers entire body.	Quickening occurs. Fetal heart rate by stethoscope possible. Fundus is at umbilicus.
6	Verxix caseosa present. Eyebrows and eyelashes present.	Chloasma and linea nigra begin to form.
7	Testes begin to descend in male.	Nest-building behaviors usually present.
8	Subcutaneous fat accumulating. Nails reach end of fingers.	Woman beginning to make plans for infant care. Interested in preparation for childbirth.
9	Movements strong. Fat continues to accumulate.	Fundus at xyphoid process. Shortness of breath acute. Vascular spiders on legs may be present. Braxton Hicks contractions may be noticeable.
10	Fetus fully developed. Nails project beyond ends of fingers.	Lightening occurs in primiparas. Frequency of urination reoccurs. Woman expresses desire for pregnancy to end.

Nursing Research Highlight

Figure Drawings

Are Figure Drawings Useful in Determining Attitudes Toward a Changing Body During Pregnancy?

During pregnancy a woman's body changes very rapidly. The woman's attitudes and her husband's reaction toward this change play an important role in her experience of pregnancy. In a study conducted by three researchers (Harris, Dombro, and Ryan, 1980), human figure drawings were collected from 39 couples during their third trimester of pregnancy. Husbands were asked to draw a picture of their wives, and the women of themselves. Because this type of test is a projective instrument, subjects are more likely to express feelings that they might not consciously verbalize or reflect the attitudes and feelings of the husbands and wives regarding their experience of pregnancy. The drawings done by the husbands ranged from extremely positive to negative feelings. In general, women tended to draw themselves so that the shape of their body underneath could be seen. In one instance, a wife drew herself as angelic; her husband drew her with a devils' tale. It can be assumed, therefore, that human figure drawings during pregnancy can be a useful diagnostic tool of marital relationships as well as an approach to therapeutic intervention.

Reference

Harris, R., Dombro, M., & Ryan, C. (1980). Therapeutic uses of human figure drawings by the pregnant couple. *J.O.G.N. Nursing, 9*(4), 233.

Table 16-7 Timetable for Physiologic Changes of Pregnancy

System	1st Trimester	2nd Trimester	3rd Trimester
Cardiovascular	Blood volume increasing ————————		
	Pseudoanemia	Blood pressure slightly decreased	
	Clotting factors increasing —————————————————————		
Reproductive			
Ovaries	Corpus luteum active	Corpus luteum fading	
Uterus	Increased growth ———————————————————————		
		Placenta forming estrogen and progesterone —————	
Cervix	Softening progressing —————————————————————————		"ripe"
Vagina	White discharge present ————————————————————————		
Musculoskeletal		Progressive cartilage softening —————————	
		Lordosis increasing ————————————	
Integument			
Pigmentation		Progressively increasing —————————	
Renal			
Kidney	GFR increasing —————————————————		
		Glycosuria ————————————————————	
	Aldosterone increased, increasing sodium and fluid		
Gastrointestinal		Slowed peristalsis —————————————	
Endocrine			
Thyroid	Increased metabolic rate ————————————————————		

Implementation

Problems related to physiologic changes of pregnancy are usually problems of worry or concern so the main implementation that solves such problems is anticipatory guidance presenting education and reassurance that such changes are normal. Even though a woman has read pamphlets or talked to her friends about physiologic changes of pregnancy, she often is surprised to see a change occurring in herself. She may say something such as "I knew I'd be tired but I never guessed I'd be this tired," or "I read about a brown line forming on my abdomen but I never expected it to become this dark." Almost everything in life seems bigger and different when it is happening to you rather than when you read about it happening to others.

Table 16-7 offers a timetable of physiologic changes of pregnancy to aid in anticipatory guidance.

Evaluation

Evaluation is an important tool to determine if a woman really "heard" teaching. Remember that people do not hear well under stress, and pregnancy is a 9-month stress period. It is not unusual for a woman to pocket information away, thinking, "I'll concentrate on what that means when it happens to me, not now," and then at the point it happens, realizing that she has forgotten what you said. Evaluation that reveals learning did not take place confirms that pregnancy is a period of stress more often than it reflects the quality of teaching.

Below is a nursing care plan concerning one physiologic change of pregnancy.

Nursing Care Planning

Mary Kraft is a 23-year-old woman you meet in an obstetrician's office. She is 16 weeks pregnant.

Assessment

Patient states, "My back aches all the time. I can trace the path of veins up my legs they ache so much."

Patient walks with a marked lordosis; wearing a 3-inch heel on shoe. Employed part-time as a librarian.

Analysis

Concern related to physiologic changes of pregnancy.

Locus of Decision Making. Patient.

Goal. Patient's comfort related to musculoskeletal and vascular changes of pregnancy will improve.

Criteria. Patient will voice less discomfort from back and leg pain.

Nursing Orders

1. Review the necessity of good posture during pregnancy to protect back ligaments.

2. Distribute pamphlet "Your Baby Inside You" and review photos of correct posture.
3. Discuss wardrobe during pregnancy and possibility of limiting amount of time spent each day on high heels.
4. Help to plan ways for daily rest with feet elevated to reduce pressure in veins of lower extremities and vulva.
5. Teach pelvic rocking to reduce back discomfort.

Questions for Review

Multiple Choice

1. Mrs. Jones is a patient you see in a prenatal clinic. Early in pregnancy she reports frequent urination. You would explain to her that this results mainly from

   a. pressure on the bladder from the uterus.
   b. decreased concentration of urine.
   c. the addition of fetal urine to her urine.
   d. decreased glomerular selectivity.

2. At her 16-week checkup, Mrs. Jones's blood pressure is slightly decreased from her prepregnancy level. You would analyze this change in relation to which of the following statements concerning blood pressure during pregnancy.

   a. Normally, blood pressure increases steadily throughout pregnancy.
   b. Blood pressure does not normally decrease until the day of delivery.
   c. A decrease in the second trimester may occur due to placental growth.
   d. Blood pressure will normally progressively decrease throughout pregnancy.

3. Mrs. Jones asks you what a "normal" weight gain is during pregnancy. You would tell her

   a. 18–20 pounds.
   b. 20–25 pounds.
   c. 25–30 pounds.
   d. 30–35 pounds.

4. Mrs. Jones often has allergic responses to drugs. She is concerned that she will be allergic to her baby or her body will reject the pregnancy. You base your reply to her on which factual statement below.

   a. Immunologic activity is decreased during pregnancy.
   b. The level of aldosterone during pregnancy reduces production of IgG antibodies.
   c. The decreased corticosteroid activity during pregnancy ensures this will not happen.
   d. The kidneys release a hormone during pregnancy to prevent this from happening.

5. Mrs. Jones's physician suggests that she eat iodized salt during pregnancy. You would explain to her that the reason for this precaution is

   a. thyroid activity, which depends on iodine intake, increases during pregnancy.
   b. because there is decreased thyroid activity during pregnancy, the thyroid does not produce as much iodine as normally.
   c. Progesterone formation is dependent on a high iodine intake.
   d. adrenal gland activity during pregnancy decreases iodine effectiveness.

6. At her 24-week checkup, you assess Mrs. Jones's urine and discover it is 1 + for sugar by a dipstick test. You would base your analysis of the finding on which statement below.

   a. Lactose may be spilling into her urine.
   b. Sugar in urine is an innocent finding in pregnancy.
   c. The decreased glomerular filtration rate is the cause.
   d. Mrs. Jones must have eaten a high-calorie meal before the test.

7. As Mrs. Jones lies on the examining table, she grows very short of breath and dizzy. This phenomenon probably happens because

   a. her cerebral arteries are growing congested with blood.
   b. the uterus requires more blood in a supine position.
   c. blood is trapped in the vena cava in a supine position.
   d. sympathetic nerve responses cause vasodilation when a woman is supine.

8. Mrs. Jones has her finger pricked for a blood cholesterol level at a health screening fair and calls to tell you that her level was very high. You could assure her that

   a. an increased cholesterol level is a normal finding for pregnancy.
   b. a high cholesterol level is necessary during pregnancy to stimulate adequate glomerular filtration.
   c. she should not have had a test done independently.
   d. a high cholesterol level is necessary during pregnancy to aid in blood volume.

9. Blood volume normally increases during pregnancy. The extent of this increase is what percent of prepregnancy volume?
   a. 10–20 percent
   b. 20–30 percent
   c. 30–50 percent
   d. 70–100 percent

10. Determining a mean blood pressure is necessary to establish whether hypertension of pregnancy exists. If Mrs. Jones's blood pressure is 120/80, her mean blood pressure is
    a. 85.5.
    b. 93.3.
    c. 100.5.
    d. 133.3.

Discussion

1. Almost all body systems accommodate to meet the requirements of pregnancy. How do respiratory adjustments aid fetal growth?
2. Fatigue in early pregnancy is a symptom that many women find distressing. What physiologic adjustments account for such extreme fatigue?
3. Some women with heart disease are unable to successfully complete a pregnancy because of the necessary cardiovascular adjustments. What are these adjustments?

Suggested Readings

Allen, E., et al. (1981). Are normal patients at risk during pregnancy? *J.O.G.N. Nursing, 10,* 348.

Bettoli, E. J. (1982). Herpes: Facts and fallacies. *American Journal of Nursing, 82,* 924.

Frankl, W. S. (1982). Hemodynamics: How it changes with pregnancy. *Consultant, 22,* 373.

George, G., et al. (1981). Exercise before, during, and after pregnancy. *Topics in Clinical Nursing, 3,* 33.

Gillespie, S. A., et al. (1981). A reference for clinicians: Discomforts of pregnancy. *Issues in Health Care of Women, 3,* 375.

Halpern, J. S., et al. (1983). Use of drugs during pregnancy. *Journal of Emergency Nursing, 9,* 160.

Hamilton, M. S., et al. (1981). Pelvic examination: Patient safety and comfort. *J.O.G.N. Nursing, 10,* 344.

Hytten, F. E. (1978). Physiological adjustments in pregnancy. In R. R. MacDonald (Ed.). *Scientific basis of obstetrics and gynecology.* Edinburgh: Churchill Livingstone.

Maring-Klug, R. (1982). Reducing low back pain during pregnancy. *Nurse Practitioner, 7,* 18.

Martin, B. J., et al. (1982). Oral health during pregnancy: a neglected nursing area. *M.C.N., 7,* 391.

Nilsen, S. T. (1984). Smoking, hemoglobin levels, and birthweight in normal pregnancies. *American Journal of Obstetrics and Gynecology, 148,* 752.

Sciarra, J. J., & Gerbie, A. B. (1978). *Gynecology and obstetrics.* New York: Harper & Row.

Sibley, L., et al. (1981). Swimming and physical fitness during pregnancy. *Journal of Nurse Midwifery, 26,* 3.

Trimmer, E. (1982). About the heartburn of pregnancy. *Midwife Health Visitor and Community Nurse, 18,* 142.

Waterfield, M., et al. (1983). Midwives, smoking and antenatal care. *Midwives Chronicle, 96,* 73.

Zacharias, J. (1983). A rational approach to drug use in pregnancy. *J.O.G.N. Nursing, 12,* 183.

17

The Diagnosis of Pregnancy

OBJECTIVES

Following mastery of the contents of this chapter you should be able to

1. Define the terms *presumptive, probable,* and *positive* in relation to pregnancy diagnosis.
2. Describe the important signs and symptoms for diagnosis of pregnancy.
3. Describe the techniques or measures used in pregnancy diagnosis.
4. Analyze the meaning of diagnosis of pregnancy to women and their support people.
5. Synthesize knowledge of pregnancy diagnosis with nursing process to achieve quality maternal-newborn nursing care.

THE DIAGNOSIS OF PREGNANCY is an important event: For many women, medical confirmation that they are pregnant makes the pregnancy real for the first time. It is also an important step in accepting the pregnancy and its eventual outcome, the newborn child.

A woman may be in a physician's office or prenatal clinic only one hour, but if her pregnancy is confirmed at that time, she invariably feels "more pregnant" when she leaves. From that day on, most women try to eat a proper diet, give up or cut down on cigarette smoking, and stop taking over-the-counter medications. A woman may not take these measures before confirmation of her pregnancy, which is a good reason for an early diagnosis. If the woman does not wish to continue the pregnancy, early diagnosis is imperative: Abortion should always be carried out at the earliest stage possible.

Pregnancy is diagnosed on the basis of the symptoms the woman reports and the signs a physician, nurse practitioner, or you elicit. These signs and symptoms are traditionally divided into three classifications: presumptive, probable, and positive.

Presumptive Signs

Presumptive signs are those that are least indicative of pregnancy; as single entities they could easily be indications of other conditions besides pregnancy. These findings are largely subjective, or ones experienced by the woman but undocumented by an examiner.

Amenorrhea

In a healthy woman who has menstruated previously, the absence of menstruation strongly suggests that impregnation has occurred. However, amenorrhea may announce the initiation of menopause rather than pregnancy, or menstruation may be delayed because of uterine infection, a change in climate, worry (perhaps over becoming pregnant), chronic illness such as severe anemia, or stress. It occurs in athletes who train strenuously. Occasionally, the spotting that may occur with implantation or at the time estrogen/progesterone secretion changes from corpus luteum–based to placenta-based is mistaken for a menstrual flow; since this "flow" occurs in the presence of pregnancy, amenorrhea is an even more unreliable sign of pregnancy.

Fatigue

Early in pregnancy, perhaps even before the first missed menstrual period, most pregnant women have episodes of fatigue and drowsiness. The rapid growth of the fetus at this stage probably uses the woman's glucose stores at a high rate, leaving her with a low blood glucose at certain times during the day. Fatigue has many causes, however—among them illness, overexertion, and depression (sadness is manifested as body fatigue).

Nausea and Vomiting

At least 50 percent of women (as many as 90 percent) experience some nausea and vomiting early in pregnancy (Alley, 1984). These symptoms often occur on rising (morning sickness) but may occur anytime during the day; in many women the acuteness of the symptoms can be correlated with fatigue or meal preparation. Morning sickness may precede the missed menstrual period but generally occurs at about the same time. It normally disappears by the end of the twelfth week of pregnancy. Like fatigue, however, nausea and vomiting have many other causes—a gastrointestinal disorder, emotional stress, infection, or anorexia nervosa, for example.

Frequent Micturition

The expanding uterus puts pressure on the base of the bladder, causing a woman to feel as though she needs to urinate frequently. A presumptive sign of pregnancy when coupled with a missed menstrual period, this could also be caused by a mild urinary tract infection or a pelvic tumor. This lack of specificity limits its value in diagnosing pregnancy.

Breast Changes

Breast changes—a feeling of fullness coupled with an increase in the diameter and darkening of the areola, the enlargement of Montgomery's tubercles, prominence of veins, and the secretion of colostrum—are most significant and noticeable in women having their first pregnancy. In a woman who has breast-fed a child during the past year, they are sometimes almost unnoticeable. They occur monthly in some women as part of premenstrual tension syndrome. Breast changes occur early, at about the sixth week of pregnancy.

Vaginal Changes

As vascular activity increases in the vagina, the walls of the vagina deepen in color, becoming violet, in contrast to the normal nonpregnant pink. Called *Chadwick's sign,* this may occur in any condition in which vaginal vascularity is increased (for example, in the presence of a rapidly growing uterine tumor). Increased color is present at the sixth week of pregnancy.

Skin Changes

Striae gravidarum (red marks on the abdomen), linea nigra (a dark pigment line on the abdomen), and melasma (pigment formation on the face) are skin changes that generally appear only with pregnancy. However, striae may occur with any rapidly expanding abdominal mass; a linea nigra may remain on the abdomen for a while following a pregnancy and so may be misleading in the diagnosis of a new pregnancy. These changes take place during the second trimester; in any event, they would rarely be the first sign noticed.

Quickening

Quickening is the woman's first perception of fetal movement. It was once believed that a child lay lifeless in a woman's body until a point in pregnancy when "soul," or life, was instilled into it. *Quick,* as used in biblical references ("the quick and the dead") means "alive"; *quickening* is the old term for the "instillation of life into the fetus."

The first time a woman feels a child move is not a true measure of movement because the fetus has been making faint, undetectable movements since early in pregnancy. Once quickening has occurred (usually at 18 to 20 weeks), the woman should continue to feel movements. The strength of the movements will vary with the thickness of the uterus and abdominal wall along with the position and strength of the fetus. Movements are generally best felt when the woman lies on her back. Any time that 24 hours pass without any discernible movement, a woman should ask to have the fetal heart sounds auscultated. If they are present, despite the decrease in movements observed, it can be assumed that the fetus is well.

Although a woman's statement that she "feels life" should be a reliable sign of pregnancy, it cannot be accepted as any more than presumptive. Occasionally, the movement of gas in the intestine may simulate such a sensation. A woman who wishes to be pregnant very much can overinterpret other body functions, such as intestinal gas, as fetal movement.

Probable Signs

Probable signs of pregnancy are, in contrast to presumptive signs, almost all objective findings or ones that can be documented by an examiner. Although also more reliable, they still are not positive or true diagnostic findings of pregnancy.

Uterine Changes

Bimanual examination (one finger of the examiner in the vagina, the other hand on the abdomen) demonstrates that with pregnancy the uterus is more anteflexed, larger, and softer to the touch than normally. About the sixth week of pregnancy (at the time of the second missed menstrual period), the lower uterine segment just above the cervix becomes so soft that when it is compressed between the examining fingers by bimanual examination the wall cannot be felt or feels as thin as tissue paper. This extreme softening of the lower uterine segment is known as *Hegar's sign* (Figure 17-1).

During the sixteenth to twentieth weeks of pregnancy, when the fetus is still small in relation to the amount of amniotic fluid present, *ballottement* (from the French word *balloter,* meaning "to toss about") may be demonstrated. On bimanual examination, if the lower uterine segment is tapped sharply by the lower hand, the fetus will bounce or rise in the amniotic fluid up against the top examining hand. This phenome-

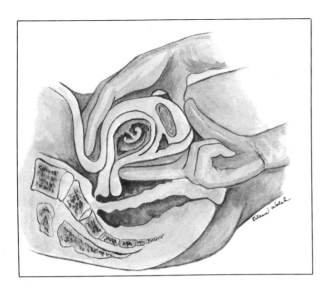

Figure 17-1 *Hegar's sign. When the lower uterine segment is compressed between the examining fingers, it feels as thin as tissue paper.*

non is interesting; it can, however, be simulated by a pedunculated uterine tumor.

As the blood supply to the cervix increases in amount, the feel of the cervix changes from something like the tip of your nose to something less hard, like an earlobe. This marked softening (*Goodell's sign*) occurs at about the time of the second missed menstrual period. The phenomenon is not diagnostic of pregnancy, though, because once again it could occur with a rapidly growing uterine tumor. (One method of remembering which name applies to which sign of pregnancy is to remember that Chadwick's, Goodell's, and Hegar's signs occur in alphabetical order from the lower reproductive tract upward—in other words, Chadwick's sign is a vaginal change, Goodell's sign a cervical change, and Hegar's sign a uterine change.)

Enlargement of the uterus at a slow steady rate is also an important sign of pregnancy. The uterus should rise above the symphysis pubis by the twelfth week, reach the umbilicus at about the twentieth or twenty-fourth week, and reach the xyphoid process at the thirty-sixth week. Although enlargement at this predictable rate rarely occurs with other phenomena, it can occur with a uterine tumor.

Fetal Outline

About the twenty-fourth week of pregnancy, the uterine wall has become thinned to such a degree that a fetal outline within the uterus may be palpated and identified by a skilled examiner. However, since a tumor with calcium deposits occa-

sionally simulates fetal outline, even this sign does not constitute a positive confirmation of pregnancy.

Braxton Hicks Contractions

Uterine contractions begin early in pregnancy, at least by the twelfth week, and are present throughout the rest of pregnancy, becoming stronger and harder as the pregnancy advances. They may be felt by a woman as periods in which hardness or tightening is felt across her abdomen. An examining hand may be able to feel the contraction as well. An electronic monitor will be able to measure the exact frequency and strength of such contractions.

These "practice" contractions are termed *Braxton Hicks contractions* or *Braxton Hicks sign*. They serve as warm-up exercises for labor and become so strong and noticeable in the last month of pregnancy that they may be mistaken for labor contractions (false labor). They can be differentiated from true labor contractions on internal examination by the absence of cervical dilation. These contractions always accompany pregnancy to some degree, but they could be caused by any growing mass in the uterus.

Sonography

As indicated in Chapter 15, high-frequency sound waves projected toward a woman's abdomen are useful in demonstrating fetal maturity. This technique may also be used to diagnose pregnancy (Figure 15-4). In the event of pregnancy, a characteristic ring, indicating the gestational sac, will be revealed on the oscilloscope as early as the sixth week of amenorrhea. This method of determination also gives information about the site of implantation and whether a multiple pregnancy exists or not. It is helpful if a woman having a sonogram for early pregnancy diagnosis drinks at least 1,000 ml of fluid prior to the assessment. A full bladder pushes the uterus out of the pelvis and also helps with transmission of the ultrasound.

Ultrasound used in this manner is a fairly recent method of pregnancy diagnosis. It is considered to be only a probable sign of pregnancy unless either fetal limb or fetal heart movement can be clearly distinguished on the screen (real-time mode).

Progesterone Withdrawal Test

In the progesterone withdrawal test, progesterone is given orally or intramuscularly to a woman. If she is not pregnant, a menstrual flow will occur within 3 to 5 days because the peaking and falling of the amount of synthetic progesterone causes a withdrawal effect, or sloughing of the endometrium. If the woman is pregnant, the corpus luteum or the placenta produces enough hormone to neutralize the effect of the declining synthetic hormone level and no bleeding occurs. Women sometimes call this test an "abortion shot" because when they fear they are pregnant, they see a physician, who gives them an injection, and within a few days they have a normal menstrual period (as if the injection interfered with the pregnancy). In reality, the physician merely demonstrated that they were not pregnant. Today, when immunologic tests can offer quick diagnostic results, progesterone withdrawal tests are rarely used. They have the potential of causing damage to a fetus by the teratogenicity of high levels of progesterone. Such a test, therefore, is used today not to diagnose pregnancy, but to diagnose that pregnancy does *not* exist.

Laboratory Tests

The commonly used laboratory tests for pregnancy are based on the presence in the urine or serum of pregnant women of human chorionic gonadotropin (HCG), a hormone produced by the chorionic villi. Because all laboratory tests for pregnancy are somewhat inaccurate, positive results from these tests are considered probable rather than positive signs of pregnancy. HCG is measured in international units (IUs). In the nonpregnant female, no units are detectable (because HCG is produced by the trophoblast cells, which are not present). HCG appears in the serum of women as early as 24 to 48 hours following implantation; by the thirtieth day following the last menstrual period, it rises to 0.1–1.0 IU per ml, a level that is measurable by common immunologic tests on serum.

Although HCG is present in the bloodstream by the eighth to tenth day of pregnancy, it may not be present in urine in quantities great enough to use for testing until the fortieth day of gestation. The level of HCG peaks between the sixtieth and eightieth day of pregnancy to levels about 100 IU per ml. Following this, the level declines again, until at term it is only 3–20 IU per ml. In the past, biologic tests were used to detect HCG, based on the principle that when urine containing HCG was injected into various animals, the hormone produced characteristic effects in the animal, indicating pregnancy. Immunologic radioreceptor assay, and radio immunoassay tests

are now preferred. Home pregnancy tests, based on these methods, are also available.

Biologic Tests

The Aschheim-Zondek test, devised in 1927, was the first laboratory test for pregnancy. Although it is rarely used today, the test has historic significance because the name is often applied erroneously to any pregnancy test. For an Aschheim-Zondek test, five immature female mice were injected with quantities of a woman's urine over a two-day period, and 100 hours from the first injection the mice were killed and their ovaries were examined. If HCG was present in the injected urine, hemorrhagic graafian follicles or corpora lutea would be present. Although an Aschheim-Zondek test was 97 percent accurate, its usefulness was limited by the number of animals required, the long waiting period for test results, and the time required by laboratory personnel to perform the test.

Other animals that can be used for biologic testing are rabbits, rats, frogs, or toads. As mentioned, none of these tests is used any longer, but they retain historical interest. Many women still refer to any positive laboratory result for pregnancy by saying, "The rabbit died." Actually, even when these tests were commonly used, the rabbit always died, whether the woman was pregnant or not: It had to be sacrificed to allow for examination of the ovaries.

Immunologic Tests

Immunoassay tests record antigen-antibody reactions in urine.

Rapid Slide Tests. Rapid slide tests take only a few minutes for results to be obtained, which makes them ideal tests to complement findings of a physical examination. The most common slide test done today uses latex particles coated with HCG and an anti-HCG rabbit serum. The anti-HCG serum is first mixed with the woman's urine, then the HCG particles are added. Failure of the mixture to agglutinate (form clumps) is a positive test; it means the urine contained HCG and the HCG in the urine neutralized (reacted with) the antiserum before the latex-coated HCG particles were added.

The test is read after 2 minutes and is 97 percent accurate. False-positive results can occur if proteinuria is present; false-negative results can occur with a low specific gravity of the urine sample. Such tests are sensitive for as little as 2 IU per ml of HCG and are accurate within 5 days after a missed menstrual period. Pregnosticon R is the brand name of a hemagglutination-inhibition test; Gravidex and Pregnosticon Slide Test are brand names for latex agglutination tests.

Tube Testing. For a tube test, a measured amount of the woman's urine is added to a tube of reagent, followed by a specified amount of diluent. The tube mixture is rotated until it is mixed well and then allowed to stand completely undisturbed in a rack for 40 to 60 minutes. At the end of this time, the bottom of the tube is examined for the presence of a circle of color. A ring of color means HCG was present in the urine sample, preventing clumping of test particles; nonagglutinated particles therefore rolled freely down the sides of the tube to form a ring. Tube tests are more sensitive than slide tests, detecting as little as 0.5–1.2 IU per ml of HCG. A high level of proteinuria (2+ and above) in the urine sample results in the formation of a colored ring but it is incomplete or uneven. Such distorted rings should be read as negative.

Immunologic tests are used to rule out an ectopic (tubal) or an intrauterine pregnancy before scheduling pelvic x-rays or administering a drug that could be harmful to a fetus.

Radioreceptor Assay

Radioreceptor assay testing is intended to detect HCG by its ability to bind to protein receptor sites. Artificial plasma membrane sites are "loaded" with radioactively tagged HCG, to which is added a sample of the pregnant woman's blood serum. If HCG is present in the serum, it will displace the radioactively tagged HCG; if no HCG is present, no displacement will occur. HCG's presence is estimated by "counting" the radioactively tagged particles after allowing a time interval for displacement.

Radioreceptor assay is extremely sensitive, detecting as little as 0.2 IU per ml of HCG. It is an effective test for pregnancy as soon as 6 days after ovulation.

Radioimmunoassay Tests

Radioimmunoassay (RIA) techniques on blood serum make it possible to demonstrate the presence of HCG earlier than ever before. With this test, pregnancy can be diagnosed as early as 8 days after implantation or at the same time as the missed menstrual flow. Radioimmunoassay tests measure the beta subunit of HCG hormone. Results can be obtained in 3 to 24 hours, and the test is sensitive to 5 IU per ml of HCG.

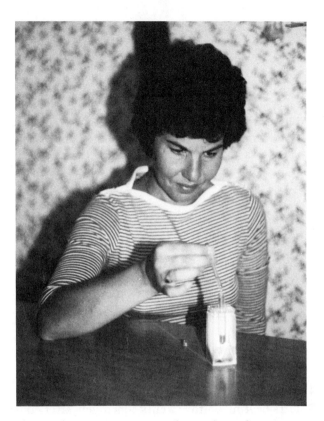

Figure 17-2 *Many women today perform their own home pregnancy tests. A dark circle is characteristic of a positive test.*

Home Pregnancy Tests

Several brand name kits for pregnancy testing based on immunologic reactions are available as over-the-counter purchases. These have a high degree of accuracy if the instructions are followed exactly. Their convenience (and privacy) allows women to avoid the anxiety and stress involved in waiting for a physician's appointment (Figure 17-2). If finances are a problem, using a home test can save a woman the cost of a physician's visit (a difference of up to $45). These are tube tests; in most brands, a positive test is indicated by the formation of a dark ring in the bottom of the test tube.

Unfortunately, one of the chief reasons women go for early prenatal care is not that they think they need a health checkup, but that they wish to have the pregnancy officially diagnosed. Women who diagnose their pregnancies at home by means of a test kit may tend not to go for prenatal care until something seems to be wrong or late in pregnancy. They need to be cautioned that prenatal care is important to safeguard pregnancy outcome: Home test kits cannot fill this role.

Women who are taking psychotropic drugs (tranquilizers) may have false-positive results on immunologic tests. Women on oral contraceptives may also have false-positive results; for such a test to be accurate, oral contraceptives should be discontinued 5 days before the test. A woman who has proteinuria, is postmenopausal, or has hyperthyroid disease may also show a false-positive result.

A woman in early pregnancy, with an incomplete or a missed abortion (see Chapter 39), or with an ectopic pregnancy, may have a false-negative result.

Positive Signs

There are only four positive signs of pregnancy: fetal heart sounds, fetal movements felt by the examiner, fetal heart movement on sonogram, and an X-ray film outline of the fetal skeleton.

Fetal Heart Sounds

Fetal heart rate usually ranges between 120 and 160 beats per minute. Although the fetal heart starts beating on the twenty-fourth day after conception, it is audible by auscultation of the abdomen with an ultrasonic monitoring system that converts ultrasonic frequencies to audible frequencies (Doppler technique) only at the eleventh week of gestation. Because a Doppler technique broadcasts the sound, this has the added advantage of allowing the woman as well as the examiner to hear the heart sounds. Hearing fetal heart sounds may be an important step in helping a woman accept the reality of pregnancy.

It is possible to hear fetal heart sounds with an ordinary stethoscope only at about 18 to 20 weeks of pregnancy. Fetal heart sounds are difficult to hear through abdomens with a great deal of subcutaneous fat or greater-than-normal amounts of amniotic fluid (hydramnios). They are heard best when the position of the fetus is determined by palpation and the stethoscope is placed over the area of the fetus's back.

An ordinary bell stethoscope may be used to auscultate heart sounds, but special fetal heart stethoscopes are available. One such stethoscope rests on the examiner's head and allows for bone conduction of the sound as well as air conduction to the eardrum. Others have a diaphragm that is larger than normal.

In addition to the fetal heartbeat, two other sounds are often heard on auscultation, the funic and uterine souffle. *Souffle* means "blowing." The *funic souffle* is the murmur of the blood rushing through the umbilical cord. Because this is part of the fetal circulation, the rate of the sound parallels the fetal heart rate. Blood moving through the distended maternal arteries creates the *uterine souffle*, which, because it represents maternal blood movement, has the same rate as the maternal pulse (about 70 to 80 beats per minute).

Fetal Movements Felt by the Examiner

Movements of the fetus perceived by the woman may be misleading. Those felt by an objective examiner are much more reliable and constitute a positive sign of pregnancy. Such movements may be felt by the twenty-fourth week of pregnancy unless the woman is extremely obese.

Fetal Heart Movement Recorded by Sonogram

By using a real-time technique of ultrasound, after a gestational sac has been identified, movement of the fetal heart may be demonstrated as early as 7 weeks of gestational age.

X-ray Outline of Fetal Skeleton

An X-ray showing the outline of a fetal skeleton is a fourth proof that pregnancy exists. Such an outline can be apparent as early as the fourteenth week of gestation; it is readily apparent after the twentieth week. Although resulting in a positive sign of pregnancy, X-rays may be teratogenic to the growing fetus; therefore, this sign is only academically, not clinically interesting because it is never used for diagnosis.

Utilizing Nursing Process

Diagnosis of pregnancy marks a major life milestone and invariably introduces a feeling of intense fulfillment and achievement—or an equally extreme crisis state if the pregnancy is not wanted.

Assessment

Most women who come to a health care facility for a diagnosis of pregnancy have already "hunched" that they are pregnant, based on a multitude of presumptive signs (Table 17-1).

Table 17-1 Time Frame for Diagnostic Findings of Pregnancy

Time from Implantation (weeks)	Positive Finding or Test
1	Serum immunologic tests positive Nausea and vomiting
2	Amenorrhea (first missed menstrual flow) Breast changes
3	Urinary frequency
6	Chadwick's, Goodell's, Hegar's signs Immunologic tests of urine positive Sonogram of gestational sac Second missed menstrual flow
7	Heartbeat by sonogram
10	Third missed menstrual flow
11	Heartbeat by Doppler technique
12	Fatigue Uterus palpable over pubis
14	X-ray of fetal skeleton Ballottement
16	Palpable fetal outline by examiner Fetal heartsounds by stethoscope
18	Quickening
20	Braxton Hicks contractions
24	Skin changes Palpation of fetal movement by examiner

Many women have already done a home pregnancy test as a prior confirmation.

When a sexually active woman is admitted to a hospital setting for diagnostic testing, such as an intravenous pyelogram that includes pelvic X-ray, you might want to suggest that she have a rapid serum pregnancy test done to rule out pregnancy first.

Urine for pregnancy tests must meet certain criteria if false-negative test results are to be avoided. Since the urine should be concentrated, ideally the woman should have nothing to drink after about 8:00 P.M. the evening before the test. The first morning voiding should be collected in a dry, clean container. If the sample will not be used for at least an hour, it should be refrigerated: HCG is unstable at room temperature. As an aid

to help interpretation of the results, it is good routine to test urines being submitted for pregnancy testing for protein count by a dipstick method (to be certain a high protein level is not present) as well as for specific gravity (to be certain the sample is concentrated).

Analysis

As a nursing diagnosis is never a diagnostic test, a pregnancy test itself is never a nursing diagnosis. A nursing diagnosis might be established, however, concerning the woman's anxiety or disappointment over the test result.

Planning

Unless there is an immediate reason for pregnancy testing—such as suspicion of an ectopic pregnancy or a scheduled X-ray procedure—it is best if a woman waits until a week after her missed menstrual period; the most frequent cause of a false-negative reading is a low level of HCG very early in pregnancy. Some women refrain from smoking or drinking alcohol when they think they might be pregnant; when they realize they are not (by a menstrual flow or a negative test result), they "binge" on cigarettes or alcohol. A false-negative report can be very destructive if it leads a pregnant woman into this type of behavior.

Implementation

Be certain when doing pregnancy testing that you follow directions accurately; they differ slightly brand name to brand name. Be certain when doing test tube analysis that the tube is allowed to set *undisturbed* for the correct time interval. Shaking it or lifting it to check on progress or even placing the settling rack next to an instrument such as a centrifuge that shakes as it runs does not allow the particles to settle out. No positive ring will then occur. Women who test their urine at home are often guilty of such inspection during the waiting period, which also results in a false-negative reading.

Evaluation

Because no pregnancy test is 100 percent accurate and ovulation may occur later in a menstrual cycle than anticipated, at times a woman who is pregnant will not be found to be pregnant on examination or test. Caution any woman who thinks that she is pregnant but has a negative result that if another week passes without menses she should return for a repeat test. She may in fact not be pregnant; but therapy may be needed for some other cause of amenorrhea, such as an ovarian tumor.

Nursing Care Planning

A nursing care plan concerning a diagnosis of pregnancy is always individualized to the woman concerned. It always includes plans for continuing or not continuing the pregnancy. Following are three examples of such care planning.

Christine McFadden is a 15-year-old who comes to a prenatal clinic for pregnancy diagnosis.

Assessment

Patient unsure of last menstrual period (about 4 months ago). Has nausea every morning; has vomited last two mornings. Has breast tenderness and feels tired. Definite increase in abdominal size. Thinks she has felt "something twisting inside me." Has been sexually active; no contraceptive used.

Uterus palpated 4 cm above symphysis pubis. Secondary areolae present on breasts; colostrum expressed from nipples. Fetal heart tones present by Doppler at 150.

Analysis

Concern related to pregnancy of about 16 weeks' length by positive sign criteria (M.D. to confirm).

Locus of Decision Making. Shared.

Goal. Patient to make firm decision on whether to continue or end pregnancy by 1 week.

Criteria. Patient to telephone health care facility with decision by Monday.

Nursing Orders

1. Mark for M.D. evaluation and physical exam.
2. Schedule for routine blood work and urinalysis.
3. Discuss plans for continuing pregnancy or abortion to end pregnancy.
4. If decision in 1 week is to end pregnancy, schedule appointment for abortion and return visit here for contraceptive counseling to prevent a second unwanted pregnancy.
5. If pregnancy will be continued, arrange appointments for prenatal care around school schedule so patient can remain in school and prenatal care can be optimal.
6. Evaluate in terms of physical, developmental, and psychological readiness for childbearing due to age.

Mary Kraft, 23 years old, is seen in an obstetrician's office.

Assessment

Last menstrual period 37 days ago. Did home pregnancy test: result positive. Some nausea in morning; some breast tenderness. "Really excited" at being pregnant.

Has been trying to conceive since surgery for endometriosis 4 months ago. Uterus not palpable above symphysis pubis. No fetal heart sounds heard by Doppler. Slight linea nigra present on abdomen.

Analysis

Concern related to possibility of pregnancy by presumptive signs of pregnancy (M.D. to confirm).

Locus of Decision Making. Patient.

Goal. Patient to continue the pregnancy.

Criteria. Patient will return for prenatal care at scheduled intervals.

Nursing Orders

1. Mark for M.D. evaluation and physical exam.
2. Schedule routine blood work and urinalysis (include serum HCG for pregnancy confirmation).
3. Arrange appointments for prenatal care around work schedule so prenatal care can be optimal.
4. Husband wants to be included in pregnancy care and be an active participant at delivery.

Angie Baco, 42 years old, is seen in a prenatal clinic.

Assessment

Last menstrual period 12 weeks ago. Was using vaginal foam for contraception. Has mild nausea in a.m.; frequency of urination, some breast tenderness. "Knows" that she is pregnant because she has been pregnant seven times before. Not "excited" about a pregnancy at this time of life, but would continue it if she is pregnant.

Uterus palpable slightly above symphysis pubis. Fetal heart tones by Doppler at 120.

Analysis

Concern related to pregnancy of 12 weeks' duration by positive sign criteria (M.D. to confirm).

Locus of Decision Making. Shared.

Goal. Patient to continue the pregnancy.

Criteria. Patient to return for prenatal appointments as scheduled.

Nursing Orders

1. Mark for M.D. evaluation and physical exam.
2. If pregnancy is confirmed, discuss impact of pregnancy for self and family to clarify its meaning.
3. Schedule routine blood work and urinalysis.
4. Schedule appointments for prenatal care around family commitments so close family support is maintained and prenatal care is optimal.
5. Refer to M.D. for any additional assessment interventions, such as sonogram or amniocentesis (age 42 years).

Questions for Review

Multiple Choice

1. Mrs. Bakowski is a woman you see in a prenatal clinic. Which of the following assessments is a probable sign of pregnancy?
   a. Chadwick's sign
   b. nausea and vomiting
   c. a positive urine pregnancy test
   d. amenorrhea

2. Which of the following is a positive sign of pregnancy?
   a. positive urine pregnancy test
   b. fetal movement felt by examiner
   c. Hegar's sign
   d. uterine contractions

3. Mrs. Bakowski is asked to bring in a urine sample for pregnancy testing. Which of the following instructions would you give her concerning this request?
   a. She should drink 1,000 ml of fluid prior to voiding.
   b. She should use a clean-catch technique.
   c. A double-voided specimen is necessary.
   d. It should be a first morning sample.

4. If Mrs. Bakowski is pregnant, what breast changes would you expect to find on assessment?
   a. slack, soft breast tissue
   b. deeply fissured nipples
   c. enlarged lymph nodes
   d. darkened areolae

5. Mrs. Henry is a woman with symptoms of urinary tract infection. She is reluctant to have pelvic x-rays because she is concerned she is pregnant. The best method to detect pregnancy prior to pelvic x-rays is
   a. X-ray of fetal skeleton.
   b. progesterone withdrawal test.
   c. radioimmunoassay test.
   d. by physical exam.

6. A friend tells you that she is going to use a home pregnancy test (a test tube technique) to determine whether she is pregnant or not. Which precaution below would you give her?
   a. "Use a dilute urine specimen."
   b. "Don't test until after two missed menstrual periods."
   c. "If the test is positive, arrange for prenatal care."
   d. "Be certain to agitate the tube during testing."

7. Which of the following statements is accurate concerning laboratory tests for pregnancy?
   a. Such tests are 100 percent accurate.
   b. Laboratory tests use urine or blood serum.
   c. Biologic pregnancy tests give quicker results than immunologic tests.
   d. A concentrated urine may give a false-negative reading.

Discussion

1. The first time a woman feels "really pregnant" is often following a positive pregnancy diagnosis. How might this new attitude affect her health practices?
2. Home pregnancy testing is now available. What are some arguments for and against home pregnancy tests?
3. The positive signs of pregnancy are few. What are these signs?

Suggested Readings ◀ ▶

Abiri, M. (1984). Ultrasound diagnosis. *Female Patient, 9,* 132.

Abrams. J. (1983). Gynecology: Urinalysis, pregnancy tests, and Pap smears in your office. *Consultant, 23,* 179.

Alley, N. M. (1984). Morning sickness: The client's perspective. *J.O.G.N. Nursing, 13,* 185.

James. P. D. (1983). Human chorionic gonadotropin and the significance of the beta sub-unit. *American Journal of Medical Technology, 45,* 99.

Patterson, J. E. (1983). Colposcopy. *J.O.G.N. Nursing, 12,* 11.

Robertson, J. R. (1983). Office endoscopy. *Female Patient, 8,* 73.

Senreich, S. A. (1983). Pregnancy testing in the emergency department. *Topics in Emergency Medicine, 5,* 62.

Sheehan, C. (1983). Current status of pregnancy testing. *American Journal of Medical Technology, 7,* 391.

Sokol, R. J., et al. (1980). Maternal-fetal risk assessment: A clinical guide to monitoring. *Clinical Obstetrics and Gynecology 22,* 547.

Trimmer, E. (1982). When your patients ask about home pregnancy testing. *Midwife Health Visitor and Community Nurse, 18,* 92.

18

Health Care: The First Prenatal Visit

OBJECTIVES

Following mastery of the contents of this chapter, you should be able to

1. Assess both psychological and physical status of a woman at a first prenatal visit in order to help ensure a safe pregnancy outcome.
2. State a nursing diagnosis related to prenatal care.
3. Plan the individualized prenatal care necessary to ensure a safe pregnancy outcome.
4. Describe implementations that should be included in a first prenatal visit.
5. Evaluate a woman's readiness and acceptance of prenatal care.
6. Analyze ways that prenatal care can be individualized to be meaningful to women.
7. Synthesize knowledge of prenatal care with nursing process to achieve quality maternal-newborn nursing care.

IDEALLY, PRENATAL CARE begins in a mother's childhood. It includes a good calcium and vitamin D intake during infancy and childhood, which helps widen a woman's pelvis and prevent contractions from rickets or other malformations. It includes a good overall diet, so that both the woman and her sexual partner enter pregnancy in the best state of health possible. It includes adequate immunization against contagious diseases during childhood, which lessens the chances of a woman contracting diseases such as rubella during pregnancy.

Prenatal care also includes the instillation of positive attitudes and concepts about sexuality, womanhood, and childbearing, so that the woman can enter pregnancy in good psychological health, unburdened by old wives' tales. Prompt and effective treatment of sexually transmitted diseases will help prevent pelvic inflammatory disease, thus protecting her fertility and making her as free as possible from such complications of childbearing as ectopic pregnancy. Also involved in prenatal care is reproductive planning information, which is intended to ensure that each pregnancy is planned and the child desired.

A woman is wise to schedule a premarital examination with a physician or nurse-midwife for reassurance about her fertility, detection of gross problems that need correction, and authoritative reproductive life planning information. If she did not have a premarital examination, a prepregnancy examination is her next wisest choice. Her hemoglobin level and blood type (including Rh factor) can be determined at this time; minor vaginal infections such as those arising from *Candida* can be corrected to ensure fertility; and the woman can be counseled on the importance of a good protein diet and early prenatal care in the event she does become pregnant. For prenatal care, a woman may choose to go to a clinic, a physician in general practice, or an obstetrician or nurse-midwife. The most important point here is early initiation of prenatal care, which can greatly lessen the risk of infant mortality.

Prenatal care is an important aspect of childbearing from a nursing standpoint because a great deal of the care involves listening, counseling, and supporting—three areas of nursing expertise. At the first prenatal visit, an extensive history is taken; a nurse skilled in the technique of patient health history taking can obtain vital information for the first visit (and succeeding ones too) at this time (Figure 18-1). A woman is also given a complete physical examination, including a pelvic examination. Specimens for blood work and a urinalysis are obtained; pelvic measurements may be taken to determine pelvic adequacy. During the first visit, a woman should be given appropriate guidance and instruction related to her history and physical examination. This advice helps make the pregnancy a safe one.

The Initial Interview

Setting and Ambience

Interviewing expectant mothers elicits a welter of contradictions. Women are likely to want to talk about their past health and present pregnancy so their interviews should go smoothly and be productive. On the other hand, some women may never have been interviewed by a health care person in depth before; they may want to talk but not feel free to do so. A woman may not regard certain information as important and answer questions about these areas vaguely; perhaps she is unaware that she is the only person who knows the answers to a number of vital questions ("How do you feel about being pregnant?" or "What have you been taking for your morning nausea?"). She may be afraid of criticism—of herself or of her

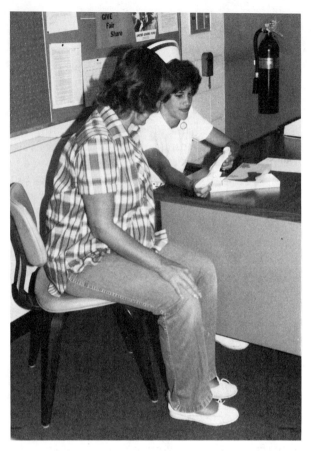

Figure 18-1 *Interviewing at prenatal visits is an important facet of care: It lays the foundation for prenatal teaching.*

views—and so resist expressing herself. Outside pressures, such as older children coming home from school, dinner preparation, or catching her bus, may take a toll on interview effectiveness. Later in pregnancy a woman may feel discomfort from having to sit still so long.

If an interview if going to be productive, all these factors must be considered and their effects modified.

Setting

Interviewing is best accomplished in a private, quiet setting. Trying to talk to a woman in a crowded hallway or a waiting room full of other patients is never effective; pregnancy is too private an affair to be discussed under these circumstances.

A woman should be invited to sit down. Your provision of a chair in a private room suggests that you have reserved this time just to talk to her. In response to your making her feel welcome, she will feel freer to describe her concerns in depth. You must also be seated. Perching on the edge of a desk or cart or leaning against a wall

suggests you have only a few minutes to spare, and she had better limit her answers to a simple yes or no to avoid trespassing on your time.

It is helpful if the receptionist in the clinic or office—or you, if you make the appointment—cautions a patient that the first visit will necessarily be a long one. This warning will prevent the woman from trying to sandwich the visit in between other errands or from having to terminate the interview because of another appointment. The fact that a woman who has been cautioned in this manner still tries to hurry matters is an interesting finding to note. Considered with other observations, it might indicate that she is trying to ignore her pregnancy or is so worried that you, the physician, or nurse-midwife will discover her pregnancy is not going well that she prefers to keep the visit short.

Establishing Rapport

Women need to feel that they are important, that what they have to say is important, before they can begin to answer questions in any depth. A private, personal setting conveys this sense of importance; calling the woman by her correct name also conveys it. Knowing what name to call patients is always a problem in nursing. If you are a student or a new graduate and the woman is older than you are, you should probably not call her by her first name. On the other hand, if the woman is close to your age (and women of childbearing years fall into a relatively young age group), ask if she would like you to call her by her first name. You will notice that obstetricians invariably call their patients by their first names. This personal, concerned touch is appreciated by most women. (As long as the woman's age or her personal preference does not interfere, this is an effective technique for you, too.)

Calling a woman by her first name may solve the problem of what to call an unmarried pregnant woman. Addressing her as *Ms.* may be an answer. A more straightforward approach is to call her *Miss,* because, contrary to what you may think, an unmarried pregnant woman usually wants you to know she is unmarried. Older unmarried women may choose to get pregnant (or not abort an unexpected pregnancy). While they have usually freely chosen their life style—and are secure in it—they may have worries such as child support and paternal role models that you need to explore. Young unmarried women often have another set of problems. An adolescent probably lives at home; her parents are angry with her because she is pregnant; her boyfriend may have disappeared; and girls she thought were her friends are shying away from her. Calling any of these women *Mrs.* will not change her response to the pregnancy, and it may convince her that you are either hard of hearing or so grossly unconcerned that you cannot remember that she is not married.

Make certain a woman knows *your* name and understands your role correctly. If she views you as a secretary, she will be willing to discuss superficial facts (name, address, phone number, and the like) but will resist discussing more intimate things (her feelings toward this pregnancy, the difficulty she has reworking old fears, how scared she is about delivery).

Do not be a "form filler-inner." If you do nothing during the interview but read questions from a form and fill in spaces, you might as well hand the woman the form and let her fill it in herself. She can establish no more rapport with you on this basis than she could achieve with the printed form itself.

Presentation of Questions

History taking is basic data gathering. It seems simple: You want an answer, and so you ask a question. *How* you ask a question, however, will affect the kinds of answers you receive. Using fact-finding and open-ended questions as well as supportive statements produces in-depth results. Vague, compound, critical, or oversophisticated questions limit your effectiveness as an interviewer.

A fact-finding question is straightforward: "How much do you normally weigh?" "What was the date of your last menstrual period?" These are questions that generally evoke a simple answer: "I weigh 110 pounds." "My last period was March 21st." An open-ended question gives the woman freedom to answer in a number of ways. A good technique is to begin and end all sections of an interview with an open-ended question, which encourages a woman to spontaneously produce information you might not have already elicited. An example of an open-ended question is "Why did you come to the office today?" A woman may answer in a variety of ways: "I'm pregnant." "I think I'm pregnant." "I hope I'm pregnant." "I'm afraid I'm pregnant." "I'm pregnant. *Do* something about it." The attitude implied by the words *think, hope,* and *afraid* would not be expressed in response to a fact-finding question such as "Are you here because you think you are pregnant?"

A vague question is an open-ended question gone wrong. It is so open-ended that the woman does not know how to answer. It baffles her and makes the interview a trying rather than a comfortable experience. "What about your general health?" is an example of such a question. The only answer a woman might give is, "What about it?" Ask exactly what you want to know about her health: "Have you ever had any serious illnesses?" "Have you ever been hospitalized?" "Are you currently being treated for any disease?"

In a multiple, or compound, question, two fact-finding questions are intertwined. "Do you have nausea and vomiting?" is such a question. If the woman has one but not the other, she is still likely just to answer yes or no because she does not want to delay matters by going into detail. Neither answer is correct. Single questions are better: "Do you have nausea?" "Do you have vomiting?"

A leading question suggests the answer by its structure. Because a woman wants to please you (you are in authority), she will answer in the manner you suggest. "You don't have any vaginal spotting, do you?" is such a question. Perhaps she actually does have spotting, but you imply she should not, so she will try to accommodate you by saying, "No, I don't." "Are you happy to be pregnant?" is another example. Because you have implied that she ought to be happy, she may feel trapped into answering affirmatively, despite her true feelings.

Supporting Statements. Many women will "toss" comments out to see if they catch your attention. This off-handed presentation generally hides strong feelings—so strong that they may need a good deal of urging to elaborate. At the same time, the comments show the women are so worried they cannot keep the concerns totally repressed. A woman in this conflict will be helped by your reassurance that she is free to discuss whatever is on her mind, that the clinic or office is interested in her entire well-being, not just her physical symptoms, blood pressure, or weight gain. Her statement might be, "This had better be a boy," followed by silence. A supportive response from you might be, "Tell me why you say that." Such a request lends weight to her statement and makes it important enough for her to discuss.

Suppose a woman says, "My first baby was stillborn." The woman looks as if she would like to say more about that pregnancy, that baby. But, after all, you are interviewing her because of a new pregnancy. Can you afford to spend time discussing that earlier pregnancy? Do you want to discuss it? Is there a place for that information on the form in front of you? You *do* have time, because how she accepts this pregnancy is going to be largely dependent on how well she handled the outcome of the earlier one. A supportive statement, such as "That must have been hard on you," will help her to express her feelings.

Transition Statements. Transitions in interviews are bridges between the parts of the interview; they allow you to move smoothly from one portion of an interview to another. Their content is basically an explanation of what is coming next. "I'm going to ask you some questions now about illnesses in your family" sets the stage and guides the woman's thoughts to that channel. It is disconcerting to jump to a new topic without such a statement. For example, if you ask, "Are you eating well?" and immediately afterward ask, "Is there any diabetes in your family?" the woman may put the two statements together and conclude that you know something about her the nurse-midwife did not discuss—namely, that she is becoming diabetic. It will be difficult for her to concentrate on any other subject when she is needlessly preoccupied with anxiety about diabetes.

Critical Remarks. If you think of history taking as simple data gathering, you can avoid making critical remarks ("You shouldn't do that"; "Why on earth do you think that?"). Such remarks made in response to a woman's comments will limit the information you can obtain at an interview. The woman did not come to the health care setting to be criticized. She came to be told she is or is not pregnant. Your judgmental attitude may make her too uncomfortable to come back; or if she does she will be careful in the future to slant her answers to obtain your approval. Remember that your eyebrows or your facial expression can reveal your disapproval just as readily as what you say. During an interview, a woman will use your facial expressions and your tone of voice as clues to your attitudes.

The Overly Sophisticated Question. An overly sophisticated question is one that contains words or concepts beyond the woman's understanding. "Have you been gravid before?" is such a question. True, gravid does mean pregnant, but it is not a term the average woman would be expected to recognize.

Parts of an Interview

An initial interview has several purposes: to gain information about the woman's physical and psychosocial health, to establish rapport, and to obtain a basis for anticipatory guidance at the conclusion of the visit.

Introduction

It is surprising how many professionals neglect to extend the simple courtesy of introducing themselves to patients. "Hello, Mrs. Smith, I'm Cynthia Harper, a registered nurse" takes less than a minute, yet identifies you and your role. It is so much simpler for patients calling a clinic or office to be able to identify you by name rather than saying, "I spoke to the little blonde girl. I don't know if she was a nurse or not."

Purpose

Women need an explanation of why they are being asked so many questions at a database interview. It is helpful if they know what areas you are going to be discussing: explaining the purpose of the interview is an important second step. "I'm going to be talking to you today in order that Dr. Weber, the physician, Ms. James, the nurse-midwife, and I can all get to know you better. I'm going to begin by asking you about any concerns you have. Then I'll ask you questions about your family, your past health, and any previous pregnancies you have had. We'll talk in detail about the reason you've come into the office today."

The Woman's Chief Concern

A woman makes an appointment at a health care facility because she has a special problem or need that is uppermost in her mind. On her way to the appointment perhaps she has rehearsed various ways of wording the problem that could precisely convey her pain, or her fear, or her hope. Until she has voiced this chief concern, it is hard for her to concentrate on other matters and give an accurate report of her history. An obstetric history therefore begins with an attempt to elicit this chief concern: "Why did you come to the clinic today?" or "Why did you make your appointment?"

After she has stated her chief concern, explore it in detail. You need to know the duration, intensity, frequency, and description of any symptoms she has, her actions with respect to them, and any associated symptoms. Suppose, for example, that her chief concern is nausea and vomiting. You need to know how long she has noticed these symptoms (duration); whether she has actually vomited or is just nauseated, and how late into the day she experiences the nausea (intensity); whether she notices it every day or only occasionally (frequency); exactly what she is describing (vomiting undigested food or bile-stained fluid) (description); what she has tried to do to relieve the nausea and vomiting (eating dry crackers, taking an over-the-counter medication) (her actions); and whether or not she has a fever or diarrhea (associated symptoms). You may discover by gathering all this information that the woman's symptoms are more suggestive of gastroenteritis than morning sickness; her problem may be a virus, not a pregnancy.

Following an in-depth look at the chief concern, ask, "Is there anything else that concerns you?" Because the woman's first response was respected and treated as important, she is likely to feel free to mention any further concerns.

Family Setting or Profile

Many physicians leave the social history or family setting history until the end of a health interview. Using this order is similar to interviewing in the dark and then switching on the light only for the last few sentences. In order to interview a woman intelligently, you need to know whether she lives alone or with a husband or family. If she lives alone, whom does she approach for emotional support or advice or help with problems? What is the source and level of her income? One of the hardest and sometimes most awkward questions to ask is, "Are you married?" One method of avoiding this question is to ask, "Who else lives at home with you?" The married woman answers, "My husband and my 4-year-old son." The single woman answers, "No one," "My parents and my brothers and sisters," or "My boyfriend." If this method of discovering marital status makes you more comfortable than a direct question, use it. Remember, however, that most unmarried women want you to know they are unmarried and will just as readily answer a direct question, "Are you married?"

It is good to know the size of the apartment or house in which a woman lives. If she is expecting a baby, you are going to be talking to her in the coming months about a bedroom or space for the baby's bed. It is important to know whether the essential rooms are on the ground floor or upstairs, since she may be restricted from climbing stairs more than once or twice a day following delivery or during the last part of pregnancy.

Before you can begin to offer a woman any more than stereotyped health care instruction, it is important to know her husband's or sexual partner's age, educational level, occupation, and shift he works on, if applicable; you also need to know her age and educational level, whether or not she is employed, and what kind of work she does (does it involve heavy lifting, long hours of standing in one position, handling of a toxic substance?).

As mentioned in Chapter 13, situations such as changing status from independence to dependence because of stopping work, chronic illness at home, the death of a significant person during pregnancy, the infidelity of a husband, geographical moves, financial hardship, or lack of support people may be injurious to a woman's ability to accept her pregnancy and child. No one in the clinic or office will be aware of these potentially harmful situations if you do not ask the questions about family setting that expose them.

Past Medical History

A number of diseases pose potential difficulty during pregnancy. These include kidney disease, heart disease (coarctation of the aorta and rheumatic fever cause problems most often), hypertension, sexually transmitted disease, diabetes, thyroid disease, recurrent convulsions, gallbladder disease, urinary tract infections, varicosities, and tuberculosis. Questions about these conditions form an important part of a woman's past history because they may become active during or immediately following pregnancy. It is also vital to find whether a woman had such childhood diseases as mumps (epidemic parotitis), measles (rubeola), German measles (rubella), or poliomyelitis. From this information you can reach an estimate of the antibody protection she has against these diseases, in case she is exposed to them during her pregnancy. If pregnant, she can be immunized against poliomyelitis by the Salk (killed virus) vaccine. She *cannot* be immunized against the others, since the vaccines contain live viruses, as does the oral Sabin poliomyelitis vaccine.

You should learn about a woman's drug sensitivities, so that prescription of drugs that might harm her can be avoided during pregnancy. A complete allergy history is vital: Women with allergies of any magnitude should probably breastfeed rather than bottle-feed their infants in order to avoid possible milk allergy in the infant. This choice is the woman's, not yours to make; however, you will need the information in order to counsel her appropriately.

Any past surgical procedures are important. Adhesions resulting from past abdominal surgery may cause difficulty with the growth of the uterus. Because of the known deleterious effect of smoking on the growth of a fetus, the woman's smoking history should be obtained. Ask about alcohol consumption, since excessive alcohol intake may lead to poor nutrition or be responsible for a fetal alcohol syndrome in the baby. Do not allow a woman to answer vaguely, "I drink socially," or "I only smoke occasionally." Ask her *exactly* what she means so you can accurately judge the frequency of these events.

Ask whether she takes any medication, prescribed or over-the-counter; the effect of these on a growing fetus will have to be evaluated. Ask about the use of illegal drugs such as marijuana or cocaine: These can also be deleterious to fetal growth. Most women answer these questions honestly during pregnancy because they are concerned about protecting the health of the fetus.

Gynecologic History

When most women had children early in life and it was unusual to care for a woman in childbirth past age 30, the number of reproductive tract or women's health problems such as breast disease that they experienced while pregnant were very few in number. Today, when women often delay conception of their first child past 30 years of age, it is not unusual to discover a woman who has had a problem with her reproductive tract or breast health.

A woman's past experience with her reproductive system has some influence on how well she accepts a pregnancy. You need to know the age of menarche and how well she was prepared for it as a normal part of being a mature woman. You also need to know the interval, the duration, and the amount of menstrual flow. Does she have discomfort? If she describes menstrual cramps as "horrible" and wonders how she "lives through them some months," imagine what her concept of labor must be like! She will need more-than-average counseling as pregnancy progresses. Some women who have extreme dysmenorrhea are looking forward to pregnancy as 9 months without discomfort; they may need counseling in the postpartal period about active ways to relieve menstrual discomfort.

Seek out information about any past gynecologic or breast surgery or any other problem in these areas. Common breast disorders are summarized in Table 18-1. Such disorders may influence breast feeding decisions. If a woman has had a tubal operation, such as surgery for an ectopic pregnancy, the risk of another tubal pregnancy becomes theoretically higher. If she has had uterine surgery, her child may have to be delivered by cesarean birth rather than vaginally. If she has had frequent dilatation and curettage of the uterus, her cervix may be incompetent or unable to remain closed for 9 months; she may deliver prematurely. Table 18-4 lists common gynecologic illnesses and their possible significance. Ask what reproductive planning methods, if any, she has been using. Occasionally, a woman becomes pregnant with an intrauterine device in place. It will have to be removed to prevent infection during pregnancy. If the woman did not realize she was pregnant, she may have continued to take an oral suppressant for some time into the pregnancy.

A problem that should also be included as part of a woman's gynecologic history is stress incontinence, which is incontinence of urine on laughing, coughing, deep inspiration, jogging, or running (the diaphragm descends with these actions, increasing abdominal pressure, which increases bladder tension and causes emptying). This problem happens so often in some women that they must continually wear a sanitary pad or plastic lined underpants. If the problem occurs often, the woman's vulva may be chronically irritated and inflamed.

Stress incontinence occurs from lack of strength in the perineal muscles and bladder supports. It is associated with difficult deliveries, the birth of large infants, grand multiparity, and instrument deliveries. Some women accept stress incontinence as a normal consequence of childbearing and so do not report it at health care assessments (because they think of it as normal).

Stress incontinence may be prevented and relieved to some degree by strengthening perineal muscles by doing Kegal exercises. Surgical correction by a low abdominal incision (a vesicourethropexy or Marshal-Marchetti operation) can be performed to fix the urethra to the fascia of the rectus muscle of the abdomen. This offers support to the neck of the bladder and decreases the tendency for easy emptying on abdominal pressure.

Questions for a complete gynecologic history are summarized in the box on page 342.

Obstetric History

Do not assume that the current pregnancy is the first simply because a woman is very young or says she has only recently been married. Ask. You need to obtain the facts about past pregnancies as well as eliciting the woman's subjective feelings about these pregnancies. You need to know the child's sex and place and date of birth for each previous pregnancy. It is good to review the pregnancy briefly. Was it planned? Did she have any complications such as spotting, swelling of her hands or feet, falls, or surgery? Did she take any medication? Did she receive prenatal care? What was the duration of gestation? What was the duration of labor? Was labor what she expected? Worse? Better? What was the type of delivery? What was the type of anesthetic used (if any)? What was the infant's birth weight? What was the condition of the infant at birth? Did the infant cry right away? Was there any blueness? Did the baby

Table 18-1 Breast Health Disorders

Structure	Possible Findings	Significance
Accessory nipples	Present at birth along mammary lines (Figure 18-2)	May increase in size at puberty or during pregnancy due to estrogen stimulation. If actual breast tissue is present under nipple, this tissue is subject to all breast diseases.
Breast hypertrophy	Abnormal enlargement of breast tissue	Breast growth continues until progesterone is being produced at mature levels; if ovulation is not fully established until late in adolescence, breast growth continues. Can lead to both physical and emotional stress from appearance. Surgical breast reduction can be accomplished. If a large portion of glandular tissue is removed, breast-feeding may not be possible later. Breast self-examination should continue.
Breast hypoplasia	Less than average breast size	Small breasts do not interfere with breast-feeding. Augmentation surgery can be accomplished by an implant of a prosthesis filled with silicon gel or saline. Caution women to continue with breast self-examination as breast tissue is not replaced. A woman may breast-feed with implants in place although she might choose not to as a breast infection (mastitis) might necessitate removal of the implant. Following a traumatic blow to a breast, the breast should be examined, because if silicon leaks from the implant, it could cause an embolus.
Sebaceous cyst	A raised, movable, non-tender nodule (Figure 18-3A)	Application of warm soaks followed by a topical antibiotic ointment 3 to 4 times a day will cause the cyst to open and drain. Caution women that a sebaceous cyst may recur and that it involves only skin tissue, not breast tissue, so is not a true breast lesion.
Nipple fissure	A crack on the nipple surface	Occurs typically with breast-feeding; if present at any other time, it may be a symptom of chronic discharge and needs a referral.
Fat necrosis	A firm well defined benign lump	Occurs following a blow to the breast. Generally recommended these be biopsied and then excised.
Galactocele	A round, centrally located painless lump	A cyst filled with breast milk. Occurs most often when breast feeding is halted abruptly. Contents can be aspirated. Should not recur.
Intraductal papilloma	Clear nipple discharge present, no tumor is palpable (Figure 18-3B)	Occurs any time after puberty. No immediate therapy is indicated because nipple discharge without a palpable tumor is rarely associated with breast carcinoma. Can be biopsied and excised.
Duct ectasia	Nipple discharge, clear, green, or black, is present; local swelling and pain	Inflammation of the terminal milk ducts. Occurs most often in postmenopausal women. Is biopsied and involved glands incised. Should not recur.
Fibrocystic disease	Painful, round, fluid-filled, freely moveable lumps; most often located in outer upper quadrants of breasts (Figure 18-3C)	Occurs from puberty to menopause. The consistency of lesions varies with the phase of the menstrual cycle; they tend to disappear during pregnancy and lactation. Taking a simple analgesic or applying warm compresses may be comforting. Reducing sodium intake may result in less fluid retention in cysts. A short-term diuretic just prior to menses may reduce fluid retention. Fluid is associated with intake of methylxanthines, present in caffeine, theophylline, and theobromine. Cysts may be aspirated. Does not lead to breast carcinoma except that carcinoma may not be palpable under fluid filled cysts.

Table 18-1 (continued)

Structure	Possible Findings	Significance
Fibroadenoma	Round, rubbery feeling well-defined lump	Occurs in response to estrogen stimulation; most frequent in young black women; rarely seen postmenopause. May increase in size during adolescence and during pregnancy and lactation or from ovulation suppressants. Can be surgically excised.
Carcinoma	A single, firm, fixed painless lesion (Figure 18-3D); retraction of skin (Figure 18-3E), nipple discharge, and nipple retraction may be present	Occurs most frequently in high-risk postmenopausal women in upper outer quadrant of left breast (Table 18-2). Most are discovered on self breast examination. Therapy is surgery (mastectomy or lumpectomy, see Table 18-3) followed by chemotherapy or radiation. Women cannot breast feed following radiation or the extensive removal of breast tissue.

Table 18-2 Characteristics of Persons at High Risk for Breast Cancer

Female
Caucasian
Over age 40
With a familial history of breast cancer
Natural menopause occurred after age 50
Nulliparous or women who had first pregnancy after age 34
Never breast-fed a child
Exposed to carcinogens
Obese
With a high fat intake
From an upper socioeconomic level
With fibrocystic breast disease

Table 18-3 Types of Breast Surgery

Type	Description
Lumpectomy	Removal of the breast lump.
Simple mastectomy	Removal of the full breast tissue.
Modified radical mastectomy	Removal of all breast tissue and skin, most or all of axillary lymph nodes.
Radical mastectomy	Removal of all breast tissue, associated pectoralis major and minor and dissection of the axilla and removal of lymph nodes.
Breast reconstruction	Plastic surgical intervention to rebuild a breast using a silicon or saline implant.

become yellow during the hospital stay? (Avoid the terms *cyanosis* and *jaundice* unless you define them as you use them: Many woman do not know what they mean.) Some mothers know the infant's Apgar score and can tell you this. Also inquire about the need for special equipment, whether the baby was discharged from the hospital with her, and the child's present state of health. What was the outcome of the pregnancy for *her*? Did she have stitches following delivery? Did she have any complications such as excess bleeding or infection?

Ask about any previous miscarriages or abortions. Did she have any complications during or following them? *Abortion* is the medical term for any pregnancy terminated before the age of viability. The *age of viability* is the earliest age at which a fetus could survive if he were born at that time, generally accepted as 20 weeks, or a fetus above 400 gm. Although you chart both induced and spontaneous pregnancy terminations in the same way, women appreciate your separating them into *miscarriage* (a spontaneous abortion) and *abortion* (used in its more limited meaning of induced or therapeutic or planned termination of pregnancy) when you are talking to them. If the woman's blood type is Rh negative, ask if she received RhoGAM immunoglobulin after miscarriages or abortions so you will know whether Rh sensitization could have occurred.

Pertinent terms of pregnancy are defined in the Nursing Care Highlight on page 342. After a history of previous pregnancies is obtained, determine a women's status with respect to the number of times she has been pregnant, including the present pregnancy (*gravida*), and the number of children above the age of viability she has previously delivered (*para*). For example, a woman

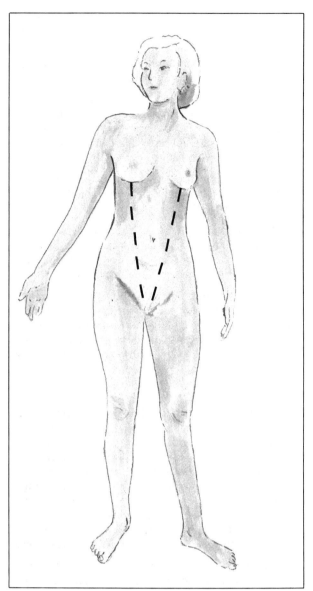

Figure 18-2 *Accessory nipples occur along mammary lines.*

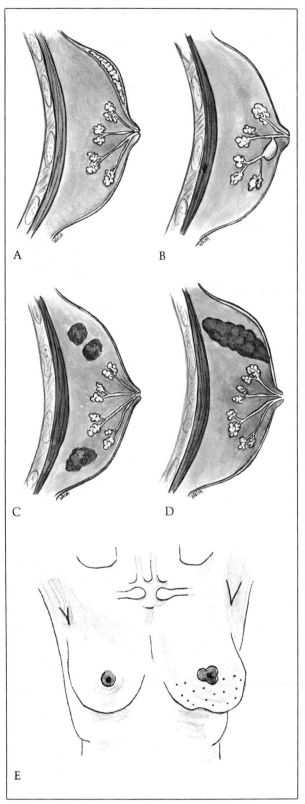

Figure 18-3 *Common breast lesions. A. Sebaceous cyst. B. Intraductal papilloma. C. Fibrocystic disease. D. Carcinoma. E. The orange peel appearance of breast carcinoma from local edema.*

Table 18-4 Gynecologic Disorders

Disorder	Possible Symptoms	Suggested Therapy
Vulva		
Cysts of Skene's or Bartholin's glands	Asymptomatic swelling at the sides of the urinary meatus or vestibule	Such cysts are surgically incised to prevent blockage and infection of the gland.
Condylomata acuminata	Cauliflower-like lesion on vulva	Tends to occur in women with chronic vaginitis. Caused by the epidermatrophic virus that causes common warts. Removed by cryocautery or knife excision.
Lichen sclerosus	Whitish papules on the vulva; asymptomatic	No need for removal; the area is biopsied because leukoplakia, a potentially cancerous condition, has an almost identical manifestation.
Leukoplakia	Thick, gray, patchy epithelium that cracks and infects easily, accompanied by itching and pain	Possibly a premalignant state. Therapy involves systemic antibiotics and frequent return visits to health care personnel (every 6 months) for observation to detect any changes suggestive of carcinoma.
Carcinoma of the vulva	A shallow vulvar ulcer that does not heal	Occurs most often in postmenopausal woman; represents only 3 to 4 percent of all reproductive tract cancer in women. Therapy is vulvectomy (vagina is left intact and sexual relations and pregnancy may be possible with cesarean birth to prevent tearing of fibrotic vulvar tissue).
Vagina and Cervix		
Adenosis	Asymptomatic vaginal cysts	Caused by diethylstilbestrol (DES) administration while in utero. Columnar rather than squamous epithelium is present on vaginal walls. Has the potential for becoming malignant (clear cell adenocarcinoma). If adenosis is present, an examination 2 or 3 times a year with a Pap test and Lugol's staining is necessary and the woman should not use estrogen sources such as oral contraceptives. If adenocarcinoma occurs, local destruction of atypical cells can be achieved by excision, cautery, or cryosurgery.
Cervical polyp	Red, vascular protruding pedunculated tissue that bleeds readily with trauma	A polyp may be discovered because of vaginal spotting on coitus, tampon insertion, or vaginal examination. Is removed vaginally by incision. Often associated with chronic cervical inflammation.
Cervicitis (erosion)	Reddened cervical tissue with a whitish exudate	Douching with a vinegar solution aids healing. May be treated with cryosurgery if extensive.
Nabothian cyst	Clear shining circles on cervix from blocked ducts of glands	No therapy necessary.
Cervical carcinoma	Postcoital spotting, unexplained vaginal discharge, or vaginal spotting between menstrual periods	Most frequent type of reproductive tract malignancy. High risk factors are coitus with multiple partners or uncircumcised males, herpes type II infections, or DES during pregnancy. Diagnosed by Pap test or colposcopy. Therapy is conization, radiation, or surgical excision. Pregnancy is possible following cervical carcinoma; cesarean birth may be necessary because of fibrotic cervical tissue.
Ovaries		
Endometrial cyst	Chocolate-brown colored cyst on tender enlarged ovary; may cause acute pain if rupture occurs	Caused by endometriosis; occurs in women aged 20 to 40 years. Therapy is surgical excision; ovary may or may not be removed depending on extent of cyst.

Table 18-4 (continued)

Disorder	Possible Symptoms	Suggested Therapy
Ovaries (continued)		
Follicular cyst	Amenorrhea and possibly dyspareunia; ovary is tender and enlarged	Follicular cysts regress after 1 to 2 months; a low-dose oral contraceptive may be prescribed for 6 to 12 weeks to suppress ovarian activity; estrogen may be continued for 6 months.
Polycystic disease	Multiple follicular cysts of both ovaries are present	There is excess adrenal supply of estrogen leading to inhibition of FSH and anovulation. Clomiphene citrate therapy to induce ovulation or wedge resection of the ovaries is used as therapy.
Corpus luteum cyst	Delayed menstrual flow followed by prolonged bleeding; ovary is enlarged and tender	A corpus luteum has persisted rather than atrophied. Most regress in about 2 months; a low-dose oral contraceptive may be prescribed for 6 weeks to suppress ovarian activity.
Dermoid cyst	Asymptomatic; ovary is enlarged on examination	Arise from embryonic tissue; may contain hair, cartilage, and fat. Most common ovarian tumor of childhood; also occurs at 30 to 50 years (Figure 18-4). Therapy is surgical resection.
Serous cystadenoma	Occur bilaterally; asymptomatic except for signs of pelvic pressure	Most common type of benign ovarian cyst; malignancy rate is high: 20 to 30 percent. Therapy is surgical resection.
Carcinoma	Asymptomatic	Arises from epithelial tissue most often in women over 50 years of age. Environmental contamination may play a role in development. Therapy is hysterectomy and salpingo-ophorectomy.
Uterus		
Endometrial polyp	Intermenstrual bleeding	Removed by dilatation and curettage.
Leiomyomas (fibroids)	Asymptomatic or with increased menstrual flow	Formed of muscle and fibrous connective tissue in response to estrogen stimulation (Figure 18-5). Increase in size during pregnancy; may cause interference with cervical dilatation and cause postpartal hemorrhage. Stress to the myometrium by uterine contractions may be the original cause of formation. Therapy is surgical resection (myomectomy) or hysterectomy if childbearing is complete.
Endometrial carcinoma	Vaginal bleeding between menstrual periods	Diagnosis is by endometrial washing, not Pap test (Figure 18-6). Therapy is hysterectomy.
Uterine prolapse	Vaginal pressure and low back pain	The uterus has descended into the vagina due to overstretching of uterine supports and trauma to the levator ani muscle (Figure 18-7). Occurs most often in women who had insufficient prenatal care, birth of a large infant, a prolonged second stage of labor, bearing-down efforts or extraction of a baby before full dilatation, instrument delivery, and poor healing of perineal tissue postpartally. Degrees of prolapse are shown in Table 18-5. Therapy is surgery to repair uterine supports or placement of a pessary, a plastic uterine support (Figure 18-8). Women with pessaries in place need to return for a pelvic examination every 3 months to have the pessary removed, cleaned, and replaced and the vagina inspected; otherwise, vaginal infection or erosion of the vaginal walls can result.

Gynecologic History Questions

Menstrual history	Age at menarche.
	Frequency and duration of menstrual periods.
	Amount of menstrual flow (document by amount of pads or tampons used).
	Discomfort (document if first day, all days, etc., and action taken to relieve it).
	Does any female sibling or her mother have dysmenorrhea also (endometriosis is familial)?
	Presence and size of clots, if present.
	Presence of premenstrual syndrome (irritability, moodiness, headache, diarrhea) on 1 or 2 days prior to menses.
	Dates of last two menstrual periods and duration and type of flow.
Reproductive tract history	Vaginal discharge (document amount and whether pad is necessary or not—include duration, frequency, description, associated symptoms, actions taken).
	Vaginal pruritus.
	Vaginal odor.
	Reproductive tract surgery.
Sexual history	Sexually transmitted diseases (include herpes, gonorrhea, and syphilis).
	Is patient currently sexually active? Heterosexually? Homosexually? Bisexually?
	Discomfort (dyspareunia) or postcoital spotting present?
	Concerns (worried over frequency, position, partner's satisfaction with coitus). Is orgasm experienced?
Contraception history	Contraceptive presently being used (length of time used, satisfaction, any problems).
	Types used in past.
Breast health	Has she ever noticed any abnormality (lump, discharge, pain)?
	Has she ever had breast surgery?
	Has she breast-fed a child?

Nursing Care Highlight

Pregnancy Status

Term	Definition
Para	A live birth
Gravida	A pregnant woman
Primigravida	A woman who is pregnant for the first time
Primipara	A woman who has delivered one live-born child
Multigravida	A woman who has been pregnant before
Multipara	A woman who has delivered two or more live-born children
Nulligravida	A woman who has never been pregnant
Nullipara	A woman who has never had a live birth

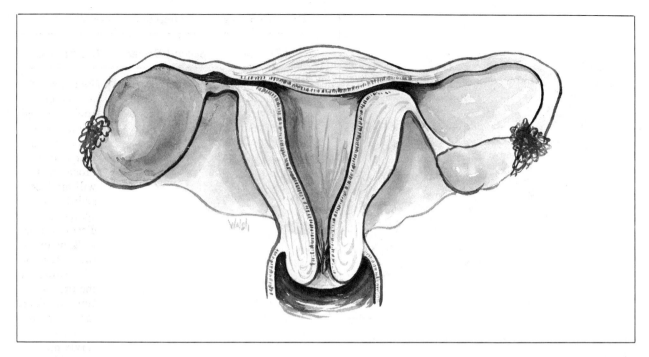

Figure 18-4 *Because they cause so few symptoms, ovarian tumors often grow to large sizes before they are discovered.*

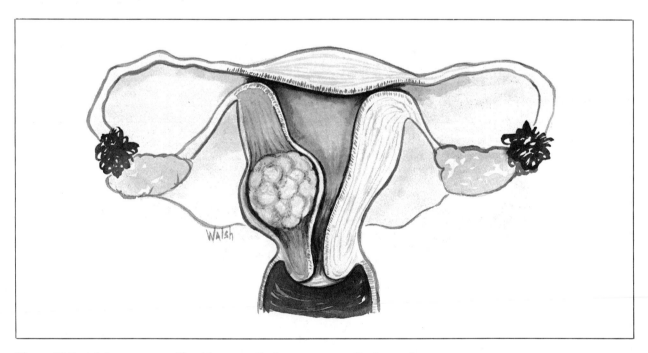

Figure 18-5 *A leiomyoma or fibroid tumor. Such tumors can displace a large uterine surface and interfere with fertility.*

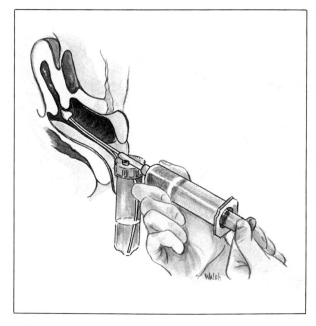

Figure 18-6 *Technique of endometrial washing to secure uterine cells for analysis.*

Table 18-5 Degrees of Uterine Prolapse

First Degree	Second Degree	Third Degree
The cervix has descended to a halfway point in the vagina.	The cervix has descended to the vagina introitus.	The entire uterus protrudes through the introitus (also termed *procidentia*). Procidentia will produce additional symptoms of discomfort on walking or sitting down due to pressure on the uterus. Chronic ulcers that form on the exposed cervix may cause bleeding.

Figure 18-7 *Uterine prolapse. A. First degree. B. Second degree. C. Third degree.*

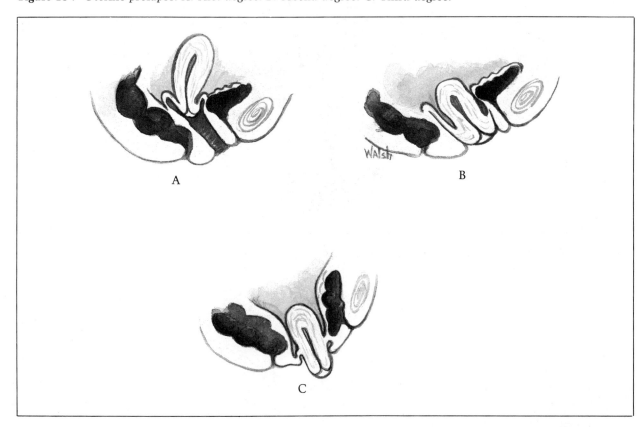

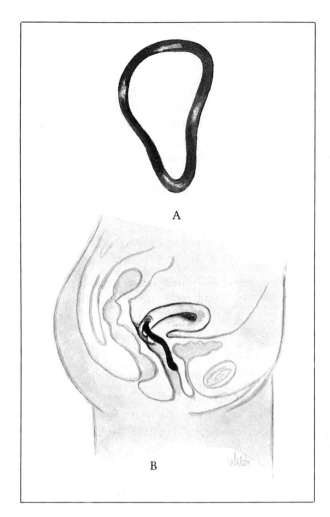

Figure 18-8 *A. A uterine pessary. B. A pessary in place, supported between the pubic bone and posterior vaginal fornix.*

who has had two previous pregnancies, has delivered two term children, and is again pregnant is gravida III, para 2. A woman who has had two abortions at 3 months (under the age of viability) and is again pregnant is a gravida III, para 0.

A newer system for classifying pregnancy status (abbreviated TPAL) attempts to further detail pregnancy history. By this system the gravida classification remains the same, but para is broken down into:

T = the number of full term infants born (infants born at 37 weeks or after).

P = the number of preterm infants born (infants born before 37 weeks).

A = the number of spontaneous or induced abortions.

L = the number of living children.

Using this system, the woman in the first example above would be gravida 3, para 2002.

A pregnant woman who had the following past history—in 1978, a boy born weighing 7 pounds, now alive and well; in 1979, a girl born weighing 7½ pounds, now alive and well; in 1982, a girl born weighing 4 pounds, now alive and well— would have her pregnancy information summarized as follows: gravida IV; para 2103.

Present Pregnancy History

It is a good idea to establish a baseline health picture at the initial visit: If on subsequent visits a symptom is mentioned, you can then check your records to see whether it is truly a new symptom. It may be that the woman is just becoming more aware of it.

You need to know whether or not a pregnancy was planned. "All pregnancies are a bit of a surprise. Is that how you reacted to this one?" is the kind of statement that will give you this information if you feel uncomfortable asking it directly. Other ways to word such a question are, "Some unmarried women want to have babies and some don't. How was it with you?" or "Some married couples plan on having children right away, some plan on waiting. How was it with you?"

Ask the date of the last menstrual period and whether the woman has had signs of early pregnancy, such as nausea, vomiting, breast changes, fatigue, and heartburn. Is she having any minor discomforts of pregnancy, such as constipation, backache, frequent urination? Has she felt quickening yet? At this point in pregnancy, how does she feel about the pregnancy? Has she reached a point where she can say she wants this child growing inside her? Is she taking any medication prescribed or over-the-counter? Has she experienced any of the danger signals of pregnancy, such as bleeding, continuous headache, visual disturbances, or swelling of the hands and face?

Day History

Information about a woman's nutrition, elimination, sleep, recreation, interpersonal interactions, and sexual activity can be elicited best not by direct questions but by asking the woman to describe a typical day of her life. The box on page 346 lists nutritional, sleep, elimination, interpersonal interaction, and sexual information that is helpful to obtain. If any of this information is not reported spontaneously as a woman describes her day, ask for additional information.

Review of Systems

A review of systems takes about 10 minutes to complete. You will be amazed at the results obtained, however, by telling a woman you are going to start at the top of her head and go through

Information Gained from a Day History

Nutritional history	Ask for a 24-hour recall of type and amount of food eaten (be certain that snacks as well as sit-down meals are described). Include how much fluid is consumed daily. Include alcohol consumption as fluid. Food preparation. Ask who cooks. What seasonings are regularly used? How is food usually cooked (fried? boiled?)? Is food eaten largely in planned settings or mainly as snacks? Difficulties. Is there any difficulty eating (nausea and vomiting? new braces?) Food allergies? Likes and dislikes? Food patterns. How many meals are eaten out daily? Weekly? Are any vitamin or vitamin supplements taken?
Sleep history	Ask about total hours of sleep each 24 hours, and sleep rituals. Any sleeping difficulty, such as insomnia, frequency of urination during the night? Has pattern changed recently (stress changes sleep patterns)? Is a medication regularly taken to induce sleep?
Recreation history	Ask what hobbies are enjoyed. How much physical activity (jogging, rollerskating, etc) is enjoyed daily?
Elimination history	Ask what is the usual pattern of bowel movements. What is urinary frequency? Has either pattern changed recently? Is anything used to aid bowel movements (laxatives, roughage in diet, enema)? Are there any problems with voiding (frequency, burning)?
Hygiene history	Ask if there is any sensitivity to soaps, skin-care preparations. Does she use feminine hygiene products? Does she douche regularly?
Interpersonal history	Ask who lives at home. How do these people interact with each other? Do they eat together or as each arrives home? Who gives psychological support to whom?

---

to her toes asking about body parts or systems and any diseases she has had. This method causes her to recall diseases she forgot to mention earlier—diseases that are important to your history.

The following body systems and conditions should constitute the minimum covered in a review of systems for a first prenatal visit:

1. *Head.* Headache? Head injury? Seizures? Dizziness? Syncope?
2. *Eyes.* Vision? Glasses needed? Diplopia? Infection? Glaucoma? Cataract? Pain? Recent changes?
3. *Ears.* Infection? Discharge? Earache? Hearing loss? Tinnitus? Vertigo?
4. *Nose.* Epistaxis (nose bleeding)? Discharge? How many colds a year? Allergy? Postnasal drainage? Sinus pain?
5. *Mouth and pharynx.* Dentures? Condition of teeth? Toothaches? Any bleeding of gums? Hoarseness? Difficulty in swallowing? Tonsillectomy?
6. *Neck.* Stiffness? Masses?
7. *Breasts.* Lumps? Secretion? Pain? Tenderness? Does she know how to do a breast self-examination? Does she do this monthly?
8. *Respiratory system.* Cough? Wheezing? Asthma? Shortness of breath? Pain? Serious chest illness such as tuberculosis or pneumonia?
9. *Cardiovascular system.* History of heart murmur? Rheumatic fever? Hypertension? Any pain? Palpitations? Any heart disease? Anemia? Does she know her blood pressure? What is her usual weight?
10. *Gastrointestinal system.* Vomiting? Diar-

rhea? Constipation? Change in bowel habits? Rectal pruritus? Hemorrhoids? Pain? Ulcer? Gallbladder disease? Hepatitis? Appendicitis?

11. *Genitourinary system.* Infection? Hematuria? Frequent urination? Sexually transmitted disease? Pelvic inflammatory disease?

12. *Extremities.* Varicose veins? Pain or stiffness of joints? Any fractures or dislocations?

Conclusion

End an interview by asking if there is something you have not covered that the woman wants to discuss. Resist explaining your clinic appointment system or giving prenatal health information until the woman has had a physical examination and a confirmation of pregnancy. If she is hoping she is not pregnant or is not ready to accept her pregnancy, she is not ready to listen to health instruction.

Because initial health history taking is time-consuming, the use of forms the patient fills in herself is often advocated. Pregnancy is such a personal experience that it seems callous to depersonalize it in this way. A better solution to the time problem is for nurses to learn good interviewing technique so they can secure thorough and meaningful health histories within a time constraint. The rapport that is established by face-to-face interviewing gives a woman the feeling that she is more than just a file card. It may be as important in bringing her back to a health care setting as her desire to be assured that her pregnancy is progressing normally.

The Father's or Support Person's Role

Because most appointments in health care settings are made for daytime hours, few husbands or prospective fathers used to accompany women for prenatal visits. Some of them regarded prenatal visits as only concerning the woman or assumed they would not be welcomed if they did go. Perhaps nurses, who set the tone in clinics and offices, did not always make them feel welcome.

Today, more and more fathers and young children are accompanying women for prenatal care. If a man is present, should he be included in an initial interview? As a whole, interviewing is most effective if it is a one-to-one interaction. A woman may be unwilling to mention certain of her concerns with her sexual partner present for fear of worrying him. A husband may not be the father of her child, and she may be unable to voice her concern over this fact or alert you to the possibility she is worried about blood incompatibility because another man is the father.

However, if childbearing is a family affair, it is just as important to determine the father's degree of acceptance of the pregnancy and of being a father as it is to establish how far the woman has come in the process of acceptance. Interviewing the woman alone and then inviting the support person and family to join her while you talk about pregnancy symptoms with them as a couple is a compromise solution. The main areas you should investigate with the father are his present health, his feelings and concerns about the pregnancy, and his knowledge of pregnancy and childbirth. He should be allowed to be in the room for the physical examination (if the woman wishes); and following the confirmation of pregnancy, he should be present when health care information is given. Providing some private interview time with a husband allows him to express worries he is reluctant to voice in front of his wife for fear of concerning or hurting her.

The Physical Examination

At the initial visit, following the health history, the woman will be given a physical assessment. She should undress and put on a gown so every body surface can be exposed during the assessment. Supply an extra cover sheet for the abdominal and pelvic examination. (Be certain that the examining room temperature is comfortable. Be certain to provide privacy. In order to prevent the spread of infection, the paper table cover should be changed between patients.) The woman should then be asked to empty her bladder. This is necessary to make the pelvic, or internal, examination comfortable for her and to allow for easier identification of pelvic organs. Save the voided urine for albumin and glucose testing and for microscopic examination to detect the presence of bacteria. Some health care settings require this urine to be obtained by a clean-catch technique; if so, give the woman good instructions on how to do this (see Procedure 18-1). A woman and her sexual partner can be taught to test the urine for albumin and glucose by a test-tape method as a way of allowing them to participate in their own health monitoring. Remember that although urine becomes for you, as a nurse, a substance frequently handled and inspected, many women regard it as dirty and any such testing objectionable. Evaluate each couple individually.

A woman should be weighed to obtain a base weight for comparison with all future weights (Figure 18-9). If she wants to, she could weigh herself with her support person's assistance. Pre-

Procedure 18-1

Obtaining a Clean-Catch Urine Specimen

Procedure

1. Wash your hands; identify the patient; explain the procedure.

2. Assess patient status; analyze appropriateness of procedure; plan modifications of procedure as appropriate.

3. Implement care by assembling supplies: commercial clean-catch urine specimen kit, or five sterile cotton balls, sterile specimen container, appropriate antiseptic solution. Provide privacy.

4. Assist patient to moisten three cotton balls in antiseptic solution and give instructions. Patient will cleanse urinary meatus with three cotton balls (washing front to back, right side of meatus, left side of meatus, directly over meatus) using each cotton ball for only one stroke and then discarding it.

5. Next, the patient will wipe away the antiseptic solution using the same technique. (Some commercial kits do not require this.)

6. Next, the patient should begin to void and dip the sterile specimen container into the urine stream to obtain a midstream urine specimen.

7. After 10 to 20 ml is obtained in specimen cup, patient may finish voiding in toilet.

8. Cap specimen container; label with patient's identification; mark "midstream" on label.

9. Evaluate effectiveness, efficiency, cost, safety, and comfort of procedure. Plan health teaching as needed such as importance of recognizing symptoms of urinary tract infection.

10. Document that specimen was obtained, amount of urine obtained, and any abnormalities with voiding or urine.

Principle

1. Prevent spread of microorganisms; promote patient safety and well-being.

2. Adults can obtain clean-catch urine specimens following careful instructions. Assess to determine level of understanding and physical ability to perform procedure.

3. Solution for cleaning differs in various health care agencies. *Thorough* cleansing appears to be more important than solution used.

4. Cleansing front to back prevents bringing rectal contamination forward in female. Discarding cotton balls also prevents this.

5. Wiping away antiseptic prevents it from entering specimen and, by germicidal action, decreasing bacterial growth and accurate analysis.

6. The flow of urine washes away bacteria from urinary meatus.

7. If intake and output is being recorded, place a bedpan on top of toilet to collect remainder of urine.

8. Most laboratory report slips accompanying specimens being sent for culture also require a list of antibiotics the person is receiving.

9. Health teaching is an independent nursing action always included as part of care.

10. Documentation of patient status and nursing care.

entering pregnancy in as good physical condition as possible. A thorough physical examination for a first prenatal visit is described below.

General Appearance

Physical examination always begins with inspection of general appearance in order to form a general impression of the woman's health and well-being. General appearance is an important assessment because people reveal how they feel by the manner in which they dress, the way they speak, and the body posture they assume.

Remove and replace, as necessary, any bandages and other dressings a woman has in place that could hide important findings. A growing problem—or perhaps one just now receiving increased recognition—is that of the battered woman. Ask how any skin abnormality such as an ecchymotic area occurred. Most marks from battering occur on the face, the ulnar surfaces of the forearms (from a woman raising her arms to defend herself), the abdomen or buttocks (from being kicked), or the upper arms (from being grabbed and held forcefully).

Expected Findings

Nonpregnant Woman. Slightly nervous; well groomed and poised.

Pregnant Woman. Excited yet slightly nervous and fatigued.

Head and Scalp Assessment

Examine the head for symmetry, normal contour, and tenderness, the hair for presence, distribution, thickness, excessive dryness or oiliness, or the use of hair dye (hair dye may be carcinogenic over an extended period of time).

Expected Findings

Nonpregnant Woman. Recently washed hair; no scalp lesions present.

Pregnant Woman. Hair growth speeds up during pregnancy due to the overall increased metabolic rate. Dryness or sparseness of hair suggests poor nutrition; excessive oiliness suggests fatigue to the extent that the woman hasn't felt well enough to wash it lately.

TEACHING POINT. Urge women during pregnancy to let some other task go and save their energy for self-care so they can continue to feel good about themselves. Dandruff shampoos may be used during pregnancy as they are not absorbed.

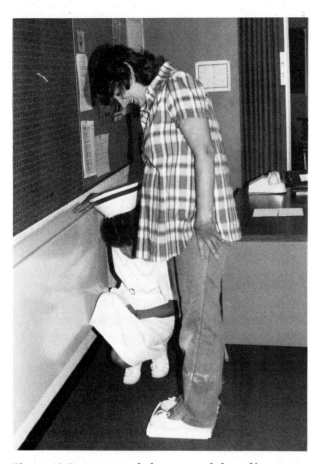

Figure 18-9 *A woman helps to weigh herself at a prenatal visit. Encouraging participation in care helps to make the pregnancy real and the woman a more informed health care consumer.*

viously, when calorie intake during pregnancy was severely restricted and women's weight gain was closely monitored, women would cheat with self-weighing. Be certain you convey an air of "accuracy is what counts," not "a minimal weight gain is important"; otherwise, their inaccuracy could make you miss a sudden weight increase, which is a signal of hypertension of pregnancy.

If you did not ask before, ask a woman her usual weight to determine how much weight she has already gained. Blood pressure, respiration rate, and pulse rate should also be measured to obtain baseline data. A sudden increase in blood pressure is also a danger sign of hypertension of pregnancy; an equally serious sudden increase in pulse or respirations may suggest bleeding. A support person can be taught the technique of blood pressure recording for added self-participation in care.

Techniques of physical examination are defined in the box on page 350. Some women may need reassurance that a full physical examination is necessary in order to ascertain whether they are

Techniques of Physical Examination

Inspection

Inspection is examining with your eyes. Smell is a lesser-used but practical second phase of inspection. The smell of stale urine, for example, suggests a woman has stress incontinence; a fishy odor suggests a trichomoniasis infection; a sweat odor suggests extreme fatigue.

Palpation

Palpation is examining by touch—either light or deep. The tips of your fingers are most sensitive to texture, vibration, consistency, and contour; the back of your hand is most sensitive to warmth.

Percussion

Percussion is the assessment of a body structure by determining the sound that you hear in response to striking the part with an examining finger. To percuss, place one finger flat on the surface to be examined and strike the first knuckle of that finger with the tip of a finger on your opposite hand (Figure 18-10). Dense body areas such as bone have a dull flat sound; those filled with air such as the lungs are resonant. If an organ is stretched (such as a distended bladder), it has a *hyperresonant* or low hollow sound. An organ stretched to an even greater point of distention has a *tympanic* or an extremely hollow ringing sound.

Auscultation

Auscultation is listening to sounds that are either discernible to the ear (coughing or heavy breathing) or magnified by means of a stethoscope. Always listen for the four qualities of sound: duration, frequency, intensity (loudness), and pitch (whether the sound is high or low).

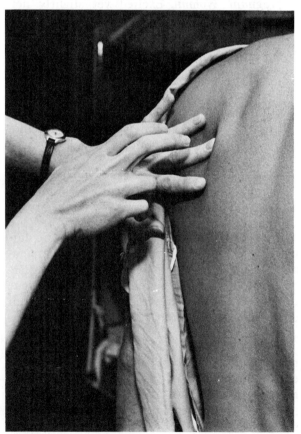

Figure 18-10 *Percussion is evaluation of sound made by tapping one finger against another.*

Eyes

Examine eyeglobes for firmness by pressing lightly against the woman's closed eyelids with your thumbs. Inspect eyebrows and eyelashes for scales or styes (*hordeolum*). Inspect whether, when the woman closes her eyes, the eyelids completely cover her eyes (edema may make eyelids too short) and whether, when she opens her eyes, the lids retract far enough that they do not obscure vision (edema may also cause this problem). Inspect conjunctiva for color and moistness (should be pink and moist). Women who have heavy menstrual flows may have anemia and may have pale appearing conjunctiva. Test for a red reflex by shining a bright light into the pupil (seeing a red circle indicates you are able to see through the pupil, aqueous humor, to the intact retina). Assess that pupil constriction is intact by shining a light on each pupil and seeing that both constrict in response to the light. Assess vision by asking the woman to read a Snellen chart (see the box on page 351) or, if not available, use print at an arm's distance.

The retina may be further inspected by means of an ophthalmoscope (Figure 18-11). With the retina focused, you should be able to discern the optic disc and the arteries and veins that supply it in close detail. Normally the margins of the optic disc are regular, and there should be no indication

Snellen Eye Testing

For Snellen chart testing, a woman stands 20 feet from the chart. Ask her to close one eye and read letters from the top down. Repeat with the second eye. In order to "pass" a line a woman must read the majority of the letters in the line correctly.

Eyesight is recorded as 20 (the distance in feet she stood from the chart) over the number corresponding to the last line she read correctly. An adult woman with normal vision standing 20 feet away from a chart can read the 20-foot line correctly, or has 20/20 vision.

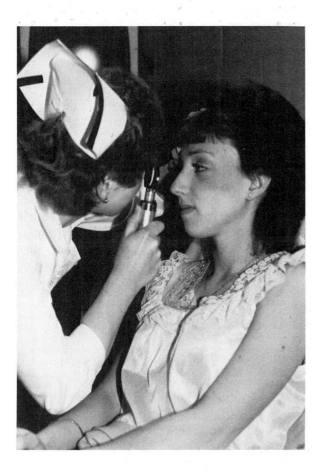

Figure 18-11 *An ophthalmoscopic examination of the eye.*

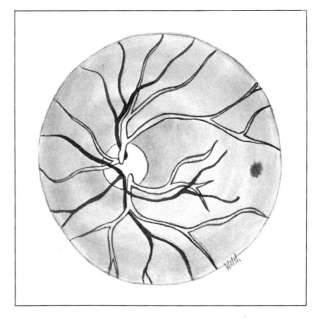

Figure 18-12 *A normal retina as seen through an ophthalmoscope.*

that it is swollen (papilledema) or compressed (occurs with glaucoma). If veins and arteries are very narrow, systemic hypertension is suggested; if copper-colored, arteriosclerosis is suggested. A normal retinal appearance is shown in Figure 18-12. Figure 36-6 shows the retina of a woman with diabetes, in which the hazy, cotton-like patches are caused by edema with infiltration around the vessel. Identifying women with diabetes is important for maternal-newborn nurses: Diabetes mellitus can interfere with a safe pregnancy outcome.

Expected Findings

Nonpregnant Woman. Many women have some degree of eyestrain from desk or computer work; their sclera may be red streaked, and they may rub their eyes or press against their temples for pain relief.

Pregnant Woman. Hypertension of pregnancy may be manifested by eye symptoms of edema in the eyelids, spots before the eyes, or diplopia (double vision). If an ophthalmoscopic examination is done, the optic disc will be swollen from edema. Help pregnant women to recognize symptoms of poor vision (danger signals of pregnancy that they should not delay reporting) rather than as symptoms unrelated to pregnancy. Caution them if they do close desk work to take a break every hour so sensations of eyestrain are not confused with danger signs of pregnancy.

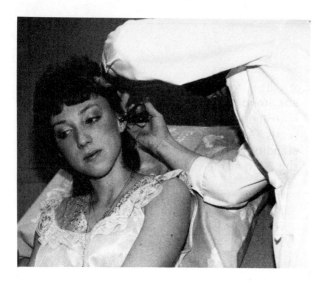

Figure 18-13 *An ear examination with an otoscope. Note how the examiner's hand rests under the instrument so if the woman should move, her ear canal will not be scratched.*

Ears

Assess ears for level (in a normal level a straight line drawn from the inner canthus of the eye through the outer canthus touches the pinna). Observe the opening to the ear canal for any discharge. Touch the pinna and watch for evidence

of pain (a sign of external canal infection). Use an otoscope to assess the tympanic membrane by first straightening the ear canal (pull upward and backward on the pinna). When inserting an otoscope tip into the external ear canal, always rest the instrument on your hand (Figure 18-13). In this position, if a woman should move her head suddenly, the otoscope will move with her, and there is no danger that the plastic tip will scratch the canal. Use the smallest size of tip possible that still gives you adequate visibility.

Assess the tympanic membrane for color (pearly gray) and landmarks (the cone of light or the reflection of the otoscope light and the outline of the middle ear malleus will be present) (Figure 18-14). A reddening or distortion of the membrane so the light or umbo are not evident suggests infection or fluid filling behind the membrane. Assess for hearing by ability to respond to a normal conversational voice.

Expected Findings

Nonpregnant Woman. Normal hearing level and normal tympanic landmarks.

Pregnant Woman. The nasal stuffiness that accompanies pregnancy due to estrogen stimulation may lead to blocked eustachian tubes and therefore a feeling of "fullness" or dampening of

Figure 18-14 *Looking through an otoscope, the malleus of the inner ear is evident through the translucent tympanic membrane. A cone of light is seen at 5 o'clock.*

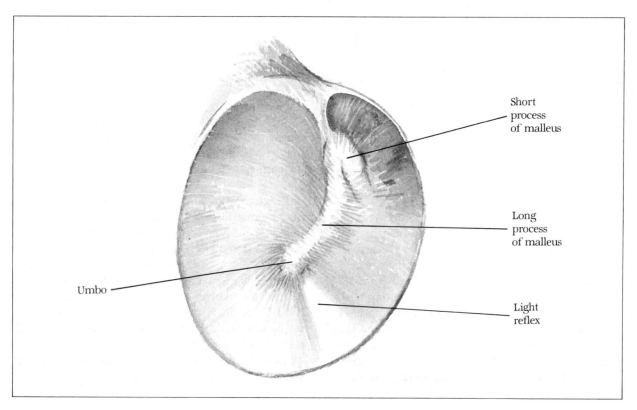

Short process of malleus

Long process of malleus

Light reflex

Umbo

sound during early pregnancy. This disappears as the body better adjusts to the new estrogen level.

TEACHING POINT. Cerumen in ear canals serves a purpose of clearing dirt from the ear canal. Teach women never to use articles such as bobby pins to clean ear canals and never to use cotton-tipped applicators to clean more than the external ear pinna or they can severely scratch the ear canal.

Nose

Observe the nose for flaring of the nostrils (a sign of need for oxygen) symmetry, drainage, midline septum, and normal color of mucus membrane. A reddened membrane with purulent drainage suggests an upper respiratory infection; a pale, "boggy" membrane with clear, watery drainage suggests an allergy is present.

Expected Findings

Nonpregnant Woman. Pink, moist mucus membrane.

Pregnant Woman. The high level of estrogen that occurs with pregnancy causes nasal congestion or the appearance of swollen nasal membranes.

TEACHING POINT. Teach pregnant women that even topical medicine such as nose drops are absorbed to some degree; a woman should avoid taking even these during pregnancy without her physician's or nurse-midwife's knowledge and consent. Teach all women how to halt nosebleeds (tip the head back, put pressure on the sides of the nose) as an emergency first-aid measure to use with young children.

Sinuses

Press with your thumbs against the frontal sinuses (over the eyebrows) and the maxillary sinuses (under both eyes) to elicit tenderness, which would suggest a sinus infection. Many women develop sinusitis in the winter time as an extension of an upper respiratory infection.

Expected Findings

Nonpregnant Woman. Nontender sinus area.

Pregnant Woman. Continuous headache is a danger sign of pregnancy (caused by cerebral edema). Tenderness over sinuses suggests that a woman's headache is sinus- rather than edema-related and, although she still needs a medical consult, she needs it for the former reason.

Mouth and Throat

Assess lips for dryness or lesions and corners of the mouth for cracking (suggests vitamin deficiency). Assess for normal color of mucus membrane and tongue and the condition of teeth and gums. Periodontal disease of the gums (reddened, swollen tissue leading to loss of teeth if unrecognized) is the leading dental problem in adults. If a woman wears a partial or full denture, ask her to remove it and inspect underneath for ulcerations or erythema. Chronic irritation from a loose or ill-fitting denture can lead to oral carcinoma. Always inspect under the tongue for any lesion: This is the first place that oral carcinoma most often occurs. A rough-textured tongue (geographic tongue) is an innocent finding although it often accompanies general symptoms of illness.

Using a tongue blade to press down on the back of the tongue, inspect the side and posterior throat for redness or drainage, and ascertain that the uvula is in the midline. If it is difficult to see tonsillar tissue at the sides of the throat, ask the woman to say, "Ah."

Expected Findings

Nonpregnant Women. Many adult women have one or more cavities in their teeth.

Pregnant Woman. The pregnant woman is prone to vitamin deficiency because of the rapid growth of the fetus; assess carefully for cracked corners of the mouth. Assess carefully for pinpoint lesions with an erythematous base on her lips; these suggest a herpes infection (a herpes lesion on the gumline is more often a shallow ulcer). Since newborns are very susceptible to herpes infection, lesions present at delivery may limit her contact with the newborn. Gingiva (gums) may be hypertrophied due to estrogen stimulation during pregnancy. They should not appear reddened, only swollen, and may be slightly tender to touch.

TEACHING POINT. Teach all women not to neglect good dental hygiene or yearly dental supervision visits (easy to do in a busy life pattern). Teach pregnant women to maintain thorough toothbrushing at least once a day (some stop thorough brushing because they notice slight blood-tinged mucus due to gingiva hypertrophy).

Neck

Examine the neck for suppleness by asking the woman to flex her neck forward and back and rotate it to both sides (women with chronic arthritis are unable to do this). Assess for a midline

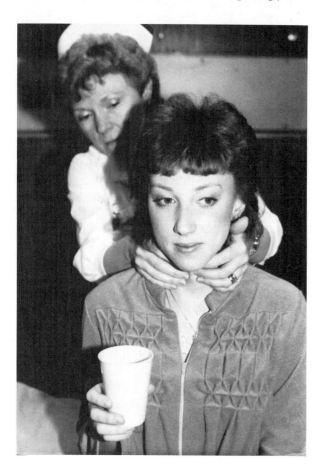

Figure 18-15 *Examination of the thyroid by palpation.*

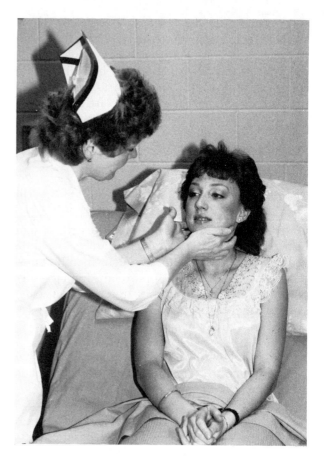

Figure 18-16 *Lymph node palpation.*

trachea (a deviated trachea suggests lung pathology). Assess the thyroid gland by palpating both sides of the trachea to determine if any lumps or tenderness is present (Figure 18-15).

Expected Findings

Nonpregnant Woman. No nodes on thyroid; midline trachea.

Pregnant Woman. Slight thyroid hypertrophy may occur with pregnancy as the overall metabolic rate is increased. Encourage a woman to continue to use iodine salt during pregnancy to supply enough iodine for thyroxin production with this increased rate (some view iodine as an unnecessary additive and discontinue using it during pregnancy).

TEACHING POINT. Teach women to eat seafood at least once weekly or to use iodized salt to ensure adequate iodine intake for thyroid health.

Lymph Nodes

Palpate lymph nodes for presence and tenderness (Figures 18-16 and 18-17). Enlarged preauricular

and postauricular nodes generally denote a recent ear infection; suboccipital nodes, a recent scalp infection; submental, a tooth infection; and submaxillary, anterior, and posterior cervical nodes, a tonsillar or throat infection.

Expected Findings

Nonpregnant Woman. No palpable lymph nodes.

Pregnant Woman. Pregnant women may develop an increased number of upper respiratory infections because of reduced immunologic resistance. They may also develop tooth abscesses from bacterial growth under hypertrophied gingival tissue and may have palpable lymph nodes.

Breasts

Breast examination has four major purposes: (a) to assess for the stage of breast development the woman has achieved (rated by the Tanner scale; see Chapter 8), (b) to assess for breast pathology such as cysts, (c) to evaluate breast readiness and competency for lactation, and (d) to provide an

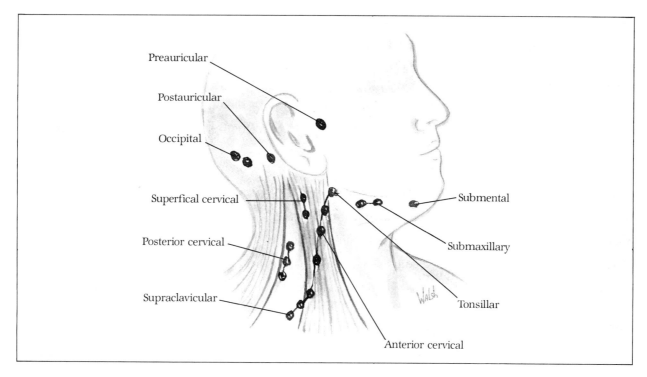

Figure 18-17 *Lymph node location.*

opportune time for teaching breast self-examination.

To assess for breast pathology, ask a woman to sit on the edge of an examining table, bed, or chair, and let her arms hang loosely at her sides. Assess for symmetry as to size, location, shape, and nipple placement. Observe for any area of dimpling and retraction that would suggest an area of tissue is firmly fixed or not freely mobile; tone (firmness or presence of pendulous tissue), presence of hair (should only be light, fine, downy); presence of veins (noticeable at about the third month of pregnancy); discharge from the nipple (clear or slightly yellow discharge is normal during pregnancy; this remains in some women who have been pregnant). Next ask the woman to raise her arms over her head and then place them on her hips, during which you repeat these observations.

Following observation of the breasts in these positions, ask the woman to lie supine on the examining table or a bed and lift her arm over her head. This movement stretches breast tissue and thins it; for a woman with a large breast, placing a small pillow or folded towel under the scapula helps to thin breast tissue even further.

Palpate quadrant by quadrant or moving in concentric circles from the nipple outward (Figure 18-18). Palpate well into the axilla as breast tissue extends to the midaxilla line. If a lesion is palpated, describe it according to the criteria in the box on page 356. Inspect the nipple for discharge; roll it gently between your finger and thumb to elicit any discharge. Be aware that many women have asymmetrical breasts (one slightly larger than the other). Supernumerary nipples may normally be present. The lower edge of each breast feels hard; do not mistake this or rib prominences underneath for more than they are.

Figure 18-18 *Breast palpation is an important assessment in women's health.*

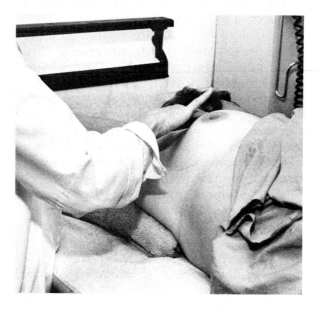

Characteristics of Breast Lesions

Characteristic	Description
Location	By breast quadrant (using the woman's right or left)
Size	Record in centimeters (estimating from the known size of your finger)
Number	Record number of lesions palpable
Consistency	Record as soft/hard or solid/cystic (spongy)
Mobility	Record as fixed or movable
Shape	Record as round or irregular
Discreteness	Record as discrete (separate) or not clearly defined
Appearance	Record erythema, dimpling, orange peel effect, retraction, or discharge of nipple
Pain or tenderness	Record as present or not

Expected Findings

Nonpregnant Woman. No masses; no nipple discharge.

Pregnant Woman. As pregnancy begins, the areola of breasts darken, Montgomery's tubercles become prominent, and breast size increases; the tone firms. Striae may occur as size increases. A secondary areola may develop surrounding the natural one; blue streaking of veins becomes prominent. Colostrum may be expelled from the nipple as early as the sixteenth week of pregnancy. A supernumerary nipple may also become darker and the woman may be concerned that this is a growing mole unless she is assured of the normalcy of this pregnancy change.

TEACHING POINT. Teach all women to do breast self-examination monthly. The day following their monthly menstrual flow is a good "marking point" to use; this is also a time when hormonal influences on breast tissue are at a low ebb, so breast tissue is normally not swollen or tender and does not cause discomfort. A woman who is currently not having a menstrual flow, for instance, pregnant women, should specify a certain day each month (the first day, the last day) for breast self-examination. Alert women that 90 percent of breast lesions are not breast cancer so if they do discover a lesion on self-examination they will report it promptly. Otherwise they might become so fearful of cancer that they are "frozen" into immobility.

Figure 18-19 shows the technique for breast self-examination.

Heart

Observe the left chest for a point of maximum impulse of the heart (the location of the left ventricle or the point where the apical heart beat can be heard best). In adults this is generally the fourth or fifth intercostal space at the midclavicular line.

There are four main points at which you should auscultate heart sounds. Although these are not the anatomic locations of heart valves, they are the listening points to which the sounds of the valves radiate and at which they can be heard best (Figure 18-20). Table 18-6 lists normal and abnormal heart sounds that may be heard on auscultation.

In order to understand heart sounds, you need to recall heart physiology. The first sound heard (S1) is that of the mitral and tricuspid valves closing and the ventricles contracting (described as a "lub" sound). The second sound (described as a "dub" sound and termed S2) is made by the closure of the aortic and pulmonary valves and atrial contraction.

With inspiration and the normal resulting increase of pressure in the lungs, the pulmonary valve tends to close slightly later than the aortic valve. This is termed *physiologic splitting* and will be heard as "lub d-dub." As long as this is

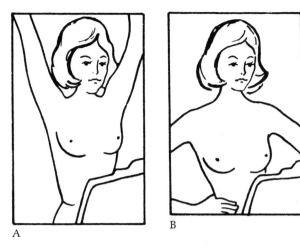

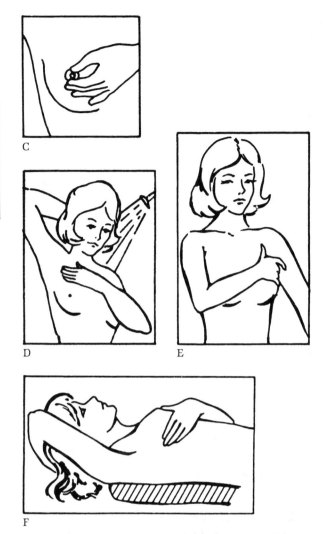

Figure 18-19 *Self breast examination technique.* Step 1. Inspection. A. In front of a mirror, look for any change in the size or shape of the breast, puckering or dimpling of the skin, or changes in the nipple. B. Inspect in three positions: (1) with arms relaxed at sides; (2) with arms held overhead; and (3) with hands on hips, pressing in to contract the chest muscles. Turn from side to side to view all areas. C. Nipple examination. Gently squeeze the nipple of each breast between your thumb and index finger, looking for any nipple discharge. Step 2. Palpation or feeling. D. In shower or bath. Fingers will glide over wet soapy skin, making it easier to feel any changes in the breasts. Check the breast for a lump, knot, tenderness, or for any change in the consistency of normal breast tissue. To examine your right breast, put your right hand behind your head, with the pads of your fingers of your left hand held flat and together; gently press on the breast tissue using small circular motions. Imagine the breast as the face of a clock. Beginning at the top (12 o'clock), make a circle around the outer area of the breast. Move in one finger width; continue in smaller and smaller circles until you have reached the nipple. Cover all areas including the breast tissue leading to the arm pit. Reverse the procedure for the left breast. At the lower border of each breast, a ridge of firm tissue may be felt. This is normal. E. Underarm examination. Examine the left underarm area with your arm held loosely at your side. Cup the fingers of the opposite hand and insert them high into the underarm area.

Draw fingers down slowly, pressing in a circular pattern, covering all areas. Reverse the procedure for the right underarm. F. Lying down. While lying flat, place a small pillow or folded towel under the right shoulder. Examine the right breast using the same circular motion as was used in the shower. Cover all areas. Repeat this procedure for the left breast. Press firmly but gently while examining your breasts, rolling the tissue between your fingers and the chest wall. (Courtesy of the American Cancer Society, New York State Division, Inc., East Syracuse, N.Y.)

associated with inspiration, it is a normal finding. Fixed splitting implies that there is always difficulty with pulmonary valve closing and suggests pathology.

A heart murmur is caused by the sound of blood flowing with difficulty or in an unusual pathway within the heart; and it can be either innocent (functional) or pathogenic (organic). If a heart is pumping with abnormal force, there may be a palpable vibration, termed a *thrill*. Palpate the precordium (area over the heart) for evidence of a thrill (feels like the sensation of a cat purring) or a *heave* (definite outward chest movement), which also denotes a struggling heart. If you hear or palpate any accessory heart sounds or movements, try to describe them with reference to the box on page 359. All additional heart sounds need further identification and investigation. Determining the cause of an abnormal heart sound requires a cardiac specialist. Determining that an abnormal sound exists, however, and securing proper referral is an important nursing role.

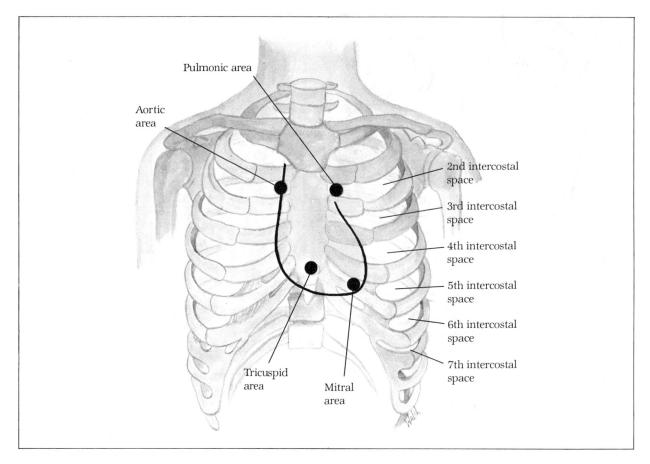

Figure 18-20 *Points at which heart sounds are best heard.*

Expected Findings

Nonpregnant Woman. Heart rate 70 to 80 beats per minute; no accessory sounds.

Pregnant Woman. It may be difficult to hear the heart beat during pregnancy because of the increase in breast size. An occasional woman will develop an innocent (functional) heart murmur during pregnancy because of the excess amount of blood her heart processes. As at all other times of

life, she needs referral for further investigation to be certain only a physiologic change of pregnancy and not a previously undetected heart condition is involved.

TEACHING POINT. Many women notice palpitation (their heart skipping a beat) during pregnancy, especially when lying supine. Teach pregnant women to always rest or sleep on the side to avoid this problem.

Lungs

Assess the rate of respirations and whether respirations are easy and relaxed or if accessory muscles are necessary for effective ventilation.

On the anterior chest lung tissue extends from above the clavicles to the sixth or eighth rib. On the posterior chest lung tissue is as low as the tenth to twelfth thoracic vertebra. Recall that a person's right lung has three lobes; the left only two. It is important when assessing lung tissue that you attempt to evaluate all five lobes: Lung disease can be specific for a lobe.

Begin lung assessment by percussing lung tissue. Normal lung sounds are resonant; overex-

Table 18-6 Heart Sounds Heard by Auscultation

Sound	Cause
S1	Closure of the tricuspid and mitral valves with the beginning of ventricular contraction (systole).
S2	Closure of the pulmonary and aortic valves with the beginning of atrial contraction (diastole).
S3	Rapid ventricular filling.
S4	Abnormal filling of the ventricles.

Description of Accessory Heart Sounds

Characteristic	*Significance*
Location	Record the listening post at which you heard the sound most distinctly.
Quality	Record the sound by a description such as blowing, rubbing, rasping, or musical.
Timing	Record where in relation to S1 and S2 you heard it. A sound superimposed between S1 and S2 is a *systolic* murmur; one between S2 and the next S1 is a *diastolic* one. Innocent murmurs (functional, denoting no pathology) are usually systolic (there are exceptions); pathologic murmurs are more apt to be diastolic.
Pitch	Record the sound as high- or low-pitched.
Radiation and thrill	Record whether you could hear it at a distant body site (radiation) or whether a thrill (a vibrating sensation) was present.
Intensity	Murmurs are graded according to the following criteria:

Grade 6: So loud it can be heard with a stethoscope not touching the chest wall; has a thrill

Grade 5: Very loud but must touch stethoscope to chest to hear; has a thrill

Grade 4: Loud; may or may not have a thrill

Grade 3: Moderately loud

Grade 2: Quiet, but easily discernible

Grade 1: Very quiet; difficult to hear

---

panded lungs sound hyperresonant; and lungs filled with fluid due to cardiovascular disease sound dull or flat. The lower anterior lobe of the right lung will sound dull, as liver covers it on the anterior surface below the fourth or fifth intercostal space.

Auscultate breath sounds by listening with the diaphragm of a stethoscope over each lung while a woman inhales and exhales (preferably with her mouth open). Listen both anteriorly and posteriorly; compare left side to right side for equal findings. Normal breath sounds are slightly longer on inspiration than expiration. Table 18-7 describes normal breath sounds as well as adventitious sounds you may hear that would reflect illness.

Expected Findings

Nonpregnant Woman. Respiratory rate of 16 to 20 breaths per minute; no adventitious sounds.

Pregnant Woman. Although lung tissue assumes a more horizontal position during pregnancy, vital capacity is not reduced. No adventi-

tious sounds such as wheezing or rales are normal. Late in pregnancy diaphragmatic excursion (diaphragm movement) is lessened because the diaphragm cannot push as low due to the distended uterus.

Abdomen

To assess the abdomen, first inspect the surface for symmetry and contour. An adult abdomen is gently depressed (scaphoid). Note any skin lesions or scars.

Auscultate the abdomen for bowel sounds before palpating, as palpating may alter bowel peristalsis and therefore disturb bowel sounds. Bowel sounds can be heard in all quadrants of the abdomen. They are high, "pinging" sounds that occur normally at time intervals of 5 to 10 seconds. If a bowel is distended, they occur more frequently; if the bowel is blocked so that there is no movement of contents, they will be absent. Listen for a full minute before you conclude that no bowel sounds are present. Auscultation for bowel sounds is more difficult as a pregnancy progresses

Table 18-7 Breath Sounds Heard by Auscultation

Sound	Interpretation and Description
Vesicular	Soft, low-pitched sound heard over the periphery of the lung; inspiration is longer than expiration.
Bronchovesicular	Soft, medium-pitched sound heard over major bronchi; inspiration equals expiration.
Bronchial	Loud, high-pitched sound heard over trachea; expiration is longer than inspiration.
Rhonchi	A snoring sound made by air moving through mucus in bronchi; normal.
Rales	A crackling (like the crackle of cellophane) made by air moving through fluid in alveoli; abnormal; denotes pneumonia, which is fluid in alveoli.
Wheezing	A whistling sound on expiration made by air being pushed through narrowed bronchi; abnormal; seen in people with asthma or foreign body obstruction.

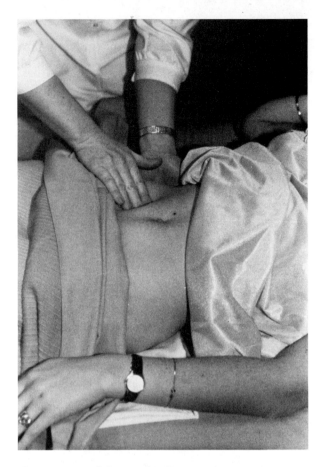

Figure 18-21 *Abdominal palpation.*

because the bowel is pushed posteriorly and laterally.

Listen along the center of the abdomen over the aorta for a bruit or the sound of blood passing through an irregular space. Palpate the abdomen in a systematic order, such as right lower quadrant, right upper quadrant, left lower quadrant, left upper quadrant. Palpate first lightly, then deeply (Figure 18-21). Ascertain whether any area is tender by watching the woman's face while you palpate; observe for "guarding," or the woman tensing her abdominal muscles to keep you from pressing deeply at that point. Note any hard area or mass.

By palpating from the right lower quadrant to the right upper quadrant, your hand will "bump" against the lower edge of the liver 1 to 2 cm below the right ribs. On the left side the lower edge of the spleen may be discernable. A liver or spleen larger than this is suspicious of disease. Liver, spleen, and bladder size can all be documented further by percussion.

Expected Findings

Nonpregnant Woman. Scaphoid abdomen; no tenderness or masses.

Pregnant Woman. At 12 weeks of pregnancy, the uterus is palpable over the symphysis pubis as a firm globular sphere; it reaches the umbilicus at 20 weeks, the xyphoid process at 36 weeks, and then returns to just over the umbilicus at 40 weeks. Palpate fundus location and measure fundal height.

Measurement of Fundal and Uterine Heights

Fundal height is measured from the notch above the symphysis pubis to the superior aspect of the uterine fundus. Uterine height should be plotted on a graph such as the one shown in Figure 18-22. If such plotting is not currently done by the prenatal care providers in your setting, it can be initiated by you as an independent nursing action.

Plotting uterine growth at each visit in this way allows variations in fetal growth to become apparent. Further investigation, such as a sonogram, can then be made to determine the cause of the growth increase or retardation.

Auscultate for fetal heart sounds (120–160 beats/minute) following the twentieth week of pregnancy (tenth week if a Doppler technique is

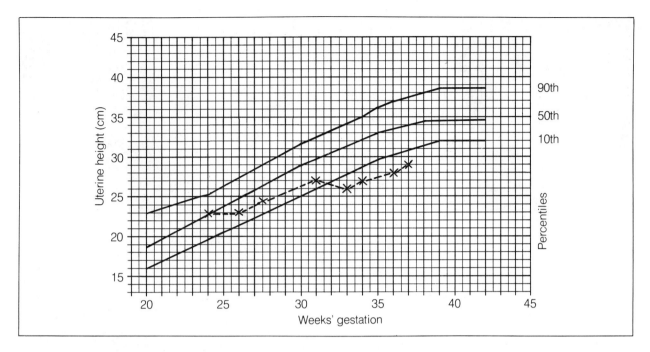

Figure 18-22 *Uterine height percentiles. Solid lines show normal percentiles. Subject whose growth is plotted was a fetus with intrauterine growth retardation. Source: Belizan, J. M., et al. (1978). Diagnosis of intrauterine growth retardation by a simple clinical method: Measurement of uterine height.* American Journal of Obstetrics and Gynecology, 131, 643.

used). Palpate for fetal outline and position after the twenty-eighth week.

Rectum

The rectum should be inspected for any protruding hemorrhoidal tissue (distended veins) or fissures. If specific symptoms are present, it is examined further. With a lubricated glove in place, a finger is inserted in the rectum and the anterior and posterior walls are palpated. This is an uncomfortable sensation of pressure for many people; if hemorrhoidal tissue is present, it can also be painful. The woman bearing down while the finger is inserted prevents the anus from being so constricted, which lessens the feeling of pressure. Following withdrawal of the gloved finger, swab a sample of feces on a paper towel and test the stool for occult blood. The presence of blood in stool is a danger signal of colon cancer.

Expected Findings
Nonpregnant Woman. No hemorrhoids; no blood in stool.

Pregnant Woman. Assess the rectum closely for hemorrhoidal tissue, which is apt to occur in a pregnant woman from pelvic pressure preventing venous return.

Extremities

Observe extremities for ease of motion, symmetry, and alignment during the entire examination. Move all joints through full range of motion. Palpate all surfaces to detect abnormal swelling or tenderness. Ask a woman to walk toward and then away from you to assess gait (easy, mobile). Assess radial and pedal pulses, the presence of edema over the tibia and the ankle, and the presence of varicose veins (blue, irregular markings on the lower extremities).

Expected Findings
Nonpregnant Woman. Full range of motion; easy gait.

Pregnant Woman. Many women develop palmar erythema and itching early in pregnancy from high estrogen level and subclinical jaundice. Assess the lower extremities of pregnant women carefully for varicosities, filling time of the toenails (should be under 5 seconds), and the presence of edema; pelvic pressure may be preventing venous return from the lower extremities. Any edema more than ankle swelling may be a danger signal of pregnancy.

Assess the gait of pregnant women to see that they are keeping their pelvis tucked under the

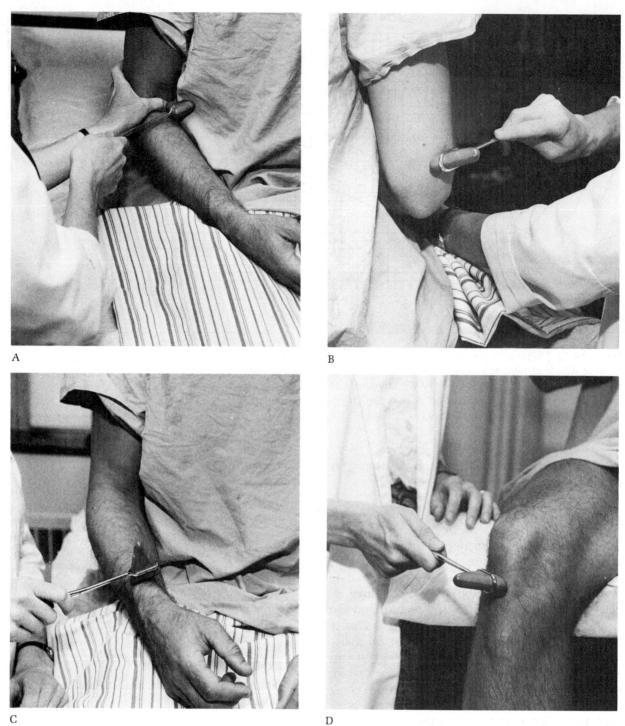

A

B

C

D

Figure 18-23 *Deep tendon reflexes: A. Biceps, B. Triceps. C. Patellar. D. Achilles. Superficial reflex: E. Babinski.*

weight of their abdomen. This position prevents them from developing muscle strains from abnormal tension on abdominal muscles. Many pregnant women have a "waddling" gait late in pregnancy from relaxation of the symphysis pubis. This development can cause pain if the cartilage is actually so unstable that it moves on walking.

Back

The back should be observed for symmetry and spinal column contour and alignment. Note any dimpling at the end of the spinal column—a common site for a dermal (pilonidal) cyst. This finding is innocent unless the cyst becomes infected or connects to deeper tissue layers. Assess for ten-

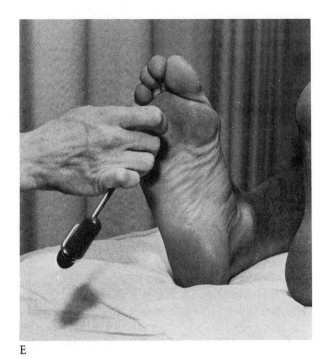

E

Table 18-8 Grading of Deep Tendon Reflexes

Grade	Interpretation
4+	Hyperactive; extremely marked reaction; abnormal
3+	Stronger than average, but within normal range
2+	Average response
1+	Less than average response but within normal range
0	No response; abnormal

derness along the spinal column by palpating each vertebra.

Expected Findings

Nonpregnant Woman. Midline spinal column; erect posture.

Pregnant Woman. The lumbar curve in pregnant women may be accentuated on standing in order to maintain body posture. This response may give a woman considerable back pain during pregnancy.

Neurologic Competence

People with neurologic disease require a complete neurologic examination, which is a detailed procedure. A general physical examination includes only testing deep tendon and superficial reflexes (involuntary responses to a stimulus) and general sensory and motor function. These findings complement findings from the general appearance assessment carried out during the entire examination.

Deep tendon reflexes test the intactness of the spinal nerve that supplies the particular body area tested. They are graded according to the scale in Table 18-8. The biceps reflex (Figure 18-23A) tests fifth and sixth cervical nerves. The triceps reflex (Figure 18-23B) tests seventh and eighth cervical nerves. The forearm will move perceptibly if these reflexes are intact.

The patellar reflex (Figure 18-23C) tests sec-

ond, third, and fourth lumbar nerves. The lower leg will move perceptibly if the reflex is intact. The Achilles tendon reflex (Figure 18-23D) tests first and second sacral nerves. The foot will move perceptibly in response to the percussion tap if the reflex is intact.

A superficial reflex that may be tested is the Babinski's reflex. Babinski's reflex (Figure 18-23E) tests first and second lumbar and sacral nerves. In a normal negative response, the toes curl downward.

Motor and Sensory Function

For a routine physical examination cranial nerves are not assessed, except for those assessed with the eye and mouth examination. Test general motor ability by asking a woman to grasp both your hands and squeeze and to push against both of your hands with her feet as she lies supine. Recall whether gait was adequate or not when you observed her walking.

To test sensory function, ask a woman to close her eyes and identify the location where you touch her on at least six different body parts.

Expected Findings

Nonpregnant Woman. Deep tendon reflexes 2+. Responsive motor and sensory function.

Pregnant Woman. Same.

Pelvic Examination

A pelvic examination is always included in a first prenatal visit. Such an examination requires the following equipment: speculum, spatula for cervical scraping, clean examining glove, lubricant, glass slides for plating the Pap smear, and culture plate and sterile cotton-tipped applicator for obtaining a cervical culture. A good examining light and a stool of correct sitting height are also necessary.

For a pelvic examination, the woman lies in a lithotomy position (on her back with her thighs flexed and her feet resting in the table stirrups) (Figure 18-24). Her buttocks should extend slightly beyond the end of the examining table. Her abdominal muscles will be more relaxed if she has a pillow under her head.

She should be properly draped (a draw sheet over her abdomen and extending over her legs). The foot of the examining table should not face the examining room door so that if someone should walk in unexpectedly the woman will not feel exposed. She should have an opportunity to talk with the person performing the examination while she is sitting up before she is placed in a lithotomy position; this consideration bolsters her self-esteem and keeps her from feeling like part of an assembly line.

It is a courtesy to a woman, especially on an initial pregnancy visit, for a nurse to be in the room with her for the pelvic examination. If she likes, her support person can remain with her at the head of the table. Women are nervous about pelvic examinations. If the pregnancy is her first, a woman may not have been in a health care setting since she finished receiving her childhood immunizations—and she may never have had a pelvic examinaton before. The many stories about how painful these examinations are, combined with natural reticence about that area of her body, make a woman tense just thinking

about the procedure. When pelvic muscles are tight and tense, not only is the examination painful, but the examiner has difficulty assessing the status of the pelvic organs.

You can help a woman relax during the examination in a number of ways. One is by remaining in the room. Having someone with her whom she knows (and following an extensive interview, the woman will feel that she knows you) is supportive. Being with her means being at the head of the table, not at its foot "where the action is." Being near to her enables you to touch her hand or cheek if she needs the support of physical contact. An explanation of what is happening or what is going to be done by the examiner is an aid to relaxation. Meaningful conversation with the woman may be helpful, but conversation with the examiner over her head is *not*. Suggesting that a woman breathe in and out (not hold her breath as she is prone to do) may help her relax (her support person can also remind her). Holding her breath will not make things easier for her; it pushes the diaphragm down and makes pelvic organs tense and unyielding.

A pelvic examination begins with inspection of external genitalia. Conditions to note include signs of inflammation, irritation, or infection, such as redness, ulcerations, or vaginal discharge. If she likes, a woman may view a pelvic examination by an overhead mirror or a mirror held by her or the examiner. Seeing vaginal or cervical pathology this way helps her to understand any problem she may have and the interventions she must use to improve it.

Figure 18-24 *A lithotomy position used for a pelvic examination. Help position a woman with her buttocks just over the edge of the table. Drape appropriately for modesty.*

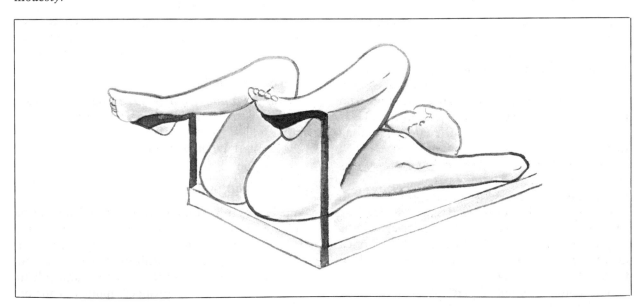

Herpes simplex II virus infections appear as clustered pinpoint vesicles on an erythematous (reddened) base. They are painful when touched or irritated by underclothing. The presence of herpes lesions on the vulva or vagina at the time of delivery will necessitate cesarean birth, in order to prevent exposure of the fetus to the virus during passage through the birth canal. Cervical cancer and herpes simplex II virus infections may be associated; therefore the presence of a herpes infection should be noted clearly in the woman's record. She should be followed in the future by cytologic smears (Pap smears) for cervical cancer.

To check whether Skene's glands are infected, the examiner inserts a sterile, gloved finger into the woman's vagina and presses it against the anterior vaginal wall, watching for any pus extruding from the openings to the glands at the urethral opening. To check for possible infection of Bartholin's glands, their sites (5 and 7 o'clock) are palpated between the vaginal finger and thumb of the same hand. If a discharge is produced from any of these gland ducts (Skene's or Bartholin's), a culture is obtained by touching the drainage with a sterile applicator tip. Infection here could be caused by something as simple as streptococci; it often is gonorrhea.

To assess whether either a rectocele or a cystocele is present, the examiner asks the woman to bear down as if she were moving her bowels while the labia is gently separated to view the vaginal walls.

To view the uterine cervix, the vagina must be opened with a speculum (Figure 18-25). No lubricant other than warm water should be used over the speculum blades; a lubricant might interfere with the interpretation of the Pap smear that will be taken. Warm water rather than cold should be used so that the woman does not contract her vaginal muscles on feeling a cold instrument.

A speculum is introduced with the blades in a closed position and directed toward the posterior rather than the anterior vaginal wall because the posterior wall is less sensitive. A speculum enters most readily if it is inserted at an oblique angle (the crease of the blades directed to 4 or 8 o'clock), then rotated to a horizontal position when fully inserted (the crease of the blades pointing to a 3 or 9 o'clock position). When fully inserted and rotated to a horizontal position, the blades are opened so the cervix is visible and secured in the open position by tightening the thumb screw at the side.

The cervix is inspected for its position (a retroverted uterus has a cervix tipped forward; an anteverted uterus has its cervix tipped posteriorly), its color (a nonpregnant cervix is light pink; in pregnancy it changes to almost purple); and any lesions, ulcerations, discharge, or otherwise abnormal appearance.

In a nulligravida, the cervical os is round and small. In a woman who has had a previous pregnancy with a vaginal delivery, the cervical os has much more of a slit-like appearance (Figure 18-26). If the woman had a cervical tear during a previous delivery, the cervical os may appear as a transverse crease the width of the cervix or a typical star-like (stellate) formation. If a cervical infection is present, a mucus discharge may be noticeable. With infection, the epithelium of the cervical canal enlarges and spreads onto the area surrounding the os, giving the cervix a reddened

Figure 18-25 *A vaginal speculum in place.*

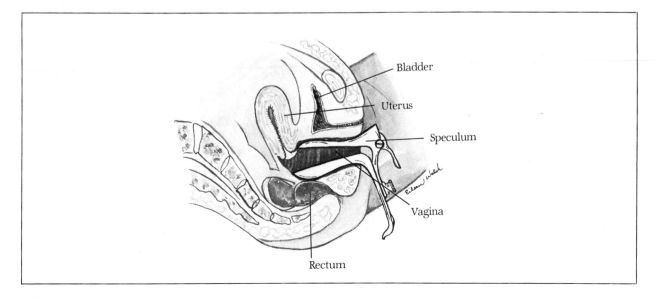

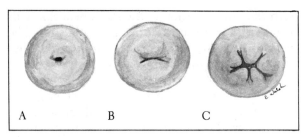

Figure 18-26 *Appearances of the cervix in nulliparous and multiparous women. A. Nulliparous cervix. B. Cervix after childbirth. C. "Stellate" cervix, seen after mild cervical tearing.*

Table 18-9 Classification of Papanicolaou Smears

Class	Description
I	Normal; no atypical cells are present
II	Normal, although there are atypical benign cells present
III	Suspicious cells, possibly malignant, are present
IV	Signs of malignancy are present
V	Definitely malignant cells are present

appearance (termed *erosion*). This area bleeds readily if it is touched.

Carcinoma of the cervix appears as an irregular, granular growth at the os. Cervical polyps (red, soft pedunculated protrusions) may also occasionally be seen at the os.

Papanicolaou Smear

Three separate specimens are usually obtained for a Pap smear: one from the endocervix, one from the cervical os, and one from the vaginal pool. For the first specimen, take a sterile cotton

Figure 18-27 *Obtaining a Pap smear from the endocervix.*

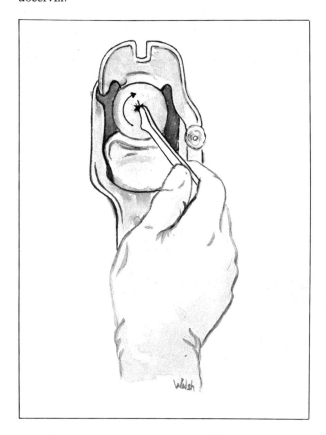

applicator, wet it with saline, and insert it through the speculum into the os of the cervix. Gently rotate it clockwise, then counterclockwise. Remove it without touching the sides of the vagina and paint a glass slide using a gentle touch so as not to destroy cells. Spray the slide with a fixative to preserve the cells.

To take the cervical specimen, press the longer end of the scraper supplied for the test on the os of the cervix; rotate it to scrape cells in a circle around the os (Figure 18-27). Smear the scraper onto a slide and spray with fixative.

For the third specimen, place a cotton-tipped applicator at the posterior fornix just below the cervix (the vaginal pool); roll it gently to pick up secretions collecting there. Remove it carefully and prepare a third slide.

The interpretation of Pap smear reports are classified according to the findings, as shown in Table 18-9. Be certain when discussing these reports with women that they do not overinterpret the classifications. Both class II and class III, for example, are not totally normal reports, yet they do not mean that cervical cancer is present. The next step would be further inspection of the cervix, usually by colposcopy.

Vaginal Inspection

Before the speculum is removed, at the time of a pelvic examination, a culture for gonorrhea is generally taken. A cotton-tipped applicator is used to gently swab the cervix, and the mucus obtained is then plated onto a special medium that allows for gonococci growth.

A speculum must be unlocked to be removed. The excessive stretching that would occur if it were removed in an open position would be very painful. If the speculum is kept partially open as it is removed, however, the sides of the vagina can be inspected as it is withdrawn. Any areas of inflammation, ulceration, lesions, or discharge can be noted. In a nonpregnant woman, vaginal walls are light pink; pregnancy turns them dark blue to purple. Such a vaginal inspection is critically important in a woman whose mother took diethylstilbestrol during pregnancy; she is prone to develop adenosis or overgrowth of cervical endothelium (possibly associated with vaginal cancer).

Trichomoniasis, a protozoal infection, generally gives signs of redness, a profuse whitish bubbly discharge, and petechial spots on the vaginal walls. Candidal (*Monilia*) infection typically presents with thick, white vaginal patches that may bleed if scraped away. Gonorrhea infection typically presents with a thick, greenish-yellow discharge and extreme inflammation, possibly along with urethral infection.

Bimanual Examination

Following the speculum examination, the examiner performs a bimanual (two-handed) examination to assess the position, contour, consistency, and tenderness of pelvic organs. The index and middle fingers of the gloved right hand are lubricated and inserted into the vagina and the walls of the vagina palpated for abnormalities. The left hand is then placed on the woman's abdomen and pressed downward toward the hand still in the vagina until the uterus can be felt between the two hands. Some examiners like a low stool supplied at this point so they can rest their right elbow against their raised knee in order to maintain enough pressure to palpate adequately.

The examiner continues to move his or her hands and identifies the right and left ovaries by the same method. Ovaries are normally slightly tender. The pressure caused by palpation may cause a woman some discomfort. Abnormalities that can be noted by bimanual examination are ovarian cysts, enlarged fallopian tubes (perhaps from pelvic inflammatory disease), and an enlarged uterus. An early sign of pregnancy (Hegar's sign) is elicited on bimanual examination. If a uterus is extremely retroverted it may not be palpable abdominally.

Rectovaginal Examination

Following a bimanual pelvic examination, the examiner withdraws the hand from the vagina and reinserts only the index finger in the vagina, the middle finger in the rectum. By palpating the tissue between the examining fingers, the examiner can assess the strength and irregularity of the posterior vaginal wall and the posterior cervix. This maneuver may be slightly uncomfortable for a woman because of the rectal pressure involved. Some examiners prefer to use a clean pair of gloves before they perform a rectovaginal examination so that they will not spread an infection from the vagina to the rectum. Following the rectal examination, if the examiner has to reexamine the vagina for any reason, a clean glove must be used in order to avoid contaminating the vagina with fecal material.

After completing the examination, tissue should be used to wipe away excess lubricant from the vaginal and rectal openings. You should perform this step if the examiner omits it before you help the woman to sit up again. Remember to wipe from front to back so that you do not carry rectal contamination forward to the vaginal introitus.

Estimating Pelvic Size

If, on this initial visit, the physician or nurse-midwife establishes that a woman is pregnant, and if she has never given vaginal birth before, pelvic measurements will usually be taken to be certain that the size and shape of her pelvis is within normal limits and will allow a child to pass safely through its bony canal at delivery. Important measurements include the anterior-posterior diameter of the pelvic inlet (diagonal conjugate) and the transverse diameter of the outlet (ischial tuberosity). These are shown and discussed in Chapter 8 along with normal pelvic anatomy.

Some care providers prefer these measurements not be taken until later in pregnancy, when a woman's perineal muscles are more relaxed and the measurements can be accomplished with a little more ease. However, there is danger in waiting too long: If the pelvis is too small, the fetal head will not deliver, and a cesarean birth will be the only safe choice for both mother and infant. So that this can be prepared for in advance, pelvic measurements must be taken at least by the twenty-fourth week of pregnancy; by that time there is danger that the fetal head is too large for safe passage.

Once a woman has given vaginal birth, her pelvis has been proved adequate, and it is not necessary to take her pelvic measurements again unless she has an intervening history of pelvic accident.

Laboratory Studies

A number of laboratory studies to confirm general health are included in assessment measures at a first prenatal visit. Normal levels for these studies are shown in Appendix G.

Blood Studies

The following blood studies are usually done at the first prenatal visit:

1. A complete blood count, including hemoglobin or hematocrit, to determine the presence of anemia. A hematocrit is a simple test that may be done in a matter of minutes in the office by a technician or nurse skilled in the technique. Black women have a blood sample taken to test for sickle cell trait or disease if they have not taken this precaution before.
2. A Venereal Disease Research Laboratories (VDRL) test or rapid plasma reagin (RPR) test to determine the presence of syphilis. Syphilis can be treated early in pregnancy before fetal damage occurs; it is important that this test be done at the first visit. A serologic test for gonorrhea is now available and may be drawn on women suspected of having the disease.
3. Blood typing (including Rh factor). This assessment allows blood to be available immediately if a woman has bleeding early in her pregnancy; it also allows care providers to prepare for the eventuality of a blood incompatibility with the fetus.
4. An antibody titer for rubella, to determine whether or not a woman is protected against the disease in case of exposure during pregnancy.

If the woman has a history of previous unexplained fetal loss, has a family history of diabetes, has had babies that were large for gestation age (9 or more pounds at term), is obese, or has glycosuria, a glucose loading or tolerance test will be scheduled toward the end of the first trimester of pregnancy to rule out gestational diabetes. Since fasting or a timed interval from meals is required before this test, arrangements for the test are usually made at the first prenatal visit.

Urinalysis

A urinalysis obtained by a clean catch technique assays albuminuria, glycosuria, and pyuria. All three of these tests can be done by means of test strips and microscopic examination of the urine. As many as 7 percent of women have an asymptomatic bacteriuria discovered at a first prenatal visit (Burrows, 1982).

Chest X-ray

If a woman is from an area where tuberculosis is a major health problem, her physician may order a tuberculin skin test to screen for this disease. It is safe to use such a test during pregnancy. Any woman who has a positive reaction would then require a chest X-ray for further diagnosis.

If a woman has a history of tuberculosis she cannot have a tuberculin skin test: The reaction would be extreme. To assess her current disease status, the physician may order a chest X-ray, which the woman may fear because she knows that radiation is harmful to a growing fetus. She needs to be assured that a lead apron will cover her abdomen to protect the fetus and that only her chest will be exposed to radiation.

It is important to screen for tuberculosis early in pregnancy because the chronic and debilitating nature of this disease increases the risk of abortion. In addition, the change in the shape of the lung tissue as the growing uterus presses on the lungs may reactivate old lesions. Fortunately, the incidence of tuberculosis in young women is declining, and few women today in this age group have this secondary complication to pregnancy.

Dental X-ray

If many dental caries are present at the time of the first prenatal examination, the woman may be referred to her dentist or a dental clinic. Carious teeth are a source of infection and should be treated before abscesses develop and cause more serious problems. Dental X-rays may be taken during pregnancy, but a woman should remind her dentist that she is pregnant and needs a lead apron to protect her abdomen.

A woman should have no extensive dental work done during pregnancy without her physician's or nurse-midwife's approval.

Expected Date of Confinement

Once a woman is told that her pelvic examination and history suggest pregnancy, she will ask when the baby is due. Her due date, or expected date of confinement (so called because at one time a long period of bed rest usually followed childbirth) is calculated by Nägele's rule: Count back 3 months from the first day of the last menstrual period and add 7 days. This date is not hard and fast, since the actual date of delivery is influenced by the date of ovulation and impregnation. For a woman with a typical 28-day menstrual cycle, the date will be relatively accurate. The woman with a 40-day cycle does not ovulate until about the twenty-sixth day of her cycle, not the fourteenth, so her child will not be ready to be born until almost 2 weeks after this date. Be certain a mother understands that delivery 2 weeks before or 2 weeks after the expected date is within normal limits.

If a woman does not know the date of her last menstrual period, the length of the pregnancy can be estimated from measurement of fundal size or by sonogram.

Risk Assessment

Following assessment at a first prenatal visit, the total findings from the health history, physical examination, and laboratory determinations are analyzed in order to estimate whether a pregnancy will continue with a good outcome or it is one that has the potential to end before term or with an unfavorable fetal or maternal outcome (a high-risk pregnancy).

Many factors enter into the categorization of high risk. A commonly used scale for risk assessment is shown in Table 18-10. A score of more than 3 identifies a fetus as being at high risk for damage. For example, the baby of a woman more than 35 years of age (score 1) in her first pregnancy (score 1) who had anemia of 10 gm or less (score 1) would, by this scale, be at high risk. Such a woman needs close observation during pregnancy and her infant will need close observation in the neonatal period until it is confirmed that he has no anomalies and is doing well. Category III is scored only after the baby is born.

The failure to identify risk potential in pregnancy leads to increased perinatal mortality. In prenatal settings in which women are scheduled for care at the rate of one every 15 minutes, a physician may not be able to deal with fetal risk assessment. Identifying fetuses at risk by using a standard scoring system such as Goodwin's can be an independent nursing function that can do much to increase the health of newborns and prevent unwanted fetal loss.

Risk assessment should be done at the first prenatal visit. An update at each pregnancy visit prevents it from losing its validity later in pregnancy.

In order that a woman can have a safe pregnancy, she needs to learn about the minor discomforts of pregnancy, its danger signals, and safe nutritional and rest and exercise considerations she will need to follow. This information is discussed in Chapter 19.

Utilizing Nursing Process

A first prenatal visit sets the tone for health care during the pregnancy. In order that women return for further health care and supervision during this important year in their life, their care must be designed to be both comprehensive and individualized.

Assessment

A first prenatal visit establishes a baseline of health information gained from the woman's history, physical assessment, and laboratory analysis; and all other findings will be compared against this data. To make these comparisons meaningful, use consistent techniques for assessment (always take blood pressure in a woman's left arm with her either lying or sitting; always secure urine samples by clean-catch technique). Be certain you assess not only a woman's present physical state but both her and her support person's readiness for a pregnancy. Assess her ability to follow prenatal instructions and what teaching style you will need to use in order to meet her individualized learning style.

Analysis

NANDA accepted no nursing diagnosis specific to prenatal care. A nursing diagnosis used in this area might be "Readiness for prenatal care related to acceptance of pregnancy," or "Potential for poor health care compliance related to inability to accept pregnancy." When establishing goals for care be certain they are realistic for a woman's life style (consider days she has a car available or days her support person could accompany her for care).

Planning

Remember when planning for a first prenatal visit to reserve sufficient time so the visit can be thorough. Optimally, care should be family centered or include the father of the child or other siblings in the visit. Be certain to appreciate the meaning of a first prenatal visit for a woman. A first prenatal visit is a major life milestone, comparable to coming of age. Respect it as such. Table 18-11 shows measures to individualize prenatal care and make it more meaningful.

Implementation

Following a health history, physical assessment, and the diagnosis of pregnancy based on probable or presumptive signs of pregnancy, a woman and her support person should be given counseling on health maintenance during pregnancy. Be certain that a woman leaving an initial prenatal visit has a firm appointment to return to the setting. Her mind is full of all the changes about to come into

Table 18-10 Antepartum Fetal Risk Score

CATEGORY I

Baseline Data (Prepregnancy)		*Reproductive History*	
Age 15 or under	1	Abortion, spontaneous	
Age 35+	1	Abortion, therapeutic	
Age 40+	2	Pelvic infection, postabortal or postpartum	
Para 0	1		
Para 5+	2	Fetal death	
Interval < 2 years	1	Neonatal death	
Isolation: 50+ miles from medical care	2	Surviving premature infant	
Weight < 100 lb (45 kg)	1	Surviving infant, low birth weight for date	
Weight 200 lb or more (90 kg)	2		
Diabetes		Antepartum hemorrhage	
Class A	1	Toxemia	
Class B, C, D	2	Difficult midforceps	
Class F, R	3	Cesarean section	
Chronic renal disease	1	Hysterotomy	
Chronic renal disease with diminished renal function	3	Myomectomy	
		Major congenital anomaly	
Preexisting hypertension		Cervical incompetence	
140+/90+	1	Large infant: 10 lb or more (4.5 kg)	
160+/110+	2	Malpresentation	
Interpregnancy cardiac failure	2		
Rh-isoimmunized mother (1:8 AHG+)		One instance of above	1
With homozygous husband	2	Two or more instances of the above (in one or more pregnancies)	2
With previously affected infant (regardless of outcome)	3		

Score (circle one)   0 1 2 3

CATEGORY II

Present Pregnancy			
Bleeding early (< 20 wk)		No antepartum care	2
Alone	1	Less than 3 visits	1
With pain	2	Heart disease: AHA functional	
Bleeding late (> 20 wk)		Class III or IV	2
Ceased	1		
Continues	2	Anemia	
With pain	3	10 gm or less	1
With hypotension	3	10 gm after 36 wk	2
Spontaneous premature rupture of membranes	1	8 gm or less	2
With latent period 24 hours	2	Megaloblastic anemia	2
Asymptomatic bacteriuria	1		
Toxemia grade I	1	Specific infections	
Toxemia grade II	3	Untreated syphilis	2
Eclampsia	3	Toxoplasmosis	2
Hydramnios (single fetus)	3	Hepatitis	1
Multiple pregnancy	2	Vaccination during pregnancy	1
Gestational diabetes		Rubella titer rising significantly	
Diagnosis before 36 wk	1	6 wk	3
Diagnosis after 36 wk	2	9 wk	2
Decreasing insulin requirement		12 wk	1
(50% + reduction in 48 hr)	3		
Maternal acidosis	3	Inhalation anesthesia (emergency)	1
Maternal pyrexia (39°C or over)	1	Abdominal operation	2
Maternal pyrexia + FHR > 160	2	Cervical suture (cerclage)	3
Rising Rh antibody titer (2 tube+)	2	Pelvic irradiation diagnostic 12 wk	1

Score (circle one)   0 1 2 3

Table 18-10 (continued)

CATEGORY III

Gestation Age Achieved

28 weeks or under	4	37 weeks or under	1
32 weeks or under	3	42 weeks or over	1
35 weeks or under	2	43 weeks or over	2

Score (circle one)   0 1 2 3 4

Total Score (0–10) =

Source: Goodwin, J. W., & Hewlett, P. T. (1973). The strategy of fetal risk management. *Canadian Family Physician, 19*(4), 54. (Modification of score devised by J. W. Goodwin, J. T. Dunne, and B. W. Thomas, *Canadian Medical Association Journal 101:* 458–464, 1969.) Reprinted by permission of author and publisher.

her life, but this setting of a date will be important the following month, when it is time for follow-up care.

During a normal pregnancy, return appointments are scheduled every month through the thirty-second week, then every 2 weeks through the thirty-sixth week, and then every week until delivery. Women who are categorized as high risk will be followed even more closely.

It is helpful to give women pamphlets or booklets about prenatal care to read later; after their initial surprise wears off, they may be in a better frame of mind to grasp the material and enjoy reading it. Be sure you have read all the printed matter you give them, to be certain the advice it contains is consistent with your oral instructions and with the views of the physician or nurse-midwife with whom you work. A beautiful picture on the cover of a pamphlet does not ensure the quality of the advice inside.

Assure a woman she may call the health care setting if she has any problems or questions during the coming month because it is important that you know about changes. Some women are raised with such awe of authority (and you represent authority as health care personnel) that they will worry about a problem for an entire month, but will not call unless you indicate beforehand that they are free to do so.

Evaluation

A first prenatal visit should be evaluated both in terms of whether the health care offered to the woman was satisfactory and whether you gathered the information necessary to formulate a plan for safe care.

Nursing Care Planning

Mary Kraft is a 23-year-old black woman you meet at her first prenatal visit. Below is a recording of an interview and physical examination you complete with her.

Assessment

Chief Concern. "I think I'm pregnant."

History of Present Illness: Has had nausea every morning for last 2 weeks. Last menstrual period 6 weeks ago (Aug. 9th). Feels "constantly fatigued."

Family Profile. Is one of fraternal twins; twin sister has Down's syndrome. Patient states she is afraid this will happen to her children. Lives in apartment with husband (married 4 years).

Works as a part-time librarian; husband is an accountant and also goes to night school for an MBA.

Past Health History. Had mumps at 10 years; fell and dislocated knee at 16 years. In cast for 6 weeks; no apparent sequelae. No major illnesses; had surgery 4 months ago for endometriosis. Neg. for sickle cell trait and disease.

Gynecologic History. Menarche at 10 years; duration of menstrual cycles: 30 days; flow for 5 days. Had a "lot of cramping" until surgery for endometriosis 4 months ago. Now "very little" pain with menses.

Obstetric History. Had a spont. abortion 2 years ago. Was unable to conceive following this. Had

Table 18-11 Current Routines vs. Suggested Alternatives for Prenatal Care

Current	Suggested
Patient records are "owned" by the health facility.	Make each mother responsible for her own obstetric folder. If her first language is not English, make provisions to record pregnancy information so she can read it.
Pregnant women are impersonally booked for their initial antenatal visit, usually by phone.	View the initial phone contact as an important communication opportunity. Have the person making phone contact convey interest, as well as information about self-care practices. Obtain preliminary assessment of risk status using a brief checklist. Give women a specific person's name as a phone contact for pregnancy-related questions. Send a follow-up welcoming letter.
The time between initial booking and the first prenatal visit is 3 to 6 weeks.	Have the pregnant woman seen within a week either in a group orientation session, individually by a health team member, or if her risk status warrants it, by a physician.
Women are seen for the first time on the examining table and are partially or completely undressed.	See the patient fully clothed and upright before physical exam. Discuss the pregnancy health history, and relevant social and psychological aspects.
Pregnant women come alone for antenatal care.	Invite and encourage family members and friends to come for antepartal visits. Allow them to enter the examination room and participate in all aspects of care to the extent they and the patient desire.
Blood pressure, weight, and urine checks are done in the waiting room or other public areas in view of others.	Provide privacy. Teach the pregnant woman and family members to do screening procedures.
Office and clinic visits are scheduled during weekdays.	Make evening and weekend hours available.
The pregnant woman sees any physician, nurse, or midwife who is available.	Try to provide continuity of care and allow some choice among care providers. Assign a primary care nurse to the family for the duration of the pregnancy to coordinate the care plan.
All women are called by their first or last names, according to established local custom.	Ask women how they would like to be addressed and record this information on their records.
Waiting time is predictable and may last as long as an hour.	Minimize waiting time by better use of care team members and careful scheduling. Plan antenatal care educational activities for waiting periods, including programs for those with special needs such as high-risk patients and non-English speakers.
Decisions about prenatal and intrapartal care are made by careproviders.	Educate pregnant women about care options and encourage them to participate in decision-making. Develop preference profiles with patients and include them in prenatal records sent to birth facilities.

Source: Mahan, C., & McKay, S. (1984). Let's reform our antenatal care methods. *Contemporary OB/GYN, 22,* 147.

an infertility series and endometriosis was discovered. Was treated with danazol (Danocrine) for 3 months, then had laparoscopy 4 months ago.

Family Medical History. No kidney, heart, or lung disease, or cancer reported. Has a twin sister with Down's syndrome.

ROS. Negative except for symptoms of chief concern.

Physical Examination

General Appearance. Well-appearing, black adult female.

Mental Status. Alert-appearing; nervous mannerism of wringing hands.

Head. Normocephalic. One "shotty" lymph node present in anterior cervical chain.

Eyes. Red reflex present; Extraocular muscles grossly intact. Conjunctiva pale.

Nose. Midline septum; mucus membrane slightly swollen and soft.

Mouth. One cavity present in left lower molar; gingiva slightly hypertrophied; pink and moist.

Neck. Supple; full range of motion.

Chest. Lungs clear to auscultation and percussion; respiratory rate: 20/minute. Heart rate: 80/minute. No adventitious sounds heard.

Breasts. Tender to touch; no masses or nipple discharge.

Abdomen. 8 cm–long surgical scar present on lower abdomen; some keloid growth present. Abdomen soft; liver palpated at 1 cm below costal margin. Femeral pulses equal bilaterally.

Genitalia. Pubic hair female distribution; slight white vaginal discharge present. Pelvic exam performed by nurse-midwife. Reported cervix as clean and slightly soft, uterus enlarged and soft, vagina purple-hued. Culture taken for gonorrhea; Pap smear obtained.

Extremities. Full range of motion; no varicosities present.

Back. No tenderness of joints; vertebrae midline and straight.

Neurologic. Biceps, triceps, patellar, and Achilles reflexes 2 +.

Analysis

Well adult black female with probable signs of pregnancy (Chadwick's and Hegar's) present.

Locus of Decision Making. Patient.

Goal. Patient to complete pregnancy within normal limits.

Criteria. Patient to complete 40-week pregnancy and deliver vaginally.

Nursing Orders

1. Blood drawn for hemoglobin, hematocrit, rubella titer, and serum HCG analysis to confirm pregnancy by nurse-midwife order.
2. Urine obtained by clean-catch for routine urinalysis. Neg. for protein and glucose.
3. Inform patient to telephone tomorrow to ask about HCG results.
4. If pregnancy test is positive, schedule for return visit for pregnancy instruction and counseling.
5. If pregnancy test is negative, advise as indicated according to nurse-midwife's further instructions.

The following is a nursing care plan in regard to prenatal care you might devise for Mrs. Kraft.

Assessment

Patient states her husband could be free on Tuesdays; would like appointments scheduled for then so he can accompany her. Interested in participating in care at visits by such actions as weighing herself and learning to take her own blood pressure; states testing urine is "not her thing."

Husband accompanied her for first visit and was supportive. Learned blood pressure taking.

Risk assessment by Goodwin's scale is 2. (Para 0 = 1; spontaneous abortion = 1).

Analysis

Woman with low risk score related to healthy life style.

Goal. Patient to participate in family-centered prenatal care for length of pregnancy.

Criteria. Both patient and husband to attend all prenatal care appointments.

Nursing Orders

1. Mark chart for Tuesday appointments.
2. Husband to attend all prenatal visits as support person.
3. Mark for self-participation at visits.

Questions for Review

Multiple Choice

1. Mrs. Smith is a 20 year old you see in a prenatal clinic. She has an accessory nipple. Which of the following teaching points would be most important to make with her?
   a. The tendency for accessory nipples is familial.
   b. Such growths fade with menopause.
   c. Bleeding from such growths is not uncommon.
   d. Such growths increase in size during pregnancy.

2. Mrs. Smith also is diagnosed as having fibrocystic breast disease. Which of the following statements is true concerning this condition?
   a. Fibrocystic breast disease is most pronounced postmenopause.
   b. Fibrocystic breast disease occurs most often in slim women.
   c. The ingestion of caffeine may increase fibrocystic lesions.
   d. Breast cancer occurs in evacuated fibrocystic lesions.

3. Mrs. Ernist is a 30-year-old woman who is having her first child. She had a breast incision and some breast tissue removed because of fat necrosis 3 years ago. She asks if she will be able to breast-feed. Your best response would be,
   a. "Breast-feeding will probably be possible."
   b. "No, you have an incision in breast tissue."
   c. "No, breast-feeding will cause you pain."
   d. "Yes, but only if you have a small baby."

4. Gynecologic health is an important part of a woman's health history. Which statement below reflects the best way to begin a menstrual history?
   a. "Discussing menstrual periods can be embarrassing. . . ."
   b. "I'd like to ask you some questions about your menstrual periods."
   c. "How old were you when you had your first period?"
   d. "How long are your menstrual periods?"

5. In light of the high incidence of some illnesses in women, which question below would be most important to include in a review of systems?
   a. "Have you ever had a heart attack?"
   b. "Do you have a peptic ulcer?"
   c. "Have you had any urinary tract infections?"
   d. "Have you had any neurologic diseases?"

6. Based on the incidence of disease in women, which assessment of lower extremities would be most important to make?
   a. lateral movement of the kneecap
   b. presence of varicosities
   c. diameter of the calf muscle
   d. blanching and refilling of toenails

7. In planning care, what two dip-stick tests are generally performed on urine at a prenatal visit?
   a. protein and sodium
   b. pH and glucose
   c. occult blood and protein
   d. protein and glucose

8. Mrs. Smith is nervous about having a pelvic examination. Which of the following suggestions would be the best technique to help her relax for the examination?
   a. "Bear down as if you have to move your bowels."
   b. "Take a deep breath and hold it."
   c. "Count from twenty to one at a steady pace."
   d. "Tense your abdominal muscles so the uterus contracts less."

9. Mrs. Smith asks if she can weigh herself at visits. The following is the rationale behind current practice:
   a. the average woman cheats at assessing her own weight.
   b. this is a nursing action that should be retained as such.
   c. self-participation in health care should be encouraged.
   d. Mrs. Smith could not appreciate the importance of a weight gain.

10. Mrs. Smith asks you to compute her expected date of confinement. Based on the fact that her last menstrual flow was July 20, her due date would be
    a. April 27.
    b. March 13.
    c. April 13.
    d. May 20.

Discussion

1. What are factors you can anticipate that might make interviewing at a first prenatal visit an easy task? What factors might interfere with a successful interview?

2. Physical assessment of women at a prenatal visit is important in order to establish baseline data. What are ways in which physical assessment can be designed to be more acceptable for women?

3. Mrs. Rodriguez has the following pregnancy history: an induced abortion in 1970, a boy born at term in 1974, a girl born at term in 1976, a spontaneous abortion in 1978, and an infant born at 32 weeks in 1980. What is her TPAL classification?

Suggested Readings

Abrams, J. (1983). Gynecology: Urinalysis, pregnancy tests, and Pap smears in your office. *Consultant, 23,* 179.

Burrows, G. N., & Ferris, G. F. (1982). *Medical complications during pregnancy* (2nd ed.). Philadelphia: Saunders.

Curling, G. (1981). Asymptomatic breast screening. *Nursing (Oxford), 1,* 348.

Davis, B. D., et al. (1982). Social skills training . . . in nursing . . . the patient profile interview. *Nursing Times, 78,* 1765.

Davis, S. R. (1983). The breast lumps that aren't cancer. *R.N., 46,* 30.

Draper, J., et al. (1983). Women's knowledge of health care during pregnancy. *Health Visitor, 56,* 86.

Estok, P. J. (1981). Balancing the power: Improving health care for women. *M.C.N., 6,* 91.

Flint, C. (1982). Where have we gone wrong? Health care for pregnant women. *Nursing Mirror, 155,* 26.

Greenberg, M. D. (1983). The pulmonary examination. *Emergency, 15,* 28.

Grossman, J. A. (1983). The complications of beautification . . . aesthetic surgery. *Emergency Medicine, 15,* 28.

Haggard, B. A. (1983). Coping with anxiety about patient interviews. *Association of Operating Room Nurses Journal, 37,* 195.

Halton, M., et al. (1983). Breast-feeding after breast reduction. *Journal of Nurse Midwifery, 28,* 19.

Hamilton, M. S., et al. (1981). Pelvic examination: Patient safety and comfort. *J.O.G.N. Nursing, 10,* 344.

Heller, B. R., et al. (1982). The nurse interview. *Nursing Outlook, 30,* 182.

Hewitt, F. S. (1981). The interview. *Nursing Times, 1,* 77.

Hytten, F. E. (1978). Physiological adjustments in pregnancy. In R. R. MacDonald (Ed.). *Scientific basis of obstetrics and gynecology.* Edinburgh: Churchill Livingstone.

King, R. C. (1982). Detailed guidelines for a thorough examination of the breast. *RN, 45,* 56.

King, R. C. (1982). Checking the patient's neurological status. *RN, 45,* 56.

Koch, S. J. (1980). Augmentation mammoplasty. *American Journal of Nursing, 80,* 1298.

Koeckeritz, J. L. (1981). The fine art of giving a physical: Organizing your plan of action. *RN, 44,* 46.

Koeckeritz, J. L. (1983). Assessing the genitalia. *RN, 46,* 52.

Leverenz, C. J., et al. (1982). Assessment of thorax and lungs. *Occupational Health, 31,* 9.

Lynch, H. T. (1980). What factors make women prone to breast cancer? *Consultant, 20,* 111.

Mahan, C. S., and McKay, S. (1984). Let's reform our antenatal care methods. *Consultant, 23,* 147.

Martin, B. J., et al. (1982). Oral health during pregnancy: A neglected nursing area. *M.C.N., 7,* 391.

Marty, P. J., et al. (1983). An assessment of 3 alternative formats for promoting breast self-examination, *Cancer Nursing, 6,* 207.

Parsons, W. D., et al. (1982). Why don't women attend for antenatal care? *Midwives Chronicle, 95,* 362.

Primrose, R. B. (1984). Taking the tension out of pelvic exams. *American Journal of Nursing, 84,* 72.

Rottenberg, R. F. (1982). Examining the joints, face and hands. *Patient Care, 16,* 177.

Shahady, E. J. (1982). Prenatal care: A strategy for healthier babies. *Consultant, 22,* 141.

Slota, M. (1982). Abdominal assessment. *Critical Care Nurse, 2,* 78.

Sokol, R. J., et al. (1980). Maternal-fetal risk assessment: A clinical guide to monitoring. *Clinical Obstetrics and Gynecology, 22,* 547.

Trimmer, E. (1983). About tender lumpy breasts. *Midwife Health Visitor and Community Nurse, 19,* 226.

Wlody, G. S. (1981). Effective communication techniques. *Nursing Management, 12,* 19.

19

Health Promotion During Pregnancy

OBJECTIVES

Following mastery of the contents of this chapter you should be able to

1. Describe minor symptoms and concerns of pregnancy.
2. Assess a woman during pregnancy for minor concerns of the period.
3. State a nursing diagnosis related to a minor concern of pregnancy.
4. Plan health promotion measures necessary throughout pregnancy to limit the minor symptoms of pregnancy.
5. Implement care to prevent or relieve the minor concerns of pregnancy.
6. Evaluate goal outcomes regarding the minor concerns of pregnancy.
7. Analyze the effect of continued prenatal care on improving the outcome of pregnancy.
8. Synthesize health promotion measures during pregnancy with nursing process to achieve quality maternal-newborn nursing care.

AFTER WOMEN LEARN that they are pregnant, some of them immediately want to know everything they should do to keep themselves well during pregnancy. Others are so surprised, so delighted, so disappointed, or so upset at the news that their only desire is to get away from the clinic or office as soon as possible to discuss it with a close friend or relative. You have to discover in each instance how receptive to instruction a woman will be. From the initial interview you have an indication of whether she is pleased or displeased with the pregnancy, and whether she intends to continue it or to take active steps to discontinue it.

Even the woman who is extremely excited and pleased to be pregnant can assimilate only so much information at any one time. You need to select from all the health information available those points that seem most relevant to her as an individual. The priority for discussing varicosity prevention, for example, would seem higher for a woman who has had varicosities in a former pregnancy than for a woman who is pregnant for the first time and is an avid sportswoman. The health measures you will teach must be maintained for an extended time: 10 lunar months. To be certain that a woman follows these measures for this long a time period, choose priorities and give meaningful, individualized health advice that will allow the woman to arrive at a plan of prenatal care that will suit her life style. This kind of advice is much more likely to be followed than that given in a standardized lecture, which a woman will instantly recognize as given to everyone and thus without particular concern for her.

Remember that a basic tenet of teaching is that people best learn information that has direct application for them. Plan to time health promotion and health maintenance information in pregnancy so those measures that are immediately applicable are taught first; those that only have relevance toward the end of pregnancy can be reserved until then.

Symptoms of Early Pregnancy

Teaching topics should include a review of the minor symptoms of pregnancy or the expected normal accompaniments of pregnancy. Be certain when discussing these with women that you remember that the term *minor* does not mean that they seem minor to the woman. A woman who is attempting to continue working, manage a household, attend to her children's needs, and participate in at least a few religious or community activities might be able to fit a pregnancy into that life with little difficulty—if she did not have nausea and vomiting and so felt little like her old self until 2:00 P.M. each day. It is reassuring to her to know that her nausea and vomiting are normal. However, they are by no means minor to her; they may be factors keeping her from enjoying and accepting this pregnancy.

In the same manner, the statement "Toothache is a normal consequence of carious teeth" is a true statement; but because it does not remove the pain, it is not helpful. Comments such as "Backache is common," "Nausea and vomiting are to be expected," "Fatigue always occurs in early pregnancy" are reassuring but also not helpful. It is as important, then, for a woman to be told how to relieve the minor discomforts or symptoms of pregnancy as it is for her to know what symptoms can be expected.

Interferences with Nutrition

A number of early symptoms of pregnancy are particularly important; active measures must be

▄▄▄ *Nursing Research Highlight* ▄▄▄▄▄▄▄▄▄▄▄

Morning Sickness:
The Woman's Perspective

The etiology of early pregnancy nausea is not agreed upon and no definitive medical treatment exists. The purpose of a study by Alley (1984) was to gather data on women's perception of how nausea and vomiting affected their life style, what factors aggravated the discomfort, what measures they tried to alleviate the problem, and whether any of those measures actually helped.

Findings of the study revealed that 36 out of 39 women who responded to the questionnaire reported having nausea and vomiting early in pregnancy. For most women the sensation lasted less than 1 hour and was first noticed during the first or second month. Only 5 women reported that the nausea and vomiting in no way affected their daily routine. Dry carbohydrates were mentioned by 20 women as helping to alleviate the nausea; clear fluid or carbohydrated beverages by 18. Salt was listed by 5 women as helpful. Interestingly, the source of information about nausea was checked as "nurse" by only 3 women.

Reference

Alley, N. M. (1984). Morning sickness: The client's perspective. *J.O.G.N. Nursing, 13,* 185.

---

taken to relieve them because they have the potential for interfering with nutrition.

Nausea and Vomiting

No definite reason has been established for the almost universal nausea and vomiting of early pregnancy. It may be due to sensitivity to the high chorionic gonadotropin hormone levels produced by the trophoblast; to high estrogen levels; to lowered maternal blood sugar caused by the needs of the developing embryo; to lack of pyridoxine (vitamin B_6); or to diminished gastric motility. Certainly it is aggravated by fatigue and possibly by emotional disturbance.

Most women have some nausea beginning as early as the first missed menstrual period and lasting during the first 3 months of pregnancy; vomiting once a day is not uncommon. The sensation is usually most intense on arising but may occur while a woman is preparing meals and smelling food. Women who work nights and sleep days often experience "evening sickness," because that is the time of day they are arising.

Increasing glucose intake seems to relieve morning sickness better than any other remedy (see the Nursing Research Highlight above). The traditional solution is for women to keep dry crackers by their bedside and eat a few before rising; sour balls may serve the same purpose. The woman should eat a light breakfast or delay breakfast until 10:00 or 11:00 A.M., past the time her nausea seems to persist. It is essential for her to maintain a good food intake during pregnancy,

so she has to compensate for a missed breakfast later in the day. It should not be skipped altogether. Drinking fluid separately from meals, and not with meals, avoiding strong smelling or fatty foods, and eating 6 small rather than 3 big meals daily are also helpful suggestions.

It is a good rule not to go longer than 12 hours between meals during pregnancy to prevent hypoglycemia, so she may need to include a late snack in her meal plans just before she retires at night. Fruit and raw vegetables may be tolerated during the morning before other foods; urge her to experiment with soups or vegetable drinks that she may not usually think of as breakfast foods but will give her early morning nutrition.

Women should be cautioned against taking home remedies, including antacids. Preparations of antacids containing sodium bicarbonate may cause fluid retention because of the sodium. A sound rule to follow is that a woman should take *no* medication during pregnancy unless her physician specifically prescribes it or her physician or nurse-midwife agrees to its use.

Morning sickness was, in the past, treated with the administration of antiemetics. (Bendectin, a drug similar to those used for motion sickness, was a common drug prescribed.) A number of drugs in this classification are now being investigated for teratogenic effects; they are no longer routinely prescribed and Bendectin has been withdrawn from production. Women may ask for a prescription because they know their mother was offered ready help by this method. Educate women that natural measures of controlling early morning nausea, such as eating a carbohydrate source on rising and delaying breakfast, are safer methods.

Morning sickness disappears spontaneously as the woman enters her fourth month of pregnancy. If it persists beyond the fourth month, or is so extreme in early pregnancy that it interferes with nutrition, its extent should be carefully investigated. It may indicate the development of hyperemesis gravidarum, a complication of pregnancy (see Chapter 39).

Pyrosis

Pyrosis (heartburn) is a burning sensation along the esophagus caused by regurgitation of gastric contents. In pregnancy, it may accompany nausea, but it may persist beyond the resolution of nausea and even increase in severity as pregnancy advances.

Pyrosis is probably caused by decreased gastric motility. It may be relieved by eating small meals frequently and by not lying down immediately after eating to help prevent reflux. Aluminum hydroxide gel and magnesium hydroxide (Maalox) or aluminum hydroxide, magnesium hydroxide, and magnesium trisilicate (Gelusil) serve to reduce gastric acidity and may be prescribed for relief. Be certain a woman understands that this "chest" pain is from her gastrointestinal tract and that, although it is called heartburn, it has nothing to do with her heart.

Gingivitis

Turgescence of the gums in association with changes in salivary pH may cause bleeding and tenderness of the gingivae (Figure 19-1). This is generally slight. However, if a woman notices bleeding when she brushes her teeth, she may fear she is bleeding inside as well, endangering her baby. She needs assurance that this problem is local, not systemic. Using a softer toothbrush will reduce gumline irritation and lessen bleeding.

Gingivitis is sometimes caused by dietary deficiencies, particularly a lack of vitamin C. Ask the woman to list all the foods she has eaten in the last two days and note whether or not she includes some citrus fruit or citrus fruit juice to assess for vitamin C intake.

Constipation

Constipation tends to occur in pregnancy as the pressure of the growing uterus presses against the bowel and slows peristalsis. If you discuss preventive measures with a woman early in pregnancy, she may be able to avoid this problem. Encourage her to evacuate her bowels regularly (many women neglect this first simple rule), to increase the amount of roughage in her diet by eating raw fruits and vegetables, and to drink extra amounts of water daily.

Some women find that an oral iron supplement leads to constipation. Help a woman find a method to relieve or prevent constipation

Figure 19-1 *Hypertrophy of the gumline can occur during pregnancy. A. Normal gingiva. B. Swollen gingiva, which makes plaque removal difficult and may cause bleeding.*

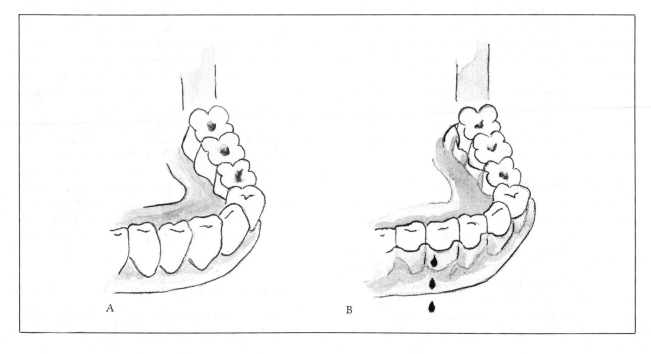

—————— Nursing Research Highlight ——————

Are Health Professionals Giving Correct Advice Regarding Alcohol and Tobacco Consumption?

Research has demonstrated that maternal alcoholism has harmful effects on infant development and fetal alcohol syndrome is now considered to be the third most common cause of mental deficiency. A total of 189 women were given questionnaires during the eighth month of pregnancy and one month later in a survey (Davidson, 1981) conducted to determine if health professionals' advice to expectant and nursing mothers is in accord with the research evidence. It was concluded that whereas the majority of women are advised against smoking during pregnancy, the same is not true for alcohol. Fewer women are given advice about alcohol consumption; and those who are, are told that it is okay in moderation or, in the postpartum period, even desirable for relaxation. This stance is not in accord with the research findings and concerns about alcohol use. Those receiving advice were primarily receiving their information from nurses and childbirth educators, with physicians being the next most frequent advice givers.

Reference

Davidson, S. (1981). Smoking and alcohol consumption—advice given by health professionals. *J.O.G.N. Nursing*, *10*(4), 256.

---

through other measures than avoiding the iron supplement: She needs this supplement in order to build iron stores in the fetus.

A woman should not use home remedies to prevent constipation, and she should especially avoid mineral oil. Mineral oil interferes with the absorption of fat-soluble vitamins (A,D,K, and E), which are needed for good fetal growth and maternal health.

Enemas should be avoided because their action might initiate labor. Over-the-counter laxatives are contraindicated, as are *all* drugs during pregnancy unless specifically prescribed or sanctioned by a woman's physician or nurse-midwife. If constipation is severe, stool softeners, mild laxatives, and evacuation suppositories may be prescribed. Some women have extensive flatulence accompanying constipation. Avoiding gas-forming foods such as cabbage or beans will help to control this problem.

Alcohol Consumption

A fetus lacks the ability to evacuate the breakdown products of alcohol, particularly acetaldehyde. This lack allows acetaldehyde to build to toxic proportions and deprive the fetus of necessary glucose and B vitamins for nervous tissue growth. Some women may have higher accumulations of acetaldehyde than others—so high that even social drinking can be harmful to a fetus (Danis, 1983). Alcohol consumption should be limited in pregnancy for all women lest these effects or a fetal alcohol syndrome develop. This syndrome (discussed in Chapter 47) includes growth retardation, mental deficiency, and craniofacial or structural musculoskeletal anomalies in the infant. The exact amount of alcohol that will lead to damage to the fetus is not well documented, but perhaps as little as 1 oz of alcohol a day during the early months of pregnancy may be damaging. Women should therefore limit their alcohol intake during pregnancy to no more than 1 oz (30 ml) of pure alcohol per day in order to prevent direct insult to fetal growth. One ounce of pure alcohol per day is comparable to 4 oz (120 ml) of wine, one mixed drink, such as a highball, or 6 oz (180 ml) of beer. It is best if a woman avoids alcohol entirely during pregnancy.

Pregnancy may be the motivation a woman needs to seek help for excessive drinking. Be certain to ask about drinking habits on an initial interview; investigate what a woman means by a term such as *social drinker*. You may discover a woman in a vulnerable, ready-to-ask-for-help moment. For more information on the health care provider's role here, see the Nursing Research Highlight above.

Interferences with Activity

Symptoms of early pregnancy that interfere with activity need to be relieved: They can lead to

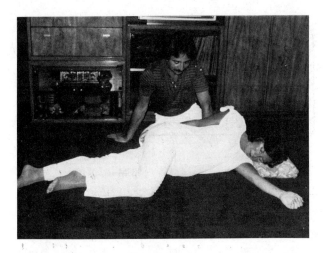

Figure 19-2 *Modified Sims' position as a rest position during pregnancy. The knees and elbows should be slightly bent, the muscles limp, and the breathing slow and regular. Notice that the weight of the fetus is resting on the floor.*

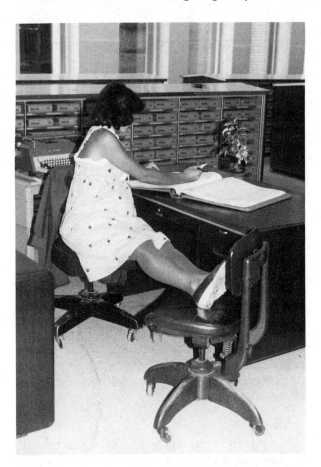

Figure 19-3 *If at all possible, women who are employed need to arrange a "feet-up" period during their workday.*

complications of pregnancy because activity is necessary to prevent stasis and thrombophlebitis in lower extremities.

Fatigue

Fatigue is extremely common in early pregnancy, probably due to increased metabolic requirements. It can usually be relieved by increasing the amount of rest and sleep. Some women are reluctant to sleep or rest during the day because they fear being perceived as lazy by their neighbors or husband. If they work, they worry about being accused of not holding their own at their job.

Explain that their changing metabolism increases their need for rest during the early months. A good resting position is a modified Sims' position, with the top leg forward (Figure 19-2). This puts the weight of the fetus on the bed, not on the woman, and allows good circulation in the lower extremities, which relieves the aching of poorly nourished leg muscles. Be certain a woman knows not to rest in a supine position or she may develop supine hypotension syndrome (faintness and hypotension from the presence of the expanding uterus on the inferior vena cava). Be certain she knows not to rest with her knees sharply bent since this adds greatly to pooling of blood in the venous system and potential thrombophlebitis.

Women who continue employment during pregnancy should be reminded that they need rest as much as the woman who stays at home. The majority of women who are working at the time their pregnancy is confirmed continue working until the ninth or tenth lunar month of pregnancy. A working woman might use a part of her lunch hour to sit in the women's room with her feet up on a chair, or at her desk with her feet elevated on an adjoining chair (Figure 19-3). After she returns home from work in the evening, she may need to modify the customary routine of cooking dinner, doing the dishes, straightening up the house, and so on, to *resting*, then cooking dinner, doing the dishes, and so on. If she has a husband, he should help with or take over dinner preparation or dish washing—part of "we are having a baby at our house" for a husband who does not usually share in chores.

Some women are reluctant to take the time out of their day for rest because they know that pregnancy is not an illness (and of course it is not), and so they proceed as usual. Rarely is there justification during a normal pregnancy for women to take extra days off from work because of their condition, but it is unrealistic to proceed as if nothing is happening to them. Fatigue can increase morning sickness so if a woman becomes too tired, she does not eat properly. If she is too

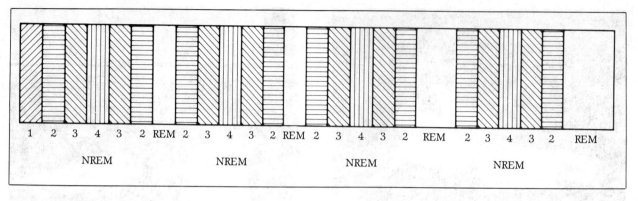

Figure 19-4 *A typical sleep pattern.*

fatigued, preparing meals becomes too great an effort, and she does not eat properly. If she remains on her feet without at least one break during the day, the tendency for varicosities to develop increases, and so does the danger of thromboembolitic complications. Ask a woman at prenatal visits whether or not she plans to have or manages to have at least *one* short rest period every day.

Sleep

Sleep is the optimal condition for body growth because growth hormone is secreted at its highest level then. A woman has to build new body cells in order to support a pregnancy, which appears to be the physiologic reason for women needing an increased amount of sleep—or at least rest—during pregnancy.

Sleep cycles are guided by biorhythms, specifically 24-hour or *circadian* rhythms. During any night, sleep is composed of repeated cycles of 60 to 120 minutes (an average of 90 minutes) in length. The average person who sleeps 7 to 8 hours a night has four to six sleep cycles during a night. As a sleep cycle begins, a person first enters non-rapid-eye-movement (NREM) sleep. As a woman falls deeper and deeper asleep, she passes from stage I to stage II, III, and IV of NREM sleep over a period of 20 to 30 minutes. Following about 30 minutes of stage IV sleep, sleep progresses back through stages III, and then II until it passes into a phase of rapid-eye-movement (REM) sleep (Figure 19-4).

The purpose of NREM sleep appears to be rest and restoration of the body. It is termed mandatory or *obligatory* sleep because, during the periods of stage III and stage IV, the secretion of growth hormone (somatotropin hormone) from the pituitary is at its highest level. Corticosteroids and epinephrine from the adrenal glands are at their lowest levels. This balance of hormones is the ideal combination for protein synthesis and cell growth. In contrast, the rapid eye movements that occur with REM sleep may serve to coordinate binocular vision; dreams that occur during this time apparently serve as a release of tension or help to integrate new knowledge and experience in the brain's memory system.

Sleep deprivation has definite destructive effects on health. Difficulty in concentrating and episodes of misperception, irritableness, marked fatigue, and anxiety occur with loss of REM sleep. People who are allowed to sleep for only short periods suffer REM-sleep deprivation, because each time they return to sleep they begin with NREM sleep and must progress through its four stages before they reach an REM-sleep stage. This is shown diagrammatically in Figure 19-5. If sleep is severely deprived, lack of NREM sleep can occur as well during pregnancy, leading to apathy and depression.

Pregnant women rarely have difficulty falling asleep at night because they have such a physiologic need for sleep. Late in pregnancy, however, a woman often finds herself awakened from sleep at short frequent intervals by the activity of the fetus. She may wake with dyspnea from oxygen want if she does not use two pillows (sleeping on a couch with an arm rest may be best for her). Because this leads to loss of REM sleep, it can leave her with a feeling of anxiety or not feeling rested even though she has slept as many hours as normally. If a woman does have trouble falling asleep or getting back to sleep, drinking a glass of warm milk is a good sleep inducer. Total relaxation exercises (lying quietly, systematically relaxing neck muscles, shoulder muscles, arm muscles—an exercise often taught in preparation for childbirth classes) can be helpful.

Exercise

Women need exercise during pregnancy to prevent circulatory stasis. For many women, teaching is centered on helping them realize the need

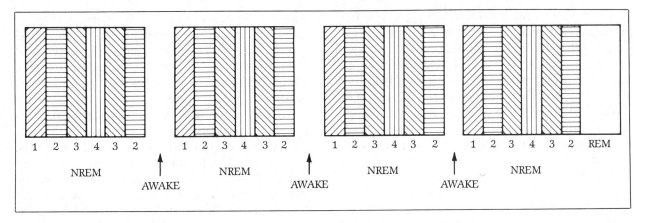

Figure 19-5 *A sleep pattern interrupted by wakefulness. Notice the decreased amount of REM sleep present.*

for exercise and urging them to get enough. Others may have to be taught to restrict exercise or participation in sports. If a woman is a competent horsewoman, for example, there is little reason for her to discontinue riding until it becomes uncomfortable (as long as she does not have a history of spontaneous abortion). However, pregnancy is no time to learn to ride, because a beginning rider is in more danger of being thrown than is an experienced one. The same principles apply to skiing and bicycling. An accomplished skier or bicycler may continue her activity in moderation until balance becomes a problem, but pregnancy is no time to learn to ski or ride a bicycle, because the lack of skill may result in many falls. Swimming is a good activity for pregnant women and, like bathing, is not contraindicated as long as the membranes are intact. Long-distance swimming to a point of fatigue, however, is difficult to justify. Sports such as volleyball, soccer, squash, tennis, golf, softball, basketball, and weight lifting may be continued until the woman no longer feels comfortable with the level of activity. Contact sports such as football (caution that volleyball, touch football, soccer, and basketball can have a degree of contact) and gymnastics other than floor exercises should be discontinued at the time the uterus rises up above the protection of the pelvic bone (about 12 weeks). As bone cartilage softens close to delivery, women may be increasingly prone to knee dislocation accidents from active sports participation late in pregnancy. Hot tubs and saunas following workouts are contraindicated because they conceivably could raise the fetal internal temperature (a teratogenic situation).

Walking is a good exercise throughout pregnancy, and women should be encouraged to take a walk daily unless many levels of stairs or an unsafe neighborhood is a contraindication.

Aerobic exercises ensure good respiratory exchange. Jogging is questionable because of the strain the extra weight of pregnancy places on the knees. In addition to the more mobile knee cartilage present, relaxed symphysis pubis movement is present; this can produce pain on jogging.

Muscle Cramps

Increased levels of serum phosphorus and, possibly, interference with circulation commonly cause muscle cramps of the lower extremities during pregnancy. This muscle cramping is best relieved by lying on the back and extending the involved leg while keeping the knee straight and dorsiflexing the foot (Figure 19-6). With the leg in this position, it may help to knead the affected muscle until the hard "knot" is gone.

Figure 19-6 *Relieving a leg cramp in pregnancy. Pressing down on the knee and pressing the toes backward relieves most cramps. A husband assists here.*

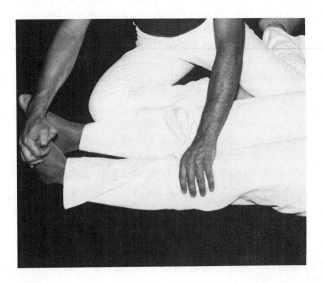

If a woman is having frequent leg cramps, her physician may prescribe aluminum hydroxide gel (Amphojel), which binds phosphorus in the intestinal tract and thereby lowers its circulating level. Lowering milk intake to only a pint daily may also help to reduce the phosphorus level (although commonly thought of as high in calcium it is also high in phosphorus). If milk is restricted, a calcium supplement may also be prescribed. Elevating the lower extremities frequently during the day to improve circulation and never stretching legs to full extension with the toes pointed may be of benefit.

Muscle cramps are a minor symptom of pregnancy, but the pain may be extreme and the intensity of the contraction can be frightening. A woman needs to be reassured that muscle cramps are normal in pregnancy and to be given instructions on how to relieve them.

Always ask at prenatal visits if this is a problem; the woman may not realize the cramping is pregnancy-related and therefore not mention it spontaneously.

Breast Tenderness

Breast tenderness is often one of the first symptoms noticed in early pregnancy. It may be most noticeable on exposure to cold air. For most women the tenderness is minimal and transient—something they are aware of, but not truly distressed by. If the tenderness is enough to cause real discomfort, encourage the woman to wear a bra with a wide shoulder strap for support and to dress to avoid cold drafts. If the pain is sharp, nipple fissure or other reason for the pain should be investigated.

Palmar Erythema

Palmar erythema or palmar pruritus occurs in early pregnancy and is probably caused by the increase in the level of estrogen; it may be related to subclinical jaundice. Constant redness or itching of the palms may make the woman think she is allergic to a new product she is using. She needs an explanation that this is normal before she spends much time and effort trying different soaps or detergents or attempting to implicate certain foods she has eaten recently. Calamine lotion may be soothing for this condition. As soon as a woman's body adjusts to the increased level of estrogen, the erythema and pruritus disappear.

Abdominal Discomfort

Some women experience uncomfortable feelings of abdominal pressure early in pregnancy. Women with a multiple pregnancy may notice this all through pregnancy. Women learn to relieve this feeling by putting gentle pressure on the uterine fundus. Pregnant women typically stand with their arms crossed in front because the weight of their arms resting on their abdomens relieves this discomfort.

When women stand up quickly, they often experience a pulling pain in the right or left lower abdomen from tension on the round ligaments. The pain is sharp and can be frightening. They can prevent this type of pain by always rising slowly from a lying to a sitting, or from a sitting to a standing, position. Because round ligament pain may simulate the abrupt pain that occurs with ruptured ectopic pregnancy (tubal pregnancy), a woman's description of sharp lower abdominal pain must be listened to carefully.

Smoking

It is well documented that *smoking in excess* (more than 10 cigarettes per day) is harmful to fetal growth because it causes carbon monoxide entrapment by the placenta. This leads to intrauterine hypoxia as the carbon monoxide unit attaches to hemoglobin more readily than does oxygen. It is often impossible for a smoker to stop if she has been smoking any length of time. She may be able to cut down on the number of cigarettes smoked per day, however, so this possibility should be explored early in pregnancy.

A nurse who does not smoke may have difficulty appreciating what a cigarette means to a smoker. If you are a nonsmoker, be aware that you are advising or asking a woman to give up something that you do not fully appreciate the need for. Behavior modification techniques—rewarding herself for not smoking (perhaps by awarding herself the money she would have spent on cigarettes to buy something else for herself)—may be suggested. Women who miss smoking may want to replace cigarettes with food snacks; review with a woman that such snacks should be fresh fruit or vegetables to avoid an excessive intake of junk food. Joining a "Stop Smoking" group is helpful. Caution her, however, that she should not particicpate in a program that uses any form of substitute medication. Health care providers should not be smoking in areas where pregnant women come for care. "No Smoking" signs should be posted in these areas so pregnant women are not exposed to cigarette smoke from women who find it impossible to quit smoking during pregnancy.

Employment

Unless a woman's job involves handling toxic substances, lifting heavy objects, other kinds of

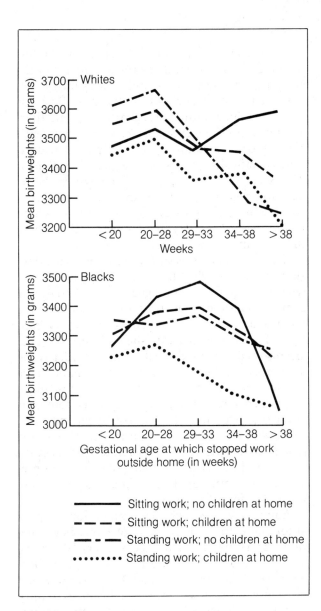

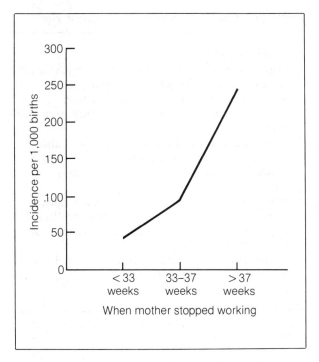

Figure 19-8 *Incidence of placental infarcts in women with stand-up jobs throughout pregnancy. From Naeye, R. L. & Peters, E. C. (1982). Working during pregnancy: Effects on the fetus. Pediatrics, 69, 724. © American Academy of Pediatrics 1982. Reprinted by permission.*

Figure 19-7 *Weeks worked during pregnancy and birthweight. From Ringler-Barman, M. (1984). Advising pregnant and postoperative working patients. Contemporary OB/GYN, 23, 80.*

excessive physical strain, or long periods of standing or having to maintain body balance, most women today continue to be employed until at least the seventh month of pregnancy. Many women continue to work until the day of delivery.

A recent study conducted in Finland (Barlow & Sullivan, 1982) reports that spontaneous abortion occurs more widely in women who work outside the home than in those who do not, regardless of occupation. The longer a woman works beyond 28 weeks of pregnancy, the lower her baby's birthweight may be (Ringler-Barman, 1984). As shown in Figure 19-7, the type of job a mother works at also influences birthweight (women with chil-

dren at home who do standing work have infants with a mean birthweight of only 3,200 gm compared to 3,600 gm in those who do sitting work with no children at home). Placental infarcts may also occur in women who continue to work during pregnancy (Figure 19-8). The meaning of such infarcts is unknown but were found in 25 percent of women who continued to hold stand-up jobs throughout pregnancy. By contrast, large placental infarcts were found in only 53 of 1,000 births of women who remained at home and in 51 of 1,000 births of women who held sedentary jobs (Naeye, 1982).

In order that women's rights could be protected during pregnancy, an employment act covering pregnant women was passed by Congress in 1978 (P.L. No. 95-555). These rights are summarized in Table 19-1. The only women not covered by this law are those who work for companies with fewer than 15 employees.

In *Standards for Maternity Care and Employment of Mothers in Industry*, the Maternal Child Health Service of the United States reports that pregnant women should not work with any of the following substances: aniline, benzene and toluene, carbon disulfide, carbon monoxide, chlorinated hydrocarbons, lead and its compounds,

Table 19-1 Employment Rights of Pregnant Women

An employer cannot

1. Deprive a woman of seniority rights, in pay or promotion, because she takes a maternity leave.
2. Treat a woman back from maternity leave as a new hire, starting over on the eligibility period for pension and other benefits.
3. Force a pregnant woman to leave if she is able to and wants to continue to work.
4. Refuse to hire a woman just because she is pregnant or fire her for the same reason.
5. Refuse to cover an employee's normal pregnancy and delivery expenses in the company health plan, or pay less for pregnancy than for other medical conditions.
6. Refuse to pay sick leave or disability benefits to women whose difficult pregnancies keep them off the job.

Source: Public Law No. 95–555, United States Congress, 1978.

mercury and its compounds, nitrobenzene and other nitro compounds of benzene and its homologues, phosphorus, radioactive substances, X-rays, and turpentine. The incidence of hospital-treated spontaneous abortion is significantly higher than usual among chemical, agricultural, construction, plastics, laundry, and machine shop workers, shoe sewers and gluers, food processors, weavers, nurses, motor vehicle and tram drivers, and metal workers in the radio and television production section of the electronics industry, especially soldering. Spontaneous abortion is higher than usual among hospital employees such as operating room nurses who work with chemical sterilizing agents, specifically ethylene oxide, formaldehyde, and glutaraldehyde (Barlow & Sullivan, 1982).

Other problems that can occur with employment are interferences in adequate rest and nutrition. Figure 19-9 shows general guidelines the American Medical Association suggests for work during pregnancy. Table 19-2 lists restrictions that physicians generally suggest for working patients with normal pregnancies (Ringler-Barman, 1984).

Remember that many women work not just for money but as a career. If they are asked to quit a job then, they are asked to give up not only money but their self-esteem. More effective than counseling women to resign from their jobs during pregnancy, then, so they do have more rest, may be counseling them to reserve periods during the day for rest and urging them to observe a proper diet in addition to continuing work.

Travel

Most women have questions about travel during pregnancy, especially as the summer months approach and they are planning vacations; many women travel throughout the year on business trips. Early in a normal pregnancy, there are literally no restrictions except that a woman susceptible to motion sickness should only take medication specifically prescribed by her physician or discussed with her physician or nurse-midwife. Late in pregnancy, travel plans should take into consideration the possibility of early labor, which would require delivery in a strange setting where the woman's obstetric history is unknown.

If a woman plans to travel to a remote location, such as a campsite, be certain that no matter what the month of her pregnancy, she knows of a nearby health care facility that could provide medical attention. If she is going to be away from home for an extended trip, she will need to make arrangements to visit a health care provider at the distant site at the times her regular prenatal visits would be scheduled. Ask her to make these plans far enough ahead of time so her records from your clinic or office can be copied to give her or for you to forward to the health care provider she will see (you need her written permission to send records). She should be certain to take enough of her prescribed vitamin supplement plus adequate prescriptions for refills as necessary.

Advise a woman who is taking a long trip by automobile to plan frequent rest or stretch periods. Every 100 miles, or at least every 200 miles, she should get out of the car and walk a short distance. This practice will relieve stiffness and muscle ache and will improve lower extremity circulation, preventing varicosities and hemorrhoids.

Women may drive as long as they fit comfortably behind the steering wheel. While pregnant, they should continue or begin to use seat belts. Occasionally, uterine rupture has been reported from seat belt use, but, overall, seat belts reduce maternal mortality in car accidents. The use of shoulder harnesses as well as lap belts should be encouraged.

Traveling by plane shortens traveling time and is not contraindicated as long as the plane has a well-pressurized cabin (true of commercial airlines, but not of all small private planes). A well-pressurized cabin is important because low oxygen concentrations may occur at high altitude if the cabin pressure is not stabilized. Low oxygen intake would lead to hypoxia, with possible brain damage to the fetus. Some airlines do not permit women who are more than 7 months pregnant on board; others require written permission from the

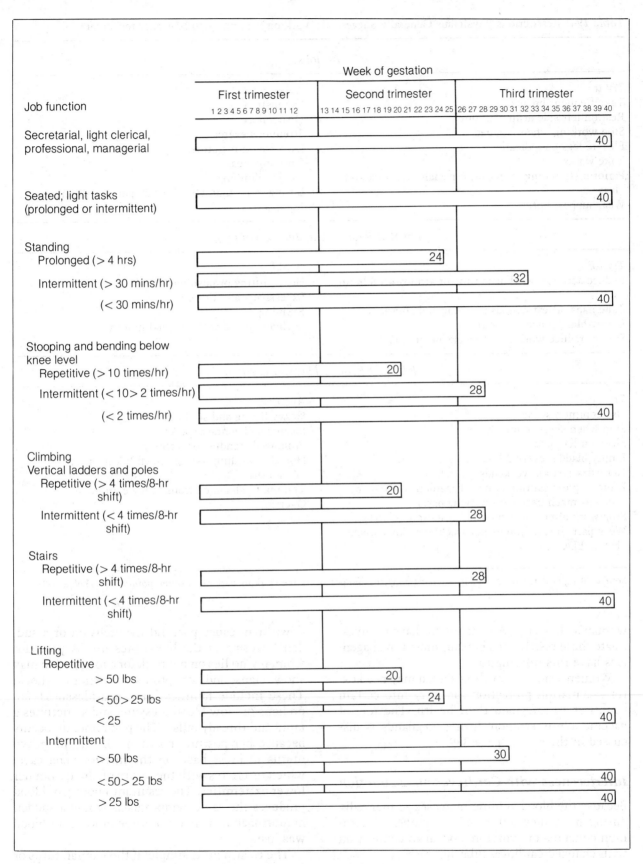

Figure 19-9 *How long may women work? General guidelines from the AMA.*
From American Medical Association, Council on Scientific Affairs. (1984). Effects
of pregnancy on work performance. Journal of the American Medical Association,
251, 1995.

Table 19-2 Restrictions Physicians Generally Suggest for Working Patients with Normal Pregnancies

All Jobs

Try to:	*Avoid:*
Take frequent breaks	Exhaustion
Rest on left side at lunch hour	Discomfort
Stop working when fatigued	Strenuous exercise
Elevate legs periodically	Extreme temperatures
Take walks	Smoking areas
Perform stretching exercises, especially for back and legs	Ladder climbing
	Lifting more than 10, 15, or 25 pounds (different responses)
Wear support hose	

Jobs that Require Standing or Walking

Try to:	*Avoid:*
Reduce activity; work part time or at most in 8-hour shifts	Heavy lifting or pushing
Take naps or rest periods morning and afternoon	Excessive stair climbing
Empty bladder every 2 hours	Running
Stop or reduce work 2 to 4 weeks before EDC	In-flight airline work in final month

Jobs that Require Physical Exertion

Try to:	*Avoid:*
Use common sense	Heavy lifting and straining
Stop when short of breath	Jogging and contact sports
Sleep on left side	Prolonged standing or walking
Empty bladder every 2 hours	Horseback riding, skiing, rough hiking after 7 months
Get extra rest on weekends	
Exercise great caution around hazardous equipment, such as machinery with moving parts	Trauma to abdomen from heavy equipment
Stop work after 7 to 8 months' gestation	Overtime
Work part time (20 hours per week) for 2 to 4 weeks before EDC	

Source: Ringler-Barman, M. (1984). Advising pregnant and postoperative working patients. *Contemporary OB/GYN, 23,* 80.

woman's physician. A woman will have to investigate these restrictions herself; most travel agencies have this information.

Women who are traveling abroad may need extra vaccination protection for entry into certain countries to safeguard their health. The role of vaccine administration during pregnancy is discussed in the box on page 389.

Interferences with Cardiovascular Function

Because the blood volume increases so markedly during pregnancy (30–50%), a number of common concerns or symptoms occur in connection with changed cardiovascular function.

Postural Hypotension

When advising women to rest during pregnancy, caution them that in late pregnancy lying down may cause postural hypotension or a sudden lowering of the blood pressure. A pregnant woman who lies on her back for a long period may show signs and symptoms of extreme shock. These include faintness and breathlessness, apprehension, low blood pressure, and sometimes a rapid and thready pulse. The phenomenon occurs because her posture (position) allows the heavy uterus to press back on the inferior vena cava, which interferes with the return of blood from her lower extremities. The resultant pooling of blood produces the same symptoms as would a sudden hemorrhage in which the same amount of blood was lost.

The treatment is simple: If the woman turns or is turned on her side, pressure is removed from the vena cava, blood flow is again adequate, and the symptoms quickly fade. When advising women to rest or sleep during pregnancy, rec-

Vaccine Administration

Vaccines are a form of medication in that they are intrusive; a woman should not take them without her physician's or midwife's knowledge and approval. Live virus vaccine administration is contraindicated during pregnancy because the virus may cross the placenta and infect the fetus. Vaccines against smallpox, mumps (epidemic parotitis), rubeola, rubella, yellow fever, or poliomyelitis (Sabin vaccine)—all live viruses—should *not* be administered to a pregnant woman. If a woman is in an area where yellow fever is endemic, or she has been bitten by a rabid animal, vaccination would be essential. Such immunization should be undertaken, however, with the understanding that fetal risk is involved.

Influenza vaccine should be avoided unless a woman has an underlying disease that makes her a high-risk candidate (such as cystic fibrosis). The vaccine against cholera contains killed bacteria and thus may be given if a woman is exposed to the infection. It does not appear to be abortifacient. Tetanus and diphtheria toxoids are apparently safe. Women may be given gamma globulin (immune serum globulin) during pregnancy; it contains antibodies, not antigens, and might be administered if the woman is exposed to hepatitis A.

The field of immunization is a constantly changing one, since new discoveries are continually being made. Before you give advice on immunizations to a pregnant woman, check with the public health authorities in your community for the most current recommendations.

Following delivery of a child, a woman should be urged to have any standard immunizations (especially rubella vaccine), she is missing so that during the next pregnancy the problem will not arise.

ommend a left side-lying position, such as a modified Sims' position, to avoid this problem (Figure 19-2).

If a woman rises suddenly from a lying or sitting position, or stands for an extended time in a warm or crowded area, she may faint from the same phenomenon (blood pooling in the pelvic area). Rising slowly and avoiding extended periods of standing prevents this problem. If a woman does feel faint, sitting with her head lowered—the same action as for any person who feels faint—will alleviate the problem.

Varicosities

Varicosities (Figure 19-10) are common in pregnancy because the weight of the distended uterus puts pressure on the vessels returning blood from the lower extremities. This causes a pooling of blood in the vessels. The veins become engorged, inflamed, and painful. Varicosities are usually found in the lower extremities; they may extend to the vulva. They occur most frequently in women with a family history of varicose veins and those who have a large fetus or a multiple pregnancy.

Women need to take precautions early in pregnancy to prevent the development of varicosities. Resting in a Sims' position or supine with the legs raised against the wall or elevated on a footstool for 15 to 20 minutes twice a day is a good precaution (Figure 19-11). Be certain that a woman does not sit with her legs crossed or her knees bent.

Some women may need the support of elastic stockings or an Ace bandage for relief of varicosities. The stocking or bandage should be put on the leg so that it reaches an area above the point of distention. The woman should apply the support before she arises in the morning; once she is on her feet, the pooling of blood has already begun, and the stockings or bandages will not be so effective. If a woman is going to buy stockings, be certain she understands they are to be medical support hose. Many panty hose manufacturers say their stockings give "firm support" and a woman may erroneously assume these to be sufficient.

Exercise is as effective as rest periods in alleviating varicosities, since it stimulates venous return. Most women state that they do not need set exercise periods during pregnancy because they work hard cleaning the house, or they have a job and get exercise there. If a woman analyzes the type of work she does, however, she will realize that a great deal of housework and office or factory work leads to stasis of lower extremity circulation. A woman remains in one position to wash dishes, to make beds, to cook dinner; to file, to run a computer, to work out an economic anal-

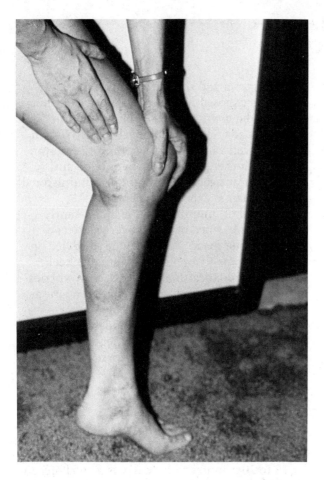

Figure 19-10 *Varicosities are distended leg veins. They occur often from pelvic pressure during pregnancy.*

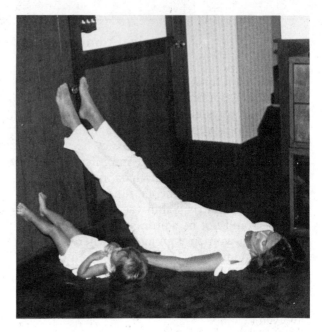

Figure 19-11 *Position to relieve varicosities. A 2-year-old daughter joins her mother in the exercise.*

ysis; to process a part on an assembly line, to teach a class. She needs to break up these long periods of standing or sitting still by a "walk break" at least twice a day.

Vitamin C may be helpful in reducing the size of varicosities as it is involved in the formation of blood vessel collagen and endothelium. Ask at prenatal visits whether or not fruits containing vitamin C are included in a woman's diet. Ask her if she takes a walk every day, weather permitting. Urge her to prevent varicosities with caution early in pregnancy; do not consider them a second trimester problem or the best you will accomplish is relieving the pain from already formed varicosities (which are permanent).

Hemorrhoids

Hemorrhoids, which are varicosities of the rectal veins, are common in pregnancy because of pressure on these veins from the bulk of the growing uterus. Preventive measures early in pregnancy may be effective in reducing their severity. Daily bowel evacuation not only helps to relieve

constipation but also helps to prevent the formation of hemorrhoids. Resting in a modified Sims' position daily is helpful. At day's end, assuming a knee-chest position (Figure 19-12) for 10 to 15 minutes is an excellent way to reduce the pressure on rectal veins. A knee-chest position tends to make a woman feel light-headed; thus, the first day, she should remain in this position for a few minutes only, gradually increasing the time day by day until she can comfortably maintain the

Figure 19-12 *Knee-chest position. This position allows for freer flow of urine from the kidneys (preventing urinary tract stasis and infection) and better circulation in the rectal area (preventing hemorrhoids), since the weight of the uterus is shifted forward.*

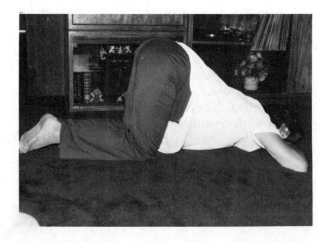

position for about 15 minutes. Stool softeners may be recommended for a woman who already has hemorrhoids. As with varicosities, *prevention* is as important as providing help for already established hemorrhoids.

Heart Palpitations

On sudden movement, such as turning over in bed, a pregnant woman may experience a bounding palpitation of the heart. This is probably due to the circulatory adjustments necessary to accommodate her increased blood supply during pregnancy. Although only momentary, the sensation is frightening because the heart seems to have skipped a beat. Slower movements will prevent its happening so frequently. It is reassuring to know that palpitations are normal and to be expected on occasion.

Interferences with Genitourinary Function

Because the endocervical and vaginal glands secrete increased amounts of mucus during pregnancy and the pH of vaginal secretions changes to a more acid level, vaginal symptoms can be anticipated.

Leukorrhea

Leukorrhea is a whitish, viscous vaginal discharge or an increase in the amount of normal vaginal secretions. It occurs in response to the high estrogen levels present and the increased blood supply to the vaginal epithelium and cervix during pregnancy. A daily bath or shower to wash away accumulated secretions and prevent vulvar excoriation should be enough to control this problem. Douching should not be necessary and should not be encouraged; it could change the pH of vaginal secretions. Some women feel they must wear sanitary pads to absorb the discharge. Women should be cautioned not to use tampons, which could cause stasis of secretions and possible subsequent infection (similar to toxic shock syndrome). Wearing cotton, not synthetic, underpants and sleeping at night without underwear is also helpful in reducing moisture and possible vulvar excoriation.

Pruritus

Any woman who has vulvar pruritus needs to be seen by a physician or nurse practitioner, since this usually indicates infection. Be certain that when she is describing pruritus-like symptoms, a woman is not really describing burning on urination, a sign of a beginning bladder infection (which also needs therapy, but of a different type).

Common vaginal infections that present with pruritus and common therapies for vulvitis are discussed in Chapter 36.

Women should not treat vaginal infections by themselves at any time, especially not during pregnancy. Some medications prescribed for these problems (metronidazole [Flagyl], in particular) are not recommended during pregnancy; they can cross the placenta and may be teratogenic. Douching is another common therapy. It is dangerous for a woman to use a bulb-type douche apparatus while she is pregnant. This design puts solution into the vagina under pressure, which can cause a circulatory embolism if the solution is pushed into the cervix and under the edge of the placenta and into maternal vessels. This is an important point to remember when talking to pregnant women about douching: Women are likely to regard the bulb-type apparatus as more convenient and will buy it if not cautioned against doing so.

A woman who is uncomfortable about discussing this part of her body or who associates vaginal infections with poor hygiene or sexually transmitted disease may be reluctant to mention an irritating vaginal discharge. Specifically ask each women at health care visits whether she has this problem.

Frequency of Urination

Frequency of urination is due to the pressure of the growing uterus on the anterior bladder. This sensation begins in early pregnancy, lasts for about the first 3 months, then disappears until late in pregnancy, when it again becomes prominent. The sensation disappears in midpregnancy because the uterus rises above the bladder; it returns in later pregnancy as the fetal head presses against the bladder.

When a woman is describing frequency of urination to you, be certain it is the only urinary symptom she has. Ask her whether she has burning on urination, or whether she has noticed any blood in her urine (signs of urinary tract infection).

There are no ways to decrease frequency of urination; the important implementation is to be certain a woman understands it is a normal phenomenon. She should not reduce her fluid intake as she needs a high fluid intake to support her circulatory volume.

Occasionally a woman notices stress incontinence (involuntary loss of urine while coughing or sneezing, or running) during pregnancy. Doing Kegal's exercises (alternatively contracting and relaxing perineal muscles) helps to strengthen urinary control and decrease the possibility that stress incontinence will occur, as well as directly strengthen perineal muscles for delivery.

Hygiene

Because pregnancy is not an illness, a woman has to take few special care measures other than to use common sense regarding hygiene. Many women, however, listen to their friends or family about what a woman can and cannot do during pregnancy and are consequently misinformed. The average woman needs some help separating fact from fiction so she can enjoy her pregnancy unhampered by unnecessary restrictions. You should know the common misunderstandings of pregnancy yourself so you can appreciate why so much health teaching is necessary. In no other area of nursing except for infant feeding are as many misconceptions or as much inappropriate information passed on to women.

Bathing

At one time, bathing was restricted during pregnancy because it was feared that bath water would enter the vagina and cervix and contaminate the uterine contents. It was also believed that hot water touching the abdomen might bring on labor. Because the vagina is normally in a closed position, or the sides approximate each other, the danger that water will enter the uterus is minimal. The temperature of the water has no documented effect on initiating labor. Sweating tends to increase with pregnancy because a woman excretes waste products not only for herself but for the child within her; and she has an abundant vaginal discharge: Daily bathing has now moved from a high place on the *don't* list to a high place on the *do* list.

As pregnancy advances, it may be hard for a woman to get in and out of a bathtub because of her problem in maintaining balance. If so, she should shower instead or take sponge baths, whichever her common sense tells her is better. If membranes rupture, or vaginal bleeding is present, bathing is contraindicated because then there *is* a danger of contamination of uterine contents. During the last month of pregnancy, when cervical dilatation may be beginning, some physicians restrict tub bathing for the same reason.

Breast Care

All women during pregnancy, whether they plan to breast-feed their baby at the pregnancy's end or not, should observe a few precautions during pregnancy in order to prevent loss of breast tone. Loss of breast tone can result in pendulous breasts later in life, which can be painful. A general preventive rule is to wear a firm, supportive bra. Wide straps spread weight across the shoulders better than narrow ones. A woman may have to buy an increased size bra halfway through pregnancy to accommodate increased breast growth.

If a woman will be breast-feeding, she can begin a simple exercise of nipple rolling once or twice a day to help toughen the nipple. Nipple rolling is the gentle process of grasping the nipple between her thumb and forefinger and gently rolling it between her thumb and finger about 10 times. If a woman's sexual partner has been using oral nipple stimulation as a part of foreplay, she may not need any exercise: Her nipples may be already conditioned. Vigorous toughening of nipples is not necessary and can lead to nipple fissures, which interfere with breast-feeding. A woman should wash her breasts with clear water only (no soap) to prevent nipple drying and cracking, which, again, can interfere with breast-feeding.

Dental Care

It is important that women continue good toothbrushing habits throughout pregnancy. Gingival tissue tends to hypertrophy during pregnancy; this means that unless the woman brushes well, pockets of plaque form readily between the enlarged gumline and teeth. Because women grow tired readily during pregnancy, brushing teeth well once a day may be more effective than trying to brush after every meal or snack but never doing a thorough job.

Tooth decay occurs from the action of bacteria on sugar. This action lowers the pH of the mouth, creating an acid medium that leads to etching of teeth. In order to keep levels of sugar in the mouth to a minimum, if a woman is going to eat candy, she should snack on a type that dissolves easily (a chocolate bar rather than taffy, which remains in the mouth a long time). Snacking on foods such as apples and carrots that are not empty calorie foods is even a better recommendation for safe dental care.

Douching

Although women have increased vaginal discharges during pregnancy, douching as a means of vaginal cleansing is not advocated (the same as it is not advocated for routine care at any time). If a woman feels that douching is necessary, her physician or nurse-midwife should specify the amount and kind of solution she may use (a mild vinegar solution—two tablespoons to a quart of water—is usually recommended). As indicated in the discussion of vaginal infections, she should never use a bulb-type syringe for douching.

Clothing

The day when a woman had to purchase a completely new maternity wardrobe to wear during pregnancy is fast disappearing. A woman today usually needs little guidance in selecting proper clothing for herself during pregnancy. Early in pregnancy, she may wear an abdominal support such as a light girdle if she wishes (for *support*, not to compress and constrict her abdomen). She should avoid garters and extremely firm girdles with panty legs; these impede lower extremity circulation. She may need to purchase larger-size bras as her breasts enlarge. If she plans on breastfeeding her newborn she might choose to buy ones suitable for breast-feeding so she can continue to use these after the baby's birth. She will have less backache if she limits her shoes to those with low heels. Otherwise, the rule is common sense and comfort.

Sexual Relations

Some women do not ask questions about sexual relations during pregnancy because they have inhibitions about broaching the subject. Most women have questions, however, about restriction of coitus during pregnancy.

Old wives' tales about sexual relations in pregnancy abound: Coitus on the date her period would have been expected (if the woman had not become pregnant) will initiate labor; orgasm will initiate labor, but relations without orgasm will not; coitus during the fertile days of a cycle will cause a second pregnancy or twins. If a woman has such concerns, she needs to voice them. Then they can be dispelled, and she will not refrain from coitus when she desires it or worry needlessly that coitus is harming her child.

Women who have a history of repeated spontaneous abortion may be advised to avoid coitus during the time of the pregnancy when the previous abortions occurred. Women whose membranes have ruptured or who have vaginal spotting should be advised against coitus until they are examined in order to prevent infection. Otherwise, there are no sexual restrictions during pregnancy.

Early in pregnancy a woman may notice a decrease in her desire for coitus due to the increased level of estrogen in her body. Breast tenderness may limit a usual pattern of sexual arousal. As pelvic congestion occurs due to the additional uterine blood supply, she may notice increased clitoral sensation; some women experience orgasm for the first time during pregnancy because of the increased pelvic congestion present.

As pregnancy advances and the woman's abdomen increases in size, she and her sexual partner may need to limit their positions for coitus. A side-by-side position, or the woman in a superior position, may be more comfortable. As vaginal secretions change, a woman may find a lubricant helpful. If she begins to experience discomfort from penile penetration, mutual masturbation or oral-genital relations might be satisfying to both partners. However, advise caution about male oral-female genital contact, since accidental air embolism has been reported from this act during pregnancy (Fatteh, 1973).

It is important that coitus during pregnancy be explored with couples during prenatal counseling. Otherwise couples who are having a problem in this area are left feeling as though there was something basically wrong with them or their relationship. They need helpful suggestions in this area as well as areas such as constipation, nausea, or bathing.

Danger Signs of Pregnancy

An important part of health teaching at a first prenatal visit involves instructing a woman about the danger signals to which she should be alert during pregnancy. Assure her you have no reason to think she is going to experience any of these things; that you have every reason to believe she is going to have a normal, uncomplicated pregnancy (assuming that is true); but that if any of these things should occur, she should inform a health care provider by telephoning immediately. Be certain you give her an alternative number to call in the event the health care facility is closed. Emphasize that if one of these danger signals should occur, it does not mean something bad has happened to her or her baby; they serve merely to alert all of you to the possibility that something *may* happen. It is important for her to report them immediately, so that they can be dealt with *before* something harmful occurs.

Vaginal Bleeding

A woman should report vaginal bleeding no matter how slight as some of the serious bleeding complications of pregnancy begin with *slight* spotting. For assessment, ask her how she discovered the spotting. If she discovered it on toilet paper after voiding, she is probably reporting actual vaginal bleeding. If she reports spotting on her underpants or spotting on toilet paper following a bowel movement, she may be reporting spotting from hemorrhoids. When a woman has spotting she needs referral to a physician or nurse-midwife for further evaluation. This person will either see her or offer her advice on the telephone, depending on the length of her pregnancy and the individual circumstances.

Persistent Vomiting

It is not uncommon during the first trimester of pregnancy for a woman to vomit once a day. Persistent vomiting that occurs more often than this is never normal; vomiting that continues past the twelfth week of pregnancy is also extended vomiting. As the nutritional supply to the fetus can be depleted with persistent vomiting, the woman needs to report the persistence of this problem.

Chills and Fever

Chills and fever, symptoms of infection, are never normal during pregnancy. They may be evidence of an intrauterine infection, which is a serious complication for both the woman and baby. They may also be symptoms of a relatively benign gastroenteritis. The woman herself cannot make an informed decision about the cause.

Sudden Escape of Fluid from the Vagina

Sudden discharge of fluid from the vagina means the membranes have ruptured; the fluid is amniotic fluid. Because this sign may be one of the first of labor, mother and fetus are both threatened: The uterine cavity is no longer sealed against infection. If the fetus is small and the head does not fit snugly into the cervix, the umbilical cord may prolapse with the membrane rupture. The head may then be compressed against the cord, and the fetus may be in immediate and grave danger. Alerting you to the happening is important for the planning of a safe and controlled delivery. Occasionally a woman mistakes stress incontinence for this escape of fluid. Vaginal examination will reveal that the membranes are still intact.

Pain in the Abdomen

Abdominal pain at any time is a signal that something abnormal is occurring. However, some women may think that it is normal in pregnancy because of the growing uterus and the deflection of other organs from their usual alignment. They are wrong—an expanding uterus expands painlessly. Abdominal pain is announcing something

else: a tubal (ectopic) pregnancy; a separation of the placenta; or something unrelated to the pregnancy but perhaps equally serious, such as appendicitis, ulcer, or pancreatitis.

When a pregnant woman stands up suddenly, particularly if she was sitting on the floor, she may experience a sharp, fleeting pain in her groin from extension of the round ligament. Most women can distinguish this sensation of pulling from other abdominal pain, but some may report it as a danger signal of pregnancy.

Pregnancy-Induced Hypertension

Four symptoms signal developing pregnancy-induced hypertension:

1. Swelling of the face or fingers.
2. Flashes of light or dots before the eyes.
3. Dimness or blurring of vision.
4. Severe, continuous headache.

It is normal for a woman to have some edema of the ankles during pregnancy, particularly if she has been on her feet for a long period of time. Swelling of the hands (ask if she has noticed that her rings are tight) or face (difficulty opening eyes in the morning due to edema of the eyelids) indicates edema too extensive to be normal. Visual disturbance or continuous headache may be a sign that cerebral edema is present or that hypertension is becoming acute. Be certain a woman is using her common sense and is not reporting symptoms she had before she became pregnant. If she had the same visual difficulties and headaches before as during pregnancy, she may need to see an ophthalmologist rather than her obstetrician.

Danger signals of pregnancy are summarized in Table 19-3.

Symptoms of Mid- or Late Pregnancy

At the midpoint of pregnancy (the twentieth to twenty-fourth weeks), a woman is usually ready for further health teaching that relates to the new developments in the latter half of pregnancy. As she starts to view the child within her as a separate person, she becomes interested in discussing and making plans for labor, delivery, and the infant's care. She should be informed of the signs and symptoms of beginning labor. At the midpoint of pregnancy it is good to review the precautions she should take to prevent constipation, varicosities, and hemorrhoids and to describe the new symptoms that may now be expected.

Table 19-3 Danger Signs of Pregnancy

Sign	Possible Importance
Vaginal bleeding	Placenta previa, premature separation of the placenta, premature birth
Persistent vomiting	Systemic infection; will lead to electrolyte and fluid disturbances
Chills and fever	Intrauterine infection
Sudden escape of fluid from the vagina	Premature ruptured membranes
Abdominal pain	Ectopic pregnancy, premature separation of the placenta, uterine rupture
Swelling of the face or fingers	Pregnancy-induced hypertension
Flashes of light or dots before the eyes	Pregnancy-induced hypertension
Dimness or blurring of vision	Pregnancy-induced hypertension
Severe, continuous headache	Pregnancy-induced hypertension

Backache

As pregnancy advances a lumbar lordosis occurs, and postural changes necessary to maintain balance will cause backache. Shoes with a moderately high heel reduce the amount of spinal curvature necessary to maintain an upright posture. Encouraging a woman to walk with her pelvis tilted forward (putting pelvic support under the weight of the fetus) is also helpful. Too often at a prenatal visit, women are only observed lying in a lithotomy position on an examining table. Make it a nursing responsibility to assess the manner in which a woman walks and what type of shoes she is wearing as she moves from the waiting room to the examining room. This assessment can reveal a lot about the cause of her backache. Advising a woman to squat and not to bend over to pick up objects, and to always lift objects by holding them close to her body, may also help. She may need a firmer mattress during pregnancy than she did before; sliding a board under the mattress serves the same purpose and is cheaper than buying a new one. Pelvic rocking or tilting, an exercise described in Chapter 21, also helps to prevent and relieve backache.

Backache can be an initial sign of bladder or kidney infection. Thus, you need a detailed account of the woman's symptoms to make certain she is describing only backache. A woman should not take muscle relaxants or analgesia for back pain without first consulting her physician or nurse-midwife.

Dyspnea

Shortness of breath occurs in pregnancy as the expanding uterus puts pressure on the diaphragm and causes some lung compression. A woman may notice this problem mostly at night, when she lies flat, and she will definitely notice it on exertion. Sitting upright, allowing the weight of the uterus to fall away from the diaphragm, will relieve the problem. As pregnancy progresses, she may require two or more pillows in order to sleep at night. She needs to limit her activities to a point before she becomes short of breath. Remember that anxiety adds to the sensation of breathlessness. Worry over dyspnea may make her more dyspneic, which is one reason this minor symptom is important to review. Distraction from the discomfort by a support person is helpful (as long as she thinks about the problem she will remain short of breath, as breathing comfortably is difficult while you are aware of your breathing pattern).

Ankle Edema

Most women experience some swelling of the ankles and feet during late pregnancy. It is most noticeable at the end of the day. Women are often first conscious of it because they kick off their shoes at a restaurant or party and then are unable to put them on again comfortably.

Ankle edema of this nature, as long as proteinuria and hypertension are not accompanying factors, is a normal occurrence of pregnancy. It is probably caused by reduced blood circulation in the lower extremities due to uterine pressure and general fluid retention. Women who spend long periods standing in one position tend to notice it most. This simple edema can be relieved best by resting in a side-lying position, which increases kidney glomerular flow rate. Sitting for half an hour in the afternoon and again in the evening with the legs elevated is also helpful. Women should avoid constricting panty girdles or knee-high stockings, as these impede lower extremity circulation and venous return.

Women need reassurance that ankle edema is normal during pregnancy. Otherwise, they worry that it is a beginning sign of pregnancy-induced hypertension. On the other hand, do not dismiss a report of lower extremity edema lightly until you are certain that the woman does not evidence any signs (proteinuria; hypertension; edema of other, nondependent parts; sudden increase in weight) that might indicate pregnancy-induced hypertension.

Frequency of Urination

Frequency of urination usually ceases after the first trimester of pregnancy. Unless a woman is cautioned that the sensation returns after lightening, she may think she has a urinary tract infection. Women who have practiced Kegal's exercises as preparation for delivery notice less of this problem.

Weight Gain

By the midpoint of pregnancy, a woman begins to gain weight faster than she did earlier in the pregnancy (a pound a week compared to about half a pound a week). The average woman finds this an encouraging sign: She interprets it to mean—as it does—that the fetus is growing and thriving inside her. If a mother is not prepared for this increase in weight, she may worry that she is gaining too much and so may miss health care appointments (for worry of being criticized) or begin a diet that lacks essential nutrients.

Alert women early in pregnancy that this increase in weight will occur and review it again at midpregnancy. When weighing women during pregnancy, remember that a sharp, sudden weight gain may indicate fluid retention or developing hypertension of pregnancy. Be careful when talking to women about weight gain that you do not put the cart before the horse. Hypertension of pregnancy does not develop because of the gain in weight; the gain in weight is evidence that hypertension and edema are developing. Teach women that a weight gain is not dangerous unless caused by an accumulation of fluid.

Contractions

Beginning as early as the twelfth week of pregnancy, the uterus "practices" contractions in preparation for labor (Braxton-Hicks contractions). Early in pregnancy, these contractions are not noticeable. In mid- and late pregnancy, the contractions become stronger, and the woman who tenses at the sensation may even experience some minimal pain similar to a hard menstrual cramp. Women need reassurance that the contractions are normal and that they are not a sign of beginning labor. They are, interestingly, however, a positive sign that her pregnancy will end. Late in pregnancy, some women feel as if they have been pregnant forever and are much in need of this type of reassurance.

Breast Changes

At about the sixteenth week of pregnancy, colostrum secretion begins in the breasts. The sensation of a fluid discharge from the breasts can be frightening unless a woman is forewarned. Instruct her to wash her breasts with clear water daily in order to wash the colostrum away and minimize the risk of infection from organisms growing in this medium.

If colostrum secretion is profuse, she may need to place gauze squares inside her bra and change them frequently to maintain dryness; constant moisture next to the breast nipple will cause nipple excoriation, pain, and fissuring. If a woman plans to breast-feed, nipple toughening, such as by nipple rolling, should be begun (see Chapter 33 for a complete discussion on preparation for breast-feeding).

Personal Care Update

An updating of personal hygiene information is helpful to women at the midpoint of pregnancy. If the physician or nurse-midwife with whom you work restricts sexual relations or bathing during the last month of pregnancy, a woman will need to be reminded of these restrictions and have the available alternatives discussed with her. She should be cautioned once more against douching, which becomes more and more hazardous the closer she comes to delivery and the beginning of cervical dilatation.

Signals of Beginning Labor

By the twenty-eighth week of pregnancy, review with a woman the events that signal the beginning of labor. These are summarized in Table 19-4 and discussed below.

Table 19-4 Beginning Signs of Labor

Lightening (settling of the fetal head into the pelvis)
Show (slight blood-streaked vaginal discharge)
Rupture of the membranes (sudden gush of clear fluid from vagina)
Excess energy
Uterine contractions

Lightening

Lightening is the settling of the fetal head into the inlet of the true pelvis. It occurs approximately 2 weeks before labor in primiparas but at unpredictable times in multiparas. The woman notices that she is not as short of breath as she was; her abdominal contour is definitely lower; and on standing she may experience frequency of urination or sciatic pain from the lowered fetal position.

Show

Show is the common term for the release of the cervical secretions (operculum) that formed during pregnancy. It consists of a mucous, often blood-streaked vaginal discharge and indicates that cervical dilatation is beginning.

Rupture of the Membranes

A sudden gush of clear fluid (amniotic fluid) from the vagina indicates rupture of the membranes. The woman should telephone the health care facility at once if labor begins this way. Following rupture of the membranes there is danger of cord prolapse and uterine infection.

Excess Energy

Feeling extremely energetic is a sign of labor that is important for women to recognize. It occurs as part of the body's physiologic preparation for labor. If they do not recognize the sensation for what it is, they will use this burst of energy for other tasks, depleting it and entering labor exhausted. If properly warned, they will conserve the energy for labor—the purpose for which nature provides it.

Uterine Contractions

For most women, labor begins with contractions. True labor contractions usually start in the back and sweep forward across the abdomen like a band tightening. They gradually increase in both frequency and intensity. Advise a woman to telephone the health care facility when contractions begin, which alerts the health care personnel that she is in labor. Inform her at what point in labor her physician or nurse-midwife will come to her home or she should come to the hospital or birthing center, but be certain she knows this is not a hard-and-fast rule. If she should become exceptionally anxious, be home alone, or have a long drive to a health care facility, she should have the option of arriving at the birthing center or hospital ahead of time.

Arrangements for Labor and Delivery

Be certain to review the arrangements a woman needs to make for labor and delivery at a midpoint in pregnancy. No matter how calm a woman seems when discussing these arrangements, all women have some fear that at the last minute they will forget what is expected of them and, for example, will go to the wrong hospital or fill in the wrong form and so have to have the baby unexpectedly alone at home. A woman who anticipates having a home birth has to organize her home and the supplies she needs to have them ready; she may have concern that her preparation will be inadequate.

Some health care providers ask women to pre-register for delivery at a health care facility, so that on the day of labor they need spend no time filling out forms. A woman needs to be certain that she knows the way to the hospital or birthing center, knows where to go when she gets there, knows who is going to drive her there, and has alternative transportation planned for if that person is not available. If she has other children, she must arrange for their care and perhaps for someone to do the cooking and housekeeping while she is away from home.

True, these are arrangements a woman has to make for herself, but asking about whether or not she has made them may be the incentive she needs to get her plans under way. Pregnancy is a stress situation and people under stress do not think as clearly or objectively as they normally do. For her safety and her new child's, if a woman seems to require assistance, help her to make some of these decisions.

Utilizing Nursing Process

Health promotion during pregnancy consists of educating women about what they can expect to happen to them during pregnancy and measures to reduce the minor symptoms of pregnancy; these steps allow pregnancy to be as rich and fulfilling an experience as they envisioned it would be. Like all successful nursing practices, health promotion during pregnancy should be based on use of the nursing process.

Assessment

Many women do not mention minor disorders of pregnancy unless specifically asked about them because they are reluctant to use a busy health care provider's time for discussing minor problems. They may spend a great deal of time worrying about these things, however. Be certain to inquire about these areas at prenatal visits. Unless they are discussed, women may not take enough precautions for preventing hemorrhoids or varicosities and have to deal with these problems later in life.

Analysis

The Fifth Annual Conference on Nursing Diagnoses accepted no diagnoses specific to the minor symptoms of pregnancy. Frequently used diagnoses in this area are "Fear related to minor symptoms of pregnancy," "Nutrition, alterations in, related to nausea of pregnancy," and "Comfort, alteration in, related to lordosis of pregnancy." When establishing goals with women concerning the minor symptoms of pregnancy, be certain that goals are realistic. You cannot expect a woman to be free of nausea of pregnancy, for example, for the first 3 months. The highest goal that you can achieve in this area is for a woman to accept or adapt to the nausea. Likewise, you probably cannot alleviate frequency of urination, backache, or fatigue.

Planning

Be certain when planning with women concerning the minor discomforts of pregnancy that you take into consideration the woman's life style. Instructions such as rest 2 hours every afternoon for a woman with three preschool children at home or a woman who works an 8-hour workday will be hard for her to follow. A plan, on the other hand, that suggests an hour of rest while preschoolers nap or during the woman's lunch hour is much more likely to be accomplished.

Implementation

The major implementation associated with the minor symptoms of pregnancy is teaching. Although the average woman is aware that such discomforts occur with pregnancy, events always seem different when they are happening to you. A woman who knew that it is normal for breast tenderness to occur may not be at all sure that the amount of breast tenderness she is having is normal; a woman who had a mental image of herself as a woman who would not gain a great deal of weight during pregnancy may be very concerned that in reality she is gaining a great deal of weight. Adolescent girls are often very uninformed about common discomforts of pregnancy and need a great deal of teaching and review in this area as their peers have had no experience with these happenings and so they have no background to relate "normal" to.

Evaluation

Many of the recommendations for decreasing minor discomforts of pregnancy are simple in nature so women may discount them as not terribly important to carry out (something to do if they have time, not daily). If they do discount these measures, minor symptoms may become much more than minor. Evaluation is an important step in seeing that this does not happen.

Nursing Care Planning

Mary Kraft is a 23-year-old woman you see in a prenatal setting. She is 13 weeks pregnant. Below are nursing care plans at 13, 14, and 17 weeks of pregnancy concerned with one minor discomfort of pregnancy.

Assessment

Patient states she has had constipation for last 2 weeks. Prepregnancy, had BM daily; now q 3rd day. Stool hard, black in color (taking iron supplement). Day history reveals she includes 2 glasses of water, fruits (apple and banana), and vegetables (greens) daily. Appears distressed when discussing problem. Concerned that "poison" from unpassed stool will affect fetus.

Analysis

Bowel elimination, alteration in: Constipation related to normal changes of pregnancy.

Locus of Decision Making. Shared.

Goal. Patient will have alleviated constipation by 1 week.

Criteria. Patient will have bowel movement QOD without pain or discomfort.

Nursing Orders

1. Assure patient that constipation is often a normal consequence of pregnancy.

2. Assure her that constipation will not affect health of fetus.
3. Encourage to include 2 additional high-fiber foods in nutrition daily (given list).
4. Encourage to rest in lateral Sims' or legs-elevated position 2× per day for 15 minutes to prevent constipation leading to formation of hemorrhoids.
5. Refer to M.D. for stool softener or additional interventions.

Mary Kraft
23 years old
Gestational length: 14 weeks

Assessment

(Telephone call). Constipation only slightly improved. Stool still hard and bowel movements have become painful. Drinking 4 glasses of water daily; has added a source of bran daily (bran cereal or bran muffin). Has not been taking stool softener prescribed by M.D. as she is concerned about taking medication during pregnancy.

Analysis

Constipation continuing related to inadequate patient compliance with medical regimen.

Goal. Unchanged.

Nursing Orders

1. Urge patient to take stool softener daily and counsel regarding safety of prescribed medication during pregnancy.

2. Reassure again that constipation is a normal occurrence in pregnancy.
3. Urge to continue program of resting in lateral Sims' or legs-elevated position daily to prevent hemorrhoid formation.
4. To call again if after taking stool softener for 1 week constipation is not relieved.

Mary Kraft
23 years old
Gestational length: 17 weeks

Assessment

Constipation no longer a problem. BM now q day; taking stool softener daily. Stool soft, no pain. Appears relaxed discussing problem.

Analysis

Problem of constipation inactive; relieved by use of stool softener and nutrition modification.

Nursing Orders

1. Assure again that this specific medication will not be harmful to fetus or her during pregnancy.
2. Urge to continue to take medication and maintain high-fiber nutrition.
3. Refer to M.D. to check if medication should be reduced to every other day or any other change necessary based on improved bowel function.

Questions for Review

Multiple Choice

1. Mrs. Allen is a patient you meet in a prenatal clinic. She states that she has a vaginal discharge and asks you about douching. A general safe rule regarding douching during pregnancy is
   a. it is never safe.
   b. a bulb-type syringe should not be used.
   c. the solution used should never be acid.
   d. a room temperature solution should not be used.

2. In discussing rest and sleep with Mrs. Allen the position you would suggest she nap in is
   a. on her stomach with a pillow under her breasts.
   b. on her side with the weight of the uterus resting on the bed.
   c. on her back with a pillow under her knees and hips.
   d. on her back with a pillow under her head.

3. Early in pregnancy you review danger signals of pregnancy with Mrs. Allen. A danger sign of pregnancy is
   a. uterine enlargement to the umbilicus by 20 weeks.
   b. severe, continuous headache.
   c. no fetal heart sounds by auscultation by 12 weeks.
   d. a whitish vaginal discharge.

4. Mrs. Allen is concerned she is nauseated every morning. The best measure you would suggest to relieve this would be
   a. take a teaspoon of baking soda before breakfast.
   b. delay toothbrushing until noon.
   c. delay breakfast until midmorning.
   d. take two aspirin on arising.

5. If constipation is a problem with Mrs. Allen, which measure below would be best to recommend?

    a. Mineral oil is a nonprescription laxative she could use.

    b. Increasing fluid intake may be beneficial.

    c. Reducing her iron supplement to every other day will help.

    d. Including more meat in her diet will provide fiber.

6. Mrs. Allen experiences frequent leg cramps. The best method for her to relieve these is to

    a. elevate her leg on two pillows.

    b. bend the knee and dorsiflex the foot.

    c. plantarflex the foot and wiggle the toes.

    d. extend the knee and dorsiflex the foot.

7. Mrs. Allen is concerned that orgasm will be harmful during pregnancy. Which advice below concerning this is most factual?

    a. Most women do not experience orgasm during pregnancy.

    b. Orgasm during pregnancy is potentially harmful.

    c. Many women experience orgasm intensely during pregnancy.

    d. Venous congestion in the pelvis makes orgasm painful.

8. Mrs. Allen is a secretary at a large corporation. She states that she wants to take a leave of absence from work but is afraid she will lose her seniority standing. You would advise her that

    a. medically, it is not wise for any woman to work past the seventh month of pregnancy.

    b. legally, her employer cannot penalize her this way.

    c. ethically, she has no right to ask for special favors.

    d. personally, she is selfish to think of herself ahead of the baby.

9. Mrs. Allen asks you about palmar erythema. Your advice would be based on the principle that palmar erythema is caused by

    a. an increased estrogen level.

    b. an allergy to fetal protein.

    c. reduced serum protein.

    d. chorionic gonadotropin hormone.

10. At a midpoint in pregnancy you review beginning signs of labor. One of the beginning signals of labor is

    a. a sudden gush of clear fluid from the vagina.

    b. excessive fatigue and headache.

    c. sharp, right-sided abdominal pain.

    d. an increased pulse rate and upper abdominal pain.

Discussion

1. A woman at a first pregnancy visit tells you that she must catch a bus and can spend only 15 minutes. What counseling information would you want to offer her as priority information?

2. Most women are able to discuss some areas of health more easily than other areas. What areas of pregnancy health care would you be certain to ask about because they are often difficult for a woman to broach spontaneously?

3. A woman's family often accompanies her at prenatal care visits. What are some ways that a husband and small children can be made to feel a part of pregnancy care visits?

Suggested Readings

Allen, E., et al. (1981). Are normal patients at risk during pregnancy? *J.O.G.N. Nursing, 10,* 348.

Alley, N. M. (1984). Morning sickness: The client's perspective. *J.O.G.N. Nursing, 13,* 185.

Barlow, S. M., & Sullivan, F. M. (1982). *Reproductive hazards of industrial chemicals.* New York: Academic Press.

Danis, R. P., & Keith, L. (1983). Fetal alcohol syndrome: Incurable but preventable. *Contemporary OB/GYN, 21,* 57.

Draper, J., et al. (1983). Women's knowledge of health care during pregnancy. *Health Visitor, 56,* 86.

Fatteh, A., et al. (1973). Fatal air embolism in pregnancy resulting from orogenital sex play. *Forensic Science, 2,* 247.

Flint, C. (1982a). Where have we gone wrong? Health care for pregnant women. *Nursing Mirror, 155,* 26.

Flint, C. (1982b). Get off the conveyor belt . . . antenatal clinic. *Nursing Mirror, 155,* 37.

Gaplerud, C. P. (1981). Drugs and pregnancy: Prescribing practices during pregnancy. *Consultant, 21,* 29.

George, G., et al. (1981). Exercise before, during, and after pregnancy. *Topics in Clinical Nursing, 3,* 33.

Gillespie, S. A., et al. (1981). A reference for clinicians: Discomforts of pregnancy. *Issues in Health Care of Women, 3,* 375.

Halpern, J. S., et al. (1983). Use of drugs during pregnancy. *Journal of Emergency Nursing, 9,* 160.

Hamilton, M. S., et al. (1981). Pelvic examination: Patient safety and comfort. *J.O.G.N. Nursing, 10,* 344.

Josten, L. (1982). Contrast in prenatal preparation for mothering. *Maternal-Child Nursing Journal, 11,* 65.

Ketter, D. E., & Shelton, B. J. (1984). Pregnant and physically fit too. *M.C.N., 9,* 120.

King, C. (1984). A personal approach to antenatal clinics. *Midwives Chronicle, 97,* 9.

Malnory, M. E. (1982). A prenatal assessment tool for mothers and fathers. *Journal of Nurse Midwifery, 27,* 26.

Maring-Klug, R. (1982). Reducing low back pain during pregnancy. *Nurse Practitioner, 7,* 18.

Martin, B. J., et al. (1982). Oral health during pregnancy: A neglected nursing area. *M.C.N., 7,* 391.

May, K. A. (1982). Three phases of father involvement in pregnancy. *Nursing Research, 31,* 337.

McGarry, J. (1983). Smoking in pregnancy—a 25 year survey. *Midwives Chronicle, 96,* 51.

Naeye, R. L., & Peters, E. C. (1982). Working during pregnancy: Effects on the fetus. *Pediatrics, 69,* 724.

Parsons, W. D., et al. (1982). Why don't women attend for antenatal care? *Midwives Chronicle, 95,* 362.

Ringler-Barman, M. (1984). Advising pregnant and postoperative working patients. *Contemporary OB/GYN, 23,* 80.

Shahady, E. J. (1982). Prenatal care: A strategy for healthier babies. *Consultant, 22,* 141.

Sibley, L., et al. (1981). Swimming and physical fitness during pregnancy. *Journal of Nurse Midwifery, 26,* 3.

Stichler, J. F., et al. (1979). Pregnancy: A shared emotional experience. *M.C.N., 4,* 153.

Trimmer, E. (1982). About the heartburn of pregnancy. *Midwife Health Visitor and Community Nurse, 18,* 142.

Waterfield, M., et al. (1983). Midwives, smoking and antenatal care. *Midwives Chronicle, 96,* 73.

Woolery, L. F. (1983). Self-care for the obstetrical patient: A nursing framework. *J.O.G.N. Nursing, 12,* 33.

Zacharias, J. (1983). A rational approach to drug use in pregnancy. *J.O.G.N. Nursing, 12,* 183.

20

Nutrition During Pregnancy

OBJECTIVES

Following mastery of the contents of this chapter, you should be able to

1. Describe the requirements for carbohydrate, protein, fat, vitamins, and minerals during pregnancy.
2. Describe the detrimental effects of caffeine, megadose vitamins, nicotine, and alcohol intake during pregnancy.
3. Describe financial assistance programs relevant to nutrition in pregnancy.
4. Assess a woman's nutritional intake during pregnancy.
5. State a nursing diagnosis related to the nutritional guidelines for pregnancy.
6. Plan health teaching for nutritional intake during pregnancy.
7. Implement health teaching regarding nutritional intake in pregnancy.
8. Evaluate goal outcomes regarding a nutritious food intake during pregnancy.
9. Analyze the effects of different life situations on nutrition patterns and nutritional health.
10. Synthesize nutrition knowledge with nursing process to achieve quality maternal-newborn nursing care.

A GOOD DIET cannot guarantee a good pregnancy outcome, but it certainly makes an important contribution. Both the nutritional state that a woman brings into pregnancy and her nutrition during pregnancy have a direct bearing on her well-being and on that of her child. The nutrition of her sexual partner is also important to ensure that healthy sperm are present for conception. Nutritional risk factors for pregnancy are shown in Table 20-1. Poor nutritional intake has such an effect it may play a part in poor neurologic and bone growth, in premature birth, and in premature separation of the placenta (abruptio placentae). There is also a correlation between inadequate protein intake during pregnancy and small-for-gestation-age newborns. A low protein intake may make a woman more prone to pregnancy-induced hypertension, one of the most serious complications of pregnancy.

Early in pregnancy, fetal growth occurs largely by an increase in the number of cells formed (hyperplasia); late in pregnancy it is mainly by enlargement of existing cells (hypertrophy). A fetus who is deprived of adequate nutrition early in pregnancy will be small for gestational age because of too few body cells; later on, retarded growth is due to a normal number but smaller-than-usual-size cells. Although both types of situations can cause direct insult to the fetus, the second appears to be more reversible after the child is born. In other words, early pregnancy nutritional deficiencies are the most harmful to a fetus. Women of childbearing age have a responsibility to always maintain themselves on a balanced diet; otherwise, in the space of time (about 6 weeks) before they recognize that they are pregnant, their poor diet and lack of important nutrient stores could seriously impair fetal growth.

The classic study of Burke and co-workers (1943) established a high correlation between maternal diet and infant health. In this study, among 284 women whose prenatal diet was evaluated, only 42 had a good or excellent diet; their infants (96%) were in good or excellent health at birth. Of 40 women rated as having a poor or very poor diet, only 8 percent had babies rated as in good or excellent health; 27 percent of their infants were in fair health, and 65 percent in poor health. Babies included in the "poor" category were stillborn, premature, or functionally immature; died within 3 days of birth; or had congenital defects at birth.

Weight Gain During Pregnancy

A weight gain of between 12 kg and 13.6 kg (25 and 30 lbs) is currently recommended as an average weight gain in pregnancy. This gain should be distributed throughout pregnancy, roughly at 1 to 2 kg (2–4 lbs) during the first trimester and then 0.4 kg (1 lb) a week during the last two trimesters. Sudden increases in weight that suggest fluid retention or a loss of weight that suggests illness needs to be carefully evaluated at prepartal visits. An underweight woman at the beginning of pregnancy should be expected to gain more than these amounts to make up for her weight deficit. A woman who is overweight prior to pregnancy should not diet during pregnancy in order to reduce the normal weight gain: This intake is necessary to supply nutrients to the fetus.

Table 20-1 Nutritional Risk Factors During Pregnancy

An obstetrical patient is likely to be at nutritional risk if, at the onset of pregnancy:

1. She is an adolescent (15 years of age or less).
2. She has had three or more pregnancies during the past 2 years.
3. She has a history of poor obstetric or fetal performance.
4. She is economically deprived (an income of poverty level or is a recipient of local, state, or federal assistance, such as Medicaid or food programs such as WIC).
5. She is a food faddist, ingesting a bizarre or nutritionally restricted diet.
6. She is a heavy smoker, drug addict, or alcoholic.
7. She has a therapeutic diet for chronic systemic disease.
8. She had a prepregnancy weight at her first prenatal visit of under 85% or over 120% of standard weight.

She is likely to be at nutritional risk, if, during prenatal care:

9. She has a low or deficient hemoglobin/hematocrit (low is Hb under 11.0 gm, HCT under 33%; deficient is Hb under 10.0 gm; HCT under 30%).
10. She has inadequate weight gain (any weight loss during pregnancy or gain under 2 pounds (1 kg) per month).
11. She has excessive weight gain during pregnancy (over 2 pounds [1 kg] per week).
12. She is planning to breast-feed her infant.

Source: Task Force on Nutrition. (1978). Assessment of maternal nutrition. Chicago: The American College of Obstetrics and Gynecologists and the American Dietetic Association.

What Is a Healthy Diet?

Based on the information discussed above, the old saying that a pregnant woman must "eat for two" is actually based in scientific fact (Figure 20-1). The question to ask if a problem arises is *what* foods should she eat for two. Many women will not have to increase the *quantity* of their intake to provide for the child forming inside them; instead, they will have to increase the *quality* of their intake.

Good nutritional counseling during pregnancy should help a woman gain an appropriate amount of weight during her pregnancy, decrease the incidence of pregnancy-induced hypertension, provide an environment in which the fetus can gain an appropriate amount of weight, prepare her body for lactation or the feeding of her new baby,

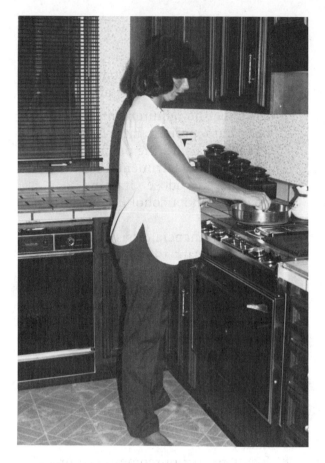

Figure 20-1 *Encourage pregnant women to eat a varied diet with a high iron and protein content.*

and acquire nutritional knowledge that she can use as her child grows into adulthood under her care.

In past years, when weight gain in pregnancy was severely limited to under 20 pounds, women were reluctant to talk about their dietary intake at prenatal visits. Some of them lied or did not eat at all the day before coming for a visit. Now that a more lenient weight gain is recommended (25 to 30 pounds), women are more relaxed about discussing what they eat and are receptive to nutritional counseling and advice.

The recommended dietary allowances (RDA) for girls and women and the requirements that pregnancy adds are shown in Table 20-2. These increases are shown diagrammatically in Figure 20-2.

Calorie Intake

The recommended daily allowance of calories for women of childbearing age is 2,000 to 2,400. As can be seen in Table 20-2, an additional 300 calories—or a total caloric intake of 2,300 to 2,700 calories—is recommended to meet the in-

Table 20-2 Maternal Daily Dietary Allowances

	Recommended Daily Allowances for Nonpregnant Women				Recommended Daily Allowances to Be Added for Pregnancy
	Age 11–14	*Age 15–18*	*Age 19–22*	*Age 23–50*	
Calories (kcal)	2,400	2,100	2,100	2,000	+300
Protein (gm)	46	46	44	44	+30
Vitamin A (μg)	800	800	800	800	+200
Vitamin D (μg)	10	10	7.5	5	+5
Vitamin E (mg)	8	8	8	8	+2
Ascorbic acid (mg)	50	60	60	60	+20
Folic acid (μg)	400	400	400	400	+400
Niacin (mg)	15	14	14	13	+2
Riboflavin (mg)	1.3	1.3	1.3	1.2	+0.3
Thiamine (mg)	1.1	1.1	1.1	1.0	+0.4
Vitamin B_{12} (μg)	3.0	3.0	3.0	3.0	+1.0
Vitamin B_6 (mg)	1.8	2.0	2.0	2.0	+0.6
Calcium (mg)	1,200	1,200	800	800	+400
Phosphorus (mg)	1,200	1,200	800	800	+400
Iodine (μg)	150	150	150	150	+25
Iron (mg)	18	18	18	18	+30–60
Magnesium (mg)	300	300	300	300	+150
Zinc (mg)	15	15	15	15	+5

Source: Food and Nutrition Board. (1979). *Recommended daily dietary allowances.* Washington: National Academy of Sciences, National Research Council.

Figure 20-2 *Additional recommended dietary allowances (RDA) for girls and women during pregnancy.*

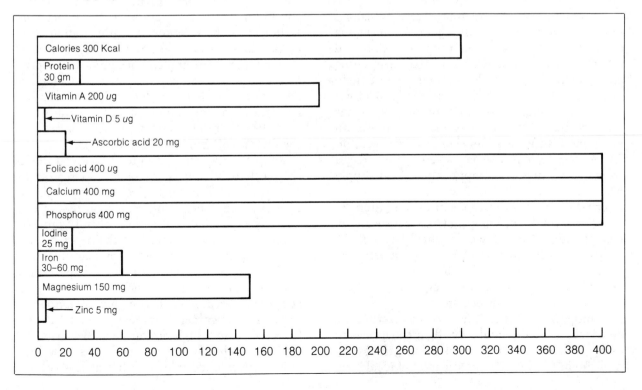

creased needs of pregnancy. In addition to supplying energy for the fetus and placenta, these calories provide for a rise in metabolic rate from stimulated thyroid function and an increased work load from the extra weight a woman must carry.

The physiologic changes of pregnancy, such as the 30 to 50 percent increase in blood volume and blood constituents that occurs, plus the addition of the fetal cells, requires an increase in the amount of protein and iron ingested. If a woman does not take in enough calories, her body will use protein for energy, thus depriving the fetus. In addition, a breakdown of protein would lead to ketoacidosis. A fetus grows poorly in an acid environment.

Even in obese women, a pregnancy diet should never contain fewer than 1,500 calories: A diet low in calories is almost automatically low in protein, which is detrimental to fetal growth. The use of saccharin as a sugar substitute is not recommended, as a woman needs the sugar to maintain carbohydrate levels (and the safety of saccharin for the population as a whole is still seriously questioned from a carcinogenic standpoint). A woman should be careful not to drink over 480 ml (16 oz) of diet soda a day or take over 10 quarter-grain tablets of saccharin a day in order to prevent ingesting a high saccharin content (Howard, 1982). Many diet sodas are now being sweetened by aspartame, rather than saccharin. Aspartame has not been associated with cancer in research studies but should be avoided by pregnant women until its safety is completely confirmed.

In helping a woman plan an increased caloric intake, be sure that she is planning on adding calories by eating foods rich in protein, iron, and other essential nutrients, rather than just eating empty-calorie foods such as pretzels and doughnuts. Effective advice often includes preparation of snacks such as carrot sticks or broccoli greens early in the day when she is not tired; these can be kept readily available in the refrigerator. Otherwise, later in the day when she is tired, a woman will snack on empty-calorie food simply because it is readily available.

Some women worry about increasing their total caloric intake during pregnancy because they fear gaining so much weight that they will be overweight permanently. If a woman merely eats more nutritious foods, thereby building mainly protein and iron stores, however, she can be assured this fear will not become real.

A more individualized method of determining an adequate calorie intake during pregnancy is to compute a nonpregnant ideal calorie intake by multiplying 40 calories per kilogram of ideal body weight and then adding the extra 300 calories required for pregnancy. For example, if a woman is 5'5", her ideal body weight (medium frame) is 132 pounds (see Appendix F), or 60 kg. Her nonpregnant calorie intake would then be 2,400 calories per day (60 kg × 40); her pregnancy caloric intake would be 2,700 calories per day.

Protein Needs

If protein needs are met, overall nutritional needs are likely to be also (with the possible exceptions of ascorbic acid [vitamin C], vitamin A, and vitamin D) because of the high incorporation of other nutrients in protein foods. If protein is inadequate in the diet, iron, B vitamins, calcium, and phosphorus will undoubtedly be inadequate also. Vitamin B_{12} is found exclusively in animal protein; its levels will be insufficient if animal protein is totally excluded from the diet (unless synthetically supplemented).

The recommended daily allowance for protein in adults is 44 to 46 gm. During pregnancy, the intake of protein should be increased 30 gm per day above normal.

Extra protein is best supplied by meat, poultry, fish, yogurt, eggs, and milk: The protein in these foods contains all eight essential amino acids, termed *complete* protein. The protein in nonanimal sources does not contain all eight essential amino acids (termed *incomplete*). It is possible, by choosing nonanimal proteins carefully, to provide all amino acids in the diet. Proteins that when eaten together provide all eight essential amino acids are termed *complementary* proteins. Examples are beans and rice, legumes and rice, or beans and wheat. Interestingly, supplying women with high-protein supplement drinks during pregnancy does not improve pregnancy outcome and actually may be harmful. Electrolyte shifts result from the high molecular content (Howard & Herbold, 1982). Protein should be incorporated into the diet, then, through usual food sources.

Remember when doing nutritional counseling that, although meat is the richest source of protein, it is also the most expensive type of food. Poultry, cheese, eggs, and peanut butter are usually less expensive, and a quart of milk provides 35 gm of protein, or one half the daily requirement. A woman who comes from a family with a tendency to high cholesterol levels (hypercholesterolemia) probably should not eat more than one egg per day because of their high cholesterol content. Caution women that cream cheese is a high-fat rather than a high-protein food. Because liver is such a rich source of protein, it is good for a woman to include it in her diet at least once a week. Women who do not like the taste of liver (and there are many who do not) can eat it as liverwurst or liver spread; include it in meatloaves; or make liver "dogs with everything," which covers the liver's taste. Lunch meats (bologna, salami) should not be included as staples in the diet because their salt content is exceptionally high.

Milk is a rich source of protein, but some women resist drinking it because it is also a high-caloric food. Skim milk, either liquid or dry, supplies the same protein as regular milk but half the calories. Thus, there is no need to eliminate this essential food to prevent too much weight gain.

Some women find it difficult to drink a quart of milk a day because they simply do not like its taste. Buttermilk can be substituted, or chocolate or another flavoring can be added to make milk palatable (buttermilk has the disadvantage of having a high salt content). Yogurt or cheese may also be substituted for milk, or milk may be incorporated into custards, eggnogs, or cream soups.

Common foods from each basic food group are contrasted by protein content in Table 20-3.

Fat Needs

There is only one fatty oil, linoleic acid, that cannot be manufactured in the body from other sources; it must therefore be consumed specifically during pregnancy. Using vegetable oils that have low cholesterol contents (safflower, corn, peanut, and cottonseed) rather than animal oils (lard or butter) is generally recommended for all adults as a means of preventing atherosclerosis. Vegetable oils have the additional advantage of containing linoleic acid.

Vitamins

The intake of vitamins as a daily dietary supplement has become so common for so many people that they underestimate the importance of them. Both fat-soluble and water-soluble vitamins are important during pregnancy, however, to support the growth of new fetal cells. Women should avoid taking megadose vitamins as the intake of such excessive vitamin levels is associated with fetal malformation in animal models. The intake of excessive vitamin A as Accutane, a medication prescribed for acne, is documented as causing congenital anomalies in humans.

Fat-Soluble Vitamins

The fat-soluble vitamins (A, D, K, and E) are so named because they are absorbed across the villi of the intestine with fat. Their storage in cells

Table 20-3 Protein Content of Common Foods

Food	Amount	Protein Content (gm)
Meat		
Beef, rib roast	3 oz	17
Bologna	2 slices	3
Chicken	1 drumstick	12
Clams (raw)	3 oz	11
Haddock	3 oz	17
Ham	3 oz	18
Hamburger	3 oz	21
Liver, beef	3 oz	22.5
Vegetables and fruits		
Carrots	1	1
Collards	1 cup	5
Corn	1 ear	3
Lima beans	1 cup	16
Peanut butter	1 tbsp	4
Peas, dried, split	1 cup	20
Spinach	1 cup	5
Apple	1	Trace
Banana	1	1
Orange	1	1
Watermelon	1 wedge	2
Breads and grains		
Bagel	1	6
Bread, rye	1 slice	2
Bread, white	1 slice	2
Bread, whole wheat	1 slice	3
Cornmeal	1 cup	11
Oatmeal	1 cup	5
Rice, white	1 cup	4
Spaghetti	1 cup	5
Dairy products		
Butter	1 pat	Trace
Cheese (American)	1 oz	7
Egg	1 whole	6
Ice cream	1 cup	6
Margarine	1 pat	Trace
Milk	1 cup	9
Yogurt	1 cup	8

Source: Nutritive value of foods. (1970). U.S. Department of Agriculture, Home and Garden Bulletin, No. 72.

with fat makes it easy to take a toxic dose of these vitamins. To ensure that they are absorbed from the gastrointestinal tract, a pregnant woman should not use mineral oil as a laxative: These important vitamins may be eliminated from the body with the mineral oil rather than being absorbed.

Vitamin A. Vitamin A promotes growth and reproduction of body cells, maintains healthy skin and mucus membrane, and is beneficial to vision (particularly night vision). It is found in large amounts in yellow and dark-green vegetables, butter, and margarine. Vegetables not only provide a good source of this vitamin but are also a good source of protein and add bulk to the diet to aid bowel movements.

Oral contraceptives may deplete vitamin A stores, so a woman who has been using oral contraceptives prior to pregnancy needs to be certain to include good sources of vitamin A in her early pregnancy diet. Table 20-4 contrasts common foods from each food group by their vitamin A content.

Vitamin D. Vitamin D is necessary for the metabolism of calcium and phosphorus. It must be present in the diet of a pregnant woman to ensure good bone growth and proper mineralization of bones and teeth in the fetus. Some vitamin D is formed by exposure of skin to sunlight, but the majority must be ingested. Fortunately, most commercial milk today is fortified with 400 IU (10 µg) of vitamin D per quart, so a quart of milk taken daily will supply most of the vitamin D a pregnant woman requires.

Vitamin K. Vitamin K promotes the formation of prothrombin and fibrin to ensure efficient blood clotting. In case a bleeding complication should occur during pregnancy, adequate levels of this vitamin will help safeguard both mother and fetus. Vitamin K is found primarily in green, leafy vegetables, soybeans, fish meal, and vegetable oils. Since it is also formed by bacterial action in the intestines, some of the vitamin is available to the body even if it is not supplied daily in the diet.

Vitamin E. The relationship of vitamin E to good nutrition has not been clearly determined. Wheat germ, nuts, eggs, and legumes are rich sources.

Water-Soluble Vitamins

Water-soluble vitamins are not stored in the body so must be taken in daily in order for an adequate level to be maintained. They are destroyed readily by boiling vegetables. Steaming and stir-frying are better food preparation methods to preserve vitamin content.

Vitamin C. Vitamin C, or ascorbic acid, is necessary for protein utilization and absorption of iron as well as the formation of bone and connective tissue. It also appears to augment resistance to infection. Found largely in citrus fruits and in tomatoes, broccoli, brussels sprouts, and cabbage,

Table 20-4 Vitamin A and Vitamin C Content of Common Foods

Food	Amount	Vitamin A (IU)	Vitamin C (mg)
Meat			
Beef, rib roast	3 oz	70	0
Bologna	2 slices	0	0
Chicken	1 drum-stick	50	0
Clams (raw)	3 oz	90	8
Haddock	3 oz	0	2
Ham	3 oz	0	0
Hamburger	3 oz	30	0
Liver, beef	3 oz	45,420	22.7
Vegetables and fruits			
Carrots	1	5,500	4
Collards	1 cup	10,260	87
Corn	1 ear	310	7
Lima beans	1 cup	0	0
Peanut butter	1 tbsp	0	0
Peas, dried, split	1 cup	100	0
Spinach	1 cup	14,580	50
Apple	1	50	3
Banana	1	230	12
Orange	1	260	66
Watermelon	1 wedge	2,510	30
Breads and grains			
Bagel	1	30	0
Bread, rye	1 slice	0	0
Bread, white	1 slice	Trace	Trace
Bread, whole wheat	1 slice	Trace	Trace
Cornmeal	1 cup	620	0
Oatmeal	1 cup	0	0
Rice, white	1 cup	0	0
Spaghetti	1 cup	0	0
Dairy products			
Butter	1 pat	170	0
Cheese (American)	1 oz	350	0
Egg	1 whole	590	0
Ice cream	1 cup	590	1
Margarine	1 pat	170	0
Milk	1 cup	350	2
Yogurt	1 cup	170	2

Source: Nutritive value of foods. (1970). U.S. Dept. of Agriculture, Home and Garden Bulletin, No. 72.

the daily amount recommended for a pregnant woman is 70 to 80 mg. The safety of taking excessive amounts of vitamin C to prevent upper respiratory infections is not well established, and it should not be tried during pregnancy. Common foods from the four basic food groups are contrasted by their vitamin C content in Table 20-4.

Vitamin B Complex. The principal B vitamins are thiamine, riboflavin, niacin, pyridoxine (B_6), folic acid, and B_{12}. They are essential for proper nerve growth, for the maintenance of good vision, and for conversion of carbohydrate to energy; they also aid in the digestion and assimilation of food. Sources are protein foods, namely, meat, eggs, enriched breads, enriched cereals, and dairy products.

Women who have been using oral contraceptives prior to pregnancy may have B_6 deficiencies and need additional supplements during pregnancy. Common foods from the four basic food groups are contrasted by their vitamin B_1 (thiamine) and B_2 (riboflavin) content in Table 20-5.

Folic Acid. Although folic acid (folacin) belongs to the B vitamin group, its importance warrants separate discussion. It was thought previously that a diet high in iron would be sufficient for adequate hemoglobin formation in the fetus. It is now recognized that folic acid is also necessary. In a pregnant woman with low levels of folic acid, a megaloblastic anemia or a low red cell count and low hemoglobin may develop. If a woman manifests such symptoms at the time she delivers, the infant may be anemic as well. In addition, low levels of folic acid in a woman may be associated with premature separation of the placenta or spontaneous abortion.

Both the woman and her infant respond well to the administration of folic acid during pregnancy. For these reasons most pregnant women are given a folic acid supplement of 400 to 800 μg per day. Oral contraceptives may deplete serum folic acid levels. Women who were taking oral contraceptives prior to pregnancy are probably most in need of supplementation.

Minerals

Minerals are necessary for new cell building in the fetus. Because they are found in so many foods and a pregnant woman seems to have increased ability to absorb them, deficiency—with the exception of calcium, iodine, and iron—is rare.

Calcium and Phosphorus

Because the skeleton and teeth of the fetus constitute a major portion of the structure (tooth formation begins as early as the eighth week; bones begin to calcify at 12 weeks in utero), extra amounts of calcium and phosphorus are needed during pregnancy. Calcium is provided by milk (a quart a day supplies three-fourths of a day's re-

Table 20-5 Thiamine and Riboflavin Content of Common Foods

Food	Amount	Thiamine (mg)	Riboflavin (mg)
Meat			
Beef, rib roast	3 oz	1.05	0.13
Bologna	2 slices	0.04	0.06
Chicken	1 drumstick	0.03	0.15
Clams (raw)	3 oz	0.08	0.15
Haddock	3 oz	0.03	0.06
Ham	3 oz	0.40	0.16
Hamburger	3 oz	0.07	0.18
Liver, beef	3 oz	—	—
Vegetables and fruits			
Carrots	1	0.03	0.03
Collards	1 cup	0.27	0.37
Corn	1 ear	0.09	0.08
Lima beans	1 cup	0.25	0.11
Peanut butter	1 tbsp	0.02	0.02
Peas, dried, split	1 cup	0.37	0.22
Spinach	1 cup	0.13	0.25
Apple	1	0.04	0.02
Banana	1	0.06	0.07
Orange	1	0.13	0.05
Watermelon	1 wedge	0.13	0.13
Breads and grains			
Bagel	1	0.14	0.10
Bread, rye	1 slice	0.05	0.02
Bread, white	1 slice	0.06	0.05
Bread, whole wheat	1 slice	0.09	0.03
Cornmeal	1 cup	0.46	0.13
Oatmeal	1 cup	0.19	0.05
Rice, white	1 cup	0.23	0.02
Spaghetti	1 cup	0.20	0.11
Dairy products			
Butter	1 pat	—	—
Cheese (American)	1 oz	0.01	0.12
Egg	1 whole	0.05	0.15
Ice cream	1 cup	0.43	2.23
Margarine	1 pat	—	—
Milk	1 cup	0.07	0.41
Yogurt	1 cup	0.10	0.44

Source: Nutritive value of foods. (1970). U.S. Dept. of Agriculture, Home and Garden Bulletin, No. 72.

quirement), cheddar cheese, and green, leafy vegetables. If a woman is eating enough calcium-rich foods daily, she invariably consumes enough phosphorus, which is found mainly in organ meats, whole grain products, milk, nuts, and eggs. In order for a woman to absorb and utilize calcium and phosphorus from these sources, she must also have adequate amounts of vitamin D.

Interestingly, calcium is absorbed more efficiently during pregnancy than normally in order to supply this great need to the fetus. If a woman cannot drink milk due to lactase deficiency, she can take a daily calcium supplement. Be certain she understands that the increased absorption rate of calcium during pregnancy could result in toxicity if she assumes "a little supplementation is good for me; a lot will be even better."

Before nutrition counseling in pregnancy became common, a woman expected to lose "a tooth a child"; she accepted that the fetus would drain calcium from her teeth with growth, destroying at least one tooth over the 9-month period. The calcium in teeth is not as readily absorbed as that of bone, however, so this loss may have been caused by poor oral hygiene rather than calcium drain. A good calcium intake during pregnancy can take whatever validity there was out of this prediction, turning it into just another old wives' tale. Common foods from the four basic food groups are contrasted by their calcium content in Table 20-6.

Iodine

Iodine is essential for the formation of thyroxine and therefore for the proper functioning of the thyroid gland. It is important that a woman ingest enough during pregnancy to supply the needs of increased thyroid gland function. If iodine deficiency occurs, the thyroid may become enlarged (goiter) in the woman or fetus; in extreme instances, it may cause hypothyroidism (cretinism) in the fetus. Thyroid enlargement, or hypothyroidism, in the fetus is serious at birth because the increased pressure on the airway may lead to early respiratory distress; hypothyroidism leads to mental retardation if not discovered at birth.

In areas where water and soil are known to be deficient in iodine, a woman should use iodized salt and include a serving of seafood in her diet at least once a week. If salt should be restricted during pregnancy (rare except for a woman with preexisting kidney disease), she may need an iodine supplement.

Iron

A fetus at term has a hemoglobin of 17 to 21 gm per 100 ml of blood. This high hemoglobin level is necessary to oxygenate the blood, since in fetal circulation venous and arterial blood are so mixed that 100 percent oxygenation of red blood cells is not attained. In addition to needing iron to build this high level of hemoglobin, after the twentieth week of pregnancy, the fetus begins to store iron in the liver. These reserves will last the

Table 20-6 Calcium Content of Common Foods

Food	Amount	Calcium Content (mg)
Meat		
Beef, rib roast	3 oz	8
Bologna	1 slice	2
Chicken	1 drumstick	6
Clams (raw)	3 oz	59
Haddock	3 oz	34
Ham	3 oz	8
Hamburger	3 oz	10
Liver, beef	3 oz	9
Vegetables and fruits		
Carrots	1	18
Collards	1 cup	289
Corn	1 ear	2
Lima beans	1 cup	55
Peanut butter	1 tbsp	9
Peas, dried, split	1 cup	28
Spinach	1 cup	167
Apple	1	8
Banana	1	10
Orange	1	54
Watermelon	1 wedge	30
Breads and grains		
Bagel	1	9
Bread, rye	1 slice	19
Bread, white	1 slice	21
Bread, whole wheat	1 slice	24
Cornmeal	1 cup	24
Oatmeal	1 cup	22
Rice, white	1 cup	21
Spaghetti	1 cup	11
Dairy products		
Butter	1 pat	1
Cheese (American)	1 oz	198
Egg	1 whole	27
Ice cream	1 cup	194
Margarine	1 pat	1
Milk	1 cup	288
Yogurt	1 cup	294

Source: Nutritive value of foods. (1970). U.S. Dept. of Agriculture, Home and Garden Bulletin, No. 72.

infant through the first three months of life, when intake will consist mainly of milk, which is low in iron. About 290 mg of iron are necessary for this hemoglobin building and iron storage. If a woman's hematocrit is under 34 percent between the twenty-fourth and thirty-second weeks of pregnancy, the fetus is probably not building sufficient iron stores.

In addition, a woman needs iron to build an increased red cell volume for herself and to replace iron that will be lost in blood at delivery.

She needs about 370 mg of iron, or a total iron intake of 660 mg (290 + 370 mg).

Women in low-income groups find it difficult to include enough iron in their diets, since the foods richest in iron (organ meats; eggs; green, leafy vegetables; whole grain or enriched breads; dried fruits) are also the most expensive. The recommended daily allowance of iron for nonpregnant women is 18 mg per day. An average diet takes in about 6 mg of iron per 1,000 calories. If a woman eats a 2,400-calorie diet daily, she therefore takes in 12 to 15 mg of iron. Since only 10 to 20 percent of dietary iron is absorbed, however, she is actually taking in less than this amount (closer to 9–10 mg). Therefore, a prenatal diet should be supplemented with 30 to 60 mg of iron per day in order to ensure that adequate iron is ingested and absorbed. Teach a woman not to regard this medication as a substitute for eating iron-rich foods; it is intended as a supplement to an iron-rich diet. Iron supplements may cause nausea for some women; those women should be advised to take their iron following meals or to try enteric-coated iron, although absorption with both methods will be less than if taken on an empty stomach.

Iron is better absorbed from the stomach in an acid environment than an alkaline one. Taking the iron supplement with orange juice (citric acid) rather than milk, for example, gives a fetus more iron to use. Oral iron compounds turn stools black and tend to cause constipation in some women. Teach a woman not to stop the iron compound because constipation occurs. Increasing fluid intake or fiber in the diet will probably relieve the constipation. Some women need a stool softener prescribed in order to be comfortable. Many women are reluctant to take a medication during pregnancy (which is a point of view that needs to be supported), so will omit the iron compound rather than add the stool softener. Stool softeners such as sodium docusate (Colace) are not associated with teratogenic action, however; they can be taken safely during pregnancy.

Common foods compared by their iron content are shown in Table 20-7.

Fluoride

Since fluoride aids in the formation of sound teeth, a pregnant woman should drink fluoridated water. In an area where water is not fluoridated either naturally or artificially, supplemental fluoride may be recommended. Fluoride in large amounts causes brown-stained teeth, so a woman must not take the supplement either more often than prescribed or if tap water in her area is naturally or artificially fluoridated.

Table 20-7 Iron Content of Common Foods

Food	Amount	Iron Content (mg)
Meat		
Beef, rib roast	3 oz	2.2
Bologna	1 slice	0.7
Chicken	1 drumstick	0.9
Clams (raw)	3 oz	5.2
Haddock	3 oz	1.0
Ham	3 oz	2.2
Hamburger	3 oz	3.0
Liver, beef	3 oz	7.5
Vegetables and fruits		
Carrots	1	0.4
Collards	1 cup	1.1
Corn	1 ear	0.5
Lima beans	1 cup	5.9
Peanut butter	1 tbsp	0.3
Peas, dried, split	1 cup	4.2
Spinach	1 cup	4.0
Apple	1	0.4
Banana	1	0.8
Orange	1	0.5
Watermelon	1 wedge	2.1
Breads and grains		
Bagel	1	1.2
Bread, rye	1 slice	0.4
Bread, white	1 slice	0.6
Bread, whole wheat	1 slice	0.6
Cornmeal	1 cup	2.9
Oatmeal	1 cup	1.4
Rice, white	1 cup	1.8
Spaghetti	1 cup	1.3
Dairy products		
Butter	1 pat	0.0
Cheese (American)	1 oz	0.3
Egg	1 whole	1.1
Ice cream	1 cup	0.1
Margarine	1 pat	0.0
Milk	1 cup	0.1
Yogurt	1 cup	0.1

Source: Nutritive value of foods. (1970). U.S. Dept. of Agriculture, Home and Garden Bulletin, No. 72.

Sodium

Sodium is the major electrolyte that acts to maintain the fluid balance in the body, because when sodium is retained rather than excreted by the kidney tubules, an equal or balancing amount of fluid is also retained. It was formerly believed that this retention of fluid led to hypertension of pregnancy; therefore, it was generally recommended that salt, because of its high sodium chloride content, be severely restricted during pregnancy in order to minimize fluid retention. Women were left to try to eat tasteless, unappetizing food. In the early months of pregnancy, when nausea and vomiting make food unappetizing at best, some women did not eat at all, and the protein content of their diets fell below the recommended level.

Contrary to this still often-voiced belief, however, sodium should *not* be seriously restricted during pregnancy. Although substantial sodium is retained during pregnancy, this adjustment to the increased intravascular and interstitial fluid volume is normal, not excessive. While the total blood volume increases during pregnancy, the functional blood volume may be less than normal because the placenta is using so much for exchange. Depleting sodium by diuretics or decreased intake may seriously reduce the blood volume to a point where the placental exchange will be compromised. It is important that enough fluid be retained in the maternal circulation to cause a pressure gradient across the placenta, which allows optimal exchange to occur. A pressure gradient also maintains the glomerular filtration rate in the mother, another important reason for sodium intake.

Unless a woman is hypertensive or has heart disease when she enters pregnancy—in which instances she would previously have been on a salt-restricted diet—she should continue to season foods as usual. Only if she is a person who always uses an excess of salt should she change her use of salt. She should, however, curtail foods that are very salty, such as lunch meats and potato chips, and avoid using additives such as monosodium glutamate, so excessive fluid, which may put a strain on her heart, is not retained.

Many women will find your teaching about salt during pregnancy contrary to what they were told during a previous pregnancy (or what their mothers tell them). They welcome the change in nutrition philosophy but question it. Be certain you have the reason salt is allowed straight in your own mind so you can explain it correctly: Salt does not cause excessive retention of fluid and therefore does not lead to hypertension of pregnancy and edema. It *does* help regulate fluid balance in the body and the fetus. The cause of hypertension of pregnancy has still not been discovered, but it is far more complex than the intake of salt during pregnancy.

Zinc

Zinc is a mineral only recently recognized as being important for cell growth. It is found in dietary staples such as milk and grains so it is un-

Table 20-8 Crude Fiber Content of Various Foods

Food	Crude Fiber (%)
Bran	10.0–13.5
Whole grain	1.0– 2.0
Nuts	2.0– 5.0
Legumes (cooked)	1.5– 1.7
Vegetables	0.5– 1.5
Fruits (fresh)	0.5– 1.5
Fruits (dried)	1.0– 3.0

usual to find a deficiency in a woman of childbearing age who has been eating a nutritious diet prior to pregnancy.

Fluids

Extra amounts of water are needed during pregnancy for good kidney function, since the woman must excrete waste products for two. Two glasses of fluid daily over and above the daily quart of milk is a recommended fluid intake (a total of six glasses).

Fiber

Eating fiber-rich foods daily is a natural way of preventing constipation, as the bulk of the fiber in the intestine aids evacuation. Fiber also lowers cholesterol levels and may remove carcinogenic contaminants from the intestine. A food has a high fiber content when it consists of parts of the plant cell wall that are resistant to normal digestive enzymes of the small intestine. Bran is the seed coat of grain kernels. Refined grains have had the bran and germ removed and have much less fiber content. Crude fiber content refers to how much fiber is left after intestinal breakdown. Table 20-8 contrasts various foods as to crude fiber content.

Amounts of Foods Needed Daily

Table 20-9 lists the quantities of each food that will supply the calories and nutrients recommended in Table 20-2. In discussing nutrition with a woman, remember that she will more readily grasp what amounts of food are required if you talk in terms of servings of food rather than about milligrams or percentages.

Foods shown in Table 20-10 can be substituted

Table 20-9 Quantities of Food Necessary During Pregnancy

Food Group	Active Nonpregnant Woman	Pregnant Woman
Meat	2 servings of meat, fowl, or fish daily; 3–5 eggs per week	4 servings of meat, fowl, or fish daily; or 1 egg and 3 servings of meat, fowl, or fish daily
Vegetables:		
Dark green or deep yellow	1 serving (at least 3 times per week)	2 servings daily
Other vegetables	1 or more servings daily	1 or more servings daily
Fruits:		
Citrus, melon, strawberries, tomato	1 serving daily	1 or more servings daily
Other fruits	1 serving daily	1 serving daily
Breads and cereals	4 or more servings daily	4 servings daily
Milk	1 pint (two 8-oz glasses) daily	1 quart (four 8-oz glasses) daily
Additional fluid	Ad lib	At least 2 glasses daily

Table 20-10 Substitute Foods

For	Substitute
1 8-oz glass whole milk	1 glass skim milk 1 glass buttermilk ½ cup cottage cheese ¼ cup nonfat or whole dry milk ½ cup ice cream 1¼ oz cheddar cheese
1 serving vegetable or fruit	1 medium potato, tomato, or piece of fruit (used whole) ½ grapefruit 1 cup tomato juice (has vitamin C content of ½ cup orange juice)
2–3 oz lean meat	2 oz poultry or fish 2 eggs 1 oz cheddar cheese 4 tablespoons peanut butter 1 cup cooked dried beans, peas, or nuts ¼ cup cottage cheese
Bread or cereal	½–¾ cup cooked or ¾ cup ready-to-serve cereal ½–¾ cup cooked macaroni, spaghetti, or rice

for those in Table 20-9. Table 20-11 shows a typical day's menu based on these foods.

Nutritional Problems in Pregnancy

Nutritional problems may occur in pregnancy as a result of a number of factors or circumstances. Nausea and vomiting are two of these problems, discussed in detail on page 378.

Cravings

Cravings for food during pregnancy are so common that they can be considered a normal part of pregnancy. Formerly these strange desires for food were considered to reflect a woman's need to call attention to the pregnancy or were a reaction to her imposed dependent state. It is true that a woman may feel helpless because she has just left her job or she may feel unattractive in her pregnant state, and she can demonstrate that she is both able to manipulate her environment and attractive in her support person's eyes if she sends him to the store for fresh strawberries she "absolutely must have."

Cravings may be the same kind of phenomenon as the thirst that occurs in patients who have been told that they can have no fluids by mouth. Previously they did not experience a sensation of being thirsty; almost as soon as they are told they cannot drink, however, their thirst becomes overpowering. Because most cravings are for high-carbohydrate foods, such as chocolate, doughnuts, and sponge cake, a craving may primarily reflect a physiologic need for more carbohydrate in the diet rather than a psychological compensation.

Now that women are allowed more calories in their daily diets and a greater weight gain in pregnancy, cravings are less of a problem. When nutrition planning with a pregnant woman, ask if she notices cravings. Allowing a few extra calories or adjusting other food choices to include the food or foods that the woman craves will prevent her from cheating on her diet. This is a more positive

Table 20-11 Sample Menus

A Typical Day's Menu

Breakfast	1 glass orange juice (8 oz)
	1 slice toast with butter or
	  fortified margarine
	1 egg
	1 serving sausage
	Supplemental vitamin, folic acid,
	  and iron capsule

Snack	1 glass milk (8 oz) 1 piece fruit
Lunch	1 peanut butter and jelly sand- wich 1 cup tomato soup 1 glass milk (8 oz)
Afternoon snack	1 glass milk (8 oz) Celery sticks and canned chick peas
Dinner	1 serving roast beef 1 medium potato 1 serving corn 1 dinner roll or 1 slice bread Green salad with French dressing Fruit Jell-O 1 glass water (8 oz)
Bedtime snack	1 glass milk (8 oz)

A Less Typical Adequate Menu During Pregnancy

Breakfast	1 orange Pieces of tuna fish
Morning snack	1 glass milk (8 oz) 1 apple 1 serving grits
Lunch	1 hamburger on a bun 1 serving cole slaw 1 serving french fries 1 serving ice cream 1 glass soft drink (noncaffeine)
Dinner	1 serving pigs' knuckles 1 serving collard greens 1 serving rice 1 glass milk (8 oz)
Bedtime snack	1 eggnog (8 oz milk) Supplemental vitamin, folic acid, and iron capsule

---

approach to nutritional counseling than leaving a woman feeling guilty because she is eating foods she desires and enjoying her pregnancy.

Pica

Some women report an abnormal craving for non-food substances (termed *pica* from the Latin "magpie," a bird who is an indiscriminate eater) during pregnancy. The commonest form of pica is a craving for clay or laundry starch or ice cubes. Eating of these substances is seen most often in women in the Southeast, but it does occur everywhere. Clay and ice cubes are fairly innocent substances if eaten, except in large quantities, which can result in a diet becoming deficient in protein, iron, and calcium. Laundry starch can not only have this effect but can also directly reduce the amount of iron absorbed from the stomach (best absorbed in an acidic environment).

Pica, like cravings, was at one time closely associated with psychological needs in pregnancy. Now it is recognized as a symptom accompanying iron deficiency anemia. Always ask women before nutritional counseling if any form of pica is present. Most women do not supply this information unless asked directly; they worry that you will find their behavior odd or they may not associate the habit with eating as much as with nervousness.

Encouraging a woman to stop eating a nonfood substance may be ineffective: If she first began this habit as an iron-deficient adolescent, by the time she reaches childbearing age, the habit may be well established. For a nurse, who is unlikely to have this type of dietary pattern, discouraging the habit presents the same problem as discouraging smoking when you are a nonsmoker: How can you understand the urge a woman feels for one of these strange substances? Do not scold or nag in counseling. Stress instead that despite the habit of eating clay or starch, her diet must be high in protein, vitamins, and iron during pregnancy.

Generally, correcting the iron deficiency anemia will automatically correct the pica; be certain that a woman is assessed for this lack. She should also understand the importance of taking the iron supplement prescribed for her. Ask at future visits if she notices any difference.

Underweight

Fashion's concentration on slim female figures makes it easy to overlook the health problem of a woman who is underweight. A woman who enters a pregnancy in this condition, however, needs dietary counseling just as much as an overweight woman or one who eats nonfood substances.

Underweight is defined as a state in which a person's weight is 10 to 15 percent less than ideal weight for height (see Appendix F). Although underweight usually occurs because of a long-standing poor nutritional pattern, it may signify underlying disease, which makes it important to recognize during pregnancy. Most people who are underweight have an accompanying iron deficiency anemia, reduced resistance to disease, and a sense of fatigue.

Underweight can occur because of poverty and the inability to buy adequate food; however, many poor women are actually obese because starch foods are inexpensive compared to protein foods. Underweight may occur due to excessive worry or stress, emotions that lead to a loss of appetite. It may be due to depression, which causes a chronic loss of appetite. It may be present as a symptom of anorexia nervosa, a condition in which a woman has developed a revulsion to food. The majority of underweight conditions occur, however, due to insufficient intake of food and chronic poor nutritional habits.

Nutritional counseling with underweight women, therefore, may not be easy: You may be asking a woman to change lifelong habits of eating, at a time when she is worried and under stress because of the pregnancy and change may be especially difficult for her. Counseling produces an extreme challenge during the first trimester of pregnancy, when fetal need is greatest. At a time when she has nausea and vomiting and wants to eat nothing, you want her to eat more than ever before.

Beginning counseling by asking a woman to list what she has eaten in the last 24 hours (a 24-hour dietary recall) is often an effective means of pointing out to her how inadequate her intake is. If you only ask her if she eats well, she will say that she does (it seems adequate to her because it is her usual pattern). When she examines the list of what she has eaten, however—and all she sees listed is a cup of coffee for breakfast, a container of yogurt and a glass of diet soft drink for lunch, a pork chop, salad, and a second cup of coffee for dinner—she can better appreciate how little this actually is; she is not even eating for one, much less two.

Total caloric intake for an underweight woman may need to be 500 to 1,000 calories above that ordinarily specified during pregnancy. Working out well-planned meals rather than depending on quick takeout foods is generally helpful for in-creasing the daily intake of calories. Additional calories might be added in the form of a concentrated formula, such as an instant liquid breakfast drink. Be certain a woman understands she should not choose a high-protein drink devised for high-protein dieting regimens. Such diet drinks deliver a concentrated solute load (breakdown products of protein) to the kidney (already working to capacity due to the pregnancy); they also provide so little carbohydrate in proportion to protein that they encourage the breakdown of protein for body energy, a process that results in acidosis. High-protein diets of this nature are not recommended for long-term use by any individual; they should be totally avoided by women during pregnancy.

A 500-calorie increase over normal requirments should result in a weight gain of an additional pound per week. Be certain when the total weight gain during pregnancy is calculated at each office visit that this additional pound per week is planned for, or the total weight gain of the woman may seem excessive when it is actually healthy.

If being underweight is making a woman feel tired, she needs to be urged to schedule adequate rest periods daily in order to feel sufficiently energetic to prepare nutritious meals and gain adequate weight during the pregnancy. She may need additional nutrition counseling in the postpartal period so that she can maintain better nutrition and enter a possible subsequent pregnancy without nutritional lack. Even when these women gain excessive weight during pregnancy, they still have a higher-than-usual incidence of low-birth-weight infants, probably because of their depleted nutrient stores at the pregnancy's beginning (Edwards, 1979).

Obesity

Obesity is a serious problem among women in the United States (approximately 20 percent of American women are overweight). Women with less education and from poverty areas tend to be more overweight than others because they may not be so aware of the comparative levels of carbohydrates in foods and because of the cheapness of many starchy foods (macaroni, spaghetti). Native American women have an exceptionally high ratio of obesity.

By definition, a person is *overweight* if she is 10 percent above the desirable weight for her height and age group; *obese* if she is *more* than 10 percent above her desirable weight (see Appendix H). Although obesity may occur from hypothy-

Table 20-12 Food Values of Common Snack Foods

Food	Protein	Calcium	Iron	Vitamin A	Vitamin C	Calories
Carbonated cola, 8 oz	0	0	0	0	0	145
Doughnut, plain	1	13	0.4	30	Trace	125
Brownie	1	9	0.4	20	Trace	85
Apple pie, 1 slice	3	11	0.4	40	1	350
Fudge, 1 piece	Trace	22	0.3	Trace	Trace	115
Cheese pizza, 1 slice	7	107	0.7	290	4	185
French fries, 1 serving	3	10	0.5	52	11.0	211
Potato chips, 10	1	8	0.4	Trace	3	115
Pretzels, 3-inch sticks, 10	Trace	2	Trace	0	0	20
Popcorn, with oil and salt, 1 cup	1	1	0.2	0	0	40

Source: Nutritive value of foods. (1970). U.S. Dept. of Agriculture, Home and Garden Bulletin, No. 72.

roidism, it most often results from excessive caloric intake and decreased energy expenditure.

Obesity becomes a problem during pregnancy because a woman's circulatory volume increases 30 to 50 percent and her metabolism must increase to meet the demands of the pregnancy; additional stress is put on a possibly already overworked body. It is often difficult to hear fetal heart tones on an obese woman; palpating for position and size of the fetus is also difficult. If a cesarean birth is needed at delivery, the excessive adipose tissue complicates reaching the uterus. Ambulating during pregnancy and immediately afterward takes more effort from an obese woman because of the increased energy expenditure necessary; therefore thrombophlebitic disease and complications such as pneumonia tend to occur more frequently.

Nutrition counseling with obese women during pregnancy may be hard to individualize: Overeating has many causes. For some women, overeating is a coping mechanism for stress because whenever they feel tense or worried, they take something "comforting" to eat. As pregnancy is a stress and a time of worry, for such women to change food intake patterns at this time may be very hard. Other women overeat because their parents did and they were raised to consume a diet over-rich in calories. Changing this pattern means changing a lifelong habit (learning that cleaning their plate may not be as important as they have always thought). If their husband or children also enjoy an excessive intake of calories, in order to effect change in a woman's diet, you have to change her whole family's eating patterns.

Dieting to reduce weight is never recommended during pregnancy, however, because if carbohydrates are reduced too much, the body will utilize protein and fat for energy. This situation will deprive the fetus of protein and can lead to ketoacidosis in the woman and an environment detrimental to fetal growth. A pregnancy diet, therefore, in even the most obese woman, should never be below 1,500 to 1,800 calories.

Overweight women tend to exercise less than those of normal weight (exercising is more awkward and more tiring, and they may feel self-conscious dressed in certain sports clothing). They need to be urged to undertake at least a minimal activity program, such as a walk around the block daily, in addition to being certain that their calorie intake represents high-protein foods.

Table 20-12 contrasts the nutritional worth of some common snack foods with their caloric totals. Helping a woman look at her diet in terms of empty-calorie versus nutritional-calorie foods may help her to eat more sensibly during pregnancy. Early in pregnancy, when she is eager to appear pregnant, she may be very resistant to any limitation of intake. She needs to understand that a fetus grows best on nutritional foods, not necessarily those with the most calories. She may need additional nutritional counseling in the postpartal period so she can prepare a more nutritional diet in the future for herself and her expanding family.

Food Allergies

Women who are allergic to specific foods should not eat them during pregnancy (nor at any other time, for that matter). Many women do not have food allergies, but certain foods make them uncomfortable when they eat them. It is good to ask what these foods are before beginning any nutritional counseling: women will not eat these foods even if you recommend them. If you know what these are for each woman, you can suggest alternative foods, which will be eaten.

Constipation

Because of the reduced activity of the gastrointestinal tract during pregnancy from pressure of the growing uterus and the placental hormone relaxin, many women experience constipation during pregnancy. This leads to a feeling of bloating or fullness and lack of appetite. Women need to include an adequate intake of fiber-rich foods in their diet; increased bulk in the intestines will promote peristalsis. Preventing constipation by nutritional intervention is preferable to treating it with laxatives or enemas.

Lactose Intolerance

The sugar in milk is lactose. In the intestine, lactose is broken down into glucose and galactose by the enzyme *lactase*. In most of the world's population lactase is present in infants but disappears by school age. A similar phenomenon occurs in dogs. Puppies can drink milk, but dogs prefer water. Blacks, Native Americans, and persons of Oriental heritage tend to have the highest percentage of lactose intolerance (about 70 percent of mature American blacks cannot drink milk). Persons most likely to be able to tolerate milk are North Europeans and their descendants.

When persons who are lactose-intolerant drink milk, they report symptoms of nausea, diarrhea, cramps, gas, and a general feeling of bloatedness. Some express these symptoms as simply, "I don't like milk."

Women who cannot drink milk may be able to eat cheese because processing changes the lactose content; some find yogurt does not affect them. They will need a calcium (1,200 mg daily) and a vitamin D (400 IU) supplement, however, as the amount of cheese or yogurt that would need to be eaten to replace the calcium of milk would be too great to be practical. Because milk is a good source of protein, you need to take a thorough diet history to assess whether, without milk, a woman is taking in enough protein.

Many baby magazines, television ads, and government pamphlets on pregnancy reiterate the importance of drinking milk during pregnancy; therefore you need to spend time reassuring women who cannot drink milk that it really is not necessary. The milk per se is never what is good for them; the nutrients of milk are what they need, and these can be provided in other ways.

A number of newborns are born lactose-intolerant and have difficulty digesting breast milk or formula. These infants have the same symptoms (watery diarrhea, cramps, irritability) as an adult. They need to be placed on lactose-free formulas so they can obtain sufficient nutrition. There is no need for a woman to worry during pregnancy that her child will be born with this problem, however, as most lactose intolerance comes with maturity, not in infancy.

Cholelithiasis

Cholelithiasis is gallbladder stone formation. Such stones form from cholesterol. Preventing gallbladder stones is important during pregnancy as an attack of gallstone formation causes extreme, sharp pain for a woman, and surgical anesthesia during a cholecystectomy poses a threat to the fetus. A woman who has had difficulty with cholelithiasis prior to pregnancy may need to reduce her intake of fat by broiling meat rather than frying, using a minimum of salad oils, and substituting margarine for butter.

Such a diet will automatically be lower in calories because oils and fats add many calories to a diet. Assess such a woman carefully for adequate weight gain during pregnancy. Be sure she includes some oil daily (perhaps as salad oil) so that she has a source of linoleic acid in her daily intake.

Phenylketonuria

Phenylketonuria is an inherited disorder in which a person is unable to convert the essential amino acid phenylalanine into tyrosine, the form in which it is used for cell growth. Without this conversion, the raw phenylalanine builds up in the person's serum and eventually leaves the bloodstream to invade body cells. Its invasion of brain cells leaves severe mental retardation and accompanying neurologic damage, which may result in recurrent seizures.

All newborn infants are tested by a simple screening diagnostic test at 3 days of life. By placing children found to have the disorder on a diet low in phenylalanine, brain and neurologic handicapping can be completely prevented. The length of time a child should remain on the diet is controversial, but is at least past age 5, the time at which 90 percent of brain growth has been reached.

A person with the disorder who returns to a regular diet will no longer be in danger of developing cell damage but will always have a high circulating level of phenylalanine. If a woman with this high a phenylalanine serum level becomes pregnant, her infant would be subjected to the destructive level all during the pregnancy. Mental retardation in the fetus would surely result.

A woman with phenylketonuria (named because the breakdown product of phenylalanine is excreted in the urine in this form) should consult her internist at the time she is planning on becoming pregnant. A low-phenylalanine diet is then planned for her. She follows this diet until she becomes pregnant, during the pregnancy, and, if she should breast-feed, during this time period.

A low-phenylalanine diet is a very restricted diet because phenylalanine is found plentifully in common foods. The woman needs support during pregnancy to follow this restrictive a diet (9 months is a long time). It is particularly disappointing for her if she does not become pregnant right away after starting the diet, as each month that she is "prepregnant" extends the time period she must follow this diet. A woman with this disorder is usually very knowledgeable about her diet. She is aware that this amino acid is destructive to developing brain cells, and cheating on the diet can leave her future child extremely mentally retarded.

Caffeine Use

Many women think of caffeine as just an incidental ingredient in beverages. Actually it is a central nervous system stimulant, capable of increasing heart rate, urine production in the kidney, and secretion of stomach acid. This stimulant effect occurs at a dose of between 150 to 250 mg. Caffeine intoxication with symptoms of heart palpatation, diarrhea, and stomach pain from local irritation occurs with a dose of 200 to 750 mg per day. Until the recent publicity on caffeine, it was not unusual for the average American woman to ingest an average of 210 mg per day (Brooten & Jordan, 1983).

Caffeine is related in chemical structure to uric acid. In animals its administration is associated with infertility and the development of structural anomalies such as cleft palate. In humans, a daily intake of caffeine of at least 600 mg (comparable to eight cups of coffee) has been associated with fetal death and birth defects (Graham, 1978). For this reason, the Food and Drug Administration (FDA) has issued a formal warning to women to limit their caffeine intake during pregnancy.

In order to follow this suggestion, women must be educated to limit not only the amount of coffee they drink but other sources of caffeine as well:

chocolate, soft drinks, tea, and many medicines. If a woman has difficulty omitting these common foods from her diet, she can still reduce the amount of caffeine she ingests by modifying the preparation of these foods. Instant coffee, for example, as a rule has less caffeine than brewed coffee; percolated coffee has less caffeine than dripped coffee. Decaffeinated coffee, as the name implies, contains almost no caffeine.

Tea, like coffee, varies in caffeine content, depending on the type and length of brewing. The longer tea brews, the more the caffeine content increases. Green tea has less caffeine than black tea. Noncaffeine tea is available but only at health food stores, not regular supermarkets, in many communities.

The cola bean that is used to make chocolate and cocoa is yet another natural source of caffeine. Chocolate tends to be low in caffeine, however, compared to coffee. Whereas a cup of coffee contains about 120 mg of caffeine, a cup of hot chocolate contains only 10 mg. Baking chocolate, used for cake frostings and glaces, has proportionately higher amounts, containing about 35 mg of caffeine per ounce.

Soft drinks do not naturally contain caffeine. It is added to them to improve the taste, the amounts depending on the brand or type. Table 20-13 lists caffeine levels in comparable brands, as well as those contained in coffee, tea, chocolate, and common medicines. Many soft drink manufacturers also offer caffeine-free brands, which a pregnant woman is advised to drink.

Yet another source of caffeine that a woman may not be aware of is the various over-the-counter drugs used as stimulants (No Doz, for example); analgesics (Excedrin, Midol); cold and sinus remedies (Coricidin, Dristan); and diuretics and weight control aids (Aqua-Ban, Dexatrim). If a woman is following the common sense rule of taking no medicine during pregnancy except that prescribed by her primary health care provider, she will not be exposed to these sources of caffeine.

Analgesics are probably the drugs most abused during pregnancy. It is easy for a woman to think that simple analgesics are harmless to her. Plain aspirin *is* free of caffeine, but compound products such as Anacin and Excedrin contain caffeine. Teach a woman to read labels of foods and any drug before she ingests it. Teach her to substitute fruit and vegetable drinks for beverages such as coffee and tea, not only because they are free of caffeine but they supply needed minerals and vitamins besides (see the Nursing Research Highlight on page 420).

Table 20-13 Caffeine Content of Common Beverages and Drugs

Foods	Caffeine Content (mg)
Coffee (5-oz cup)	
Decaffeinated	2
Instant	66
Percolated	110
Drip	146
Tea	
Black	20–30 (1 min brewing)
	40–50 (5 min brewing)
Green	10–20 (1 min brewing)
	25–35 (5 min brewing
Soft drinks (12-oz can)	
Coca Cola	64.7
Dr. Pepper	60
Mountain Dew	52
Tab	44
Sunkist Orange	42
Pepsi Cola	37
Royal Crown Cola	36
7-Up	0
Sprite	0
Fresca	0
Chocolate	
Hot chocolate (180 ml)	10
Milk chocolate (1 oz)	6
Baking chocolate (1 oz)	35
Chocolate syrup (2 tbsp)	13

Drugs	
Stimulants	
No Doz	200
Vivarin	200
Analgesics	
Anacin	64
Excedrin	130
Midol	65
Aspirin	0
Cold and sinus remedies	
Coricidin	30
Dristan	32
Sinarest	30
Triaminicin	30
Weight reduction aids	
Aqua-Ban	200
Dexatrim	200
Dietac	200

Source: Manufacturers' literature.

Adolescent Pregnancy

Good nutrition is often a problem with pregnant teenagers because of the dual demand of pregnancy and adolescence. A girl must take in enough food to provide not only for fetal growth but for her own growth as well. A part of adolescents' search for identity involves a turning away from foods that their mothers see as important for them (milk, warm cereal, vegetables, fruit). Teenagers indulge themselves instead in foods that their mothers usually disapprove of, such as pizza, Coca-Cola, or potato chips. In helping an adolescent plan a diet for pregnancy, you must respect her right to reject traditional foods as long as her diet includes sufficient nutrients. Pizza with pepperoni and cheese is a lunch that provides all basic food groups. A cheese hot dog "with everything" provides the same nutrition. Stress too, the importance of eating well in order to maintain a healthy and attractive body after pregnancy. Adolescents will respond to this argument.

Toward the end of pregnancy, when a girl is tired, she may begin to eat more and more junk food for snacks: Preparing nutritious snacks seems to take more and more effort. Good advice for her is to prepare some nutritious snacks such as carrot strips or cheese bites early each day and put them in the refrigerator for later on.

Counseling with adolescents may be very difficult because they often are not responsible for cooking the food they eat. You may need to speak to the mother about foods to prepare before you can alter an adolescent's diet pattern.

A pregnant adolescent needs a high caloric intake (2,400–2,700) to supply energy for her high level of activity and growth. The nutrients most poorly supplied by a typical adolescent diet tend to be calcium, iron, and vitamin A, along with total calories. Look for sources of these nutrients when analyzing a teenage pregnancy diet. Caution a girl about drinking caffeine-rich soft drinks (substitute fruit or vegetable drinks or caffeine-free forms instead) and diet drinks that contain saccharin or aspartame.

Fast Food Sources

Many women brown bag a lunch for school or work or eat at a cafeteria or fast food restaurant. Assess whether she is maintaining an adequate intake with these. The difficulty with using fast food restaurants is the limited choice of food available (the woman may grow tired of the same thing and therefore eat very little) and, unless there is a salad bar, a limited menu of fruits and

======= *Nursing Research Highlight* =======

Caffeine—Does It Affect the Outcome of a Pregnancy?

Although there have been many studies on the effects of caffeine on reproduction in animals, few studies have examined the effects of caffeine on reproductive outcomes in humans. The few studies that have been done have shown conflicting outcomes. This article (Brooten & Jordan, 1983) reviews related research in this area. Nutritional status is an important determinant of the course and outcome of pregnancy, and risk to the fetus has not been proven or disproven. Therefore, pregnant and childbearing–

aged women should be advised to limit their caffeine intake to what is considered to be a safe level until studies prove otherwise. Nurses in all health care settings need to be made aware of the possible dangers so they in turn can counsel and educate their clients.

Reference

Brooten, D., & Jordan, C. (1983). Caffeine and pregnancy—A research review and recommendations for clinical practice. *J.O.G.N. Nursing, 12*(3): 190.

---

vegetables. In most places, french fries are prepared in hydrogenated fat so are very high in saturated fat. Fast food restaurants have also been associated with outbreaks of streptococcal B infections due to undercooked hamburger. This leads to severe gastrointestinal infection with vomiting and diarrhea and possible electrolyte imbalance. As hot dogs contain little meat, eating one for lunch should not be counted as a good meat source.

A packed lunch lends few problems in pregnancy as long as a woman uses some degree of creativity in preparation so she doesn't grow so tired of packed lunches that she reduces her noon intake. Packing a lunch at bedtime rather in the morning when she possibly feels nauseated (and therefore packs very little because nothing looks good) is a good recommendation early in pregnancy. Late in pregnancy, a woman may feel too tired at bedtime to do this and so should change to preparing it in the morning when she has more energy. Including a thermos with a cream soup is a good way to add milk and calcium to the diet. Lunch meat used daily should be avoided as it tends to be high in salt. Packing carrots, sliced cucumbers, tomatoes, or apples not only makes the lunch nutritious but these also can be used for midmorning or midafternoon snacks.

The Mature Gravida

A woman who is past 30 years of age and having her first child has traditionally been termed an elderly primipara. In light of a growing tendency for women to have children later in life, many women are over 30 by the time they choose to have their first child. Many are over 30 when they

have their second or third child. The nutritional needs of this age group of women have been poorly studied, but because metabolic rate begins to slow at about 30 years of age, a woman in this category may need about 10 to 15 percent fewer calories to maintain an adequate pregnancy weight gain than would a younger woman. As kidney efficiency is slightly decreased, she needs to maintain a good fluid input in order to remove waste products both for herself and for the fetus. Many women in this age group have delayed childbearing in order to establish a career; they may be used to depending for at least part of their nutrition each week on packed or fast food lunches. They need counseling on maintaining adequate nutrition during pregnancy based on this life style.

Decreased Nutritional Stores

A woman with high parity or a short interval between pregnancies, or one who has been dieting rigorously to lose weight prior to pregnancy, may have depleted her nutritional reserves to such an extent that she has little to draw on during the first part of pregnancy, when she may not be able to eat well because of nausea and vomiting. Women who used diuretics for a dieting program may be potassium-deficient. Women who have been on oral contraceptives may have decreased folate stores. Women who were using IUDs or have menorrhagia may be iron-deficient from excessive blood loss with menstrual flows. Women who drink alcohol excessively may be thiamine-deficient. A woman who is a frequent and recent blood donor could be anemic.

Women with these decreased nutritional stores

need to be identified early in pregnancy through history taking so that nutritional counseling can begin early. They may need additional supplements during pregnancy to restore a particular nutrient.

Multiple Pregnancy

In a multiple pregnancy, the growing demands of multiple fetuses may overtax a woman's nutritional reserves. It is important that multiple pregnancy be recognized early and dietary supplements added as needed.

Smoking, Alcoholism, and Drug Dependency

The specific effects of alcohol, cigarette smoking, and drug dependency on fetal growth are discussed in Chapter 40. In addition to specific teratogenic fetal effects, these substances lead to general nutrition problems.

A woman should stop smoking cigarettes during pregnancy. If this is not possible, she should reduce her daily intake to under 10 cigarettes daily and none within 48 hours of delivery. Women who continue to smoke excessively have more low-birth-weight infants than those who do not smoke. They may eat less than nonsmokers because they finish their meals with a cigarette rather than with dessert. They may smoke a cigarette rather than eat a snack. Smoking may dull their taste sense, and so foods seem less appetizing. In contrast, women who stop smoking (and many women do decrease or stop smoking during pregnancy) snack excessively. In nutritional counseling, it is important to analyze a day's intake for both smokers and new nonsmokers. If you cannot control a woman's snacking, encourage her to eat nutritious ones. Women who drink alcohol excessively may develop specific nutritional deficiencies if they ingest alcohol in place of eating. In order to metabolize large quantities of alcohol, a woman's body must use large quantities of thiamine (vitamin B_1). These women need to take a thiamine supplement over and above the usual pregnancy supplement and to eat foods high in this vitamin during pregnancy (whole and enriched grains, as examples).

During pregnancy women should discontinue the intake of any drug not prescribed or approved by their primary care provider. Women who are drug-dependent and so do not discontinue drug use may have difficulty both supporting their drug habit and buying nutritious food. If they are dependent on a hallucinogen or euphoric drug,

they may not feel hungry at regular intervals and so may skip meals for entire days. Enrolling these women in drug withdrawal programs such as a methadone program, where a drug is supplied for them daily, helps them to be able to afford food. It also keeps them in contact with health care personnel who can urge them to continue prenatal care and follow improved nutritional patterns.

Concurrent Medical Problems

Any medical condition that requires rigid salt, protein, or carbohydrate restriction poses a potential fetal nourishment problem during pregnancy. Women who have medical problems such as kidney disease, diabetes, or tuberculosis need special dietary considerations during pregnancy; specific metabolic disorders can occur with these diseases. Nursing implementations including nutrition interventions for women with these medical problems are discussed in Chapter 36.

Cultural Influences

Adults tend to eat the foods they ate as children. Women during pregnancy do not want to change from these comfortable patterns of food preparation. For many women, because they prepare foods for their husbands and families—or their husbands share cooking duties—changing to different foods involves changing the food patterns of other people besides themselves. In nutritional counseling, therefore, you need to be aware of the cultural patterns of the population with which you work. You can then suggest foods that fit within these personal preferences. A few of these patterns are outlined below.

Chinese Diet Patterns

There are four main areas in China, and the diet pattern in each area is different. People from the *Mandarin*, or northern, area eat a diet rich in sweet and sour dishes, with noodles as a staple. *Shanghai* is the coastal region, and fish and seafood are popular dishes there. In the southern, or *Cantonese* area, pork, chicken, and dumplings filled with meat (dim sum) are popular. Inland China, or the *Szechwan* area, is known for hot foods, highly seasoned with pepper.

Chinese philosophy holds that, in order for life to be peaceful, there must be contrast or balance of all things, illustrated by the concepts of yin and yang. Foods are classified as yin or yang (hot or cold), not based on their temperature but on generally accepted beliefs about the food. Many green vegetables, for example, like mustard greens, asparagus, and bean sprouts, are yin foods. Many meats, eggs, and nuts are yang foods. In order to urge a woman to eat more of one type of food, you may also have to stress that she eat a counterbalance number of the opposite type—or she will be uncomfortable following your suggestions.

Most people in the United States with a Chinese heritage eat a diet rich in vegetables (bean sprouts, broccoli, mushrooms, bamboo shoots) stir fried (cooked quickly) so they retain their nutrients. Since meat is served mixed with these vegetables, the proportion of meat eaten daily may be small. Generous portions of complementary protein, such as rice and beans, can avoid a protein lack. Rice, rather than potatoes or bread, is a staple. Encourage pregnant women to eat enriched rice if possible for its added vitamin content. Milk is not a popular beverage because of lactose intolerance in Oriental people. Bean curd (tofu) is a good source of protein and calcium, eaten often to take the place of milk. Soybeans, mustard greens, collard greens, and kale are vegetables with high calcium. Ice cream is an enjoyable source of calcium.

Many Chinese restaurants use monosodium glutamate liberally in cooking for additional flavor. High in sodium content, this substance dilates blood vessels, leading to sensations of tingling, flushing, dizziness, and tachycardia if ingested in large amounts (termed *Chinese restaurant syndrome*). Most people do not use the additive in their home, however, so it is not a usual dietary concern.

Japanese Diet Patterns

Japanese diets include little milk or cheese. Eggs, bean curd (tofu), spinach, broccoli, mustard greens, tomatoes, and eggplant are typical sources of protein and calcium. As with a Chinese diet pattern, meat is generally served with vegetables; the small amount of protein taken in may be a problem in pregnancy unless intake is supplemented with generous portions of complementary protein.

Vietnamese Diet Patterns

Rice is the staple of the Vietnamese diet. Many tropical fruits such as bananas, pineapple, and mangos are used. As with other Asian diets, small portions of meat and seafood are combined with rice and vegetables. Dried beans are a good source of protein used often. Tomatoes, squash, and spinach are common vegetables. Milk and milk products are seldom included because of lactose intolerance. Check that a woman is eating generous quantities of green vegetables during pregnancy in order to supply calcium and that she is using complementary protein sources. Vitamin D may need to be supplemented.

A woman who has recently arrived from Vietnam may have been on an almost starvation diet in her home country and have poor nutritional stores. She needs to be sure to not let a period over 12 hours go by without eating because she does not have a supply of "back-up" nutrients. Many Vietnamese people do not have what the Western world thinks of as a typical breakfast, but eat a soup (pho) containing noodles, vegetables, meat, and rice. This type of breakfast is actually less apt to cause morning nausea.

Puerto Rican Diet Patterns

In many Puerto Rican homes, the midday meal is the large meal of the day. A hot-cold division of food categories characterizes this diet as it does the Chinese. Although many types of meat are eaten, they are often cooked as stews, so individual portions of meat or protein may be small. Beans and rice are often cooked together, a good source of complementary protein. Many Puerto Rican women do not drink milk (lactose intolerance) but do add some to coffee (cafe con leche). Black malt beer (malta) is a nonalcoholic beverage thought to be nutritious and hence popular during pregnancy. Folic acid deficiency may be a problem for Puerto Rican women; encourage them to eat green, leafy vegetables, liver, fish, meat, poultry, legumes, and whole grains. Sugar is used liberally, while lard is a fat source. These, along with starchy vegetables, cause obesity to be a common nutritional problem.

Mexican-American Diet Patterns

The Mexican-American diet is a blend of Spanish, Native American, and Anglo-Saxon diet patterns. Corn is the basic grain. Tortillas (flat cakes made from ground corn) are a staple; these are called enchiladas and tacos when filled with beans, meat, or cheese. Since meat is generally combined with beans (pinto and garbanzo) or tomato sauce, individual portions of meat may be small. Milk is limited because of lactose intolerance although it is used in custards and rice puddings. During pregnancy, vitamin A and folic acid deficiency may be problems, as is obesity.

Black Diet Patterns

Black diet patterns vary greatly; many black Americans prepare "soul food." The meat is often pork (pigs' feet, ham hocks, chitterlings, or spareribs). Vegetables are often cooked with salt pork for long periods, so water-soluble vitamins are lost. Mustard greens, collards, black-eyed peas, corn, and sweet potatoes are popular vegetables. Grits, cornbread, and rice are staples. Little milk is consumed (due to lactose intolerance), but large quantities of cheese may be eaten, as in macaroni and cheese. Problems that a pregnant woman may encounter are low hemoglobin levels from the sparsity of meat, obesity, and chronic hypertension from an increased sodium intake from salt pork.

Jewish Diet Patterns

The Jewish dietary laws (kashruth) are followed to varying degrees in Jewish homes. Orthodox Jewish families follow them strictly; reform Jewish families give them no real emphasis; Conservative families practice at varying levels. The word *kosher* means "fit or clean." Grains, fruits, and vegetables are kosher. Meat and poultry are not kosher unless the animal is properly slaughtered and the meat is soaked in salted water to remove all blood. With the exception of poultry, only animals that have split hooves and chew their cud are acceptable (beef and lamb). Pork and fish without scales and fins, such as shellfish, are prohibited. Milk and meat cannot be eaten together (such as in creamed meat soups). Yom Kippur (Day of Atonement) is a 25-hour period of fasting.

A nutritional problem of following a Jewish diet may be increased cholesterol due to high levels of saturated fat and hypertension from a high salt intake. A woman is excused from fast days during pregnancy so this is not a problem.

European Diet Patterns

Diet patterns vary widely in persons from European cultures. Diet faults tend to cluster around overcooked vegetables, with less-than-desirable levels of water-soluble vitamins, lack of fresh fruits, and excessive bread or pasta. In pregnant women, lack of vitamin C and obesity may be common nutritional problems.

Fad Diets

Every year new diets to help people lose weight painlessly are introduced. As a rule of thumb, pregnant women should not be on reducing diets, so there is no place for these in pregnancy nutrition. It is helpful to be familiar with some of the basic principles of these diets, however, as many women enter pregnancy on them or have recently been on them.

Natural Food Diets

Foods that remain in their natural state with a minimum of processing and contain no artificial ingredients are "natural foods." There can be no harm in eating only natural foods.

Organically Grown Food Diets

Foods grown without the use of pesticides, fumigants, or synthetic fertilizers and containing no preservatives or synthetic coloring agents are "organically grown foods." These must be purchased in specialty shops and are 30 to 100 percent more expensive than other foods because of low crop yields. Women who eat only organically grown food may be reluctant to take vitamin supplements during pregnancy. You can explain that, chemically, natural and synthetic vitamins are the same: Buying them at a health food store does not improve the quality.

Zen Macrobiotic Diet

Macrobiotic means "large or long life." The combination of a macrobiotic diet and a pseudo-Oriental philosophy seems to appeal to younger women and teenagers. Foods are chosen on the basis of yang (hot, masculine) or yin (cold, feminine) properties. There are ten levels of diets. The simplest level includes cereal, vegetables, fruits, seafoods, desserts, and very limited fluid. The strictest level is composed only of brown rice and, again, very limited fluid. Women ingesting a macrobiotic diet for long periods run the risk of scurvy from vitamin C deficiency, anemia, hypoproteinemia, hypocalcemia, and emaciation due to starvation. It is certainly not an adequate pregnancy diet.

Stillman Diet

The Stillman diet allows a person to eat unlimited amounts of meat, fish and eggs; eight glasses of water and a vitamin supplement are taken daily. It is an unbalanced diet, high in saturated fat, and not recommended in pregnancy.

Mayo Diet

The Mayo diet includes a high protein intake along with a generous supply of grapefruit, which supposedly has a fat-dissolving capability. There is no scientific basis for the diet, and it is not adequate during pregnancy.

Atkins Diet

The Atkins diet includes no carbohydrate sources the first week to promote ketosis. It is high in saturated fat. Ketosis, which is teratogenic to a growing fetus, should be avoided during pregnancy.

Scarsdale Diet

The Scarsdale diet provides special menus for 14 days that must be followed without substitutions. It is a diet low in total calories, iron, calcium, and thiamine.

Liquid Protein Diet

A liquid protein diet requires a woman to drink only high-protein liquid formula. Such a diet causes a high solute load (breakdown products of protein) to the kidneys and results in the woman using protein for energy, leading to acidosis. A number of deaths have been reported in young adults from such diets, probably from extreme acidosis.

Cambridge Diet

The Cambridge diet is a formula diet that relies strongly on fixed intake portions. It has not been proven to be nutritionally sound for any person, much less a pregnant woman.

Vegetarian Diets

There are many different types of vegetarian diets. Some people on vegetarian diets eat no animal or dairy products (vegans); some allow milk and eggs (lacto-ovo vegetarians); some eat fish and chicken but no red meat. A vegetarian diet can be complete if the person is knowledgeable about complementary proteins and includes these in the diet. Concerns for a pregnant woman on this diet include lack of vitamin B_{12} (meat is the chief source), perhaps calcium (encourage dark green vegetables as sources), and vitamin D (fortified milk is the main source). Most women who are vegetarians are very knowledgeable about their diets and are able to point out to you what foods are high in various nutrients and how they incorporate these in their diet.

Programs to Provide Financial Aid with Nutrition

A number of federally funded programs are available to help women meet the high cost of providing nutritious meals for themselves and their families (see the Nursing Research Highlight on page 425).

Food Stamp Program

Under the Food Stamp program, a family of low income can buy stamps that can be redeemed at grocery stores for any food item but alcohol or pet food. The cost of stamps varies, but they can increase a family's buying power by as much as $150 a month.

The advantage of this type of program is that food supplementation is provided with almost no restrictions on what foods can be selected and purchased. Rules concerning eligibility for these programs vary from time to time. With the help of stamps, a family with low income can switch from a high-starch diet to being able to eat meat daily. Just because a family can afford a better diet does not mean the members automatically eat better; assess that food stamps are used wisely.

Supplemental Food Program for Women, Infants, and Children (WIC)

Pregnant and lactating women, infants, and children up to 5 years of age who live in selected project areas and are at nutritional risk qualify for this program. A family is given a voucher, which can be exchanged for milk, orange juice, eggs, iron-fortified cereal, iron-fortified formula, or cheese.

An important part of this program is periodic, scheduled health care visits that must be kept in order to continue to qualify for the program. These checkups further protect the health of these high-risk groups.

School Lunch Programs

Millions of adolescent girls qualify for free or reduced-price school lunches. Some qualify for a free school breakfast program as well. A federally funded school lunch provides one-third of a child's RDA for a day. Pregnant adolescents from a low income family may well qualify for this

Nursing Research Highlight

Do High-Obstetric Risk Low-Income Women Have Poor Diets?

Nutritional status assessment has been an area of increasingly renewed interest in the past several years especially for high-risk populations such as low-income pregnant women and children. Low-income pregnant women are especially susceptible to nutritionally related problems and could be potentially benefited from health care and nutrition programs. But first the food consumption patterns that often account for poor nutritional status must be understood and evaluated for specific population groups. Several researchers (Bowering, Lowenberg, and Morrison, 1980) conducted a survey on 346 low-income, pregnant women attending a clinic for high-risk obstetric patients. The clients were selected by several maternal risk criteria, such as previous obstetric history, age over 35 years, and anemia coupled with low socioeconomic status. Several observations that could be tentatively linked to ethnic backgrounds, age, and related obstetric history were made regarding the dietary and nutritional status of this group of low-income, pregnant women. Data indicated that the older women may be at greater risk of having poor diets than younger women. The greater number of demands placed on them because of larger families prevents them from focusing attention on themselves. It is clear that multifaceted programs that combine obstetric care and nutrition education must be planned.

Reference

Bowering, J., Lowenberg, R., & Morrison, M. (1980). Nutritional studies of pregnant women in east Harlem. *The American Journal of Clinical Nutrition, 33,* 1980.

---

service. Check that a girl is actually eating the lunch and not "trading off" so she receives the full benefit of the program.

Additional Buying Power

A suggestion often made for improving a food dollar is to shop for specials or sales. This approach may be difficult for a woman late in pregnancy because she becomes tired easily. She may choose to limit the number of stores she visits in order to conserve energy, even while knowing that she is probably spending slightly more money.

Another suggestion is to buy in large lots. Whether a woman can follow this advice depends on her food storage room and the degree of creativity she lends to food preparation. Also some women enjoy frequent shopping trips as a form of socialization; they would dislike buying large amounts, which automatically reduces the frequency of shopping.

Using coupons from newspapers or other food purchases saves money, but only if the food purchased is something the woman was going to purchase anyway. Buying frozen carrots at a discount price when she hates carrots will not save her money because they will be wasted if not eaten.

Utilizing Nursing Process

Helping a woman plan a nutritious diet during pregnancy is a good example of how nursing process can be used to promote health.

Assessment

Socioeconomic level is not a good criterion for judging good nutritional intake. Some women with ample money actually feed their families less nutritionally than those who live on a marginal budget. Each family and woman must be assessed individually. Most people think that they eat nutritionally or at least adequately. Before you can begin to talk to a woman about improving her diet, you may need to demonstrate to her that her diet needs some revamping. One method is to ask her for a "typical day" history, or a 24-hour dietary recall. Ask first if yesterday was a typical day. If it was, ask her to list for you all the food she ate within the past 24 hours. Be certain she includes all the foods she ate as snacks as well as sit-down meals. This method of history taking yields much more accurate information about actual intake than if you ask questions such as how often during the week she eats citrus fruit, or how much milk she drinks every day. A woman who does not know what citrus fruit is cannot answer the first question, but she *can* tell you she had an orange for breakfast. A woman who knows how much milk she ought to drink a day will probably say she drinks a quart a day during pregnancy. However, if asked to list the foods she ate the day before, she may report that she drank only one glass of milk all day.

After you have a day's list of food, compare the types and amounts on the list with those shown in Table 20-9 to see if all food groups are included. Plotting foods from a person's 24-hour recall onto a wheel graph (Figure 20-3) is a helpful way of showing people that what they thought was a "perfect" intake is not perfect, or what they thought was a "little" problem involves the loss of an important food group (the graph shows that the woman who knew she did not eat many vegetables also eats no fruit, so omits a total food group; the woman who says she knows she is chronically tired eats almost nothing from the meat group). "A picture is worth a thousand words" is an old saying but important for nutrition counseling; once a person sees that an actual defect exists, she is ready to move to setting goals to improve nutrition. Such a picture also offers a reward for the woman who already has adequate intake.

Also ask a woman if she thinks she has any problems with nutrition. The woman may already know her problem—such as never eating vegetables—but has never done much to correct her fault before. The crisis of pregnancy may be the opportunity for change.

In addition to actual food intake, assess circumstances of eating, such as who prepares food and how many meals are eaten outside the home weekly. Table 20-14 summarizes this type of additional information.

To accompany history findings, assess a woman's prepregnancy weight in reference to her height according to an ideal weight chart or growth chart (Appendix F). People with poor nutrition begin to evidence physical signs as their body can no longer function adequately with missing nutrients. Table 20-15 lists important physical examination assessments that suggest a good nutritional intake.

Hemoglobin or hematocrit determinations are also important assessments of good nutrition. Women have these taken early in pregnancy and then usually repeated close to term and at delivery. A urinalysis also is important as a finding; the specific gravity of urine can suggest a disturbed fluid balance.

Analysis

The North American Nursing Diagnosis Association accepted three diagnoses in reference to nutrition: "nutrition, alterations in: less than body requirements;" "nutrition, alterations in: more than body requirements;" and "nutrition, alterations in: potential for more than body requirements." They need to be altered only slightly ("nutrition, alteration in: less than body requirements for pregnancy") in order to be relevant to maternal-newborn nursing.

Planning

Plans made for improving nutrition patterns must take into account a person's life style, financial resources, customs, habits, and personal desires. Otherwise, the person will not maintain a changed eating pattern longer than a week (Figure 20-4).

Since pregnancy lasts 9 months, the woman herself must make the choices of specific foods in the various food groups you indicate are important in pregnancy. Without this freedom, your health care setting will be full of women who give lip service to good nutrition ("I'm eating everything you say"), but who are not eating well at all.

Food is costly. In order to provide the extra servings required during pregnancy, you are asking a woman to spend more on food for herself per week than she is used to spending. Women generally view this increased expense as an investment in their child's health and so do not regard it as a burden. The family on a marginal income, however, may be willing to shoulder the additional cost but will have trouble finding the money. A woman with this problem needs a review of her diet to make certain she is not buying only starchy foods. She needs help in securing any financial assistance that is available, such as food stamps or nutrition aid programs.

Despite a health course in high school that described the necessity for good nutrition, the average woman may know less than you realize about what foods are the best sources of particular nutrients. Planning for nutrition counseling, then, invariably begins with education on what is a good diet and in consultation with the woman, on how she is going to improve her nutrition habits.

A woman who eats no meat, for example, could solve her problem in two ways—either by agreeing to try to include meat in her diet daily or working out with you combinations of com-

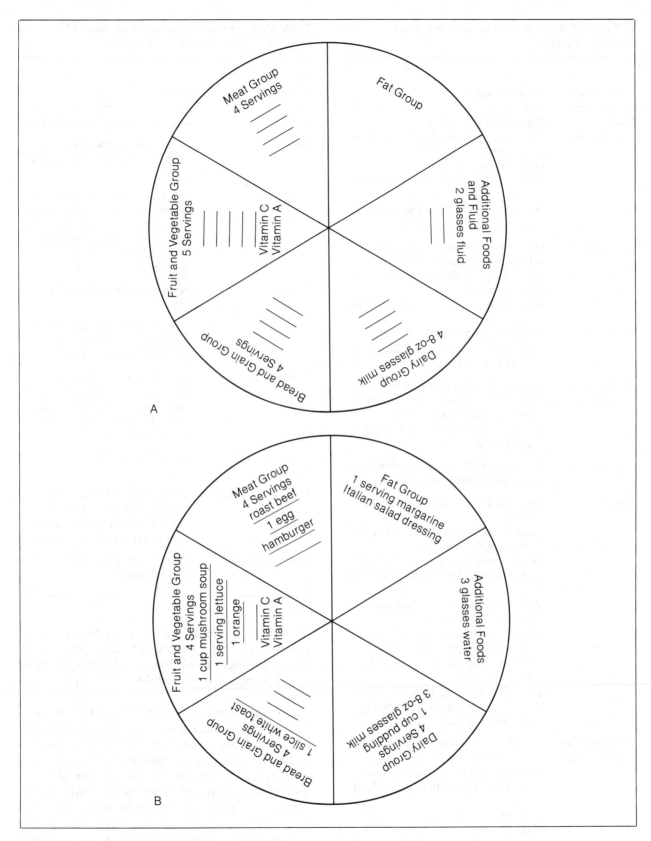

Figure 20-3 *A. Graph for analysis of pregnancy food intake. B. This example of a graph for food group analysis shows a 24-hour recall deficit in 1 serving meat group, 1 serving fruit and vegetable group (no strong source of vitamin A), and 3 servings bread and grain group.*

Table 20-14 Areas to be Assessed for a Total Nutrition History

Area of Assessment	Pertinent Questions
Food preparation	Who does the cooking? How many persons does the woman cook for? How are foods usually prepared? What are spices or condiments commonly used? What type of oil is used for frying (saturated or unsaturated)?
Food pattern	How many meals are eaten a day? Which is the biggest meal? How many snacks are eaten a day? What are they? How many meals are eaten outside the home? Where are they eaten? Cafeteria? Fast food store? Restaurant? Bagged lunch?
Financial concerns	Is there enough money for food? Would the woman eat differently if more money was available? Is any supplementary financial program used?
Activity level	Is she normally active or sedentary? (Could increase calorie need.)
Health	Does she know of any allergies to food? Does she have any trouble with chewing or digestion? What is bowel movement frequency? Does she take any medication? What type? Was she taking oral contraceptives prior to pregnancy? Does she take supplemental vitamins? What type? How many? Does she drink alcohol? What type? How much? Does she smoke cigarettes? What is her stress level? Does this affect her appetite?
Personal food preferences	Are there any foods she particularly enjoys or dislikes? Are there any foods she feels are harmful or particularly beneficial to her? Are there any cultural or religious preferences?
Family dietary patterns	Does anyone in the family eat a special diet? Is anyone obviously over- or underweight? Does the family eat meals together? Is mealtime a social time?

Table 20-15 Physical Signs and Symptoms of Adequate Nutrition During Pregnancy

Area of Assessment	Findings
Hair	Shiny; strong with good body.
Eyes	Good eyesight, particularly at night; conjunctiva moist and pink.
Mouth	No cavities in teeth; no swollen or inflamed gingiva; no cracks or fissures at corners of mouth; mucous membrane moist and pink; tongue smooth and nontender.
Neck	Normal contour of thyroid gland.
Skin	Smooth, with normal color and turgor; no ecchymotic or petechial areas present.
Extremities	Normal muscle mass and circumference; normal strength and mobility. Edema limited to slight ankle involvement; normal reflexes.
Finger and toenails	Smooth; pink.
Height and weight	Within normal limits of ideal weight chart prior to pregnancy; following normal pattern of pregnancy weight gain.
Blood pressure	Within normal limits for length of pregnancy.

plementary proteins that will supply high-level protein and iron. Remember that eggs and legumes are meat group foods. Incorporating these in a diet increases the number of meat group portions.

Establish priorities where nutrition seems to be most deficient. Do not ruin your gain at that point by saying, "You must drink more milk. Add a glass at breakfast and another for dinner." The woman may hate milk, and she may feel that you are forcing health care values on her without considering her preference. State instead, "You need to eat more calcium every day. Let's look at a list of foods high in that and you can pick one or two you'd like to add more of. Could you drink more milk? Have you ever tried yogurt?"

Implementation

In many health care settings, nutrition counseling has become largely the province of the dieti-

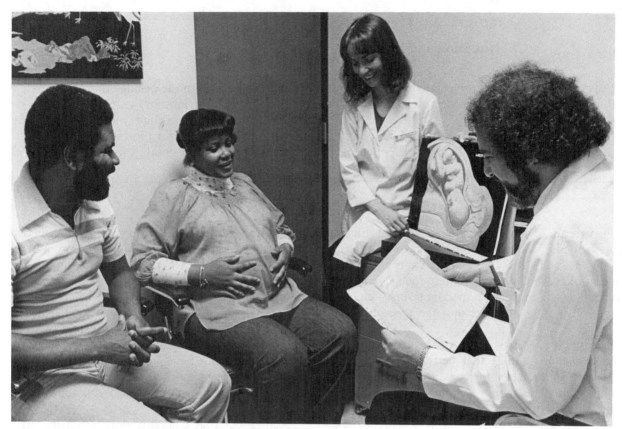

Figure 20-4 *Learning about fetal growth helps a pregnant woman eat more nutritionally. (Courtesy of Harvard Community Health Plan, Boston.)*

tian. You order the diet, and it comes from the facility kitchen fully prepared and labeled. The dietitian discusses possible exchanges or alterations with the patient. In an ambulatory setting, such as a prenatal clinic or physician's office, you often do not have the luxury of a dietitian nearby. Even if you do, it is advantageous to use her as a resource person and do the nutrition counseling yourself. Doing all other counseling—talking about bathing, exercise, clothing, travel, rest—and then passing nutrition counseling on to another person gives nutrition a different value from the other health topics. It makes it seem complicated (if you cannot handle it, how can a woman alone in her kitchen?), impersonal (you see the woman month after month; she sees a dietitian once or twice), and unimportant (it was not important enough for you to do). Do you want to imply these values?

Implementation of a changed dietary pattern can be a lonely and seemingly unrewarding endeavor. People often need support by a telephone call or person-to-person contact in order to eat a different lunch than others around them are eating; to be motivated enough to get up 15 minutes earlier in the morning to prepare breakfast rather

than just dashing to work without anything more than coffee; or to resist a soft drink with their fast food dinner and drink orange juice instead. Asking people to list what foods they eat daily and to bring in the chart to show you at a health maintenance visit is an effective motivating technique for many people (the same effect as doing well on tests because the success is reported on a report card). In research studies, this is called a *Hawthorne effect* (people who are being watched do better than those who are not). With this system, the average person will eat better so the list looks better when she presents it. Hopefully, as soon as she appreciates that better eating patterns make her feel better, she will continue them indefinitely.

Be familiar with the usual dietary pattern in the part of the country or the ethnic groups of women with whom you are working. Collard and dandelion greens, for example, may not appeal to you as vegetables, but nutritionally they compare favorably to spinach or broccoli, two vegetables you may customarily recommend. There is no reason to try to convert women to your eating habits if their way is only "different," not inadequate.

Nursing Care Highlight

Nutrition and Pregnancy

1. Advise women during pregnancy not to go longer than 12 hours between meals to avoid hypoglycemia.
2. Be certain women regard vitamins as medication and follow the medication rule concern-

ing them: Take none besides those recommended by their primary care provider.
3. Nutrition during pregnancy should be high in calories to provide for protein sparing and high in protein for fetal growth.

Be careful of statements such as "Eat high-protein foods." These are meaningless for many women as food, after all, does not come from the supermarket labeled "high-protein food." Women need advice given in more specific terms—for example, "Eat three servings of some type of meat every day."

The word *diet* has come to mean a form of unpleasant food denial. It is better to talk about the "foods that are best for you during pregnancy" or "pregnancy nutrition" rather than a "pregnancy diet." The first two phrases have a positive sound and are closer to what you will be encouraging the woman to eat. A list of prenatal instructions listing proper foods is good to distribute to women as long as it is short and clear, like Table 20-9. Complicated lists of foods or a list of *don'ts* will land in the wastepaper basket rather than be used and followed. The Nursing Care Highlight above stresses important guidelines to remember.

Evaluation

When evaluating whether an improved nutrition pattern has been successful or not, rely on your most important assessments: weight, energy level, general appearance, bowel function, and as you have access to them, hemoglobin and urinalysis findings.

Urge people to be honest about whether they are actually following a new nutritional pattern or not. If they are not, it is not a crime (who is perfect?); it simply means that the plan you arrived at must not have somehow fitted their life style or degree of motivation. You cannot know this unless they are honest with you about their success.

Remember that changing nutritional patterns is difficult. People always have some degree of back-sliding at holidays and special events. Respect this as a fact of human nature. If it is crucially important that such a phenomenon does not occur on the next holiday, you will need to help the woman make concrete plans about how it can be avoided or your next evaluation will reveal the same problem.

Be certain to comment on the things the woman is doing correctly. This is an elemental rule of teaching that almost every teacher forgets in his or her zeal to create a perfect student.

Nursing Care Planning

Nursing care plans concerning nutrition must be individualized, as foods that people eat and their nutrition patterns are so different. Below are three nursing care plans individualized for different women during pregnancy.

Christine McFadden
15 years old

Assessment

Patient is student in high school; no previous pregnancies. Lives at home where food is prepared by mother. Eats breakfast at home, lunch at high-

school cafeteria, dinner often at fast-food takeout on way to part-time job. Culture: English-Irish. States she does not exercise but "is always on the go."

24-hour diet history:
Breakfast: 2 slices toast, 1 glass orange juice.
Lunch: grilled cheese sandwich, 1 glass milk.
Dinner: 1 hamburger, 1 serv. french fries, 1 cup coffee.
Snacks: 6–8 cookies, 1 bag pretzels, 1 glass cola.
Does not dislike milk or vegetables; just does not eat them.
Admits to being poor medicine taker.
Prepregnancy weight: 115; appropriate for height.

Weight today (last menstrual period about 16 weeks ago): 122.
Appears pale, although hemoglobin is 11 gm.

Analysis

Nutrition, alteration in, less than body requirements related to inadequate food intake (little protein, no vegetables except french fries, little milk, high caffeine).

Locus of Decision Making. Shared.

Goal. Patient to complete pregnancy within good nutritional parameters.

Criteria. Patient:

1. Pregnancy weight gain to total 25–30 pounds.
2. Hemoglobin to remain above 11 gm.
3. Able to describe adequate pregnancy nutrition at next visit.
4. To take vitamin and iron supplement daily.

Nursing Orders

1. Diet to be 2,700 calories (to allow for teenage growth).
2. Counsel concerning pregnancy nutrition and difficulty with cafeteria and fast food sources.
3. Help to design a compliance chart to record vitamin and iron supplement daily for increased compliance.
4. Review nutrition next visit (to bring up any problems she encounters).
5. Offer strong support following improved nutrition (few support people around her to reinforce actions).

———————

Mary Kraft
23 years old

Assessment

Patient is housewife; part-time job in public library. Cooks for self and husband; "not a good cook." Often cooks just for herself as husband attends night school. Culture: black. One previous pregnancy that ended in spontaneous abortion 2 years ago. Finances "adequate." Walks to work or store daily. Has "always" had a weight problem" she keeps under control by "eating almost nothing."

24 hour diet history:
Breakfast: 1 cup black coffee.
Lunch: None.
Dinner: 1 serv. macaroni and cheese; 1 serv. greens, 1 cup coffee.
Snacks: 2 glasses milk, 1 candy bar.

Prepregnancy weight: 110 (10 pounds under desirable weight).
Weight today (last menstrual period 9 weeks ago): 111.
Appears thin, hemoglobin 11 gm.

Analysis

Nutrition, alteration in, less than body requirements related to low food intake (low total calories, low protein, no fruit, high caffeine).

Locus of Decision Making. Patient.

Goal. Patient to complete pregnancy within good nutrition parameters.

Criteria. Patient:

1. Pregnancy weight gain to total 35–40 pounds (10 pounds underweight prepregnancy).
2. Hemoglobin to remain above 11 gm.
3. Can describe adequate pregnancy nutrition at next visit.
4. To take vitamin and iron supplement daily.

Nursing Orders

1. Diet to be 2,900 calories daily (500 additional calories to increase weight).
2. Counsel concerning pregnancy diet and need to increase intake.
3. Return in 1 week for nurse appointment for further nutrition review and suggestions.
4. Patient to bring suggestions that might make cooking for herself in evening or at noon easier or more fun.
5. Respect cultural influences on nutrition; wants to raise children with knowledge and appreciation of black culture.

———————

Angie Baco
42 years

Assessment

Patient is housewife; cooks for 5 children (ages 20, 19, 18, 15, and 7) and husband. Enjoys cooking; has won prizes at county fair for cakes and pies. Exercises little.
Culture: Italian. Is reluctant to take an iron supplement because it might cause constipation; no objection to vitamins. Finances adequate. Had weight gain of 50 pounds last pregnancy, mild gestational diabetes.

24 hour diet history:
Breakfast: 1 serv. oatmeal with milk and honey, 1 glass orange juice, 2 slices cinnamon toast with butter.

Lunch: 1 serv. tomato soup, bacon and cheese sandwich, 2 pieces cherry pie, 1 glass lemonade. Dinner: 1 serv. spaghetti and meatballs, 1 serv. green salad, 2 slices bread and butter, 2 pieces carrot cake, 1 glass milk, 1 cup coffee. Snacks: 2 slices cinnamon toast, 2 oranges. Prepregnancy weight: 144 (30 pounds above ideal weight). Weight today (12 weeks since LMP): 150. Hemoglobin 11.5 gm.

Analysis

Nutrition, alteration in, more than body requirements, related to excessive food intake (high total calories and questionable protein intake, little milk).

Locus of Decision Making. Patient.

Goal. Patient to complete pregnancy within good nutritional parameters.

Criteria. Patient:
1. Weight gain to be 30–40 pounds.
2. To increase level of exercise daily.
3. Hemoglobin to remain above 11 gm.
4. Able to describe adequate pregnancy nutrition at next visit.
5. To take vitamin and iron supplement daily.

Nursing Orders
1. Pregnancy diet to be limited to 2,400 calories.
2. Counsel concerning pregnancy nutrition and need to limit high-calorie but not high-protein foods.
3. To try vitamin and iron supplement for 1 week and see if constipation occurs.
4. Husband to accompany her at next visit to talk about family's cooperation in limiting high-calorie foods.
5. Give generous support for attempts at compliance; difficult for her to change diet pattern.
6. Encourage her to attempt a walk daily to increase exercise level.

Questions for Review

Multiple Choice

1. Mrs. Marvin is a woman you meet in a prenatal setting. What is the most effective way to assess her usual food intake?
   a. Assess a list she makes describing a good diet.
   b. Ask her to describe her total intake for a week.
   c. Assess her skin for hydration and mucus membrane for color.
   d. Ask her to describe her intake for the last 24 hours.

2. You plot Mrs. Marvin's breakfast on a food graph. Which of the following would you *not* plot as a source of complete protein?
   a. a fried egg
   b. a slice of whole grain toast
   c. a ham slice
   d. a glass of milk

3. You analyze Mrs. Marvin's diet as being low in iron. Which food below is *not* rich in iron
   a. milk
   b. legumes
   c. grains
   d. beef

4. Mrs. Marvin enjoys drinking tea. Advice you would give her regarding this is that
   a. tea is irritating to the stomach due to tannic acid.
   b. tea contains caffeine so should be avoided during pregnancy.

   c. tea is soothing for the nausea and vomiting of early pregnancy.
   d. only if she drinks over four cups a day will tea cause a problem.

5. Mrs. Marvin tells you she wants to avoid saturated fat. Which food below contains saturated fat?
   a. corn oil
   b. lean roast beef
   c. vegetable oil
   d. potato skins

6. The B vitamins are important in a pregnancy diet. Which of the following foods is the best source of vitamin B_{12}?
   a. carrots
   b. hamburger
   c. milk
   d. cottage cheese

7. In order to ensure a good intake of vitamin A, which advice below would you give Mrs. Marvin?
   a. boil all vegetables well
   b. eat green leafy vegetables
   c. eat yellow vegetables
   d. eat fresh fruit

8. A month after teaching Mrs. Marvin about good nutrition in pregnancy you evaluate her intake and discover she is still not eating adequate protein daily. An adequate protein intake during pregnancy may prevent which complication of pregnancy?
   a. hypertension of pregnancy
   b. congestive heart disease

c. urinary frequency

d. nausea and vomiting

9. Protein is basically found in meat. How many meat servings are recommended for women during pregnancy daily?

    a. 2

    b. 4

    c. 6

    d. 8

10. Mrs. Marvin is eligible for WIC program funding. With this assistance program, she could receive

    a. a community-prepared lunch.

    b. reduced prices at the supermarket.

c. free meat and designated poultry.

d. free cheese and milk.

Discussion

1. Many women know little about nutrition planning even though they prepare all their family's meals. What nutrition planning would you want to discuss with a woman at the beginning of pregnancy?

2. Ingesting enough iron during pregnancy may be a major problem for women. How would you help a woman avoid this problem?

3. Many women never drink milk. How can you encourage an adequate calcium intake under these circumstances?

Suggested Readings

Abrams, B. (1981). Helping pregnant teenagers eat right. *Nursing (Horsham), 11,* 46.

Barwell, B. (1982). Phenylketonuria . . . a problem in pregnancy. *Health Visitor, 55,* 345.

Brooten, D., & Jordan, C. (1983). Caffeine and pregnancy—A research review and recommendations for clinical practice. *J.O.G.N. Nursing, 12,* 190.

Burke, B. C., et al. (1943). Nutritional studies during pregnancy. *American Journal of Obstetrics and Gynecology, 46,* 38.

Danis, R. P., & Keith, L. (1983). Fetal alcohol syndrome: Incurable but preventable. *Contemporary OB/GYN, 21,* 57.

Deskins, B. B., et al. (1982). The community health nurse's nutrition guidelines: A trimester approach for expectant mothers. *M.C.N., 7,* 202.

Diebel, P. (1980). Effects of cigarette smoking on maternal nutrition and the fetus. *J.O.G.N. Nursing, 9,* 333.

Edwards, L., et al. (1979). Pregnancy in the underweight woman: Course, outcome and growth of the infant. *American Journal of Obstetrics and Gynecology, 135,* 297.

Gould, S. F., et al. (1981). Obesity and pregnancy. *Perinatology Neonatology, 5,* 49.

Graham, D. M. (1978). Caffeine—its identity, dietary sources, intake and biological effects. *Nutrition Review, 36,* 97.

Henley, E. C., et al. (1982). Nutrition across the woman's life cycle: Special emphasis on pregnancy. *Nursing Clinics of North America 17,* 99.

Howard, R. B., & Herbold, N. H. (1982). *Nutrition in Clinical Care* (2nd ed.). New York: McGraw-Hill.

Jacobson, H. N. (1983). Diet therapy and the improvement of pregnancy outcomes. *Birth, 10,* 29.

Karvetti, R. L. (1981). Effects of nutrition education. *Journal of the American Dietary Association, 79,* 660.

Korczowski, M. M., et al. (1981). Strengthen the nurse's role in nutritional counseling . . . guidelines for charting. *Nursing and Health Care, 2,* 210.

Labson, L. H. (1981). Assuring good nutrition prenatally. *Patient Care, 15,* 20.

Langford, R. W. (1981). Teenagers and obesity. *American Journal of Nursing, 81,* 556.

Lechtig, A. (1982). Studies of nutrition interventions in pregnancy. *Birth, 9,* 115.

Lemasters, G. K. (1981). Zinc insufficiency during pregnancy. *J.O.G.N. Nursing, 10,* 124.

Leonard, L. G. (1982). Twin pregnancy: Maternal-fetal nutrition. *J.O.G.N. Nursing, 11,* 139.

Lind, T. (1984). Would more calories per day keep low birthweight away? *Lancet, 1,* 501.

Mandelbaum, J. L. (1983). The foodsquare: Helping people of different cultures understand balanced diets. *Pediatric Nursing, 9,* 20.

Metzler, S., et al. (1981). Teaching prenatal nutrition in an outpatient clinic: A change project. *Issues in Health Care of Women, 3,* 341.

Riordan, J., et al. (1980). Preparation for breast-feeding and early optimal functioning. *J.O.G.N. Nursing, 9,* 277.

Roberts, B., & Weigle, A. (1983). Caffeine and pregnancy outcome. *J.O.G.N. Nursing, 12,* 21.

Seifrit, E. (1983). Nutrition and the older primigravida. *Journal of the American Dietetic Association, 82,* 529.

Stephens, C. J. (1981). The fetal alcohol syndrome: Cause for concern. *M.C.N., 6,* 251.

Tull, M. W., et al. (1981). Effects of caffeine on pregnancy and lactation. *Pediatric Nursing, 7,* 51.

Veninga, K. S. (1982). An easy recipe for assessing your patient's nutrition. *Nursing (Horsham), 12,* 57.

White, J. H., et al. (1981). When your client has a weight problem. *American Journal of Nursing, 81,* 549.

Winick, M. (1984). Nutrition and pregnancy. *Female Patient, 9,* 21.

Worthington-Roberts, B. S., et al. (1981). *Nutrition in pregnancy and lactation.* (2nd ed.). St. Louis: Mosby.

Wynn, M., et al. (1982). The importance of maternal nutrition in the weeks before and after conception. *Birth, 9,* 39.

21

Preparation for Parenthood

OBJECTIVES

Following mastery of the contents of this chapter, you should be able to

1. Describe the purpose and content of expectant parents' classes.
2. Describe the advantages of prepared childbirth.
3. Compare common methods of prepared childbirth.
4. Describe common exercises that are effective for strengthening muscles for childbirth.
5. Describe the Lamaze (psychoprophylactic) method of prepared childbirth.
6. Describe the Dick-Read method of abdominal breathing as an advantageous technique to teach unprepared women in labor.
7. Analyze the role of the nurse in providing information for both expectant parents' and prepared-childbirth classes.
8. Synthesize the principles of prepared childbirth with nursing process to achieve quality maternal-newborn nursing care.

ALTHOUGH PARENTHOOD is the occupation most closely involved in protecting the physical and mental health of the next generation, it is one of the few occupations that require no formal course of instruction, no examination to test a person's competency, and no refresher course to ensure that a parent is following up-to-date concepts of childrearing.

Every pregnant woman, whether primipara or grand multipara, should be asked during the prenatal period whether or not she would be interested in participating in a course that will help to prepare her for giving birth or raising her child. In most communities today, such courses are available for prospective parents. You should be familiar with the material of these courses so that you can be certain the ones you are advocating present adequate and accurate information and to help parents differentiate the two types of courses offered. Nurses are the people in the community most often asked to conduct educational programs for prospective parents, and thus you may be asked to present such a program. If there are no preparation-for-parenthood classes in your community, you *should* organize and teach such classes; preparation-for-childbirth classes are usually taught by childbirth educators or nurses with special preparation in one or more forms of prepared childbirth (see the Nursing Research Highlight on page 436).

Prospective parents usually are not ready for participation in such a program early in pregnancy. They need time to accept the pregnancy, to work through what it feels like to be having a child, to think about being a mother or father. At the time of quickening, when they can feel the child stir and move, attending classes may become part of nest building. Mention early in pregnancy that such courses are available; at quickening (18 to 20 weeks) suggest the concrete opportunities available.

The programs offered are of two principal types: in one (expectant parents' classes) the course of normal pregnancy and beginning childcare are discussed, and in the other active preparation for childbirth is taught.

Expectant Parents' Classes

Parents, like all students, learn best when material is presented in a variety of ways. Some topics, such as childbearing anatomy, are best taught by lecture. A topic such as the psychological aspects of pregnancy is best taught by group interaction. Imagine how you, if you were pregnant, would respond to a nonpregnant nurse standing in front of a classroom telling you how it feels to be pregnant. You would want to tell *her* how it feels. You would want to talk to the other pregnant women in the group and see if they feel as you do, to assure yourself that you are responding normally to this pregnancy. Some topics are best taught if both men and women are present; others, such as the man's feelings toward pregnancy, might be best handled in a group attended only by prospective fathers. Principles of teaching/learning apply to group presentations as well as individual teaching situations. These are shown in the box on page 437.

Course Planning

Most preparation-for-parenthood programs are planned to cover 4 to 8 hours of time spaced over a 4 to 8 week period. Both women and their support people are included. The curriculum should be individualized for the group and that group's

Nursing Research Highlight

Does Childbirth Preparation Increase Maternal Attachment?

Interesting answers to this question were postulated in a study by Croft (1982). This nurse researcher followed 61 primiparous women. These mothers were scored on maternal-infant attachment at 1 day postpartum and 1 month postpartum. While no significance was found at one day postpartum, the mothers who had childbirth preparation scored lower in maternal-infant attachment at 1 month. Several factors may explain these interesting results. It is suggested that the mental activities of attention focusing and controlled breathing to decrease pain may distract mothers from their own bodies and, therefore, may detach them from their infants during the childbirth process. Many thought-provoking questions are posed by this study.

Reference

Croft, C. (1982). Lamaze childbirth education—implications for maternal-infant attachment. *J.O.G.N. Nursing, 11,* 333.

---

particular needs. If all the women in the group already have children, for example, they may not feel a need for a tour of a maternity unit as part of the program; instead, they may want a review of what is new in baby food or child care. If all the women are teenagers, they may be most interested in what is going to happen to their bodies during pregnancy, or what sports activities are safe to continue during pregnancy. They probably will want a tour of the maternity unit included. If all the women in the class work, at least part-time, they will want "brown bag nutrition" discussed and how to include rest periods during work hours.

It is good to begin a first class by passing out cards to the members of the group and asking them to write down the topics they most want to hear discussed at sessions. Asking members to put their interests in writing is often more productive than asking the group for oral suggestions. Some people are not willing to admit before a group of strangers that they do not know very much about childbirth or children. However, they will express their needs in writing: "Tell us how to space babies better." "Does the baby feel anything when it's being born?" "Do I *have* to eat liver?"

Some people have not thought through what they expect or want from the course. They have come because they want to learn, assuming the course would consist of a series of preplanned lectures. They need help in selecting topics that will be of interest to them. Review with them topics that other groups have asked to have discussed or the time-honored concerns in pregnancy. This introduction will stimulate individual ideas.

Some group leaders like to proceed without any set plan, just asking at every meeting what the group would like to discuss that evening. Use this technique judiciously unless you are skilled in group dynamics. Otherwise, every week the topic will be decided by the most talkative members of the group, and less voluble members will sit through eight sessions with few of their questions answered.

Collecting the topics that people would like to hear discussed, then organizing the material for presentation, is a good compromise between an entirely open group and formal, stiff lectures. It assures everyone in the group that his or her topic will be discussed. It assures you that the essential information of pregnancy and childbirth will be covered and allows you time to prepare for classes—and preparation is necessary if you are to cover a topic thoroughly.

A typical course plan for 8 weeks might be as follows.

Lesson 1: Group Introduction

Because members of the group learn as much (perhaps more) from interaction with each other as from an instructor, they first need to become acquainted with one another. Arrange your classroom so the chairs are in a circle, not in rows. Provide noncaffeine drinks or fruit if at all possible within your setting and budget.

Begin by suggesting that couples introduce themselves, giving their names, indicating whether or not this is their first baby, and mentioning anything else interesting about themselves that they want to share with the group. Fathers will usually identify themselves at the first meeting by their occupation: "I'm Bob Jones, a teacher. This is our first baby." Women, too,

Principles of Teaching/Learning

Principle	*Example*
TEACHING	
Know your subject	Because maternal-newborn nursing is a rapidly changing field, you constantly have to read new articles and research studies to be certain that what you thought was current information has not become obsolete.
Know your audience	Teaching techniques differ depending on an audience. Material presented and style of presentation for an adolescent audience might be very different from that presented to women having their third or fourth child.
Know your ability	Identify teaching strategies that are comfortable for you (role-playing, for example, may not be right for everyone).
Define teaching goals	Goals serve as guidelines that help you sift through all you know about a subject in order to select the parts you will teach and to help determine the teaching order.
Teach from the simple to the complex	People cannot grasp complex material until they have learned the fundamental information.
Provide adequate time and space for learning	Learning takes place best in an environment that is free from distraction.
Be consistent	People can become confused if they are told two or three different ways of doing something.
Recognize that nonverbal teaching is as effective as verbal teaching	Your gestures and facial expressions teach as much as your spoken words.
Teach principles, not Do-as-I-say actions	Teaching a principle allows a woman to modify actions to an alternative method as long as the principle is followed.
Teach what women should do, not what they should not do	Teaching from a positive standpoint makes learning more enjoyable.
Include evaluation as a final step	Evaluation is the process whereby you can measure whether or not learning has taken place.
LEARNING	
Learning occurs only when a person is ready to learn	Most women are anxious to learn during pregnancy because they are interested in their pregnancy.
Learning occurs most quickly if the woman can see how the new information will benefit her	Most women learn pregnancy information quickly because they can understand its personal relevance.
Learning occurs best if rewards, not penalties, are offered	Praising a woman for demonstrating that she has learned is more effective than scolding her for not knowing.
People learn best by active participation	Having a woman actually bathe a newborn is better than doing it for her.
People learn best in a non-stressful environment	Teaching a woman breathing exercises for labor during pregnancy is more effective than teaching her during the stress of labor.

Learning ability plateaus	People learn to a point of saturation, then stop. Space teaching to allow for a time of processing before further information can be absorbed.
Learning occurs at widely varied rates and abilities	Teaching must be varied in order to meet the entire range of needs and abilities present in any group.

generally introduce themselves in terms of occupation (listen for "I'm *only* a housewife"; such a woman may need assurance that she is a worthwhile person who is capable of carrying a pregnancy to completion) and sometimes in terms of interests: "Hi, I'm Betty Jones. I'm an accountant. My hobby is making dollhouse furniture."

Introductions are helpful in breaking the ice, and they provide a background for you and the other group members against which to evaluate each other's opinions. Betty Jones, for example, throughout the course, might ask questions like "What costs more, a diaper service or disposable diapers?", "Does anyone here think it's worthwhile to buy an expensive crib?" "How much is the hospital bill likely to be?" As an accountant, she might be oriented toward money, or thoughts gravitating to that value first. Her husband, on the other hand, might express more concern with feelings. He says, "I don't think I could watch my baby being born. I'd be too scared." "Do you think dogs get jealous of new babies?" "Sometimes I wish I were the one who was pregnant."

Listening to introductions and being aware of what values people are placing on things helps you to answer questions more pertinently during the course. When Betty Jones asks the group or you, "Which is better, using or not using an anesthetic?" she may actually mean, "Is there a difference in cost?" Her husband, asking the same question, might mean, "Which is better for the baby?"

If a group member has raised a question that is obviously of interest to the group, the topic should be explored following introductions. If not, a review of female anatomy and the growth of the fetus in utero is a good place to begin. It is always surprising how little many men and women know about their own bodies (how much did you know before you took anatomy and physiology?).

Many old wives' tales will surface during the discussion: Is it true a baby carried in the upper part of the uterus is a boy, and one carried in the lower part is a girl? How do I know the baby is growing where it's supposed to and isn't lost in the abdomen somewhere? Don't women produce an egg for a girl one month, an egg for a boy the

next? How does a baby breathe when it's in all that fluid? These are concerns that mothers-to-be and fathers-to-be carry with them throughout the pregnancy if they do not have an opportunity to voice them and have them clarified.

Lesson 2: Personal Care

A discussion on personal care should begin with the physiologic changes that happen in a woman's body as the basis for changes in personal care. In discussing personal care during pregnancy, you will present material that will be essentially what you give to women at prenatal visits. The difference in parents' classes is that the woman's support person is present, while he may not have been at a prenatal visit. He hears of the need for rest periods, better nutrition, and planned exercises. For couples who go to physicians who do not include teaching as part of prenatal visits, this will be new and extremely welcome information.

Lesson 3: Feelings Toward Pregnancy

It is as important for a male partner to appreciate how a woman feels about being pregnant as it is for him to talk about how *he* feels about her being pregnant. It is equally important for a woman to learn that pregnancy is a stress for her sexual partner as well as for herself.

After it has been brought out by you or the group that pregnancy is a stress period, that wives become irritable and perhaps cry easily, it is not unusual for a man to slump back in his chair, tremendously relieved, and say, "I thought it was something I did. You mean it's normal for her to act that way?"

You may find it easier to talk about the physical aspects of pregnancy, so there is a tendency to omit a class on feelings about pregnancy when planning a program for prospective parents. Remember that parents protect the mental health of the next generation. They cannot do this well unless they themselves are in good mental health. Marital discord is not conducive to sound child-rearing and mental health. Initiating a discussion about the psychological changes in women and men during a pregnancy should help to lay a foundation for better parent-child relations and is a good mental health measure.

Lesson 4: Labor and Delivery

Primiparas are always anxious to have the signs of beginning labor and each step of what they can expect in labor reviewed one more time. They are often worried that they will sleep through labor and deliver the infant at home. Some primiparas arrive at the labor wing of a hospital or an alternative birthing center on the day of delivery completely exhausted because they have been afraid to sleep soundly for the past month. It helps to be reassured that *no one* sleeps through active labor. The alternative settings for delivery should be discussed, being certain that personal preferences do not prejudice the group. These alternatives are discussed along with their advantages and disadvantages in Chapter 26.

Medication in Labor. Most women today are aware that they will have a say about the amount of medication they will be given for discomfort in labor and about the type of anesthesia that will be used for delivery. In order for a woman to be able to make a responsible choice as to whether she wants pain relief in labor or not, she needs to have the options for analgesia and anesthesia explained to her in this class.

More and more women are choosing a prepared method of childbirth so they need little analgesia in labor; your encouragement in this direction should include both the advantages of the woman and her support person being able to participate in labor and the benefits of her child's not receiving drugs. Be sure a woman and her partner understand two general rules of thumb concerning analgesia and labor: Usually, no analgesia is given in labor until the cervix is dilated 3 to 4 cm (so dilatation is not halted). It is also not given if delivery is anticipated within an hour (so the infant will not be affected at birth). With this knowledge, a woman will understand why she cannot always have pain relief at the exact time she wants it during labor. Be certain that women realize that relaxation is one of their greatest assets in the first stage of labor; pushing is reserved for the second stage.

Dilatation and Effacement. It is good to discuss the terms that apply to the progress of labor. Let women know that cervical dilatation is measured by (a) effacement and (b) dilatation. If during labor a physician or nurse-midwife reports that she is making little progress in dilatation, tell her to ask how she is doing in effacement. A positive response prevents her from becoming discouraged because nothing appears to be happening.

Health Care Facility Regulations. Familiarize yourself with the policies of the various settings where the women will deliver. Will the father of the child be allowed in the delivery room? Will he be able to hold the baby immediately after birth? Will she be allowed to breast-feed her baby in the delivery room? Is a birthing room available? Will she be able to have rooming-in in the postpartal period? How soon could she be discharged? Some women are not aware that all these options are available to them; therefore, because they do not ask for them, the women do not receive a form of care they would have liked very much.

Exercises and Breathing Techniques. Every woman should learn muscle-strengthening exercises as well as breathing techniques to limit the amount of discomfort she will have in labor. As indicated, analgesia is not given in labor until the cervix is dilated 3 to 4 cm. Meanwhile, contractions have been bitingly painful for an hour or more. Even when medication is given, it will only take the edge off the pain. Thus, common sense dictates that if a woman can take away the rest of her discomfort by correct breathing patterns she would be foolish to enter labor without learning these patterns.

All women need to learn muscle strengthening exercises during pregnancy in order to strengthen perineal muscles. Women who show an interest in additional types of preparation for labor should be enrolled in a series of classes specifically designed for labor preparation following the completion of expectant parents' classes. A woman should be cautioned that this training is basic preparation for minimizing her discomfort and helping to shorten the length of labor. It will not make her knowledgeable enough to supervise her own labor and delivery. In the event a deviation from the normal occurs, she must be ready and willing to place herself entirely in her physician's or nurse-midwife's hands for both her safety and that of her child.

Lesson 5: The Postpartum Period

The postpartum period does not seem very important when a woman is pregnant. It seems too far away to be real, and her imagination carries her only as far as the day of delivery. It will be helpful to discuss what she can expect in the hours after delivery, however. Knowing that she will stay in a birthing room or go to a recovery room for a period of time and that she will be under close observation there saves both her and her husband unnecessary worry. Knowing that the baby will be taken to a special observation or careful-watch nursery for the first 8 to 12 hours, if that is hospital policy, relieves anxiety about the infant's welfare.

The members of the group will probably be timid at first in discussing what it will feel like to be a new parent. All they can do is project how they think they will feel. In most groups, however, there is at least one person who is sure what it will be like. Remembering that this person said, "I think I'll be *scared.* I think I'll feel so *responsible*" will be reassuring to every couple the day they bring their baby home from the hospital or birthing center or spend the first hour alone with the infant if they deliver at home. They will know that they are experiencing a common apprehension.

Lesson 6: Infant Care

As a woman passes the point of quickening, she becomes interested in childcare. She wants to know the kinds of things she needs to buy and how many of each item should be purchased. She appreciates a baby bath demonstration, as it makes a pregnancy and a coming child seem very real. Thoughts such as "I wouldn't be sitting here watching a woman demonstrate how to bathe a baby unless I'm going to have one, right?" and "I'm really going to have a baby" are going through her mind.

About the fifth month of pregnancy, women make a choice as to whether they will breast-feed or bottle-feed their infants. In order to make an informed decision, they should know all the ramifications of both methods. There is a current feeling that a woman (as well as health care providers) must be either for breast-feeding or against it, as though there were a fence between the two methods and everyone must get firmly on one side or the other. Although you should advocate breast-feeding, be certain that you are not giving off unnecessary signals as to which side of the fence you are on. You can help women make this decision but the woman and her infant are the ones who have to live with it, and it has to be the right one *for them.*

Lesson 7: Plans for Birth

Allow time for open discussion of whatever topic the group chooses. Conclude the evening with a discussion of what the woman will need to take to the hospital or birthing center with her and a tour of a maternity or birthing center or a review of what arrangements a couple will need to make if they plan a home birth (Figure 21-1). In

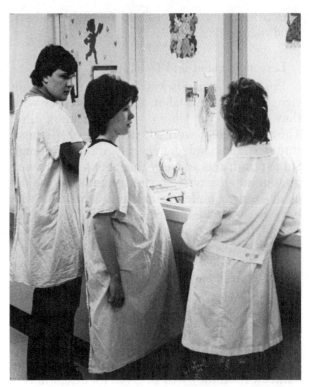

Figure 21-1 *An enjoyable part of a preparation-for-parenthood class is touring a maternity service. (Courtesy Department of Medical Photography, Millard Filmore Hospital, Buffalo, N.Y.)*

some courses the parents might be asked to complete their hospital or birthing center admission forms at the time of a tour. Doing this beforehand prevents the father from having to be separated from the mother at the time of hospital admission.

Lesson 8: Reproductive Life Planning

A review of the various methods of reproductive life planning available is helpful as the last class. Although couples are not yet ready to think about this information at this point, in the immediate postpartal period when it is time to think about it, their minds are so filled with new baby care that they have difficulty making these decisions. Knowing what options are available helps them to make informed decisions. If they choose an option such as having an IUD inserted immediately following delivery, they can alert their physician or nurse-midwife to their preference.

Many couples have difficulty terminating the last class. They put on their coats, yet stand by the doorway, reluctant to say good-bye. They are saying, without words, that the series of meetings was worthwhile; that they were scared, confused, and concerned and now are grateful because you took the time to listen to them and to respect

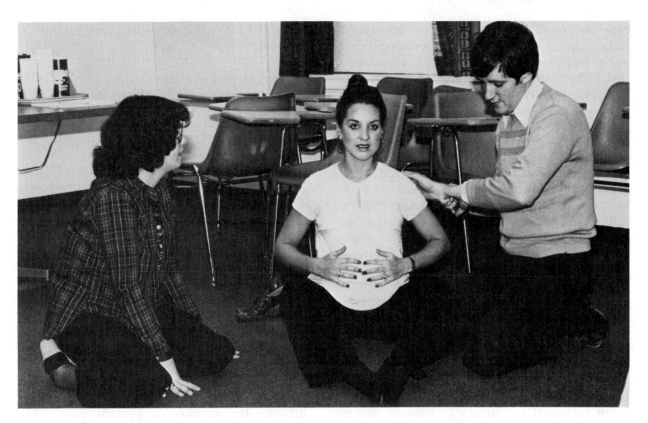

Figure 21-2 *Every woman needs to be well prepared for birth. Here a couple practices breathing patterns in a preparation-for-childbirth class. (Courtesy of the Department of Medical Photography, Children's Hospital, Buffalo, N.Y.)*

their fears. They may leave the meeting room without saying thank you. They are, after all, young, and not fully aware themselves why they are standing there so long. As the women's abdomens have expanded over the past 8 weeks, their self-esteem and their ability to cope with this new experience have grown as well. You have filled an important aspect of health supervision in their lives.

Preparation-for-Childbirth Classes

Preparation-for-childbirth classes are specifically designed to teach a woman and her support person a way to reduce the discomfort of labor contractions so she needs a minimum of analgesic administration (Figure 21-2). Parents who experience labor after one of these classes often find the birth more satisfying and the event more "natural."

Some unfortunate connotations have come to be associated with the term *natural childbirth*. In the 1950s, when almost all women delivered children with a maximum amount of anesthesia, women who chose this method of delivering rather than being administered a general anes-

thetic were labeled "fanatics" or "martyrs." Women who entered labor saying they wanted to deliver naturally, then asked for analgesia or an anesthetic, were "failures." These connotations prevented many women from attending classes in preparation for childbirth. They would have liked to be as prepared for childbirth as possible, to have their child as naturally as possible, to limit discomfort, if possible; on the other hand, they did not want to be trapped into having to "tough it out" if labor contractions were more uncomfortable than they anticipated. It seemed easier just to give up the idea altogether. Today it is generally accepted that being prepared for childbirth is not just a nicety reserved for a very few; it is every woman's right and there is no such thing as "failure."

A great deal of confusion regarding preparation for childbirth classes would be cleared away if the terminology used to describe the process was always consistent. The term *natural childbirth* should be reserved for instances in which a woman wants no analgesic, no anesthetic, no instruments used, no health care personnel in attendance, and no health care facility environment. A woman who chooses to prepare herself for childbirth but still wants to deliver in the secure environment of a hospital or alternative birth center, with health care personnel and safety equipment surrounding her, who agrees that if deviations from the normal occur during labor and delivery she will follow her physician's judgment as to analgesia or anesthesia, is choosing *prepared childbirth.* This term puts matters in the proper perspective. In prepared-childbirth classes, a woman learns exercises to strengthen her pelvic and abdominal muscles and make them more supple and exercises to help her manage her discomfort in labor. She is under no commitment to go a step farther than she wishes. She is not putting her wishes above those of the physician or nurse-midwife or other health care personnel but is only aiding them in helping her to deliver her child safely.

Being prepared for childbirth does not necessarily make childbirth less hazardous as it does not prevent such complications as hemorrhage, infection, and pregnancy-induced hypertension. (Does that trigger a flash of recognition? Those are the three main causes of maternal mortality.) Prepared childbirth may actually call for more labor room personnel in attendance because women who want to participate in their labor but are unsure of themselves need the presence of a competent health care provider as well as their usual support person.

What prepared childbirth does change is the attitude of the labor room nurse from "Bite the bullet" to "Let me show you how you can minimize the bite of that contraction"; or from "You're having a baby, what did you expect?" to "Let me teach you what you can expect."

Exercises for Childbearing

The purposes of doing exercises during pregnancy are to promote comfort, facilitate labor and delivery by allowing for ready stretching of the perineal muscles, and strengthen muscles so that they will revert to their normal condition and functioning quickly and efficiently following childbirth.

A woman may begin exercise periods as early in pregnancy as she likes but most women are not interested in these activities until the time of quickening (because the pregnancy does not seem real until then). Beginning at this midpoint of pregnancy, they are then less inclined to lose interest before delivery and thus defeat the purpose of the exercises they have done. Women who enroll in Lamaze prepared programs generally begin the program and therefore the exercises in the last 6 weeks of pregnancy. Although this time frame is advantageous from the position of learning the

Table 21-1 Safety Precautions for Exercises During Pregnancy

1. Never exercise to a point of fatigue.
2. Always rise from the floor slowly to prevent orthostatic hypotension.
3. To rise from the floor, roll over to the side first and then push up to avoid strain on the abdominal muscles and round ligaments.
4. For leg exercises, to prevent leg cramps, never point the toes (extend the heel instead).
5. Do not attempt exercises that hyperextend the lower back (to prevent muscle strain).
6. Do not hold your breath while exercising as this increases intraabdominal and intrauterine pressure.
7. Do not continue with exercises if any danger signal of pregnancy occurs.
8. Do not practice second-stage pushing. Pushing increases intrauterine pressure and could rupture membranes.

conditioned responses of Lamaze preparation necessary for prepared labor, it has a drawback of also limiting the number of perineal exercises a woman performs.

A woman has to use common sense in exercising. First, she should set aside a specific time each day for the task; otherwise her participation will be sporadic. Initially, she should do each exercise only a few times, gradually increasing the number she does at each session. She should not participate in an exercise program without her physician's or nurse-midwife's approval. She should not attempt exercise if any of the danger signals of pregnancy appear, and she should never exercise to a point of fatigue. Common safety precautions to use for doing exercises in pregnancy are summarized in Table 21-1.

Because many of these exercises can be incorporated into daily activities, they take little time from a woman's day. If practiced during pregnancy, because they strengthen abdominal and perineal muscles, they can make a real difference in the length and the comfort of labor. They can hasten perineal healing and abdominal support following childbirth.

The following exercises are designed to stretch the perineal muscles and to make them more supple. A supple perineum offers less resistance to the fetal head at delivery and is more likely to stretch rather than to tear.

Tailor Sitting

All kindergarten children know how to tailor sit. Women have to be retaught. To do this correctly, so the perineum stretches and blood sup-

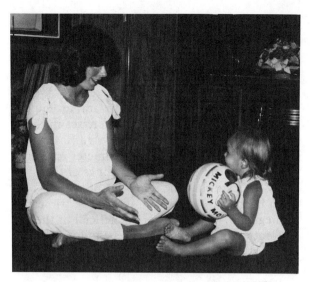

Figure 21-3 *Tailor sitting strengthens the thighs and stretches perineal muscles. Notice that the legs are parallel so that one does not compress the other. A woman should use this position for television watching, telephone conversations, or here, playing with an older child.*

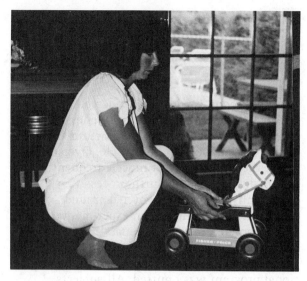

Figure 21-4 *Squatting helps to stretch the muscles of the pelvic floor. Notice that the feet are flat on the floor for optimum stretching.*

ply to the lower legs is not occluded, the woman should not put one ankle on top of the other but should place one leg in front of the other (Figure 21-3). As she sits in this position, she should gently push on her knees (pushing them toward the floor) until she feels her perineum "stretch." This is a good position to use to watch television, to read, or to talk to friends. It is good to plan on sitting in this position for at least 15 minutes every day. By the end of pregnancy, the woman's perineum should be so supple that when she tailor sits her knees will almost touch the floor if pushed to that position.

Squatting

Squatting (Figure 21-4) also stretches the perineal muscles. A woman should practice this position for about 15 minutes a day. Women in nonindustrial cultures squat many times a day—to tend a fire, to pick up a child, to wash vegetables—but women in the United States rarely squat. Most women need a demonstration of squatting. Otherwise, they have a tendency to squat on tiptoes, a more ladylike position. In order for the pelvic muscles to stretch, a woman must keep her feet flat on the floor. A woman can assume this position while watching television, talking on the telephone, reading, or perhaps peeling potatoes. Incorporating squatting into daily activities reduces the amount of time a woman has to devote to her daily exercises.

Pelvic Floor Contractions

Pelvic floor contractions can be done during the course of daily activities as well. While working around the house or sitting at her desk, the woman should tighten the muscles surrounding her urethra, relax, tighten the muscles surrounding the vagina, relax, tighten the muscles surrounding her rectum, relax, tighten her entire perineum, relax. She can repeat this sequence 50 to 100 times daily. Another method is to start to void, then tighten the perineum until the urine stream stops, begin again, stop again. Perineal muscle-strengthening exercises, often called *Kegal's exercises*, are helpful in the postpartum period as well to promote perineal healing, to increase sexual responsiveness, and to help prevent stress incontinence (see the Nursing Research Highlight on page 444).

Abdominal Muscle Contractions

Abdominal muscle contractions help strengthen abdominal muscles during pregnancy and therefore help retain abdominal shape following pregnancy. Strong abdominal muscles contribute to effective second-stage pushing during labor and help to prevent constipation in the postpartal period. These contractions can be done in a standing or lying position along with pelvic floor contractions. A woman merely tightens her abdominal muscles, then relaxes, and she can repeat the exercise as often as she wishes during the day.

Another way to do the same thing is to practice "blowing out a candle." A woman takes a fairly

Nursing Research Highlight

Prenatal Teaching of Kegal's Exercises—Is It Effective?

An experimental study by Henderson (1983) was conducted to evaluate the effectiveness of a prenatal teaching program on postpartum regeneration of the pubococcygeal muscle. Overstretching of the pubococcygeal muscle frequently occurs during the childbirth process. Specifically, this study centered around perineometer readings of an experimental group of 32 women receiving a prenatal teaching program for the use of Kegal's exercises with a control group of 30 women for whom the instructional program was omitted. All subjects received postpartum instruction from a pre-existing program presented by hospital staff. Data analysis suggests that women in the experimen-

tal group who were offered a prenatal teaching program for the use of Kegal's exercises in the third trimester of pregnancy had significantly higher mean postpartum perineometer readings than the control group. The findings of this study indicate that the inclusion of such a program in the care of women in the last trimester of pregnancy would be very beneficial in the restoration of the pubococcygeus following childbirth.

Reference

Henderson, J. S. (1983). Effects of a prenatal teaching program on postpartum regeneration of the pubococcygeal muscle. *J.O.G.N. Nursing, 12*(6), 403.

---

deep inspiration, then exhales normally; then, holding her finger about 12 inches in front of herself as if it were a candle, exhales forcibly, pushing out residual air from her lungs. Try it. You can feel your abdominal muscles contract as you reach the end of your forcible exhalation.

Pelvic Rocking

Pelvic rocking (Figure 21-5) helps to relieve backache during pregnancy and early labor by making the lumbar spine more flexible. It can be done in a variety of positions: on "all fours," lying

Figure 21-5 *Pelvic rocking is helpful in relieving backache during pregnancy and labor. The woman lies on her back and hollows it to lift it off the floor. Her husband checks the exercise here.*

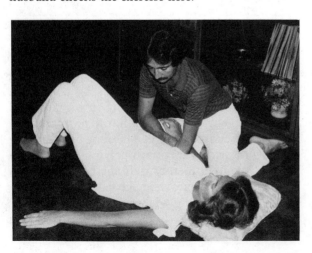

down, sitting, or standing. To do it in a supine position, a woman tightens her buttocks and flattens her lower back against the floor, trying to lengthen or stretch her spine. She holds the position for a minute, then hollows her back or raises the lumbar spine off the floor. The woman should do this exercise at the end of the day about five times to relieve back pain and make herself more comfortable for the night.

Methods of Minimizing the Discomfort of Childbirth

Remember a dance or a celebration in high school that you planned and made paper flowers for by the thousands? Remember staying up all night to help decorate? Were you ever so exhausted and yet so satisfied before or since? Your *active* participation in the event made it meaningful to you. Active participation in childbirth can have the same effect. Prepared childbirth gives a woman the means to participate in the event because she is intellectually, emotionally, and physically involved.

There are a number of approaches to prepared childbirth: The Lamaze, or psychoprophylactic, method is the most popular in the United States. All methods are based on three premises. First, discomfort during labor can be minimized if a woman comes into labor informed about what is happening and prepared with breathing exercises to use during contractions. In classes, therefore, a woman learns about her body's response in labor

Nursing Research Highlight

The Birth Experience— Can It Be Painless?

A newspaper article commenting on painless childbirth in a South India community led Genest (1981) to some interesting research. He reviewed recent studies on pain and psychoprophylaxis in relation to preparation for childbirth. He found that childbirth preparation classes lowered anxiety levels and altered the mothers' assessments of their impending labors. The prepared mother had lowered perceptions of pain and more positive feelings toward birth.

Reference

Genest, M. (1981) Preparation for childbirth—evidence for efficacy. *J.O.G.N. Nursing, 11,* 82.

---

and the mechanisms involved in childbirth and practices breathing exercises during the months of pregnancy prior to delivery. Second, discomfort during labor can be minimized if a woman's abdomen is relaxed and the uterus is allowed to rise freely against the abdominal wall with contractions. Methods differ only in the manner by which they achieve this relaxation. Third, pain perception can be altered by distraction techniques or by a *gating theory* of pain perception.

According to the gate control theory of why people experience pain, as soon as the endings of small peripheral nerve fibers detect a stimulus, they transmit it to cells in the dorsal horn of the spinal cord. Impulses pass through a dense, interfacing network of cells in the spinal cord (substantia gelatinosa) and, immediately, a synapse occurs that returns the transmission to the peripheral site through a motor nerve (you touch a candle flame; the impulse travels to the spinal cord and back, and you lift your hand away from the flame). Following this short-circuit synapse, the impulse then continues in the spinal cord to reach the hypothalamus and cortex of the brain. There, the impulse is interpreted and perceived as pain. Gating mechanisms in the substantia gelatinosa are capable of halting an impulse at the level of the spinal cord so the impulse is never perceived at the brain level as pain—a process similar to closing a gate takes place. You can assist gating mechanisms by three techniques: cutaneous stimulation, distraction, and reduction of anxiety.

Cutaneous Stimulation. If large peripheral nerves next to an injury site are stimulated, the ability of the small nerve fibers at the injury site to transmit pain impulses appears to decrease. Therefore, rubbing an injured part or applying heat or cold to the site are effective maneuvers to suppress pain. Effleurage or light massage used in

the Lamaze method is a form of cutaneous stimulation.

Distraction. If the cells of the brain that register an impulse as pain are preoccupied with other stimuli, a pain impulse will not register. Distraction, or having a person focus on some pattern or action, accomplishes this goal. Different preparation-for-childbirth classes use different breathing techniques or focusing for this purpose.

Reducing Anxiety. Pain impulses are perceived more quickly if anxiety is also present. Thus, the third technique of gating is to reduce patient anxiety as much as possible. Teaching a woman what to expect during labor is a means of achieving this goal (see the Nursing Research Highlight above).

The Lamaze Method (psychoprophylaxis)

The Lamaze or psychoprophylactic method of prepared childbirth is the method most often taught in the United States today. The word *psychoprophylaxis* is a combination of the words describing what is attempted by the method: preventing pain in labor (prophylaxis) by use of the mind (psyche). It is based on the theory that through stimulus-response conditioning women can learn to use controlled breathing automatically and therefore to reduce pain sensation during labor. The method was developed in Russia but was popularized by a French physician, Ferdinand Lamaze. Formal classes are organized by the American Society for Psychoprophylaxis in Obstetrics (ASPO) or the International Childbirth Education Association (ICEA). The most popular book on the subject (*Thank you, Dr. Lamaze*) was written in the 1960s by Marjorie Karmel, who had personally used the method.

When the method was first introduced in the United States in the 1950s, it met with a great deal of resistance from health care personnel. Women themselves objected to what they considered as being placed in the same category as dogs (the experiments of the Russian physiologist Ivan Pavlov with dogs are the basis for psychoprophylactic childbirth).

A woman using this method was perceived by many as a zealot who would be ready to jeopardize her child's health if necessary to prove the worth of the system. She tended to view any health care person who was telling her that she needed an anesthetic for delivery as someone bent on undermining her beliefs rather than a conscientious person trying to explain, for example, that her particular complication (placenta previa) required that forceps and therefore a spinal anesthetic be used for delivery to ensure her child's safety. With people working so far apart from each other and viewing each other as enemies rather than partners in an enterprise, it is a wonder that the method survived. Because of this early negative beginning, you may still hear people say that they do not believe the method is effective or that women coached in the method are stubborn or difficult in labor.

Recent studies document that the Lamaze method of prepared childbirth not only reduces pain in labor but appears to have fetal benefits as well. In a study of 500 patients (Hughey, 1978), Lamaze-prepared women had one fourth the number of cesarean births, one fifth the amount of fetal distress, and one third the number of postpartal infections as control women without Lamaze preparation.

Three main premises are taught these women in the prenatal period: (a) pain does not have to occur with contractions; (b) sensations such as uterine contractions can be inhibited from reaching the brain cortex and registering as pain; and (c) conditioned reflexes are a positive action to use to replace pain sensations in labor. A great deal of time in classes is spent reviewing or teaching reproductive anatomy and physiology and the process of labor and delivery. Thus a couple is familiar with what will happen to the woman in labor and the nature of contractions. The implications for nurses caring for a Lamaze-prepared woman in labor are that the woman is usually very aware of the normal course of labor; she is likewise very aware, when a complication begins to develop, that something out of the ordinary is happening. Women who use a Lamaze method of preparation for childbirth arrive at the hospital in good control of contractions and, because they are so knowledgeable about what is to happen during labor, extremely cooperative and helpful.

Time at classes is also spent on learning conditioned reflexes. While conducting studies of salivation in dogs, Pavlov noticed that every time he put out food for his dogs, the dogs salivated. To learn more about this phenomenon, he tried ringing a bell each time he presented food and found that after a time the dogs salivated at the sound of the bell even when meat was not offered. This is called a *conditioned response.* The same training technique is applied to the birth process in the Lamaze method. A woman is conditioned to relax automatically on hearing a command ("contraction beginning") or on the feel of a contraction beginning. Learning by conditioning is especially applicable to basic simple responses, such as those in childbirth, in which it works wonderfully well.

In order to use the second premise in labor, that sensations coming into the brain can be inhibited from registering, a woman is taught to concentrate on her breathing patterns and focus on a specified object, blocking out other phenomena. The effectiveness of focusing can be observed in athletes who hurt themselves in basketball or football games but do not feel the pain until after the game because of intense concentration on winning. A mother, running to scoop her child away from danger, will manifest the same inhibition phenomenon: she will not even be aware that she has wrenched her ankle in the process of rescuing her child until the child is safe.

In order to use the Lamaze method, the responses to contractions must be recently conditioned to be effective (since conditioned responses die out if not reinforced). It is generally recommended, therefore, that women do not begin classes in this method before the twenty-sixth week of pregnancy. They then continue the classes or at-home practice to the end of pregnancy. Such timing corresponds nicely to that of the psychological nest building that occurs at about the same time.

A woman is required to bring a support person who will act as her coach in labor with her to class. Classes are kept small so there is time for individual instruction attention with each couple. Breathing exercises taught vary from teacher to teacher, especially in terms of complexity, but have common features. Typical exercises taught are the following:

The Cleansing Breath. To begin all breathing exercises, a woman breathes in deeply and then exhales deeply, a "cleansing breath." To end each exercise she repeats this step. It is an important one to take as it limits the possibility of hyperventilation with rapid breathing patterns; it also ensures a full fetal oxygen supply.

Conscious Relaxation. Conscious relaxation is learning to deliberately relax body portions, which prevents a woman from unknowingly remaining tense and causing unnecessary muscle strain and fatigue during labor. She practices relaxation during pregnancy by deliberately relaxing one set of muscles, then another and another until her body is relaxed. A support person concentrates on noticing symptoms of tenseness, such as a wrinkled brow, clenched fists, or a stiffly held arm. By either placing a comforting hand on the tense body area or telling the woman to relax that area, he helps her to achieve relaxation during contractions.

Consciously Controlled Breathing. Breathing exercises involve chest breathing. Shallow breathing done in specific patterns prevents the diaphragm from descending fully and therefore prevents it from putting pressure on the expanding uterus. To practice, a woman lies on her back on the floor with a pillow under her head and a small one under her knees, if she needs it for comfort. She inhales comfortably but fully, then exhales, with her exhalation a little stronger than her inhalation. She practices breathing in this manner at a controlled pace; she uses different breathing rates in labor depending on the intensity of contractions.

1. Level 1, or A, is slow or rhythmic chest breathing. Slow chest breathing consists of comfortable but full respirations at a rate of 7 to 8 breaths per minute (Figure 21-6A). This level is used for early contractions.

2. In level 2, or B, shallow chest breathing is lighter breathing than in level A. The rib cage should expand, but the diaphragm barely moves. The rate of respirations is up to 30 per minute. This is a good level of breathing for contractions when cervical dilation is between 4 to 6 cm (Figure 21-6B).

3. Level 3, or C, breathing is even more shallow, mostly at the sternum. The rate is 50 to 70 breaths per minute. As the respirations become faster, the exhalation should be a little stronger than the inhalation for good air exchange and to prevent hypoventilation. If a woman practices saying "out" with each exhalation, she almost inevitably will make exhalation stronger than inhalation. The woman uses this level for transition contractions. Keeping the tip of her tongue against the roof of her mouth prevents oral mucosa from drying during such rapid breathing.

4. At level 4, or D, the woman uses a "pant-blow" pattern, such as taking three to four quick breaths (in and out), then a forceful exhalation.

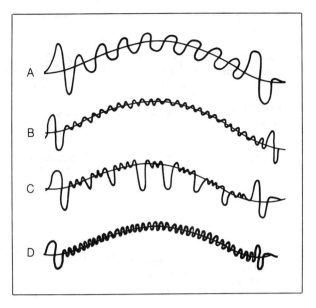

Figure 21-6 *A. Rhythmic chest breathing. B. Shallow chest breathing, 30 per minute. C. Pant-blow breathing. D. Shallow chest panting. Notice the deep cleansing breath at the beginning and end of each type of breathing.*

Because this type of breathing sounds like an imitation of a train (breath-breath-breath-huff), it is sometimes referred to as "choo-choo" breathing (Figure 21-6C).

An alternative method is for the woman to concentrate on a tune inside her head and tap the rhythm on her abdomen, concentrating on nothing but her breathing and the rhythm and the tune.

5. Chest panting is continuous, very shallow panting (Figure 21-6D). It can be used during very strong contractions or during the second stage of labor to prevent the mother from pushing before full dilatation.

Some programs stop at the point a woman has mastered the levels of breathing; others have her learn to shift from one level to another on command, or at the point she feels a need for more pain relief. To do this, at the sound of "contraction beginning," she first takes a cleansing breath, then breathes at 12 breaths a minute; at the sound of "contraction getting harder," 30 breaths a minute; "harder still," 70 breaths a minute, and so on, imitating basic shifts she will use in labor.

Once a woman has learned to do breathing exercises in a reclining position, she needs to practice them standing—while she is doing dishes, cooking, running a duplicating machine. Once labor starts, she should begin to use the technique with the first contraction. The advantage of being able to use it effectively in a standing position is

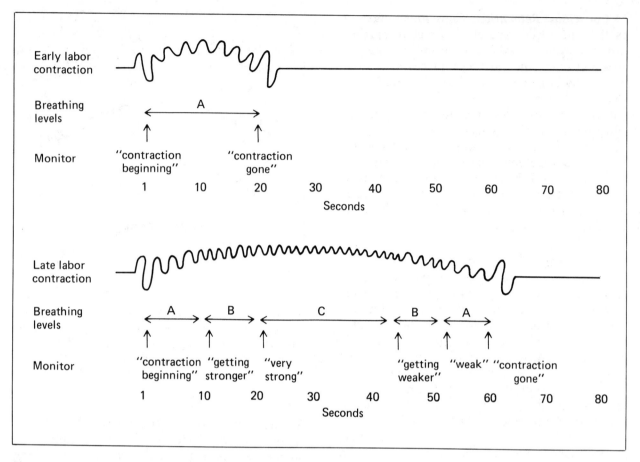

Figure 21-7 *Examples of Lamaze breathing patterns.* A, B, *and* C *are levels of breathing.*

that she can handle her contractions and yet continue with the normal activities that women are engaged in when labor begins (picking up around the house, packing a suitcase, cooking, and so on). She should not save the techniques for use later in labor, when contractions become more intense, since at that time the local tenderness of the uterus and the awareness that contractions are starting to hurt may make it difficult for her to relax. Using breathing with the first contraction is rewarding. It puts a woman immediately in control of a new, potentially frightening situation.

In connection with breathing levels, a woman is taught a role-playing drill for labor. She maintains all her muscles in a state of relaxation except for one specific muscle group, which she contracts. This effort is similar to what she must undertake in labor; when her uterus is contracted, all her other muscles must be relaxed. This type of drill is carried out as follows.

The woman contracts her left arm, and with her coach telling her when to change, takes three breaths of slow chest breathing, then four to six breaths at level 2, then 15 to 20 breaths at level 3.

She then comes down through levels back to slow chest breathing. She practices the same shifting of breath levels using different muscle groups to represent the uterus: the right arm and right leg, the left arm and right leg, the right arm and left leg. A woman who can successfully perform the various levels of breathing and change from one to another on command is prepared to handle all labor contractions up to the pelvic division of labor.

Figure 21-7 illustrates the use of levels of breathing. An early labor contraction is mild. When the contraction begins, the person with the woman (the coach) says, "Contraction beginning." The woman breathes at level A; she feels no bite from the contraction and so does not need to change to a more involved breathing pattern. Later in labor, the contraction is stronger and longer. Now, at the sound of "contraction beginning," the woman begins level A breathing (3 breaths), shifts to level B (4–6 breaths), then to level C (10 breaths). The contraction is lessening. She shifts down to level B (4–6 breaths), then to level A (3–4 breaths). The contraction is gone. Her coach tells her when to shift breathing levels, depending on his estimation of the strength of the

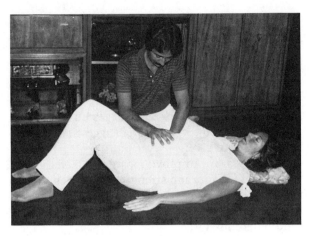

Figure 21-8 *Practicing controlled breathing.*

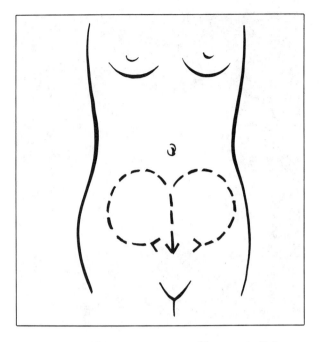

Figure 21-9 *Effleurage patterns. Effleurage is light massage, performed with only enough pressure to avoid tickling. It desensitizes the abdominal skin, in turn relaxing the underlying muscles. During uterine contractions, a woman traces the pattern on her bare abdomen with her fingers.*

contraction: "Contraction beginning, getting stronger, stronger, getting weaker, weaker, almost gone, gone" (Figure 21-8). These words indicate to her when to shift up or down (or she naturally varies rhythm or effort depending on the strength of the contraction she feels). In the space of time before transition, when contractions are longest and strongest, the woman will need to utilize her level D breathing or continuous light panting as well.

A woman needs practice during pregnancy to perfect different levels of breathing. Because of the practice required, this method cannot be taught readily to unprepared women in early labor. Teaching simple abdominal breathing (discussed below), which is easier to master and does not lead to as much hyperventilation, may be better in these situations.

Effleurage. One further exercise in the Lamaze technique is effleurage, which is light abdominal massage, done with just enough pressure to avoid tickling. It is used in connection with breathing levels. To ensure that she is maintaining a steady rhythm for massage, a woman should trace a pattern on her abdomen with her fingertips such as the one shown in Figure 21-9. The rate of effleurage should remain constant, even though breathing rates change. Effleurage decreases sensory stimuli transmission from the abdominal wall and so helps prevent local discomfort. Spreading talcum powder on her abdomen prevents irritation.

Focusing. Focusing intently on an object is another method of keeping sensory input from reaching the cortex of the brain. A woman brings with her into labor a photograph of her sexual partner or children, a graphic design, or just something that appeals to her (Figure 21-10). She con-

centrates on it during contractions. Be careful that you do not step in her line of vision during a contraction and break her concentration.

Pushing. Once the transition stage is over and the pelvic division of labor begins, a woman feels she has to push. She needs no further breathing exercise at this point except to be certain not to hold her breath while she pushes as pushing feels good by itself. Holding her breath is contrain-

Figure 21-10 *A woman chooses what object she wishes to use to focus on during labor. Here, a woman explains the meaning of a chosen picture to a birthing room nurse.*

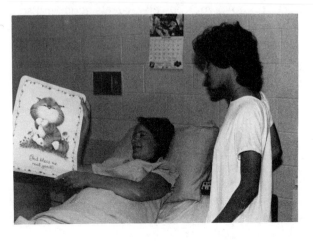

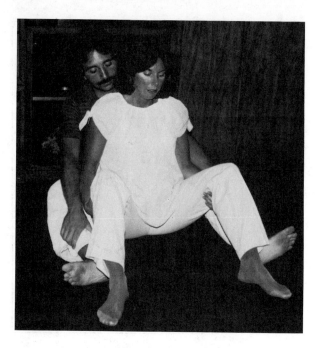

Figure 21-11 *Practicing pelvic division pushing. Note the woman's open mouth as she breaths out to avoid a Valsalva maneuver. Caution women not to really push with practice during pregnancy; the increase in intrauterine pressure could possibly rupture membranes.*

dicated as this increases intrathoracic pressure and prevents good blood return from the vena cava (a Valsalva maneuver). She should, instead, continually breathe out as she pushes (Figure 21-11). This can be practiced in class except that the woman should not actually push (an increase in intrauterine pressure could rupture fetal membranes). When the fetus is at the pelvic floor close to delivery, it is better for a woman not to push if the baby's head is to be born easily, between contractions. In order to stop pushing, the woman may need to pant (small, short breaths that prevent her from using her abdominal muscles to push). The sensation of pushing can be compared to the sensation you feel when you have a strong urge to move your bowels; it feels good, and so it is almost impossible not to push. Panting must be shallow, or the woman will hyperventilate, become dizzy, and may even faint. Panting, like active pushing, is an activity that can be taught when it is needed.

The typical content of a series of Lamaze classes is shown below:

Class One. The first class generally begins with an introduction of couples to each other and a review of the course objectives by the instructor. Stressed is the concept that the goal of classes is to make childbirth a satisfying experience and

that there is no failure in prepared childbirth. Anatomy and physiology of the reproductive system and the process of pregnancy from fertilization to term are reviewed. Common discomforts of pregnancy such as constipation, backache, and urinary frequency are reviewed and tips on avoiding the problems are suggested. Nutrition for pregnancy is reviewed and suggestions for improving it are given.

Exercises to improve posture, decrease the chance of fatigue, and strengthen muscles used in labor—such as Kegal's exercises, pelvic rocking, and tailor sitting—are discussed, demonstrated, and redemonstrated.

A number of neuromuscular control exercises to introduce the concept of concentration-relaxation are explained, demonstrated, and practiced. A major goal early in teaching is to increase a woman's ability to respond to verbal commands and to establish a feeling of close communication between her and her support person who will coach her in labor.

Class Two. For the second class, exercises for body strengthening and neuromuscular control are reviewed and the woman and her support person are moved a step further by means of a presentation of the stages of labor. Following this, a breathing technique (slow chest breathing) to be used in the first stage of labor and effleurage are introduced, demonstrated, and practiced.

Class Three. For a third class, stages of labor and the principles of breathing with contractions using effleurage are reviewed. Other breathing patterns that allow a woman to accelerate and decelerate breathing and panting during the delivery phase of labor are demonstrated and practiced. Variations of labor (such as back labor) and how to avoid and correct hyperventilation are stressed.

Class Four. Class four begins with the usual review of past material. More variations of breathing, such as pant-blow, are taught. Pushing without holding the breath is included, as are effective measures to decrease the length of the second stage of labor such as maintaining a semi-Fowler's position or squatting. Women should not practice pushing during pregnancy: Increased abdominal pressure can cause enough intrauterine pressure to possibly rupture membranes.

Class Five. For the fifth class, past material is reviewed and questions are answered; new material concerning analgesia and anesthesia, other variations such as malpresentations, forceps delivery, cesarean birth, and the role of fetal and uterine monitoring is introduced. The use of a uterine monitor can be helpful for the prepared woman in labor, because it can help to alert her when a contraction is beginning (a monitor registers uterine tightening before she feels the tightening).

Class Six. For a final class, a complete run-through of a simulated labor and delivery is staged. Events of the postpartal period are presented. The role of breast-feeding in the immediate postpartal period and uterine involution are also included.

The Psychosexual Method

The psychosexual method of childbirth was developed by Sheila Kitzinger in England during the 1950s. The method stresses that pregnancy, labor, delivery, and the early newborn period are all important continuing points in a woman's life cycle. It includes a program of conscientious relaxation and levels of progressive breathing that encourage a woman to "flow with" rather than "struggle against" contractions of labor.

The Wright Method

Erna Wright described a method of prepared childbirth in her 1966 text *The New Childbirth.* The Wright method focuses on conscious relaxation techniques and progressive chest-breathing exercises. Stressed is the ability of a woman to prepare herself for childbirth with the aid of a support person or by herself; therefore, no matter what the circumstances of labor, she will be able to reduce discomfort.

The Dick-Read Method

The Dick-Read method is based on the approach proposed by Grantly Dick-Read, an English physician. Although this method of reducing pain in labor was proposed by Dr. Dick-Read as early as the 1930s, twenty years passed before it became accepted as a workable method of pain reduction in labor. The premise of the method is that fear leads to tension, which leads to pain. If you can prevent this chain of events from occurring, or break the chain between fear-tension or tension-pain, you can reduce the pain of childbirth contractions.

Relaxation during labor, therefore, is an important part of the Dick-Read method. Most labor rooms during the 1950s were structured for this approach to childbirth; some hospital labor rooms still retain this decor. The rooms were non-stimulating (few accessories, plain walls), as a woman was expected to rest or even sleep be-

tween contractions. A support person does not have a major role in this method because a woman can begin the breathing pattern by herself and rests between contractions. The presence of a support person in the room is still comforting, however. Although not as popular a method of instruction for prepared childbirth as the Lamaze method in the United States today, the Dick-Read breathing techniques are often easier to teach to women who appear at the door of a labor room totally unprepared; being familiar with the method allows you to give them some quick help in labor.

Whole-Body Relaxation Exercise. A relaxation position that is generally taught during pregnancy is a modified Sims' position. A woman lies on her side, with a pillow under her head. She allows the weight of her abdomen to rest against the mattress or floor. No body part should rest on another, but each should be supported by the mattress or floor. In order to become thoroughly relaxed, a woman practices contraction and relaxation similar to that initiated in Lamaze preparation. With all muscle groups relaxed, many women can fall instantly asleep in this position. They can use the technique during labor to sleep or nap between contractions to prevent exhaustion.

After resting in this position, a woman should never rise quickly or she will become extremely light-headed and dizzy. To rise from the floor after practice, she should first push herself up onto her hip with her hand and elbow, then over onto her hands and knees, then finally up onto her feet. This should be done slowly, as in a slow-motion film.

When caring for a woman who has been prepared for labor by the Dick-Read method, you will generally find that she assumes this position between contractions. The drawback is that you cannot hear the fetal heart sounds with the woman in this position. If you are going to auscultate for the sounds with a stethoscope, you may have to ask the woman to turn on her back.

Some women dislodge an external fetal heart monitor as they turn to this position. If a woman has been taught to use the position, however, it is important to encourage her to maintain it. It reduces pressure from the uterus against the vena cava and actually is the preferred position for all women in labor.

Abdominal Breathing. Abdominal breathing is the form of distraction that women are taught by a Dick-Read method. Abdominal breathing not only prevents a woman from tensing her

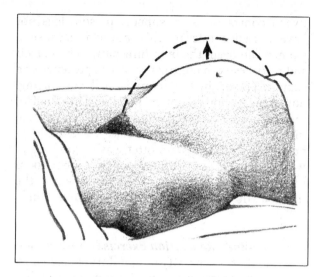

Figure 21-12 *Abdominal breathing. When a woman inhales using her abdominal muscles, she can feel her abdominal wall rise.*

whole body (because she is busy concentrating on what she is doing) but also forces the abdominal muscles to rise, giving the uterus room to rise freely and easily with a contraction and maintaining a good blood supply to the uterus. (One theory proposed to account for the pain of contractions is that contractions cause ischemia of the uterus and thus pain, in the same way that poor lower extremity circulation causes ischemia of a leg and leg cramps.) Removing the pressure of the abdominal wall also prevents the uterus from bumping against it with each contraction, presumably reducing local tenderness and so pain.

To do abdominal breathing, a woman lies on her back and inhales slowly, using her abdominal muscles. If she is truly using them, her abdominal wall will rise with the inhalation. She then exhales slowly, allowing the abdominal wall to return gradually to its normal position (Figure 21-12). When a woman first begins to learn abdominal breathing, she finds she can breathe this way for only about 20 seconds (a 10-second inhalation and a long, sustained 10-second exhalation). (Try it. Unless you are an accomplished swimmer, you will find it hard work to maintain abdominal control longer than 20 seconds.)

If a woman begins doing this exercise 10 times a day at about the fifth month of pregnancy, by the end of pregnancy she will be able to maintain a well-paced 30-second inhalation and a well-paced 30-second exhalation. The inhalation-exhalation time should be built up gradually during pregnancy: 20 seconds total time (inhalation and exhalation) the first week; 25 seconds the fol-

lowing week; 30 the third week, and so on until the total time is 60 seconds. She should count as she breathes, so that she knows it is taking 60 seconds. A woman has to concentrate on exhaling steadily; this is hard to do and there is a tendency to hurry it.

In early labor, the total length of uterine contractions is about 20 seconds. As labor increases in intensity, the contractions grow longer, ultimately 50 to 60 seconds. Thus, a woman who can handle a 60-second controlled breath can reduce discomfort in labor up through transition, until she experiences the welcome and wonderful compulsion to push with contractions. Abdominal breathing up to 70 seconds' duration gives a woman extra assurance that she will be able to handle her longest contractions. However, few women can achieve this much control. While the woman is learning this technique, it is important that she put her hand on her abdomen and actually feel the abdominal wall rise. Otherwise, she cannot be sure that she is breathing correctly.

Abdominal breathing can be taught to a woman who comes into labor totally unprepared as an emergency method of reducing labor discomfort. However, a woman so taught is not able, without practice, to maintain more than a 20-second total breath. By the time she arrives at the hospital, she is already tense and frightened and dreads the next contraction so much that she may have difficulty relaxing enough to give the method a fair try. Although she can do no more than 20-second breaths, she can lengthen their period of effectiveness by attempting to repeat the abdominal breathing pattern immediately after finishing one cycle. This is difficult to do, because as she finishes her first breath, the contraction is still strong. Thus, she may be unable to keep her mind on concentrated breathing and inhale regularly again. Such a woman needs a support person with her.

Abdominal breathing patterns are diagrammed in Figure 21-13.

The Bradley Method (husband-coached)

The Bradley method of childbirth (originated by Dr. Robert Bradley in the 1960s and described in the book *Husband Coached Childbirth*) is based on the premise that childbirth is a joyful, natural process. The important role of the husband during pregnancy, labor, and the early newborn period is stressed. During pregnancy a woman performs muscle-toning exercises and limits or omits foods that contain preservatives, animal fat, or a high salt content. Pain is reduced in labor by abdominal breathing similar to the

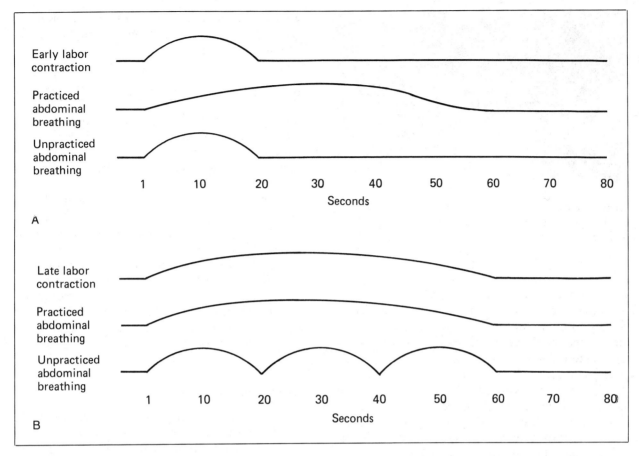

Figure 21-13 *Abdominal breathing patterns. A. The woman who practiced before childbirth and uses practiced abdominal breathing can effectively breathe through contractions. B. A woman who learns the technique in labor (unpracticed abdominal breathing) will still be able to reduce the discomfort of contractions.*

Dick-Read method. In addition, the woman is encouraged to walk during labor and to use an internal focus point as a dissociation technique.

The Bradley method is used widely in some areas of the United States or at specific centers. A woman who needs internal fetal monitoring will have difficulty ambulating following insertion of the monitor and you may need to assure the woman that her breathing exercises can be just as effective in a reclining position.

Preparation for Cesarean Birth

The fact that cesarean birth may be necessary in order to ensure a safe delivery is covered in most preparation-for-childbirth classes. A woman who knows that she is to have a cesarean birth (due to a pelvic abnormality or because she is a candidate for a repeat cesarean birth) needs specific preparation. Because part of the getting ready is prepara-

tion for the surgery itself, this topic is discussed in Chapter 42.

General Rules for Supporting a Woman in Labor

The types of prepared childbirth that are taught vary from community to community, and the complexity of different types of preparation varies within a community. No matter which prepared childbirth method a woman is using, general rules for helping her during labor apply (Figure 21-14).

Eating

Women are usually cautioned not to eat once they begin labor, which prevents vomiting and aspiration in the event a general anesthetic has to be used to ensure a safe delivery. Women using a

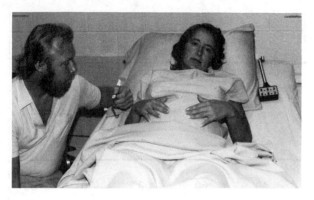

Figure 21-14 *Using prepared childbirth in labor. A coach times contractions; the woman is using a light effleurage technique.*

prepared technique, however, have often been instructed to continue to eat, or at least to drink, during labor in order to maintain their energy level; sips of orange juice, oranges, and lollipops are suggested for maintaining a good energy level. These suggestions are not out of line in the healthy woman who anticipates being able to complete labor as she planned without surgical interruption. Probably all women need calories during labor. Why not provide them with lollipops instead of the traditional ice chips?

Occasionally a woman eats a full meal when she realizes that she is in labor as a deliberate means of preventing a physician from using a general anesthetic. This method of manipulation should be thoroughly discouraged: Digestion slows during labor and no woman can be certain that a general anesthetic will not be necessary. Eating a complete meal early in labor appears to be an unnecessary handicap to a physician. Any woman who does not trust her physician's judgment and fears an unwarranted general anesthetic will be "sneaked in" on her should use the more positive approach of changing physicians.

Rest and Sleep

Remember that a woman prepared by the Lamaze method is taught not to rest between contractions, but instead to be alert and ready to respond to her next contraction. She will want the lights on, possibly a radio on. Do not urge her to rest or sleep. She may not even want to lie down, since she may incorporate a pant-blow type of breathing for contractions just before transition that involves her sitting upright. She may want to walk during early labor or sit on the floor with her head resting on a chair seat. She may feel most in control if she squats. Teach the woman how to read

the uterine monitor if one is in place to alert her to a beginning contraction long before she can tell by a hand on her abdomen.

Respect for the Role of a Labor Coach

A further role of the nurse during labor is supporting the coach. Do not take over when he is hesitant. Instead, teach him or review with him what to do. Compare this situation with a nursing instructor doing something you want to do rather than taking the time to show you how to do it.

Orient a couple to the unit, and point out where supplies such as towels and washcloths and ice chips a coach might need are stored so he can get them as necessary. Review procedure for the delivery room so he can be assured early in labor that he will be welcome there. Offer praise not only for the woman but for the coach. Relieve a coach as necessary so he can get something to eat or visit with older children.

Offer Support as a Coach

Women who write articles on Lamaze childbirth in women's magazines invariably begin their articles with "Labor began when my husband, who was to serve as my coach, was out of town." The article then recites page after page of unkind, unsympathetic, or ill-mannered statements made to them during labor by nurses. When a woman is depending on a support person to be with her, not only because of the novelty of the experience (lying on the living room rug practicing contractions is *not* the same as having the real labor contractions), but also because she believes his presence will enable her to reduce labor pain—and then that person is not available—surely everything that comes after that moment could easily be viewed as unkind, unsympathetic, and ill-mannered.

A Lamaze coach, however, can be *anyone* who knows the methods and the correct words to say. Every nurse who works on a labor unit should be as skilled in the technique as she is at listening to fetal heart sounds. Often, if a woman has to be admitted without her coach, a course instructor will come if requested. If not, offer your services. If a woman has forgotten to bring her focusing object with her, help her to find a substitute one, such as a drawing of a baby from a teaching aid. Ask her what specific words her husband or coach uses as "breathing cues." Stay with her and say them: "Contraction beginning, contraction getting stronger, stronger, on the top, getting weaker now, still weaker. That's it. Contraction gone."

The words are not magic or complicated. Being able to assist a woman in labor is not magic or complicated. It is merely demonstrating the essence of nursing: caring and concern.

Respect Contraction Time

It is important not to interrupt women doing exercises in labor. Once their concentration is disrupted, they feel the bite of the contraction, and when they have been using breathing exercises and so reducing pain sensations, suddenly feeling the real force of a contraction is frightening. The woman tenses, the pain becomes worse as she becomes more frightened, and she may doubt her ability to breathe constructively in the face of such sharp pain. Allow a woman to finish breathing with her contraction, then ask your question or announce what procedure you need to do next. Or ask your question, but wait patiently for 60 seconds for the answer.

Prevent Hyperventilation

Hyperventilation is a state of respiratory alkalosis that occurs when a woman exhales more deeply than she inhales ("blows off") extra carbon dioxide. This situation can occur when a woman is practicing breathing exercises in preparation for labor but is more apt to occur during actual labor. She feels light-headed and may have tingling or numbness in her toes and fingertips. If allowed to progress, hyperventilation can cause coma.

To correct hyperventilation, a woman should be taught to practice breathing exercises with a paper bag nearby. She can correct symptoms of hyperventilation by breathing in and out into the paper bag. This technique causes her to rebreathe the carbon dioxide she exhales and so replaces the amount lost. If a paper bag is not available, she can use her cupped hands.

The best means of handling hyperventilation is to prevent it from occurring. Be certain that when women are breathing rapidly they are not hyperventilating. Be certain they end all breathing sessions with a long, cleansing breath that helps to restore carbon dioxide balance.

Respect Supplies

Many childbirth education instructors advise couples to pack a bag of supplies to bring to a hospital or birthing center for use during labor (often referred to as a "goody" bag—Figure 21-15). Typical supplies are shown in Table 21-2. Be certain that a coach and the woman know that these same supplies are available on a labor unit or at a

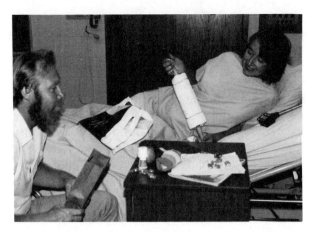

Figure 21-15 *A couple in early labor unpacking a "goody" bag of supplies for labor.*

birthing center if they should arrive without them.

Do Not Expect Prepared Childbirth to Achieve Miracles

Some women believe that, by using a prepared childbirth method, they will have a totally painless labor. When they realize that this hope is not going to be totally realized, they panic and then are unable to use their breathing preparations. Some coaches are far too nervous during labor to be the supportive person they imagined they would be, and a woman may be more nervous than she thought she would be in labor. In order to reduce anxiety or take the edge off of contractions, an injection of meperidine (Demerol) might be effective. With this degree of relaxation, a woman is then able to return to effective breathing exercises. In other instances, simply the support of a person like yourself—someone confident that breathing can be effective in reduc-

Table 21-2 Supplies to Prepare for Labor

Chapstick—for dry lips
Mouthwash—for rinsing dry mouth
Toothbrush and toothpaste—for dry mouth
Warm socks—comfort
Small rolling pin covered with soft cloth—back massage
Focal point—to increase concentration
Busy work (knitting, magazines)—to pass time
Paper bag—to prevent hyperventilation
Extra pillow—for semi-Fowler's position in labor
Watch—for timing contractions
Talc—for reducing friction of effleurage
Lollipops—for energy and dry mouth
Snacks (apples, potato chips)—for coach

ing the discomfort of labor—is all a woman needs to use her preparation effectively.

The time will come when *all* women will participate in some kind of prepared childbirth. This prediction does not imply that all women will lie in birthing rooms and breathe with their contractions in special ways. All women should not be expected to react this way during childbirth anymore than all women should be expected to react the same way to any stress situation. All women should be offered the option of prepared child-birth, however, so that those who want to use these techniques and participate actively in the birth of their children can do so. Women who come to a hospital ready to use these techniques in labor should have the support of health care personnel. Nurses who are serving as community instructors and nurses in the hospital and birthing centers need to work in harmony, so that each knows what the other is doing. Such cooperation would benefit both parents and the children about to be born.

Utilizing Nursing Process

Nursing care for a laboring woman must be designed with careful thought in order that labor can be a fulfilling experience for her and her support person.

Assessment

All women should attend a preparation-for-childbirth program during pregnancy so they can learn the normal processes of labor and can prepare themselves as much as they choose for labor. Some women may be too frightened by the thought of labor to really hear what is told them, however, and some women assume that attending the classes will be enough and so do not practice exercises. They arrive at a health care facility in labor with no real ability to use breathing preparations. Assess each woman individually for what she wants to know about labor and how well prepared she actually is.

Analysis

The Fourth Annual Conference on Nursing Diagnoses accepted no diagnosis specific to labor preparation. The nursing diagnosis "Knowledge deficit related to preparation for childbirth" is a common one used. Be certain when setting goals with a woman concerning labor preparation or knowledge deficit that the goals are realistic for her. Not all women want to participate in childbirth; they might prefer to accept a level of analgesic as a means of comfort in labor.

Planning

Planning for preparation for childbirth should include an individual woman's needs. Some women learn better in groups, some individually. If a woman is going to use a childbirth preparation that requires a support person to be with her, she may need to make plans for an alternative person if there is a possibility her main support person will be unavailable at the time of labor.

Implementation

Preparation-for-childbirth methods differ among sections of the country, especially in the complexity of breathing exercises taught. Being certain that such programs are offered and adequate support for women in labor who want to use such preparation is available are nursing responsibilities. Always try to reinforce the method a woman has already learned; if at all possible, do not try to teach a new method during labor.

Evaluation

Evaluation of whether a woman is adequately prepared for childbirth should be carried out during the last prenatal visits before labor. If a woman arrives in labor without good preparation, it may be possible to refresh or review the breathing patterns she learned in order to make them effective. If she is totally unprepared, teaching abdominal breathing may be the most efficient method for instant preparation.

Nursing Care Planning

Christine McFadden is a 15-year-old you meet in a prenatal clinic.

Assessment

Patient states, "I'm really scared thinking about labor but I don't want to take a course if I'm going to end up having a c-section" (possible because of small pelvic size).

Analysis

Lack of preparation for labor related to lack of interest.

Locus of Decision Making. Shared.

Goal. Patient will be familiar with process of birth by thirty-sixth week of pregnancy.

Criteria. Patient will:

1. Voice knowledge of normal process of labor and delivery.
2. Perform muscle-strengthening exercises for postpartal healing.
3. Be familiar with anesthetic options and cesarean birth process by thirty-sixth week of pregnancy.

Nursing Orders

1. Encourage Kegal's exercises and abdominal strengthening exercises at prenatal visits.
2. Include labor and delivery information in prenatal discussion at thirtieth week of pregnancy as no formal class will be taken.
3. Include newborn expectations and care at thirty-sixth week of pregnancy.
4. Mention possibility of more preparation or a specific cesarean preparation program later in pregnancy in hopes she changes her attitude toward preparation.

———————

Mary Kraft is a 23-year-old you meet in an obstetrician's office.

Assessment

Patient states, "Both my husband and I want to know everything we can learn about labor. I want to use a prepared method. He wants to be there for the whole thing."

Analysis

Knowledge deficit related to preparation for childbirth.

Locus of Decision Making. Patient.

Goal. Patient and husband will both be well-informed, active participants in labor and delivery.

Criteria. Patient:

1. Can voice normal patterns of labor and delivery and means to control pain of labor.
2. To complete formal preparation course.

Nursing Orders

1. Explain differing preparation-for-childbirth courses available to couple.
2. Patient to call if any difficulty enrolling in chosen course.
3. Provide discussion space at prenatal visits for questions that may arise from course information.
4. Mark chart for M.D. discussion of analgesia and anesthesia as couple want to be well informed, but probably will not use in labor.

———————

Angie Baco is a 42-year-old you meet at a prenatal clinic.

Assessment

Patient states, "I want as much medicine as possible in labor, so I'm as sleepy as possible." Husband expresses no interest in seeing child born. States, "I didn't see any of the others."

Analysis

Knowledge deficit related to modern preparation for childbirth options.

Locus of Decision Making. Patient.

Goal. Patient will be prepared within the limits acceptable to her by thirty-sixth week of pregnancy.

Criteria. Patient will:

1. Voice full range of options, including a prepared childbirth method.
2. Express satisfaction in chosen level of participation in labor.

Nursing Orders

1. Discuss full range of preparation options for labor beginning at next visit.
2. Include labor and delivery information in prenatal visits at thirtieth week of pregnancy if no formal class will be taken.
3. Encourage Kegal's exercises and abdominal strengthening exercises at prenatal visits.
4. Mark chart for M.D. discussion of analgesia and anesthesia for labor if patient desires to use medication in labor.

Questions for Review

Multiple Choice

1. Mrs. Madison is a woman interested in preparation for childbirth. She asks you why you stress tailor sitting as an exercise for pregnancy. Your best response would be that it

   a. improves the blood supply to the uterus.
   b. strengthens abdominal muscles.
   c. decreases respiratory effort.
   d. stretches perineal muscles.

2. Pelvic rocking during pregnancy

   a. should hurt or it will not be effective.
   b. stretches perineal muscles.
   c. relieves backache.
   d. may cause mild abdominal cramping.

3. To teach Mrs. Madison to do Kegal's exercises, you would teach her to

   a. practice starting and stopping a urine stream.
   b. clasp her hands on her abdomen and push.
   c. tighten perineal muscles and hold for 10 seconds.
   d. tighten abdominal muscles while whistling.

4. A rule for exercising in pregnancy you would want Mrs. Madison to be aware of is that

   a. she should expect to feel abdominal pain with exercises.
   b. she should not point her toes while exercising.
   c. she should include pushing as an exercise.
   d. she should not do abdominal strengthening exercises.

5. Mrs. Madison is going to take a Lamaze preparation-for-childbirth course. Which of the following statements is a principle of Lamaze preparation?

   a. Abdominal breathing allows the uterus to expand freely.
   b. Distraction aids pain reception in the brain cortex.
   c. Chest breathing prevents the diaphragm from descending.
   d. Labor can be made pain-free.

6. Which of the following is true concerning Lamaze preparation?

   a. A cleansing breath is taken every 10 minutes.
   b. A woman should eat a full meal to provide energy in labor.
   c. Kegal's exercises should not be used as part of preparation.
   d. Conditioned response training is started late in pregnancy.

7. If Mrs. Madison experiences symptoms of tingling and dizziness while doing breathing exercises, you would teach her to

   a. rebreathe using her hands cupped.
   b. exhale more forcibly with each breath.
   c. ask for oxygen supplementation.
   d. exhale into a paper bag.

8. Mrs. Madison's husband wants to act as her coach during labor. You would explain a coach's role as

   a. an important participant in a successful labor.
   b. an observer who must take careful notes.
   c. a person convenient for furnishing supplies.
   d. an auxiliary person to assist as necessary.

9. Mrs. Madison also is planning to take an expectant parents' class during pregnancy. Material you would expect her to learn from this course would be

   a. chest-breathing exercises to use in labor.
   b. beginning newborn care.
   c. how to use a uterine monitor during labor.
   d. ways to use abdominal breathing.

Discussion

1. The acceptance of prepared childbirth by nurses in the United States was slow in coming. What are some reasons for this?
2. A coach in labor can easily feel unwelcome on a busy maternity service. What are definite ways you could make such a person feel welcome?
3. Preparation for parenthood classes vary depending on the individual people in attendance. What modifications would you make if a class was mostly teenage girls? Career women?

Suggested Readings

Bernau, K. M., et al. (1983). Integrating parent education into the hospital setting: A childbirth education program. *M.C.N.*, 8, 13.

Christiani, K. (1983). Training for childbirth. *Nursing Times*, 79, 58.

Cogan, R., et al. (1982). Effect of childbirth education communication skills training on postpartum reports of parents. *Birth and Family Journal*, 9, 241.

Cogan, R. (1983). Variations in the effectiveness of childbirth preparation. *Perinatal Press*, 7, 51.

Croft, C. A. (1982). Lamaze childbirth education: Im-

plications for maternal-infant attachment. *J.O.G.N. Nursing*, 11, 333.

Dick-Read, C. (1972). *Childbirth without fear: The original approach to natural childbirth*. (4th ed.). H. Wessel and H. F. Ellis (Eds.). New York: Harper & Row.

Dzurec, L. C. (1981). Childbirth education: Childbirth educators . . . are they helpful? *M.C.N.*, 6, 329.

Fawcett, J. (1981). Needs of Cesarean birth parents. *J.O.G.N. Nursing*, 10, 372.

Hughey, M. J. (1978). Maternal and fetal outcome of

Lamaze prepared patients. *Obstetrics and Gynecology, 51,* 653.

Jimenez, S. M., et al. (1979). Prenatal classes for repeat parents: A distinct need. *M.C.N., 4,* 305.

Kitzinger, S. (1979). *Education and counseling for childbirth.* New York: Schocken.

McCraw, R. K., et al. (1981). Selection factors involved in the choice of childbirth method. *Issues in Health Care of Women, 3,* 359.

McCraw, R. K., et al. (1982). Motivation to take childbirth education: Implications for studies of effectiveness. *Birth and Family Journal, 9,* 179.

Manderino, M. A., et al. (1984). Effects of modeling and information on reactions to pain: A childbirth preparation analogue. *Nursing Research, 33,* 9.

Melzack, R., et al. (1984). Severity of labor pain: Influence of physical as well as psychologic variables. *Canadian Medical Association Journal, 130,* 579.

Meredith, S. (1983). Natural childbirth. *Midwife Health Visitor and Community Nurse, 20,* 228.

Moore, D. (1983). Prepared childbirth and marital satisfaction during the antepartum and postpartum periods. *Nursing Research, 32,* 73.

Roberts, J. E. (1983). Factors influencing distress from pain during labor. *M.C.N., 8,* 62.

Shearer, M. (1981). Teaching prenatal exercise: Posture. *Birth and Family Journal, 8,* 105.

Shrock, P., et al. (1981). Teaching prenatal exercises. *Birth and Family Journal, 8,* 167.

Sweet, P. T. (1979). Prenatal classes especially for children. *M.C.N., 4,* 82.

Vinal, D. F. (1982). Childbirth education programs: A study of women participants and non-participants. *Birth and Family Journal, 9,* 183.

Webster-Stratton, C., & Kogan, K. (1980). Helping parents parent. *American Journal of Nursing, 80,* 240.

Whitley, N. (1979). A comparison of prepared childbirth couples and conventional prenatal class couples. *J.O.G.N. Nursing, 8,* 109.

V

The Period of Parturition

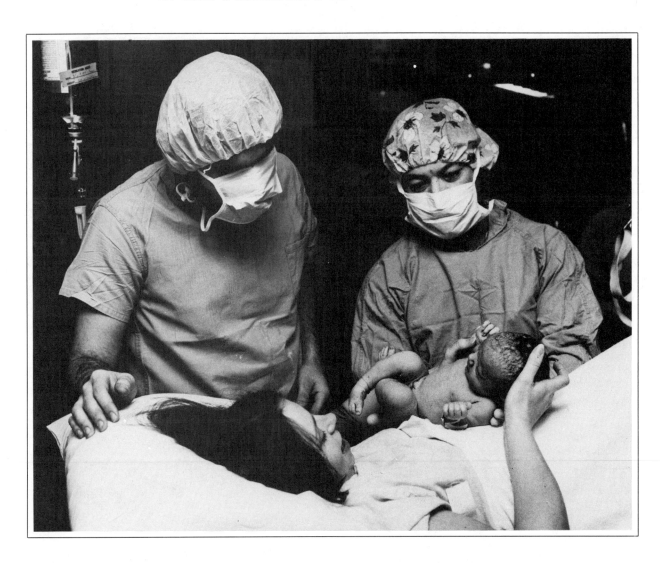

22

Psychological Aspects of Labor

OBJECTIVES

Following mastery of the contents of this chapter, you should be able to

1. Describe the common psychological phenomenon of "readiness for labor" that occurs at the end of pregnancy.
2. Describe common psychological reactions to labor.
3. Assess the woman for psychological changes that occur as labor progresses.
4. State a nursing diagnosis related to psychological aspects of labor.
5. Plan care to meet the changing emotions that occur with labor.
6. Implement care to reduce stressors and make labor a satisfying emotional experience for a woman and her family.
7. Evaluate goal criteria to see if goals were accomplished.
8. Analyze strategies of care that support the psychosocial reactions during labor.
9. Synthesize knowledge of psychosocial aspects of labor with nursing process to achieve quality maternal-newborn nursing care.

FEAR OF THE UNKNOWN is a universal fear, and labor is an unknown. Whether a pregnancy is the first, second, or fifth a woman has experienced, it is the first time she has been in labor with that child. Even though it may not be her first labor, then, it is still an unknown.

There are countless stories about how awful labor is. A woman who discovered that labor was not all bad with a first birth may begin to worry, therefore, that she experienced the exception, not the rule, her first time. She may fear her next labor will surely be a horrible one.

Not only is labor an unknown, but for most healthy women a hospital admission or an overnight stay in a birthing center to have a baby is their first health care facility admission. Sights and sounds that are routine to other types of hospital patients, such as gatch controls for beds,

call-light buttons, or the rattle of a food tray in the hallway, are strange. A woman needs comprehensive care so she can be assured that, although she is in a strange place and what is happening to her internally feels strange, she is not among strangers.

Readiness for Labor

A woman's readiness for labor has a great deal to do with how she perceives labor. At the time of quickening, women begin to view being pregnant in a positive light. They begin the psychological work of thinking of themselves as pregnant, of adjusting to their changing body image. They begin to like the sensation of seeing themselves in this new way.

At about the twenty-eighth week of pregnancy, women move into a new phase—that of not thinking of themselves so much as being pregnant, but of thinking of themselves as having a child. They change from thinking about clothing for themselves to thinking about clothing for a baby. Again, this is an enjoyable step in pregnancy.

Late in pregnancy, as their due date approaches, thoughts change once more. A woman moves from anticipation and planning for a baby to desire to get the pregnancy over. She is like a person who has stayed at the prom too long and recognizes that the lavender and gold boughs she first walked under are not as grand as she thought, but actually purple and yellow crepe paper hanging from basketball hoops. The baby is a weekend guest who has stayed well past Monday morning.

These feelings bring odd sensations and questions. What kind of mother will she be if she is tired of the child and the child is not even born yet? What kind of woman is she no longer to enjoy being pregnant?

Having such thoughts lowers her self-esteem at a time when it needs to be bolstered because she is shortly going to be exposed to sensations she has never felt before (and so difficult to describe that no matter how many books she reads about childbirth she will never truly be prepared for it until she experiences it). Reassurance that the feeling of entertaining an unwelcome guest is normal is helpful in maintaining self-esteem.

The Stress of Labor

Ability to tolerate stress (to cope adequately) depends on a person's perception of the event, support people available, and past experiences with coping (see Chapter 1). Women who have attended preparation-for-labor classes and are knowledgeable about the physiologic process of labor are better prepared to perceive the birth process factually than are those who know little about what will happen to them. By teaching such classes, nurses contribute greatly to helping women tolerate the stress of labor.

Fatigue

By the time her due date approaches, a woman is generally tired from the burden of carrying an extra 20 to 30 pounds of weight with her every second of her day. Most women do not sleep well during the last month of pregnancy because they have backache in a side-lying position; they turn on their back and the fetus kicks and wakens them; they turn to their side and their back aches—and so on. As mentioned previously, some women do not sleep well the last 2 weeks of pregnancy because they are afraid they will sleep through labor contractions and the baby will be born at home, away from professional supervision.

Sleep hunger makes it difficult for them to perceive situations clearly or to adjust rapidly to new situations. It makes the process of labor loom as an overwhelming experience they surely will not be able to endure. It makes a little deficiency—a wrinkled draw sheet—appear as a threatening discrepancy in their care.

Pain

Women who arrive at a labor wing of a hospital or at a birthing center are in pain. It is an extremely organized woman who can finish locating shirts so her husband has something to wear during the time that she will be away from home, ride in the car while she and her husband drop off a crying 2-year-old at her mother's home, ride further to the health care facility, then walk from the parking lot into the building and still remember to breathe at a prepared rate through contractions. Once she is in a birthing room in an environment free from outside interferences, she can quickly begin to control breathing patterns and reduce the pain of labor contractions to a feeling closer to irritation than pain. But at the door to a labor unit, she is in pain. Pain reduces the ability to cope with everything and may make her quick-tempered and quick to criticize anything around her.

Fear

Women enjoy a review of physiologic happenings in labor because they like to be reminded that this is not a strange, bewildering experience but a well-known and documented process. This description puts a fence around it, controlling the enormity of it. A good explanation of what will happen in labor and a review for those who have had classes in preparation for labor, explaining that contractions are a certain length and a certain firmness and are following the expected course, is always gratefully received.

Being taken by surprise—labor moving faster than she thought it would or slower than she thought—is frightening to a woman. It brings to her mind any horror stories of labor that she has heard from her mother or friends. A television drama or novel in which a woman died in childbirth is suddenly recalled. This might be the day, the time, the hour, *she* is to die. Women also worry that their infant may die or be born with an abnormality; they may be afraid they will not meet their own behavior expectations.

Fear increases when women are left alone. You cannot realistically be at the bedside of all the women on a labor unit all the time if you are the only nurse assigned to the unit. You can convey the feeling to patients, however, that your concern is with them even when you are physically absent. Saying that you are going to be gone for a few minutes and then being gone for only a few minutes, returning promptly, making it obvious that you are checking often, is a reassuring intervention.

Reducing Stress in Labor

Ways to reduce stress in labor center around helping a woman to perceive labor clearly despite her fear, pain, and fatigue that make this difficult and around providing support people for her, either from her family or friends or from health personnel.

Support People

The husband or the father of the child or someone else that the woman chooses (in alternative birthing centers this includes other children) should be admitted to the labor or birthing room with the woman. He or she should be able to follow the woman into the delivery room or remain with her in a birthing room through delivery. Having

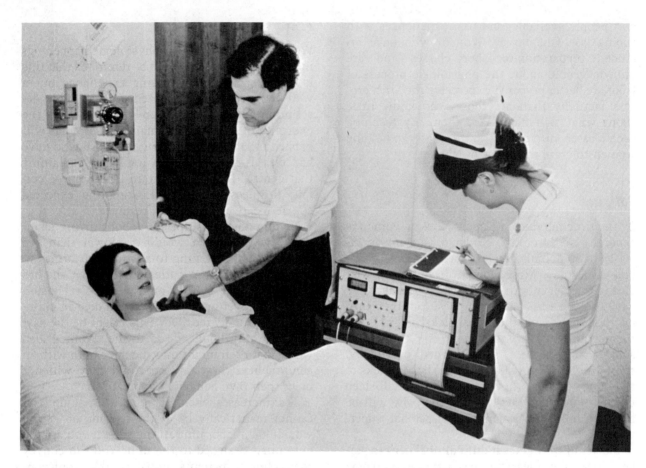

Figure 22-1 *A support person serves an undeniably important function during labor. (Courtesy of the Department of Medical Photography, Children's Hospital, Buffalo, N.Y.)*

someone with her is important to a woman in early labor; later, as contractions become intense and hard, her interest turns inward to the functioning of her body and she may actually be unaware that anyone else is in the room. This is an important point to remember. As contractions grow harder and more intense (the transition or pelvic stage of labor), being in the room becomes more and more important for the husband or father. He may not view being with his wife in early labor as that important. To the woman, the beginning of labor, when everything is still so new and she is still so unused to the sensation of contractions, may be the time she needs a support person the most (Figure 22-1).

Teaching

Familiarity is always comforting. Nothing feels like coming home. It is helpful if a woman has had a tour of the health care facility where she will deliver. She then has some idea in advance about the physical aspects of the unit and knows some of the personnel. If for some reason she has

not seen the unit before, you need to make her feel at home promptly on admission.

Introduce yourself. Be certain that all who care for her introduce themselves and explain what they will be doing. Women under stress are very aware of social amenities, of friendliness or the lack of it. They are *afraid* of being alone with strangers when their child is born. If all personnel on a labor unit wear scrub dresses or suits with only small badges for identification, introductions become extremely important. If a woman needs help in labor, she wants to be certain that the person she calls is a nurse, not a technician or a nurse's aide.

Ask whether a woman has attended classes on labor and how much she knows about labor. Fill in needed information well in advance of when it is needed. It is good practice to ask whether there is anything about labor that concerns her particularly. Women often respond with a question such as "Is it really as bad as everyone says?" Despite attendance at preparation-for-labor classes, most prominent in her mind at this point is what her mother told her 10 years ago. Knowing in early

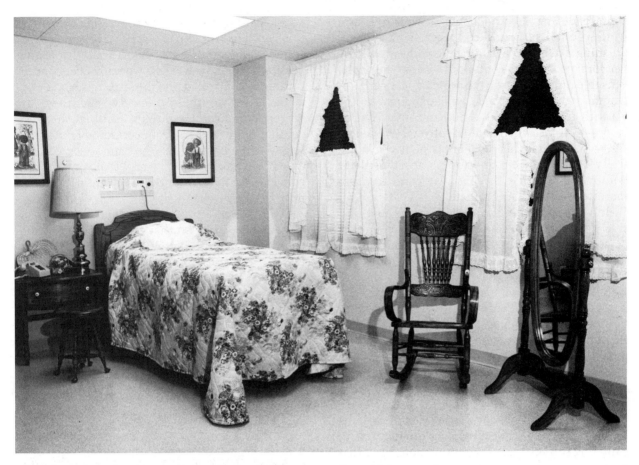

Figure 22-2 *A birthing room. Notice the home-like surroundings. (Courtesy of the Department of Medical Photography, Children's Hospital, Buffalo, N.Y.)*

labor what her misbeliefs are leaves time to try to correct them before labor gets so intense that listening to explanations becomes difficult.

In one study (Levy and McGee, 1975) investigators reported that if a mother communicated all positive aspects of labor to her daughter, the daughter was unprepared for the intensity of labor and therefore had a difficult labor. If the mother's description of labor was very bad, the daughter was unable to relax enough to appreciate what was happening to her and so also viewed labor as very difficult.

A middle ground seems to be the appropriate answer to how bad labor contractions are. They do hurt, but with a few simple breathing exercises, a positive approach, and caring support people, labor becomes an event to be cherished rather than dreaded.

Labor rooms are traditionally kept free of articles that collect dust so that they can be easily cleaned. Consequently they seem bare and unwelcoming. A woman needs to be told why labor rooms are structured to be functional rather than beautiful. Women protect their unborn children

against threat—a psychological reaction to pregnancy. They may react badly, therefore, to having their child born in dreary, tasteless surroundings. Fortunately, more hospitals are providing birthing or perinatal rooms for women in labor, and these are decorated in a home-like and comfortable atmosphere (Figure 22-2).

Women in labor need to have their call bell answered promptly. They are very aware of how many minutes elapse between their ring and a response. An intercom system saves steps for nursing personnel, but it is a poor excuse for communication on a labor service. A voice from a wall offers little comfort. It conveys instead a feeling that walking the 20 steps to the room is an effort. Perhaps the woman only wants her supply of ice chips replenished. But what, she wonders, if she begins hemorrhaging acutely (the imagination can work overtime when one is in labor); how will the voice from the wall appreciate the seriousness of her condition? Suppose she dies while the voice from the wall asks, "Can I help you?"

There is no substitute for personal touch and

contact during labor. Patting a woman's arm while you tell her that she is progressing in labor, brushing a wisp of hair off her forehead, wiping her forehead with a cool cloth—these are indispensable methods for conveying concern. A woman who is touched, who experiences the warmth and friendliness of human contact during labor—a time when she is physically dependent—will handle her newborn (who is also physically dependent and undergoing an adjustment not unlike the one she has just gone through) more warmly and affectionately.

Be wary of making careless remarks just outside the door. Because a woman and her support person are so concerned with what is happening to them, they interpret anything they hear as relating to them. "We've got a problem" said outside the door is interpreted as meaning *they* are having a problem. Laughter outside a door is interpreted as laughter *at them*. A whisper about the terrible food in the hospital cafeteria is interpreted as a whisper *about them*. Avoid this kind of situation by remaining alert to the sensitivities of a woman in labor.

When coping levels are low, it is easy to be frustrated with things such as hospital forms. Being asked to wait while a woman fills in forms or a nursing shift changes is an intolerable delay that no professional nurse should ever be a part of. If forms are necessary, the husband or whoever accompanies the woman can be asked to fill them in. He can be invited to join his wife in her room as soon as they are completed. If a woman has no one with her, she can fill in the forms after the physical admission procedures have been carried out. If she is in active labor, she can fill in the forms after the baby is delivered.

Stages of Labor

Labor has three separate time periods—the time from beginning cervical dilatation through full dilatation (the preparatory, dilatational, and deceleration sequence); the time from full dilatation until the fetus is pushed through the birth canal and born (the pelvic division or traditional second stage); and the time during which the placenta is delivered (the placental stage)—and each stage feels so different that it evokes a different reaction. Care must be individualized for each woman, depending on the stage of labor she is in.

Cervical Dilatation

The time span during which cervical dilatation occurs is the longest time interval in labor (about 12 to 14 hours in a nullipara, 8 hours in a multi-

para). At first it is exciting to feel labor contractions. They are little more than menstrual cramps; they project a this-is-really-happening quality. Soon, however, if a woman is not concentrating on controlled breathing exercises, they become biting in their intensity, and they last longer and longer. Despite the fact that she is becoming more and more uncomfortable, nothing seems to be happening. She cannot see cervical dilatation. She begins to worry that something is going wrong. Nine months are over; victory is so near, yet it is escaping her.

Women need to be given reports in labor on what is happening so that they do not grow discouraged or fearful at the seeming lack of progress.

Control

A woman wants to remain in control of herself during labor. She is most comfortable, after all, if she is in control of her emotions at the supermarket or in her own kitchen or at her office and would like to be now as well. Women respond to stressful and painful situations differently, however. Some women handle the stress of labor by being extremely quiet. Others feel most comfortable when they can show their emotions. There is no reason that women all have to react the same in labor. Your role is to help each woman express her feelings in the way she chooses, without concern that she must be pushed into a mold or will be reminded later that she screamed instead of breathed with labor contractions.

Do not be fooled into thinking that all women who appear calm during labor are in control of their emotions. Intense fear also calms people into immobility, but quietness from fear will not foster a good mother-child interaction later on. It is an outward projection of good behavior at the expense of mental health.

Feelings of Responsibility

The feeling of what having a child means may become real for a woman for the first time during the first stage of labor. Some women want to talk about what it will be like to have a child beginning today. Often during their pregnancy they have talked about what it will be like to have a child, but never before about having a child *today*. Thoughts arise such as "Never again for 18 years will I sleep soundly through a night. Never again will I be able to choose a job with just my and my husband's careers in mind, soak for hours in a tub, take off for a weekend trip at a moment's notice. After *today*, a child will always be there, needing to be dressed and fed and cared for. Am I really ready for this?"

The mother who already has a child at home may worry that she will not have time to care for this new child. She seems to be busy every moment with her one child! How can she be sure she has a big enough heart to love two children? How can she love them equally? These thoughts were present in pregnancy also, but never before did she have to consider them important until *today.*

During early labor a woman may begin to worry about the sex of the child she is having. All during pregnancy she relied on the tried and true cliché "as long as it's healthy, I don't care" as her answer to which sex she preferred. And it did not matter because having the child was too far down the road to be real. Today, in a matter of hours, it will matter. She and her husband will either be very happy or at least moderately disappointed, perhaps very disappointed. In pregnancy she could control many things: How carefully she ate, how much rest and exercise she managed, the quality of her prenatal care. Now she may feel frustrated that she had no control over the sex of her child, a difference that can be important to her. *Today.*

These feelings of increased responsibility coupled with fatigue and pain increase her anxiety. They may make her view her support person sitting in a chair by her bed—smiling and seemingly enjoying himself, stretching lazily, chatting and joking with nurses—as taking this process too lightly, irresponsibly. She may worry that the task of childrearing will fall to her alone, the responsible person here.

Remembering that the first stage of labor is a time for introspection helps you to plan nursing care (Figure 22-3). A woman needs time just for working through a final rounding out of pregnancy tasks (throwing aside the daughter role; after today she is a mother, not a daughter); she also needs time to talk about those things that can be worked through best by talking (magically, mothers are no more busy with two children than they were with one; even if she feels unready to be a mother, in the next day or two she will be with her baby under the supervision of knowledgeable people to help her get ready). She needs time alone with her support person to discuss how she feels about having this child. She may need time without her support person to voice worries she does not want to burden that person with.

Each labor is different. Each woman in labor reacts differently to the process depending on her background and her personality. For most women, the dilatational time of labor has two common entities: It is long, and it is frustrating when nothing seems to be happening. Any intervention aimed toward helping a woman under-

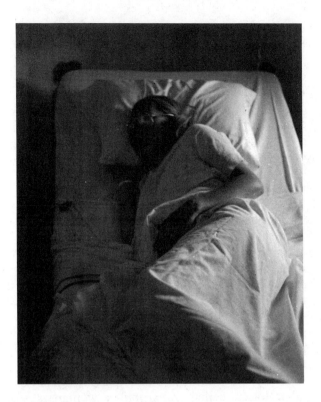

Figure 22-3 *Labor is a time for introspection, for asking, "What kind of mother will I be?" Be certain to leave some time for this private thinking-through work.*

stand what is happening and reducing stress is therapeutic in the first stage.

Pelvic Division or Second Stage

With full dilatation, the second stage of labor begins. During this stage the fetus is pushed through the birth canal. Now the nature of contractions changes, from a crescendo-decrescendo pattern that caused dilatation to an overwhelming desire to push or bear down as if to move the bowels. The feeling is so intense there is nothing a woman can do to stop it.

Even women who take preparation-for-labor classes are surprised at the intensity of this form of contraction. An instructor spent some time in class telling them they would have to push to expel the fetus. They are still not prepared for the sensation that they are not doing or controlling the pushing; their uterus is controlling it, whether they are ready or not. The worry about having *this baby today* can reach a point of panic with the second stage of labor.

Because the feeling of pushing is so strong, most women react by tensing their abdominal muscles, trying to resist, which makes the sensation painful and even more frightening. They expect this new form of contraction to be even more painful than the type they have had before. It takes a few minutes for them to appreciate that if they relax or push with the contraction all pain disappears. The process can be compared to that of a swimmer, whose muscles ache so with fatigue that he feels he cannot take another stroke, suddenly realizing he has his second wind and stroking is pain-free. It is the same as sliding down the other side of a mountain after the arduous climb to the top.

Women need to have someone with them as they enter this stage of labor to reassure them that what they are going through is normal; that in another minute, as soon as they get used to this sensation of pushing, having the baby can be fun.

Some women react to this change of contractions by growing increasingly argumentative or angry, by crying or screaming. Family support people may not be adequate at this point. The woman momentarily wants someone with her to give more knowledgeable support that everything is all right than a family member may be qualified to give.

In the first moments of the pelvic division of labor (often called *transition*) a woman is so acutely attuned to what is happening to her body that she does not hear instructions well. If she is going to be moved from a labor room to a delivery room at this time, it is difficult for her to understand your request, "Move over to the cart." She may ignore her husband's questions as if he had said nothing. It is good for her to know that these are typical reactions; it is important for family support people to know that this inward turning is a normal part of labor. Being aware of these responses reduces the impact of the strange abdominal sensation to an acceptable, conquerable level.

Placental Stage

The third stage of labor is delivery of the placenta. Expulsion of the placenta may be effected by the mother's bearing down as she did during the second stage of labor, or the physician or nurse-midwife may exert gentle pressure on the uterine fundus to aid in delivery.

Following the delivery of the placenta, any perineal stitches needed are put in place. The suturing of the perineum is a long, tedious procedure from the mother's perspective. Everyone else in the delivery room seems to be involved in something else. The physician and assistant are occupied with the stitching, which is an important repair, requiring careful inspection to avoid overlooking a cervical or vaginal laceration that could lead quickly to postpartum hemorrhage. You are busy with care of the newborn. The father is looking at the bassinet off to the side rather than at his wife. The job is over, tension is gone, the staff members begin to talk among themselves, ignoring the mother.

The mother may feel rejected, perhaps like the discarded packing crate in which a new appliance arrived. The health care personnel seem to be much more interested in trying out the new "appliance," commenting on its lusty cry, its weight, or its sex, than in seeing to the "carton" that allowed the appliance to be shipped safely.

A woman is as vulnerable to hurt in the immediate postpartum period as she was during pregnancy and early labor. Be certain that she is included in explanations, that you appreciate how anticlimactic she feels (an "after-the-prom" feeling). Otherwise, the "postpartum blues" can begin minutes after birth.

The Father and Labor

It is well documented that fathers of children offer a high degree of support during labor, and it should not be a health care facility policy to exclude them. A professional nurse should not associate herself with a labor unit in which such an obsolete policy is still followed.

A father is awkward in a health care facility. Remember, this may be the first time he has been in one. He will push a chair into a corner and sit there out of the way unless he is urged to pull it up to the woman's bedside. He will say too little or too much, as people do when they are nervous. He may attempt to act unconcerned by reading a newspaper or book.

A father is as vulnerable as his sexual partner during labor—perhaps more so because he is helpless to do anything to aid in the progress of labor. He may be used to being all doer, all decision maker, and for the next 12 hours he will be forced into the role of an observer. This may make him quick-tempered and irritable. He is also probably as fatigued as the woman. She has not slept soundly for the past month, but neither has he. There may be things at work that need his supervision. Part of his attention may be on them. For the next three days any other children are his responsibility. Part of his attention may be on wondering how they are. He is drawn in many directions, trying to give support in a process he does not fully understand. No wonder fathers have such bad reputations in labor rooms. It is their nervousness and their fatigue, not their unwillingness or inability to help, that are at fault.

The father needs as much reassurance as the woman that everything is going well in labor. A frequent "Your wife is fine, she's doing great" is very reassuring to a man who knows more old wives' tales than you do and all of them are about the terrible things that happen to women in childbirth. He needs to be included in explanations of progress: "Mary is in early labor. Her contractions are about 40 seconds long and 10 minutes apart. The bottom of the uterus, the part called the cervix, is just beginning to open, to dilate." Like every father, he wants to know how long it will be before the baby is born. Give him an approximation of time based on the averages but stress that each labor is unique (otherwise, he may hold you accountable if it takes longer; he may be used to working within honored time limits).

If a father is unprepared for labor, he can be given some tasks to do while the woman is in labor. He can time the duration and frequency of contractions. He can rub his partner's sacral area if that part of her back is causing a great deal of discomfort. He will recognize these chores as being little more than the modern health care provider's way of assigning him "water to boil," but nonetheless, he generally welcomes having something to do.

Do not feel compelled to keep him busy, however. His most important contribution is just to be there, to be a supportive, comforting, loving presence. If he does nothing more than hold his wife's hand for the 12 hours she is in labor, he has contributed in a unique way to the birth of his child. He has provided a caring atmosphere for his child to be born into. In a world of plastic plants and pervading uninvolvement such contributions cannot be discounted.

The father whose sexual partner is going to deliver by a prepared method of childbirth has an active role to play: He serves as her coach throughout labor. Be certain to reassure him that, although he will take an active part, you will also be readily available as a support person. It is frightening for him to think that the good or bad outcome of this labor rests solely on him.

It may be difficult for a father to appreciate how important it is for his partner to have him with her in labor. If she is using breathing exercises and has reduced the pain of labor to controllable stinging sensations, he may view this as an easy time free from stress. He may need a reminder that although the pain is gone from labor contractions the banding or tightening feeling remains; the unknown aspect of labor is still present. And these feelings are just as stressful as pain.

He may fail to realize that personality changes during the second stage of labor are normal and may reprimand the woman for not cooperating or for growing agitated. A warning ahead of time is helpful.

The feeling of responsibility that engulfs the woman in labor may be experienced by the father at this time also. He may not like his job very much. If he were free, or if only he and his wife were concerned, he would quit work that day and try something new. But after today there will be a baby to support too. He is not as free to take chances as he was yesterday. Life is closing in on him *today*, making him grow up whether he is ready or not.

He needs time alone with the woman during labor for the opportunity to share with her his feelings about his child—his feelings of being a father. On the other hand, he may need talk time with health care personnel and generally appreciates having someone present in the room with him who knows more about labor than he does. It is difficult for him to be supportive when he is concerned about his sexual partner's safety.

One interesting study (Bradley, 1962) showed that when fathers were present during labor the first stage of labor for primiparas was 3½ hours shorter and the first stage for multiparas was 1½ hours shorter than in control labors where fathers were not present. The first stage progresses most rapidly if the mother is relaxed, and this decrease in labor time probably reflects the degree of relaxation that an effective support person can help supply.

The Unsupported Woman in Labor

If women have no support person with them in labor, they need to be able to use you as their support person. Often young girls are not aware that they could have asked the father of their child to accompany them. They may want to phone him to tell him they are in labor and that he can come to be with them. The fact that he chooses to include himself in the labor experience shows his commitment as a support person and his value to the woman as an important person in her life.

Young girls may need a review of anatomy so they are certain they understand what happens in labor. They may be worried that the baby will tear them because they are not yet fully grown. They require frequent reassurance that everything is going well and not only the baby but they too are safe from harm.

Unmarried women should have time during labor to complete their pregnancy work just as married women do: to think about what it will be like to be a mother, to care for a child. If they have made a decision to place the baby for adoption, they need time to think about whether this is still what they want now that the day of birth has arrived. It is much easier to decide to place a baby for adoption during pregnancy when the event seems far away than during labor when the decision involves something that is happening *today*.

Because the acceptance of the pregnancy may have come late in pregnancy for unmarried women who did not plan on having a child, they may not have completed the psychological tasks of pregnancy by the time they are in labor. Not being ready for a baby may make labor more difficult. In a study of 48 women (Davids, 1961) it was shown that women who were not ready for childrearing had longer labors (16.8 hours) than women who were ready (7.3 hours).

Labor Closure

A new stage in life cannot proceed until a former one is closed. Almost everyone, for example, can remember a day they "grew up" or closed out being a child. Most nurses can remember a day they "earned their wings" or changed from being a student to being a practicing nurse. A military term for this closure is "debriefing." Labor and delivery is such a unique experience that a couple needs time following it to talk about the experience in order to integrate it into other life experiences and allow bonding and childrearing to proceed. Be certain to provide time for this immediately after delivery and again in the next few days to facilitate the process.

Home Births

Because labor units of hospitals were for many years managed with operating room–like efficiency, warmth and humaneness were sometimes overlooked in favor of routines or rules. This circumstance has made delivering a baby at home, where warmth and familiarity are the chief ingredients, an attractive alternative. Home birth is discussed in Chapter 26. When a woman delivers at home, unfortunately, she sacrifices the safety of having backup equipment and care available should something be wrong with her infant at birth or happen to herself during labor or delivery.

Nurses can be instrumental in making the milieu of hospital units or alternative birth centers so accepting and humane that women do not have to choose an unsafe alternative in order to have their baby surrounded by the people important to them. Understanding the psychological reactions to labor and delivery in order to give helpful support in labor is vital to creating an atmosphere where women do feel comfortable and want to come for care.

Utilizing Nursing Process ——————————————

As the emotional outcome of labor influences parent-child bonding and future childbearing, it is important that care during this time be planned by use of nursing process to ensure that it is comprehensive.

Assessment

An important part of assessment for psychological reactions to labor is assessment of a woman's knowledge of the process of labor: Women are less fearful of a process they are familiar with than a process that is foreign to them. As a rule, women who attended a preparation-for-childbirth course are more knowledgeable than those who did not, but a great deal depends on the quality of the course and whether the woman attended all the sessions. Ask about a woman's past experience with childbirth; the woman who had a great deal of anesthesia or analgesia during a past labor may remember almost nothing about it or remember facts out of proportion to their actual occurrence.

Some women are reluctant to reveal how frightened they are by labor because this revelation makes them feel vulnerable to threat. Some women may be "supporting" their support person and feel a need to be the strong member during labor. An introductory statement such as "A lot of women find the thought of labor very frightening. How do you feel?" may be helpful as it gives the woman "permission" to admit to being afraid.

Use observation to detect signs of tension such as clenched fists or jawline, excessive talking or silence.

Analysis

Two nursing diagnoses accepted by the Fourth Annual Conference on Nursing Diagnoses (NANDA) were "Fear" and "Knowledge, deficit of." These diagnoses certainly apply to the labor experience. Do not discount the possibility that a well diagnosis of "adequate psychological adjustment to labor related to preparation for labor" could be more accurate. When establishing goals with a woman in labor be certain that they are realistic to the situation. You are working within a relatively short time frame (12 hours), so goals must be geared to this time period. Appreciate also the magnitude of the labor experience. It will probably not be possible to alleviate all fear or all anxiety: Labor is so unusual an experience that the average woman does not have coping resources large enough to deal totally with it.

Planning

Planning during labor should be done with the awareness that a woman is under stress and that with stress, problem solving, in particular, is reduced. For effective planning, you may need to suggest alternatives rather than ask her to try to devise them.

Implementation

Implementations with the woman in labor are always family-centered; you need to think of the family unit as your patient, rather than just a woman. This philosophy automatically includes the father of the child in care and enlarges his role in support during labor.

Evaluation

The evaluation of a labor experience may not reveal that it was everything a woman hoped it would be because its uniqueness makes it unlikely that she was able to imagine what it would actually be like. "Debriefing," or allowing a woman and her support person time to talk about the labor experience in the next 2 or 3 days, helps to put the experience into perspective. This implementation is important in the immediate postpartal period.

Nursing Care Planning

Christine McFadden is a 15-year-old patient (gravida 1, para 0, premature 0, abortion 0, living children 0) you care for in labor.

Problem Area. Psychological adjustment to labor.

Assessment

States, "I hate this. I didn't want this baby. I don't want to go through with this. I just want a c-section to get this over." Has been told that her pelvic measurements are borderline and a cesarean birth may be necessary. Grandmother purchased baby items to be ready for birth; Chris did not participate in preparation. Attended no preparation-for-labor classes. Appears tense, frightened; cheeks stained with tears.

Analysis

Fear related to ineffective preparation for labor.

Locus of Decision Making. Shared.

Goal. Patient will complete labor within bounds of emotional health.

Criteria. Patient:

1. Will learn ways to participate in labor rather than be a passive observer.
2. Is able to accept labor by vaginal delivery if possible.
3. Is able to accept c-birth decision if this decision is made.

Nursing Orders

1. Assess knowledge of labor and fill in gaps of knowledge.
2. Teach abdominal breathing for pain relief and as a self-participation measure.
3. Give good explanations for all equipment used, procedures done.
4. Offer opportunity to discuss feelings about labor and coming child.
5. In postpartal period assess adequacy of maternal-child relationship because of poor preparation for labor.

Problem Area. Lack of support during a significant life crisis.

Assessment

States, "I hate Mark [father of child] for putting me through this. I hate my parents." No support person with her. Asked that father of child specifically not be notified of labor.

Analysis

Inadequate support during significant life crisis.

Locus of Decision Making. Shared.

Goal. Patient to identify one person as adequate support person.

Criteria. Patient to ask for a family member or health care provider to serve as support person.

Nursing Orders

1. Ask if a family support person should be called.
2. Provide continuous nursing support until this person arrives.
3. Support family member if one chosen because relationship is not optimal.
4. Offer opportunity to discuss feelings about ability to handle this level of stress by herself and advantage of relying on others for support.

Mary Kraft is a 23-year-old patient (gravida 2, para 0, premature 0, abortion 1, living children 0) you care for in labor.

Problem Area. Psychological adjustment to labor.

Assessment

States, "I thought labor would be worse than this; so far this is all downhill." Using breathing exercises learned in prenatal class; has husband with her for support person. Baby planned; has clothing, etc., ready for baby. States she does not care about sex of child. Asked for birthing room; husband wants to be with her for delivery as well as labor. Appears relaxed, but tired.

Analysis

Primapara psychologically prepared for labor and new child related to readiness for childbearing.

Locus of Decision Making. Patient.

Goal. Patient will complete labor within bounds of psychological well-being.

Criteria.

1. Patient will participate in labor rather than be passive observer.
2. Couple will complete labor as a family unit.

Nursing Orders

1. Offer support and relief of coach as necessary.
2. Offer additional nursing support as necessary.
3. Offer education of labor happenings as necessary.
4. Encourage rest to prevent exhaustion from level of excitement.
5. Assess mothering ability in postpartal period as routine (no problem anticipated).

Angie Baco is a 42-year-old patient (gravida 7, para 6, abortion 0, premature 0, living children 5) you care for in labor.

Problem Area. Psychological adjustment to labor.

Assessment

States, "Well, here I am, all the way to 37 weeks." Seems sad that labor will be induced this morning because of gestational diabetes but happy that pregnancy came this far. States that she knows more about labor than everyone here (six previous labors) but seemed grateful for explanation of admission procedures. Baby not planned initially, but has baby items ready, name for baby chosen. Says she wants a girl but boy would be "okay." She wants to deliver in a delivery, not a birthing, room *"in case the baby isn't all right."* Husband not sure he wants to see delivery; says "we'll see when time comes." Did not see any previous births. Couple's last child had congenital heart disease, died 4 days after birth.

Patient appears relaxed although bites lip when not actively engaged in conversation.

Analysis

Fear related to poor outcome of previous pregnancy.

Locus of Decision Making. Shared.

Goal. Patient to complete labor within bounds of psychological well being.

Criteria. Couple:

1. To complete labor as a family unit.
2. Is able to face and accept a possible poor outcome of pregnancy.

Nursing Orders

1. Provide adequate support because of anxiety.
2. Support husband as necessary (he is not certain he is ready for poor outcome to pregnancy).
3. Reassure frequently that labor is going well and fetus is doing well (as appropriate).
4. Assess mother-child relationship in postpartal period because of mother's perception that infant may be ill.
5. Assess mother-child relationship in postpartal period if child is a boy (having boy only "okay," not desired).

Questions for Review

Multiple Choice

1. Mrs. Timaldi is admitted to a labor unit in active labor. Which of the following assessments would make you worry that she might have difficulty accepting this child?

   a. She says she is tired of being pregnant.
   b. She says she hasn't slept well lately.
   c. She says she wants a boy.
   d. She says she is exhausted.

2. The first stage of labor is often a time of introspection. In light of this fact, which of the following nursing care statements would be true?

   a. A woman should be left entirely alone during this period.

b. A woman will rarely speak or laugh during this period.

c. A woman may spend time thinking about what is happening to her.

d. No nursing care should be done during this time.

3. During the second stage of labor (pelvic stage) a woman generally

   a. cannot tell the difference in contractions.

   b. is frightened by the change in contractions.

   c. falls asleep from exhaustion.

   d. starts to feel hungry and unsatisfied.

4. During this second stage of labor a woman is generally

   a. very aware of activities immediately around her.

   b. anxious to have people around her.

   c. no longer in need of a support person.

   d. turning inward to concentrate on body sensations.

5. The use of a birthing room in place of a traditional labor room can be an effective comforting implementation during labor because

   a. birthing rooms have softer mattresses.

   b. they have a homelike familiar atmosphere.

   c. bright colors distract from pain of contractions.

   d. they offer the woman something to think about during labor.

Discussion

1. Preparing women for psychological changes during labor is as important as the preparation for physiological changes. In a preparation-for-labor class, what would you teach concerning psychological changes of labor?

2. A woman is often afraid to be alone while in labor. What are ways in which you could convey a caring attitude if you could not physically remain with her during every minute of labor?

3. In an alternative birth center, a woman's older children may accompany her to the center. How might the presence of other children affect a woman's psychological changes during labor?

Suggested Readings

Bradley, R. A. (1962). Fathers' presence in delivery rooms. *Psychosomatics, 3,* 474.

Cranley, M. S., et al. (1983). Women's perceptions of vaginal and cesarean deliveries. *Nursing Research, 32,* 10.

Davids, A., et al. (1961). Psychological study of emotional factors in pregnancy: A preliminary report. *Psychosomatic Medicine, 23,* 93.

Freeman, M. H. (1979). Giving family life a good start in the hospital. *M.C.N., 4,* 51.

Levy, J., & McGee, M. (1975). Childbirth as crisis. *Journal of Perspectives on Social Psychology, 31,* 171.

Mercer, R. T., et al. (1983). Relationship of psychosocial and perinatal variables to perception of childbirth. *Nursing Research, 32,* 202.

Raphael-Leff, J. (1984). Varying needs . . . women vary greatly in their response to birth. *Nursing Mirror, 158,* v.

Roberts, J. E. (1983). Factors influencing distress from pain during labor. *M.C.N., 8,* 62.

Shannon-Babitz, M. (1979). Addressing the needs of fathers during labor and delivery. *M.C.N., 4,* 378.

Sullivan, J., et al. (1980). The Utah Test appraising mothers, revised . . . to predict those who will be above average in positive response to labor and delivery. *Issues in Health Care of Women, 2,* 31.

23

The Labor Process

OBJECTIVES

Following mastery of the content of this chapter, you should be able to

1. Describe the common theories explaining the onset and continuation of labor.
2. Describe four stages of labor.
3. Describe the role of the passenger, the passage, and the force in the labor process.
4. Describe the signs and symptoms that occur with differing stages of labor.
5. Differentiate between true and false labor.
6. Analyze the effects of physiologic changes during each stage of labor.
7. Synthesize knowledge of normal labor with nursing process to achieve quality maternal-newborn nursing care.

LABOR IS THE SERIES of events by which the products of conception are expelled from the woman's body. The terms *childbirth, accouchement, confinement, parturition,* and *travail* are all synonyms for labor. *Labor* is an apt term because a great deal of work is involved in the process of birth. For the woman and the fetus alike, it is a time of change, both a time of ending and a time of beginning.

Whether the process of labor is successful or not depends on three integrated concepts: whether the woman's pelvis (the *passage*) is of adequate size and contour; whether the *passenger* (the fetus) is of appropriate size and in an advantageous position and presentation; and whether the force of labor (*power*, or uterine factors) is adequate. It has become popular to add a fourth *P*—the psyche—to these factors. Although it is true that the psyche, or the woman's reaction to labor, is important, one of the problems that causes psychological stress in labor is that, ready or not, on a certain day at a certain time, labor as a physiologic process will begin. The process and stages of labor are discussed below.

Process of Labor

The Passage

The passage refers to the route the fetus must travel from the uterus through the cervix and vagina to the external perineum; because these organs are contained inside the pelvis, the fetus must also pass through the pelvic ring. Pelvic anatomy and the maternal pelvic measurements that are taken to predict the adequacy of the maternal pelvis are discussed in Chapter 8. Important measurements are the inlet, midpelvis (level of the ischial spines), and outlet. Remember that the narrowest diameter of the pelvis at the inlet is the anteroposterior diameter; at the outlet, the transverse diameter (Table 8-2).

In most instances of disproportion, the pelvis is the organ at fault. Even when the fetus is causing the problem, it is often because the fetal head is presented to the birth canal at more than its narrowest diameter, not because the head is actually too large.

This is an important point to understand when discussing with parents why an infant cannot be delivered vaginally. It is one thing to learn that a child cannot be born vaginally because the mother's pelvis is too small and another to learn that the infant's head is too large. The first fact is merely unfortunate; the second implies that something is seriously wrong with the baby. A thought of that kind can interfere with the establishment of the good maternal-child relationship that is necessary for the child's sound mental health.

The Passenger

The head is the body part of the fetus with the widest diameter, or the part most likely to be unable to pass through the pelvic ring. Whether a fetal skull can pass or not depends on both its structure and alignment with the pelvis. In order to understand how such a presentation occurs, you must have some acquaintance with the bones, fontanelles, and suture lines of the fetal skull (Figures 23-1 and 23-2).

Structure of the Fetal Skull

The *cranium* (the uppermost portion of the skull) is composed of eight bones. The four superior—the frontal bone, the two parietal bones, and the occipital bone—are the important bones in terms of obstetrics. The frontal bone is actually two fused bones; the area over the bone is referred to for obstetrical purposes as the *sinciput*. The area over the occipital bone is referred

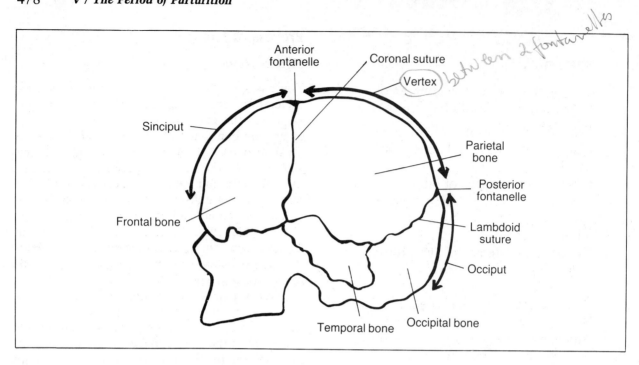

Figure 23-1 *The fetal skull (lateral view).*

to as the *occiput*. The other four bones of the skull (sphenoid bone, ethmoid bone, and two temporal bones) do not play a large part in obstetrics, since they lie at the base of the cranium and therefore are never presenting parts. The chin can be a presenting part. For obstetrical purposes it is referred to by its Latin name *mentum*.

The two parietal bones of the skull are joined by a membranous interspace, the *sagittal* suture line. The *coronal* suture line is the line of junction of the frontal bone and the two parietal bones. The *lambdoid* suture line is the line of junction of the occipital bone and the two parietal bones. The suture lines are important in delivery

Figure 23-2 *The fetal skull (from above).*

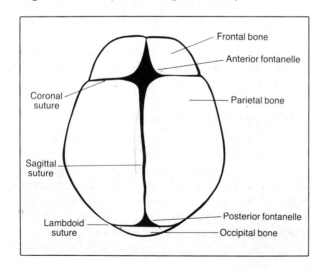

because they allow the cranial bones to move and overlap, thus molding or diminishing the size of the skull so that it can more readily pass through the birth canal.

At the junction of the main suture lines are significant membrane-covered spaces, the fontanelles. The *anterior fontanelle* lies at the junction of the coronal and sagittal lines. Because the frontal bone consists of two fused bones, four bones (counting the two parietal bones) are actually involved at this junction, making the anterior fontanelle diamond-shaped. It measures approximately 3 to 4 cm in its anteroposterior diameter and 2 to 3 cm in its transverse diameter. For obstetric purposes the anterior fontanelle is often referred to as the *bregma*.

Three bones (the two parietal bones and the occipital bone) are involved at the junction of the lambdoid and sagittal suture lines; thus the *posterior fontanelle* is triangular. It is smaller than the anterior fontanelle, measuring about 2 cm across its widest part. Fontanelle spaces compress during delivery to aid in molding of the fetal head. Their presence can be assessed on manual examination of the cervix after it has dilated during labor to establish the position of the fetal head and whether it is favorable for delivery. The space between the two fontanelles is referred to for obstetric purposes as the *vertex*.

Diameters of the Fetal Skull

The diameter of any structure refers to the distance across it. The shape of a fetal skull causes it

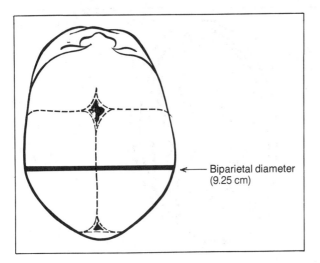

Figure 23-3 *Biparietal diameter.*

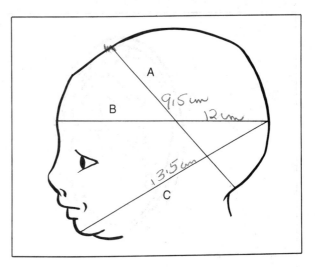

Figure 23-4 *Anteroposterior diameters of the skull. A. Suboccipitobregmatic diameter (9.5 cm). B. Occipitofrontal diameter (12 cm). C. Occipitomental diameter (13.5 cm).*

to be wider in its anteroposterior diameter than in its transverse diameter. To fit through the birth canal, the fetus must present the smaller diameter (the transverse diameter) to the smaller diameter of the maternal pelvis; otherwise progress will halt and birth cannot be accomplished.

At the pelvic inlet, for example, the fetus must present the narrowest diameter, the biparietal diameter (about 9.25 cm) (Figure 23-3) to the anteroposterior diameter of the pelvis (a space about 11 cm wide). At the outlet, this narrow diameter must be presented to the transverse diameter, a space about 11 cm wide. If the anteroposterior diameter of the skull (a measurement wider than the biparietal diameter) is presented to the anteroposterior diameter of the inlet, engagement, or the settling of the fetal head into the pelvis, may not occur. If the anteroposterior diameter of the skull is presented to the transverse diameter of the outline, arrest of progress may occur at that point.

The diameter of the anteroposterior fetal skull depends on where the measurement is taken. The narrowest diameter (about 9.5 cm) is from the inferior aspect of the occiput to the center of the anterior fontanelle (the *suboccipitobregmatic* diameter). The *occipitofrontal* diameter, measured from the bridge of the nose to the occipital prominence, is about 12 cm. The *occipitomental* diameter, which is the widest anteroposterior diameter (about 13.5 cm), is measured from the chin to the posterior fontanelle. These diameters are shown in Figure 23-4.

Which one of these anteroposterior diameters is presented to the birth canal depends on the degree of flexion of the fetus's head. In full flexion, the head flexes so sharply that the chin rests on the thorax, and the smallest anteroposterior di-

ameter, the suboccipitobregmatic, will be presented to the birth canal. If the head is held in moderate flexion, the occipitofrontal diameter will be presented. In poor flexion (the head hyperextended) the largest diameter, the occipitomental, will be presented.

This anteroposterior diameter must fit through the transverse diameter of the pelvic inlet, a space of about 12.4 cm to 13.5 cm; and at the outlet, through the anteroposterior diameter of the pelvis, a space of 9.5 to 11.5 cm. It follows that a fetal head presenting a diameter of 9.5 cm will fit through a pelvis much more readily than if the diameter is 12.0 or 13.5 cm. This relationship is shown in Figure 23-5. Diameters of the fetal skull are summarized in comparison with pelvic diameters in Table 23-1.

Molding. Molding is the change in the shape of the fetal skull that occurs during labor to reduce the engaging diameters and make passage of the fetal head easier.

Molding is produced by the force of uterine contractions pressing the vertex against the not-yet-dilated cervix. The change in shape is possible because the bones of the fetal skull are not yet completely ossified and therefore do not form a rigid structure. Skull bones overlap so that the head becomes narrower but longer.

At birth, the overlapping of the sagittal suture line and generally the coronal suture line can be easily palpated in the newborn skull.

In a brow presentation, there is little molding because frontal bones are fused. Because molding does not occur readily in brow presentations, the

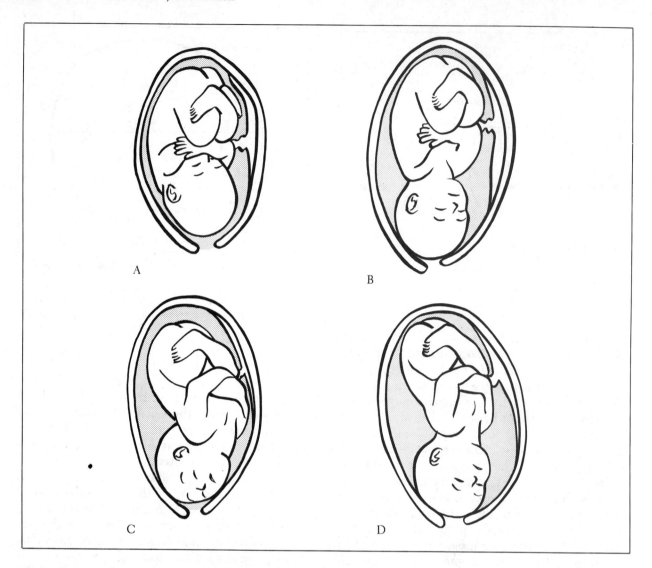

Figure 23-5 *Fetal attitude. A. Fetus in full flexion presents smallest (suboc-cipitobregmatic) anteroposterior diameter of skull to inlet in this good attitude. B. Fetus is not as well flexed (military attitude) as in A and presents oc-cipitofrontal diameter to inlet. C. Fetus in complete extension presents wide (oc-ciptomental) diameter. D. Fetus in partial extension (brow presentation).*

labor will undoubtedly be arrested and the fetus be unable to pass through the pelvis. In a breech presentation, no skull molding occurs, and so the fetal head may present a delivery problem.

Fetal Presentation and Position

In addition to being familiar with the component parts and diameters of the fetal head, you should be able to use with understanding the terms describing fetal presentation and position.

Attitude. Attitude describes the degree of flexion the fetus assumes or the relation of the fetal parts to each other (Figure 23-5). A fetus in *good* attitude is in complete flexion: the spinal column is bowed forward; the head is flexed forward so much that the chin touches the sternum; the

arms are flexed and folded on the chest; the thighs are flexed onto the abdomen; and the calves of the legs are pressed against the posterior aspect of the thighs. This is a normal "fetal position." A good attitude is advantageous for delivery not only because it helps the fetus present the smallest anteroposterior diameter of the skull to the pelvis but also because it puts the whole body into an ovoid shape, occupying the smallest space possible.

A fetus is in moderate flexion if the chin is not touching the chest but is in an alert, or "military," position (Figure 23-5). This position causes the next widest anteroposterior diameter to present to the birth canal, the occipitofrontal diameter. A fair number of fetuses assume a military position at the early part of labor. This position

Table 23-1 Diameters of Fetal Skull Compared to Female Pelvic Diameters

Diameter	Measurement	Average Diameter (cm)
Anteroposterior fetal skull diameter		
Suboccipitobregmatic	Inferior aspect of occiput to center of anterior fontanelle	9.5
Occipitofrontal	Bridge of nose to occipital prominence	12.0
Occipitomental	Chin to posterior fontanelle	13.5
Transverse fetal skull diameter, biparietal	Distance between parietal prominences	9.25
Anteroposterior pelvic diameters		
Diagonal conjugate	Inferior margin of symphysis pubis to sacral promontory	12.5
True conjugate	Internal aspect of symphysis pubis to sacral promontory	11.0
Transverse pelvic diameter, ischial tuberosities	Between ischial tuberosities at the level of the anus	11.0

does not usually interfere with labor because one of the mechanisms of labor (descent and flexion) causes the fetus's head to fully flex at that point in labor.

If a fetus is in poor flexion, the back is arched, the neck is extended, and the occipitomental diameter of the head is presented to the birth canal. This is an unusual position; it presents too wide a skull diameter to the birth canal for normal delivery. Such a position may occur if there is less than normal amniotic fluid present (*oligohydramnios*), which does not allow the fetus adequate movement, or it may reflect a neurologic abnormality that is causing spasticity.

Engagement. The presenting part of the fetus is said to be engaged when it has settled far enough into the pelvis to be at the level of the ischial spines, a midpoint of the pelvis. Descent to this point means that the significant diameter of the presenting part of the fetus (the biparietal diameter in a cephalic presentation; the intertrochanter diameter in a breech presentation) has passed through the pelvic inlet or the pelvic inlet is adequate for delivery. Saying that engagement has occurred is another way of saying that lightening has occurred. Nonengagement of the head at the beginning of labor in a primipara indicates a possible complication: An abnormal presentation or position, abnormality of the fetal head, or a cephalopelvic disproportion may be preventing the head from engaging. In multiparas, engagement may or may not be present at the beginning of labor. A presenting part that is not engaged is said to be "floating." One that is descending but has not yet reached the ischial spines is said to be "dipping." Whether engagement has occurred or

not is assessed by vaginal and cervical examination.

Station. Station refers to the relationship of the presenting part of the fetus to the level of the ischial spines (Figure 23-6). When the presenting part is at the level of the ischial spines, it is at a 0 station (synonymous with engagement). If the presenting part is above the spines, the distance is measured and described as −1 cm (−1 station), −2 cm (−2 station), and so on. If the presenting part is below the ischial spines, the distance is determined (+1 cm, +2 cm, and so on) and designated as a +1 station, a +2 station, and so on. At a +3 or +4 station the presenting part is at the perineum and can be seen if you separate the vulva (synonymous with *crowning*).

Figure 23-6 *Station (anteroposterior view). Station, or degree of engagement, of the fetal head is designated by centimeters above or below the ischial spines. At −5 station, head is "floating." At 0 station, head is "engaged." At +5 station, head is at outlet.*

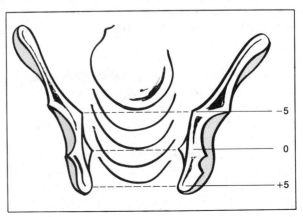

Table 23-2 Types of Cephalic Presentations

Type	Lie	Attitude	Description
Vertex	Longitudinal	Good (full flexion)	The head is sharply flexed, making the parietal bones or the space between the fontanelles (the vertex) the presenting part. This is the most common presentation and allows the suboccipitobregmatic diameter to present to the cervix.
Brow	Longitudinal	Moderate (military)	Because the head is only moderately flexed, the brow or sinciput becomes the presenting part.
Face	Longitudinal	Poor	The extension of the fetus's head makes the face the presenting part. From this position, extreme edema and distortion of the face may occur. The presenting diameter (the occipitomental) is so wide delivery may not be possible.
Mentum	Longitudinal	Very poor	The complete hyperextension of the head causes the presentation of the fetal chin. The widest diameter (occipitomental) is presenting. Pressure on the presenting part may cause such edema of the mouth that sucking following delivery will be unsuccessful. As a rule, the fetus cannot enter the pelvis in this presentation.

To remember whether a plus or minus station is below the spines, think what you are trying to accomplish (move the fetus from above the pelvic ring to below it). As the fetus passes further toward the goal of being born (beyond the midpelvis) the stations become plus designations. When describing what the terms *engagement* and *station* mean to parents, be certain to include an explanation that ischial spines are dull bony protrusions. No parent likes to think of her child transversing through needle-sharp "spines."

Fetal Lie. Lie is the relationship between the long (cephalocaudal) axis of the fetal body and the long (cephalocaudal) axis of a woman's body, that is, whether the fetus is lying in a horizontal (transverse) or a vertical (longitudinal) position. About 99 percent of fetuses assume a longitudinal lie (with their long axis parallel with the long axis of the woman). Longitudinal lies are further classified as *cephalic* (the head is the presenting part, i.e., first contacts the cervix) or *breech* lie (the breach, or buttocks, is the portion to contact the cervix first).

Fetal Presentation. A fetal presentation denotes the body part that will first contact the cervix or deliver first. This is determined not only by the fetal lie but by the degree of flexion (attitude).

CEPHALIC. Cephalic presentation is the most frequent type of presentation (presenting as much as 95 percent of the time). The four types of cephalic presentation—vertex, brow, face, and mentum—are shown in Table 23-2. The area of the fetal skull that contacts the cervix often becomes edematous during labor due to continual pressure against it (called a *caput succedaneum*). In the newborn infant, the point of presentation can be analyzed from the location of the caput.

BREECH. Breech presentations occur in only a small number of births, about 3 percent. A good attitude of a breech presenting fetus brings the knees up against the umbilicus; a poor attitude does not. Breech presentations always present a degree of difficulty with delivery; the presenting part influences the degree of difficulty. Three types of breech presentation are possible; these are shown in Figure 23-7 and described in Table 23-3.

SHOULDER. In a transverse lie, the fetus is lying horizontally in the pelvis, or its long axis is perpendicular to that of the mother (Figure 23-8). One or other of the shoulders (*acromion process*) usually becomes the presenting part, although this part could be an iliac crest or a hand or elbow. Only a very few fetuses (under 1%) lie transversely. This usually occurs due to relaxed abdominal walls from grand multiparity, which allow the uterus to be unsupported and fall forward; pelvic contraction, which causes there to be more horizontal then vertical space; or placenta previa, in which the placenta is located low in the uterus and obscures some of the vertical space. Most infants in a transverse lie must be delivered by cesarean birth as they are unable to deliver nor-

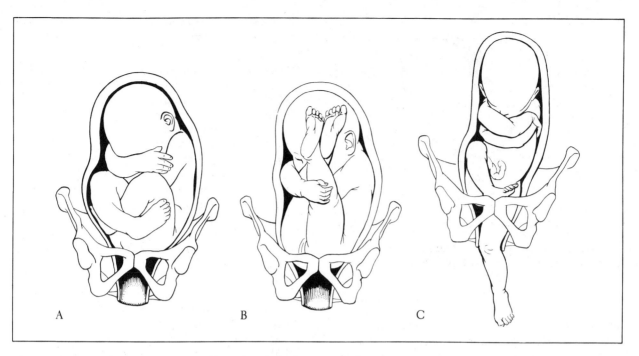

Figure 23-7 *Breech presentation. A. Complete breech. B. Frank breech. C. Footling breech. (From Clinical Education Aid, No. 18, Ross Laboratories, Columbus, Ohio, 1958.)*

mally from this "wedged" position. With this presentation, the usual contour of the term abdomen is distorted or is fuller side to side rather than top to bottom. Discovering a shoulder presentation is an important assessment: It almost automatically identifies a delivery position that puts both mother and child in jeopardy unless skilled health care personnel are available to safely deliver the child by cesarean birth.

Fetal Position. Position is the relationship of the presenting part to a specific quadrant of the woman's pelvis. For convenience in defining position, the maternal pelvis is divided into four quadrants: right anterior, left anterior, right posterior, and left posterior (the mother's right and left, not the examiner's). Four parts of the fetus have been chosen as points of direction in order to describe the relationship of the presenting part to one of the pelvic quadrants. In a vertex presentation, the occiput is the chosen point; in a face presentation, it is the chin (mentum); in breech presentations, it is the sacrum; in shoulder presentations, it is the scapula or the acromion process. A position is marked by an abbreviation of three or four letters. The middle letter denotes the fetal landmark (O for occiput, M for chin, Sa for sacrum, A for acromion process). The first letter defines whether the landmark is pointing to the mother's right (R) or left (L). The last letter

Table 23-3 Types of Breech Presentations

Type	Lie	Attitude	Description
Complete	Longitudinal	Good (full flexion)	The fetus's thighs are tightly flexed on the abdomen; both the buttocks and the tightly flexed feet present to the cervix.
Frank	Longitudinal	Moderate	Attitude is moderate because the hips are flexed, but the knees are extended to rest on the chest. The buttocks alone present to the cervix.
Footling	Longitudinal	Poor	Neither the thighs nor lower legs are flexed. If one foot presents, it is a single footling breech; if both present, it is a double footling breech.

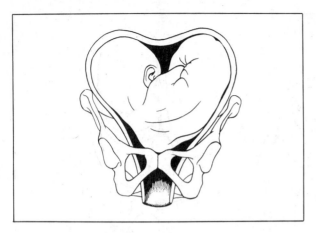

Figure 23-8 *Transverse or shoulder presentation. (From Clinical Education Aid, No. 18, Ross Laboratories, Columbus, Ohio, 1958.)*

Table 23-4 Possible Fetal Positions

Vertex presentation
LOA = Left occipitoanterior
LOP = Left occipitoposterior
LOT = Left occipitotransverse
ROA = Right occipitoanterior
ROP = Right occipitoposterior
ROT = Right occipitotransverse
Breech presentation
LSA = Left sacroanterior
LSP = Left sacroposterior
LST = Left sacrotransverse
RSA = Right sacroanterior
RSP = Right sacroposterior
RST = Right sacrotransverse
Face presentation
LMA = Left mentoanterior
LMP = Left mentoposterior
LMT = Left mentotransverse
RMA = Right mentoanterior
RMP = Right mentoposterior
RMT = Right mentotransverse
Shoulder presentation
LSCA = Left scapuloanterior
LSCP = Left scapuloposterior
RSCA = Right scapuloanterior
RSCP = Right scapuloposterior

defines whether the landmark points anteriorly (*A*), posteriorly (*P*), or transversely (*T*).

The fetal position is left occipitoanterior (LOA), for example, in a vertex presentation (the fetus is in good attitude in a vertical cephalic lie) when the occiput of the fetus points to the left anterior quadrant of the mother. When the occiput points to the right posterior quadrant, the position is right occipitoposterior (ROP). LOA is the most common fetal position and right occipitoanterior (ROA) the second most frequent position. Table 23-4 presents a summary of possible positions. Common positions in cephalic presentations are depicted in Figure 23-9. Position is important because it influences the process and efficiency of labor. A fetus delivers fastest from a ROA or LOA position. Labor is considerably extended if the position is posterior; it may be more painful as the rotation of the fetal head puts pressure on the sacral nerves and causes sharp back pains. Figure 23-10 depicts how a fetal head in ROA and ROP appear from an outlet view.

Determining Fetal Presentation and Position

The vertex is the ideal presenting part because the skull bones are capable of molding so effectively to accommodate the cervix; it may actually aid in cervical dilatation; and it prevents complications such as a prolapsed cord (cord passing between the presenting part and the cervix and entering the vagina before the fetus). When a body part other than the vertex presents, labor is invariably longer due to ineffective descent of the fetus, ineffective dilatation of the cervix, and irregular and weak uterine contractions. Labor is often extended by being less effective, tiring the mother and reducing the excitement of the experience. If an operative delivery has to be accomplished, the mother has a longer hospitalization,

and more pain and more disability following the delivery. If the fetus delivers vaginally, she has a greater chance of having perineal tears or cervical laceration, again, increasing her disability and decreasing her chance of problem-free future childbearing. Threatening and unsatisfactory labor can interfere with maternal-child bonding.

The presentation of a body part other than the vertex puts the fetus at a risk because of the increased chance of proportional difference between the fetus and pelvis, making a cesarean birth necessary and the membranes more apt to rupture early (increasing the possibility of infection). The fetus is more apt to suffer anoxia and meconium staining, complications that lead to respiratory distress at birth.

There are four methods by which the fetal position, presentation, and lie can be established: (a) combined abdominal inspection and palpation, (b) vaginal or rectal examination, (c) auscultation of fetal heart tones, and (d) sonography or X-ray examination. These methods are discussed in Chapter 24.

The Power

The power of labor is supplied solely by the fundus of the uterus until cervical dilatation. Follow-

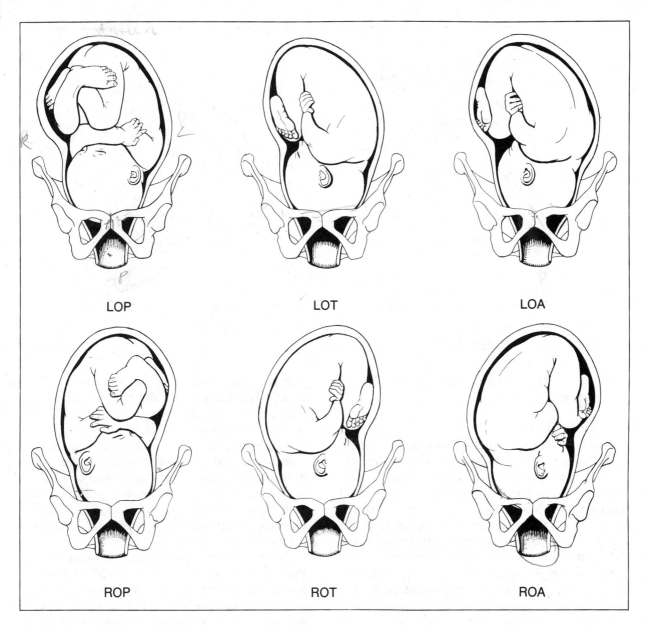

LOP LOT LOA

ROP ROT ROA

Figure 23-9 *Fetal position. All are vertex presentations. A = anterior, L = left, O = occiput, P = posterior, R = right, T = transverse. (From Clinical Education Aid, No. 18, Ross Laboratories, Columbus, Ohio, 1958).*

ing full dilatation, this primary power is supplemented by the use of the abdominal muscles. It is important for women to understand not to use abdominal muscles as power until the cervix is dilated: They can impede the primary force and cause fetal and cervical damage.

Labor normally begins when a fetus is sufficiently mature to cope with extrauterine life, yet not too large to cause mechanical difficulties in delivery. However, the trigger that converts the random, painless Braxton Hicks contractions into strong, coordinated, productive labor contractions is obscure. In some instances, labor begins before the fetus is mature (premature birth); in others, labor is delayed until the fetus and the placenta have both passed beyond the optimum point for birth (postmature birth). A number of theories of why labor occurs follow.

Uterine Stretch Theory

Any hollow body organ stretched to capacity will contract and empty. A distended bladder empties by incontinence. A distended stomach empties by vomiting. By analogy, a uterus stretched to capacity by a mature fetus may also be "ripe" for emptying. This is an old theory of the cause of labor onset. Stretch may play a role in the initiation of labor, but by itself it does not seem an adequate precipitating cause. It is true that labor generally begins earlier in multiple than in single gestations, but in a single premature birth the uterus empties before it is stretched

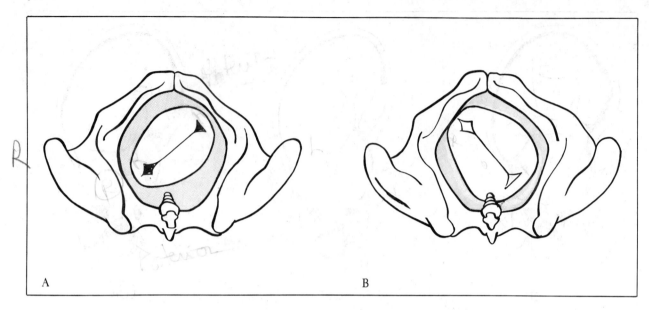

Figure 23-10 *Fetal presentation views from the outlet. A. Right occipitoanterior (ROA). B. Right occipitoposterior (ROP).*

to capacity. Thus, some additional or different mechanism must be involved.

Oxytocin Theory

A second long-accepted theory is that oxytocin, a hormone released by the posterior pituitary gland, initiates labor contractions. It is well established that oxytocin administered to a woman at term will initiate labor; if administered during labor, it acts to strengthen uterine contractions, assisting labor. It can also be demonstrated that at about the thirty-seventh week of pregnancy the uterus becomes increasingly sensitive to oxytocin. (Oxytocinase, an enzyme produced by the placenta that apparently inhibits the action of oxytocin on uterine tissue, decreases at this time.)

Oxytocin is present in maternal blood during labor. Interestingly, however, it is also present under other stress situations. Thus, it may be present in the bloodstream because labor is a stress, not because it *initiates* contractions.

Animal studies have shown that despite destruction of the posterior pituitary so extensive as to preclude the production of oxytocin, labor still occurs at the end of the normal gestation period. Oxytocin appears to have its effect by raising uterine muscle calcium levels to a point at which the myometrium is capable of contraction (Huszar, 1981).

Progesterone Deprivation Theory

It is well known that progesterone is essential for maintaining a pregnancy. When the corpus luteum of pregnancy is removed in rabbits, prompt delivery of the products of conception occurs. Progesterone levels, according to this theory, fall just prior to the onset of labor. This change is not well documented, however, except by the observations of Haskins (1954) that the placentas of women delivered by cesarean birth in whom labor did not occur contain twice as much progesterone as the placentas of women who had been in labor; and by the findings of Kumar et al. (1963) that in the majority of premature births the placenta contains less progesterone than those of infants delivered at term.

Exactly how progesterone can prevent contractions is puzzling. Daniel et al. (1960) suggest that progesterone tends to maintain a high concentration of potassium and a low concentration of sodium chloride and water in the myometrium at the placental site. This high level of potassium may cause a myometrial block. As progesterone production falls, the block lessens, and efficient, coordinated uterine contractions occur. It can be demonstrated that with a high progesterone level present, alpha receptor sites (stimulation sites) in the myometrium are not responsive to epinephrine.

It is well documented that estrogen serum levels rise near term. The decline in progesterone that allows labor to begin, therefore, may not be as much an acute decline as a discrepancy in the estrogen/progesterone ratio that is interpreted as a decline in progesterone.

Fetal Adrenal Response Theory

Interestingly, in 400 B.C., Hippocrates wrote that the fetus initiated labor. Two thousand years later, new research has begun to suggest that his hunch was accurate. In experiments in lambs, when a fetal lamb had its pituitary gland removed in utero, labor did not begin. Labor could be initiated, however, by injecting the lamb fetus with either adrenocorticotropin (ACTH) to stimulate the adrenals or an adrenal hormone. Removal of both adrenal glands in the fetal lamb produced the same threat to labor as removal of the pituitary. Labor in these pregnancies could be initiated by the administration of cortisol. Fetal adrenal glands, therefore, appeared to be responsible for the "trigger" that initiated labor.

Cortisol is not the single trigger for labor, however, because when cortisone is given to mothers to hasten fetal lung maturity, it does not begin uterine contractions. Cortisone, however, probably does play a role in prostaglandin synthesis through its contribution to the production of placental estrogen (see below).

Findings that support this theory in humans are that the adrenal glands in babies born by spontaneous labor are heavier than those of infants born by cesarean birth or by induced labor.

Prostaglandin Initiation Theory

A precursor from the fetal adrenals is conjugated in the placenta into estrogen from early in pregnancy. At term as estrogen formed by fetus and placenta reaches a peak, maternal decidua may begin to synthesize and produce prostaglandin PGF2a. Prostaglandins are formed from arachidonic acid, an essential fatty acid. This may be released by fetal membranes at term and conjugated into prostaglandins by the uterine decidua. Prostaglandins stimulate the myometrium (smooth muscle) to contract; they may play a role in reducing the progesterone level. A low progesterone level causes the uterine muscle to be sensitive to oxytocin. Inhibitors of prostaglandin synthesis such as aspirin may delay labor in women. PGF2a and its immediate precursor are found in increased amounts in amniotic fluid during early spontaneous labor. That prostaglandins can initiate uterine contractions has been established by the usefulness of prostaglandins in induced abortion.

Systemic Effects of Labor on the Mother

Although labor is a local process in that it involves the abdomen and reproductive organs, it is such an intense process that it also has systemic effects.

Cardiovascular System

Labor is hard effort: During this period of activity, cardiac output, blood pressure, and pulse rate all increase. During the second stage (pushing stage) the cardiac output may be increased as much as 40 percent above the prelabor level. Central venous pressure will also rise to reflect the peripheral resistance created by the contracting uterus.

As the fetus is delivered, there is a blood loss averaging 300 to 500 ml. Because a woman's blood volume increases 30 to 50 percent during pregnancy, this blood loss is not detrimental to the average woman but actually plays a role in reducing her blood volume to prepregnancy levels. Immediately following delivery of the fetus, with the weight and pressure removed from the pelvis, blood from the peripheral circulation may "flood" into the pelvic vasculature, momentarily dropping the pressure in the vena cava. This is quickly compensated for; actually a heavy load of blood is then delivered by the vena cava to the heart, which has implications for the mother who has a cardiac problem at the time of birth.

Hemopoietic System

The major change in the blood-forming system is the development of leukocytosis, or a sharp increase in the number of circulating white blood cells. At the end of labor an average woman has a white blood count (WBC) of 25,000 to 30,000 mm^3, compared to a normal of 5,000 to 10,000 mm^3. This response is due to the effect of strenuous exercise. Being alert that the rise occurs prevents you from interpreting an elevated WBC during this time as a suggestion of infection.

Respiratory System

Whenever there is an increase in cardiovascular parameters, there is an accompanying increase in respiratory rate in order to supply additional oxygen for the bloodstream to carry. The woman develops slight hyperventilation. Total oxygen consumption increases much as it would in a person performing strenuous exercises such as running.

Temperature Regulation

The increased muscular activity associated with labor has a tendency to elevate the woman's temperature a degree. In order to prevent excessive temperature increases, diaphoresis occurs with accompanying evaporation to cool and limit warming.

Fluid Balance

Insensible water loss increases during labor because of the increase in rate and depth of respirations (which causes moisture to be lost with each breath) and the presence of diaphoresis. The average woman eats nothing during labor and her fluid intake is reduced to only sips of fluid and ice cubes or hard candy. The combination of increased losses during this time and decreased intake may make supplemental fluid by intravenous therapy necessary. It is important that women recognize the administration of fluid during labor as prophylactic rather than curative. Otherwise they misinterpret fluid administration as an indication that something is going very wrong (television programs use the sight of intravenous fluid as an instant clue that a person has become suddenly very seriously ill) when it is actually being used to ensure that everything will go well. Women also need to be fully informed that intravenous therapy does not hurt once the needle is inserted and will not interfere with ambulation or turning. Otherwise they interpret it as something that will interfere with and make labor an unendurable situation for them.

Elimination

With the decrease in fluid intake during labor and the increased insensible water loss, the kidneys begin to concentrate urine to preserve both fluid and electrolytes (specific gravity will rise to a high normal level of 1.020–1.030). It is not unusual for there to be a trace of protein in urine from the breakdown of protein due to increased muscle activity (trace to 1+). Pressure of the fetal head as it descends in the birth canal against the anterior bladder reduces bladder tone or the ability of the bladder to sense filling. If a woman is not asked to void about every 2 hours during labor, her bladder can overfill and leave her in the postpartal period with lessened bladder tone.

Gastrointestinal System

The gastrointestinal system becomes fairly inactive during labor, probably due to a shift in blood away from it to more life-sustaining organs and to pressure on the stomach and intestine from the contracting uterus. Digestive and emptying time of the stomach is prolonged (the reason eating during labor is usually restricted). Some women experience a loose bowel movement as contractions grow stronger, similar to what may occur with painful menstrual cramps.

Neurologic System

The neurologic responses that occur during labor are related to pain (increased pulse and respiratory rate). Early in labor, the contraction of the uterus and dilatation of the cervix cause the discomfort. Uterine and cervical nerve plexus registers at the 11 and 12 thoracic nerves. At the moment of delivery, the pain is centered on the perineum as it stretches to allow the fetus to move past it. Perineal pain is registered at S2–4.

Pain in labor is not constant; it rises to an acute, wave-like peak, subsides, and then is completely gone until it occurs again. Perineal pain is only a short burning or tingling pain lasting under a minute's time. The more a woman knows about the pattern of the pain, the better able she is to combat it.

Reproductive System

The uterus undergoes the most change during labor in order to effectively expel the fetus to the external world. Related changes occur in the vaginal and perineal muscles.

Perineum

The perineum undergoes thinning as labor progresses so by the time the cervix is dilated and the fetal head begins to descend through the vagina, the depth of the perineal musculature has been reduced to only a 1 cm thickness (from a normal thickness of 4–5 cm). In the thinned state it is easily stretched and mobile, thus allowing the distal end of the vagina to stretch to a distance of 10 cm. The pressure of the fetal head causes so much pressure on the perineum as the thinning and vaginal dilatation occurs that sensory nerve endings are blocked (natural anesthesia of the perineum). This anesthesia is so complete that if the perineum should tear the woman would not even be aware that sensitive body tissue has been injured.

Perineal thinning can be observed during labor. With each contraction, the levator ani muscle and its accompanying fascia draw the vagina and rectum upward, gradually shifting muscle mass away from the birth canal.

Uterus

The mark of labor is regular, gradually progressive uterine contractions that effectively dilate the cervix. Muscle contracts because of actomyosin, a protein substance; adenosine triphosphate (ATP), the substance that supplies the energy for contraction; and adenosine triphosphatase, an enzyme necessary to activate adenosine triphosphate. The formation of adenosine triphosphatase is dependent on the presence of vitamin B complex. A premenopausal woman has more of this contractive substance present in the uterus than

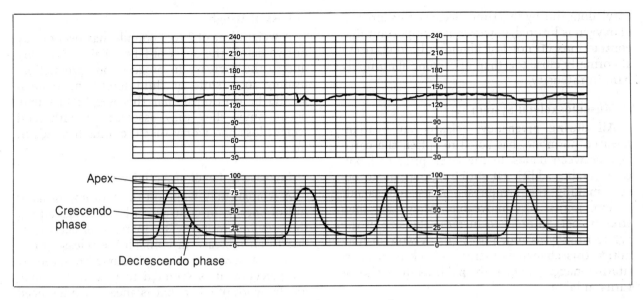

Figure 23-11 *Three phases of a uterine contraction as shown on an electronic uterine monitor. The upper recording line is a fetal heart rate.*

does the postmenopausal woman; it is in even greater amounts in the pregnant than the non-pregnant uterus. The progressive rise in estrogen during pregnancy is probably the influencing factor for adenosine triphosphate being present at the time of labor to maintain contractions.

Uterine contractions have three phases: a first phase during which the intensity of the contraction increases (the increment, or crescendo phase), a second phase during which the contraction reaches its height (apex), and a third phase during which the intensity decreases (decrescendo). The first phase is longer than the other two phases combined. A uterine contraction is diagrammed in Figure 23-11.

Uterine contractions can be palpated by placing your hand on the woman's fundus. They should be assessed in terms of three characteristics: duration, intensity, and frequency.

Duration. The duration of a contraction is the length of the contraction from the time you can feel it on the uterus until the uterus can be felt to relax again. A woman will not feel it as soon as you do, but determine time from your objective view, not hers, for consistency.

If labor is being electronically monitored, the duration of a contraction is measured from the point at which it reaches 20 mm Hg on the monitor screen or tape until, after increasing, it returns to 20 mm Hg again. The woman feels the contraction when the pressure reaches about 25 mm Hg. In early labor, the duration of contractions is about 20 seconds. At the end of labor they are 60 seconds long.

Intensity. Intensity is the strength of a uterine contraction. Contractions are *mild* if the uterus can be easily indented with your fingers at the height of a contraction, *moderate* if indentation is becoming difficult, and *strong* if the uterus cannot be indented by examining fingers. Always feel for intensity gently; the fundus grows sensitive to manipulation as labor progresses, and the feel of probing fingers becomes painful.

Normally the resting pressure of the uterus is 0 to 15 mm Hg. If an internal uterine monitor is being used, a mild contraction is one in which pressure is about 30 mm Hg. A strong contraction has a pressure reading of 50 mm Hg. Moderate contractions, therefore, are those with pressures between 30 to 50 mm Hg. Contractions gradually intensify during the first stage of labor, beginning as mild contractions and then becoming strong.

Frequency. Frequency is the rate at which contractions are occurring. Frequency is timed from the *beginning* of one contraction to the *beginning* of the next. The interval may be 40 to 50 minutes at the beginning of labor but gradually decreases until contractions are no more than 2 minutes apart in the second stage of labor. It is important that a relaxation interval always be present, even if it is only a minute in length, to allow time for uterine blood vessels to fill and continue to supply adequate nutrients and oxygen to the fetus during labor.

During a contraction, both uterine veins and arteries are compressed to some extent, causing poor blood flow into and away from the placental cotyledons. The fetus draws on the oxygen in the cotyledons during this time. Because this amount of oxygen is limited, however, it is important that contractions do not last abnormally long, occur abnormally close together, or become abnormally hard in intensity.

Musculoskeletal System

All during pregnancy, relaxin, an ovarian-released hormone, has acted to soften the cartilage between bones. In the week prior to labor, considerable additional softening appears to occur, making the symphysis pubis and sacral/coccyx joints very moveable. They can then stretch apart in order to increase the size of the pelvic ring by as much as 2 cm. A woman may notice this change as increased back pain or irritating, nagging pain at the pubis as she walks or turns in labor.

Signs of Labor

During the 40 weeks of gestation, subtle physiologic and psychological changes have taken place in the gravid woman preparatory for labor. At the same time, fetal growth and development progress, finally, bringing the fetus to the point where he can survive in an extrauterine environment.

By the end of pregnancy, women feel so short of breath, have so many minor discomforts (backache, frequency of urination), and have planned for so long that, however much they may dread the beginning of labor, they rarely fail to feel relief on realizing that the time for labor is at hand.

Preliminary Clues

Lightening

In primiparas, lightening or settling of the fetal presenting part to the level of the ischial spines occurs about 10 to 14 days before labor begins. It changes the shape of the woman's abdominal contour as the uterus is lower and more anterior. Lightening gives the woman relief from the diaphragmatic pressure and shortness of breath she has been experiencing. The woman may have shooting pains in her legs from pressure on the sciatic nerve following lightening. She will certainly notice an increase in frequency of urination from the increased pressure on the bladder. Walking may be awkward and waddling from the lower center of gravity. Lightening probably occurs early in primigravidas because of tight abdominal muscles. In multiparas, lightening is not as dramatic and usually occurs on the day of labor or even after labor has begun.

Loss of Weight

A weight loss of 2 to 3 pounds may occur a day or two before the onset of labor. This is probably due to the decrease in progesterone production, leading to a shift in fluid retention. Women should be cautioned that this weight loss may occur, since they may associate it with fetal weight loss and worry that the fetus has died in utero.

Increase in Level of Activity

A woman may wake on the morning of labor full of energy, in contrast to her feelings during the previous month. The increase in activity is due to an increase in epinephrine release, initiated by a decrease in progesterone produced by the placenta; it is secreted to prepare her body for the work of labor that is ahead. Women need to be told that this energy is to assist them in labor; you do not want them to arrive at the hospital exhausted from other activities and unable to participate fully in labor. If a woman is extremely fatigued when she enters labor, uterine contractions cannot be maintained and she may need medication to help her achieve adequate contractions.

Braxton Hicks Contractions

In the last week or days before labor begins, the woman usually notices extremely strong Braxton Hicks contractions, which she may interpret as true labor contractions. They can be differentiated from true labor contractions in the ways summarized in Table 23-5.

Table 23-5 Differentiation Between True and False Labor Contractions

False Contractions	True Contractions
Begin and remain irregular.	Begin irregularly but become regular and predictable.
Felt first abdominally and remain confined to the abdomen.	Felt first in lower back and sweep around to the abdomen in a wave.
Often disappear with ambulation.	Continue no matter what the woman's level of activity.
Do not increase in duration, frequency, or intensity.	Increase in duration, frequency, and intensity.
Do not achieve cervical dilatation.	Achieve cervical dilatation.

Women, particularly primiparas, have great difficulty in distinguishing between the two forms of contractions. A woman sometimes comes to the hospital or a birthing center and is admitted to the labor unit because the false contractions so closely simulate real labor. It is discouraging for a woman who is having discomfort (and false or not, strong Braxton Hicks contractions cause discomfort) to be told that she is not in true labor and should return home to wait for true contractions to begin. It is something like waking Christmas morning and being told that Christmas has been postponed for a week. Such women need sympathetic support. They do not find their situation amusing. They can be assured that misinterpreting labor signals is a natural mistake. They can be told that if false contractions have become so strong that they can be mistaken for true labor, true labor must not be far away.

Ripening of the Cervix

Ripening of the cervix is an internal sign, of which a woman is not aware; it is seen only on pelvic examination. The physician, nurse-midwife, or nurse practitioner will look for this sign at the pregnancy's predicted term. All during pregnancy, the cervix feels softer than normal and has the consistency of an earlobe (Goodell's sign). At term, the cervix becomes still softer, until it can be described as "buttersoft," and tips forward. This is ripening, an internal announcement that labor is close at hand.

Rupture of the Membranes

Labor may begin with rupture of the membranes, which the woman experiences as either a sudden gush or scanty, slow seeping of clear fluid from the vagina. Women worry when labor begins with rupture of the membranes because of old wives' tales that such labors are "dry" and thus difficult and long. Actually, amniotic fluid continues to be formed until delivery of the membranes, after the child is born: No labor is ever dry. Early rupture of the membranes causes the fetal head to settle snugly into the pelvis and may actually shorten labor.

A woman who experiences rupture of the membranes as a sudden gush of fluid should lie down with her feet elevated. Someone should telephone her physician or nurse-midwife, who will probably instruct her to come into a hospital or birthing center so that it can be determined whether the fetal head is firmly engaged and fitting snugly into the pelvic brim. If it is not, the umbilical cord may prolapse into the vagina after the membranes supporting it are ruptured. A pro-

lapsed cord may be compressed by the fetal head, and the fetus's oxygen supply may be compromised.

If membranes rupture more than 24 hours prior to the delivery of the child, intrauterine infection is a possible consequence. Labor is generally induced at the end of 24 hours following membrane rupture if it has not begun spontaneously by that time, provided a woman is estimated to be at term. An antibiotic may be ordered for the woman to protect the fetus against infection, although there is no established proof that amnionitis will be prevented by such a measure.

Show

The pressure of the descending presenting part of the fetus causes rupture of minute capillaries in the mucous membrane of the cervix. This small amount of blood mixes with mucus and is evident as a pink or brown (old blood) vaginal discharge when the mucous plug (operculum) that has filled the cervical canal during pregnancy is released. Show should be no more than a pinkish discharge. Fresh bleeding accompanying the operculum discharge is abnormal and is a danger sign of labor, usually signaling placental bleeding. Show is proof that cervical dilatation is beginning; with dilatation, the operculum can no longer be contained in the canal.

True Labor

Uterine Contractions

The surest sign that labor has begun is the initiation of effective, productive uterine contractions. Uterine contractions are not unlike atrial or ventricle cardiac contractions. They are involuntary. The woman has no more control over their duration, intensity, or progress than she does over her heartbeat. This is frightening in early labor until a woman realizes that she can control the degree of discomfort contractions give her if she uses the exercises she has learned in preparation-for-labor classes.

Labor contractions appear to begin at a "pacemaker" point in the myometrium of the fundus near one or the other uterotubal junctions. Perhaps contractions begin in the fundus merely because the bulk of myometrial cells are there. Once it begins, each contraction sweeps down over the uterus as a wave. After a short rest period, another contraction is initiated and the downward wave begins again.

In early labor, the uterotubal pacemakers or the spontaneous initiation of contractions may not be working in a synchronous manner; in this event contractions are sometimes strong, sometimes weak, and not very regular. This mild incoordination of early labor improves after a few hours, however, as the cells become more attuned to calcium concentrations and begin to function smoothly.

In some women contractions appear to originate in the lower uterine segment rather than in the fundus. These are reverse, ineffective contractions, which actually cause contraction rather than dilatation of the cervix. Initiation of contractions in a reverse pattern is difficult to tell from palpation. It can be suspected if a woman tells you that she feels pain in her lower abdomen before the contraction is readily palpated at the fundus. It is truly revealed only when cervical *dilatation* does not occur.

Other women seem to have additional pacemaker sites or the initiation of contractions in other portions of the uterus, in which situation, severe incoordination of contractions will occur. Uncoordinated contractions slow labor and may lead to failure to progress in labor and fetal distress because they do not allow for adequate placental filling. Evaluating the rate, intensity, and pattern of uterine contractions is an important nursing responsibility with a woman in labor.

As labor contractions progress, the uterus is gradually differentiated into two distinct portions. The upper portion becomes thicker and active, preparing it to exert the strength necessary to expel the fetus when the expulsion phase of labor is reached. The lower segment becomes thin-walled, supple, and passive, so that the fetus can be pushed out of the uterus easily.

As the lower segment thins and the upper segment thickens, the boundary between the two portions becomes marked by a ridge on the inner uterine surface, the *physiologic retraction ring.*

In addition to this change in the contour of the uterine wall is a change in the contour of the overall uterus. The contour changes from a round ovoid to a structure more markedly elongated in a vertical than horizontal diameter. This lengthening of the body of the uterus serves to straighten the body of the fetus and place it in better alignment to the cervix and pelvis. Round ligaments move with the uterus as it contracts and keep the fundus forward, again to assist with placing the fetus in good alignment with the cervix. The elongation of the uterus causes it to press against the diaphragm and causes the often expressed sensation that a uterus is "taking over control" of a woman's body.

In a difficult labor, particularly in obstructed labor, when the fetus is larger than the birth canal, the round ligaments of the uterus may become tense during dilatation and expulsion and

may be palpable on the abdomen. The normal physiologic retraction ring may become prominent and observable as an abdominal indentation. Termed a *pathologic retraction ring*, or *Bandl's ring*, this danger sign of labor signifies impending rupture of the lower uterine segment if the obstruction to labor is not relieved.

Cervical Changes

Even more marked than uterine body changes are the two changes that occur in the cervix: effacement and dilatation.

Effacement. Effacement is the shortening and thinning of the cervical canal from its normal length of 1 to 2 cm to a structure with paper-thin edges in which no canal distinct from the uterus appears to exist. It is illustrated in Figure 23-12, and occurs because of longitudinal traction from the contracting uterine fundus.

In primiparas, effacement is accomplished before dilatation begins. This is an important phenomenon to point out to a woman during her first labor. She will become discouraged if, for example, at 12:00 noon her physician reports to her that she is 2 cm dilated—and again at 4:00 P.M. that she is still 2 cm dilated. Absolutely nothing has seemed to happen in 4 hours. Effacement is what is happening; when effacement is complete, dilatation will then progress rapidly.

Figure 23-12 *Effacement and dilatation of cervix. A. Beginning labor. B. Effacement is beginning; dilatation is not apparent yet. C. Effacement is almost complete. D. After complete effacement, dilatation proceeds rapidly.*

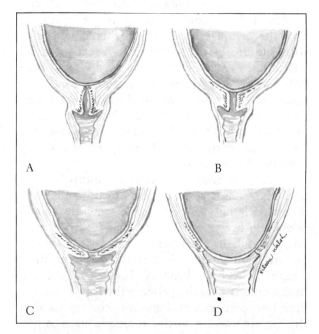

In multiparas, dilatation may proceed before effacement is complete. Effacement must occur at the end of dilatation before the fetus can be safely pushed through the cervical canal, or cervical tearing may result.

Dilatation. Dilatation (Figure 23-12) denotes the enlargement of the cervical canal from an opening a few millimeters wide to one large enough to permit passage of the fetus (about 10 cm).

Dilatation occurs for two reasons: uterine contractions gradually increase the diameter of the cervical canal lumen by pulling the cervix up over the presenting part of the fetus, and the fluid-filled membranes press against the cervix. If the membranes are intact, they push ahead of the fetus and serve as an opening wedge; if they are ruptured, the presenting part will serve this same function. Excessive pressure against the cervix, such as would occur if a woman pushed during this stage, interferes with dilatation by causing edema of the cervix. The best action of a woman during the stage of dilatation is to relax, so that she does not push with contractions.

There is an increase in the amount of show as dilatation begins, since the last of the operculum is dislodged and minute capillaries in the cervix rupture.

Stages of Labor

Labor has traditionally been divided into three stages: a first stage of dilatation beginning with true labor contractions and ending when the cervix is fully dilated; a second stage from the time of full dilatation until the infant is born; and a third or placental stage from the time the infant is born until following the delivery of the placenta.

Some authorities term the first 1 to 4 hours following delivery of the placenta the *fourth stage* of labor, to emphasize the importance of the close observation needed at that time to ensure safety of the mother. This is a helpful term in regard to planning nursing interventions except that active nursing intervention to ensure safety of the mother should be engaged in during the entire pregnancy, labor and delivery, and the postpartal period, not just in the first hour after birth and as other health care personnel do not use the term, it makes communication with others difficult. Newer terminology in reference to labor makes use of this term obsolete.

Friedman (1978) has classified the first and second stages of labor into divisions according to the objective being accomplished during each time interval. These new divisions are a *preparatory* division, a *dilatational* division, and a *pelvic* division, followed by delivery.

The Preparatory Division

The preparatory division is a time during which the cervix is readied for dilatation as uterine contractions become regular and coordinated. It consists of two phases: a latent phase and an acceleration (active) phase (Figure 23-13).

During the latent phase (that period of labor beginning at the onset of regular perceived uterine contractions and ending at the point where rapid cervical dilatation begins), contractions are mild and short (20–30 seconds in length). They gradually increase in duration and intensity. Cervical effacement occurs and the cervix dilates from 0 to 2 cm during this phase. The phase lasts about 6 hours in a nullipara, 4.5 hours in a multipara. A woman who enters labor with a "non-ripe" cervix, or one that is not soft, will have a longer-than-usual latent phase.

Analgesia given too early in labor will prolong this phase. The latent phase can also be prolonged when a cephalopelvic disproportion exists. In a woman who is psychologically prepared for labor and who does not tense at each tightening sensation in her abdomen, latent phase contractions cause only minimal discomfort. A woman can continue to walk about and make preparations for birth, such as last-minute packing of her suitcase for the hospital or birthing center or preparing her children for her departure and giving instructions to the person who will take care of them while she is away.

The acceleration phase is the remainder of the first division of labor. During this phase, cervical dilatation begins to be accomplished more rapidly; contractions are stronger (30–45 seconds long; 3–5 minutes apart). This phase lasts about 3 hours in a nullipara, 2 hours in a multipara. Show and perhaps spontaneous rupture of the membranes occur. Although this is a difficult time for a woman in labor (contractions begin to bite, or cause true discomfort), it is also an exciting time because she realizes that something very dramatic is happening. It may be a frightening time as she realizes that labor is truly progressing; she can never go back to being a child-free adult again.

The Dilatational Division

The dilatational, or second, division of labor is that time period during which cervical dilatation proceeds at its most rapid pace (also termed the

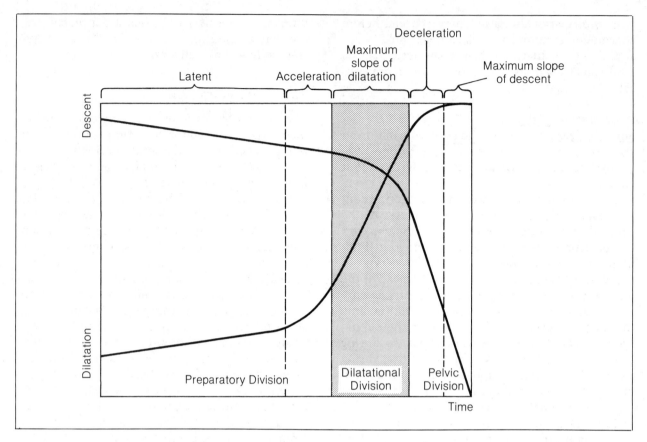

Figure 23-13 *Divisions of labor. From Friedman E. (1978).* Labor, clinical evaluation and management. *(2nd ed.). New York: Appleton-Century-Crofts.*

period of maximum slope). Analgesic administration has little effect on progress at this point. Cervical dilatation proceeds at an average rate of 3.5 cm per hour in nulliparas, 5.9 cm per hour in multiparas.

Most women assume that dilatation occurs at a steady rate throughout labor. They may grow discouraged at realizing that in the 10 previous hours (the latent and acceleration phases) their cervix has only dilated 4 cm. They imagine that labor will last at least 15 hours more. In nulliparas, however, cervical dilatation from 4 to 8 cm will take only 1 to 2 hours more; in multiparas, it may be as short as half an hour. During this division, contractions grow strong, hard, and frequent (45–60 seconds in duration with 2- to 3-minute time intervals). Some women attempt to speed labor during this period by bearing down or pushing. Teach them it is important *not* to do this until full dilatation has occurred or the cervix will grow edematous and labor will slow.

The Pelvic Division

The pelvic division includes a deceleration phase and a fetal descent phase. Deceleration is a mis-

nomer in that the progress of labor does not actually slow at this point; the final degrees of cervical dilatation are achieved and the cervix retracts over the presenting part. Contractions are so hard that the uterus feels like wood at the peak of a contraction, and they are quite long (60 to 70 seconds in duration). If the membranes have not previously ruptured or been ruptured by amniotomy, they will rupture as a rule at full dilatation. If it has not previously occurred, show will be present as the last of the operculum is released. This phase averages about 1 hour in a nullipara, one-half hour in a multipara.

With full dilatation and retraction of the cervix over the presenting part, fetal descent and negotiation of the pelvis occurs rapidly. A woman may experience momentary nausea or vomiting, since pressure is no longer exerted on the stomach because of the downward movement of the fetus. Contractions change from the characteristic crescendo-decrescendo pattern she has grown accustomed to, to an overwhelming, uncontrollable urge to push or bear down with contractions as if she were moving her bowels. She pushes with such force that she perspires and the blood vessels in her neck become distended. As the fetus de-

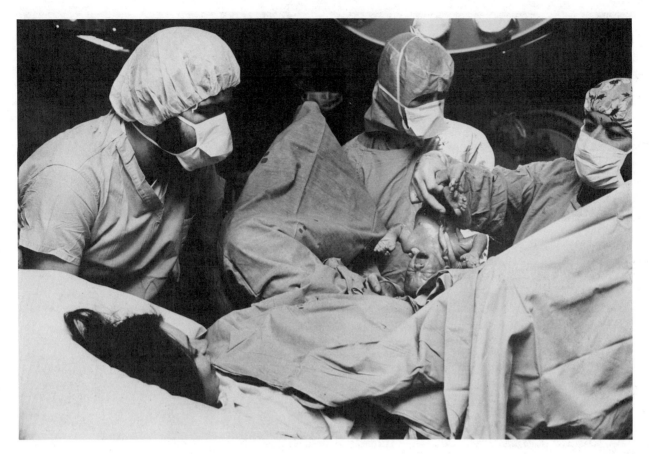

Figure 23-14 *New parents watch their baby being born. (Courtesy of the Department of Medical Photography, Children's Hospital, Buffalo, N.Y.)*

scends in the pelvic ring, being pushed beyond the open cervix, the woman's perineum begins to bulge, the labia begin to part, the vaginal introitus to stretch apart, and the presenting part of the fetus to be evident (termed *crowning*). There may be additional blood-tinged show as cervical mucus is pushed ahead of the fetus.

As these changes in the pattern of labor occur, a woman may experience a feeling of panic or acute anxiety and become argumentative or irritable. Up to this point, she may have felt in charge of her labor, aware that she could control the degree of pain or discomfort by breathing exercises. Now the sensation in her abdomen is so intense that it may seem as though labor has taken charge of her. A few minutes before, she enjoyed having her forehead wiped with a cool cloth; now she may knock your hand away. A minute before, she enjoyed having her husband rub her back; now she may resist his touch or thrust him away.

It takes a few contractions of this new type for a woman to realize that everything is still all right, just different; to appreciate that it feels good, not frightening, to push with contractions. In actuality, the need to push becomes so intense

that she cannot stop herself from pushing. She barely hears the conversation in the room around her. She does not hear your instructions. All of her energy, her thoughts, her being are directed toward delivering her child.

A woman may have sharp cramps in the calves of her legs as the fetus is pushed against pelvic nerves. These cramps are relieved in the same way as are the cramps that tend to occur during pregnancy, namely by straightening the leg and dorsiflexing the foot. The cramp may recur with the next contraction, however. As she pushes, using her abdominal muscles and the involuntary uterine contractions, the fetus is pushed out of the dilated uterus through the birth canal (Figure 23-14).

Delivery

Delivery occurs because the pressure of the presenting part on the perineum causes final stretching of the vaginal introitus. In a vertex presentation, gentle pressure for a moment on the perineum allows the head to slip out easily; following external rotation (described below) the shoulders also deliver readily following gentle

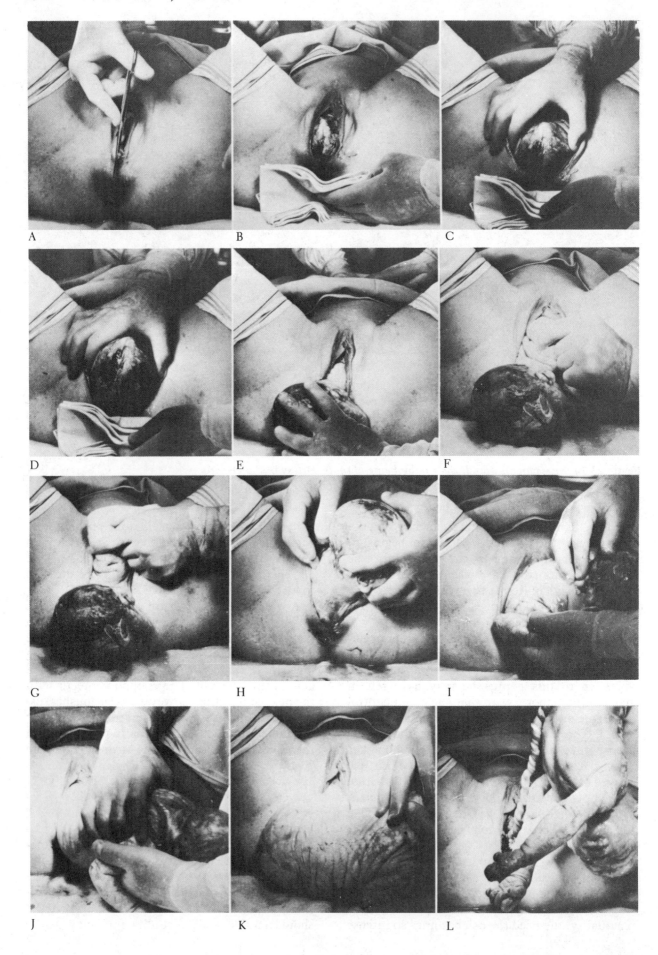

A

B

C

D

E

F

G

H

I

J

K

L

Table 23-6 Principal Clinical Features of the Divisions of Labor

Characteristic	Preparatory Division	Dilatational Division	Pelvic Division
Functions	Contractions coordinated, polarized, oriented; cervix prepared	Cervix actively dilated	Pelvis negotiated; mechanisms of labor; fetal descent; delivery
Interval	Latent and acceleration phases	Phase of maximum slope	Deceleration phase and second stage
Measurement	Elapsed duration	Linear rate of dilatation	Linear rate of descent
Diagnosable disorders	Prolonged latent phase	Protracted dilatation; protracted descent	Prolonged deceleration; secondary arrest of dilatation; arrest of descent; failure of descent

Source: Friedman, E. (1978). *Labor, clinical evaluation and management.* (2nd ed.). New York: Appleton-Century-Crofts.

traction on the head. The remainder of the child's body then slides outward without any further opposition (Figure 23-15).

The principal clinical features of the divisions of labor are shown in Table 23-6. The newer method of dividing labor and relevant characteristics are contrasted to the traditional stages of labor in Table 23-7. Divisions of labor are shown diagrammatically in Figure 23-13.

Fetal Response to Labor

Although the fetus is basically a passive participant in labor, the effect of pressure and circulatory changes cause detectable physiologic differences, as well as position changes.

Systemic Changes

Neurologic System

The pressure exerted by uterine contractions on the fetal head can be detected by the change in fetal cardiac rate during contractions. The fetal heart rate typically decreases by 5 mm Hg at the height of a contraction as soon as contraction strength reaches 40 mm Hg. This is the same response that occurs in any instance of increased intracranial pressure.

Cardiovascular System

The average fetus has such mature response ability to cardiovascular change that he or she is unaffected by the continual slowing (bradycardia) and the return to normal (baseline) levels of heart rate that occur with labor. During a contraction, the arteries of the uterus, which are corkscrew in contour, are sharply constricted. Filling of cotyledons therefore almost completely halts during a contraction. The amount of nutrients exchanged during this time is reduced, causing a slight hypoxia. The corresponding increase in blood pressure, which occurs from increased intracranial pressure, serves to keep circulation from falling below normal during the time of labor.

Integument

The pressure involved in birth is often reflected in minimal petechiae or ecchymotic places on the fetus (particularly the presenting part). Edema (a caput succedaneum) will also invariably be present.

Musculoskeletal System

The uterine contractions tend to force the fetus into a position of full flexion. As this is the position assumed during pregnancy, it causes no discomfort or difficulty for the fetus.

Respiratory System

The process of labor appears to aid in the maturation of surfactant production by alveoli of the lung. The pressure applied to the chest clears it of lung fluid so the infant born by vaginal birth tends to be able to establish respirations easier than the fetus born by cesarean birth.

Position Changes

Passage of the fetus through the birth canal involves a number of different position changes to

Figure 23-15 *Birth of a baby. From Danforth, D. (Ed.). (1971).* Textbook of obstetrics and gynecology. *(2nd ed.). New York: Harper & Row.*

Table 23-7 Divisions of Labor

| Assessment | Preparatory Division | | Dilatational Division | Pelvic Division | |
	Latent Phase	Acceleration Phase	Phase of Maximum Slope	Phase	Fetal Descent
Time interval	6.1 hours nullipara	3.4 hours nullipara	1–2 hours nullipara (3.5 cm/hr dilatation rate)	0.7 hour nullipara	0.7 hour nullipara (3.6 cm/hr rate)
	4.5 hours multipara	2.1 hours multipara	½–1 hour multipara (5.9 cm/hr dilatation rate)	0.3 hour multipara	0.3 hour multipara (7.0 cm/hr rate)
Contractions Duration Frequency Intensity	20–30 seconds 5–20 minutes Mild (30 mm Hg)	Contractions increasing in frequency, intensity, and duration	30–60 seconds 3–5 minutes Moderate–strong (30–50 mm Hg)	60–70 seconds 2 minutes Strong (50–100 mm Hg)	
Fetal descent	Station 0 in nullipara Station 0 to + 2 in multipara	+1 to +2	+2 +1 to +2	+2 to +4 +2 to +4	
Cervical dilatation	0–4 cm	4–8 cm	8–10 cm		

├──────── Traditional first stage ────────┤ Traditional transitional period ├── Traditional second stage ──┤

Source: Adapted from Friedman, E. (1978). *Labor, clinical evaluation and management.* (2nd ed.). New York: Appleton-Century-Crofts.

keep the smallest diameter of the fetal head (in cephalic presentations) always presenting to the smallest diameter of the birth canal. These position changes are termed the *cardinal movements of labor*. They are *descent, flexion, internal rotation, extension, external rotation,* and *expulsion* (Figure 23-16).

Descent

Descent begins with engagement. In primiparas, descent occurs approximately 2 weeks before labor. In multiparas, it occurs with the beginning of labor or with the pelvic division. Descent is the downward movement of the biparietal diameter of the fetal head to within the pelvic inlet. Full descent occurs when the fetal head extrudes beyond the dilated cervix and touches the posterior vaginal floor. This causes the mother to experience a pushing sensation (the pressure of the fetus on the sacral nerves causes the sensation). The fetal heartbeat should be recorded at this point in labor, since this is a particularly dangerous point

for the fetus; the movement downward into the birth canal may cause compression of the cord, compromising blood supply. Descent occurs because of pressure on the fetus by the uterine fundus; full descent may be aided by abdominal muscle contraction.

Flexion

As descent occurs, pressure from the pelvic floor causes the head to bend forward onto the chest. The smallest anteroposterior diameter (the suboccipitobregmatic diameter) is the one presented to the birth canal in this flexed position. Flexion is aided by the abdominal muscle contraction during pushing.

Internal Rotation

During descent, the head enters the pelvis with the fetal anteroposterior head diameter in a diagonal or transverse position. The head flexes as it touches the pelvic floor, and the occiput rotates until it is superior, or just below the symphysis

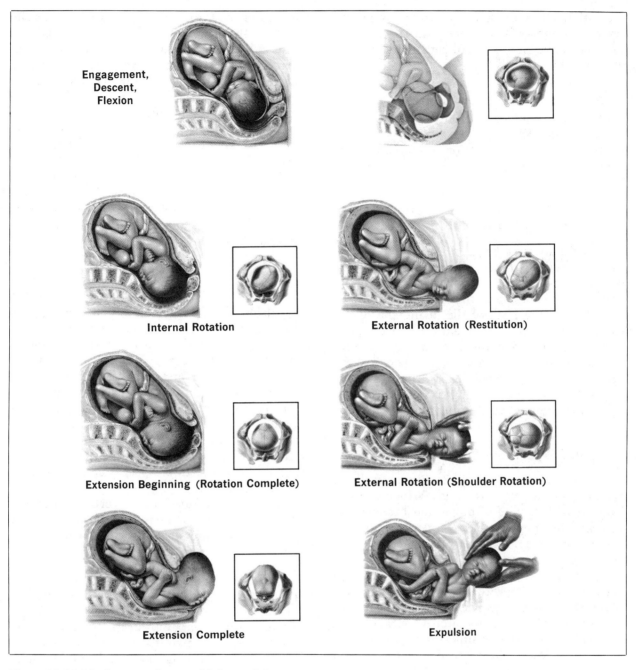

Figure 23-16 *Mechanism of normal labor in left occipitoanterior position. (From Clinical Education Aid, No. 13, Ross Laboratories, Columbus, Ohio, 1964.)*

pubis, bringing the head into the best diameter for the outlet of the pelvis (the anteroposterior diameter is now in the anteroposterior plane of the pelvis). This movement brings the shoulders, coming next, into the optimum position to enter the inlet or puts the widest diameter of the shoulders (a transverse one) in line with the wide transverse diameter of the inlet.

Extension

As the occiput is born, the back of the neck stops beneath the pubic arch and acts as a pivot for the rest of the head. The head thus extends, and the foremost parts of the head, the face and chin, are born.

External Rotation

In external rotation, almost immediately after the head of the infant is born, the head rotates from the anteroposterior position it assumed to enter the outlet, back to the diagonal or transverse position of the early part of labor. The after-coming shoulders are thus brought into an anteroposterior position, which is best for entering the outlet. The anterior shoulder stops under the symphysis pubis, allowing the posterior shoulder to be delivered first, assisted perhaps by upward flexion of the infant's body.

Expulsion

Once the shoulders are delivered, the rest of the baby is delivered easily and smoothly because of its smaller size. Expulsion is the end of the pelvic division of labor.

Placental Stage of Labor

The placental stage begins with delivery of the infant and ends with the delivery of the placenta. Two separate phases are involved: a placental separation phase and a placental expulsion phase.

Following the birth of the infant, the uterus can be palpated as a firm, round mass just inferior to the level of the umbilicus. After a few minutes of rest, uterine contractions begin again, and the organ assumes a discoid shape. It remains this new shape until the placenta has separated, about 5 minutes after delivery of the infant.

Placental Separation

Placental separation takes place automatically as the uterus resumes contractions. With a contraction, there is such a disproportion between the placenta itself and its attachment site as the uterus contracts down on an almost empty interior that folding and separation of the placenta occur. Active bleeding on the maternal surface of the placenta begins with separation; the bleeding helps to separate the placenta still further by pushing it away from its site. As separation is completed, the placenta sinks to the posterior aspect of the lower uterine segment or the upper vagina.

The occurrence of separation is suggested by a number of signs: a sudden gush of blood from the vagina; the extension of the umbilical cord 3 or more inches out of the vagina; a change in the uterus as it becomes firmer and round in shape again and rises high in the abdomen to the level of the umbilicus.

If the placenta separates first at its center and last at its edges, it tends to fold on itself like an umbrella and presents at the vaginal opening with the fetal surface evident (Figure 23-17A). It appears shiny and glistening from the fetal membranes. This is called a *Schultze presentation.* About 80 percent of placentas separate and pre-

sent this way. If the placenta separates first at its edges, it slides along the uterine surface and presents at the vagina with the maternal surface evident (Figure 23-17B). It looks raw, red, and irregular because its cotyledons show. This is a *Duncan presentation.* The two presentations have long been remembered by nurses by their associating "shiny" (the fetal membrane surface) with Schultze and "dirty" (the irregular maternal surface) with Duncan (Figure 23-18).

Bleeding occurs with placental separation as part of the normal consequence of the process, before the uterus can contract enough following placental delivery to seal maternal sinuses. The normal blood loss is 250 to 300 ml.

Placental Expulsion

Expulsion of the placenta may be effected by the mother's bearing down as she did during the second stage of labor; or, if she is anesthetized, by the physician's or nurse-midwife's gentle pressure on the fundus of the uterus (after it is first established that the uterus is firm and contracted). This is termed a *Crede's maneuver.* If *pressure is applied to a uterus in a noncontracted state, it may evert (turn inside out).* This is a grave complication of delivery; in an everted uterus, the maternal blood sinuses are open, and gross hemorrhage occurs.

If the placenta does not deliver spontaneously, it can be removed manually. With delivery of the placenta, the third stage of labor is over.

Danger Signals of Labor

There is a wide variation in the pattern of labor contractions and maternal response to labor and delivery. Certain signals alert you that the course of events is deviating too far from normal. These are summarized in the box on page 502.

Fetal Signals

Fetal Heart Rate

As a rule of thumb, fetal heart rates over 160 beats per minute (marked fetal tachycardia) or below 100 beats per minute (marked fetal bradycardia) are signals that the fetus is experiencing distress. Stage II and variable dipping patterns (see Chapter 24) on fetal monitors are just as important signs of fetal distress as tachycardia or bradycardia. The fetal heart rate may return to within

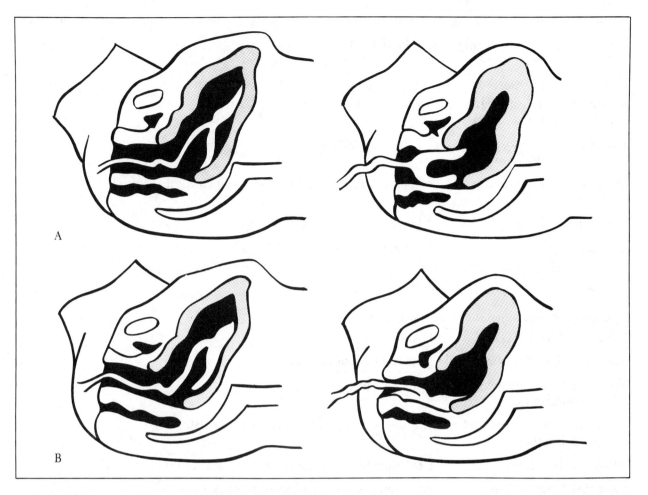

Figure 23-17 *Delivery of the placenta. Note the change in contour of the woman's abdomen after separation of placenta. A. Placenta separates first at center and delivers with fetal surface in evidence (Schultze presentation). B. Placenta separates first at edge and delivers with maternal surface in evidence (Duncan presentation).*

Figure 23-18 *Maternal (left) and fetal (right) surface of the placenta. (From Clinical Education Aid, No. 2, Ross Laboratories, Columbus, Ohio, 1960.)*

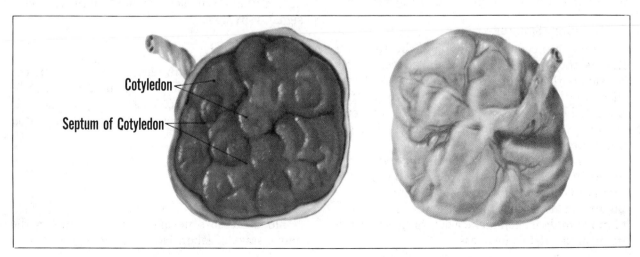

Danger Signals of Labor

Fetal Danger Signals	Probable Cause
Decreasing fetal heart rate (below 100 beats/minute).	Hypoxia is developing.
Increasing fetal heart rate (above 160 beats/minute).	Hypoxia is developing.
Abnormal fetal monitoring patterns.	Hypoxia from cord compression or placental insufficiency.
Meconium staining.	Anoxia with vagal stimulation.
Hyperactivity.	Hypoxia.
Fetal acidosis (fetal blood pH below 7.2).	Hypoxia.

Maternal Danger Signals	Probable Cause
Decreasing blood pressure.	Hemorrhage.
Increasing blood pressure.	Hypertension of pregnancy.
Increasing pulse rate (over 100 beats/minute).	Hemorrhage.
Contractions longer than 70 seconds duration.	Uterine tetany (fetal hypoxia will result).
Pathologic retraction ring.	Cephalopelvic disproportion (uterine rupture is imminent).
Abnormal lower abdomen contour.	A full bladder is in danger of rupture.
Increasing apprehension.	Psychological trauma or oxygen want.

101 to 159 beats per minute between these patterns and give you a false feeling of security if you are relying only on the first rule of thumb.

Meconium Staining

Although meconium staining of the amniotic fluid is not always a sign of fetal distress, its correlation with fetal distress is high. It may indicate that a vagal reflex of the fetus, due to hypoxia, has increased bowel motility and caused loss of rectal sphincter control, leading to the escape of meconium into amniotic fluid.

Meconium staining may be normal when the presentation is breech, since pressure on the buttocks can cause meconium loss. Meconium staining should always be reported, so that a physician or nurse-midwife can make a determination as to its meaning and seriousness.

Hyperactivity

Ordinarily, a fetus is quiet and barely moving during labor. Hyperactivity of the fetus may be a signal of hypoxia.

Fetal Acidosis

When blood determinations are made on the fetus during labor by use of a scalp capillary technique, the finding of acidosis (blood pH below 7.2) is a certain sign that fetal well-being is becoming compromised.

Maternal Signals

Blood Pressure

Blood pressure normally rises slightly in the pelvic stage of labor. How high is high or low is low depends on what blood pressure is normal for the woman in her nonpregnant state. A rule of thumb in labor is to report a systolic pressure over 140 mm Hg and a diastolic pressure over 90 mm Hg, or an increase in the systolic pressure of 30 mm Hg or diastolic pressure over 15 mm Hg (the basic criteria for pregnancy-induced hypertension). A falling blood pressure is just as essential to report as an increasing one, since it may be the first sign of an occult intrauterine hemorrhage. A falling blood pressure is often associated with other clinical signs of shock, namely, apprehension, increased pulse rate, and pallor.

Pulse

Most women during pregnancy have an average pulse rate of 70 to 80 beats per minute. Pulse normally increases slightly during the pelvic division of labor because of the exertion involved in this division. A maternal pulse more rapid than 100 beats per minute during the normal course of labor is unusual. In general, pulse rates over 100 should be reported as possible indications of hemorrhage.

Contractions

Uterine contractions become more frequent, more intense, and longer in duration as labor progresses. Contractions becoming less frequent or less intense or shorter in duration may indicate uterine exhaustion (inertia). This problem must be corrected or a cesarean birth performed if delivery is to be achieved.

A period of relaxation must be provided between contractions if the intervillous spaces of the uterus are to fill and maintain an adequate supply of oxygen and nutrients for the fetus. As a rule of thumb, uterine contractions lasting longer than 70 seconds may begin to compromise fetal well-being and should be reported. The physician or nurse-midwife can then make a determination, based on the fetal heart sounds and the stage of labor, as to the effect, if any, of these long contractions on fetal or maternal well-being.

Pathologic Retraction Ring

An indentation across a woman's abdomen where the upper and lower segments of the uterus join may be a sign of impending uterine rupture, or at least of uterine distress. For this reason, it is important to observe the contours of the woman's abdomen periodically during labor. If you are auscultating the fetal heartbeat by stethoscope, observation of the woman's abdomen is automatic. If an electronic monitor is in place, you have to remember to make these observations.

Abnormal Lower Abdomen Contour

A full bladder during labor may be manifested as a round, protruding bulge on the lower anterior abdomen. This is a danger signal for two reasons: the bladder may be injured by the pressure of the fetal head, or the pressure of the full bladder may not allow for descent of the fetal head.

Increasing Apprehension

Warnings of psychological danger during labor are as important to consider in assessing maternal well-being as are the traditional physical signs. A woman who is so frightened that she cannot cooperate in delivery needs more anesthetic than does the woman who is secure that everything that is happening to her is within normal expectations. The more anesthetic that is used, the greater the risk to woman and fetus. A woman who is becoming increasingly apprehensive despite clear explanations of unfolding events may be close to the pelvic division of labor. She may also have a concern that you have not met. Try an approach such as "You seem more and more concerned. Could you tell me what it is that is worrying you?" Seek consultation to investigate this apprehension as you would for a physical danger signal. Increasing apprehension can also be a signal of oxygen want or internal hemorrhage.

Utilizing Nursing Process

In order that nursing care during the period of labor is designed to make the process safe and optimally the enriching experience for a couple that it can be, care must be planned using nursing process.

Assessment

Women need careful observation during labor so danger signals of labor can be recognized at the first moment they occur. If a woman is using pre-pared childbirth, a coach may be timing contractions. Be certain that you also periodically time and evaluate contractions so the woman's assessment remains complete.

Analysis

A nursing diagnosis is always an action that can be managed by a nurse. The physiologic happenings of labor are never, by themselves, therefore, nursing diagnoses. A woman's concern or discomfort caused by these happenings are frequently used nursing diagnoses in this area. Be certain when establishing goals with a woman and her support person that you do not project a definite time for labor to be completed. The time of labor can vary greatly from person to person and still be within normal limits.

Planning

When planning care in labor, both the woman and her support person must be included in planning as the experience should be a shared one for the couple. Planning may include review and education of the normal process of labor: Even though a couple learned this during pregnancy, at the moment that it is really happening it may seem very different from what they imagined.

Implementation

Nursing care for the woman in labor is based on the physiologic and psychological happenings of that point in labor. This care is discussed in detail in Chapter 24.

Evaluation

Evaluation of care for a labor experience should consist of not only whether the labor was safe from both maternal and fetal standpoints but whether it fulfilled the expectations of the couple. A labor experience introduces a child and parents for the first time, and it is unfortunate when this first impression is a negative one due to some factor that could have been eliminated or improved.

Nursing Care Planning

Mary Kraft is a 23-year-old woman you care for in labor. An admission nursing care plan you might establish with her would be the following.

Assessment

Breathing regularly with contractions; lies supine to do breathing.

Temperature 99.2, pulse 74, respirations 20, BP 110/78. Contractions 45-second duration, 5-minute frequency, moderate intensity. Labor began 7 hours ago. Effacement 70%; dilatation 2 cm. Station −1; vertex presentation, position LOA, FHR 120. Moderate amount pink-tinged show; membranes ruptured spontaneously just prior to coming to hospital. Fluid clear, no blood or meconium staining. States "I'm scared for the baby. I didn't want a dry birth."

Analysis

Para 0, gravida 2 in latent stage of labor with fear related to early rupture of membranes.

Locus of Decision Making. Shared.

Goal. Patient to complete labor within normal time limits and free of complications.

Criteria.

1. Labor and delivery to be accomplished without medication or anesthetic interventions; to use breathing exercises for contraction discomfort.
2. Fetal assessments to remain within normal limits.
3. Husband to be active coach during labor and delivery.

Nursing Orders

1. Admit to birthing room.
2. Place external fetal and uterine monitors and teach her to use these to detect contractions' beginning.
3. Encourage to lie on side, not back, for labor to prevent supine hypotension syndrome.
4. Notify private M.D. and house officer of admission.
5. Keep nonambulatory until checked by M.D. because of ruptured membranes.
6. Assure her that ruptured membranes are normal at this point.

Questions for Review

Multiple Choice

1. Ms. Laport is a patient you care for in labor. She asks you why labor begins. Which statement below is a possible explanation of this?
   a. Progesterone level rises at term to initiate contractions.
   b. The ovary releases additional estrogen at term.
   c. Prostaglandins may be the causative factor of labor.
   d. Calcium is drawn from bones to block relaxation fibers.

2. If the fetus is in an ROA position during labor, you would interpret this to mean the fetus
   a. is in a longitudinal lie facing the left posterior.

b. is facing the right anterior abdominal quadrant.

c. is in a common breech delivery position.

d. is presenting with the face as the presenting part.

3. The fetus is at a −1 station. You would interpret this to mean that

a. the fetus is at the ischial spines.

b. the fetus is engaged.

c. the fetus is "floating."

d. the fetus is "crowning."

4. In order for a fetus to best traverse the birth canal, the smallest head diameter must be presented to the birth canal. Which of the following is the smallest anteroposterior cranial diameter?

a. suboccipitobregmatic

b. biparietal

c. occipitomental

d. occipitofrontal

5. If your evaluation of Ms. Laport revealed all the following, which would be a danger signal of labor?

a. blood-tinged vaginal discharge at full dilatation

b. meconium-stained amniotic fluid

c. maternal pulse of 90 to 95 beats per minute

d. fetus presenting in an LOA position

6. During labor, effacement of the cervix is defined as

a. widening of the cervical os.

b. turning "inside out" of the cervical os.

c. molding and elongation of the cervix.

d. thinning and shortening of the cervix.

7. Dilatation follows effacement in the primipara. Full dilatation is a usual distance of

a. 3–4 cm.

b. 7–8 cm.

c. 8–10 cm.

d. 12–14 cm.

8. In teaching Ms. Laport about labor you would explain that the force that propels the fetus through the vagina is basically

a. a combination of fundal and abdominal pressure.

b. mainly gravitational from the superior fetal lie.

c. cervical contractions beginning with full dilatation.

d. abdominal and perineal muscle contractions.

9. Labor contractions may originate from a pacemaker point. In the average woman, this point is located

a. just superior to the cervical os.

b. laterally at the level of the bladder.

c. at one or the other uterotubal junctions.

d. at the uterine wall under the placenta.

10. In Ms. Laport, the placenta presents with the maternal surface evident. Which statement below is a true statement concerning this presentation?

a. This is a common placental delivery presentation.

b. This is an abnormal placental delivery presentation.

c. The uterus does not contract well following this presentation.

d. This presentation reflects a placental abnormality.

Discussion

1. Most women think of labor as a local process, but it also involves systemic changes. What are cardiovascular changes that occur with labor? Respiratory changes?

2. The terms effacement and dilatation are often confusing to women in labor. How would you explain these terms?

3. A fetus must make positional changes in order to navigate a birth canal. What is the physiologic reason for these maneuvers?

Suggested Readings

Beal, M. W. (1984). Nurse-midwifery intrapartum management: patterns of care given by nurse-midwives and physicians. *Journal of Nurse Midwifery, 29*, 13.

Beard, R. W. (1979). Controlling and quantifying uterine activity. *Contemporary Obstetrics and Gynecology, 13*, 75.

Bowe, N. L. (1981). Intact perineum . . . a slow delivery of the head does not adversely affect the outcome of the newborn. *Journal of Nurse Midwifery, 26*, 5.

Brown, L. K. (1984). Physiology of labour. *Nursing (Oxford), 2*, 600.

Carr, K. C. (1980). Obstetric practices which protect against neonatal morbidity: Focus on maternal position in labor and birth. *Birth and Family Journal, 7*, 249.

Daniel, E. E., et al. (1960). Electrolytes in the human myometrium. *American Journal of Obstetrics and Gynecology, 79*, 417.

Flood, B., and Naeye, R. L. (1984). Factors that predispose to premature rupture of the fetal membranes. *J.O.G.N. Nursing, 13*, 115.

Friedman, E. (1978). *Labor, clinical evaluation and management.* (2nd ed.). New York: Appleton-Century-Crofts.

Haskins, A. L. (1954). The progesterone content of placentas before and after the onset of labor. *American Journal of Obstetrics and Gynecology, 67*, 330.

House, M. J. (1981). Episiotomy: Indications, technique and results. *Midwife Health Visitor and Community Nurse, 17*, 6.

Huszar, G. (1981). Biology and biochemistry of myometrial contractility and cervical maturation. *Seminars in Perinatology, 5*, 216.

Kesby, O. (1982). A case for the birthing chair. *Nursing Mirror, 155*, 37.

Klein, R. P., et al. (1981). A study of father and nurse

support during labor. *Birth and Family Journal, 8,* 161.

Kumar, D., et al. (1963). Studies in human premature births. *American Journal of Obstetrics and Gynecology, 81,* 126.

Liggins, G. C. (1979). What factors initiate human labor? *Contemporary Obstetrics and Gynecology, 13,* 147.

May, K. A. (1982). The father as observer. *M.C.N., 7,* 319.

McKay, S. R. (1981). Second stage labor: Has tradition replaced safety? *American Journal of Nursing, 81,* 1016.

Monheit, A. G., et al. (1983). Perinatal risk assessment: A look at the record of some established systems. *Perinatology Neonatology, 18,* 124a.

Pillay, S. K., et al. (1980). Fetal monitoring: A guide to understanding the equipment. *Clinical Obstetrics and Gynecology, 22,* 571.

Redshaw, M., et al. (1982). The influence of analgesia in labour on the baby. *Midwife Health Visitor and Community Nurse, 18,* 126.

Roberts, J. E. (1979). Maternal positions for childbirth: A historical review of nursing care practices. *J.O.G.N. Nursing, 8,* 24.

Roberts, J. E. (1983). Factors influencing distress from pain during labor. *M.C.N., 8,* 62.

Sasso, S. C. (1983). Prostaglandins for OB-GYN. *M.C.N., 8,* 107.

Sciarra, J. J. (1978). *Gynecology and obstetrics.* New York: Harper & Row.

Stewart, N. (1982). Postscript patience: A critique of current third stage practices. *Midwives Chronicle, 95,* 293.

Warwick, C. (1984). Management of labour: Basic principles. *Nursing (Oxford), 2,* 603.

Wilkerson, V. A. (1984). The use of episiotomy in normal delivery. *Midwives Chronicle, 97,* 106.

24

Nursing Care During the Labor Experience

OBJECTIVES

Following mastery of the contents of this chapter, you should be able to

1. Describe assessment measures of a woman in labor, including the use of fetal and uterine monitors.
2. Analyze problems of a woman in labor and construct a nursing diagnosis.
3. Assist a woman in labor to establish realistic goals and criteria for progress in labor.
4. Plan implementations that foster a safe, comfortable, and successful labor.
5. Evaluate the established goals and reassess or continue implementations based on goal attainment.
6. Analyze whether present nursing care measures truly meet the needs of women in labor.
7. Synthesize knowledge of nursing care in labor with nursing process to achieve quality maternal-newborn nursing care.

IMPLEMENTATIONS TO MAKE labor safe, comfortable, and effective are important because labor and delivery are enormous emotional and physiologic accomplishments for a woman and her support person. This is true whether it is a first labor and everything is new and unexpected or a second or third labor: No two labors are identical.

Most physicians or nurse-midwives ask a woman to telephone them when she first believes that she is in labor and to come to the hospital or birthing center when her contractions are 5 to 10 minutes apart. At the health care facility, assessment, analysis, and planning of care need to be begun immediately. Steps of this are summarized in Procedure 24-1 on page 509.

Initial Assessment of a Woman in Labor

A woman plans well if she has a suitcase packed by 2 weeks before her expected delivery date, since 2 weeks before or after the expected date of confinement is a normal time for labor to begin. Despite all the situation comedy programs to the contrary, however, unless she is a grand multipara, she has ample time once labor begins to finish packing and make a safe trip to a hospital or birthing center.

It is reassuring to a woman to know what health care facility entrance she should use. She is under stress, and people under stress are sensitive to annoyances that otherwise would not concern them. For the same reason, health care forms should be simple; preferably, just a signature should be required. It is equally helpful if a woman has had a tour of the labor and delivery unit during her pregnancy in conjunction with a preparation-for-labor class so that she can feel "at home" or at least that she is not among strangers. Check to see whether she has a support person with her and, if so, admit both the woman and her support person to a labor or birthing room as a unit.

Initial Interview

Certain information must be obtained so that the extent of a woman's labor, her general physical condition, and her preparedness for labor and delivery can be evaluated and you can plan comprehensive nursing care. This procedure must take place quickly in order to recognize a woman in very active labor or with a history of precipitous deliveries. Nevertheless, interviewing skill and tact must be practiced lest you leave the impression that you are more interested in the information than in the woman.

Ask about her expected date of confinement; then you and medical personnel can be alerted to the possibility of a premature birth. Ask questions to determine the stage of labor and whether any abnormality is readily apparent. You need to know the frequency, duration, and intensity of her contractions; the amount of and character of show; and whether or not her membranes have ruptured. Ask when she last ate, to establish risk in case a general anesthetic must be planned. Ask whether she has any known allergies to drugs; then you will know if there will be an immediate problem with medication administration. Ask what pregnancy this is for her (gravida and para). If she had any previous pregnancies ask the outcome and any complications at labor or delivery she experienced.

This information is scant but distinguishes the woman who is in very active labor and needs immediate care from the woman who has arrived at the hospital or birthing center at the average time and will need paced interventions.

Procedure 24-1

Summary of Admission Procedures

Procedure	*Rationale*
1. Orient both woman and support person to birthing room.	1. Birth is a family-centered event. Familiarity leads to relief of stress.
2. Take and record temperature, pulse, respirations, and blood pressure.	2. Establish baseline values.
3. Take nursing history.	3. Establish risk factors.
4. Perform physical examination.	4. Establish risk factors.
5. Perform Leopold's maneuvers and take FHR.	5. Establish fetal presentation, position, and well-being.
6. Perform vaginal examination.	6. Establish effacement, dilatation, fetal presenting part, and station.
7. Obtain urine specimen.	7. Test for protein, glucose, and specific gravity.
8. Obtain necessary blood samples.	8. Send for hemoglobin, hematocrit, blood type, and VDRL for syphilis.
9. Explain and connect any fetal or uterine monitoring equipment to be used.	9. Safeguard fetal well-being during labor.

Birthing Rooms, Labor Rooms

Traditionally, women completed their dilatational or first stage of labor in a labor room (a bare, easy-to-clean patient room), then at the pelvic or second stage of labor were transferred to a delivery room (designed as an operating room). In newer hospitals (or redesigned labor units) or birthing centers, labor rooms have been replaced by birthing or perinatal rooms where a woman remains for all three stages of labor—and the immediate period postpartum or fourth stage of labor as well.

In the beginning of labor, the birthing room appears as a comfortable bedroom. At the second stage of labor, cupboards at the sides are opened to reveal sterile packs of supplies; a screen or folding partition at the end of the room opens to disclose newborn care equipment; if a woman chooses to deliver in a lithotomy position or that is her physician's preference, the bed converts into a delivery platform. Many women choose a semi-Fowler's or sitting position, so such a bed can also be converted to simulate a birthing chair (Figure 24-1). If a woman chooses to deliver from a side-lying or dorsal recumbent position, sterile linen is merely added to cover the bed surface.

Nurse-midwives tend to use alternative birth positions rather than a lithotomy position. With less tension on the perineum, women may have fewer perineal tears from these positions. An epi-siotomy can be made in alternative positions, though suturing is more difficult. The advantage of an upright position is that the baby's own weight aids in delivery.

The advantage of a birthing room is that a woman does not need to be transferred in the middle of labor. Also, the home-like atmosphere allows her and her support person to relax and fully participate in this rare life event.

Initial Assessment and Preparation Procedures

In order to establish a woman's physical well-being, her temperature, pulse, respiration, and blood pressure, as well as the fetal heartbeat, should be taken and evaluated. Though you have the woman's stated report of contractions, assess them yourself. Always take her blood pressure between contractions as blood pressure may rise 5 to 10 mm Hg during a contraction.

Length of Contractions

If you rest your fingers on a woman's abdomen at the fundus of the uterus *very gently*, you can determine the beginning of a contraction by the gradual tensing and upward rising of the fundus. You are usually able to feel this tensing about 5 seconds before the woman is able to feel the contraction. Therefore, do not rely on her to tell you

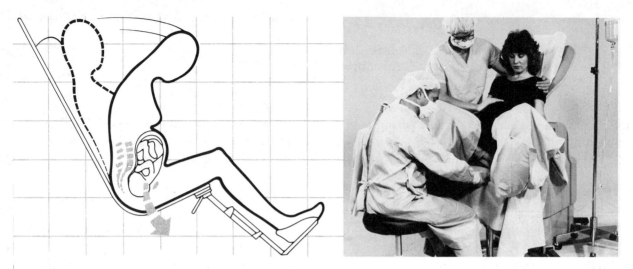

Figure 24-1 *A birthing chair.*

when a contraction is beginning or you will underestimate the length of contractions. (You are able to feel a contraction when the intrauterine pressure reaches about 20 mm Hg. The pain of a contraction is not felt until pressure reaches about 25 mm Hg.) The duration of a contraction is timed from the moment the uterus first tenses until it has relaxed again.

Intensity of Contractions

In addition to observing the duration of contractions, you need to make an estimation of intensity, or the strength of the contraction. Contractions are rated as mild (the uterus is contracting but does not become more than minimally tense), moderate (the uterus feels firm), or strong (the contraction is so intense the uterus feels as hard as wood at the peak of the contraction). The uterus cannot be indented by your fingertips in a strong contraction.

When estimating the intensity of contractions, check the fundus at the conclusion of the contraction to determine whether it relaxes or becomes soft to the touch. If it does, you know that the uterus is not in continuous contraction but is providing a relaxation time during which its blood

vessels can fill to supply the fetus with adequate oxygen.

Frequency of Contractions

Next, time the frequency of contractions. The frequency is timed from the *beginning* of one contraction to the *beginning* of the next. Be certain you are not timing from the end of a contraction to the beginning of the next or you will report contractions as being closer together than they actually are. You need to time three or four contractions before you have any picture of the frequency at which they are occurring. The duration and frequency of contractions are depicted diagrammatically in Figure 24-2.

Use as light a touch as possible on a woman's abdomen while you are timing contractions or estimating their strength (Figure 24-3). The fundus of the uterus becomes sore if it has to push against extra weight with each contraction—unnecessary discomfort for a woman in labor.

Rupture of Membranes

In as many as 25 percent of labors, labor begins with spontaneous rupture of the fetal membranes. In most instances with rupture of mem-

Figure 24-2 *Duration and frequency of contractions.*

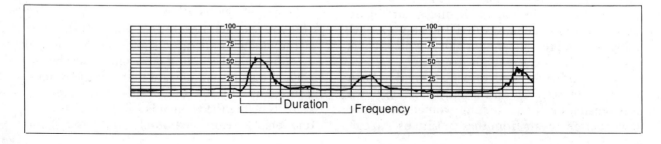

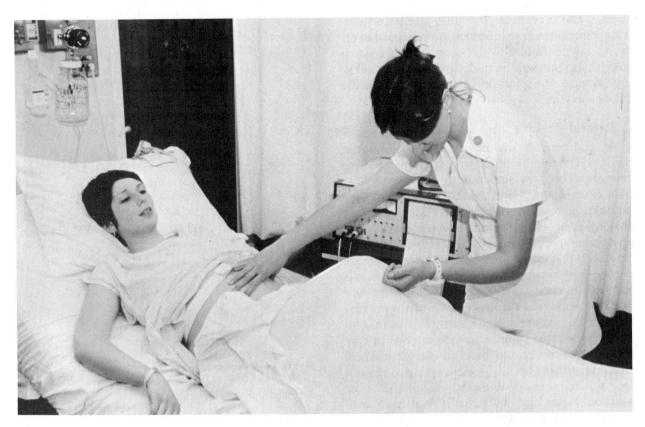

Figure 24-3 *Observing the frequency, duration, and strength of contractions. Note how the nurse's hand rests lightly on the woman's abdomen. She stands away from the bed so she does not obstruct the woman's line of vision as the woman studies a geometric wall picture to help her to concentrate on a breathing pattern, a help to women prepared in the Lamaze method of childbirth. (Courtesy of the Department of Medical Photography, Children's Hospital, Buffalo, N.Y.)*

branes, there is a sudden gush of amniotic fluid from the vagina. Women are startled by this sensation (it feels as if they have lost bladder control). It may happen while they are shopping or in a public place, and they may be embarrassed before they realize that the warm, moist fluid on their perineum and legs is not urine but the announcement that labor is beginning. In other women, rupture of membranes is not a dramatic event but only a slow loss of fluid, and there is a question whether membranes have ruptured.

If there is a question as to whether or not the membranes have ruptured, a simple test with Nitrazine paper may supply the answer. Vaginal secretions are acid; amniotic fluid is alkaline. If amniotic fluid has passed through the vagina recently, the pH of the vagina will probably be alkaline if tested by Nitrazine paper. An additional test is a fern test. Because of its high estrogen content, amniotic fluid will show a fern pattern when dried and examined under a microscope; urine will not.

To obtain amniotic fluid, insert a sterile, cot-ton-tipped applicator deeply into the vagina and then touch it to a strip of Nitrazine paper or a glass slide. For a Nitrazine test, compare the paper with the chart accompanying it. If the paper indicates a pH below 6.5, the membranes are probably still intact. A pH over 6.5 indicates leakage of amniotic fluid. A false reading may occur in women with intact membranes who have a heavy, bloody show, since blood is also alkaline. Ask the woman whose membranes ruptured at home what the color of the amniotic fluid was. It should be clear as water.

Yellow-stained fluid may indicate a blood incompatibility between mother and fetus (the amniotic fluid is bilirubin-stained from the breakdown of red blood cells). Green-colored fluid indicates meconium staining. Meconium staining is often normal in breech deliveries because of buttock compression, which expels meconium into the fluid. In a vertex presentation, meconium staining generally indicates that the fetus has suffered anoxia in utero and the anoxia has led to spontaneous sphincter relaxation (a vagal response) and meconium loss into amniotic fluid. Immediate physician intervention is needed in order to safeguard fetal well-being. In either situation, the infant will be in danger following delivery because of aspiration of meconium into the trachea or lungs.

Perineal Washing

At one time it was customary to shave the pubis and perineum of all women preparatory to delivery. The area surrounding the vagina was then cleaned and disinfected to help prevent contamination of the birth canal. Today, whether shaving is necessary or not is controversial. If a physician or nurse-midwife does not anticipate that an episiotomy (perineal incision) will be needed, just cleansing the perineum is all that is required. In even those instances when some hair must be removed, a minishave or just removing the hair immediately surrounding the vaginal introitus is all that is necessary. Some health care agencies specify cotton balls to use for perineal cleaning; others specify sterile sponges, disposable washclothes, or reusable washclothes. The solution varies also, but usually is a mild antiseptic. Be certain to separate the labial folds with washing so that any secretions in the folds are removed. Wash from front to back, cleaning the anal area last to prevent bringing contamination forward from the rectum.

Provide privacy for a woman during the procedure. Remember, again, that she is very sensitive to the feeling tone of people caring for her. If she begins to experience a contraction while you are completing a perineal preparation, stop and wait until it has passed. On a busy labor service, it is easy to think, "I haven't time to wait. I have a dozen other things to do in this half hour." However, labor contractions at their strongest rarely last more than 60 seconds. Surely you can wait 60 seconds for someone's comfort.

After a woman's perineum has been cleansed, instruct her not to touch the area to keep it as clean as possible during labor.

Perineal Shaving

Perineal shaving, if done, is simple; but because it will be one of your first interactions, the procedure can color the woman's impression of the health care facility and of your care of her (Figure 24-4).

You will need a good light source in order to see exactly what you are doing. The perineal hair should be well lathered prior to shaving so that the shaving is not painful and skin cuts can be avoided. The shaving solution used will vary from institution to institution, from green soap to

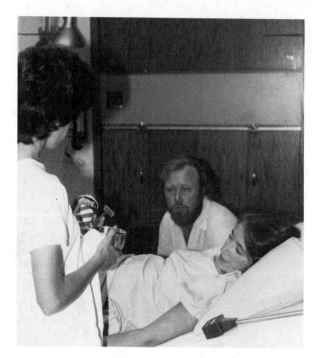

Figure 24-4 *Be certain to give good instructions to women in labor. Here a nurse describes what a mini-perineal shave will involve.*

shaving cream to a mild dishwashing detergent mixed with warm water. The perineum is very sensitive to hot and cold, so be careful that the water is at a comfortable temperature. Cold water will cause abdominal tension and discomfort if a woman should experience a contraction during the procedure. Despite the advantageous cumulative bacteriocidal and bacteriostatic properties of hexachlorophene, it should be avoided as a lathering agent until the long-range effects of absorption of this compound have been documented.

After the perineal hair has been well lathered, begin at the level of the clitoris and stroke from above downward with a safety razor, around the vulva to the base of the perineal body. Be certain to stretch the skin from above as you work, so that the skin is taut and allows the razor to move easily. Use single strokes, front to back, rinsing the razor head after each stroke, so that pathogens from the anal area are not carried forward to the birth canal.

After the anterior portion of the perineum has been shaved, ask the woman to turn on her side to allow you to shave any hair surrounding the anal area. With the upper part of the woman's leg well flexed, you have a good view of the anal area in this side-lying position. After all hair on the perineum has been shaved away, the perineum is then washed thoroughly.

Some women choose to shave perineal hair by themselves at home before coming to a health care agency. This practice should be discouraged: Without being able to view the area well, a woman has a tendency to shave away more than is necessary or to knick sensitive skin and leave a portal of entry for infection.

Urine Specimen

A urine specimen to be tested immediately for protein and glucose and then sent to the laboratory for a complete urinalysis should be obtained next. A woman is able to void most easily if she is allowed to use the bathroom. A bedpan or receptacle placed on the toilet will allow for comfort and also will permit any material passed by the vagina to be preserved. If a woman describes any symptoms that suggest urinary tract infection (burning on urination, blood in her urine, extreme frequency, flank pain), you will need to obtain a clean-catch urine for culture. Women who report ruptured membranes should not be ambulated until it is confirmed that the fetal head is engaged so that the umbilical cord cannot slip past the loosely fitting head and prolapse during voiding, causing fetal distress.

Enema Administration

At one time every woman was given an enema in early labor. It was thought that cleansing the bowel at this point avoided the excretion of stool at the time of delivery and possible contamination of the birth canal. Moreover, it was hoped that the peristaltic action of the bowel would increase uterine contractions and possibly speed labor; it emptied the lower bowel of stool, so perhaps allowed quicker descent of the fetal head. As some enema solution was retained in the lower bowel, however, because of pressure of the fetal head against the lower bowel, there was invariably some stool excretion at the time of delivery. Whether enema administration speeds labor or fetal descent is debatable. An enema is therefore no longer a routine procedure.

If it should be ordered under an individual circumstance, an enema is not given to a woman who is near the pelvic division of labor for fear that as she bears down to expel the enema she will expel the fetus as well. Enemas are not given to women after membranes have ruptured because of the danger of contamination of the then unprotected birth canal and fetus from fecal contaminants.

Enemas are uncomfortable procedures to women not in labor; to a woman in labor they are doubly uncomfortable. A Fleet enema (Figure 24-5) is not only the most convenient type of enema

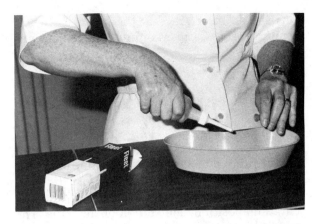

Figure 24-5 *If an enema is to be administered during labor, a Fleet enema is the simplest type because of the small amount of fluid necessary.*

to administer but the most comfortable for the woman because of the small amount of fluid that is injected and the speed with which it can be given. It may be difficult to insert an enema tip into a woman's rectum because of the pressure of the presenting part on the anal area and the presence of hemorrhoids that have developed during pregnancy. Be certain to provide privacy and explain that you are aware that this is something the woman is not looking forward to. Assure her that you will be as gentle as possible and that if she tells you when she is beginning to have a contraction or any abdominal cramping you will stop the flow of fluid until her discomfort passes. Be certain the enema dispenser tip is well lubricated to allow it to pass hemorrhoidal tissue without pain.

Following administration of an enema, allow a woman to get up and go to the bathroom to expel it. Remind her to wipe herself from front to back following expulsion of the enema, so that she does not carry fecal material forward to the birth canal. After she returns to bed, the perineal area should be rewashed to eliminate the possibility of fecal contamination. Recheck fetal heart tones because pressure from expelling the enema could compress the fetal cord.

Other Procedures

Next, blood is drawn for hemoglobin or hematocrit reading, VDRL (serologic test for syphilis), and blood typing. Thus everyone dealing with the woman can be assured that she is in good physical health, and the blood laboratory is alerted that a woman with a certain blood type is in labor or if a blood incompatibility is likely to exist in the newborn.

Ideally, a fetal monitor to record fetal heart sounds and a monitor to record uterine contractions should be attached at this point to ensure accurate fetal assessment during the remainder of labor.

Health Assessment of a Woman in Labor

The next level of assessment needed includes a more definitive history and performing of a vaginal or rectal examination to determine the presence of effacement, degree of dilatation, and presentation, position, and station of the fetus. The nurse who can assess a woman in labor this thoroughly is an indispensable asset to the physician or nurse-midwife who uses the labor unit where she works. Since neither physicians nor nurse-midwives can realistically stay with all their patients throughout labor, a nurse assumes the major part of the responsibility for assessment and for safeguarding both mother and child during labor.

History Taking

The history taken at this point should include a review of a woman's pregnancy, both physical and psychological events, and a review of past pregnancies, general health, and family medical information.

If the woman is in active labor, the history taken on arrival may be the only history obtained until after the baby is born. However, most women get to the hospital or birthing center in time for thorough history taking.

Current Pregnancy History

To determine the woman's health during this pregnancy, begin with an open-ended question such as "How did your pregnancy go?" or "How has your pregnancy been?" This type of question allows a woman to answer in any of a number of ways: "Too long," "Terrible," "Good, except that I worried so much . . . ," "All right, after I decided there wasn't much I could do about it," "Great." If you begin with a question such as "Any problems during this pregnancy?" you limit a woman to concrete problems (spotting, injuries) and thereby limit the amount of information you will obtain.

If a woman answers your opening inquiry with a noncommittal "Good" or "Fine," pursue some specific areas of the pregnancy: When was her last menstrual period? How many days does her average period last? How long is the interval between periods? (This helps to document the due date. If she has 40-day cycles, she will probably be in labor 2 weeks after her due date.) Did she have prenatal care? When did she first go for care? It is important to ask her the reasons for her actions. If she went exceptionally early, even before she missed a period, what was the reason? Was she frightened? Did she anticipate trouble with the pregnancy? If she went unusually late, why was that? Was she so secure in her own judgment that she did not feel a need for care? Was she hoping she was not pregnant and trying to delay the diagnosis to avoid facing the pregnancy? Was money such a problem that she could not afford care? The answers to these questions will be important in planning postpartal nursing implementations because she could be elaborating situations that will interfere with optimal mother-child bonding or future health care.

How often did her physician or nurse-midwife ask her to come to the office or clinic during pregnancy? This is a good question to validate her first response; that is, a woman who made weekly rather than monthly prenatal visits either has an extremely conservative obstetrician or nurse-midwife or has not had a "fine" pregnancy, despite what she says. Did she keep all her scheduled prenatal appointments? If not, why not? Financial or transportation problems? Was she afraid the physician or nurse-midwife would discover something wrong (no news is good news)? Was she fearful something would be wrong? Does she have a friend or relative who has a child with a defect? Did she feel the office or clinic personnel were not interested in her, that she was only a number on a chart? Does that influence her feelings about this health care agency staff? It is frightening to feel alone in labor even with people around you because a previous experience led you to believe that health care personnel are indifferent to you.

Ask about and explore any medical problems a woman had during pregnancy. Did she have any spotting? When? How long did it last? What did she do? If she called her physician or nurse-midwife, what did she say to do? Did she follow the instructions? What happened? How does she feel about the episode? Did it frighten her? Did her physician or nurse-midwife assure her that spotting in early pregnancy is usually benign? Is she still worried about it?

Did she notice any swelling of her hands or feet during pregnancy? If she had edema, what was its extent? Just in her ankles at bedtime? In her face when she awoke in the morning? What was her prepregnancy weight? How much weight did she gain during pregnancy? Was her physician or nurse-midwife happy with that weight gain?

Did she have any falls? When? How did she

fall? How far did she fall? Did she have any aftereffects? Almost all women have a fall of some sort during pregnancy. If a woman delivers a healthy child, the incident will be as nothing. If she delivers a child with a congenital defect, she may blame herself for the problem. This kind of information prepares the health care personnel who will be caring for a woman after delivery to help her work through her adjustment to a child who is not the perfect child she imagined she carried.

Did she have any infections? A rash that might suggest rubella (a pink macular rash lasting 2 or 3 days)? Herpes lesions?

Did she take any medication during pregnancy? What kind? Did she drink alcohol? Does she smoke cigarettes? Drink caffeine beverages? It is realistic to ask a young woman whether she took any hallucinogens or euphoric drugs during pregnancy or whether she smoked marijuana. If you convey the impression that you are interested in her welfare and that of her child (and such questions are important to the immediate welfare of the infant if the woman is addicted to drugs such as heroin or barbiturates), most women will answer truthfully.

Was the woman ill in any way during pregnancy? Did she have influenza? A bladder infection? Back pain? Varicosities? Hemorrhoids? When did she have the illness? What did she do about it? Did she take medication? Is she aware of a blood incompatibility? Does she know her blood type? Did she take vitamins or iron or folic acid during pregnancy? (If not, the hemoglobin of her child may need special attention to be certain it is adequate.)

Interviewing women in labor is difficult because you both are constantly interrupted by labor contractions. Impatience shows: Remember that the longest contraction is rarely more than 60 seconds. A woman may concentrate so intently on a breathing exercise that a question asked just prior to a contraction is completely driven from her mind. As the contraction subsides, repeat the question as if you had not asked it before or as if you do not mind asking it again.

At the same time you are asking about the early part of pregnancy, ask whether or not the pregnancy was planned. You may find this an awkward question. It is not. It is a good question here because the manner in which a woman accepted her pregnancy has a great deal to do with how she will accept her child. You might word the question: "Most pregnancies come as a surprise—how was this one for you?"

If she states that the child was unplanned, ask whether or not she was using a birth control measure. Many young women have inaccurate birth control information and will need counseling in the postpartum period to provide themselves with better protection in the future.

As you pursue the history of the remainder of the pregnancy, attempt to identify a point at which a woman changed her mind about wanting a baby. Do not be naive. Not all children are wanted. It is normal not to want a baby if your circumstances make it difficult or impossible to supply all the love and care the child needs. Be careful that you do not sound judgmental. If you imply that the correct answer to the question "Did you plan this pregnancy?" is "I want this baby very much. I love him already," that is the answer you will get. This is not eliciting information; it is asking for compliance.

Does she remember at what month in pregnancy she felt the child inside her move? The month quickening occurred helps you document the due date. The woman who is worried that her child may not be all right will probably remember exactly when she felt life. The woman who has four normal children at home and has every reason to think this child will also be normal may not have been sufficiently aware of quickening to time it accurately. Ask her to think in terms of holidays as a way of jogging her memory. She may recall that she felt the fetus move while she was at a Fourth of July picnic or on vacation.

Ask the woman who said she did not want the pregnancy whether feeling the child kick inside her made any difference. Many women will say that it did. "I guess that was the first time the pregnancy was real. I started to plan after that." If quickening did not change her attitude, can she name a point where it did change? Has she made everything ready for the baby? When did she begin to prepare for the baby? A woman who says she has done nothing has been so worried that her child would be born imperfect or dead that she could not begin to look at tiny shirts or gowns, has divorced herself from emotional attachment to the baby, or has no money for baby clothing. She cares too much or too little or needs financial help.

It is good to ask her about the attitude of the father of the child toward the pregnancy. How did he feel about her being pregnant? How has he acted since she started labor? Is he supportive when she is worried, or too "manly" to display emotions and consequently of little help to her?

Did she attend any classes on preparation for parenthood or labor? If she wants an anesthetic for delivery, does she prefer a particular type? Listen to her reply. Does she say a "general" because she is terrified of the pain her mother warned her of? Or because she is afraid the baby will be born dead and she wants to delay the inevitable? Has she heard scare stories about spinal anesthesia and is afraid of it even though she would like to be awake during the baby's birth? Does she want "nothing" because she really believes that is the way to have children, or is she determined to prove something to her husband or herself?

Make certain a woman understands that her physician or nurse-midwife will have the ultimate say about whether an anesthetic is needed and the kind of anesthetic she receives, but that if there is a choice her wishes will be respected. If she indicates that she wants to be awake but wonders how she will react to the situation, assure her that seeing the birth of her child is an event that will happen only a few times in a lifetime. It is a moment to be treasured, and she will be among friends, who will not be critical of her reactions, no matter what they are.

Ask next about her plans for the coming baby. Has she chosen a pediatrician? Does she plan to breast-feed or bottle-feed? It is important to know this because if she is going to breast-feed she should not receive a lactation suppressant after delivery.

It is preferable to interview a woman in a private setting without her support person present. True, this is his child also, but her thoughts about the pregnancy are *her* thoughts. Whether or not she wants this child and what she is concerned about are things she can choose to share or not to share with the child's father. If you interview her with the child's father present, she may have to make a choice: either to give you wrong information or to admit a particular thought to her support person unwillingly. It is always poor judgment and poor health interviewing technique to force people to reveal confidences or to be untruthful.

Women who come into labor with concerns about the health of their unborn child may need extra help in the immediate postpartum period "binding in" or claiming their infant. Questions concerning psychological adaptation to pregnancy are therefore as important as those that deal with the woman's physical well-being throughout the pregnancy.

Past Pregnancy History

Ask, have you ever been pregnant before? If so, what was the outcome? How were her other children born? Vertex? Breech? Cesarean birth? What was the reason for cesarean birth? What was the infant's birth weight? Were there any complications at birth? Was any special equipment used? Did the infant go to the regular nursery? Did the infant go home from the hospital or birthing center with her? Did the infant have any jaundice or cyanosis? What is the present state of health of her child or children?

Were any of her children stillborn? Any prematurely born? Any miscarriages? Any abortions? (Women generally differentiate miscarriages from abortion and appreciate categorizing these separately.) Any complications for herself following any delivery? If there was infection or cervical tearing following previous childbirth, the cervical dilatation you are hoping for here may not occur with ease. It is best to be forewarned of this possibility. Ask a woman whether her blood type is Rh negative and whether she received Rh (D antigen) immune globulin (RhoGAM) following an abortion, a stillbirth, or a past delivery.

Past Health History

Ask, have you ever had any surgery (surgical adhesions might interfere with free fetal passage); heart disease or diabetes (women with heart disease and diabetes need special precautions during labor and delivery); iron deficit or sickle cell anemia (blood loss at delivery may be more important than normally); tuberculosis (tuberculosis lung lesions may be reactivated at delivery by changes in lung contour); kidney disease or hypertension (blood pressure will need to be watched even more carefully than normally); sexually transmitted disease (the infant may be exposed to the disease by vaginal contact if the disease is still active); or herpes lesions (these can be transmitted to the fetus at birth if vaginal lesions are present)?

Family Medical History

Because some diseases are transmitted by genetic patterns and others tend to be multifactorial, it is important to know whether any of these diseases are in either the mother's or the father's family. Adequate preparation for a child born with a disease can then be made. Does any family member have a heart disease, a blood dyscrasia, diabetes, kidney disease, cancer, allergies, seizures, congenital defects, or mental retardation?

Maternal Physical Examination

Following history taking, a woman needs a thorough physical examination, including a pelvic examination, to confirm the presentation and position of the fetus and determine the stage of dilatation.

Physical assessment during labor begins, as does all physical assessment, with a woman's overall appearance. Does she appear tired? pale? ill? frightened? Is there obvious edema or dehydration? Are there open lesions anywhere? Assess for abdominal scars as abdominal or pelvic surgery can leave adhesions. Assess skin turgor for dehydration.

Assess by palpation any enlargement of lymph nodes. Is there any suggestion of infection? Inspect the mucous membrane of the mouth and the conjunctiva of the eyes for color. Does the color (paleness) suggest anemia? Does she wear contact lenses (they will have to be removed if a general anesthetic becomes necessary for delivery)? What is the condition of her teeth? Are they carious? Do any teeth appear abscessed (such a condition might account for a postpartum temperature)? Does she have a bridge or dentures or retainers (which might have to be removed if a general anesthetic becomes necessary)?

Is there evidence of erythema in the posterior pharynx? A streptococcal throat infection will require treatment to prevent transmission to the child. Does she have rhinitis? Any other upper respiratory tract symptoms? Examine the outer and inner surfaces of her lips carefully. Does she have herpes lesions (pinpoint vesicles on an erythematous base)? Type II (genital) virus is lethal to newborns. If herpetic lesions are present, anywhere, a woman will probably be isolated from her child until the lesions crust.

Are her lungs clear to auscultation? Does she have normal heart sounds and rhythms? Many pregnant women at term have a heart murmur evident as a grade II or III systolic ejection murmur from the extra volume of blood that must cross heart valves. Inspect and palpate her breasts. Are they free of cysts or lumps? Does she inspect her own breasts monthly? Do not try to teach breast self-examination while a woman is in labor; she will be unable to concentrate on what you are saying. If she needs instruction in this area, indicate it on her chart, so that the postpartum nursing staff (or yourself) can provide it before she leaves the hospital or birthing center.

Mark the chart also of a woman who has a palpable mass in her breasts for reexamination following labor and delivery. Such a woman should not receive an estrogen lactation suppressant until the mass is ruled out as a malignancy (it is probably an enlarged milk gland).

Estimate fetal size by fundal height (should be at the level of the xyphoid process at term) and presentation by Leopold's maneuvers (discussed below). Palpate and percuss her bladder area (over the symphysis pubis) to detect a full bladder. Even though a woman has just voided, she might not have emptied her bladder sufficiently (retention) because of pressure of the fetal head. A full bladder is uncomfortable during labor and may impede the descent of the fetus. In addition, an overdistended bladder can be injured in labor under pressure of the fetus; this can cause urinary retention in the postpartum period.

Inspect the lower extremities for edema and varicose veins. Women with large varicosities are prone to thrombophlebitis following delivery. Some physicians prefer not to use delivery room stirrups if varicosities are prominent during labor, since the stirrups may press against them. Severe edema suggests hypertension of pregnancy, so the extent and intensity of edema must be assessed and recorrelated with the woman's blood pressure.

Leopold's Maneuvers

Leopold's maneuvers (Figure 24-6) are a systematic method of determining fetal position. Begin by observing a woman's abdomen. Ask yourself: What is the longest diameter in appearance? Is it horizontal or vertical? If the fetus is active, where is the movement apparent? The long axis is the length of the fetus. The activity probably reflects the position of the feet.

If a woman empties her bladder before palpation is begun, she will be more comfortable and the results more productive, since the fetal contours will then not be obscured by a distended anterior bladder.

In Leopold's maneuvers, as in any form of palpation, best results are obtained if the palpation is done systematically. A woman should lie in a supine position with her knees flexed slightly so that her abdominal muscles are relaxed. Be certain your hands are warm (by washing them in warm water first if necessary); cold hands cause abdominal muscles to contract and tighten. Use gentle but firm motions.

First Maneuver

Palpate the superior surface of the fundus (Figure 24-6A). What is the consistency? A head feels more firm that does a breech. What is the shape? A head is round and hard; the breech is less well defined. What is the mobility of the palpated part? A head moves independently of the body; the breech moves only in conjunction with the body. Form an opinion of what portion of the fetus lies in this fundal area.

Second Maneuver

Palpate the sides of the uterus to determine which direction the fetal back is facing (Figure 24-6B). This maneuver is accomplished most suc-

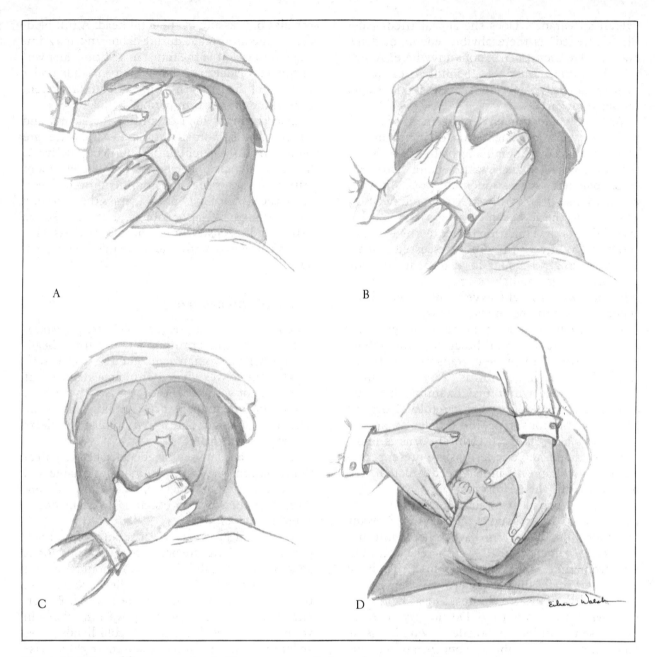

Figure 24-6 *Leopold's maneuvers. A. First maneuver. B. Second maneuver. C. Third maneuver. D. Fourth maneuver.*

cessfully if the left hand is held stationary on the left side of the uterus while with the right hand you palpate the opposite side of the uterus from top to bottom. Next, hold the right hand stationary to immobilize the uterus, and palpate top to bottom on the left side. You will find one side a smooth, hard, resistant surface (the back), while on the opposite side you will feel a number of angular nodulations (the knees and elbows of the fetus).

Third Maneuver

Next, palpate to discover what is at the inlet of the pelvis (Figure 24-6C). Gently grasp the lower

portion of the abdomen just above the symphysis pubis between your thumb and index finger and try to press your thumb and finger together. If the presenting part moves upward to allow you to press your hands together, the presenting part is not engaged (not firmly settled into the pelvis). Is it firm (the head)? Or is it soft (the breech)?

Fourth Maneuver

The fourth maneuver is more difficult than the first three and causes some discomfort for the mother. For the maneuver, assuming you have found the fetus to be in a cephalic presentation, you will want to determine the fetal attitude (degree of flexion). Place your fingers on both sides of the uterus about 2 inches above the inguinal ligaments (Figure 24-6D). Press downward and inward. The fingers of one hand will slide along the uterine contour and meet no obstruction; this is the back of the fetal neck. Your other hand will meet an obstruction an inch or so above the ligament; you are touching the fetal brow. The position of the fetal brow should correspond to the side of the uterus you have designated as containing the elbows and knees of the fetus. If the fetus is in a poor attitude, you will meet an obstruction on the same side as the fetal back; that is, your fingers will touch the hyperextended head.

Some information as to the infant's anteroposterior position may also be gained from this final maneuver. If the brow is very easily palpated (as if it lies just under the skin), the fetus is probably in a posterior position (the occiput is pointing away from you).

Leopold's maneuvers therefore tell you about the presentation, presenting part, position, and attitude of the fetus, which are all important facts to know to help predict the course of labor. It is difficult to palpate fetal contour in an obese woman or one with hydramnios (excessive amniotic fluid).

Vaginal Examination

Vaginal examination is necessary to determine the extent of cervical effacement and dilatation and to determine the fetal presentation, position, and degree of descent. At one time the majority of examinations done during labor were done rectally because it was thought that the risk of spreading pathogenic bacteria from the distal vagina to the cervix was thereby reduced. If careful technique is used, however, and vaginal examinations are kept to the few required, they do not increase the incidence of infection. They may actually *reduce* the spread of infection, because to assess rectally, it is necessary to press the posterior vaginal wall against the cervix; this can spread organisms to the cervix from the vagina. Further, they give more accurate and useful information than rectal examinations. The key words in pelvic examinations are *careful technique* and *few in number*. The technique for a vaginal examination in labor is described in Procedure 24-2 on page 520.

Women usually have an advantage over men in doing vaginal examinations in that their usually narrower fingers cause less pressure and less discomfort on vaginal examination (Figure 24-7). Be certain your fingernails do not extend beyond the edge of the fingertips of your examining fingers,

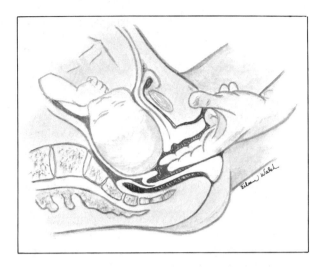

Figure 24-7 *Technique of vaginal examination.*

so that there is no danger of piercing an examining glove.

Vaginal examination may be done either between contractions or during contractions. More fetal skull may be palpated during a contraction as the cervix retracts more at that time, but examining during a contraction is more painful and so rarely justifies the additional amount of information gained. Palpating membranes during a contraction when they are under pressure may cause them to rupture.

Women are anxious to have frequent progress reports during labor, assuring them that their work is not in vain. Tell the woman immediately after the examination about the progress of dilatation. Most women are aware of dilatation but not the word *effacement*. Just "no further dilatation" is a depressing report. "You're not dilated a lot more, but a lot of thinning out is happening and that's just as important" is the same report given in a positive manner.

Vaginal examinations are never done in the presence of fresh bleeding, since this may indicate a placenta previa (implantation of the placenta so low in the uterus that it encroaches on the cervical os). Performing a vaginal examination might tear the placenta and cause hemorrhage, with resultant danger to both mother and fetus. If in doubt, err on the side of postponing a vaginal examination until a consultant arrives.

Assessment for Pelvic Adequacy

Pelvic adequacy by means of an internal conjugate and ischial tuberosity diameters is generally done during pregnancy so that by the thirty-second to thirty-sixth week of pregnancy, the nurse-midwife or physician is alerted to the prob-

=== *Procedure 24-2* ===

Vaginal Examination in Labor

Purpose: Determine cervical readiness and fetal position and presentation.

Procedure

1. Wash your hands; explain procedure to patient. Provide privacy.

2. Assess patient status; analyze appropriateness of plan; adjust plan to individual patient need.

3. Implement plan by assembling equipment: sterile examining glove, sterile lubricant, antiseptic solution. Ask the woman to turn onto back with knees flexed (a dorsal recumbent position). Pull sterile examining glove on to dominant hand.

4. Discard one drop of clean lubricating solution and drop an ample supply on tips of gloved fingers.

5. Pour antiseptic solution over vulva using nongloved hand.

6. Place ungloved hand on the outer edges of the woman's vulva and spread her labia so you can inspect the external genitalia for lesions such as occur with primary syphilis or herpes infections.

7. Look for escaping amniotic fluid or the presence of umbilical cord or bleeding.

8. If there is no bleeding or cord visible, introduce your index and middle fingers gently into the vagina, directing them toward the posterior vaginal wall.

9. Touch the cervix with your gloved examining fingers. Palpate for cervical consistency and rate it *firm* or *soft*. Measure the extent of dilatation; palpate for an anterior rim or lip of cervix.

Principle

1. Prevent spread of microorganisms; ensure patient cooperation and compliance.

2. Care is always individualized according to a patient's needs.

3. Position allows for good visualization of perineum. A sterile glove prevents contamination of birth canal.

4. To ensure that quantity you use will not be contaminated.

5. Prevent the spread of organisms from perineum to birth canal.

6. Allow for good perineal visualization. Look for red, irritated mucous membranes; open, ulcerated sores; clustered, pinpoint vesicles.

7. Amniotic fluid implies membranes have ruptured and umbilical cord may have prolapsed. Bleeding may be a sign of placenta previa. *Do not do a vaginal examination if a possible placenta previa is present.*

8. The posterior vaginal wall is less sensitive than the anterior wall. Stabilize the uterus by placing your ungloved hand on the woman's abdomen.

9. The cervix feels like a circular rim of tissue around a center depression. Firm is similar to the tip of a nose; soft is as pliable as an earlobe. The anterior rim is usually the last portion to thin.

   You should measure the width of your fingertips on a centimeter scale if you are going to do vaginal examinations so you know how wide your index and middle fingers are at the tip. An index finger averages about 1 cm; a middle finger about 1½ cm. If they can both enter the cervix, the cervix is dilated 2½ to 3 cm. If there would be room for double the width of your examining fingers in the cervix, the dilatation is about 5 to 6 cm. When the space is four times the width of your fingertips, dilatation is complete—10 cm.

10. Estimate the degree of effacement.

10. Effacement is estimated in percentage. A cervix before labor is 2 to 2½ cm thick. If it is only 1 cm thick now, it is 50 percent effaced. If it is tissue paper thin, it is 100 percent effaced. It is difficult to feel for dilatation with a 100 percent effaced cervix because the edges of the cervix are so thin; it is difficult to be certain whether you are touching fetal scalp or brushing against an edge of the paper-thin rim of the cervix. Practice is necessary.

11. Estimate whether membranes are intact.

11. The membranes (with a slight amount of amniotic fluid in front of the presenting part) are the shape of a watch crystal. With a contraction, they bulge forward and become prominent and can be felt much more readily.

12. Locate the ischial spines. Rate the station of the presenting part. Identify the presenting part (confirm what you suspect from doing Leopold's maneuvers).

12. Ischial spines are palpated as notches at the 4 and 8 o'clock positions on the pelvic outlet. Station is the number of centimeters the presenting part is above or below the spines. Differentiating a vertex from a breach may be more difficult than would first appear. A vertex has a hard smooth surface; buttocks feel softer and give under fingertip pressure. Fetal hair massed together and wet may be difficult to appreciate through gloves, however. Palpating the two fontanelles, one diamond-shaped and one triangular, helps the identification. You can identify the anus because the sphincter action will "trap" your index finger.

13. Establish the fetal position.

13. The fontanelle you are able to palpate is invariably the posterior one because the fetus maintains a flexed position, presenting the posterior not the anterior fontanelle. In a right occipitoanterior (ROA) position, the triangular fontanelle will point toward the right anterior pelvic quadrant.

   In a left occipitoanterior (LOA) position, the posterior fontanelle will point toward the left anterior pelvis. In a breech presentation, the anus can serve as a marker for position. When the anus is pointing toward the left anterior quadrant of the woman's pelvis, the position is left sacroanterior.

14. Withdraw your hand. Wipe the perineum front to back to remove secretions or examining solution. Leave patient comfortable and turned to side.

14. Use as gentle a technique with withdrawal as insertion. Wipe front to back to avoid moving rectal contamination forward to the vagina. Side-lying is the best position to prevent supine hypotension syndrome in labor.

15. Evaluate effectiveness of procedure. Record procedure and assessment findings.

15. Document nursing care and patient status.

16. Inform the woman of labor progress and graph the new findings on a labor graph.

16. Providing knowledge is a prime method of reducing anxiety during labor. Graphing progress is a part of risk assessment.

lem that a possible cephalic disproportion will occur. Women with this potential problem are cautioned not to attempt a home birth or use a birthing center without nearby hospital facilities.

Pelvic capacity can be reassessed during early labor although these procedures involve excessive vaginal manipulation and discomfort (and do not change from the diameters obtained during pregnancy) so do not need to be retaken routinely. Procedures for these estimates are described in Chapter 8.

Assessing the mobility of the coccyx by grasping it between the thumb and finger (one finger in the rectum and one in the vagina) is helpful as this is a measurement that may change with increased relaxation close to delivery. If the coccyx is not mobile, it can decrease the pelvic outlet by at least 1 cm.

Midpelvic Adequacy

If ischial spines protrude into the pelvic cavity they allow for less room in the cavity than if they are only subtle ridges. To locate the spines, on a vaginal exam, locate the sacrospinous ligament first (a firm ridge of tissue running laterally from the sacrum to insert at the spine). Follow it laterally with your finger until you bump against a node of bone (the ischial spine). Estimate both the length of the ligament and the size of the spine. The sacrospinous ligament is normally 3 to 4 cm in length. A shorter distance suggests a smaller-than-usual posterior angle or perhaps a small midpelvis. The sacrum should feel hollow or convex, increasing the size of the midpelvis.

Outlet Determination

Estimate the angle formed by the posterior surface of the symphysis pubis (the suprapubic angle) by placing your thumbs along the slope of the bone and approximating the angle they form. Normally this angle is 85° to 90° (a right angle). This can also be estimated by placing your fingers vaginally and pressing up against the pubic arch. If your fingers cannot be separated in this position, the angle is unusually steep (less than 90°). An unusually steep pubic arch may prevent the fetal head from delivering freely and increase the possibility that the perineal tissue may tear during delivery as it is pushed posteriorly.

X-ray Pelvimetry

Women who have a pelvis of questionable normal measurements may have X-ray pelvimetry ordered. Be certain to assure the woman and her support person that X-ray at term is not teratogenic and X-ray determination yields more specific information than can be gained from manual examination not only as to the shape and size of the pelvis but fetal size and position in relation to the pelvis.

In addition to women who have questionable measurements, women who may have diameters rechecked by pelvimetry are women with dysfunctional labor, who will be administered an oxytocic to induce or assist labor, who are suspected of carrying a fetus in an abnormal position, who have a past history of a difficult delivery or who have had a pelvic fracture or injury. Primiparas also fall in this category when the fetal head is "floating" or has not engaged.

Be certain that someone accompanies a woman in labor to the X-ray department and that the X-ray is taken promptly and she is returned to the labor wing, again promptly. Take fetal heart rate every 15 minutes while the woman is away from a fetal monitor; if the woman is near the pelvic division of labor, take a sterile delivery pack as well.

Sonography

Sonography may be used at term to determine the diameters of the fetal skull and to determine presentation, presenting part, position, flexion, and degree of descent of the fetus. It has the advantage of not involving X-ray but unfortunately does not offer as clear an estimation of diameters as does X-ray pelvimetry, and the long term effects of sonography are not yet known.

Fetal Physical Assessment

On admission to a labor unit, specific steps of fetal assessment need to be undertaken. Although passive in labor, a fetus is subjected to extreme pressure by uterine contractions and during passage through the birth canal. Compression of the umbilical cord and placenta by uterine contractions may compromise the fetal blood and oxygen supply during these times. Being certain that the fetal heart rate remains within normal limits is an important assessment to ensure that labor is not too strenuous for an individual fetus.

Auscultation of Fetal Heart Sounds by Stethoscope

A typical type of stethoscope for listening to fetal heart rate is shown in Figure 24-8. Fetal heart sounds are transmitted through the convex portion of the fetus, since that is the part lying in close contact with the uterine wall (Figure 24-9). In a vertex or breech presentation, fetal heart sounds are best heard through the fetal back; in a face presentation, the back becomes concave, and

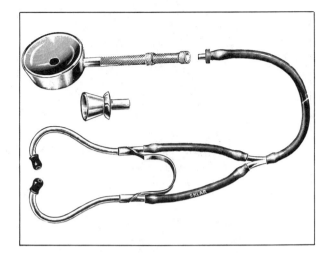

Figure 24-8 *Leff stethoscope with weighted bell. Such a stethoscope conducts FHR well because of its large surface. (From J. Sklar Manufacturing Company Inc., Long Island City, NY 11101, with permission.)*

so they are best heard through the more convex thorax.

In breech presentations the sounds are heard most clearly high in the uterus at a woman's umbilicus or above. In cephalic presentations, they are heard loudest low in the abdomen. In ROA position, the sounds are heard best in the right lower quadrant; in LOA position, in the left lower quadrant. In posterior positions (left or right occipitoposterior—LOP or ROP—the heart sounds are loudest at the maternal side. Figure 24-10 shows typical sites where heart sounds can be heard.

Hearing the fetal heart sounds in these positions provides confirmatory information about fetal position. Conversely, recognizing the fetal position aids you in locating fetal heart sounds.

Fetal heart rate (FHR) should be counted every 30 minutes during beginning labor, every 15 minutes during active labor, and every 5 minutes during the second stage or pelvic division of labor. Use a fetoscope or a Leff stethoscope while auscultating fetal heart rate during labor as these stethoscopes are much more effective and allow you to obtain a more accurate rate. Auscultating by stethoscope is never the preferred method of continual monitoring of FHR in labor, however, as fetal distress occurs in about 10 percent of normal labors. Until irreparable damage has occurred, it is difficult to diagnose fetal distress with the standard methods of monitoring fetal heart rates, such as listening every 15 to 30 minutes to fetal heart sounds by means of a stetho-

Figure 24-9 *Taking fetal heart rate by auscultation. Nurse checks fetal heart rate before beginning continuous electronic monitoring. Strap on abdomen is external tokodynamometer to record uterine contractions. Stethoscope used is a headscope model (a fetoscope); it transmits sound by bone as well as air. (Courtesy of the Department of Medical Photography, Children's Hospital, Buffalo, N.Y.)*

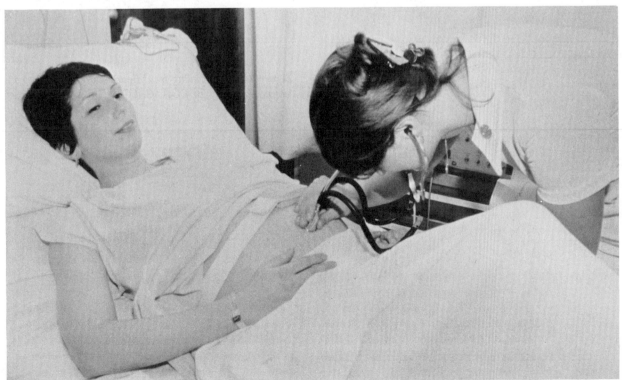

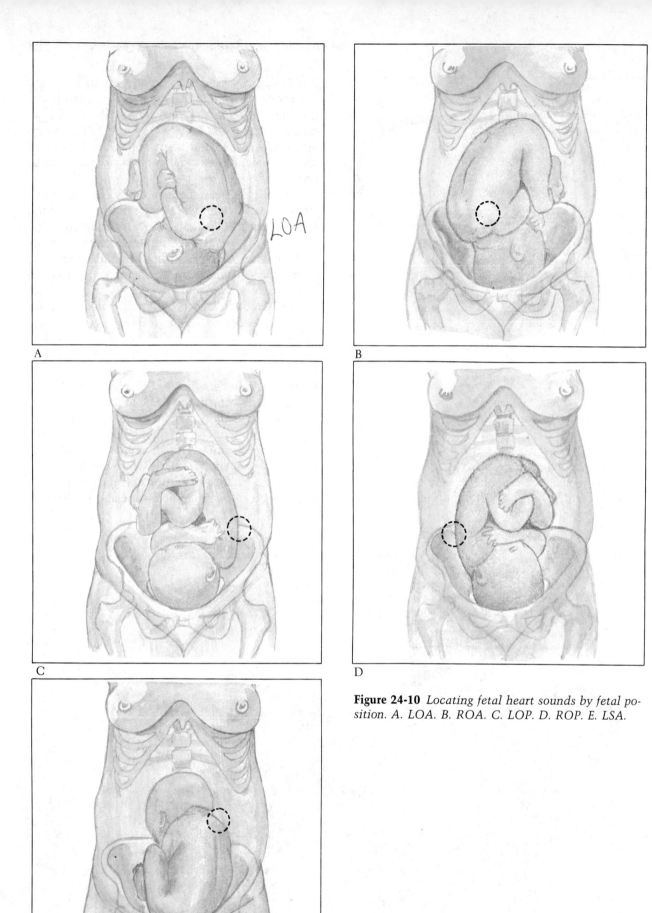

Figure 24-10 *Locating fetal heart sounds by position. A. LOA. B. ROA. C. LOP. D. ROP. E. LSA.*

scope. Errors in counting rates occur because the rate is so rapid. Periodic heart-rate sampling may miss a pattern of change for up to half an hour, during which time irreversible damage or death may take place. It is difficult to hear fetal heart sounds by an auscultatory method during a contraction; thus, essential information on what is happening to the fetal heart rate during contractions is unavailable, further limiting the usefulness of the auscultatory method.

If stethoscope monitoring is the only method available in a particular instance, Bonica and Hon (1972) suggest that this procedure be followed: Count fetal heart rate for at least 20 consecutive periods. Start the count before the onset of a uterine contraction and continue for at least 2 minutes after the uterus is fully relaxed. Rest for 5 seconds and begin a count again. Record the average fetal heart rate for each period and the relationship of each period to a uterine contraction. Given these data, you can plot the relationship of the fetal heart sounds to the peak of uterine contractions. Fetal heart monitoring by electronic or ultrasonic techniques is always preferable to this method, however.

Fetal Heart Monitoring Devices

Recording fetal heart rates during labor offers information on the fetal heart rate both between contractions (the baseline rate) and during contractions. Normal patterns and their descriptions are shown in Table 24-1; patterns that reflect fetal distress are described in Table 24-2. Figures 24-11 and 24-12 illustrate these patterns.

Figure 24-13 is a diagrammatic sampling of a labor room fetal heart rate record. At 10:00 A.M., the fetal heart rate averages 150 beats per minute. Any dip in the rate is slight, occurs with contractions, and disappears at the end of the contraction (type I deceleration, a normal fetal heart rate pattern). As labor progresses, the deceleration pattern becomes type II (at noon). Deceleration begins late in the contraction and lasts beyond it; tachycardia is also present. The woman is turned on her side and oxygen is administered. At 12:10 P.M., 10 minutes later, no noticeable improvement is observed. At 12:15, the record shows a fetus in extreme distress. The late deceleration pattern continues. The baseline fetal heart rate is falling. This is the graph of a fetus dying. Ten minutes later, an infant, alive and well and with a 1-minute Apgar score of 9, was delivered by cesarean birth. This is a common, everyday success story when monitoring equipment is correctly used.

Several types of monitoring devices are now

Table 24-1 Normal Fetal Heart Rate Patterns

Pattern	Importance
Baseline rate	This is the rate of the fetal heart between contractions (Figure 24-11A). It should be between 120 and 160 beats per minute.
Baseline variability	Baseline rate fluctuates slightly (5 to 15 beats per minute) as the fetus moves or sleeps (Figure 24-11A). If no variability is present, it means the natural pacemaker activity of the heart (effect of the sympathetic nervous systems) has been affected. Narcotics can cause this response, as can barbiturates administered to a woman in labor; but fetal hypoxia and acidosis must also be investigated. Baseline variability increases when the fetus is stimulated; it slows when the fetus sleeps. Very immature fetuses will show diminished baseline variability because of immature overall nervous system stimulation and immature cardiac node function.
Beat-to-beat variability	This pattern refers to the difference between successive heartbeats. It is governed by the parasympathetic nervous system. A fetus who is withstanding the effects of successive labor contractions well has both beat-to-beat and baseline variability (sometimes referred to as *short-term* and *long-term* variability) (Figure 24-11A).
Early deceleration (Type I)	During a uterine contraction there may be a brief deceleration in fetal heart rate, probably due to head compression leading to mildly increased intracranial pressure and decreased cerebral blood flow. This leads to vagal stimulation and a momentary decreased FHR. The rate rarely falls below 100 and returns quickly to between 120 and 160 beats per minute at the end of the contraction (Figure 24-11A).
Acceleration	These are transient increases in FHR caused by fetal movement. They indicate fetal well being and adequate oxygenation. They may occur with contractions as the fetus moves in response to uterine pressure.

Table 24-2 Fetal Heart Rate Distress Patterns

Pattern	Importance
Fetal tachycardia	A fetal heart rate over the normal rate of 160 is fetal tachycardia. A rate of 161 to 180 is moderate tachycardia; higher than 180, marked tachycardia. A fetus in distress often has an increased heart rate of this nature before the heart rate begins to fall. Transient tachycardia occurs with fetal movements.
Fetal bradycardia	A fetal heart rate below the normal limit of 120 is fetal bradycardia. A rate of 100 to 119 is moderate bradycardia; under 100, marked bradycardia. Bradycardia almost always signifies fetal hypoxia.
Late deceleration	Late deceleration identifies decelerations that are delayed until 30 to 40 seconds after the onset of the contraction and continues beyond the end of the contraction (Figure 24-11B). This is an ominous pattern in labor because it suggests uteroplacental insufficiency or decreased blood flow through the intervillous spaces of the uterus during uterine contractions. Late decelerations often accompany baseline tachycardia. The pattern is caused by either a rising lactic acid level or myocardial depression from poor oxygenation. This high level of lactic acid activates chemoreceptors in the fetus to increase blood pressure and pulse. Such a condition may occur with marked hypertonia or with abnormal uterine tonus caused by the administration of oxytocin. Immediate steps to correct the situation must be instituted; if oxytocin is being used, slowing the rate of administration or stopping it altogether; changing the woman's position from supine to lateral (to relieve pressure on the aorta and vena cava and supply more blood to the uterus); or administering intravenous fluids or oxygen to the woman may be helpful.
Variable pattern	The variable pattern of deceleration occurs at unpredictable times during contractions and indicates compression of the cord, which is an ominous development in terms of fetal well-being (Figure 24-11C). However, because the pattern is variable, it can be completely missed if monitoring is not continuous. If this pattern is recognized on the monitor, changing the woman from a supine to a lateral position or to a Trendelenburg's position is recommended. Administering oxygen to the woman may be helpful. If these measures do not correct the fetal heart pattern, a cesarean birth may have to be performed to save the fetus's life.
Sinusoidal pattern	In a fetus who is severely anemic or hypoxic, central nervous system control of heart pacing may be so impaired that the fetal heart rate pattern resembles a frequently undulating wave. Although the cause of this pattern is poorly understood, it is being recognized as a pattern as equally ominous as a late deceleration or variable deceleration pattern.

available for recording fetal heart rate and uterine contractions. In high-risk situations, techniques for analyzing fetal blood composition in order to establish blood oxygenation may also be used. Some important studies done recently on fetal monitors are summarized in the Nursing Research Highlight on page 530.

The fetal heart rate should be screened on all women in early labor by an electronic monitoring system. Women who are categorized as high risk for any reason or who have oxytocin stimulation should have the monitor left in place for continuous monitoring.

External Monitoring

In a breech presentation or before a woman's cervix is sufficiently dilated—or because of a physician's or nurse-midwife's preference—fetal heart rate can be monitored reliably by means of a Doppler ultrasonic system (measures the returning sound wave from blood in the fetal heart), by

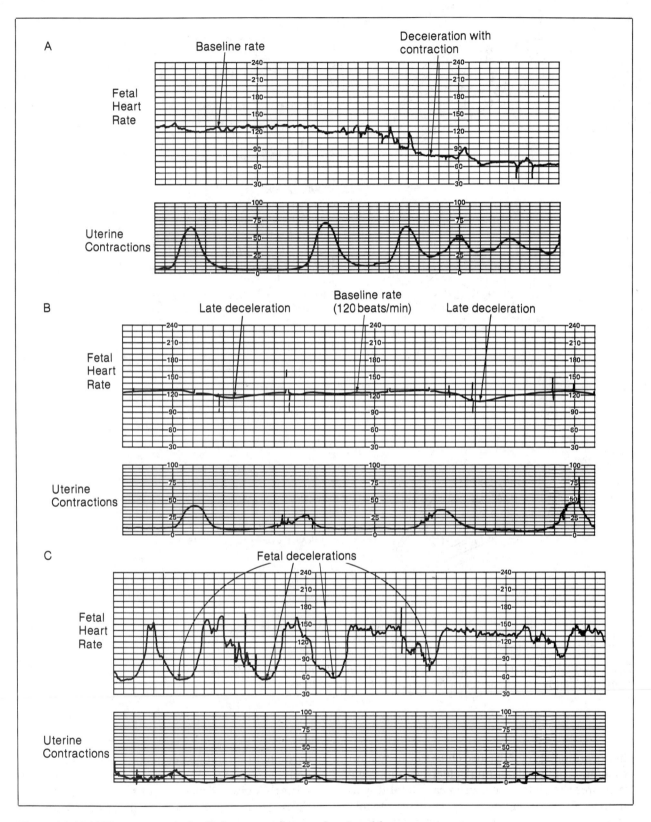

Figure 24-11 *FHR patterns. A. Both short-term (beat-to-beat) and long-term (change in baseline rate) variability are present. B. Late decelerations. Note that the fetal decelerations (arrows) occur after the uterine contractions. C. Variable decelerations. Notice that the fetal deceleration (arrows) occur at unpredictable times in relation to contractions. From Paul, R. H. (1971) Fetal intensive care. Los Angeles, California: LAC/USC Medical Center.*

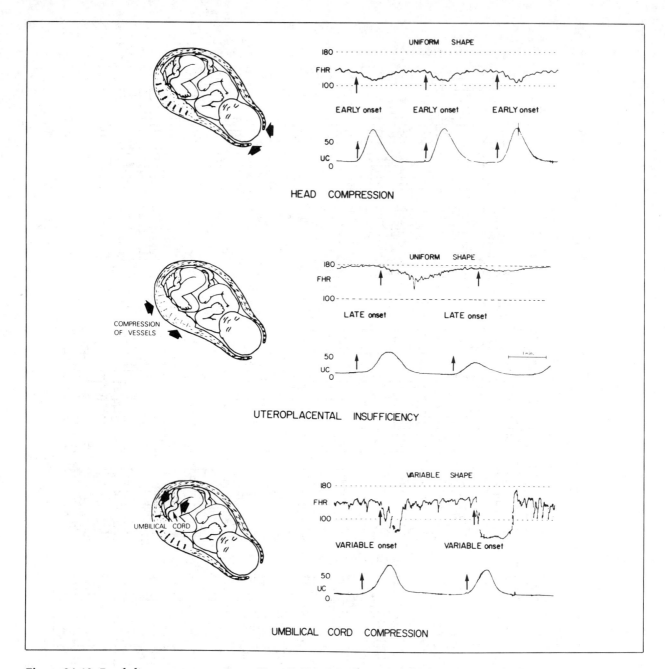

Figure 24-12 *Fetal distress patterns. From Hon, E. H., & Paul, R. H. (1970).* A primer of fetal heart rate patterns. *New Haven, CT: Harty Press.*

phonocardiography (measures heart beat by a microphone), or by abdominal electrocardiography (measures the distance between each fetal R wave on an ECG strip). Figure 24-14 shows a Doppler ultrasonic monitoring sensor, one of the types most frequently used. When held in place against a woman's abdomen by a cloth strap, a small Doppler unit converts fetal heart movements into audible beeping sounds. The sounds may be translated into electronic impulses and plotted on a

permanent graph paper record. An external tokodynamometer transducer used in connection with this gives a printout of the uterine contractions. Such a unit is held in place on a woman's abdomen by a cloth strap.

External monitoring has the advantage of being noninvasive and easily applied; it can be begun early in labor because it does not depend on cervical dilatation or on the fetus being well descended (Figure 24-15). It is not as reliable as internal mon-

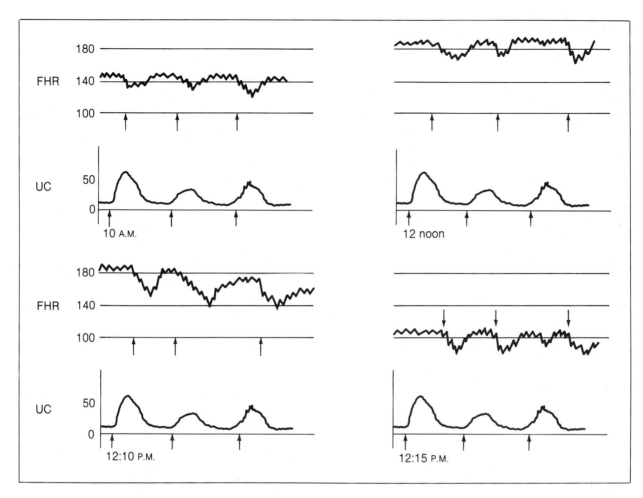

Figure 24-13 *Data recorded by fetal monitor. Note that by 12:15 P.M. the fetal heart rate (FHR) baseline is falling and the late deceleration pattern with uterine contractions (UC) continues.*

itoring in that a change of maternal or fetal position may interfere with the quality of the tracing.

Internal Monitoring

The most reliable method of recording fetal heart sounds is by the use of a fetal scalp electrode. When the fetal head is engaged, the woman's cervix is dilated 3 cm, and the membranes have ruptured, the woman's vulva is washed with an antiseptic, and a fetal scalp electrode is inserted vaginally and attached to the fetal scalp (this will leave a break in the skin visible at birth). The electrode wire threads vaginally and attaches to a leg plate; from here wires attach to the monitor. The fetal electrocardiograph signal obtained is amplified and fed into a cardiotachometer. The output from the cardiotachometer is then recorded on a permanent graph paper record. Although internal monitoring provides a clearer printout of fetal heart rate, because it is intrusive

and carries with it the risk of uterine infection, it is not used as frequently as external monitoring. It is reserved for a woman who is categorized as high risk during labor.

Uterine Contractions by Monitor

If the fetal heart rate alone is being recorded, the difference between a type I (head compression) and type II (late) deceleration cannot be observed. It is as important, therefore, to record uterine contractions during labor as it is to record the fetal heartbeat.

Uterine contractions may be monitored by an internal or external system. For external monitoring a pressure transducer (a tokodynamometer) is placed against the abdomen over the uterine fundus by an adjustable strap. The transducer then converts the pressure registered into an elec-

Nursing Research Highlight

Fetal Monitors

Fetal monitors are often a source of tension for the pregnant woman. Very often the psychological impact a monitor has on a woman is viewed as secondary compared to the valuable information it obtains. However, many recent research studies have explored this important aspect.

1. Sonography—Is it a simple procedure to the pregnant woman? Ultrasonography was first used in the United States in 1964 in many areas of medicine including obstetrics. A study by Milne and Rich (1981) examined the cognitive and affective aspects of the responses of pregnant women to ultrasound procedures. The subjects consisted of 20 women in their second or early third trimester. They found that prior to the procedure there were high levels of anxiety experienced regarding the implication of the knowledge that it would reveal. During the procedure a feeling of excitement was experienced as the woman were able to construct a personal mental image of the baby. Milne and Rich found subsequent to the sonography the subjects experienced an enhanced awareness and personal knowledge of the baby in utero, which they hoped would lead to a further desire to relate to the baby.

2. Radiotelemetric fetal monitoring—Is it better? While all nurses caring for laboring women must accurately maintain technical instruments such as fetal monitors, they also must care for their psychological needs. The traditional fetal heart monitors often limit a mother's freedom and comfort. This in turn limits her ability to maintain control. Radiotelemetric fetal monitoring involves no restraints or cables. The mother is able to move about freely while the fetus's heart rate is continuously monitored. Hodnett (1982) found in her study that placing a laboring woman at the center of control over her experience has implications for nursing practice

and education. Hodnett states that adaptation of existing technology, so that it fulfills its purpose both physiologically and psychologically during the labor experience, may ensure a satisfying and safe childbirth experience.

3. Nurses' attitudes toward fetal monitoring— Do they feel it is necessary? For many years the only method of monitoring the fetus's heart rate was through periodic auscultation. Now electronic devices allow for a better understanding of the fetal condition during labor. There are many diverse opinions among nurses and physicians regarding continuous use of electronic devices during the labor experience. Some feel electronic monitors attempt to replace the personal attention needed by the woman in labor. However, the nurse who is familiar and comfortable with the monitor may convey these feelings to the patient and allow for a more satisfying intrapartal experience. Cranston (1980) found in her study of 124 registered nurses that 52 percent of the nurses felt that routine continuous monitoring of all patients in labor would be ideal. Many felt that the electronic devices allow the nurse more time for intrapartal teaching. While fetal monitoring enables a sophisticated means of fetal surveillance it also seems to reassure the mother. If nurses can convey these positive attitudes they can make the labor experience a safer and more satisfying experience.

References

Cranston, C. S. (1980) Obstetrical nurses' attitudes toward fetal monitoring. *J.O.G.N. Nursing, 9*(6), 344.

Hodnett, E. (1982). Patient control during labor: Effects of two types of fetal monitors. *J.O.G.N. Nursing, 11*(2), 94.

Milne, L. S., & Rich, O. J. (1981) Cognitive and affective aspects of the responses of pregnant women to sonography. *Maternal Child Nursing Journal, 10*(1),15.

---

tronic signal so it can be recorded on graph paper. Transducers must be placed over the uterine fundus so that they register the area of greatest contractility.

The quality and frequency of uterine contractions may be monitored by means of a Teflon

catheter passed through the vagina into the uterine cavity (Figure 24-16). The catheter is filled with sterile water and attached to a pressure recorder. As each contraction puts pressure on the uterine contents, the pressure exerted on the catheter is recorded. A correlation can then be

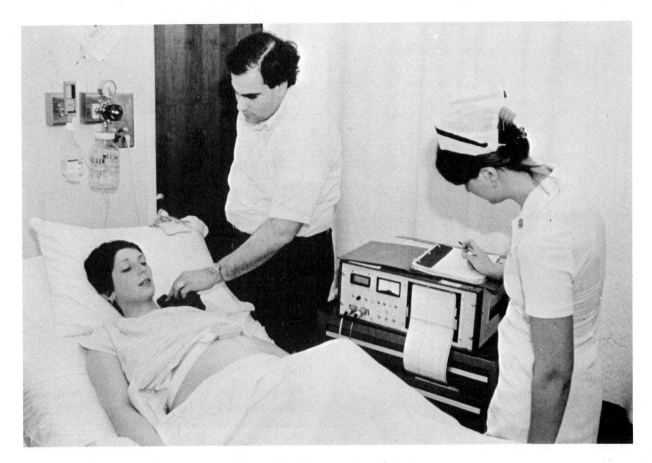

Figure 24-14 *External electronic monitoring of fetal heart rate and uterine contractions. Husband wipes perspiration from his wife's neck as she nears second stage of labor. Oxygen mask lies ready on pillow in case fetal heart rate pattern shows inconsistencies remediable by oxygen administration. The monitor for uterine contractions is evident; the external fetal heart monitor is obscured by the bed cover. (Courtesy of the Department of Medical Photography, Children's Hospital, Buffalo, N.Y.)*

Figure 24-15 *Placement of external monitor leads for fetal heart rate and uterine contractions.*

Figure 24-16 *An internal fetal heart rate monitor in place. Uterine contractions are monitored by the intrauterine catheter.*

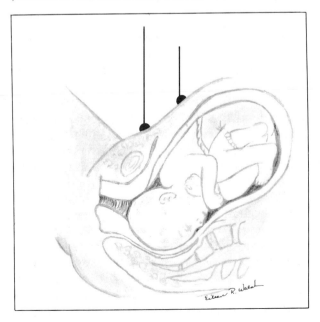

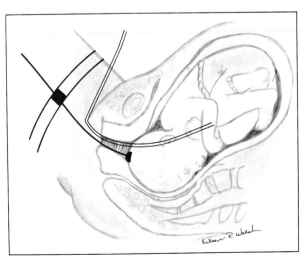

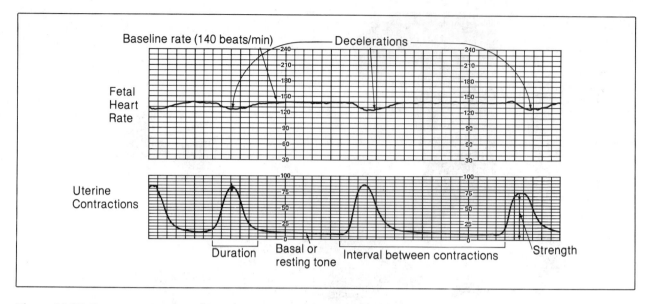

Figure 24-17 *Common terms used in reference to monitoring strips.*

made between the fetal heart rate and uterine pressure from contractions.

When uterine contractions are being monitored by an internal pressure gauge, the frequency, duration, baseline strength, and peak strength of contractions all can be evaluated. Strength of the contraction is evaluated by the size of the peak of the contraction of the tracing. Equally important to evaluate is the return of the uerine tone to baseline strength between contractions. This ensures placental filling between contractions.

With latent contractions, the baseline level is under 5 mm Hg; with active contractions, it is about 12 mm Hg; during the second stage or pelvic division of labor, the baseline may be as high as 20 mm Hg. If baseline readings do not return to 20 mm Hg or below, uterine hypertonia and a compromise of fetal well-being are indicated. External monitors record only the frequency and duration of contractions. Common terms used in reference to monitoring strips are shown in Figure 24-17.

Telemetry

A telemetry system of monitoring allows monitoring of both FHR and uterine contractions to be done free of connecting wires to a monitor. For this method, an internal pressure uterine lead is inserted and a fetal scalp electrode is attached; a miniature radio transmitter is placed in the vagina. The radio transmitter broadcasts the FHR and uterine contraction findings to a distant monitor. The major advantage of telemetry is that it allows a woman to ambulate while being monitored.

Fetal Blood Sampling

By monitoring fetal blood composition, damage to the fetus may be determined before it is apparent on an ECG or an external monitoring system. Changes in blood composition are the cause of the alterations in fetal heart rate.

Fetal blood can be monitored by analysis of small samples of blood droplets, collected from the fetal scalp as it presents to the cervix. It is not necessary or practical to monitor all fetuses by blood sampling during labor. The procedure is generally reserved for high-risk fetuses and is therefore discussed in Chapter 43.

Nursing Responsibilities During Monitoring

A woman and her support person need a good explanation of why monitoring equipment is necessary. Most people associate monitors with intensive care units and thus with critical illness. A woman may interpret the presence of monitoring equipment at her labor bedside as a sign that something is going terribly wrong, that she or her baby is in grave danger. If she wants labor to be "natural," she may interpret a monitor as "clinical" and interfering.

Assure both parents about the routineness of this procedure. Tell them that the equipment provides more accurate information about the fetal heart beat than a stethoscope does. If parents are informed that monitoring equipment is good for the welfare of their child, they will not only tolerate its presence but welcome it. A woman who is worried that something will happen to her child during labor is reassured by listening to the beeping sound of the fetal heart. Many women ask for a graph tracing to save for their child's baby book.

Occasionally, a woman feels discomfort from the strap that holds an external monitoring unit in place, or the snugness of the sensor head limits her ability to breathe deeply, as in abdominal breathing. Spreading talcum powder on the abdomen may make the strap more comfortable. Taking off the sensor periodically and allowing for a position change is helpful. If a woman changes her position herself (and she will change position during labor because she is human, not a machine), repositioning the sensor will be necessary. Remind her that this will happen—not so she will lie frozen in one position during labor, but so she will not think her baby's heart has stopped when her change of position shifts the beam of the sensor.

Women do not need to lie on their backs for monitoring so it does not increase the likelihood of supine hypotension syndrome. Be careful that you do not fall into the habit of nursing the equipment and not the patient, communicating with the monitor and not the woman and her support person. Monitoring equipment frees you from the task of listening to fetal heart rates every 15 to 30 minutes—not to spend more time at your desk or in the supply room or looking at the monitor, but to spend more time giving emotional support in labor.

Some nurses tend to be resentful of or resistant to using monitoring equipment for observation of the fetal heartbeat. Many perceive such equipment as unnecessary. Such a response can be compared to that of the nurse who resisted thermometers when they were first introduced because she was used to determining temperature by feeling brows; or to the response of the nurse who resisted blood pressure cuffs when they were first introduced because she found reading the dial and interpreting two figures too complicated. It has been documented that fetal heart monitoring is more accurate than intermittent stethoscope listening, and nurses have proved to be capable of interpreting the graphed patterns correctly. Therefore, opposition to the use of monitoring devices is difficult to justify except that it is always difficult to change.

It has also been proposed that the woman herself will object to a monitor. If she does, she is probably responding to the attitude of the nurse in the room, who is making it clear that she does not like the monitor. Surely no one doubts that a woman prefers to deliver a healthy, normal baby rather than a dead or mentally retarded one. If a monitor can make the difference—and monitors can—how can women object to them? Monitors and sensors do not interfere with the "natu-

ralness" of labor; they can actually be helpful to the woman who is using breathing exercises with contractions in that a monitor can alert her when a contraction is beginning. In addition they strengthen the "naturalness" of having healthy children.

Risk Assessment

Following initial assessment procedures, a woman is categorized as being at low, moderate, or high risk to have difficulty in labor herself or to deliver a newborn who will need special care at birth. If a risk assessment scale (see Chapter 18) was used during pregnancy, it should be updated at this time and new factors gained from the labor assessment added. The Nursing Care Highlight on page 534 lists factors you might discover about a woman in labor that are high risk. If any of these are present, both woman and infant need close observation during labor and the postpartal period.

Graphing Labor Progress

Graphing labor progress can be an independent nursing function. If a health care agency does not have commercial graph forms, you can use simple square-ruled graph paper. Number the left side of the graph 1 to 10 (representing centimeters of cervical dilatation). Number the bottom line to represent hours of labor. Number the right side of the graph -3 to $+4$ to represent the station of the fetal presenting part.

After each cervical examination, plot the extent of cervical dilatation and the fetal descent on the graph. The pattern of cervical dilatation when graphed in this way is typically an S-shaped curve. The descent pattern of the fetus typically forms a downward curve. The sharp downward slope of fetal descent should cross the dilatation line at the same time as maximum cervical dilatation occurs (phase of maximum slope). A typical labor graph is shown in Figure 24-18.

Plotting the duration of labor phases offers another assessment area or way to recognize any indication that something is wrong with the labor. Various abnormal patterns that may be detected are shown in Figure 24-19 and defined in Table 24-3.

Implementations During Preparatory and Dilatational Divisions of Labor

Following the initial assessment comes the planning of assessment measures to ensure the continued health of both fetus and mother. A time-

======== *Nursing Care Highlight* ========

High Risk Factors for a Woman in Labor

Abnormal fetal position or presentation

Abnormal fetal heart rate pattern

Anemia

Chronic illness in the woman such as cardiac disease or diabetes.

History of previous precipitous birth

Hydramnios

Hypertension

Lack of support person

Maternal age over 35 or under 16

Meconium stained amniotic fluid

Multiple gestation

Premature labor

Potential blood incompatibility

Previous cesarean birth

Prolonged pregnancy

Rupture of membranes more than 24 hours earlier

Temperature elevation (possible infection)

Vaginal infection or vaginal herpes lesions during pregnancy

---

table for these and other nursing interventions during the first stage or preparatory and dilatational divisions of labor is shown in Table 24-4.

Temperature

The temperature of a woman in labor should be recorded on admission to the labor suite. This safeguard rules out active infection, which would necessitate isolation procedures to protect the other women in the unit and the newborn. Temperature should be repeated every 4 hours during labor. Temperatures over 37.2°C (99°F) should be reported to the attending physician or nurse-midwife, as the sign may indicate the development of infection. It is more likely, unless there are accompanying symptoms, that it reflects dehydration in a woman who is taking no fluids by

Figure 24-18 *Normal labor graph.*

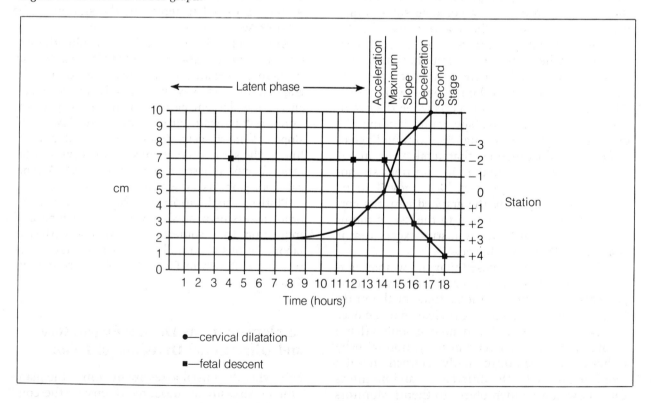

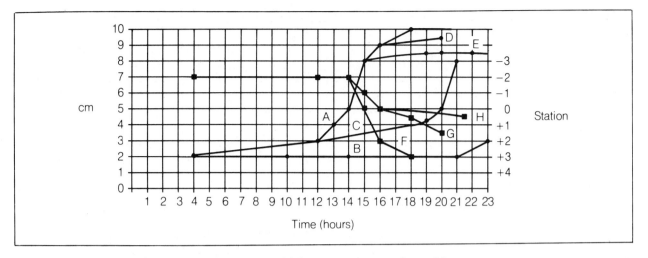

Figure 24-19 *Abnormal labor graph. A = normal labor curve, B = prolonged latent phase, C = protracted active-phase dilatation, D = prolonged deceleration phase, E = protracted descent, F = secondary arrest of dilatation, G = normal descent, H = arrest of descent.*

Table 24-3 Abnormal Phases of Labor Detectable by Graphing

Phase	Definition
Prolonged latent phase	A latent phase that is more than 20 hours in a nullipara and 14 hours in a multipara is a prolonged latent phase.
Protracted active-phase dilatation	If the phase of maximum slope occurs at a rate less than 1.2 cm per hour for multiparas and 1.5 cm per hour for nulliparas, it is a protracted or abnormally extended phase.
Prolonged deceleration phase	If a deceleration phase is longer than 3 hours in a nullipara, 1 hour in a multipara, the phase is abnormally long or protracted.
Protracted descent	The slope of fetal descent is normally greater than 1 cm per hour in nulliparas, 2 cm per hour in multiparas. A descent under these limits is considered a protracted descent.
Secondary arrest of dilatation	This is cessation of progressive dilatation in the active phase before full dilatation.
Arrest of descent	This is cessation of progressive linear descent occurring in the pelvic division.

mouth (a different situation but one that still requires some intervention). Following rupture of membranes, temperature should be taken hourly as the possibility for infection increases markedly after this time.

Pulse and Respiration

Pulse and respiration rate should be taken and recorded every hour during labor. A woman's pulse may be rapid on admission because she is nervous and anxious. After she has become better acquainted with her surroundings and has been assured that everything is going well, it should be in a range of 70 to 80 beats per minute. A persistent pulse rate over 100 suggests tachycardia from dehydration or hemorrhage. Respiration rate during labor is 18 to 20 breaths per minute. Do not count respirations during contractions as women tend to breathe rapidly during contractions from pain. If a woman is using controlled breathing to decrease pain in labor, you are counting controlled, not actual respirations.

Observe for hyperventilation (rapid, deep respirations). Prolonged hyperventilation will result in "blowing off" carbon dioxide and symptoms of dizziness and tingling of hands and feet. Rebreathing into a paper bag and reassurance to reduce anxiety is necessary to reverse this process.

Blood Pressure

Blood pressure also should be taken and recorded every hour during labor. If a woman receives an

Table 24-4 Time Intervals for Nursing Interventions During First Stage of Labor (Preparatory and Dilatational Divisions)

		Continued Frequency	
Intervention	Admission	Latent Phase	Active Phase
Assess and Record:			
Temperature	X	q4h (unless membranes are ruptured, then q1h)	q4h (unless membranes are ruptured, then q1h)
Pulse	X	q1h	q1h
Respirations	X	q1h	q1h
Blood pressure	X	q1h	q1h
Voiding	X	q2–4h	q2–4h
Fetal heart rate	X	Continuously by monitor or q30min	Continuously by monitor or q15min
Contractions	X	Continuously by monitor or q30min	Continuously by monitor or q15min
Provide:			
Ambulation	Until membranes rupture		
Support	X	Continuously	Continuously

analgesic agent that tends to be hypotensive (such as meperidine), check the woman's blood pressure about 30 minutes after administration to be certain that the medication's effect is not causing hypotension. Blood pressure should be recorded between contractions, both for the woman's comfort and for best accuracy, since blood pressure tends to rise 5 to 10 mm Hg during a contraction. An increase in blood pressure may indicate the development of pregnancy-induced hypertension occurring during labor and delivery. A decrease in blood pressure or a decrease in the pulse pressure (the difference between the systolic and diastolic pressures) may be indicative of hemorrhage.

A blood pressure over 140/90 is suggestive of hypertension of pregnancy. If a woman knows her prepregnancy blood pressure (unfortunately few women do), a systolic elevation of 30 mm Hg or a diastolic elevation of 15 mm Hg over the prepregnancy level can also be used as a suggestion of hypertension of pregnancy developing.

Food and Fluid Intake

How much fluid or solid food a woman should ingest during labor is controversial. When it may be necessary for delivery to take place under general anesthesia, she should have nothing to eat or drink during labor except ice chips or lollipops in order to prevent aspiration with anesthesia administration.

On many labor services, every woman in labor is treated as if she were awaiting a general anesthetic. One reason for continuing such a policy is that there is always a chance that a woman may ultimately require this type of delivery assistance; a policy of no food for anyone covers all eventualities. A second reason is that digestion in the stomach is slowed during labor and thus no woman needs great amounts of food at this time. Some women experience a very dry mouth and lips during labor from mouth breathing. Applying a cream to her lips and allowing her hard candy or ice chips to suck on are generally enough to relieve this discomfort.

Women in prolonged labor need to maintain an adequate fluid and caloric intake in order to prevent secondary uterine inertia (a cessation of labor contractions), as well as generalized dehydration and exhaustion. If oral fluids are contraindicated by the delivery plan, intravenous glucose solutions may be administered to maintain caloric reserve.

Bladder Care

A woman should be asked to void every 2 to 4 hours while in labor. She needs to be reminded to do so because she is concentrating on so many new sensations in her abdomen that she may misinterpret the discomfort of a full bladder as part of labor. A full bladder can best be discerned by percussion of the bladder area (an empty bladder percusses as a dull sound; a full one as resonant). A

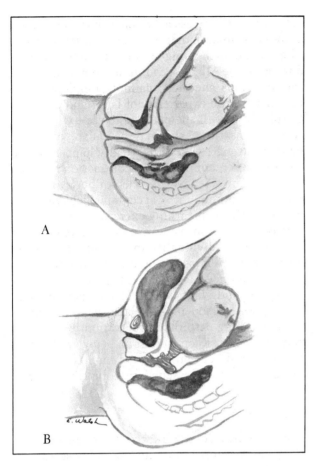

Figure 24-20 *Relationship of a full bladder to ease of descent of fetus. A. Empty bladder. B. Full bladder blocks descent.*

ara. If analgesia cannot be given when a woman first enters the hospital because dilatation has not progressed sufficiently, she should be told why the medication is being withheld. Most women believe that an analgesic given in labor will take away all their discomfort. In most instances, the woman will still feel the tension of contractions along with some discomfort. The analgesic does take the biting edge off the contraction and make it bearable, enabling her to work better with contractions, however. The analgesics and anesthetics used in labor and delivery are discussed in Chapter 25.

Position of a Woman During Labor

In early labor, a woman may be out of bed walking or sitting up in bed or in a chair, whatever position she prefers. Because the main piece of furniture in a traditional labor room or even a birthing room is a bed, most women assume that they are expected to lie in bed and so must be assured otherwise (Figure 24-21). A woman

Figure 24-21 *Walking during labor may increase the strength of contractions as the weight of the fetus is against the cervix. Sitting up in bed or a chair accomplishes this same action.*

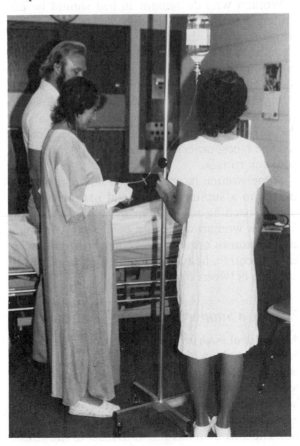

woman should be encouraged to void spontaneously if possible. If she cannot void and the bladder is distended, she may need to be catheterized. Catheterizing a woman in labor is uncomfortable for her and difficult for you because the vulva is edematous from the pressure of the fetal presenting part, causing the urethra to be difficult to locate and the urethral canal to be stretched downward. Use a small catheter (number 12-14F) and insert the catheter between contractions. Use extremely careful aseptic technique so the risk of urinary tract infection is not increased. The relationship of a full bladder to easy descent of the fetus is shown in Figure 24-20.

Analgesics

Many women who plan to receive an analgesic for labor think that the minute they arrive at a health care facility they will be given something for their discomfort. In order not to impede the progress of labor, however, analgesics are not routinely given to women until cervical dilatation has reached 3 to 4 cm in a primipara and 4 to 5 cm in a multip-

whose membranes have ruptured should be kept flat until a fetal monitor shows good baseline variability and no variable decelerations or she has been checked by a physician or nurse-midwife: Unless the head of the fetus is well engaged (firmly fitting into the pelvic inlet), an umbilical cord may prolapse into the vagina if she walks about.

Following the administration of medication such as a sedative or narcotic, a woman should lie down so that if she becomes dizzy she will not fall. As labor becomes advanced, lying down or squatting is her best position so that if delivery is precipitous the infant will not be born while she is walking upright and suffer an injury. A squatting position is effective in that it helps to align the fetal presenting part with the cervix and also uses the fetal weight to help effect cervical dilatation.

Women with fetal heart monitors in place often assume that they must lie in bed so the monitor works properly. With external monitors, they may sit up in a chair by the side of the bed or walk about as long as the machine connections are long enough to reach that far. With an internal monitor in place, they may sit in a chair and, unless monitoring is continual, they can be ambulatory if the monitor is periodically disconnected from the insertion catheter.

Women who do remain in bed should be encouraged to lie on their side during labor. This position causes the heavy uterus to tip forward away from the vena cava, allowing free blood return from the lower extremities and adequate placental filling and circulation.

Most women are comfortable in this position and adjust to it readily. Check that the chair for the woman's support person is on the side of the bed she faces; otherwise, she will keep turning to her back to talk.

Some women have learned to do breathing exercises in a supine position and may need additional coaching to do them in a side-lying position. If a woman must turn to her back during a contraction in order to make her breathing exercises effective, help her to remember to return to her side between contractions.

Role as a Support Person

A great deal is written about the nurse's responsibility to help women maintain control during labor, as if labor and delivery are like an afternoon tea where a woman's manners are observed and her white gloves are inspected for spots. Labor, however, is not like a tea party. It is a stress situation and a woman has a right to react to the stress.

A better approach to helping a woman in labor is to reduce the stress as much as possible, which allows a woman to maintain her own self-control. There is no such thing as unacceptable behavior during labor. All the reading a woman does, all the questions she asks, cannot completely prepare her for the experience of labor and delivery. Despite how well she planned to cope with these strange sensations, she may be caught off guard by their strength when they really happen. If she chooses to scream with each contraction as a way of coping and screaming works for her (it is a distraction technique), it is acceptable behavior during labor. Doing breathing exercises to reduce the pain of contractions is more constructive for most women, but individuality in care should provide for those who choose to be unconventional.

A woman needs a clear explanation of what is happening and what is going to happen. Include her support person in the plans. Help a woman with breathing patterns or relaxation techniques. Stay with her. Keep her from being frightened. You will find her "problem" of maintaining control in labor to be lessened, or gone altogether.

Amniotomy

If membranes do not rupture spontaneously, a physician or nurse-midwife may choose to perform an amniotomy (rupture of the membranes) during the first stage of labor. After pulling on a sterile glove, the physician introduces a blunt, pointed hooked instrument (an amniohook) into the vagina and touches it against the pouching membranes. The membranes are ruptured to open them and allow amniotic fluid to drain vaginally.

It is more dangerous for a baby to be born with membranes intact than with them ruptured. If they are intact, the infant will be born surrounded by amniotic fluid, which allows a quantity of the fluid to be aspirated with the first breath. There are stories of babies born with the membranes intact (born "under the caul")—considered at one time to be good luck or an omen that the child was a special, protected child (Hamlet was born this way). In reality, a child born this way is more likely to have aspiration pneumonia than special powers.

Rupture of the membranes almost always makes labor proceed faster, since the head fits more snugly into the cervix and contractions seem to become more effective. The color of the amniotic fluid should be carefully noted (green or blackish green indicates meconium staining; yellow suggests blood incompatibility with hemolysis; pink or red staining suggests bleeding). Cloudiness suggests infection. Odor is also important; an odor suggests infection. Amount should also be judged to rule out hydramnios. Amount is very difficult to judge as the fluid spilled onto the pad under a woman is quickly absorbed.

Since the membranes contain no nerve endings, amniotomy is not a painful procedure. A woman will experience some discomfort from the gloved hand in the vagina, as she would in a pelvic examination during labor.

One possible complication of rupturing membranes (or when they rupture spontaneously) is that the umbilical cord may prolapse and then as the presenting part enters the cervix be tightly compressed, which compromises circulation to the fetus. Fetal heart rate should be taken before and immediately following amniotomy to detect this complication. Prolapsed cord is rarely overt (the cord extends so far into the vagina it is evident on the perineum). A prolapse will be revealed first by a decrease in fetal heart rate (bradycardia) of the baseline value or variable decelerations on a monitor.

Implementations During Pelvic Division of Labor

If the membranes have not previously ruptured, the transition (deceleration phase) into the second stage or the pelvic division of labor may be marked by a gush of amniotic fluid from the vagina resulting from the rupture of the membranes as the fetus is pushed into the birth canal. Show becomes prominent as the last of the operculum is released.

A woman needs someone with her as she enters the second stage of labor. The change in the nature of contractions from the crescendo-decrescendo pattern to the almost violent urge-to-push type is frightening. She may have cramps in the calves of her legs as the fetus compresses pelvic nerves and she may need help in relieving them by dorsiflexion of her feet.

Fetal heart sounds should be counted at the beginning of the second stage to be certain that the start of the baby's passage into the birth canal is not occluding the cord and interfering with fetal circulation. A timetable for interventions during the second stage of labor is shown in Table 24-5.

Effective Second-Stage Pushing

For pushing during the pelvic division of labor to be most effective, a woman must push *with* contractions and rest between them. Pushing is best done from a semi-Fowler's position or squatting rather than lying flat. Place one or two pillows under a woman's head and let her flex her thighs on her abdomen. She will achieve the best effect if she grasps her legs just below the knees and pushes as a contraction begins, as if she were starting to move her bowels. Her effort should be as sustained as possible; short pushes do not move the fetus forward well. To prevent her from holding her breath during pushing she should continue to breathe out during a pushing effort. Holding her breath causes a Valsalva maneuver or temporarily impedes blood return to the heart because of increased intrathoracic pressure. This could conceivably interfere with blood supply to the uterus during this time.

Pushing is exhausting but exhilarating. Best of all, when a woman is pushing, *really* pushing, the contractions become painless—a welcome relief

Table 24-5 Time Intervals for Nursing Interventions During Second Stage of Labor (Pelvic Division)

Intervention	Beginning of Second Stage	Continued Frequency	After Birth of Infant	After Delivery of Placenta
Assess and Record:				
Temperature		q2h		X
Pulse	X	q1h	X	X
Respirations	X	q1h	X	X
Blood pressure	Following anesthetic administration	q1h	X	X
Fetal heart rate	X	Continuously by monitor or q5min		
Contractions	X	Continuously by monitor or q5min		
Provide:				
Support	X	Continuously	Continuously	Continuously

after the long, hard, uncomfortable ones that proceed transition. At first she may be reluctant to push with contractions; she is afraid that pushing will hurt, and she has had enough pain. A few tentative pushes, however, will convince her that this stage holds for her the same exhilaration that a marathon runner feels with "second wind." Pushing with contractions feels good.

As descent, flexion, internal rotation, and extension occur, the anus of the woman appears everted; stool may be expelled from the pressure exerted on it. As the fetal head touches the internal perineum, the perineum begins to bulge and appear tense. As the fetal head is pushed still tighter against the perineum, the fetal scalp becomes visible at the opening to the vagina. At first this is a slit-like opening, then oval, then circular. The circle enlarges from the size of a dime to that of a quarter to that of a half dollar. When the head has descended so far that the biparietal diameters are completely encircled by the vaginal opening, *crowning* has occurred.

To keep the second stage from moving too fast in a multipara, it may be necessary to prevent her from pushing. The best way to accomplish this goal is to have her pant with contractions. Since it is difficult to push effectively when she is using her diaphragm for panting, she stops pushing. Remember that pushing is involuntary. No matter how much she wants to cooperate with you, stopping this overwhelming urge to push is amost beyond her power. Demonstrating "panting like a puppy" and panting with her may be most effective. Be sure that she is inhaling adequately or she will hyperventilate and become light-headed. Have her take deep breaths between contractions. Breathing into a paper bag also helps hyperventilation as it causes the woman to rebreathe carbon dioxide.

The multipara is generally taken to a delivery room, or the birthing room is converted into a delivery room, when the cervix reaches 7 to 8 cm dilatation. As a rule, a primipara remains in a labor room and pushes with contractions until the baby's head has crowned the size of a quarter or half dollar (full dilatation and descent).

Fetal Heart Monitoring

The fetal heartbeat should be continually monitored during the pelvic stage of labor.

Before Delivery in a Birthing Room

If a woman has been admitted to a birthing room or is at a birthing center, she completes delivery in the same room. The room is converted to a delivery room by the addition of sterile packs of supplies on waiting tables; the partition at the end of the room is opened to reveal the "baby island," or newborn care area. The infant equipment available should include a radiant-heat warmer, equipment for suction and resuscitation, and supplies for eye care and identification of the newborn. This equipment is the same as that included in a delivery room; its appearance, however, is more home-like and friendly. The radiant heat warmer should be turned on well enough in advance so the bottom mattress is pleasantly warm to the touch at the time of delivery. If sterile towels and a blanket are placed on the warmer, these will also be warm to use to dry and cover the infant.

Drapes and materials used for delivery are sterile so no microorganisms are accidentally introduced into the uterus. A table with equipment is set up far enough in advance that preparation does not need to be hurried. Covered, a table set up in this way can be left up to 8 hours. Equipment usually provided on an instrument table is listed in Table 24-6. In addition, a sterile gown

Table 24-6 Delivery Equipment and Supplies

For Preparation of Mother
Prep cup for antiseptic
4 × 4 sponges
Sponge forceps
Buttocks pad
Leg drapes
Towels
Abdominal drape
Towel clips
Needle holder
#14 urinary catheter
Basin for urine

Episiotomy and Perineal Repair
Pair episiotomy scissors
Pair suture scissors
Thumb forceps with teeth
Suture material
Kelly clamps
Allis clamps

For Placental Delivery
Basin for placenta

For Newborn Care
2 bulb syringes
Cord clamp
3 cord blood tubes
Baby blanket

For Safety
Vaginal packing

and gloves and sterile towels to dry the hands should be provided for the person who will deliver the infant.

What is going to happen in the next hour involves sensations that are difficult to appreciate unless they are experienced. All the preparations will not be enough to sustain a woman unless she has a support person with her. It will be important later that this person shared this moment with her; in years to come a couple will talk of it often. Delivery is such a new phenomenon for most people that much of a support person's effectiveness may be lost during delivery. Health personnel who know what is happening and can give assurance that everything is going the way it should are indispensable in a birthing or delivery room at the second stage of labor.

You need to scrub your hands for 3 minutes at a sink and to pull on a clean gown over your labor room uniform, a cap over your hair, a mask over your nose and mouth. If anesthesia is going to be used, you may need cloth "boots" over your shoes to prevent static electricity. The support person who is going to stay with the woman for the delivery must follow the same gowning procedure. Offer help to a support person with gowning and masking or a person who wants to see his child born very much may change his mind rather than admit he does not know if he can touch the mask or the front of the gown after he has it in place.

A support person should be as welcome at the time of delivery as he was in a labor room. Fathers do not faint any more often than do student nurses or medical students, and a woman needs the support during this final phase of childbirth as much as she did during the previous phases. Do not feel compelled to keep a father busy during the delivery phase with tasks such as continuing to time contractions. Sitting on a high stool at the head of the bed where his wife can see him and he can see the delivery in the table mirror is his most satisfying position. His role is support, not busy work.

Perineal Cleaning

The perineum is cleaned with an antiseptic by the physician, nurse-midwife, or the scrub nurse and then rinsed with a designated antiseptic solution prior to delivery. Use a sterile glove and sterile compresses impregnated with whatever specific cleansing solution is designated by health care agency procedure. Use warm water (set a bottle of sterile water in a warm water basin) as cold water could cause uterine cramping. Cleaning should be done from the vagina outward, using a clean compress for each stroke. A wide area including vulva, upper inner thighs, pubis, and anus is included. Figure 24-22 shows a typical pattern for cleaning. Following cleaning, sterile drapes are placed around the perineum.

Fecal material may be expelled from the rectum as the rectum is compressed by the pressure of the fetal head. This is sponged away by the physician or nurse-midwife to prevent contami-

Figure 24-22 *Pattern for cleaning perineum prior to delivery. That cleaning is done from birth canal outward is an important consideration.*

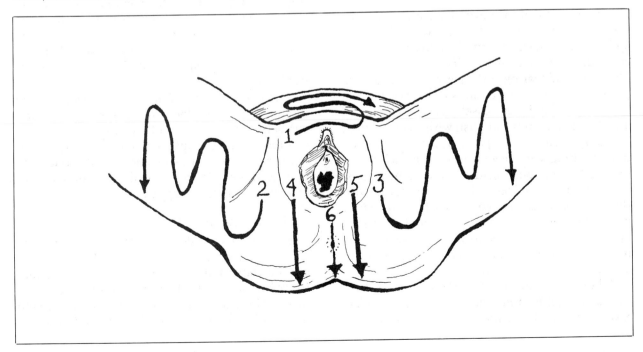

nation of the birth canal. As soon as the head of the fetus is prominently visible (about 8 cm across), the physician or nurse-midwife may place a sterile towel over the rectum and press forward on the chin of the fetal head while pressing the other hand downward on the fetal occiput (a Ritgen maneuver). This helps the fetus achieve extension, so that the head is born with the smallest diameter presenting; it also controls the rate at which the head is born. Pressure should never be put on the fundus of the uterus to effect delivery. This may rupture the uterus.

A woman who has not had anesthesia experiences the birth of the head as a flash of pain or a sensation of heat as if someone had poured hot water on her perineum. It is a fleeting sensation and is not particularly uncomfortable.

Checking the Position of the Umbilical Cord

Immediately following delivery of the head, the physician or nurse-midwife determines whether or not a loop of umbilical cord is encircling the neck by passing fingers along the occiput to the newborn's neck. It is not uncommon for a single loop of cord to be positioned this way. If such a loop is felt, it is gently loosened and drawn down over the fetal head. If it is too tightly coiled to allow for this procedure, it must be clamped and cut before the shoulders of the infant are delivered. Without such care, interference with the fetal oxygen supply or tearing of the umbilical cord can result.

Birth

A mother is asked to continue pushing until the occiput of the fetal head is firmly at the pubic arch; then the head is actually delivered between contractions to prevent it being expelled too rapidly and avoid tearing of the perineum and a rapid pressure change in the infant's head (which could rupture cerebral blood vessels). A woman may be asked to deliberately not push with a contraction. To comply, she should pant, which prevents her from pushing with her abdominal muscles. She may be asked to push again between contractions to deliver the shoulders. She is so involved with the coming birth that you often have to repeat instructions for her. Her coach, even if in control up to this point, may be as overwhelmed by the magic of birth as she is: Support and a feeling of confidence must come from you.

Following expulsion of the fetal head, restitution and external rotation occur. The shoulders and the remainder of the newborn must now be delivered to free the chest for the first breath. Gentle pressure is exerted downward on the side of the infant's head, and the anterior shoulder is born. Slight upward pressure on the side of the head allows the anterior shoulder to nestle against the symphysis and the posterior shoulder to be born. The remainder of the body then slides free without any further difficulty.

The child is considered born when the whole body is delivered. This time should be noted and recorded as the time of birth—a nursing responsibility. (Most physicians and nurse-midwives regard it as their responsibility or pleasure to announce the sex of the infant.)

Cutting and Clamping the Cord

The infant is held with the head in a slightly dependent position to allow secretions to drain from the nose and mouth; the mouth may be gently aspirated by a bulb syringe to remove more secretions. The infant may be held at the level of the maternal uterus or laid on the abdominal drape of the mother while the cord is cut. A cord continues to pulsate for a few minutes after birth and then the pulsation ceases. There are a number of theories as to the optimum time for cutting the cord and the best position for the infant. Delaying the cutting until pulsation ceases and maintaining the infant at a uterine level allows as much as 100 ml of blood to pass from the placenta into the fetus. This addition may help to prevent iron deficiency anemia in infants. On the other hand, late clamping of the cord may cause overinfusion with placental blood and the possibility of polycythemia and hyperbilirubinemia in the infant. Raising the infant on the abdomen may modify the amount of blood infused as well as allow the parents a free, unobstructed view of the new child. The timing of cord clamping will therefore vary, depending on the individual physician or nurse midwife.

The cord is clamped 8 to 10 inches from the infant's umbilicus by two Kelly hemostats and cut between them. A cord blood sample is taken as a ready source of infant blood if blood typing or other emergency measures need to be done. The vessels in the cord are counted. An umbilical cord clamp or tie is then applied.

First Respirations

Within 20 seconds after birth, the average infant draws a first breath and cries. The most important transition to the outside world, the establishment of independent respirations, has been made. The baby will be handed to a nurse, who receives him or her in a sterile blanket. Use a firm

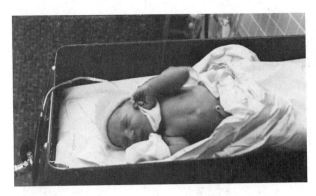

Figure 24-23 *A newborn baby minutes after birth. Notice the knit cap to decrease heat loss. A cord clamp is also in place.*

grip with newborn babies in the first few minutes of life because they are slippery with amniotic fluid. Lay the infant on the radiant warmer and dry with a warmed towel. Cover the head with a wrapped towel or cap; and, if the infant was not laid on the mother's abdomen so she could see her new child, and if respirations are good, wrap the baby snugly and take him or her to the head of the table to show to the mother and father. It is easy to omit this step in the excitement of the moment, the excitement of feeling that you and the physician or nurse-midwife have delivered the baby. Do not forget whose baby it is you have delivered. With birth of the infant, the second stage of labor is complete (Figure 24-23).

Introducing the Infant

There is evidence that the immediate period following birth is a sensitive period during which the parents are "ripe" or most responsive to beginning attachment or "bonding" with the infant (Klaus & Kennell, 1982).

Both mother and father usually want to touch their newborn (to prove to themselves that he or she is *real*). They want to have a complete look at the baby (to prove to themselves there are no defects). Remember the fall the mother had at the fifth month? Remember the day she did not feel the baby move for hours? She needs to be assured that nothing she did during pregnancy, or that happened to her during pregnancy, has hurt the baby. This is important reassurance for parents if the parent-child relationship is to get off to a good start.

A mother should be encouraged to hold her baby following birth but do not leave her alone with the infant because she is more tired than she realizes. She might fall instantly asleep. If she

wishes to breast-feed, this is an optimal time for her to begin. An infant sucking at the breast stimulates release of endogenous oxytocin, which aids in uterine contractions and involution or the returning of the uterus to its prepregnant stage. Many parents ask that prophylactic eye drops not be administered to the infant until after they have had a chance to see the infant (and the infant has had a chance to see them). There is no reason to rush with eye drops so this practice should become the routine rather than the exception to the rule.

Use of a Delivery Room

If a woman is high risk for any reason, the physician may choose to use a delivery room rather than allow the mother to remain in the birthing room for delivery. A delivery room table makes the mother and birth canal more accessible for surgical procedures and the room invariably holds many more emergency supplies than does a birthing room.

If a delivery room will be used, a woman must be moved at the beginning of the second stage of labor to the room. Transfer to a delivery room at this point is awkward as her interest is on what is happening inside her. Also, she has grown used to the labor room surroundings, and being transferred to a sterile-appearing operating room is intimidating. Her support person may feel particularly threatened by the strange, obviously surgical surroundings in a delivery room.

A delivery room's dominant piece of furniture is the delivery table, a stainless steel obstetrics platform. An instrument table stands at its foot and holds the sterile instruments and supplies required during a delivery. A second table or stand with basins is also at the foot of the table; one basin will receive used sponges and the other will receive the placenta (Figure 24-24).

If a woman is to be transported to a delivery room, it is easiest for her to be taken in her labor room bed. This way she will not have to slide onto a cart in the labor room and again onto the delivery table in the delivery room. Once in the delivery room, the woman should be helped to slide over onto the delivery table. Delivery rooms are kept at about 68°F to reduce the danger that the gases used in some deliveries might explode. A woman may complain that the room or the sheets on the delivery table seem cold. More often, though, she is too involved in the final climactic moments of labor to notice the change in temperature. Help her make the transfer from the bed or cart to the table between contractions,

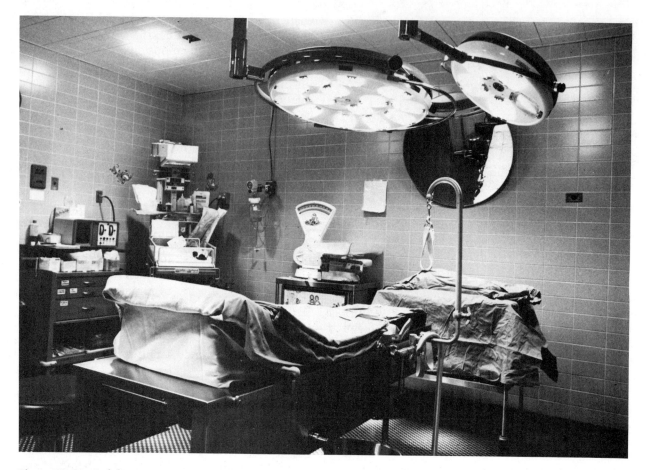

Figure 24-24 *A delivery room. Notice the bolster on the table that allows a woman to maintain a semi-Fowler's position for effective pushing during delivery. (Courtesy of the Department of Medical Photography, Children's Hospital, Buffalo, N.Y.)*

so that it is most comfortable for her; be certain the bed is held snugly against the delivery table so that she feels secure in the move. Since contractions will now be coming about every 1 to 2 minutes, this transition must be done quickly and efficiently, yet without seeming to rush.

Anesthesia

If a low spinal or a saddle block anesthetic is to be administered, a woman is asked to sit up on the side of the delivery table or bed or to turn on her side, depending on the anesthesiologist's preference. If she is going to do the former, she needs support; she is "front-heavy" and with a contraction becomes extremely uncomfortable. Her back should be held rounded and her head flexed forward on her chest to provide the anesthesiologist the widest possible exposure to the vertebral canal. Ask her to lean her head against your shoulder for support. Plant your feet firmly; she is

exhausted and may lean harder against you than you anticipate.

As soon as the anesthetic is injected, the anesthesiologist will wait a specified number of seconds (about 30) and then ask you to help the woman to lie down again. It is important that she lie down immediately; if she sits up too long, the anesthetic will not rise high enough in the spinal canal, and adequate anesthesia will not be achieved. On the other hand, if she lies down too soon, before the anesthesiologist says it is all right, the anesthetic may rise too high in the spinal canal, causing respiratory paralysis. This situation is the exception to the fundamental rule that you should always wait for contractions to pass before you reposition or talk to a woman. Ignore a beginning contraction if it is time to change position after the administration of a spinal anesthetic.

If a woman is to receive a general anesthetic,

she remains supine on the table. Local or pudendal blocks are generally administered close to delivery, after a woman's feet are placed in a lithotomy position.

Positioning for Delivery

In the United States, most physicians prefer a lithotomy position for delivery. When the physician has masked and scrubbed and donned a sterile gown and gloves, the woman's legs are covered by sterile cloth leggings to her thighs. Her legs are raised to the table stirrups. It is important that both legs be raised at the same time to prevent strain on back and lower abdominal muscles. It is also important that the strap holding the leg in the stirrup is secured snugly but not so tightly that it causes constriction. Stirrups are currently perceived by women as an unnatural position for delivery. Stirrups, however, are not uncomfortable and provide the most advantageous position for accomplishing an episiotomy, an operative delivery, or viewing the perineum in order to detect lacerations or other problems at delivery. Pad stirrups with abdominal pads if a woman has ankle edema; be certain that there is no pressure on the calf of her leg in order to prevent a thrombophlebitis.

Lying for longer than an hour's time in a lithotomy position leads to intense pelvic congestion as blood flow to the lower extremities is difficult. For this reason, legs should be placed in lithotomy position only at the last moment. Pelvic congestion may lead to an increase in thrombophlebitis in the postpartal period. It may also contribute to excessive blood loss with delivery and placental loosening.

Delivery room tables have metal handles on their sides that a woman can grasp to continue her pushing effort. If a nurse is going to be in attendance at the head of the table (and one should be), there is no need to use wrist straps. It is frightening and demeaning to be strapped down to a table and may leave bitter memories of a delivery that otherwise would have been a fulfilling experience. The purpose of the straps is to prevent the woman from touching sterile drapes. This concern is not really a problem: Wrist straps should be obsolete for the sake of human dignity.

Because pushing becomes ineffective in a lithotomy position, the top portion of the table can be raised to a 30 to 60° angle so the woman can continue to push effectively. Once a woman is placed in a lithotomy position by means of the table stirrups, the table is "broken" (its lower half is folded downward) so that the physician can be in close proximity to the birth outlet. Never leave the foot of a broken delivery room table until you are replaced by the physician or nurse-midwife so that if birth occurs precipitously, the infant will not be injured.

Episiotomy

An episiotomy (Figure 24-25) is a surgical incision of the perineum in order to prevent tearing of the perineum and to release pressure on the fetal head during delivery. An episiotomy incision is made with blunt-tipped scissors in the midline of the perineum (a midline episiotomy) or begun in the midline but directed laterally away from the rectum (a mediolateral episiotomy). Mediolateral episiotomies have the advantage over midline cuts in that, if tearing occurs beyond the incision, it will be away from the rectum with less danger of complication from rectal mucosal tears. However, midline episiotomies appear to heal more easily, cause less blood loss, and result in less discomfort to a woman in the postpartal period.

Episiotomies were once done only when tearing seemed imminent but are now considered a part of a normal delivery. They substitute a clean cut for a ragged tear, minimize pressure on the fetal head, and shorten the last portion of the second stage of labor.

The pressure of the fetal presenting part against the perineum is so intense that the nerve endings in the perineum are momentarily deadened. Thus, an episiotomy may be done in a woman who has received no anesthesia without her feeling the cut. There is a slight loss of blood at the time of the incision, but the pressure of the presenting part serves to tampon the cut edges and keep bleeding to a minimum. The fetal head generally moves forward considerably with the tension on the perineum relieved.

Forceps

Forceps are metal instruments that may be used during normal labor to extract the fetus from the birth canal. The use of low or outlet forceps for this purpose is so common (especially when a woman has had anesthesia that is making second-stage contractions ineffectual) that it can be considered a routine procedure in delivery. The use of forceps shortens the second stage of labor, prevents excessive pounding of the fetal head against the perineum, prevents exhaustion from a woman's pushing effort, and can speed delivery in the event of fetal distress.

Forceps used to extract the head gently are ap-

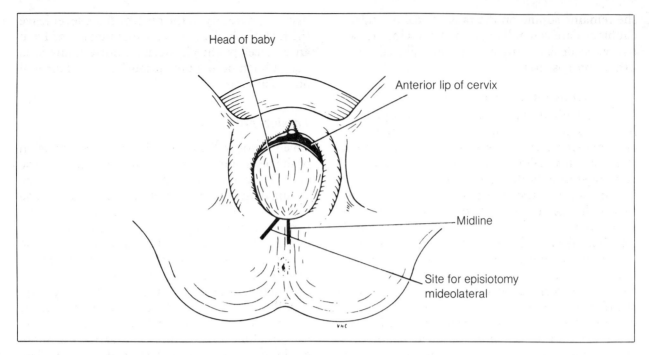

Head of baby

Anterior lip of cervix

Midline

Site for episiotomy
mideolateral

Figure 24-25 *Position of episiotomy incision in a woman during second stage of labor. Baby's head is presenting at vaginal orifice (crowning). From Snell, R. S. (1981).* Clinical anatomy for medical students, *2nd ed. Boston: Little, Brown.*

plied when the fetal head is at the perineum (+3 or +4 station) and the sagittal suture line of the fetal head is in an anteroposterior diameter in relation to the outlet. Simpson's or Elliot forceps are the most common type of outlet forceps used. The blades of the forceps are slipped alongside the fetal head in the birth canal (they are designed to mold to the contour of a fetal head), and the handles of the instrument are joined and locked. Gentle traction is then exerted along the pelvic axis to deliver the head (Figure 24-26).

In order for forceps to be used safely, it must be ascertained that the woman's pelvis is adequate,

Figure 24-26 *Application of outlet forceps.*

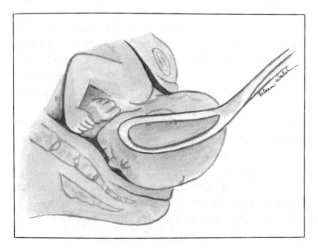

effacement is complete, the cervix fully dilated, and the membranes are ruptured. Anesthesia must be used to attain sufficient perineal relaxation and prevent pain. Before the application of forceps, the physician must be certain of the position of the fetus to apply the forceps properly.

There are as many scare stories about the use of forceps as there are about the use of saddle block or spinal anesthetics. When forceps were first designed and used, some of these stories were undoubtedly true. With improvements in their design, and in the hands of a skilled obstetrician, forceps are now an adjunct rather than a deterrent to safe childbirth. Although forceps appear hard and cold and as if they should put pressure on a fetal head, they are so designed that pressure is put on the shank, not on the blade, and so they actually reduce pressure to the fetal skull. Forceps marks from the pressure of a blade against an infant's cheek may be noticeable for 24 to 48 hours after delivery. These marks, which are usually no more than a linear ecchymosis, are normal and are not a complication of forceps use.

Implementations During the Placental Stage

Following birth of the infant, there is a short space of time (3 to 5 minutes) during which the uterus rests, and then it resumes contractions in order to deliver the placenta. If a complication such as a severe cervical or perineal tear has occurred or the infant is not breathing well so other health care personnel are involved in other care, you may be asked to observe for this moment. Signs that the placenta are loosened and is ready to deliver are a lengthening of the umbilical cord, a sudden gush of vaginal blood, or a change in the shape of the uterus.

The placenta is delivered either by the natural bearing-down effort of the mother or by gentle pressure on the contracted uterine fundus by the physician or nurse-midwife. *Pressure is never applied to a uterus in a noncontracted state or it may evert and hemorrhage.*

Once the placenta is delivered, oxytocin or ergonovine or one of its derivatives, is generally administered IM or IV on the physician's or nurse-midwife's order. These medications increase uterine contraction and therefore minimize uterine bleeding.

One of the most widely used drugs is methylergonovine maleate (Methergine), a semisynthetic derivative of ergonovine. Methergine produces strong and effective contractions, and its effect lasts several hours. The usual dose is 0.2 mg (1 ml) given intramuscularly or intravenously. Another drug often used today is the synthetic oxytocin preparation Syntocinon. The usual dose is 10 units (1 ml) given intravenously or intramuscularly. Syntocinon does not have the sustained action of Methergine.

The administration of these drugs is the nurse's responsibility in most health care facilities. She either administers the drug intramuscularly or adds it to an established intravenous line. Medication should not be given until the delivering physician or nurse-midwife indicates that it is appropriate. She or he may want it given as the fetal anterior shoulder is delivered or may want to inspect the placenta first, to be certain that it is intact and without gross abnormalities and that none of its cotyledons remain in the uterus. Both ergot derivatives and oxytocins cause hypertension by vasoconstriction, so a baseline blood pressure should be determined before administration. They should not be used with women with elevated blood pressure. Be certain that intramuscular oxytocin administered in the delivery or birthing room is recorded on the maternal record. The next dose of medication to maintain contraction cannot be given closer than 3 to 4 hours to this dose or severe hypertension can occur: Exact timing of administration is important (and an easy point to forget in the excitement of seeing an infant born). Intravenous administration of a synthetic oxytocin such as Pitocin may be continued for up to 8 hours after delivery.

If the placenta does not deliver spontaneously, the physician or nurse-midwife will need to remove it manually by inserting a gloved hand into the uterus. He or she needs fresh sterile gloves for this procedure in order not to introduce pathogens into the uterus. The placenta is inspected following delivery to be certain that it is intact and is normal in appearance. If unusually large or small it may be weighed (normally a placenta is one sixth the weight of the infant).

If suturing of an episiotomy is done immediately after the delivery of the placenta, a woman who delivered without the aid of an anesthetic will theoretically still have so much natural pressure anesthesia of the perineum that she will not require an anesthetic. In actual practice, enough time has usually passed before the placenta is delivered (about 5 minutes) so that the woman needs injection of a local anesthetic in order to be comfortable during this procedure. Women who received a local block anesthetic such as a pudendal block or those who have had spinal or general anesthesia do not need additional medication.

Take vital signs (pulse, respirations, and blood pressure) and palpate the uterus fundus for size, consistency, and position. Pulse and respirations may be fairly rapid (80–90 beats per minute and 20–22 respirations per minute) and blood pressure slightly elevated due to the excitement of the new mother and the recent oxytocin administration. Vital signs will be required every 15 minutes for the first hour and the second set taken is probably a better baseline.

Transfer to Recovery Room

When the episiotomy repair is complete (usually in about 10 minutes although it seems to the mother like half an hour), remove the drapes covering her, ask for help, and with extreme care lower both of the woman's legs from the table stirrups simultaneously. Check the fundus height and consistency again. Check vital signs once more. Cleanse the woman's vulva and perineum of any secretions (clean front to back) with warmed sterile water and a sterile compress, dry with a sterile towel, and apply a sterile perineal pad held by a sanitary belt to absorb vaginal discharge (lochia).

If the delivery was in a birthing room, the birthing bed is returned to its original position. Offer a clean gown and a warmed blanket because a mother often experiences a chill and shaking sensation 10 to 15 minutes after delivery. This may be due in part to the low temperature of a delivery room but is primarily the result of exhilaration and exhaustion. It is a normal phenomenon, but it is frightening to the mother. She gets the same feeling as she did in labor, that her body is taking over and she is no longer in charge. She may associate the shaking chill with fever or infection and worry that she will be ill at a time when she most wants to be well to care for her new child. Reassure her that this is a normal happening. Fortunately, the sensation is transitory.

If a woman delivered in a delivery room, help her to slide to a recovery room bed or cart for transfer to the recovery room. If the father has not been in the delivery room, be certain the mother and he have an opportunity to talk together alone right after she leaves the delivery room. They have a great deal to discuss and fulfilled dreams to share (or crushed hopes if the child was the unanticipated sex or was born with a health deviation).

This is the beginning of the postpartal period or the fourth stage of labor (Figure 24-27). It is one of the most hazardous periods of childbirth because the uterus may be so exhausted from labor that it cannot maintain contraction and therefore hemorrhages. In addition, a woman is so exhausted she generally falls asleep almost im-

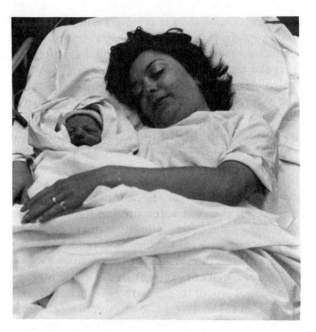

Figure 24-27 *A mother and infant shortly after delivery. Notice the satisfied yet exhausted expression on the mother's face.*

mediately, thereby losing all self-protection. Specific assessments done during this time are continued throughout the postpartal period; these are discussed in Chapter 29 with other aspects of postpartal care.

Utilizing Nursing Process

Labor and delivery of a child calls for all the psychological and physical coping methods that a woman has available to her. No matter how much preparation for childbirth she has had, the experience itself is bigger than and different from what she anticipated. She is venturing into the unknown as surely as a man taking a first step on the moon. Individualized nursing care planning is necessary to provide for the needs of a woman during such an overwhelming experience. Do not try to use "standard" nursing care plans: It is easy to miss the significance of the experience for the individual woman.

Assessment

Assessment of a woman in labor must be done with a degree of speed but also with gentleness. The woman is keenly aware of words spoken around her, the manner with which procedures are carried out with her; and she protects her body against invasion. She may perceive a venipuncture as an excessively painful experience rather than a simple momentary pain. She may have difficulty relaxing for a vaginal examination be-

cause she is worried that any pressure on the fetal head will cause pain for her.

Analysis

The Fourth Conference on Nursing Diagnoses chose no diagnosis specific to childbirth but many of the symptoms that occur with childbirth (pain, fear, blood loss) can be used and adapted to diagnoses. Be certain that goals established during labor are realistic (not all pain can be alleviated; not all fear controlled in such a short time frame).

Planning

Plans for nursing implementations must be adjustable so that they can change with any change in labor progress and are adjustable to the needs of the individual woman and her support person.

Implementation

Implementations in labor must always be done between contractions if that is possible so the woman is free to use a prepared childbirth technique to limit the discomfort of contractions.

This need calls for good coordination of care between health care providers and planning with the woman and her support person.

Evaluation

Evaluation must be included as a continual step of care for a woman in labor so the safety of both herself and her about-to-be born child is protected. It is advantageous to talk to women in the early postpartal period about their labor experience both as a means of evaluation of nursing care during labor and as a chance for the woman to work through this overwhelming an experience and bring it down to a manageable size in her life.

Nursing Care Planning

Mary Kraft is a 23-year-old woman you care for in labor.

Problem Area. Blood loss.

Assessment
BP:110/78; p-84; R-20. Slight pink-tinged show present.

Analysis
Potential for hemorrhage related to blood loss from placental site.

Locus of Decision Making. Patient.

Goal. Patient to complete labor and delivery without excessive blood loss.

Criteria. Blood loss at delivery will be 250–300 ml; BP and pulse will remain within normal limits.

Nursing Orders
1. Take BP, pulse, and respirations q1h. Notify physician if BP is below 100/70; pulse is above 100; respirations are above 22.
2. Observe and record perineal appearance for bleeding q1h.
3. Assess color of amniotic fluid for pink or red tinge.
4. Assess FHR q30 minutes latent phase; q15 minutes pelvic division of labor.

Problem Area. Elimination.

Assessment
Mother states she has been constipated during last month of pregnancy. No BM for last 3 days. Has noticed extremely frequent voiding for last week; no pain on voiding.

Analysis
Difficulty with elimination, related to pressure of fetal head at term pregnancy.

Goal. Patient to maintain normal voiding pattern during labor and delivery.

Criteria. Patient to complete bladder emptying without need for bladder catheterization.

Nursing Orders
1. Ask patient for midstream urine specimen and test for glucose, ketones, protein, and S.G. Report 1+ ketones, protein over a trace, protein over 1+, S.G. over 1.030.
2. Ask to void q2h. Can use bathroom until membranes rupture.
3. Fleet enema administered per nurse midwife orders. To walk to bathroom to expel enema solution.
3. Assess extent of diaphoresis and provide washcloth and clean gown and bedding as needed.
6. Check bladder distention q2h.

Problem Area. Contraction estimation.

Assessment
Contractions 45 seconds duration, 5 minutes frequency, moderate intensity. Duration of labor: 7 hours. Effacement 70%; dilatation 2 cm. Station: 0. Vertex presentation, position LOA, FHR 120; mod. amt. pink-tinged show; membranes intact.

Analysis
Potential for prolonged labor related to ineffective contractions.

Goal. Patient will complete labor within normal time frame.

Criteria. Dilatation and effacement will proceed within normal parameters.

Nursing Orders
1. Plot baseline labor progress and fetal station on Friedman graph.
2. Repeat vaginal examination when contractions are 60 seconds long (active phase).
3. Apply fetal and uterine monitors; assess contractions for duration, intensity, and frequency q15 minutes.
4. Allow to ambulate until membranes rupture.

Problem Area. Fetal well-being.

Assessment

Fetus is in LOA position, Station 0. FHR 120 baseline. No deceleration patterns on monitor.

Analysis

Potential for fetal status interference related to stress of labor.

Goal. Patient will complete labor with fetal parameters remaining within normal parameters.

Criteria. FHR remains 120–160; no meconium staining or deceleration monitor patterns present.

Nursing Orders

1. Apply external fetal monitor for 15 minutes for baseline reading.
2. Assess FHR for baseline rate and variable pattern, presence of late decelerations.
3. If membranes rupture, observe fluid for color and odor.

Problem Area. Hydration.

Assessment

Patient had 1 cup chicken soup 1 hour ago; no further food or fluid to eat or drink. Skin turgor good; S.G. of urine 1.014.

Analysis

Potential for nutrition deficit related to labor.

Goal. Patient completes labor without fluid or nutrition deficit.

Criteria. Patient's urine specific gravity and skin turgor remain normal during labor.

Nursing Orders

1. Keep NPO except for clear candy lollipops or ice chips.
2. Assess S.G. of urine q2h with voiding.
3. Assess skin turgor by subcutaneous lifting of skin.
4. Mouth care (brushing teeth, rinsing with mouthwash), petroleum jelly to lips as necessary for comfort.
5. Assess temperature q4h for elevation.

Problem Area. Pain.

Assessment

Using controlled Lamaze breathing technique. Lies supine for breathing pattern. Uses geometric design to concentrate on.

Analysis

Potential for alteration in comfort related to labor contractions.

Goal. Patient to utilize Lamaze method of prepared childbirth during labor.

Criteria. Patient to complete labor without need for medication administration.

Nursing Orders

1. Admit to birthing room.
2. Encourage to lie on side for breathing exercises.
3. Husband to act as coach.
4. Change pads frequently, provide other supplies for comfort as necessary.
5. Support or relieve coach as necessary.

Questions for Review

Multiple Choice

1. Mrs. Herman is a woman you care for in labor. To assess the frequency of her labor contractions, you would time
   a. the beginning of one contraction to the beginning of the next.
   b. the end of one contraction to the beginning of the next.
   c. the time interval between the acme of contractions.
   d. how many contractions occur in a 5-minute time span.

2. Although the time frame for labor differs with individual women, which time period would you find excessive for a nullipara woman?

   a. a latent phase of labor of 24 hours
   b. a deceleration phase of 2 hours
   c. a phase of maximum slope of 1.5 cm per hour
   d. a fetal descent slope of 1 cm per hour

3. You place an external fetal monitor on Mrs. Herman. Which instruction should you give her concerning this?
   a. to lie supine so the tracing does not show a shadow
   b. to not flex her knees so her abdomen is not tense
   c. to lie on her side so she is comfortable
   d. to not use her call bell to avoid interference

4. If the fetus is not receiving enough oxygen during labor because of uteroplacental insufficiency,

which monitor pattern would you anticipate you would see?

a. a shallow deceleration occurring with the beginning of contractions
b. variable decelerations, too unpredictable to count
c. fetal baseline rate increasing at least 5 mm Hg with contractions
d. fetal heart rate declining late with contractions and remaining depressed

5. If the monitor pattern of uteroplacental insufficiency is present, which of the following would be your *first* action?

a. help the woman to sit up to a semi-Fowler's position
b. turn the woman or ask her to turn to her side
c. administer oxygen at 3 to 4 L by nasal prongs
d. ask the woman to pant with the next contraction

6. Mrs. Herman asks if she can walk with her husband while she is in labor. Which of the following would cause you to question the wisdom of this?

a. She received a narcotic analgesic 3 hours ago.
b. Membranes have ruptured and the fetal head is not engaged.
c. Mrs. Herman is currently in the latent stage of labor.
d. The fetus is in an ROA position and a vertex presentation.

7. Mrs. Herman states she is hungry and would like to eat something. Which of the following would be your best response?

a. "You could have some hard candy to suck on."
b. "Stomach-emptying time increases during labor."
c. "Most women in labor need to drink a protein supplement."
d. "Eating during labor slows the frequency of contractions."

8. Mrs. Herman's physician has told her he wants to use an episiotomy for delivery. She asks you what is the purpose of an episiotomy. Your best answer would be,

a. "It prevents distention of the bladder."
b. "It relieves pressure on the fetal head."
c. "It aids contraction of the uterus following delivery."
d. "It allows the placenta to deliver with the fetus."

9. As Mrs. Herman enters the second stage of labor, her membranes spontaneously rupture. At this occurrence, which of the following would be your *best* action?

a. Test a sample of amniotic fluid for protein.
b. Ask her to bear down with the next contraction.
c. Elevate her hips to prevent cord prolapse.
d. Assess fetal heart rate.

10. To deliver her infant, Mrs. Herman is asked to push between contractions. Which of the following is the most effective pushing technique?

a. lying supine with legs in lithotomy stirrups
b. squatting while holding the breath
c. head elevated; grasping knees; breathing out
d. lying on side; arms grasped on abdomen

Discussion

1. Many women are unsure whether they want an electronic monitor used with them in labor. How would you explain the advantages of a monitor to a couple?
2. A woman in labor is under stress because of pain. What are methods that you could use to make a woman feel relaxed in an unfamiliar setting such as a labor room?
3. When fetal membranes rupture spontaneously, special care is needed. What steps of care would be important immediately following this?

Suggested Readings

Bernardine, J. Y., et al. (1983). Neuromuscular control of childbirth: Prepared women during the first stage of labor. *J.O.G.N. Nursing, 12,* 105.

Bonica, J. J., & Hon, E. H. (1972). Fetal distress. In J. J. Bonica (Ed.). *Principles and Practice of Obstetric Analgesia and Anesthesia.* Philadelphia: Davis.

Brodish, M. S. (1981). Perinatal assessment. *J.O.G.N. Nursing, 10,* 42.

Brown, C. (1982). Therapeutic effects of bathing during labor. *Journal of Nurse Midwifery, 27,* 13.

Dening, F. (1982). Alternative positions in childbirth. *Midwives Chronicle, 95,* 256.

Finch, J. (1983). Ask mothers first . . . the rights of women in labor. *Nursing Mirror, 13,* 156.

Haddad, F. (1982). Alternative positions in labor. *Midwife Health Visitor and Community Nurse, 18,* 290.

Harr, B. D., et al. (1981). Parturition care planning. *J.O.G.N. Nursing, 10,* 54.

Hodnett, E. (1982). Patient control during labor. Effects of two types of fetal monitors. *J.O.G.N. Nursing, 11,* 94.

Howe, C. L. (1982). Physiologic and psychosocial assessment in labor. *Nursing Clinics of North America, 17,* 49.

Kesby, O. (1982). A case for the birthing chair. *Nursing Mirror, 155,* 37.

Kirkham, M. J. (1983). Admission to labour: Teaching the patient to be patient? *Midwives Chronicle, 96,* 44.

Klaus, M. H., & Kennell, J. H. (1982). *Maternal-infant bonding* (2nd ed). St. Louis: Mosby.

Klein, R. P., et al. (1981). A study of father and nurse

support during labor. *Birth and Family Journal, 8,* 101.

McKay, S. R. (1980). Maternal position during labor and birth: A reassessment. *J.O.G.N. Nursing, 9,* 288.

McKay, S. R. (1981). Second stage of labor: Has tradition replaced safety? *American Journal of Nursing, 81,* 1016.

McKay, S. (1984). Squatting: An alternate position for the second stage of labor. *M.C.N., 9,* 181.

Molloy, P. (1982). Collection of umbilical cord blood specimens at the time of delivery. *Midwives Chronicle, 95,* 205.

Pridham, I. F. (1981). Infant feeding and anticipatory care: Supporting the adaptation of parents to their new babies. *Maternal Child Nursing Journal, 10,* 111.

Quistad, C. (1984). Getting mothers and newborns off to a good start. *R.N., 47,* 39.

Stiles, D. (1980). Technique for reducing the need for an episiotomy. *Issues in Health Care of Women, 2,* 105.

Stradling, J. (1984). Respiratory physiology during labour . . . effects of voluntary overbreathing. *Midwife Health Visitor and Community Nurse, 20,* 38.

Trandel-Korenchuk, D. M. (1982). Informed consent: Client participation in childbirth decisions. *J.O.G.N. Nursing, 11,* 379.

Trevathan, W. R. (1983). Maternal "enface" orientation during the first hours after birth. *American Journal of Orthopsychiatry, 53,* 92.

Whitley, N., & Mack, E. (1980). Are enemas justified for women in labor? *American Journal of Nursing, 80,* 1339.

Yeates, D. A., et al. (1984). A comparison of two bearing-down techniques during the second stage of labor. *Journal of Nurse Midwifery, 29,* 3.

25

Analgesia and Anesthesia in Labor and Delivery

OBJECTIVES

Following mastery of the content of this chapter, you should be able to

1. Describe the physiologic basis for pain in labor and delivery.
2. Compare and contrast the action of local, regional, and general anesthesia as used in childbirth.
3. Assess a woman for her degree and type of pain and her ability to cope with it effectively.
4. State a nursing diagnosis regarding the effect of pain in labor.
5. Plan nursing implementations to relieve pain in labor.
6. Describe common measures used for pain relief in labor and delivery.
7. Evaluate goal criteria to be certain labor is a satisfying experience.
8. Analyze ways to make analgesia and anesthesia administration safe in childbirth.
9. Synthesize knowledge of analgesia and anesthesia administration with nursing process to achieve quality maternal-newborn nursing care.

THE CONTRACTIONS OF THE UTERUS are unique among involuntary muscle contractions in that they cause pain (contractions of the heart, stomach, and intestine involve involuntary muscles also but do not cause pain). The pain that accompanies uterine contractions in labor probably occurs for several reasons. Uterine contractions cause temporary anoxia to uterine and cervical cells as the blood supply to the cells is impaired by the stricture of blood vessels. This anoxia causes pain in the same way that blockage of the cardiac arteries causes the pain of a heart attack. As labor progresses and contractions become longer and harder, the ischemia to cells increases, the anoxia increases, and the pain intensifies.

A second major source of pain is caused by stretching of the cervix and perineum. This phenomenon is the same as that causing intestinal pain when intestines are stretched by gas. At the end of the transitional point in labor, when stretching of the cervix is complete and the woman begins to feel she has to push, pain from the contractions often magically disappears as long as she is pushing, until the fetal presenting part causes the final stretching of the perineum.

Additional discomfort in labor may stem from the pressure of the presenting part of the fetus on tissues, including pressure on surrounding organs: the bladder, the urethra, and the lower colon. The majority of pain at delivery is basically pain from stretching of the perineal tissue.

Both analgesia and anesthesia implementations may be used with women in labor in order to reduce discomfort. *Analgesia* refers to the absence or diminished awareness of pain. *Anesthesia* refers to the complete loss of sensation, regional (loss of sensation just to particular body parts) or general. With general anesthesia, there is accompanying loss of consciousness.

Many women in labor need some analgesia or anesthesia in order to reduce the pain that accompanies labor to an endurable level. It may be used to replace the use of prepared-childbirth breathing exercises or to complement them; some women are able to use prepared-childbirth exercises to take the bite or edge off contractions so successfully that no other pain relief measures are needed, while others find that they need some medication to take enough edge off contractions so they can begin to breathe effectively and make their prepared-childbirth exercises work.

The Perception of Pain

Sensory impulses from the uterus and cervix synapse at the spinal column at the level of T10, T11, T12, and L1. Pain relief for the first stage of labor, therefore, must be either systemic relief or medication that blocks these upper synapse sites. For relief of the pain from cesarean birth, T6 to T8 level receptors must be blocked.

Sensory impulses from the perineum are carried by the pudendal nerve to join the spinal column at S2, S3, and S4. Pain relief for delivery, therefore, when the perineum is initiating the pain, must be provided either systemically or regionally to block these lower receptor sites. This is an important point to remember when talking to women in labor about pain relief. Some interventions relieve pain for both first *and* second stages of labor; others for first *or* second stage but not for both.

Pain is apparently transmitted by small-diameter nerve fibers. These small nerve fibers can be blocked by stimulation of large-diameter nerve fibers lying near them. This is why rubbing the skin (an almost involuntary action on your part when you stub a toe or bump a knee) reduces pain. Pain sensation may also be reduced by the use of distraction or by changing the interpretation of pain for that particular person. Prepared-childbirth methods incorporate all these methods (gating theories of pain relief) into plans for reducing pain in labor: gently massaging the abdomen, focusing on a fixed object, and asking for explanations of what is happening so a woman can understand clearly what a new pain or a different pain sensation means.

Pain evokes a general stress response (a fight or flight syndrome) which releases epinephrine (leading to peripheral vasoconstriction). Because the uterus is a peripheral organ in regard to this response, the release of epinephrine must cause some vasoconstriction in the uterus. Helping a woman to relax in labor through either planned breathing exercises or the use of medication for pain relief improves blood supply to the uterus by preventing this vasoconstriction.

Responses to the Perception of Pain

The amount of discomfort a woman experiences from contractions differs according to her expectations and preparation for labor, the length of her labor, the position of the fetus, the unique character of her labor, and the availability of support people around her (Figure 25-1). The discomfort she experiences with labor becomes compounded when fear and anxiety are also present.

People respond to stress or pain in different ways based on sociocultural expectations and individual reactions. Some people with discomfort want everyone around them to know how uncomfortable they are; others prefer to keep their feelings to themselves. Some women view labor and childbirth as an illness and expect to act ill and in distress in labor. Others regard childbirth as a wellness activity and expect to remain quiet and calm throughout the process. Some women are reluctant to show that labor contractions are painful for fear of influencing a young nursing student with them against childbirth.

Pain may be perceived differently by people not only because of psychosocial responses to pain, but because of physiologic ones as well. When pain is perceived by the body, opiate-like substances to reduce pain appear to be produced by the body. The level of these naturally occurring substances—endomorphins—or the body's ability to produce and maintain them may influence a person's overall pain threshold or the amount of pain perceived at any given time.

Women who come into labor believing it will be horrible are usually surprised afterward to

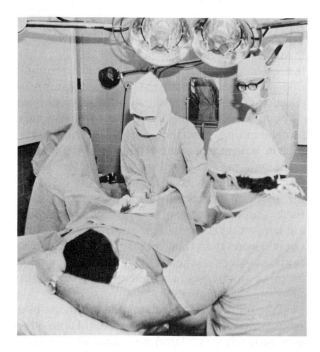

Figure 25-1 *Having a support person present during labor has a great influence on decreasing pain in labor. Here a husband sits with his wife moments before birth. (Courtesy of the Department of Medical Photography, Children's Hospital, Buffalo, N.Y.)*

realize that the agony they expected never materialized. Expectations of pain to come, however, make women so tense during labor that the pain of their contractions is worse than it would be if they were relaxed. No one can relax simply because another person tells her to, however. Some additional intervention must be used.

Implementations to Minimize Discomfort

Careful explanation of what is happening or going to happen during labor goes a long way toward alleviating anxiety and thereby reducing some of the discomforts of labor. When you are a student, the process of explaining everything that is happening seems natural and comfortable, because it is new to you, too, and you appreciate its novelty. After you have cared for the hundredth woman in labor, however, it is easy for explanations to grow fewer and fewer. You begin to think that surely there is no one in the world who does not know that the rupturing of membranes is painless, that a pink-stained show is normal, or that contractions change in character at the pelvic division of labor. A woman having her first child, however, *does not know;* a woman having her seventh child *does not remember* what it was like the last time or perhaps finds it different enough this time (although still within normal limits) to frighten her. Be certain to give explanations to a woman's husband or other support person as well as to her. It does no good to reassure her that everything is fine when her support person has not been reassured and begins to transmit his anxiety to her.

Women in labor relax best if they have a clear understanding that labor contractions are rhythmic in nature; they come and *go*, come and *go*, come and *go*, and when a contraction ends, the discomfort ends with it. This seems to be a simple enough explanation to offer women, who already should be aware of it, since the contractions are happening *to them*. A woman may not be entirely aware that this is the nature of contractions, however, or she may fear that it will change as labor progresses: she tenses with each one, dreading the unknown.

This on-off effect differentiates the pain of labor contractions from that of a toothache or severe headache. The latter are unbearable because they are sharp and continuous. Labor contractions become sharp, but intermittent; just knowing that the pain will soon vanish can make even a high level of pain easier to tolerate.

A great deal has been written in nursing literature about calling labor contractions "contractions" and not "labor pains." The theory is a sound one, not only because the sensation a woman feels truly is a contraction but also because a woman who anticipates pain becomes tense, and tension magnifies pain. Remember, however, that renaming a happening does not change its basic nature. By any name, discomfort accompanies labor. Fortunately many nursing interventions can help to reduce pain and allow labor to be as fulfilling and rewarding an experience as a woman hopes it will be.

Provide Ordinary Comfort

Anyone can stand a little discomfort from a backache. Anyone can stand being thirsty and having dry lips. Anyone can stand having a leg cramp. Few people can stand feeling all these things at once or feeling even one of them while experiencing labor contractions.

Use the ordinary comfort measures with labor patients that you would use with all patients. A woman needs ice chips to suck on or a wet cloth to wipe her lips or Vaseline to apply if they are dry during labor. She needs a cool cloth to wipe perspiration from her forehead. Rubbing or massaging her sacral area often alleviates back pain. Pressing against her sacral area during a contraction may help. Pelvic rocking between contractions may relieve tense back muscles.

Help a woman to find a comfortable position. In early labor, before membranes have ruptured,

the mother may find either sitting in a chair or walking about her most comfortable position. After membranes have ruptured, if the fetal head is not engaged, there is a danger in walking about; the cord might prolapse and fetal circulation might be impaired, so she should remain in bed. Urge women not to lie on their back during labor to avoid supine hypotensive syndrome.

Be aware of what is happening to a woman's bedclothes. Wrinkles form rapidly if she is uncomfortable and moving about a great deal. The waterproof pad under her buttocks, soiled with vaginal secretions, becomes hot and sticky. Her hospital gown becomes wrinkled and sticks to her because she is perspiring. Change the waterproof pad frequently. Never use sanitary pads in labor. Although they absorb vaginal secretions well, they tend to move out of place and may carry pathogens from the rectal area forward to the vaginal opening. Halfway through the first stage of labor, clean sheets and a clean gown give a woman a fresh, ready-to-go-again feeling. Think of comfort measures for a woman's support person as well. Is the chair by the side of the bed comfortable? Does he need a stretch or a coffee or bathroom break? He cannot comfort well if he is uncomfortable himself from hours of sitting still in one position.

Transcutaneous Electrical Nerve Stimulation

Transcutaneous electrical nerve stimulation (TENS) offers a new method of pain relief in labor. With TENS, two pairs of electrodes are taped to a woman's back to coincide with the T10–L1 nerve pathways. Low intensity electrical stimulation is given continuously or applied as a contraction begins by the woman herself. This stimulation blocks afferent fibers or prevents pain sensation from traveling from the uterus to the spinal cord synapses. As labor progresses and the pelvic division begins, the electrodes are moved to stimulate the S2–S4 level. High intensity stimulation is generally needed during the pelvic stage of labor in order to control pain.

TENS can be an effective method for pain relief in labor and has no known fetal effects, but many women object to the use of monitors during labor because of the need to be "tied down"; the same objection applies to TENS equipment. TENS may be most helpful for a woman who has extreme back pain with labor as this type of pain is difficult to relieve with controlled breathing exercises.

Prepared-Childbirth Exercises

A woman's best analgesia for labor is breathing exercises. Help a woman who is prepared to use her breathing patterns. Teach an unprepared woman a breathing pattern such as abdominal breathing (see Chapter 21).

Medication for Pain Relief During Labor

For practical purposes, all medication given during labor crosses the placenta and has some effect on the fetus. Thus, it is important that a woman receive as little medication as possible during labor. On the other hand, labor should not test a woman to the limit of her endurance. She is in labor to be a mother, not a martyr.

The history of pain relief in labor is interesting because the pattern of intervention for pain relief has swung from a feeling that none was necessary to a feeling that too much was necessary to a modern-day approach of individual consideration for a woman's needs and preferences. For centuries, offering pain relief in labor was thought to be amoral because, according to the biblical account, God commanded Eve, "I will greatly multiply thy sorrow and thy conception; in sorrow thou shalt bring forth children . . ." (Genesis 3:16). In the witch-burning period of American history, the concept that childbirth should be painful was so strong that women were burned as witches for providing comfort to other women in labor.

With the discovery of ether and chloroform in the 1800s, it became apparent that childbirth could be made completely pain-free. Unfortunately, this goal was achieved by means of complete anesthesia or unconsciousness during labor and delivery. In an account describing the first time a woman was delivered under chloroform by Sir James Simpson, in 1847, he wrote, "Shortly after her infant was brought in by the nurse from the adjoining room, it was a matter of no small difficulty to convince the astonished mother that labor was entirely over and the child presented to her was really her own living baby" (Lichtiger and Moya 1978). Aside from the physiologic risk to women from general anesthesia, this inability to accept the event of birth, to change from "being pregnant" to "being a mother" is a major disadvantage of general anesthesia or too much intervention in childbirth.

A suitable medication for use during labor must relax the woman and relieve her pain, yet have minimal effect on her systemically, on uterine contractions, on her pushing effort, or on the fetus. Whether a drug has a fetal effect or not depends on its ability to cross the placenta. Drugs with a molecular weight over 1,000 cross poorly; those with a molecular weight under 600 cross very readily. Drugs with highly charged molecules or which are strongly bound to protein cross more slowly than others; fat-soluble drugs cross most easily. A preterm fetus is generally more affected by drugs than a term fetus: An immature liver is unable to metabolize or inactivate drugs. If a drug causes a systemic response such as hypotension in a woman, there will be a decreased PO_2 gradient across the placenta, causing fetal hypoxia. If it causes confusion or disorientation in a woman, she will not be able to work effectively with labor and labor may be prolonged. If a medication causes changes in the fetus, such as a decreased heart rate or central nervous system depression, so that it is difficult for the newborn infant to initiate respirations at birth, the child will be severely compromised in the important first minutes of life.

Once labor is well under way, medication to relieve discomfort can speed labor progress because the woman is better able to work with, not against, contractions. Medication given too early tends to slow or even stop labor contractions. A rule of thumb is not to give an analgesic to a primipara before she is dilated at least 3 cm; a multipara should be dilated 4 cm before receiving analgesia.

Unfortunately, there is no perfect analgesic agent for labor or delivery that has no effect on labor, the mother, and the fetus. Medications used during labor vary among different health care agencies, and the effectiveness of new drugs is constantly being explored. Thus, it is impractical to memorize a list of drugs that are safe. It is better to remember the criteria that a drug must fulfill to be used in labor and expand the rule of basic medication administration from "Never give any drug unless you know it is safe for your individual patient" to "Never give a drug in labor without knowing it is safe for both your patients—the mother and the fetus." A timetable for administration of analgesics and anesthetics in labor is shown in Table 25-1. The Nursing Care Highlight on page 558 lists important measures to consider before administering a medication in labor.

Narcotics

Narcotics are given in labor because of their potent analgesic effect. As a category, all these drugs cause fetal central nervous system (CNS) depression and should be questioned when ordered for a woman in premature labor. A premature infant may have extreme difficulty standing the added insult of respiratory depression from CNS depression.

Morphine sulfate is an example of a narcotic formerly used a great deal in labor. It is less popu-

Nursing Care Highlight

Analgesia and Anesthesia in Labor

Before administering any medication during labor consider if it has the following desirable characteristics:

1. Is it safe pharmacologically for both mother and fetus?
2. Will it allow the woman to continue to participate in labor?
3. Will it allow the woman to remember the labor experience?
4. Will it allow labor contractions to continue effectively?
5. Will it allow the mother to push effectively during the pelvic stage of labor?

---

lar today because of its tendency to reduce maternal respiratory rates and to cause severe respiratory depression in the infant. A new technique for administration of morphine sulfate is by an intrathecal or epidural route. This method gives good pain relief for the first stage of labor; unfortunately, a woman may have severe nausea and vomiting and intense itching as side effects. Because of sustained action in the postpartal period, severe bladder distention can result if a woman is not carefully assessed. Fentanyl (Sublimaze) may be used at some centers. It has the advantage of being one hundred times as strong as morphine but with a short duration of 20 to 30 minutes.

Meperidene hydrochloride (Demerol) is a synthetic narcotic commonly used in labor today. Demerol is advantageous because it not only is an analgesic but has sedative and antispasmodic action as well. Thus it is effective in relieving pain and also helps to relax the cervix and give a feeling of euphoria and well-being. Demerol may be given either intramuscularly or intravenously. An advantage of intravenous administration is that the effect occurs sooner, and the drug is metabolized faster. The dose is 25 to 75 mg depending on a woman's weight. Action begins in about 30 minutes; duration of action is 2 to 3 hours.

Table 25-1 Timetable of Administration of Analgesics and Anesthetics in Labor

Preparatory Division	Dilatational Division	Pelvic Division	
Early (1–3 cm dilatation)	Mid (4–8 cm dilatation)	Late (8–10 cm transition) or Deceleration	Second Stage (Delivery)
Independent nursing interventions (back rub, clean bedding, etc.)	Analgesics such as Demerol →	Narcotic antagonists such as Narcan	→
Barbiturates alone (to induce relaxation and sleep) →	Analgesics such as Demerol → and a tranquilizer such as Phenergan in combination		
Tranquilizers alone (to induce relaxation and to reduce apprehension) →			
	Paracervical blocks _____	_____ →	
	Epidural blocks _____	_____ →	
	Gas analgesic such as _____ Trilene		Pudendal block →
			Saddle block
			General anesthesia

Since Demerol crosses the placenta minutes after being administered to the mother it may cause depression in the fetus. The fetal liver takes 2 to 3 hours, however, to activate the drug, so the effect will not be registered in the fetus for 2 to 3 hours after administration. For this reason, it is best if Demerol is given when the woman is more than 3 hours away from delivery (thus the peak action time of the drug in the fetus will have passed by the time of delivery). It is often a paradox to see a sleepy baby delivered to a woman who was given Demerol 2 hours before delivery and a wide-awake baby delivered to a woman who had Demerol within 1 hour of delivery. In the second instance the peak effect has not yet been reached in the infant; he will need careful assessment for the next 4 hours as the maximum effect is reached.

Alpharodine (Nisentil) is a narcotic with a shorter onset of action and longer duration than Demerol. Since the maximum fetal drug concentration is unpredictable with Nisentil, neonatal depression may occur even if the drug was administered more than an hour away from delivery. Some fetuses show a sinusoidal rhythm on a fetal monitor after Nisentil administration. For this reason Nisentil has become less popular as a medication in labor.

Whenever a narcotic is given during labor, a narcotic antagonist, such as naloxone (Narcan), should be available for administration to the infant at birth. If severe infant respiratory depression is suspected, Narcan can be given to the mother just before delivery. It crosses the placenta readily and may increase the chance for spontaneous respiratory activity by interfering with or competing for binding sites. Narcan is preferable as a narcotic antagonist to nalorphine (Nalline) or levallorphan (Lorfan); the latter two products tend to have depressant effects on neonates. Observe an infant who receives Narcan in the immediate birth period carefully: When the Narcan effect wears off, the infant may become severely depressed again.

Women who are addicted to narcotics may be given methadone in labor. Care of the narcotic-addicted woman is discussed in Chapter 36.

Other Analgesics

Pentazocine lactate (Talwin) is a comparatively new synthetic agent that may be used to alleviate pain in labor. It is usually administered as a single dose of 30 mg given intramuscularly. The effect begins in 15 to 20 minutes; unfortunately, Talwin does not seem to be as efficient at relieving labor pain as hoped when it was first introduced.

Caution women not to take acetylsalicylic acid (aspirin) for pain in labor. Aspirin interferes with blood coagulation and can lead to increased bleeding in the newborn or mother. Using alcohol as an analgesic is not recommended as, although it offers relaxation, alcohol interferes with the effectiveness of contractions (high serum levels of alcohol can actually be used to halt premature labor) and the infant can be born intoxicated.

Barbiturates

In the past, when a woman came into labor with contractions that, although perhaps frequent, were not strong, she was given a short-acting barbiturate such as secobarbital sodium (Seconal) to allow her to sleep until contractions became stronger and more effective. Barbiturates used in labor this way must be short-acting and should never be given close to delivery as they cross the placenta readily and cause respiratory depression in the newborn. Because barbiturates submit the fetus to a chemical insult, they are rarely used in labor today. They may prolong labor. Narcotic antagonists are not effective in reducing oversedation from barbiturates.

Tranquilizers

Tranquilizers may be given as adjunctive therapy in labor because they reduce apprehension and complement narcotics to such an extent that lower doses of narcotics can be used. Promethazine hydrochloride (Phenergan), hydroxyzine hydrochloride (Vistaril), and propromazine (Largon) are brands often used. Phenergan has a long effect (up to 8 hours) and so must not be repeated at more frequent time intervals during labor. Diazepam (Valium) is a tranquilizer that must be used with caution as its sodium benzoate base may compete with bilirubin-binding sites in the fetal circulation and therefore increase the risk of kernicterus (brain damage from high bilirubin levels) in the newborn; it may also cause hypotension and hypothermia in the mother.

Amnesics

At one time, a medication combining scopolamine, an alkaloid of belladonna, and morphine sulfate was used extensively in labor. The anesthesia and amnesia effected by this combination caused a woman to be in deep sleep all during labor (thus the term *twilight sleep* for the therapy). Although a woman shrieked and thrashed with each labor contraction, she reported afterward that she felt little or no pain. Unfortunately, she also reported that she did not remember anything that happened; it was difficult for her to believe that she had delivered a baby. In addition, the medication causes reduced beat-to-beat variability, fetal bradycardia, and narcosis and apnea in the infant. It is little used today but is mentioned because of its historical significance.

Gas Anesthesia

In the past, self-administered gas anesthesia such as trichloroethylene (Trilene) to produce analgesia was a popular pain relief method for labor. Trilene is a liquid that vaporizes readily; it may be used for pain relief during the latter part of the first stage of labor or during the second stage of labor. Trilene is administered by a specially designed mask that straps to a woman's wrist. When she feels she needs pain relief, such as at the peak of a contraction, she takes a deep breath of the gas. She feels giddy, the pain fades, and her arm falls away from her face. She repeats the action again with the next contraction if necessary.

Although self-administered analgesia seems ideal, it is not totally satisfactory in actual practice. Women under stress think less clearly and make decisions less easily than those free of stress. They enjoy having decisions made for them and having help given to them, rather than actively helping themselves. For this reason, self-administered Trilene may be an unsatisfactory method of pain relief for some women.

It is highly unlikely that a woman will receive too much of a self-administered gas when it is used as described and for inducing analgesia, not anesthesia. However, there is always a possibility that her hand will not fall away but will remain close to her nostrils, with inhalation of the gas continuing until she becomes anesthetized. This continuation results in an irregular pulse and increased respirations in the woman and hypoxia and CNS depression in the fetus. Thus, constant attention is required while a woman is using Trilene. It should not be administered for more than 4 hours during the course of labor as prolonged as well as intense administration may lead to fetal depression.

Methoxyflurane (Penthrane) is a second inhalant that may be self-administered during labor. As with Trilene, there is no significant neonatal depression when the inhalant is used at analgesic levels. Neither of these gases interferes with uterine tone, as may happen with other inhalation agents such as ether or chloroform. With extensive use (more than 15 ml of liquid), renal toxicity may occur with methoxyflurane.

Regional Anesthesia

Regional anesthesia is the injection of a local anesthetic to block specific nerve pathways. It achieves pain relief by blocking sodium and potassium flux in the nerve membrane and so stabilizes the nerve in a polarized resting state, unable to conduct sensations.

Because regional anesthetics are not introduced into the maternal circulation, it was once believed that they had no effect on the fetus. Now it has been demonstrated that there is some uptake of these drugs by the fetus (possibly resulting in symptoms of flaccidity, bradycardia, hypotension, and convulsions in the newborn). Effects on the fetus are minimal compared to those of systemic anesthetic agents, however, and they allow a woman to be completely awake and aware of what is happening during delivery. Since regional anesthetics do not depress uterine tone, they leave the uterus capable of optimal contractions following delivery, which is an important concern in the prevention of postpartal hemorrhage.

If an infant should be born with symptoms of toxicity from a regional anesthetic, an exchange transfusion at birth will remove the anesthetic from the bloodstream. Gastric lavage will also remove a great deal of anesthetic because anesthetics have a strong affinity for acid mediums such as stomach acid.

Depending on the region anesthetized, a woman may or may not continue to be aware of contractions following administration. Injection sites of various regional anesthetic procedures are shown in Figure 25-2.

Epidural Blocks (Peridural Blocks)

The spinal nerves in the cord are protected by a number of layers of tissue. The pia mater is the membrane adhering to the nerve fibers; surrounding this is the cerebral spinal fluid (CSF); next comes the arachnoid membrane and outside that, the dura mater. Outside the dura mater is a rather vacant space (the epidural space), and beyond it is the ligamentum flavum, yet another protective shield to the vulnerable spinal cord.

An anesthetic agent introduced into the area of the CSF (the subarachnoid space) is a *spinal* injection, or spinal anesthesia. An anesthetic placed just inside the ligamentum flavum in the epidural space is an *epidural* or peridural anesthetic, or block. Anesthetic agents placed in this space block not only spinal nerve roots in the space but also the sympathetic nerve fibers that travel with them. Such a block will provide pain relief for both labor and delivery. It may actually increase

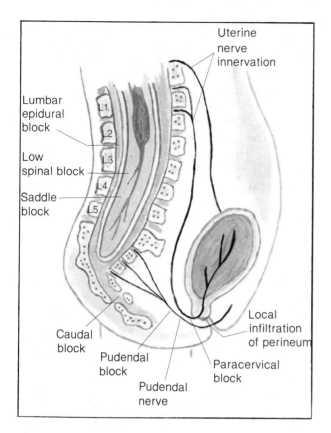

Figure 25-2 *Sites of injection for regional anesthesia for labor and delivery.*

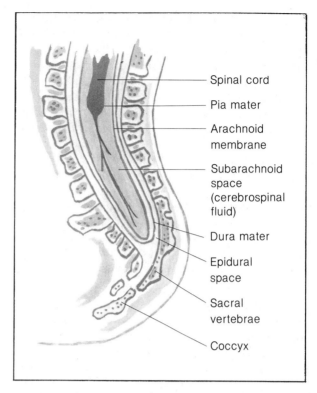

Figure 25-3 *Anatomy of the spinal canal.*

contraction strength and blood flow to the uterus because, as the woman does not experience pain any longer following the injection, the release of catecholamines (epinephrine) with a beta-blocking effect from a pain response is decreased. Anatomy of the spinal canal illustrating these spaces is shown in Figure 25-3.

The two anesthetic agents of choice for this type of regional anesthesia are chloroprocaine (Nesacaine 1.5–3%) and bupivacaine (Marcaine 0.25–0.5%). These agents appear to have the least effect on the newborn.

Women will not have "spinal headaches" following epidural anesthesia because those headaches are caused by leakage of CSF or air in CSF and the CSF space is not entered with this technique.

If hypotension occurs, turn the woman to her left side to protect vena cava return; intravenous fluid and vasopressors may be necessary to stabilize cardiovascular status. A severe reaction can cause convulsions, which small amounts of short-acting barbiturates or diazepam (Valium) will control. Such reactions are very rare but should be kept in mind when you are caring for persons receiving large amounts of regional anesthetics, such as women in labor.

Epidural blocks are advantageous for women with heart disease, pulmonary disease, diabetes, and sometimes severe pregnancy-induced hypertension: They make labor virtually pain-free, and stress from the discomfort of labor minimal. As a woman does not feel contractions, she does not push with the pelvic stage of labor, which preserves her physical energy. Epidural blocks are acceptable for use in premature labor because the drug has scant effect on the fetus. They allow for a controlled and gentle delivery with less trauma to an immature skull. If hypotension occurs, however, this can be detrimental in high risk situations, because with heart disease, diabetes, or hypertension of pregnancy, circulatory compensation may be limited.

The second stage of labor may be prolonged by the use of an epidural block because with the woman unaware of contractions and not pushing with them, descent will be slowed. A major problem is that relaxation of the levator ani muscle may impede internal rotation of the fetal head and further slow labor or make it necessary for forceps to be used to effect rotation.

Lumbar Epidural. Lumbar epidural anesthesia is begun when the cervix is dilated 3 to 4 cm. A woman is turned on her side. The lumbar area of her back is cleaned with an antiseptic solution. A local anesthetic is injected into the skin to form a wheal over the L3–L4 vertebra. A special 3- to 5-inch needle is then passed through the L3–L4 space into the epidural space. Following needle placement, a polyethylene catheter is passed through the needle into the space and the needle is then withdrawn, leaving the catheter to be taped in place. A closed system (a syringe is attached) is established to prevent infection through the catheter.

A test dose of about 2 to 4 ml of a local anesthetic solution is injected through the catheter. Assess the woman's pulse and blood pressure. If the anesthetic was accidentally placed in a blood vessel, toxic symptoms of hypotension, jitteriness, and rapid pulse will be present. Five minutes after the injection, inspect the woman's legs for flushing and warmness, evidence that the anesthetic is in the epidural space (peripheral dilatation is beginning from anesthesia of the sympathetic nervous system). Ask the woman to demonstrate that she can move her legs and that she has sensory perception or can feel a pinprick in her legs. If she can, this is evidence that the catheter is indeed in the epidural space and has not been accidentally placed in the fluid of the spinal canal. If it were in the spinal canal, she would feel numbness and not be able to move her legs (would have spinal anesthesia).

Following assurance that the anesthetic is epidural, an initial dose of about 12 to 16 ml of anesthetic is then given by the catheter. This produces anesthesia up to the level of the umbilicus. The effect of the anesthetic is unfortunately short-lived (40 minutes to 2 hours). Periodically, therefore, another dose of anesthetic must be administered to keep the woman free from discomfort (called a "top-up" dose).

Slow absorption of the drug into the maternal circulation may result in toxic reactions of drowsiness, loss of coordination, slurred speech, jitteriness, and/or anxiety. In extreme reactions, convulsions, hallucinations, and loss of consciousness can occur. Women who begin such reactions need to be provided with an airway and oxygen administration. Before a top-up dose is administered, ask the woman to both write and say out loud a consistent phrase three times, such as "I can do it." The new dose should be withheld if she is unable to do this small task as this shows lack of fine motor coordination and slurred speech.

Epidural anesthesia may be given in a "segmented" fashion. With this technique, following the test dose, only a small dose (about 4 ml) is given. This provides anesthesia for uterine contractions but not perineal relaxation. Close to delivery, if the woman sits up and an additional dose is given, perineal anesthesia will result. Leaving the lower anesthesia for late in labor allows for better internal rotation of the fetal head, as the perineal muscle is not lax, and lessens the chance that forceps for rotation will be necessary.

The chief problem with epidural anesthesia is its tendency to induce hypotension in a woman due to the blocking effect on the sympathetic fibers in the epidural space. This blocking leads to decreased peripheral resistance in a woman's circulatory system; blood flows freely into peripheral vessels and a pseudohypovolemia registering as hypotension occurs. This effect can be largely prevented by being certain that the woman is well hydrated before the anesthetic is given, usually achieved by administration of intravenous fluid such as lactated Ringers. Be certain that a woman does not lie supine but remains on her side to prevent supine hypotension syndrome. Although not usually a part of protocol, a prophylactic dose of ephedrine to maintain blood pressure may be administered before the procedure.

A nurse should be in continuous attendance when an epidural anesthetic is given. To detect hypotension, blood pressure should be taken every minute for the first 15 minutes after each new injection of anesthetic. Blood pressure should be monitored throughout the time the anesthetic is in effect to be certain the systolic pressure does not fall below 100 mm Hg or decrease 20 mm Hg in a hypertensive woman. A greater magnitude of drop may be life-threatening to the fetus unless prompt, effective corrective measures are undertaken. If such measures are instituted quickly, fetal outcome will not be compromised by the event.

Hypotension may be corrected by the prompt elevation of a woman's legs (to increase blood flow in upper body areas), by turning her to her left side (to free the vena cava from the pressure of the uterus and increase blood flow), by increasing the rate of flow of the intravenous fluid, or by the administration of a vasopressor such as ephedrine. Oxygen administration by a face mask will decrease the possibility of hypoxia in the fetus.

With an epidural block, a woman loses sensation of her bladder filling; careful observation and assessment will prevent extreme bladder distention.

Caudal Anesthesia. The epidural space at the base of the spinal canal is termed the *caudal canal*. Injection of a local anesthetic into the caudal canal (the space level with the last sacral vertebra) acts by locally blocking the low sacral nerves that leave the caudal canal at this point

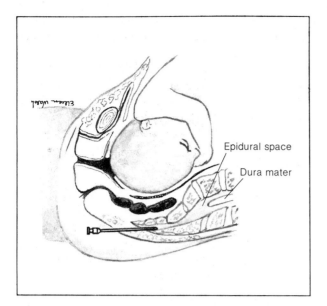

Figure 25-4 *Administration of caudal anesthesia.*

(Figure 25-4). After injection of the needle into the space, a physician may want an extra glove to palpate the woman's rectum to be certain that the needle has not penetrated forward into the rectum. There is a lesser risk of dura puncture with a caudal injection than a lumbar epidural; however, caudal anesthesia produces early perineal anesthesia, so fetal head rotation is more of a problem than with a segmented lumbar epidural block.

Because of the risk of infecting the caudal canal, a caudal anesthetic should not be used if a woman has an old pilonidal sinus or an infection over the sacral area. Lumbar epidural anesthesia is preferred today over caudal anesthesia because of the difficulty of invading the caudal space.

Paracervical Block

In a paracervical block, an anesthetic solution such as chloroprocaine (Nesacaine) is injected through the vagina into the cervical fornices at the 4 and 8 o'clock positions (Figure 25-5). This action blocks the sympathetic nerve pathway from the uterus, but not the pudendal nerve—which explains why it is used as a regional anesthetic for labor, but not for delivery. The drug is injected at 4 to 6 cm dilatation. If the fetal head is at a plus station, paracervical blocks are very difficult to perform because the fetal head is pressing so strongly on the injection points.

A woman should void prior to insertion of the drug to allow the anesthesiologist maximum vaginal space for positioning the needle. She should be on her back with her knees flexed as she would be for a vaginal examination. A paracervical needle is long and may be frightening if a woman is not warned that it is long in order to reach the

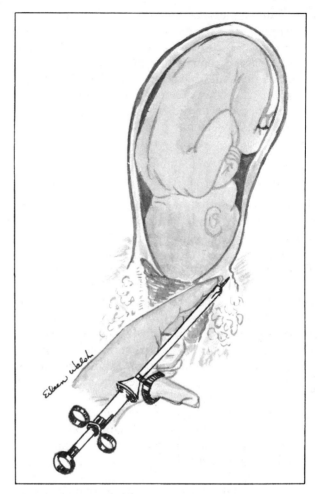

Figure 25-5 *Paracervical block.*

length of the vagina and its destination, not because it is going to be injected that far into her flesh.

Following injection, pain relief occurs within 5 minutes. Local anesthetics are short-acting, however, so as with an epidural block, repeated injections may be needed approximately every hour during a lengthy labor. In a woman who receives a paracervical block, a fetal heart monitor should be continuously in place. An increased incidence of fetal bradycardia follows administration of the medication due to a depressant effect on the fetal myocardium. Fetal heart rates sometimes fall as low as 90 per minute from this effect. If a fetal monitor is not available, fetal heart rate must be assessed frequently (every minute for the first 5 minutes after the injection). Fortunately, the bradycardia is usually transitory and the fetal heart rate returns to normal (120 to 160 per minute) in a few minutes. If the fetal heart rate should remain depressed, emergency birth of the infant may be considered. Symptoms that the mother has received a toxic effect of anesthesia are heart palpatations, a metallic taste in her mouth, tinnitis, drowsiness, confusion, and ultimately convulsions.

A paracervical block gives good pain relief during labor and, coupled with a local anesthetic such as pudendal block given at delivery, it can produce the always-hoped-for "painless childbirth." Because of the risk of fetal bradycardia, however, it is used infrequently today and always with caution.

Hypnosis

Hypnosis is another method of achieving pain relief during labor and delivery. However, only one in four people is capable of responding to hypnotic suggestion so it does not work for all women. If a woman is in this category, prior to delivery she makes a number of visits to her obstetrician or the person who will perform the hypnosis. The hypnotist either gives her a posthypnotic suggestion during a visit, so that when she enters labor she will be unaware of the pain of contractions, or arranges to meet her when she is in active labor to give her the suggestion at that time.

A woman under hypnosis will go through labor and delivery without feeling pain. The concept seems ideal, except that the effect of hypnosis is like that of twilight sleep; a woman is not aware of anything that went on following her entry into hypnosis. Thus she is uninvolved in the process of birth, and the entire process may not seem real to her afterward. The child she holds in her arms does not feel like "hers." Until she can convince herself that labor and delivery are over and accept a new phase of her life, she is not ready to be a mother. Hypnosis also excludes the father from active participation in birth as a labor coach; Hypnosis is not a family-centered approach to childbirth.

Medication for Pain Relief During Delivery

As the sensory pathways that control pain to the perineum may not be blocked by anesthetics given for labor pain relief, additional medication may need to be given to reduce the pain of delivery.

Natural Anesthesia

The simplest form of pain relief for delivery is the pressure anesthesia that results when the fetal head presses against the stretching perineum. This natural anesthesia is adequate to allow an episiotomy to be done without concern that a woman will feel the cut. The pain she experiences as the fetal head is delivered, though intense and hot, is not particularly unpleasant, occurs suddenly, and is quickly over. After the hours of hard contractions a woman has come through, this flash of pain seems almost too easy to be real. However, if a physician wishes to use forceps for better control of the fetal head, the woman will have to be given a delivery anesthetic.

Low Spinal Anesthesia (Subarachnoid Block)

In spinal anesthesia, a local anesthetic such as tetracaine (Pontocaine) is injected into the spinal fluid in the subarachnoid space of the spinal column. Spinal injection for childbirth is usually at the L3 or L4 level. Anesthesia up to the umbilicus and including both legs is achieved.

There are many scare stories about women whose legs were paralyzed after spinal anesthesia or who had "bad backs" or continuous headaches ever afterward. Possibly once someone did suffer paralysis following a spinal anesthetic; but with current administration techniques, this injury is a remote possibility because of the anatomic relationship of the spinal column and the space into which the anesthetic is injected. The spinal cord ends at the first or second lumbar vertebra; however, the dural cavity with spinal fluid continues downward to the fourth or fifth lumbar vertebra, where the injection is made into the subarachnoid space. It is almost as if the vertebral column was designed to include a place for lumbar puncture or spinal anesthesia injections. It is good practice to explain this natural phenomenon to women and their support persons during labor if they show the slightest apprehension about a spinal anesthetic or bring up one of the scare stories that are so prevalent.

Some women do experience "spinal headaches" following this type of anesthesia. The accepted theory to account for them is that there is leakage of spinal fluid from the point of needle insertion or a small amount of air is injected with the puncture. The shift in the pressure of CSF on the cerebral meninges initiates pain. The incidence of such headaches can be reduced if a small-gauge needle is used for the injection (so less air can enter and less leakage can occur) and the woman remains flat in bed for 8 to 12 hours following delivery (so any air present will not rise to the cerebral meninges) and she drinks a quantity of fluid. A high fluid intake allows for replacement of spinal fluid most rapidly. Be certain the woman understands that she must remain flat, not merely remain in bed (only a flat pillow allowed) and drinking fluid consists of about 3,000 ml per day. Lying prone may help in reducing spinal fluid leakage.

The major complication with spinal anesthesia that will occur is sudden hypotension from sympathetic blockage in the lower extremities that leads to vasodilatation and a drop in central blood pressure. This is the second most common cause of maternal death from anesthesia administration (the first is aspiration following a general anesthetic). If hypotension occurs, placental blood perfusion is suddenly compromised. The woman needs to be turned on her left side to reduce vena cava compression. The anesthesiologist will quickly increase the rate of intravenous fluid to increase blood volume; a vasopressor such as ephedrine and oxygen may be given. Do not place a woman in the Trendelenburg position following spinal anesthesia in order to help restore blood pressure: The anesthetic will rise high in her spinal column and stop uterine contraction or respiratory function.

In order to reduce the effect of hypotension, most women are administered intravenous fluid such as lactated Ringers prior to the injection so they are fully hydrated. If a woman is to receive a low spinal anesthetic, she either turns on her side with her back flexed or sits up on the side of the delivery table. The anesthesiologist locates the proper vertebra and, after testing to determine that the needle is in the canal (return of clear fluid through the needle), injects the anesthetic. The effect is almost immediate. No more contractions will be felt. The woman's legs become insensitive to feeling almost at once and motor control to lower extremities is lost.

A woman should use a pillow following administration of a spinal anesthetic to prevent the anesthetic from rising too high in the vertebral canal. The anesthetic normally reaches the level of T10. If it rises above T7, the motor nerves of the uterus will be blocked, and uterine contractions will cease. If it rises above T4, respiratory function in the woman will cease. An anesthesiologist protects against the anesthetic's rising in the spinal fluid canal by mixing or "loading" the anesthetic with a heavy glucose (10% dextrose) solution. This combination causes the anesthetic to sink in the CSF rather than rise. Epinephrine may be added to the injection to prolong the duration of the anesthetic, but this procedure is not routine as epinephrine may decrease blood supply to the uterus due to beta cell blocking.

Low or outlet forceps are generally needed for delivery following a spinal anesthetic: Since the woman no longer feels contractions and has lost abdominal muscle control, coordinated second-stage pushing is difficult.

Spinal anesthesia is used for cesarean birth today, but rarely for an uncomplicated vaginal delivery because of the "snowball" effect produced (because of the anesthesia, an IV and forceps are needed; because of the forceps, an episiotomy is needed; because of the increased episiotomy pain, a woman has difficulty enjoying her newborn . . .).

Saddle Block Anesthesia

The terms *low spinal anesthesia* and *saddle block anesthesia* are often used interchangeably. In the strict sense saddle block anesthesia is injection of an anesthetic into a low lumbar space. It causes anesthesia of the parts of the body that would be in contact with a saddle: the perineum, the upper thighs, and the lower pelvis—or anesthesia only to the L1 to L5 and S1 to S4 levels. Saddle block anesthesia is administered to the woman close to delivery while she sits on the side of the delivery room table. This sitting position for administration ensures that the anesthetic will not rise high in the spinal canal. When a woman sits up on the side of the delivery table you must support her in that position or, unbalanced (front-heavy because of the pregnancy), she might fall. Let her lean forward against you and rest her head on your shoulder. In this position she is not only supported but there is the widest expanse between vertebrae for easy injection of the anesthetic. The anesthesiologist will ask you after 2 to 5 minutes to move the woman to a supine position, which must be done immediately. If she sits up too long, the anesthetic will not rise high enough in the canal to effect pain relief (on other hand, she must not lie down before this time or the anesthetic will rise too high in the canal). Following a saddle-block anesthetic, a woman can bear down more effectively than with a routine spinal anesthetic. Like a low spinal anesthetic, it is much less used today because of the same snowballing effect.

Local Anesthetics

Local anesthesia is the simplest type of anesthesia used for childbirth.

Pudendal Nerve Block

A pudendal nerve block (Figure 25-6) is the injection of a local anesthetic into the right and left pudendal nerve at the level of the ischial spines. The injection is made through the vagina with the woman in a lithotomy or dorsal recumbent

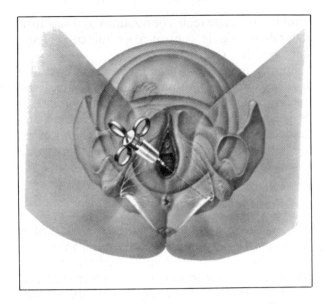

Figure 25-6 *Pudendal block. (From Clinical Education Aid, No. 17, Ross Laboratories, Columbus, Ohio, 1971.)*

position to allow for relief of perineal pain during delivery. Anesthesia achieved with this method is sufficiently deep to allow for the use of low forceps during delivery and an episiotomy repair. Although the injection is only a local one, check FHR and the mother's blood pressure immediately following the injection in case maternal hypotension occurs. The onset of a pudendal nerve block is 2 to 10 minutes; the effect lasts for about 60 minutes.

Local Infiltration

Local infiltration is the injection of an anesthetic such as Xylocaine into the superficial nerves of the perineum by the placement of the anesthetic along the borders of the vulva. Local infiltration is used for episiotomy incision and repair.

General Anesthesia

Anesthesia is the fifth most common cause of death in childbirth (hemorrhage, infection, pregnancy-induced hypertension, and heart disease are the first four causes). Half the obstetrical deaths due to anesthesia are attributed to the inhalation of vomitus following general anesthesia.

Inhalation of vomitus may be fatal because of occlusion of a woman's airway due to the foreign matter. Also, stomach content has an acid pH and so causes chemical burns and secondary infection of the respiratory tract.

In addition to this maternal insult, a general anesthetic may cause narcosis in the fetus. It may impair the establishment of an early mother-child

relationship. All during pregnancy, it is hard for a woman to believe the pregnancy is really happening. The proof that it is real, that she is a mother, that she has a baby is given at the moment of birth; if she is fully anesthetized at this time, she may continue to have difficulty accepting the child.

Being told when she regains consciousness that she has delivered a baby makes the child no more real than did being told she was pregnant. Even later, when she holds the infant in her arms, the baby may still seem like a stranger. If she believed she carried a boy and hours after delivery she is handed a girl, she may wonder whether it is hers. If she pictured a plump little girl with black, curly hair (like her own in her baby pictures) and is handed a stringy, bald-headed boy instead, she may think someone has made a terrible mistake. Suppose the child has a congenital defect. How can she be sure this is the same child she carried inside her? Doubts of this kind hamper effective mother-child interaction.

Gas Anesthesia

There are a number of volatile gases that give pain relief for delivery. All present some hazard and should, like regional anesthetics, be given only by skilled anesthetists or anesthesiologists. They are not used for uncomplicated vaginal birth as the possibility of aspiration with a general anesthetic during pregnancy is so great. They may be used when an emergency cesarean birth or version for a vaginal delivery is necessary.

Possible gases used are nitrous oxide ("laughing gas"), cyclopropane, and halothane. Ether and chloroform, once previously used extensively, are rarely used today. Queen Victoria received chloroform anesthesia for the birth of her son, Prince Leopold, in 1853, advancing chloroform's popularity and resulting in its being called "queen's anesthesia." Prolonged administration of chloroform, however, can cause necrosis of the liver; along with ether, it causes marked uterine atony, which can result in severe hemorrhage in a mother in the postpartal period.

All women who receive a general anesthesia must be observed closely in the postpartal period because of the possibility of uterine atony and the possibility of hemorrhage.

Intravenous Anesthesia

For complete and rapid anesthesia during childbirth, sodium thiopental (Pentothal), a short-acting barbiturate, is usually the drug of choice. Pentothal causes rapid induction of anesthesia and minimal postpartal bleeding. Its short action makes it readily controllable. Following induction with Pentothal, a woman is intubated and anesthesia is then generally maintained by nitrous oxide and oxygen.

Pentothal crosses the placenta rapidly. Infants born of a woman anesthetized by this method, therefore, may be slow to respond at birth and may need resuscitation. However, in view of the degree of barbiturate intoxication demonstrable in the infant, the baby's ability to respond and alertness at birth are always surprising.

Preparation for the Safe Administration of Anesthetics

The analgesia and anesthetic preparations frequently used in labor and delivery are shown in Table 25-2. Women should be well prepared for the type of anesthetic they will receive during labor and delivery, how the anesthetic will be administered ("you'll need to lie on your back; sit up on the side of the delivery table") and what she can expect to happen following the medication ("not only will you no longer be able to feel pain but your legs will feel numb too"; or whatever). Women in labor are under stress, and surprising body sensations happening to them because of lack of preparation can be very frightening—the "straw" that defeats their coping mechanism. For a woman to be struggling against anesthetic administration because of a lack of understanding of what is going on adds to the risk of anesthesia.

The delivery room or birthing room should be checked before every delivery to be certain that adequate equipment is available for the safe delivery and safe administration of anesthetic agents.

The anesthesiologist needs a minimum of six drugs readily available: ephedrine (to use in the event blood pressure falls after regional anesthetic administration), atropine sulfate (to dry oral and respiratory secretions to prevent aspiration), sodium thiopental (for rapid induction of a general anesthetic in an emergency), succinylcholine (to achieve laryngeal relaxation for intubation following a general anesthetic), diazepam (to control convulsions, a possible reaction to regional anesthetics), and isoproterenol (to reduce bronchospasm if aspiration should occur). In addition to these medications, an adult laryngoscope, an endotracheal tube, a breathing bag with a source of 100 percent oxygen, and a suction cathether and suction source should be at hand. Although the anesthesiologist checks these supplies, they are such important safeguards of the mother's health—particularly the suction and oxygen sources—that checking their presence is a nursing responsibility too.

Women should be cautioned during prenatal visits against eating more than sips of fluid once labor begins so the stomach is as empty as possible at delivery in case an emergency arises and a general anesthetic is necessary. A woman who is categorized as high risk may be instructed to eat nothing after labor begins. Regional anesthetics are safer than general anesthesia and should be used whenever possible. When a general anesthetic is chosen, a woman must be treated as a surgical patient and anesthesia induced only by a skilled anesthesiologist. Thiopental anesthesia is used when rapid induction is necessary; a gas anesthesia such as halothane may be used when rapid uterine relaxation (such as during the necessity to version a second twin) is necessary.

For general anesthesia administration, a woman should be intubated with a cuffed endotracheal tube after a rapid induction period. In order to prevent gastric reflux and aspiration before intubation is achieved, pressure on the cricoid cartilage (which seals off the esophagus by compressing it between the cricoid cartilage and the cervical vertebrae) must be applied. Pregnant women are particularly prone to gastric reflux because of increased stomach pressure from the full uterus beneath. The gastroesophageal valve may be displaced also and so may not be functioning properly.

Some anesthesiologists may order an antacid to be given to a woman before general anesthesia is administered to reduce the level of acid in stomach contents in case aspiration does occur. Explaining to the woman why she is receiving this precaution is often difficult (you have told her not to drink anything and now you are offering her something to drink.) Explain briefly that you know this seems to be a contradiction of what you have said but reducing the acidity of gastric secretions prior to anesthesia is important. If it is known that a delivery anesthetic will be used, a woman may have antacid ordered every 3 hours during labor.

In order that hypotension from anesthesia does not occur and to establish a line for emergency medications, intravenous fluid is usually begun. A woman is usually administered atropine sulfate to dry respiratory secretions as a preoperative injection and succinylcholine with induction to decrease respiration function (the anesthesiologist will use a breathing bag to breathe for her during the course of anesthesia). The moments of induction of general anesthesia before the endotracheal tube is safely in place are critical ones for the anesthesiologist. Respect the necessity to concentrate on the task at hand until this is achieved. Some women may comment after the use of a

Table 25-2 Analgesics and Anesthetics Commonly Used in Labor and Delivery

Type	Drug	Usual Dose	Effect on Mother
Narcotic analgesic	Meperidine (Demerol)	25 mg IV, 50–100 mg IM q3–4h	Effective analgesic Feeling of well-being
	Alaphaprodine (Nisentil)	10 mg IV, 20–40 mg SQ q3–4h	Effective analgesic
	Morphine sulfate	8–15 mg IM q4–5h	Effective analgesic Slows respiratory rate Can be constipating
Sedative hypnotics	Secobarbital (Seconal)	100–200 mg IM or PO, 50 mg IV	Reduces apprehension Induces lethargy and sleep (Used early in labor to encourage rest)
	Pentobarbital (Nembutal)	100–200 mg IM or PO, 50 mg IV	Same as secobarbital
Tranquilizers	Diazepam (Valium)	5–10 mg IV, IM, or PO	Reduces apprehension Induces relaxation
	Promethazine (Phenergan)	25–50 mg IM or PO	(When used with a narcotic analgesic, less analgesic is needed for effect)
	Promazine (Sparine)	25 mg IM or PO	May cause hypotension that responds poorly to vasopressors
	Hydroxyzine pamoate (Vistaril)	5–15 mg IM or PO	
Gas analgesics	Trichloroethylene (Trilene)	Self-administered by taking a breath of gas at peak of contraction	Effective pain relief for first and second stages of labor Some dizziness or light-headedness Some increase in respirations
	Methoxyflurane (Penthrane)	Self-administered by taking a breath of gas at peak of contraction (as with Trilene, only safe when self-administered; should not be given by support person)	May cause hypotension, slowed respirations Effective pain relief for first and second stages of labor
Regional anesthetics Saddle block	Local anesthetic	Administered for delivery with mother in sitting position; given between contractions Injection at L3–L4 or L4–L5 into CSF	Rapid onset in minutes Lasts about 2 hours Numbness and loss of sensation in perineum and thighs Loss of pushing sensation Maternal hypotension Postpartum headache
Caudal block	Local anesthetic	Administered for first stage of labor With continuous caudal, anesthesia will last through delivery Injected into epidural space at caudal hiatus	Rapid onset in minutes Lasts 60–90 minutes Loss of pain perception for labor contractions and delivery Maternal hypotension
Lumbar epidural block	Local anesthetic	Administered for first stage of labor With continuous block, anesthesia will last through delivery Injected into epidural space at L3–L4	Rapid onset in minutes Lasts 60–90 minutes Loss of pain perception for labor contractions and delivery Maternal hypotension

Effect on Labor Progress	*Effect on Fetus or Newborn*
Relaxation may aid progress as cervical relaxation occurs Will halt labor contractions if given too early	Should be given 3 hours away from delivery to avoid respiratory depression in newborn
May weaken contractions for short period Used in women with irregular contractions sometimes to reduce uterine irritability Minimal effect if used in early labor Large doses may impair strength of contractions	Causes serious respiratory distress in newborn Should be given 3 hours away from delivery to avoid respiratory depression Sleepiness for first 48 hours
None apparent	Valium may interfere with bilirubin binding in susceptible infants All tranquilizers may cause slight delay in onset of newborn respirations
None apparent	Not depressant when used in analgesic proportions Can become depressant if used over 3–4 hours
None apparent	Not depressant when used in analgesic proportions
Progress halts (used just prior to delivery, and delivery managed with outlet forceps)	None apparent
Loss of need to push with contractions; can be coached to push with contraction or delivery will be managed by low forceps May slow labor if given too early	May cause transient behavior changes in newborn for first few days of life
Will slow labor if given too early Obliterates pushing feeling so second stage may be prolonged	May be some differences in response in first few days of life

Table 25-2 (continued)

Type	Drug	Usual Dose	Effect on Mother
Paracervical block	Local anesthetic	Administered for first stage of labor Injected into vaginal fornices	Rapid onset in minutes Lasts 60–90 minutes Possible hypotension
Local anesthetics Pudendal block	Local anesthetic	Administered just prior to delivery for perineal anesthesia Injected through vagina	Rapid anesthesia of perineum
Local infiltration of perineum	Local anesthetic	Injected just prior to delivery for episiotomy incision and repair	Anesthesia of perineum almost immediately
Gas anesthetics	Ether	Administered by open-drip method for delivery	Irritating to respiratory tract May cause vomiting in recovery period Good relaxation
	Cyclopropane	Administered by closed system Highly inflammable	Rapid anesthesia, so is used in emergency situations May cause cardiac arrhythmias
	Halothane	Administered just prior to delivery by closed system	Rapid anesthesia, so is used in emergency situations
	Nitrous oxide	Administered just prior to delivery by allowing mother to take a few breaths at a time	Good analgesic; light anesthesia. Both induction and recovery are rapid
General intravenous anesthetic	Thiopental	Administered IV by anesthesiologist	Rapid anesthesia; also rapid recovery

general anesthetic that their throat feels raw or sore. This pain is from the insertion of the endotracheal tube and is normal. Sipping cold liquids (as soon as safe after general anesthesia) relieves the discomfort.

If aspiration of vomitus occurs in the delivery room, prompt attention is essential. The trachea is suctioned by the anesthesiologist to remove as much foreign material as possible; the woman is intubated if she was not previously and given 100 percent oxygen. She will be given a medication such as isoproterenol intravenously to reduce bronchospasm and a corticosteroid intravenously to reduce an inflammatory reaction. Positive pressure ventilation may be started. Blood gases and a chest X-ray film will be taken to demonstrate the degree of aeration she is capable of.

A woman will be kept on mechanical ventilation until the chest X-ray films, blood gases, and her overall clinical condition improves. She is critically ill at the time of aspiration and often will be transferred to an intensive care unit for the special care she requires to survive this occurrence.

During her intensive care period, she needs to be kept informed of her baby's progress and, if possible, allowed to see the baby. The infant's physical presence helps to assure her that, although she is ill, the baby was delivered and is doing well (if that is the circumstance). If she is transferred to another section of the hospital (to the intensive care unit) and taking the baby to her is not practical, being able to see a Polaroid snapshot of her infant is very helpful.

The Risk of Anesthesia

If a difficult birth is anticipated, a general anesthetic may be the method of choice to achieve a safe outcome for both mother and child. However, general anesthesia should never be considered routine in childbirth because of the risk if the fetus does not breathe spontaneously and

Effect on Labor Progress	*Effect on Fetus or Newborn*
Effect varies widely; sometimes labor slowed, other times shortened	Fetal bradycardia may result If bradycardia is persistent (over 15 minutes), rapid delivery of the fetus may be considered
None apparent	None apparent
None apparent	None apparent
Extreme uterine relaxation Uterine contractions will be decreased with complete anesthesia Uterine atony will persist into third stage	If deep anesthesia achieved, there is depression of the newborn
Extreme uterine relaxation Allows for rapid intrauterine manipulation Uterine atony will persist into third stage	If baby is born within 8 minutes after administration, there is minimal newborn depression (it takes over 8 minutes for fetal concentrations to reach those of mother)
Extreme uterine relaxation Uterine atony will persist into the third stage	Some neonatal depression
Uterine relaxation not enough to perform uterine manipulations	If nitrous oxide used in conjunction with 20% oxygen, newborn depression is minimal
Forceps required as abdominal pushing is no longer possible	Infant will be born with depression

needs resuscitation, the resultant threat to the mother-infant relationship, and the risk to the mother's life from laryngeal spasm on aspiration.

The risk of anesthesia correlates with the amount and the length of time anesthesia is used. Because of possible aspiration of vomitus, a general anesthetic during delivery carries a much greater risk to both mother and infant than does regional anesthesia such as a pudendal block.

It became customary to rely heavily on the use of analgesia during labor and anesthesia during delivery during the 1940s because at the time these were introduced, women were deprived of their support person in labor and delivery, and surrounded by nurses who were technically skilled but not prepared to handle their feelings of fright and loneliness. Since physicians came to the hospital only in time for delivery, not before, they provided no support. Is it any wonder that women screamed and fought procedures and needed anesthesia? A woman protects her body from intrusive or hurtful procedures all during pregnancy. This protective reaction does not stop until after delivery, when it shifts to the body of the newborn. When contrasted with the scene of a woman screaming and thrashing during delivery because she was unprepared for the experience, general anesthesia seemed like a panacea.

However, when nurses are educated to offer psychological support to patients in labor, a great deal of the fear and fright of childbirth can be handled by words and supportive actions rather than by medication. With a woman's fear controlled, and her lying alert and cooperative at delivery, the risk of general anesthesia far outweighs any advantages.

Nurses can contribute enormously to making childbirth safer than it is currently by using all the professional skills of nursing to ensure that women are well informed and feel secure because they have a meaningful support person with them as well as skilled persons who are concerned about and looking after their best interests.

Utilizing Nursing Process

As analgesia and anesthesia are risks for mother (hypotension and aspiration) and the fetus (bradycardia) and perhaps for the family if the method reduces the ability of the father to participate in the birth, its use must always be balanced against the risk for the mother (asking her to endure pain) and the family (turning the birth into a negative rather than a positive growth experience). In order that planning of such balancing is done with thoroughness, it must be done by using the nursing process.

Assessment

Remember that pain thresholds cause the amount of pain that people experience to be very different in amount. Remember also that pain is a subjective symptom. No one but the woman herself can describe or know how much or how extensive is her pain.

Assess how much discomfort a woman is having in labor by what she voices. Look also for subtle signs of pain such as facial tenseness, flushing, or paleness; fisted hands; rapid breathing; or rapid pulse rate. Knowing the extent of a woman's discomfort is a guide to the choice of medication or intervention she needs in labor.

Analysis

Pain is a diagnosis accepted by NANDA. Even though you do not usually refer to the discomfort of labor as "pain" but as "contractions," do not omit the word *pain* from a nursing diagnosis: The term strengthens the depth of the problem you are describing. Some women are not as concerned with the actual pain they are having as they are with their reaction to it. A diagnosis of "Loss of self-esteem related to inability to use prepared-childbirth method" or "Fear related to pain during labor" is possible.

When planning goals with a woman in labor, be certain that they are realistic. A plan to reduce all pain during labor is unrealistic; a plan to minimize or reduce pain is very realistic.

Planning

A major area of planning for the discomforts of labor is how to educate women about the discomfort of labor so their perceptions of it are realistic. In planning care, be certain to include planning for comfort measures such as changing a wrinkled sheet or offering Vaseline for dry lips.

Implementation

Offering analgesia or assisting with anesthesia administration during labor or delivery requires knowledgeable skills of administration in addition to a caring presence that allows a woman to accept analgesia when she needs it and encourages other women to experience a labor without heavy sedation. Some women require analgesia or anesthesia because a complication of labor develops. Helping these women to understand why the medication is necessary calls for equal care and skill.

Evaluation

Evaluation should reveal that a woman found labor and delivery to be an experience that was not only endurable but allowed her to grow in self-esteem and the family to grow through a shared experience. Asking women to describe their labor experience in relation to pain is not only evaluative but aids women to work through this emotional period of life and integrate it into their previous experiences.

Nursing Care Planning

Mary Kraft is a 23-year-old woman (gravida 2, para 0) you care for in labor.

Assessment

Patient states, "I don't want any drug for labor or delivery." Last ate 2 hours ago (roast beef, potatoes, jello). Has lollipops with her to suck on during labor. Knowledgeable of Lamaze method for control of discomfort in labor; husband will be support person and coach.

Using breathing exercises effectively with contractions. Focuses on photo at foot of bed for distraction. Husband is effective coach.

Analysis

Potential for alteration in comfort, pain, related to labor.

Locus of Decision Making. Patient.

Goal. Patient to complete labor and delivery without undue discomfort.

Criteria. Patient to complete labor and delivery using prepared childbirth without medication or anesthetic intervention.

Nursing Orders

1. Reassure that her wishes will be respected as to the amount of medication desired.
2. Support breathing pattern efforts as needed.
3. Respect necessity to focus during contractions (do not block vision).
4. Offer husband relief as desired from position as coach.

Interim Assessment. 3:00 P.M. Beginning pelvic division of labor.

Assessment

Patient states, "It feels good to push. Don't give me any anesthetic." Pushing effectively with contractions; not as prepared for this stage as first stage of labor; husband continues to be supportive but also not as knowledgeable.

Analysis

Unchanged.

Goal. Unchanged.

Criteria. Unchanged.

Nursing Orders

1. Continue to support pushing efforts (tends to hold breath).
2. Support decision to have no delivery anesthetic.

———————————

Angie Baco, 42 years old (gravida 7, para 6) is another woman you care for in labor.

Assessment

Asking questions about what will happen in terms of analgesia and anesthesia. Wants "a shot for pain, but no spinal." Had severe spinal headache following last delivery 7 years ago. States it made the entire labor experience "just one big headache." Last ate 4 hours ago. Attended no preparation-for-labor classes.

Most comfortable on left side; uses short frequent breaths with contractions (learned this last time while in labor). Husband appears supportive but not well informed about labor. Physician has spoken to her about having an epidural block as blood pressure slightly high (130/90) and he does not want her stressed and uncomfortable.

Analysis

Potential for alteration in comfort, pain, related to labor and delivery.

Locus of Decision Making. Patient.

Goal. Patient to complete labor and delivery within limits of pain tolerance and safety.

Criteria. Patient to accept an epidural block for pain relief in labor.

Nursing Orders

1. Observe closely for hyperventilation (short catchy breaths make her prone to this).
2. Keep NPO in case general anesthesia is necessary (high risk for cesarean birth as she is a gestational diabetic).
3. Educate as necessary as soon as method of pain relief is established as to its benefit.
4. Support husband as necessary and keep him informed of progress. (Patient relies on him to be calm.)
5. Explain that at her early stage of labor (2 cm dilated) it is too soon to give medication for pain relief.

Interim Assessment. Lumbar epidural block given at 3:30 P.M.

Assessment

Patient states, "I don't feel a thing. Is anything still happening?" Voices fear of baby being "stuck" inside her because she does not feel contractions.

Blood pressure has remained 130/90–124/88 since anesthesia injection. Appears noticeably tense; biting fingernails; startles at sound of young girl in next labor room crying.

Analysis

Unchanged.

Goal. Unchanged.

Criteria. Unchanged.

Nursing Orders

1. BP, P, and R q 15 min. as epidural protocol.
2. Encourage to lie on left side to minimize possible supine hypotensive syndrome.
3. Maintain NPO status although epidural is expected to be delivery anesthetic as well.
4. Assure that dilatation is progressing even though she is now unaware of contractions.
5. Husband has decided to view delivery; support husband as this is new experience for him and patient relies on him to calm her.

Questions for Review

Multiple Choice

1. Mrs. Adams is to have a paracervical nerve block for pain relief in labor. Which of the following would *not* be part of your preprocedure preparation?

   a. Explain that the method will provide pain relief for both labor and delivery.
   b. Explain that the needle looks long but the injections will be almost painless.
   c. Explain that the injection will be made from the vagina.
   d. Explain that the woman will lie on her back for the injection.

2. You take an injection of Nisentil into Mrs. Brown's room for pain relief during labor. As you are about to give it, she asks you for a bedpan because she has to move her bowels. Your best action would be to

   a. give the injection, then offer the bedpan; abdominal comfort will help her move her bowels.
   b. hold the injection until you evaluate her labor progress.
   c. give the injection first, then offer the bedpan in order to complete a clean procedure before a contaminated one.
   d. give the bedpan before you give the injection because Nisentil is constipating.

3. Mrs. Carol refuses to have a lumbar epidural block because she does not want to have a spinal headache after delivery. Your best teaching point concerning this would be,

   a. "The anesthesiologist will do her best to avoid this."
   b. "The pain relief offered by the procedure will compensate for the discomfort afterward."
   c. "Spinal headache is not a complication of epidural blocks."
   d. "Your doctor knows what is best for you."

4. Following a lumbar epidural block, Mrs. Carol's blood pressure suddenly falls to 90/50. Your *first* action would be to

   a. raise her head off the bed.
   b. ask her to inhale deeply at least five times.
   c. administer oxygen by face mask.
   d. turn her on her left side.

5. Mrs. Downs states that she does not want any medication for pain relief during labor. Her doctor has approved this for her. Your best statement to her concerning this choice would be,

   a. "That's wonderful; medication during labor is not good for fetal well-being."
   b. "Your doctor [a man] has never been in labor; he may be underestimating the pain you will have."
   c. "I respect your preference whether it is to have medication or not."
   d. "Let me get you something for relaxation if you don't want anything for pain."

Discussion

1. A number of women still ask for a general anesthetic in labor. What would you want to teach a woman who says she "wants to be asleep for the whole thing"?
2. Nursing interventions for regional block anesthesia administration are important to know. What are important actions to take preceding and following an epidural anesthetic?
3. Paracervical anesthesia was thought at one time to be the ultimate answer to painless childbirth. What are the reasons this method is no longer extensively used?

Suggested Readings

Beck, W. W. (1973). Prevention of the spinal headache. *American Journal of Obstetrics and Gynecology, 115,* 354.

Brodsky, J. B. (1983). Exposure to anesthetic gases: A controversy. *Association of Operating Room Nurses Journal, 38,* 132.

Brownridge, P. (1982). A 3-year survey of an obstetric epidural service with top-up doses administered by midwives. *Anaesthesiology and Intensive Care, 10,* 298.

Gartside, G. (1982). Easy labour—a personal experience of childbirth under hypnosis. *Nursing Times, 78,* 2187.

Heidrich, G., et al. (1982). Helping the patient in pain. *American Journal of Nursing, 82,* 1828.

Jacobi, A. G. M. (1982). Obstetric anesthesia and the cardiac patient. *Perinatology/Neonatology, 6,* 51.

Jacobs, P. Epidurals in labor and delivery rooms. *Canadian Nurse, 78,* 42.

Johnson, J. M. (1980). Teaching self-hypnosis in pregnancy, labor and delivery. *M.C.N., 5,* 98.

Knuppel, R. A. (1980). Recognizing teratogenic effects of drugs and radiation. *Contemporary Obstetrics and Gynecology, 15,* 171.

Larin, J. M. (1982). Drug and obstetric medication effects on infant behavior as measured by the Brazelton Neonatal Behavioral Assessment Scale. *Physical and Occupational Therapy in Pediatrics, 2,* 75.

Latham, J. (1983). Complications . . . pain control . . . risks involved when carrying out nerve blocks. *Nursing Times, 79,* 36.

Lichtiger, M., & Moya, F. (1978). *Introduction to the practice of anesthesia.* (2nd ed.). New York: Harper & Row.

MacLaughlin, S. M., et al. (1981). Epidural anesthesia for obstetrics patients. *J.O.G.N. Nursing, 10,* 9.

Mattia, M. A. (1983). Hazards in the hospital environment: Anesthesia gases and methylmethacrylate. *American Journal of Nursing, 83,* 72.

Moquin, T. F. (1982). The anesthetic management of uncomplicated labor and delivery using the segmental technique of continuous lumbar epidural analgesia. *American Association of Nurse Anesthetists Journal, 50,* 372.

Nicolls, E. T., et al. (1981). Epidural anesthesia for the woman in labor. *American Journal of Nursing, 81,* 1826.

Ratigan, T. R. (1983). Anatomic and physiologic changes of pregnancy: Anesthetic considerations. *American Association of Nurse Anesthetists Journal, 51,* 38.

Redshaw, M. (1982). The influence of analgesia in labour on the baby. *Midwife Health Visitor and Community Nurse, 18,* 126.

Reisner, L. S. (1983). Obstetric analgesia and anesthesia: Current concepts: The first stage of labor. *Perinatology/Neonatology, 7,* 27.

Reisner, L. S. (1983). Obstetric analgesia and anesthesia: Current concepts: The second stage of labor. *Perinatology/Neonatology, 7,* 39.

Roberts, J. E. (1983). Factors influencing distress from pain during labor. *M.C.N., 8,* 62.

Rogers, A. G. (1983). What to expect from the most common analgesics . . . guide to therapeutic potency. *R.N., 46,* 44.

Santangeli, B. (1984). Control of pain in labour. *Nursing Mirror, 158,* 30.

Sigg, L. V., et al. (1983). Recognizing hypoventilation in the recovery room. *Association of Operating Room Nurses Journal, 38,* 270.

Stein, J. M., et al. (1983). Local anesthetics: Principles of safe use. *Hospital Practice, 18,* 73.

26

Alternative Birth Settings

OBJECTIVES

Following mastery of the contents of this chapter, you should be able to

1. Compare and contrast four common alternative birth settings as to advantages and disadvantages, safety, patient participation, and patient satisfaction.
2. Assess a woman's preparedness for birth in an alternative birth setting.
3. State a nursing diagnosis related to birth in an alternative setting.
4. Plan nursing implementations that are appropriate for alternative birth settings.
5. Implement care in alternative birth settings including an emergency delivery setting.
6. Evaluate goal outcomes as to whether an alternative birth setting was safe and satisfying.
7. Analyze ways that birth safety and patient satisfaction can be improved related to all alternative birth settings.
8. Synthesize knowledge of alternative birth settings with nursing process to achieve quality maternal-newborn nursing care.

THE USUAL SETTING for childbirth varies from country to country depending on tradition, health care facilities available, and the extent to which women make their preferences for birth settings known. In pioneer America, birth was supervised by midwives at home. In the 1800s, it became a physician-supervised event and was moved into hospital settings. Today, birth may be supervised by a nurse-midwife or a physician; the setting may be a home, an alternative birth center, or a hospital. Due to circumstances beyond a woman's control it also occurs in unplanned settings such as taxis.

Home Birth

Home birth is the usual mode of delivery in developing countries. Under the supervision of nurse-midwives, it is a popular choice for birth in Europe. There has been a small group of activists for home birth in the United States for the last 10 to 15 years as part of the overall consumer awareness movement and as a protest by women against unyielding hospital rules and regulations. You might have an opportunity as a student or later in a job to work with a physician or nurse-midwife who encourages and supervises home births. The Maternity Center Association of New York City and the Frontier Nursing Service of Kentucky are two examples of organizations who maintain an active program of out-of-hospital birth. Possible advantages and disadvantages of home birth are shown in Table 26-1.

To be a candidate for a home birth, a woman must be in good health and have an adequate system of support people that will sustain her during labor and assist her for the first few days of the postpartal period. She needs a home that has basic necessities such as running water, adequate heat, and cooking and sewer facilities. The windows should have screens so a multitude of flies or other vectors are not present. The pregnant woman must be able to adjust easily, or be able to change with circumstances.

A woman who chooses home birth early in pregnancy should be able to feel that she can change her mind later on without losing face or disappointing health care personnel who advocate home birth. The woman should know her blood type and normal blood pressure and should be kept informed of changes that occur in pregnancy. She must agree that, if for some reason a complication of pregnancy such as hypertension or placenta previa is present, she will agree to go to a hospital for labor and care.

Reasons for Choosing Home Birth

Many women who choose home birth are from well-educated and middle-income families. It is interesting to explore with a couple their reasons for choosing a home birth as these reasons probably reflect their degree of maturity and readiness for parenthood and also will help you to appreciate how the couple will respond if, due to a complication of mother or infant, hospitalization for basic safe care is needed. Exploring with a couple the reason for their motivation for home birth helps them to make a more informed decision. It can reveal that a couple plans a home birth for a reason such as they do not have reliable transportation (no car or undependable car) or the route to the nearest hospital is one that entails bumper to bumper traffic. They feel safer planning a home

Table 26-1 Home Birth Advantages and Disadvantages

Advantages	Disadvantages
1. The woman must be knowledgeable about the birth process. 2. The woman must be well prepared for controlling the discomfort of contractions. 3. The woman should consider breast-feeding to aid uterine contraction postpartally. 4. The woman has the greatest freedom for expressing her individuality. 5. There is no separation of the family at birth.	1. Adequate equipment other than first-line emergency equipment is not available. 2. Health care personnel may have difficulty relating to the couple if hospitalization is required. 3. A sense of guilt may occur if the child is born with a health problem. 4. Exhaustion of the woman and support person may occur because of the responsibility placed on them. 5. Interference with taking-in phase may occur because the woman must "take-hold." 6. Dissatisfaction may result with a support person who is not as strong as hoped for.

birth than having to worry about not being able to get to the hospital on time when the woman is in labor.

Such a couple might be better served by helping them analyze their support system. Perhaps they have a friend or neighbor or family member who would be happy to furnish transportation for them. In many communities the fire or police department will furnish transportation for a woman in labor; in others, a paramedic or ambulance service will respond. In still others, friendship house or community health centers will lend their vans for this service. Couples need to be educated that labor—with few exceptions—is not a sudden process. It involves hours of time. Once they realize they will have time and transportation, they can see that use of a hospital or alternative birth center also becomes an option for them (see the Nursing Research Highlight on page 579) for the most common reasons that families chose home birth. A number of these considerations are discussed below.

When a Health Care Facility Is Unavailable

The tradition of home birth is maintained in developing countries as the best level of care available. With no health care facility in the area (or the closest health care facility over a hundred miles away) home birth is preferable to a long transport over rough roads, which might result in the infant being born in the back of a car or truck and the umbilical cord being torn from a sudden, twisting motion. Rarely is this a primary reason for choosing home birth in the United States, but families in a very mountainous or rural area could have this problem.

The Danger of Infant Mortality

In the 1800s, before the germ theory was discovered by Lister, hospitals had frightening mortality records of infections in both mothers and infants: Microorganisms spread from health care providers to parturient women. As late as the 1940s, there were outbreaks of infection in newborn nurseries that killed all the babies in those nurseries. For these reasons, home birth can be viewed as a method of safeguarding both mother and infant from nosocomial infection. In all fairness, however, home birth is not conducted with as many safeguards for sterility as are used in a more formal setting; a mother or an infant could still contract an infection.

Expense of a Home Birth

In a country like Sweden, which provides free health care for all citizens, home birth is a cheaper method of health care (no nurses must be paid for round-the-clock care of the mother and infant, no hospital food must be paid for) than are health care settings. In the United States, where the average person subscribes to a third party insurance plan, the financial situation reverses. It will cost a couple almost nothing to have a child in a hospital; it will cost them $200 to 300 to have the child at home if their insurance policy does not pay for services outside a health care setting. For the couple who are unemployed and receiving medical assistance, the birth may also be paid for in a health care setting but not at home.

There are some individuals who do not subscribe to insurance who choose home birth because for them it will be much more economical ($200 to 300 compared to $1,000). For such cou-

Nursing Research Highlight
Alternative Birth Settings

Why Do Women Choose Home Birth?

In a study by Searles (1981), a questionnaire was designed to determine and prioritize the reasons women decide to have a home birth. Of the 59 women receiving the questionnaire 33 responded. Findings indicated that women chose home birth primarily because they have very negative feelings about the hospital setting, such as fear of what will happen there, loss of control, disliking routines and the general environment. Also, they felt the home offered many qualities not available in the hospital. Examples of statements included wanting to be close to the baby without any interference, wishing to be in control of one's body, preferring the more relaxed atmosphere of home, and believing that birth is a natural normal phenomenon and home is the natural setting if there are no medical problems. The study provides maternity care personnel with insight and understanding of the factors involved in women's decision for home birth.

Reference

Searles, C. (1981). The impetus toward home birth. *Journal of Nurse Midwifery, 26*(3), 51.

---

ples, choosing home birth is not actually a free choice, however; their finances have determined it for them. Such a couple might be well advised to begin to save money for a health care setting or make arrangements with the health care agency for delayed payments so they truly have a choice. Planning for expenses for childbirth is a mark of maturity, responsibility, and readiness for parenting (the parent who believes that the expenses at birth will be the last childcare expense is not well prepared for childbearing).

Family Integrity Issues

Home birth allows for family integrity in that there is no separation of the woman and her family. On the other hand, it puts the responsibility on the woman to prepare her home for the delivery (difficult if she is exhausted toward the end of pregnancy) and to take care of the infant at birth and assess the baby's wellness. Many women, passing through a "taking-in" phase postpartally, are happy to hold the infant, but continue with a dependent passive role during this time in relation to the infant's actual care. Home birth also requires support people to truly be that; unfortunately, some people are not able to come through in a crisis situation such as childbirth.

Expression of Individuality

Some women choose home birth because they want to use an alternative birth position, such as side-lying, or want the birth to be by the Leboyer method (use of a quiet, semi-darkened room with soft music followed by an immediate warm, soothing bath for the infant). It is true that a home birth will allow a woman to choose these things. Most hospitals and physicians or nurse-midwives also allow women to enjoy these procedures (with the understanding that, if a complication occurs, she agrees to modify her requests according to the new needs of the situation).

Other people ask for a home birth because they do not want their infant spanked at birth (they can be assured that *no one* spanks infants at birth anymore and knowledgeable birth attendants have not done it for 20 years or more). Others want home birth because they do not want any analgesia or anesthesia; they are worried that, once they are in a hospital, health care providers will immediately push syringes into them. They may need their rights as a patient and citizen reviewed with them: No one can touch another's body unless that person gives permission. If they do not want any medication or anesthesia in a hospital setting, no matter what the reason for admission, they will not receive any. It is only a matter of making their wants known. Other people say they know that is true but they don't want the "hassle" of having to "fight city hall." Parents who decide to deliver at home need good coping abilities in order to be able to handle this unusual time in their life; if their inability to make their wants known results from poor coping ability, they may not be good candidates for home birth.

Birth as a Wellness Event

When hospitals were thought of as settings where only the very ill were treated, then a wellness event such as birth was out of place in a hospital setting. When you consider the modern

Table 26-2 Factors That Create a High-Risk Status

Abnormal fetal presentation or position.
Maternal age over 35 or under 15 years.
Bleeding during pregnancy.
Drug or alcohol dependence.
Hydramnios.
Hypertension of pregnancy.
Infection in mother.
Maternal illness.
Past history of difficult delivery.
Past cesarean birth.
Potential for blood incompatibility.

role of hospitals as settings to promote health as well as restore health, however, the setting is not incongruous for birth at all. Couples need to understand that home birth is not realistic when the woman or fetus is categorized as high risk for any reason. Possible high-risk categories are shown in Table 26-2.

Preparation for Home Birth

When a couple has had an opportunity to discuss the situation with knowledgeable health care personnel and choose among the alternatives available to them, only a small number of couples actually feel that home birth is the only acceptable option for them.

Prenatal Care Still Needed

Be certain that a couple does not equate home birth with lack of prenatal care. A woman who plans on delivering at home needs the same level of prenatal care as other women. In order that she be knowledgeable about childbirth, she needs to have read extensively or have attended a preparation-for-childbirth class. She needs careful screening for risk factors because their presence will make plans for home birth unrealistic and unsafe. Home Oriented Maternity Experience (HOME) and the International Childbirth Education Association (ICEA) both teach special series on home births.

Stress that during the prenatal period the mother should do perineal exercises such as Kegal's exercises and tailor sitting because no episiotomy will be used for delivery. If her perineum is not supple and does not retract readily, severe tearing could result.

Children and Home Birth

A home birth allows other children to view birth (Figure 26-1). The couple may need to limit who will be able to view the birth. If older chil-

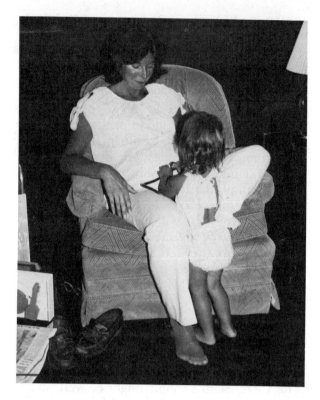

Figure 26-1 *Home birth may be an alternative birth method chosen in order that a family not be separated by a hospitalization. Here an older sibling listens to the new baby's heart beat during early labor.*

dren will be present, a person separate from the mother's main support person needs to be designated. She will need to plan to provide entertainment for older children (timing contractions for over 10 minutes is not interesting) and to provide explanations and food and sleep. Most mothers feel that they can manage both things—supervise older children and concentrate on labor contractions—and they are usually mistaken. It is particularly important that the mother not be expected to provide for these needs during labor when she becomes introverted and has concern only for herself.

"Another hand" to cook for, entertain, and generally supervise older children is indispensable. This extra person could be a grandparent, a neighbor, friend, or other relative. The main support person should not accept these roles because he or she needs to be free to support with undivided attention. Persons should be chosen who will not be so awed by the birth that they find themselves watching the birth instead of older children. A child who is without supervision during this time can remember the experience as an unpleasant, alienating one rather than the pleasant one anticipated for him.

A woman needs to ask herself if the experience

would be enjoyable for an older child. Would the sight of her in pain and undressed be only bewildering? Allowing the child to witness the birth of kittens or puppies might be more appropriate for many families as a way of exposing the child to birth.

Health Care Providers' Role

Home birth may be supervised by a physician, but a nurse-midwife is more commonly involved. She works in consultation with a physician and refers women who develop a complication of labor and delivery and therefore are no longer candidates for home delivery.

Requirements

The couple is responsible for providing supplies necessary other than those the birth attendant will bring with her, such as sterile gloves. Supplies and equipment they need to organize are shown in Table 26-3.

Prenatal Home Visit

Before the plans for a home birth are formally made, at least one visit should be made to the home to confirm that the house will be an acceptable and safe place for a birth. This opportunity also aids you in evaluating the degree of preparedness and commitment of the woman for this experience and detects any special problem that might occur due to home environment or structure.

At the visit, the birth process and how the equipment the couple will provide will be used is reviewed and any questions the couple has about the experience answered. Particularly important is a stress on the events of early labor, such as when and how the woman should telephone the birth attendant team (preferably as early as she realizes that she is in labor); how to time contractions and danger signals she should be alert to before the birth attendant arrives, such as rupture of membranes, vaginal bleeding, or no relaxation between contractions. The couple will be relying on their own judgment during this time interval so they are taking an increased chance unless they can adequately safeguard the maternal and fetal health during this time. Reviewing an emergency birth procedure in case traffic or another delay prevents the birth attendants from arriving or the labor is precipitous is necessary. Plans for other children should be finalized. One of the advantages of a home birth is that the mother can choose what delivery position she prefers, whether she wants options such as her support person to cut the cord, and whether she wants a

Table 26-3 Supplies Necessary for a Home Delivery

For the Mother

A delivery place. This could be a bed or the floor. If a bed is used it should be firm. Placing a wooden door or piece of plywood under a mattress can make it firmer.

Plastic protection for bed (such as a shower curtain or plastic tablecloth) during the delivery.

Blankets to pad the floor if the floor surface will be used.

Clean towels and wash clothes.

Two dozen disposable plastic pads to use as buttocks pads.

2 dozen sterile 4 × 4s.

A bowl for the placenta.

1 Fleet enema.

A flashlight with new batteries for an examining light.

Two pillows (to prop against for pushing).

Newspaper (to protect the floor from splashing amniotic fluid and use to wrap placenta for disposal).

A trash receptacle with plastic bag.

Paper towels and hand soap for hand washing.

Antiseptic solution for hand washing.

A telephone to call for emergency help (if this will be a public telephone, correct change for the call).

A mirror (dresser or standing or hand held) so the woman can view the birth.

Warmed olive oil (to lubricate perineum).

Honey or sugar cubes (to promote energy).

For the Infant

A rubber bulb syringe to suction mouth at birth.

Alcohol and cotton balls for cord care.

A tape measure.

A receiving blanket.

Diapers.

A baby gown.

For Postpartal Care

Vitamin A&D ointment or lanolin for breast care.

One box sanitary pads (unopened).

One nursing bra.

Extra gauze squares or pieces of cotton for bra pads.

quiet, darkened Leboyer birth. Review these requests with her so they can be communicated to the birth attendant. A woman delivering at home should also agree to breast-feed as the natural release of oxytocin from breast-feeding is her best protection against postpartal hemorrhage.

As a final step of preparation, you need to review with the couple the ultimate goal of a home delivery: a safe birth. Refresh the agreement that, if complications should occur, the couple will consent to immediate transfer to a hospital for care for either the mother's or infant's safety. Refusal when the infant's health is at stake can be interpreted as a form of child abuse. The telephone number of the community emergency service must be posted conspicuously by a telephone; if the house has no telephone the couple needs to have a car (with a full gas tank) present on the day of birth.

The Day of Delivery

Beginning with the thirty-eighth week of pregnancy the woman must be certain that the room that will be used for the delivery is clean and prepared for the birth except for the delivery bed itself. Encourage damp dusting in the room and vacuuming or damp mopping every day to keep down the microorganism count from accumulating dust. When the woman realizes that she is in labor, she needs to make the final preparations for a labor bed. She spreads out the plastic sheet, shower curtain, or table cloth to protect the mattress and covers that with a freshly washed, clean sheet. This sheet will become badly stained so it is practical to choose an old one. Be certain that the woman does not interpret "old" as soiled. In order to keep the level of microorganisms low, it should be freshly laundered. Some women make up a delivery bed with an additional top and bottom sheet under the plastic shower curtain. This is convenient following birth because at that time the plastic sheet and soiled cover sheet can be removed and a fresh, clean bed is ready with no further effort. Caution the woman that she will need to continue to use a plastic pad/sheet (more than just disposable squares) for the first week postpartum or the bed mattress will surely be stained from lochia discharge.

When she notifies the birth attendant team that she is in labor and reports her contraction pattern, the woman will be encouraged to continue with daily activities as much as possible (but to stop short of fatigue) to make the time of labor seem shorter—similar advice to that given a woman who is planning on delivering at a birthing center or hospital. When labor contractions are moderate in intensity and have a regular pattern, the birth attendant team arrives.

As one of these people, wash your hands and set up equipment necessary for a physical examination. The nurse-midwife or physician with the team will examine the woman in a manner similar to a health assessment in a health agency setting. Blood pressure, pulse, respirations, and temperature are assessed. Leopold's maneuvers are done to determine the fetal position and presentation. Duration, frequency, and intensity of contractions are verified. Note specifically the degree of pain the woman is having and how effectively she is able to breath with contractions. If contractions appear to be more painful than their strength would seem to indicate or are unusually sluggish for the time she has been in labor, some degree of dystocia (difficult labor) may be present. A disadvantage of home birth is that you do not have X-ray or sonography available to reveal if this problem is being caused by a cephalopelvic disproportion.

When timing contractions manually, rest your hand on the woman's abdomen and leave it there, a technique much less distracting than removing it and reapplying it repeatedly. Listen for FHR through at least five contractions to see if you can detect a bradycardia that lasts beyond the contraction (late deceleration). Use of a Doppler instrument for FHR detection is convenient because it gives immediate feedback to the couple as well as yourself that the fetus is doing well.

A pelvic examination is done to determine cervical effacement and dilatation. Sterile technique for a pelvic examination is just as important in the home as in a health care agency. Use an antiseptic solution, sterile gloves, and sterile lubricating jelly.

Promote and support breathing exercises with contractions. Encourage the couple to play cards or a board game, watch television, or read—whatever activities they enjoy to help time pass. Be certain the woman stays on her left side to keep the uterus free of the vena cava so supine hypotension syndrome does not become a problem. Because the woman will not be having any anesthetic, most women can drink carbohydrate-rich fluid such as orange juice or eat easily digested foods such as chicken broth, yogurt, or jello early in labor. Keep amounts small so nausea caused by the contracting uterus pressing on the stomach does not occur.

It is not necessary to stay with a woman continually during early labor, and she usually enjoys having time alone with her support person. Come prepared with an activity such as reading material for yourself so the couple does not feel they need to entertain you; if the woman called early in labor, labor will last for 12 to 18 hours. Do not be hesitant to nap nearby so you can be awake later on when labor becomes active.

When active labor does begin (cervical dilatation is progressing rapidly) take the FHR every 15 minutes. Encourage controlled breaths with contractions. Discourage any food intake because digestion almost completely stops at this point. Moisten the woman's lips with Vaseline if necessary; put a cool towel on her forehead if she is perspiring freely. Check the temperature of the room and raise it if necessary so the infant will not be born into a cool climate. Recheck supplies and ready delivery packs.

Delivery

As the woman enters the transition stage of delivery, encourage a squatting or sitting position for effective pushing. Take the FHR as frequently as every 5 minutes. Observe the technique the woman uses for pushing and correct it as necessary. Abdominal pushing should be a secondary action; an "assist," not the entire effort. Many women think of pushing as the entire force and so exert more pressure than is necessary with a pushing effort, an action that can lead to increased intrauterine pressure on the fetus. Encourage grunting with pushing (this has the same effect as a tennis player grunting while serving) to prevent breath holding and hypoxia to the fetus from a Valsalva maneuver. Be certain the woman ventilates well following a contraction to correct her oxygen–carbon dioxide balance. With crowning, recheck supplies. Place two baby blankets in a 150° oven to warm. Caution: Do not use a hotter oven or they will burn. If the woman has a microwave oven, one or two minutes on a medium setting will warm blankets adequately.

Because no episiotomy will be done, it is more important at home birth that the perineum draws back or it will tear. A warm compress or warmed olive oil applied to the perineum may be helpful to allow the perineum to stretch effectively. As the head crowns, set up a sterile field on the bed surface with a sterile towel, 4 × 4s, rubber bulb syringe, cord clamps, and cord scissors. Slide a clean, disposable pad under the woman's buttocks. Spread newspapers on the floor around the bed to protect against splashing amniotic fluid.

The head is delivered solely between contractions. You need to support the woman's efforts to pant during contractions so she does not push any further during these. The infant's mouth and nose are suctioned as the head is delivered; the head is held slightly downward immediately after it is born and the back rubbed. As soon as the infant has taken in a breath, he or she is laid on the woman abdomen's for warmth. Cover with a warmed baby blanket and pat the baby dry. The cord can be cut and the baby brought up to nurse at the mother's breast. The placenta is delivered gently.

Following this, one of the most dangerous periods for the woman begins. Because she will not be receiving an oxytocin to contract her uterus, there is a much greater possibility of uterine atony and massive hemorrhage than in an alternative birth center or hospital delivery setting. Following delivery of the placenta, someone (nurse, midwife, support person) should put their hand on the fundus of the uterus and rest it there with gentle but firm pressure for the next full hour. This should not be the woman herself as she may fall soundly sleep following delivery. Take maternal pulse and blood pressure every 15 minutes for the first hour following delivery as another gauge of hemostasis.

Encourage the infant to breast-feed because this action releases maternal oxytocin, which will assist uterine contractions. The infant will usually suck hungrily in this period of first reactivity. As soon as the infant wakes again (1 to 2 hours), breast-feeding should be tried again. Make certain that the woman realizes these efforts are for her health, not solely for infant nutrition.

The perineum and vagina need to be inspected for tearing following delivery. A gooseneck light is helpful for providing visibility. If this is not available, you will need to hold a flashlight so the birth attendant can inspect all walls of the vagina. If a tear did occur, it can be sutured immediately without anesthesia due to natural perineal anesthesia, or a local injection of xylocaine will alleviate the pain of suturing.

Care of the Infant

The infant at a home birth needs a thorough physical assessment. Wash away obvious blood but leave clean vernix in the folds of the groins and axilla, because these aid in skin lubrication. Keep the infant warmly wrapped. Eye prophylaxis is mandatory at home births the same as in a hospital setting. Delay this action until the mother falls asleep, if she wishes, so she can interact with her infant. At a home birth infants do not receive vitamin K as a rule, so they must be observed more carefully in the next 3 days for ecchymotic bleeding (which can lead to extreme jaundice as the blood is absorbed).

Observe that the infant sucks vigorously so you can be assured he will receive adequate nutrition after you leave.

The Postpartal Period

Birth attendants usually remain with the couple for 2 or 3 hours after the birth because the couple is so exhausted that they both may fall asleep. The mother may silently hemorrhage or the infant aspirate mucus during this unobserved time. Be certain before you leave the home that the woman understands the responsibility for safe self-care during the postpartal period: checking fundal height every morning to determine that the fundus is gradually decreasing in height, changing perineal pads frequently to reduce bacterial counts (a woman who chose home birth to save money may omit this precaution), breast-feeding every 2 to 3 hours during the first 24 hours (to encourage uterine involution), drinking extra fluid and eating protein-rich meals, and avoiding heavy lifting. The woman should call the birth attendant if any of the following occur in herself: temperature over 101.6° orally, saturation of a perineal pad in under 15 minutes, passing of large clots, inability to void by 8 hours after delivery or pain or frequency on urination. Similar danger signs in the infant include: jaundice, erythema around the cord, excessive mucus, no voiding or meconium by 24 hours, inability to suck at breast, and excessive bruising.

If a woman had perineal sutures placed, sitz baths three times a day beginning 12 hours after birth are comforting (she can use a regular bathtub after it has been well cleaned).

Be certain the couple understands the responsibility for seeing that the birth is registered and that they do receive a birth certificate for the infant. If they chose home birth because they are opposed to "rules," they might also find this type of regulation offensive. Later on, when they have trouble enrolling the child in school or establishing citizenship, they will wish they had been more careful.

The mother should telephone the birth attendant at 12 hours after birth (or vice versa) to assess her progress. A home visit is usually made at 18 to 24 hours. Important mother-child assessments to make at this time are shown in the box on page 742. A mother may become extremely exhausted following a home birth because she must awaken every 2 hours to breast-feed, and she may feel a need to immediately return to a full level of activity to prove that birth is a natural process (so home birth is the natural place for it). She may need to be reminded that in pioneer America, when all births were at home, a woman expected to be confined to bedrest (where the term *expected date of confinement* originated) for a month because she was so exhausted afterward (or that because birth is natural does not mean that it is not exhausting; labor is called *labor* because it is hard work).

It is suggested that a mother keep in close contact with the birth attendant during the next 2 weeks and then return for a postpartal checkup and reproductive life planning at 4 to 6 weeks. She needs to establish contact with a pediatrician or a well child conference for infant care. Many pediatricians like to see an infant within 24 hours if they are going to follow the child. This preference poses a problem: The father, usually unsure of baby care at this time, will have to take the infant to the doctor's office.

Complications and Home Birth

The couple agreeing to home birth must understand that, although the average healthy woman will have an average healthy child, unexpected complications do occur in about 15 percent of all births. If a complication such as cord prolapse should occur during a home birth, the risk to the child is greater than if such an occurrence happens in a hospital setting. Having a number for emergency transport available and having a skilled birth attendant present decreases this risk, but it is still above that of a general hospital setting.

If an infant should be stillborn or die within the first 24 hours of birth because inexperienced parents were unable to evaluate his or her condition correctly, they are apt to have an extreme guilt reaction; if one partner wanted the home birth more than the other, the resulting resentment may end the marriage or relationship between the couple. Of particular concern is that a couple appreciates that hemorrhage in the mother or jaundice in a newborn can be lethal; jaundice may be more difficult to evaluate in a home setting than a nursery because of less lighting and distorted color analysis due to wallpaper. Some anti–home birth groups are so concerned with this lack of adequate infant assessment they have gone so far as to label home birth *child abuse*: They feel it does not respect the rights of the fetus to choose the safest place for birth.

At the present time home birth is chosen by only a small segment of the population and, despite predictions that the rate will increase, is not growing in numbers. When present at a home birth, nurses have a responsibility to make the birth as safe as possible by guarding the fetal health during labor, ensuring that sterile supplies are used at delivery, and making an immediate health assessment of the newborn. Perhaps an even more important role is being an activist to suggest that hospitals extend privileges to nurse-midwives, to make hospital birth more natural, and to suggest alternative birth centers as a compromise setting for safe birth.

Alternative Birth Centers (ABCs)

Alternative birth centers are wellness-oriented facilities: Birth is their prime function and they provide more safeguards for care than are offered by home birth. They are designed to move childbirth, because it is a wellness phenomenon, out of acute care hospital settings, yet create a setting that still provides emergency care should a complication of labor and delivery arise. Such a setting is established near a hospital or within easy transport distance.

Reasons for Choosing an Alternative Birth Center

The basic reasons for choosing an ABC is promotion of a nonstructured environment for birth.

A woman who is rated as high-risk for any reason (see Table 26-2) is not eligible to deliver in an ABC. If a complication occurs during labor or delivery, she or the newborn is transferred immediately to the back-up hospital for care.

Reduction of Infant Mortality

Delivery in such a setting reduces the chance of spread of infection from an acute care area; it can proceed without the number of set rules that must be maintained in a high-risk setting. In addition to a home-like atmosphere, safety precautions for the child and mother are maintained because of the presence of skilled health care providers and emergency equipment.

Financial Considerations

Use of more health care resources than are necessary is what makes a hospital birth expensive and eventually not in the best interest of women during childbirth, if such settings limit their decision-making ability and self-care ability due to rules meant for ill persons. Many third-party payment plans pay for alternative birthing center costs as well as in-hospital birth; so for the couple with medical care insurance, these centers are an economical setting. If the couple does not have a third-party payment plan, they are more economical than an in-hospital birth.

Family Integrity

Alternative birth centers have separate labor rooms into which a woman and her support person can feel free to invite as many friends and siblings as they choose. In some centers a central play area for siblings and cooking facilities are available. Family integrity can therefore be maintained in such a setting.

Expression of Individualism

Alternative birth centers encourage a woman to use a prepared method of childbirth. She may bring to the center music she wants played and in many centers the father can perform such tasks as cutting the umbilical cord if he chooses.

Birth as a Wellness Event

The use of an ABC can be compared to the greater use of ambulatory clinics in almost all health care areas or the availability of ambulatory surgery sites for procedures such as eye surgery or tonsillectomies (that are wellness oriented).

Prenatal Care

An ABC may provide prenatal care, reproductive life planning counseling, postpartal health care, and infant well-child care; or it may not actually provide them, but refer couples to these services.

Not all health care providers believe that alternative birth centers are safe enough facilities in which to give birth. One of the ways that they can be made safe is that women who deliver at such settings receive quality prenatal care and are screened for possible complications prior to labor.

Delivery

One reason that home birth became obsolete was because it was impossible for a physician to attend all home births that were happening at once. Women were asked to come to hospitals so they could be observed. A birthing center supplies both advantages. Birth can be supervised by a health care person yet the woman does not have to be admitted to a hospital. A woman is expected to labor and deliver using preparation-for-childbirth methods rather than relying on analgesia for comfort. A minimum of anesthesia is used for delivery.

A woman goes to a center when her contractions are about 5 minutes apart and regular; she remains for a few hours of close observation following delivery (perhaps as long as 24 hours) before returning home. Many physicians, nurse-midwives, or nurses who work at alternative birth centers may also work or have privileges at the hospital that serves for back-up and referral.

Postpartal Care

A woman has the opportunity to rest following delivery before she is discharged. The alternative birth center initiates contact with the woman at 24 hours after birth (or asks the woman to make contact) and as often as daily for the following week.

Advantages and disadvantages of alternative birth centers are listed in Table 26-4.

Table 26-4 Advantages and Disadvantages of Alternative Birth Centers

Advantages	*Disadvantages*
1. The woman is encouraged to be prepared to control the discomfort of labor. 2. The woman is encouraged to be knowledgeable about the labor process. 3. The woman should consider breast feeding to aid uterine contraction postpartally. 4. Family integrity can be maintained because the family may accompany her to the birthing center. 5. The woman is attended by skilled professionals during labor and delivery. 6. Emergency care is immediately available.	1. Extended high-risk care is not immediately available. 2. The woman may be fatigued following birth because of the early discharge.

Hospital Birth

A hospital is still the most common setting for birth in the United States. Major hospitals have the advantage of having ready supplies and expert personnel if the mother or fetus or newborn should have a complication of birth. A small community hospital, however, that maintains its specialists such as an anesthesiologist or neonatologist only on an on-call basis may be no more prepared to deal with an emergency than an alternative birth center.

Women who are high risk for any reason are urged not to deliver at home and are refused permission to deliver at a birthing center so are candidates for this setting. Many women who have every reason to think they are risk-free choose a hospital environment because of the greater confidence they feel being near an area well equipped with skilled personnel. Many communities do not have ABCs so a woman's options are limited.

In evaluating studies that compare the complications of birthing centers or home births to hospitals, be sure to keep in mind that high-risk mothers deliver their children at hospitals so, of course, mothers and newborns at hospital settings have more complications. These complications do not arise because of the hospital setting, however, but because the mothers brought these problems with them to the hospital.

Hospital birth in the past became a problem for many couples because hospitals deal with a great many patients and so in order to keep things running smoothly, enforce a large number of rules. The person who is in a hospital because he is extremely ill is not aware of all the rules being enforced—or finds them comforting because they serve as assurance that the many caregivers will perform therapies the same way. For a woman who is not ill the rules of hospitals can be annoying and interfering. To alleviate this problem, most hospitals divide their maternity care into two categories: care for the high-risk mother or fetus and care for the well woman and fetus.

Care of the High-Risk Mother or Fetus

Prenatal Care

High-risk mothers are under the care of a physician during pregnancy although they may also be seen by a nurse-midwife for health supervision and education during pregnancy. A mother who has been rated as high-risk during pregnancy may be hospitalized for the length of her pregnancy; many are hospitalized for the last month of pregnancy. Others remain at home during pregnancy but come for more than the usual number of prenatal visits for care.

In discussing labor and delivery with them, be certain that they are aware of what the usual course for a woman with their specific condition entails. They should attend a preparation-for-parenthood and a preparation-for-childbirth course so they are prepared for parenthood and are as knowledgeable as possible about the process of labor and delivery. Due to their special circumstance, they may not be able to complete labor without analgesia or anesthesia, but the knowledge gained in a class helps them to understand how these medications work and their particular need for them.

Labor and Delivery

For labor, high-risk women are admitted to the labor wing of the hospital. In the 1960s when the Dick-Read method of childbirth was used (mothers were expected to sleep between contractions) or a high level of analgesia or amnesia was common, labor rooms were very sparse-looking rooms. Unfortunately, some hospitals still maintain this stripped-down appearance. Some women find this environment depressing, although they can also appreciate that a room stripped of extra furniture allows emergency equipment to be brought to the bedside faster.

At the hospital admission, the support person is usually separated from the woman and sent to the admissions department to fill in the appropriate forms. A couple can circumvent this separation by preregistering at the hospital so that on the day of admission only the woman's signature on a consent form is necessary (a consent signed in advance is not an informed consent because it was not signed when the current circumstances were in effect). If a period of separation is unavoidable, you should use the time constructively for history taking, which requires a private setting anyway.

Women who are high-risk can expect to be monitored for uterine contractions and fetal heart rate continuously during labor (and should welcome this care because they are not "usual" mothers). They may have intrauterine monitoring used, which restricts their movement more than external monitoring does. They usually have intravenous fluid therapy begun to provide energy and fluid and also as an emergency route for drug administration. As they near delivery, they are transferred to a delivery room. If it is necessary to use forceps for the delivery, they can expect to receive an anesthetic such as a low spinal or epidural so this manipulation can be done without discomfort. They can expect to have an episiotomy done if instruments are used to protect the perineum from tearing.

Teach women to use monitors as a means of alerting themselves to when a contraction is beginning. Teach them the safety of forceps use for high-risk situations and the advantages of regional anesthesia (pain-free, they can enjoy the last moments of labor and the baby's birth). Advocate that hospital rules allow a woman's support person to remain with her in the labor room and follow her to the delivery room if at all possible. Even if a cesarean birth is selected as the method to best deliver a well infant, a support person should be able to be present.

Be aware, however, that when a woman is critically ill or very concerned for the fetus's well-being, she may prefer not to have a support person with her but to rely on health care personnel during this time. Not all support people are ideal at giving support. In a crisis situation she does not want to have to be supporting this person as well as handling the crisis.

Postpartal Care

Following the delivery, a woman is transported to a recovery room for the immediate postpartal period (1 to 4 hours) and then to a postpartal unit where she is hospitalized for 3 to 4 days before discharge. Her infant may be taken to a recovery or intensive observation nursery and then remain in her room or a nearby nursery for the length of her hospital stay. If ill at birth, the infant will be cared for in an intensive care nursery or transported to a regional center for safe care. A recovery room is a suitable step for the mother because she is high-risk; every infant of a high-risk mother is a high-risk infant until ruled otherwise, so a recovery room for the infant is also suitable. A longer postpartal recovery period is wise because the mother has had some insult to her health or she would not have been categorized as high-risk. She may have greater-than-usual difficulty bonding to the infant because of the stress of birth and so need added supervision and role modeling of well-child care, which can be provided by skilled health care providers.

This system of childbirth is obviously a long way from "natural" and is the reason that hospital birth is so opposed by some individuals. People need to be educated that these procedures are designed for the high-risk woman and are necessary to fulfill for her the ultimate goal of all childbirth: a healthy family and a healthy infant.

Care of the Well Mother and Fetus

Prenatal Care

Well mothers are cared for by either physicians or nurse-midwives during pregnancy, or both working in complementary fashion. All well women should attend a preparation-for-parenthood and a preparation-for-childbirth course during pregnancy so they are prepared for parenthood and can control the discomfort of labor contractions with a minimum of analgesia and anesthesia. At a first prenatal visit a woman should ask her obstetrician, physician, or nurse-midwife his or her philosophy of prenatal and delivery care; if it is not as lenient as she wishes, the woman should feel free to choose a physician who will allow her the choices in labor she wants. In defense of a philosophy of care in which women are given few choices, remember that not all woman *want* to be active consumers of health care. For the woman who normally has difficulty with problem solving, pregnancy may compound her problems so much that she is unable to make

Nursing Research Highlight

Choosing Birth Settings

The Concept of Control and Birth Setting

A sample of 41 out-of-hospital subjects and 65 in-hospital subjects was used by Fullerton (1982) to assess whether the concept of control functions in the choice of an in-hospital or an alternative birth environment. It was demonstrated in this study that choices of the childbirth experience are related to the degree of control that one expects to exert over specific life events (the more control one desires, the more an out-of-hospital setting is desired).

Birthing Rooms—An Account of Consumer Satisfaction

Due to local increases in home births and consumer requests for more choice and control of their birthing experience a birthing room concept was developed and implemented in a Midwestern city hospital. After a 1½-year period an evaluation questionnaire was distributed to all consumers using it during a 1-year period. There was an 89.3 percent return rate of the 122 deliverable questionnaires. The overall response to the birthing room concept was rated as positive by 98.2 percent of respondents (Kieffer, 1980).

References

Fullerton, J. T. (1982). The choice of in-hospital or alternative birth environment as related to the concept of control. *Journal of Nurse Midwifery, 27*(2),17.

Kieffer, M. J. (1980). Part II: Consumer satisfaction during one year. *J.O.G.N. Nursing, 9*(3), 155.

---

choices. Some women enjoy the security of knowing that the "system" works and is taking care of them.

Labor and Delivery

A well mother comes to the hospital when her contractions are about 5 minutes apart and regular. If she has preregistered at the hospital, she is admitted to a labor room or birthing room without any separation from her support person. A birthing room is decorated in a home-like atmosphere like those used at alternative birth centers; the bed is one that can be used as a labor bed until delivery, when it can be converted into a birthing chair or a lithotomy position. Labor rooms, as mentioned, tend to be decorated much more simply, although all hospitals are making an effort to improve labor room decor. A well woman is expected to use a prepared method of childbirth with a minimum of analgesia and anesthesia for delivery (although an advantage of a hospital birth is that these are readily available if she needs them). Her support person can stay with her for the entire labor and delivery experience. (In the 1950s, maternity services had small waiting rooms for fathers because they were unwelcome; in the 1960s, they created large waiting rooms to show they were welcome; in the 1970s, they converted back to small waiting rooms because the support person is never separated from the woman in a waiting room.)

Most hospitals screen a woman in early labor with an external monitor for both fetal heart rate and uterine contractions. If the fetal heart rate is good, the monitor can usually be removed and used only for periodic screening as labor progresses. A woman may have intravenous fluid started as a prophylactic measure. This can be begun in a dorsal hand vein, however, which causes little discomfort and inconvenience for her.

At the time of delivery, the woman is transported to a delivery room if a labor room was used; if a birthing room was used, the room is converted into a space for baby care and delivery. Transport to a delivery room at this time is awkward; it is the step that makes a birthing room so much more enjoyable (see the Nursing Research Highlight above).

Postpartal Care

Following delivery, eye care for the infant can be delayed until the parents have a chance to become acquainted. The woman remains in a birthing room for about 4 hours; she could be discharged from there or remain in the hospital on a postpartal unit for 24 hours or as much as 3 or 4 days. A woman who used a delivery room is transferred to a recovery room for an hour afterward and then admitted to a postpartal unit for 24 hours to 3 or 4 days' stay. On a postpartal unit, rooming-in where the infant remains in the mother's room for the major amount of the day should be advocated. Demand feeding for infants should be the rule rather than the exception. Visiting from the major support person should not have any restrictions; siblings of the newborn should be allowed to visit at least once and touch

Table 26-5 Advantages and Disadvantages of Hospital Birth

Advantages	Disadvantages
1. The woman is encouraged to be prepared to control the discomfort of labor.	1. Separation of the family occurs if the woman stays for 3 or 4 days of postpartal care.
2. The woman is encouraged to be knowledgeable about the labor process.	2. The woman may feel intimidated into agreeing to more procedures than she wishes.
3. The woman should consider breast-feeding to aid uterine contraction postpartally.	3. Her physician may not be present during her entire labor and delivery, fragmenting her care.
4. Emergency care and extended high-risk care are immediately available.	

and become acquainted with the newborn. A postpartal stay has the disadvantage of separating the mother from her children and her support person. It has the advantage of allowing a few days of maximum rest so when a mother does return home she is well rested and able to cope with the responsibility of integrating the newborn into her family.

Advantages and disadvantages of hospital birth are shown in Table 26-5.

Choosing a Birthing Setting

The setting for birth that a woman chooses depends on her health and that of the fetus she carries and her preferences as to how much supervision she desires at the time of birth. It is important to remember when discussing alternative birth settings that a philosophy of care rises basically from what women want from care. In the 1800s, birth moved into hospitals not because physicians were forcing anesthesia on women, but because women *wanted* anesthesia for childbirth. After Queen Victoria delivered an infant under chloroform, receiving anesthesia for childbirth was a status symbol. Once women began to insist on anesthesia for childbirth, they could no longer push effectively during the pelvic division of labor and so it became necessary to use a lithotomy position and an episiotomy and forceps for delivery.

Physicians, being mainly men and never having given birth, overinterpreted the pain of childbirth, believing it to be totally excruciating and missing the exhilarating and fulfilling or orgasmic part of the experience. This attitude led to the belief that anesthesia for the delivery stage was the most important; in actuality pain relief during the hours of labor is more welcome by most women, as the pain at delivery is very fleeting.

As women became assertive in the 1960s about what the pain actually consisted of and when the pain relief was most important, birthing practices began to change. Birthing practices will continue to change if women continue to make their wants known; if women choose obstetricians, physicians, or hospitals who subscribe to lenient birth practices. The overall standard of care in communities will also change to accommodate the average wants of women in that community (the addition of birthing rooms to hospitals has humanized maternity care for mothers laboring in regular labor rooms as well). As most nurses are women, nurses are in a strong advocate position for making childbirth for the well woman a "natural" process. Nurses also have a strong responsibility to not be led astray by fads or other rituals undertaken in an effort to make birth natural but that are against safe care.

Table 26-6 lists ways that nurses can help to improve hospital birth.

Alternative Methods of Delivery

In any setting, the actual method of infant birth varies depending on circumstances present.

The Leboyer Method of Birth

Frederick Leboyer is a French obstetrician who proposed in 1975 in a book *Birth Without Violence* that the shock of moving from a warm, fluid-filled intrauterine environment to a noisy, air-filled, brightly lit delivery room is a major shock to a newborn and so birth attendants should make every effort to reduce this contrast. With the Leboyer method, the birthing room is darkened so there is no sudden contrast in light; it should be pleasantly warm, not chilled. Soft music or at least no harsh noises should be present. The infant should be handled very gently,

Table 26-6 Ways to Improve Hospital Birth

1. Teach women to be active consumers of health care so they ask questions about their care and are not slotted into a "routine."
2. Teach women to use health care providers who honor their individuality and allow them maximum ability to make decisions for themselves.
3. Teach women to ask what medications they are being administered and to insist that they receive only a minimum of analgesia and anesthesia for labor and delivery.
4. Teach women to ask for explanations of procedures and what alternatives are available for them.
5. Insist that a woman's support person be allowed to accompany her through all steps of pregnancy and birth and the postpartal period.
6. Allow women to keep their newborns with them for a major part of each day so they can become acquainted with each other.
7. Allow siblings to visit and hold the newborn to become acquainted.
8. Individualize care whenever possible so that birth is a fulfilling experience for each woman.
9. Teach women to insist that their physician remain with them during labor rather than arrive at the hospital only at the last moment for delivery (continuity of care).

including late cutting of the cord and immediately after birth being placed into a warm water bath.

These principles received a great amount of publicity in the public press as being new and different. In reality the concept that infants should be handled gently at birth has always been practiced. Surely no one questions that soft music, gentle handling, and a welcome atmosphere are important ingredients for all birth attendants to try to incorporate into birth. Dim lights (or at least not bright, glaring lights) could be given more consideration in most institutions. Some neonatologists question the wisdom of a warm bath as it may reduce spontaneous respirations and allow a high level of acidosis to occur. Late cutting of the cord may lead to excess blood addition to the newborn and result in polycythemia in some infants. The Leboyer method of childbirth, however, is accepted by most authorities as an alternative method of managing a delivery.

Birth Under Water

In some communities, couples have taken the concept of warm water being soothing to a newborn to the extent of the woman sitting in a tub of warm water during delivery and allowing the in-

fant to be born under water. This technique is thought to reduce the abrupt change from the intrauterine fluid-filled environment to a bright, air-filled extrauterine one. Although such deliveries have been reported as successful in the popular press, it is easy to analyze the possible dangers: uterine infection for the woman and aspiration of water by the infant. Theoretically, as long as the placenta is still attached and the cord is not cut, the infant does not breath and is safe under water; in reality, some newborns take their first inspiration as soon as the chest is delivered because the abrupt change in pressure causes rapid lung expansion. Theoretically also, the placenta does not deliver for 5 minutes following the infant's birth so the infant does not need to breath for this length of time; in reality, this action can occur with the very next uterine contraction—or within seconds.

As bathtubs are not sterile vessels, even if the water used is boiled and then cooled, it would not be sterile. As a mother often expels fecal material with final contractions, the water could contain a high level of potentially infectious agents. A spread to the cervix and uterus could result in a severe infection for her; by aspirating water, the infant could develop a severe pneumonia, aside from suffering the danger of tracheal spasm from aspiration.

Birth under water is not an accepted method of safe delivery and supports the principle that a little knowledge is a dangerous thing.

Emergency Delivery of an Infant

Occasionally, a woman enters a birthing center or hospital so far advanced in labor or with a birth canal that offers so little resistance that delivery occurs before a birth attendant arrives. A community health nurse may find herself summoned to assist at an unplanned home delivery. At any public event, a nurse may be called on to perform this service. In catastrophic circumstances transportation may not be available and you may need to assist a woman to give birth at home. Every nurse should have the knowledge and the ability to deliver a baby in an emergency situation. Firemen, policemen, and taxicab drivers, who have much less knowledge of the birth process than a nurse, do this all the time.

The first requirement for assisting at a birth is calmness. Of all infants born, 95 percent are in a vertex presentation, and the majority are in an advantageous position (LOA or ROA). Thus, the probability is high that the delivery will be uncomplicated. Calmness on your part conveys to the woman (and her support person) that there is reason for her to be calm as well. Relaxed, she can assist you—and the woman must assist; it is, after all, she, not you, who actually delivers the baby.

Place a coat or any soft material on the floor so the woman can lie down. It is best if the woman does not push but pants with contractions as soon as the fetal head crowns, so that the fetal head will be born gently, without undue pressure. This limits tearing of the perineum and injury to the fetal head. Wash your hands with soap and water or a disposable alcohol wipe and rest your hand on the fetal head to help control the fetus's progress; this method prevents perineal tearing or an abrupt pressure change to the fetal head. External rotation generally occurs spontaneously once the head is delivered; allow it to occur naturally. Have the mother pant with any more contractions once the head is born to allow you time to check the neck of the infant for a loop of cord and to prevent the shoulders from being born too rapidly. If a loop of cord is present and slides free easily (and it usually does), pull it over the infant's head and free it; if it does not, it must be clamped or tied twice (with string ligatures, such as boiled shoelaces), then cut between the ties with boiled or alcohol-wiped scissors before the remainder of the child is delivered.

Take a clean piece of cloth and swab excess mucus from the infant's mouth. If it seems necessary, press down slightly on the side of the head until the superior shoulder impinges on the symphysis. A little upward pressure on the head delivers the inferior shoulder. With the inferior shoulder delivered, the superior shoulder slides out rapidly, and the remainder of the child's body is delivered smoothly. Be careful. The baby is very slippery so slides from your hands easily.

Do not put traction on the cord as the body is delivered or you may cause a maternal hemorrhage by tearing or dislodging the placenta before it is ready to be delivered.

Hold the infant with the head slightly lowered, so that secretions drain from the mouth and throat. In a few moments the infant will draw in a quick breath and cry. The cry guarantees that the baby is breathing, because the sound is caused by the passage of air over the vocal cords. If the infant does not cry spontaneously (this is unlikely, since the mother has had no anesthesia to cause narcosis in the infant), do not attempt to spank him, tub him, jackknife him, or perform any of the actions you may have seen tried in movies. Rub the back gently. If this is not effective in initiating respirations after 2 minutes, begin artificial respiration by mouth-to-mouth breathing (see Chapter 47).

If the infant is crying well and needs no special measures, do not attempt to cut the cord. Remember that the fetal vessels end in dead-end villi; the infant will not bleed from the placenta when the placenta is born. An infant can bleed from an insecurely tied cord, however, and cord ties are not as easy to tie as they look. The cord is wet, your hands are wet, and the string slips. The infant is perfectly safe with the umbilical cord left uncut.

Lay the infant on the mother's abdomen, face down, and wait for the signs that the placenta has separated: an extension of the umbilical cord, a spurt of new blood, a rising upward of the uterus against the abdominal wall. When these signs are evident, with gentle tension, remove the placenta from the vagina. *Do not attempt to push on the uterus to expel the placenta or you may cause inversion of the uterus.* As soon as the placenta is delivered, the uterus will rise upward and contract against the abdominal wall. Wrap the infant with the cord and placenta still attached in a warm blanket and encourage the infant to breastfeed. This action will release natural oxytocin and help in uterine contraction. Arrange for transportation of infant and mother to a health care facility for follow-up care. Since no oxytocin will be given, you will have to keep a hand on the fundus of the uterus, gently massaging it to help it to remain contracted until another health care provider relieves you.

Utilizing Nursing Process

If nursing process is a system that is adequate for nursing care, it must be adequate in both wellness and illness settings. Its application to a home birth setting is proof that it is an effective system of planning nursing care.

Assessment

Assessment for a home birth involves both physical and psychological assessment. Much of this assessment can be done informally at a class for preparation for birth, or teaching controlled breathing exercises for labor; other assessment is done more formally at a 38-week home assessment and during the time of labor and delivery and a postpartal visit. One of the reasons that hospital-based care is sometimes not as fulfilling as it could be for you is that you work in a prenatal setting and so follow a woman all through pregnancy, but then on the day of labor and delivery do not see her—or you work in a labor and delivery setting, and so see her only during that time. Making assessments for a home birth, therefore, normally is a time when you not only gain important information for a safe birth but a fulfilling time for job satisfaction as you grow to know this couple you will follow through all stages.

Analysis

Nursing diagnosis statements related to home birth are similar to those constructed for a hospital or alternative birth setting. Some examples might be: "Ineffective uterine contraction pattern related to maternal exhaustion," "Pain related to uterine contractions" or a wellness diagnosis of "Ability to complete home birth related to active preparation and presence of support person." If a nursing diagnosis reveals a lack of support people or lack of knowledge of newborn care, you need to consider whether the woman is a candidate for home birth as the presence of support people and responsibility for newborn care are two critical requirements. Be certain in helping the couple to set goals that a healthy mother and healthy child are the ultimate goals established. If they cannot envision this broad a concept but insist that an inexpensive birth or a side-lying birthing position is their ultimate goal, you may need to reconsider the appropriateness of home birth; the couple may need to reevaluate their level of maturity and readiness to be parents. A parent who is not mature enough to sacrifice a small goal for a larger one will be unable to become a successful parent.

Planning

Planning with a couple for home birth is rewarding because the couple is committed to making the event safe and fulfilling: They follow preparation instructions well. An occasional couple may be proceeding with making the birth so natural that they postpone buying supplies such as disposable pads, which seem so "clinical" or hospital-associated. You may need to review with them that even the least experienced mother prepares a nest as nest building is a natural step in making the transition from "being pregnant" to "having a child." Friends of a couple who are planning to have a home birth may give them a shower of supplies they need in preference to baby clothes. This is helpful if finances are a problem and usually educates the friends about home birth—making them better childbirth health consumers. Be certain the couple establishes a plan for continuing newborn health supervision. Most communities have services for free or reduced-fee child care if finances are a problem.

Implementation

Nursing implementations at home birth are a fulfilling type of implementation because they are done with informed health care consumers who are very committed to taking an active role in childbirth and assessment and self-care. Because you have no usual emergency backup service of a resident staff and extensive resuscitation equipment, it is necessary for you to be very familiar with normal pregnancy, labor, delivery, and postpartal findings before assisting at a home birth. If the mother must be transferred to a hospital because of a complication, you will need to serve as an advocate for the couple (some health care providers may let their feelings about home births being an unsafe form of childbirth be apparent).

Evaluation

The final evaluation of the couple's goals is the same as that of a hospital delivery: The birth outcome should be a healthy one for mother and baby. If the outcome is not favorable, new assessment and new plans must be made. It may be difficult for the couple to accept routine health care for the infant (one reason they chose home birth was because they oppose the system). Fortunately, their overriding concern for the health of the child will enable them to make plans and compromise values and achieve success that in the beginning they had no idea they could achieve (a definition of a parent).

Nursing Care Planning

Carla is a 26-year-old primigravida who with Bob, a 28-year-old, has decided on having a home birth. They have a son Zak who was born under a general anesthetic 4 years ago. Since then, Carla has become a vegetarian who eats only natural foods and allows no foreign substances to enter her body. You make a home visit at a midpoint in pregnancy and design the following care plan.

Problem Area. Psychological preparation for home birth.

Assessment

Patient is very committed to home birth "to avoid a hospital admission" so no foreign substances or medication are used with her. Her support person is interested in home birth so son can view birth.

Analysis

Couple with questionable motivation related to home birth.

Locus of Decision Making. Patient.

Goal. Couple will reexamine motivation for home birth by 3 weeks' time.

Criteria. Couple will express a healthy mother and healthy child as their goal for birth.

Nursing Orders

1. Urge couple to discuss plans so their goals are congruous.
2. Ask mother to locate a caretaker for Zak during birth.
3. Sign contract to stipulate financial arrangements and agree to allow emergency hospital care.
4. Urge registration at preparation-for-childbirth classes.

Problem Area. Adequate supplies for home birth.

Assessment

Mother states she has bed supplies readied; having some difficulty purchasing other supplies because of finances.

Analysis

Inadequate preparation for home birth related to lack of supplies.

Goal. Couple will provide adequate supplies by thirty-eighth week of pregnancy.

Criteria. Couple will have prepared supplies on written list reviewed with them.

Nursing Orders

1. Urge couple to make bed more firm (take kitchen door off hinges and use as bedboard).
2. Begin to save money weekly for purchasing supplies.

3. Sink in bathroom is broken. Buy a gallon of distilled water for hand washing.
4. No rug in room. Urge mother to damp dust floor daily with wet cloth attached to broom.
5. No telephone in apartment. Arrange for neighbor to remain home during labor to give access to emergency telephone.
6. Couple has a Volkswagen Beetle; advised to keep it over half filled with gasoline after thirty-eighth week of pregnancy for emergency transport.

Problem Area. Physical preparation for childbirth.

Assessment

Mother following vegetarian diet. Diet reviewed by nutritionist and found to be adequate except for iron content. Patient has prenatal vitamins she takes "not very regularly." Has attended no preparation-for-childbirth classes. Has read on subject and feels this will be adequate.

Analysis

Questionable physical preparation for childbirth related to lack of formal preparation-for-childbirth classes.

Goal. Patient to self-prepare for labor by thirty-eighth week of pregnancy.

Criteria. Patient voices commitment to perineal and abdominal exercises.

Nursing Orders

1. Review vegetarian pregnancy nutrition. Stress supplemental prenatal vitamins with iron.
2. Stress perineal exercises: Kegal 4× daily, squatting for household tasks, tailor sitting.
3. Stress daily walking exercises and Sims' position to prevent varicosities.
4. Urge to practice controlled breathing for pain relief in labor.

Questions for Review

Multiple Choice

1. You are at a sports event when a woman begins a precipitous delivery. You volunteer to assist until further help arrives. As the fetal head delivers, your best action would be to

   a. ask the woman to bear down strongly.
   b. support the head with your hand.
   c. apply a cold compress to the perineum.
   d. not touch the perineum or fetal head.

2. The infant cries immediately and is not in obvious respiratory distress. Following delivery of the placenta, your *best* action would be to

   a. cut the cord using a flamed pocket knife.
   b. place the infant on the mother's abdomen.
   c. hold the infant with the head elevated.
   d. encourage the infant to breast-feed.

3. You volunteer to accompany the mother in the am-

bulance to a hospital. During this transport, your best action would be to

   a. continuously rest your hand on the uterine fundus.

   b. encourage the mother to sleep to restore energy.

   c. keep the infant from crying to conserve strength.

   d. remind the woman that her next birth may be precipitous.

4. Beth is a woman who is considering a home birth. Which statement below would lead you to believe she is a good candidate for this?

   a. "I want to have a baby without boring prenatal care."

   b. "All women in my family have had easy labors."

   c. "The main thing I want is to have a healthy baby."

   d. "I know nothing about birth so a hospital intimidates me."

5. Beth asks you about the advantages of an alternative birthing center. You would explain to her that

   a. no physicians will care for her.

   b. a birthing center maintains birth as a wellness event.

   c. she will be encouraged to breast-feed her infant.

   d. a birthing center has no advantages over home birth.

6. Beth asks about the advantages of a hospital birth. You would explain that

   a. what was right for her mother will be right for her.

   b. a hospital's primary function is promotion of health.

   c. having anesthesia administered will shorten labor.

   d. she'll have the security of knowing emergency equipment is on hand.

Discussion

1. The home is an alternative setting for birth. Under what circumstances would you *not* advise a couple to consider this option?

2. You are asked to serve on a committee to explore the feasibility of building an alternative birth center in your community. What are the advantages and disadvantages of such a setting?

3. Hospitals are frequently criticized in today's press for dehumanizing childbirth. What are concrete measures nurses can take to make hospital birth more family centered and satisfying?

Suggested Readings

Adamson, D. G. (1980). Home or hospital births? *Journal of the American Medical Association, 243,* 1732.

Ballard, R. A. (1983). The essence of an alternative birth center. *Birth, 10,* 97.

Baster, O. S., et al. (1982). Labor/delivery/recovery room blends best of birthing styles. *Modern Healthcare, 12,* 150.

Declercq, E. R. (1983). Public opinion toward midwifery and home birth: An exploratory analysis. *Journal of Nurse Midwifery, 28,* 21.

DeVries, R. G. (1983). Image and reality: An evaluation of hospital alternative birth centers. *Journal of Nurse Midwifery, 28,* 3.

Gillespie, S. A. (1981). Childbirth in the 80s: What are the options? *Issues in Health Care of Women, 3,* 101.

Hewitt, M. A., et al. (1981). Nurse-midwives in a hospital birth center. *Journal of Nurse Midwifery, 26,* 21.

Hogan, K. A. (1980). Home versus hospital delivery: Issues and perspectives. *Issues in Health Care of Women, 2,* 11.

Hughes, M. (1921). The "birthing room" alternative. *Dimensions in Health Service, 58,* 32.

Jennings, B. (1979). Emergency delivery: How to attend to one safely. *M.C.N., 4,* 148.

Jennings, B. (1982). Childbirth choices: Are there safe options? *Nurse Practitioner, 7,* 26.

Jorgensen, A. J. (1982). Home births. *Journal of Nursing Care, 15,* 14.

Lubric, R. W. (1983). Childbirth centers: Delivering more for less. *American Journal of Nursing, 83,* 1053.

May, K. A., et al. (1984). In-hospital alternative birth centers: Where do we go from here? *M.C.N., 9,* 48.

Searles, C. (1981). The impetus toward home birth. *Journal of Nurse Midwifery, 26,* 51.

Strane, S. (1982). Childbirth—yesterday and today. *Journal of Nursing Care, 15,* 22.

VI

The Postpartal Period: Parenthood

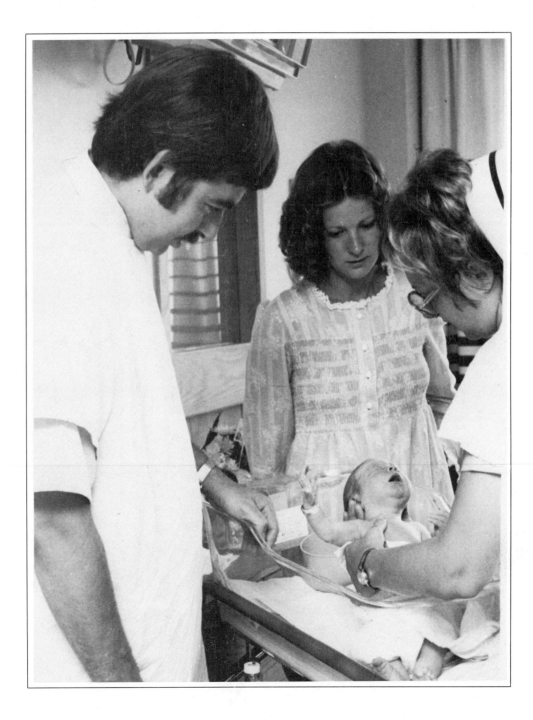

27

Psychological Aspects of the Postpartal Period

OBJECTIVES

Following mastery of the contents of this chapter, you should be able to

1. Describe the usual psychosocial reactions that occur during the puerperium.
2. Assess a woman during the puerperium for psychosocial changes.
3. State a nursing diagnosis in relation to psychosocial aspects of the puerperium.
4. Plan nursing care to meet the special needs of a woman and her growing family during the postpartal period.
5. Implement care of a woman during the postpartal period that is specific to her psychosocial needs at that time.
6. Evaluate goal outcome in relation to psychosocial aspects of the period.
7. Analyze ways to make the postpartal period a time of growth rather than of ending for a woman and her family.
8. Synthesize knowledge of psychosocial aspects of the postpartal period with nursing process to achieve quality maternal-newborn nursing care.

THE TERM *PUERPERIUM* is from the Latin *puer*, "child," and *parere*, "to bring forth." It refers to the 6-week period following the birth of a baby and delivery of the placenta and membranes. This 6-week puerperium, or postpartal period, is a time of retrogressive changes, when the uterus, vagina, and ovaries return to the nonpregnant state. It is also a period of progressive change, since the normal reproductive cycle is restored and breast tissue is prepared for milk production (lactation). Psychological changes occur too as a woman begins to experience her new role as a mother.

Nursing care during the puerperium has long been considered routine, and postpartal mothers have been regarded as women with many complaints and few care problems. In fact, the contrary of each of these two descriptions is true. The wonder is how *little* a new mother complains, in view of everything that is happening to her. The tremendous psychological and physiologic events of this period demand nursing care that is anything but routine.

For every mother, whether she has just had her first or her tenth child, whether the child was wanted or unwanted, something in the experience has unique meaning. She wants the personnel who care for her to feel the same level of excitement, the same passion, she feels. To a large extent, how she reacts to her new child—tenderly, compassionately, or routinely—will mimic the way health care personnel react to her during this time.

The physical care a mother receives postpartum can influence her health for the rest of her life. The emotional support she receives can influence the mental health of her child or be felt in the next generation.

Parental Love

Every woman worries during pregnancy as well as when she finally holds a newborn in her arms about her ability to be a "good" mother. Some women seem able to recognize a newborn's needs immediately and to give care with confident understanding right from the start. More often, a woman enters into a relationship with her newborn tentatively and with qualms and conflicts that she has to correct before the relationship can be meaningful.

Fathers may have even more difficulty than mothers in "claiming" an infant or feeling fatherly toward the child. A father's ability to reach out can be strengthened by allowing him time to touch and spend time with his new child in the first few days of life.

Parental love is only partly instinctive. A major portion develops gradually, in stages: planning the pregnancy, hearing the pregnancy confirmed, feeling the child move in utero, birth, seeing the baby, touching the baby, finally, caring for the baby. Many women work through these steps slowly and do not have maternal feelings for their infants for days or even weeks after giving birth. Some fathers admit they do not feel love until as late as 3 months or so after birth, when the child can smile or coo and interact with them.

Forming a strong bond with a child is not a problem only for first-time parents; experienced ones can have just as much difficulty. A mother knows she loves 4-year-old Johnny and 2-year-old Sue at home. She worries that her heart may not be big enough to love a new child also.

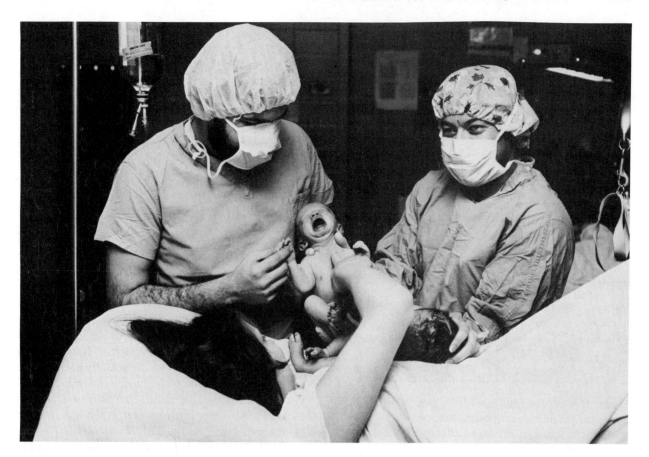

Figure 27-1 *A mother beginning interaction with her twins immediately after birth. Note the way she touches with only a fingertip. (Courtesy of the Department of Medical Photography, Children's Hospital, Buffalo, N.Y.)*

You need to provide an environment free of stringent rules if good parent-child relationships are to develop. To help parents sort out their feelings about being a mother or father and about their new responsibility, you need to provide a supportive presence and be able to offer anticipatory guidance where necessary.

Before a mother can begin to concentrate on her child, she requires adequate rest and sleep and concerned attention to the relief of her physical discomfort. The more she is ministered to during this time period, the easier it seems for her to minister to her new child. The more she is touched and nourished, the more readily she seems to reach out and touch and nourish her infant.

Few mothers show genuine warmth the first time their infants are brought to them. Even though a mother carries an infant inside her for 9 months, she approaches her newborn as she would a stranger. The first time the infant is shown to her in the delivery room or brought to her in her postpartal room, she may decline to touch her baby. She may hold him or her so she touches only the blanket and never makes physi-

cal contact. If she unfolds the blanket to examine the baby or count the fingers or toes, she uses only her fingertips, as strangers accidentally touch each other on a crowded elevator and immediately apologize and draw back (Figure 27-1).

Gradually, as a mother holds her child more and more, she begins to express more warmth. She touches the child with the palm of her hand rather than with her fingertips. She holds her newborn tighter, in a more motherly way. She smooths the baby's hair, brushes a cheek, plays with toes, lets the baby's fingers clasp hers, as sweethearts might on a date. Soon, she feels comfortable enough to press her cheek against the baby's or kiss the infant's nose or mouth; she has become a mother tending to her child. This identification process is termed *claiming*, or *binding-in*, her child (Rubin, 1977). Another term is *bonding* (Klaus, 1982). The length of time a mother takes to bond with her child depends on the circumstances of the pregnancy and delivery, the wellness and ability of the child to meet the parents' expectations, and the opportunities the mother has to interact with her child. A mother looking directly at her newborn's face, with direct

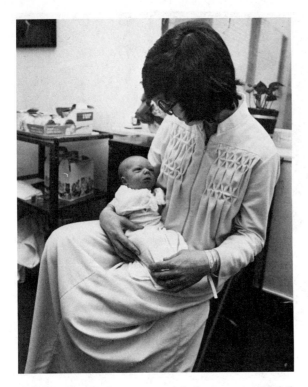

Figure 27-2 *Mothering a new baby is a responsibility. It takes time and exposure to each other for mother-child interaction to be effective. At 2 days, this mother still does not truly cuddle her child. Notice the "en face" position, however. (Courtesy of the Department of Medical Photography, Children's Hospital, Buffalo, N.Y.)*

eye contact (termed an "en face" position), is a sign that she is beginning effective interaction (Figure 27-2).

If you are to be a help to a mother, it is important for you to determine how much she knows and understands about babies. Many new mothers today have never held an infant. They have no younger family members, and their baby-sitting was confined to caring for toddlers and older children. They read everything on childcare they could find during their pregnancy, but now that they actually have a baby, the many childrearing theories they have read only confuse them.

A mother who is unfamiliar with newborns may be disappointed because her baby does not smile or laugh at her or tends to lose her moving finger with his or her eyes. She may not understand why the infant spits up on her or cries while being held. All these questionable interactions may lead her to believe that the baby does not respond to her, that she is not a "good" mother.

You may notice that a mother who is uncertain with her newborn is always in the bathroom or talking on the telephone when it is time to care for her baby. It is easy to assume that this mother

is not interested in her child. In reality, she may be too *frightened* to care for her newborn. It is easier for her to be "busy" than to reveal how little she knows about holding and soothing babies.

You need to assure a mother that the things her baby is doing are normal. Here, anticipatory guidance would involve instructing the mother in the fundamentals of normal infant development. It is a fallacy to equate the level of formal education a mother has achieved with her ability to give good child care. A mother may have graduated from college and have several advanced degrees, yet know nothing about babies. She may have gone only through grade school, yet have a feeling for children's needs. You have to evaluate each mother individually and adjust your teaching accordingly.

Teaching in the postpartal unit does not have to be formal. You can teach without lecturing by making such comments as: "Notice how large all newborns' heads seem" while you are bathing the baby, or "Babies like to be bundled firmly" while you are dressing the child, or "Notice how uneven newborn respirations are" when the mother is observing the baby. This kind of instruction will save the mother many anxious moments when she is at home.

Jealousy

Most new mothers, if given the opportunity, admit to feeling abandoned following delivery. Only hours before, a mother was the center of attention. Everyone asked about her health and her well-being. Suddenly, her baby is the chief interest. Everyone asks how the baby is. The gifts are all for the baby. Even her obstetrician, who made her feel so important for the last 9 months, may ask during a visit, "How's that healthy 8-pound boy?" She feels confused by a sensation very close to jealousy. How can a "good" mother be *jealous* of her own baby?

You can help the mother by verbalizing the problem. "How things have changed! Everyone's asking about the baby today and not about you, aren't they? How strange, even uncomfortable, that must make you feel." These are welcome words for a mother to hear. It is reassuring to know the sensation she is experiencing is normal.

When a newborn comes home, the father may have much the same feelings. He may become resentful over the time the woman has to spend with the infant. Perhaps the two used to sit at the table after dinner discussing the day or the future. Now she hurries away to feed the baby. She used to watch the late show with him at night. Now she goes to bed earlier because she knows she will be up again at 2:00 A.M.

This is a good subject to discuss with new parents. Both motherhood and fatherhood involve some compromising in favor of the baby's interests. Examination of competitive feelings should start during pregnancy or early in the postpartal period.

Disappointment

Another common feeling a mother may experience is disappointment in her baby. All during pregnancy she pictured a chubby-cheeked, curly-haired, smiling girl. She finds she is handed a skinny boy, without any hair, who is crying instead.

If a mother is awake during the delivery and sees the baby being born, the realization that her baby does not meet her expectations is easier to accept than if she was under anesthesia during the delivery. In the latter situation the mother may feel that a mistake has been made and wonder if babies were accidentally switched in the nursery. It may take her as long as 3 or 4 days to stop referring to the child by the wrong sex.

It is a loss of face for a mother to deliver a child who does not meet her expectations. Even though she objectively understands that the father is responsible for determining the sex of the child, subjectively she may feel it is her fault. If the child is scrawny-looking and definitely not as cute as the infant in the next crib, a mother may remember her adolescence, when she felt gangly and unattractive, and she may experience the inadequacy she felt then all over again.

You can never hope to change the size or sex of a child, but in the 3 or 4 days that you care for a postpartal mother and her child, you can change a mother's feelings about the infant's sex and appearance. Handle the child as if you find the infant satisfactory or even special. Comment on the child's good points: long fingers, lovely eyes, good appetite, and so on. During periods of crisis like childbearing, it is possible for a key person to offer support that can tip the scale toward acceptance, or at least help the persons involved to take a clearer look at their situation and begin to cope with the new circumstances.

The Neonatal Perception Inventory

The Neonatal Perception Inventory is a rating scale designed by Broussard (1970) as an early case-finding tool to detect potential disturbances in a child's developmental course and to promote the mental health of both a newborn and the mother.

A mother's background—how she feels about herself, the quality of mothering that she received, her total life experiences, and her cultural values—influences how she perceives her new baby. An infant who is not perceived as being better than average by his or her mother is at much higher risk for the development of subsequent emotional difficulties than the infant who is viewed as better than average. Broussard has shown that 46.5 percent of mothers rate their babies as above average on the first or second day postpartum. Rating a baby under average may reflect lowered self-esteem in the mother or may indicate her lack of knowledge of newborns (situations that can be aided by nursing interventions).

The rating scales used for the Neonatal Perception Inventory are shown in Figures 27-3 and 27-4. Six behavior items—crying, spitting up, feeding, elimination, sleeping, and predictability—are rated.

The form shown in Figure 27-3A is given to a new mother on her first or second day postpartum with an explanation such as: "We are interested in learning more about the experiences of mothers and their babies during the first few weeks after delivery. The more we can learn about mothers and their babies, the better we will be able to help other mothers with their babies. We would appreciate it if you would help us by answering a few questions. Although this is your first baby, you probably have some ideas of what most little babies are like. Will you please check the blank you *think* best describes what *most* little babies are like."

When the mother has completed the first form, she is given the second (Figure 27-3B) and told, "While it is not possible to know for certain what your baby will be like, you probably have some ideas of what your baby might be like. Please check the blank that you think best describes what *your* baby will be like."

When a mother has completed both forms, they are scored. Each item on the scale is scored on a five-point basis. "A great deal" equals 5, "a good bit" equals 4, "a moderate amount" equals 3, "very little" equals 2, and "none" equals 1. Each form is scored separately. Then the total score of the Your Baby form is subtracted from the total score of the Average Baby form (Figures 27-3A and 27-3B). A plus or positive score indicates that a mother sees her baby favorably; a minus or negative score suggests that the mother sees her baby as less than average.

At 1 month of age, the Neonatal Perception Inventory may be used again (Figure 27-4A and 27-

NEONATAL PERCEPTION INVENTORY II

AVERAGE BABY

How much crying do you think the average baby does?

| a great deal | a good bit | moderate amount | very little | none |

How much trouble do you think the average baby has in feeding?

| a great deal | a good bit | moderate amount | very little | none |

How much spitting up or vomiting do you think the average baby does?

| a great deal | a good bit | moderate amount | very little | none |

How much difficulty do you think the average baby has in sleeping?

| a great deal | a good bit | moderate amount | very little | none |

How much difficulty does the average baby have with bowel movements?

| a great deal | a good bit | moderate amount | very little | none |

How much trouble do you think the average baby has in settling down to a predictable pattern of eating and sleeping?

| a great deal | a good bit | moderate amount | very little | none |

A

NEONATAL PERCEPTION INVENTORY II

YOUR BABY

How much crying has your baby done?

| a great deal | a good bit | moderate amount | very little | none |

How much trouble has your baby had feeding?

| a great deal | a good bit | moderate amount | very little | none |

How much spitting up or vomiting has your baby done?

| a great deal | a good bit | moderate amount | very little | none |

How much difficulty has your baby had in sleeping?

| a great deal | a good bit | moderate amount | very little | none |

How much difficulty has your baby had with bowel movements?

| a great deal | a good bit | moderate amount | very little | none |

How much trouble has your baby had in settling down to a predictable pattern of eating and sleeping?

| a great deal | a good bit | moderate amount | very little | none |

B

Figure 27-3 *Neonatal Perception Inventory I. A. Average baby. B. Your baby. From Broussard, E. R., & Hartner, M. S. Further considerations regarding maternal perception of the first born. In J. Hellmuth (Ed.). (1970). Exceptional infant: Studies in abnormalities (vol. 2). New York: Brunner/Mazel.*

NEONATAL PERCEPTION INVENTORY I

AVERAGE BABY

How much crying do you think the average baby does?

| a great deal | a good bit | moderate amount | very little | none |

How much trouble do you think the average baby has in feeding?

| a great deal | a good bit | moderate amount | very little | none |

How much spitting up or vomiting do you think the average baby does?

| a great deal | a good bit | moderate amount | very little | none |

How much difficulty do you think the average baby has in sleeping?

| a great deal | a good bit | moderate amount | very little | none |

How much difficulty does the average baby have with bowel movements?

| a great deal | a good bit | moderate amount | very little | none |

How much trouble do you think the average baby has in settling down to a predictable pattern of eating and sleeping?

| a great deal | a good bit | moderate amount | very little | none |

A

NEONATAL PERCEPTION INVENTORY I

YOUR BABY

How much crying do you think your baby will do?

| a great deal | a good bit | moderate amount | very little | none |

How much trouble do you think your baby will have feeding?

| a great deal | a good bit | moderate amount | very little | none |

How much spitting up or vomiting do you think your baby will do?

| a great deal | a good bit | moderate amount | very little | none |

How much difficulty do you think your baby will have sleeping?

| a great deal | a good bit | moderate amount | very little | none |

How much difficulty do you expect your baby to have with bowel movements?

| a great deal | a good bit | moderate amount | very little | none |

How much trouble do you think that your baby will have settling down to a predictable pattern of eating and sleeping?

| a great deal | a good bit | moderate amount | very little | none |

B

Figure 27-4 *Neonatal Perception Inventory II. A. Average baby. B. Your baby. From Broussard, E. R., & Hartner, M. S. Further considerations regarding maternal perception of the first born. In J. Hellmuth (Ed.). (1970).* Exceptional infant: Studies in abnormalities *(vol. 2). New York: Brunner/Mazel.*

DEGREE OF BOTHER INVENTORY

Crying	a great deal	somewhat	very little	none
Spitting up or vomiting	a great deal	somewhat	very little	none
Sleeping	a great deal	somewhat	very little	none
Feeding	a great deal	somewhat	very little	none
Elimination	a great deal	somewhat	very little	none
Lack of a predict-able schedule	a great deal	somewhat	very little	none
Other (specify):				
_____	a great deal	somewhat	very little	none
_____	a great deal	somewhat	very little	none
_____	a great deal	somewhat	very little	none
_____	a great deal	somewhat	very little	none

Figure 27-5 *Degree of Bother Inventory. From Broussard, E. R., & Hartner, M. S. Further considerations regarding maternal perception of the first born. In J. Hellmuth (Ed.). (1970). Exceptional infant: Studies in abnormalities (vol. 2). New York: Brunner/Mazel.*

4B) to determine whether the mother's perceptions have changed. A mother receives the same instructions as previously for the first form. To acquaint her with the second form, explain, "You have had a chance to live with your baby for a month now. Please check the blank you think best describes your baby."

This age is also appropriate for the third form, Degree of Bother Inventory (Figure 27-5), which may be given with something like the following explanation: "Listed below are some of the things that have sometimes bothered other mothers in caring for their babies. We would like to know whether you were bothered by any of these. Please place a check in the blank that best describes how much you were bothered by your baby's behavior in regard to these."

The Neonatal Perception Inventory is a simple tool that can be used on postpartal units to try to identify mothers with unreal expectations of newborns or mothers who lack knowledge of newborns. Effective nursing interventions can then be structured to attempt to correct these situations and promote better mother-infant relationships. It is a helpful tool for community health nurses who make newborn visits.

Phases of the Puerperium

In terms of physical and psychological happenings, the puerperium may be divided into two separate phases. The first of these, called the *taking-in* phase (Rubin, 1977), encompasses the first 2 or 3 days; while the following phase—called *taking-hold*—is usually a time of renewed action on the part of a woman following this.

Taking-In Phase

The taking-in phase is a time of reflection for a woman. During this period she is largely passive. She relies on the nurse to initiate action. She prefers having the nurse minister to her, to get her a bath towel or a clean nightgown, arrange flowers for her, and make decisions for her rather than doing these things herself. This dependence is due partly to her physical discomfort from possible perineal stitches, afterpains (see Chapter 28), or hemorrhoids; partly to her uncertainty in caring for a newborn; and partly to the extreme exhaustion that follows delivery.

As a part of thinking about and pondering her new role, a mother usually wants to talk about her pregnancy, especially about her labor and delivery. She was pregnant for so long, looked forward to her baby's birth for so long, and imagined the baby being born for so long that now that the baby is actually here, it seems almost impossible to believe. She holds the child with a sense of wonder. The birth seems almost anticlimactic compared to her visions of the event. Can this child really be hers? Is delivery really over? She needs time to rest to regain her physical strength and time to calm her swirling thoughts.

Taking-Hold Phase

Following 2 or 3 days of passive dependence, a woman begins to initiate action herself. She prefers to get her own washcloth, to make her own decisions, and may even walk to the nursery to get her baby.

Some women seem overly concerned with their bodily functions during these days, for example, worrying about bladder and bowel control. This type of worry is a part of normal taking-hold, since bowel and bladder control is necessary for independence. A woman may express impatience with perineal stitches that still feel uncomfortable or breast tissue that still feels tender. She wants to be doing things for her newborn. She wants to go home and is impatient because she does not feel physically strong enough to be on her own.

During the taking-in period a mother may have expressed little interest in caring for her child. Now she begins to take a strong interest in caring for her baby. She realizes she has only a short time to learn and wants all the practice she can get. It is frustrating for her to watch a nurse change, feed, and bubble her baby while she merely watches. It is better if a mother is given brief demonstrations of baby care and then allowed to care for the child herself—with watchful guidance.

Even though a mother's actions suggest strong independence, she often feels insecure about her ability to care for her child. She needs praise for the things she does well: supporting the baby's head, feeding the correct amount of fluid, bubbling, and so on. Before she leaves the hospital she needs to be confident of her ability to care for and make decisions for her baby.

Neither rush a mother through the phase of taking-in nor prevent her from taking-hold during the last days of her hospitalization. For many young mothers, learning to make decisions about their child's welfare is one of the most difficult phases of motherhood. A mother needs practice in making such decisions in a sheltered setting rather than first taking on the responsibility when she is on her own.

A *letting-go* phase follows this and allows the mother to finally redefine her new role. This process is extended and occurs during the child's growing years.

Rooming-In

The more time a mother has to spend with her baby, the faster a mother-child relationship can develop. Because the average postpartal hospital stay is no more than 3 days (often only 24 hours), a mother today has very little time to become acquainted before she takes her newborn home. If the infant stays in the room with her (called *rooming-in*) rather than in a central nursery, she can become better acquainted with the infant and begin to feel more confidence in her ability to care for her child after discharge.

Complete rooming-in implies that a mother and child are together 24 hours a day. In *partial* rooming-in, the infant remains in the mother's room for part of the time, perhaps from 10:00 A.M. to 9:00 P.M., after which he or she is taken to a small nursery near the mother's room or returned to a central nursery.

With both complete and partial rooming-in, the father, after washing and donning a hospital gown, can hold and feed his infant.

Many new mothers find complete rooming-in too great a strain both physically and psychologically. Every time the baby stirs or hiccups or takes a deeper-than-usual respiration their worrying gets them out of bed. They do not sleep soundly at night because they are trying to remain alert in case the baby cries. At a time when they need to receive comfort, to take rather than to give, they feel overwhelmed by the degree of responsibility the hospital is giving them.

Many hospitals tried complete rooming-in when the concept was first introduced, found that mothers were unhappy with it, and returned to a central nursery concept, with the infants brought to the mothers only for a half hour every 4 hours for feeding.

Partial rooming-in seems to incorporate the best of the two systems. A mother can be with her baby during the day and yet can sleep soundly at night, knowing the infant is being looked after. On discharge the mother is more confident and more comfortable at home than if she had seen her new infant only briefly a few times a day.

Not only does rooming-in allow mother-child and father-child relationships to develop more rapidly, but anticipatory guidance and instruc-

Table 27-1 Signs of Poor Mother-Child Adaptation

Speaks of infant as ugly and unattractive.
Upset by vomiting, drooling, etc.
Does not hold baby warmly.
Does not make eye contact.
Juggles and plays roughly.
Picks up baby without warning.
Thinks that the infant does not love her.
Thinks that the infant judges her.
Concerned that the infant has a defect even though this possibility has been ruled out.
Cannot find any physical or psychological attribute to admire.
Cannot discriminate between signs of hunger, sleep, etc.

Source: Bishop, B. (1976). A guide to assessing parenting capabilities. *American Journal of Nursing, 76,* 1784.

tions in newborn care seem to be retained better when a nurse demonstrates bathing, feeding, changing, and so forth on a couple's own child. Anxious calls from parents concerning child care are fewer if a mother is discharged feeling confident in her ability to care for the baby and comfortable with the new responsibility because she has been allowed to have the infant with her during most of her hospital stay. Klaus and Kennell (1982) have demonstrated that extra hours of mother-infant contact affect mother-infant bonding positively.

A mother's failure to adapt well to caring for her infant is often evident by observing her and talking to her about her infant. Signs of poor mother-child adaptation are shown in Table 27-1.

Concerns of the Postpartal Period

Traditionally, most of a mother's concerns in the postpartal period have been assumed to be with care of her infant. Classes in the postpartal period have centered around teaching how to breast-feed and bathe infants. Although these are concerns for many mothers, they are not necessarily their chief problems. A woman has come through a tremendous psychological experience during pregnancy and birth of a child. She has made a complete role change from being a daughter to being a mother. It is only to be expected, then, that some of her attention and some of her interest during this time will be with herself as she tries to view herself in this new role.

Gruis (1977) asked mothers to identify their chief concerns in the postpartal period. Each mother in this study delivered a normal infant who was discharged from the hospital with her.

Table 27-2 Percentages of Mothers Noting Specific Concerns During the Puerperium

Area of Concern	Mothers Concerned (%) Degree of Concern Minor	Major	Total
Return of figure to normal	30	65	95
Regulating demands of husband, housework, children	42	48	90
Emotional tension	48	40	88
Fatigue	28	55	83
Infant behavior	47	33	80
Finding time for self	45	33	78
Sexual relations	53	20	73
Diet	33	40	73
Feelings of isolation; being tied down	42	28	70
Infant's growth and development	45	25	70
Family planning	25	43	68
Exercise	23	45	68
Infant feeding	43	25	68
Changes in relationship with husband	35	25	60
Physical care of infant	45	13	58
Infant safety	33	25	58
Discomfort of stitches	33	20	53
Breast care	40	10	50
Constipation	35	15	50
Setting limits for visitors	27	23	50
Interpreting infant's behavior	27	23	50
Breast soreness	35	13	48
Hemorrhoids	25	23	48
Labor and delivery experience	28	20	48
Father's role with baby	22	23	45
Lochia	35	5	40
Other children jealous of baby	27	13	40
Other children's behavior	25	15	40
Infant's appearance	18	20	38
Traveling with baby	27	8	35
Clothing for baby	20	10	30
Feeling comfortable handling baby	15	8	23

Source: Gruis, M. (1977). Beyond maternity: Postpartum concerns of mothers. *M.C.N., 2,* 82.

None had any complication that required an extended hospital stay, and each was living with the father of the child at the time of the study. The findings of this study are given in Table 27-2.

Notice that 95 percent of mothers were concerned about regaining their figures. It is difficult to begin a new role if you do not feel at your best.

Notice how many were concerned about finding time for themselves (78 percent). Mothers are interested in learning newborn care during this period, but they are also interested in having someone appreciate the difficulty of the step they are taking in their life. Responsibilities have greatly changed. These women need time for introspection to begin thinking through their new role and to find constructive ways to deal with their new life. (See the Nursing Research Highlight on page 608 for some additional information on postpartal concerns.)

Postpartal Blues

During the puerperium, as many as 80 percent of women experience some feelings of overwhelming sadness that they cannot account for (Pitt, 1973). They burst into tears easily and are irritable over trifles. This temporary feeling after birth has long been known as the *baby blues.*

This phenomenon is probably largely the result of a let-down feeling, an "after-the-prom" feeling. A mother looks forward to the birth of her baby so long that the actual event seems anticlimactic compared with her expectations. This level of depression may also be due to hormonal changes, particularly the decrease in estrogen and progesterone that occurs with the delivery of the placenta. For some women it may be a response to dependence caused by exhaustion, being away from home, physical discomfort, and the tension engendered by assuming a new role. The syndrome is evidenced by tearfulness, feelings of inadequacy, mood lability, anorexia and sleep disturbance.

A woman needs assurance that her sudden crying jags are normal; otherwise, she will not understand what is happening to her. Her support person also needs such assurance or he may think that she is unhappy with him or with the baby or is keeping some terrible secret about the baby from him.

Individualized nursing attention, or making certain that a mother is treated as if she, not the child, is the important patient, helps to alleviate postpartal blues. It is also important to give a mother a chance to verbalize her feelings: "There's absolutely no reason for me to be crying but I cannot stop."

Remember however that not all woman crying on a postpartal unit have the baby blues. A woman sometimes has real reasons to feel sad during this time. Perhaps problems at home have become overwhelming. Her husband may have been laid off just when they most need the money. Her mother may be ill, a child at home may be ill, and so on. Open lines of communica-

tion with postpartal mothers are important to help you differentiate problems that respond best to discussion and concerned understanding from problems that should be referred to the hospital social service department or to a community health agency.

Occasionally, serious depression that requires psychiatric care occurs during the postpartal period. This postpartal psychosis is discussed in Chapter 44.

Sexual Relations

At one time, women were cautioned not to resume sexual relations after birth of a baby until their check-up at 6 weeks. There is no apparent physiologic reason, however, to delay sexual relations this long. For most couples, coitus may be begun as soon as lochia serosa (the uterine discharge after birth) has stopped—about 2 weeks after delivery.

Sex may be painful if begun this early; tissue at the episiotomy site may be sensitive. Because vaginal epithelium is still thin at this point in time, vaginal tenderness may be noticed; use of a lubricant will help any mucosal dryness. A female-superior position is suggested because it allows a woman to control the depth of penile penetration.

Women can be cautioned that their degree of exhaustion may make them less receptive to sexual arousal than before. They may feel self-conscious about remaining stretch marks or lax abdominal tone. A woman who is breast-feeding will notice that milk is released from her nipples with sexual arousal.

A little forewarning that problems in this area may occur is helpful in preventing them. (See the Nursing Research Highlight on page 608.)

The Unwed Mother

The average unwed woman on a maternity service today is planning on keeping and rearing her child or she would not have allowed the pregnancy to come to completion. For some young couples, conceiving children without marriage is a definite, planned part of their lifestyle. For other couples, the pregnancy was not planned, but by the end of the pregnancy, they are certain they will raise the child.

An unwed woman may need more postpartal teaching than her married counterpart because her network of support people is apt to be less secure. Ask, Where will she be living after discharge? Who will actually be caring for the baby? What will be the source of finances? If the mother

=== *Nursing Research Highlight* ===

Postpartal Psychology

What Are the Concerns of First-Time Mothers After 1 week at Home?

To answer this question, Bull (1981) had 30 new mothers complete a checklist questionnaire on the third day postpartum and again after 1 week at home. In this studied sample, both the frequency and intensity of concerns related to physical discomfort decreased after 1 week at home. The intensity and frequency of concerns related to emotional self increased after 1 week at home. There was no significant difference in the number or intensity of concerns related to physiological change. The researcher suggests that with the increasing trend toward early discharge, there is a need for collaboration with community resources to address these areas of concern.

Reference

Bull, M. (1981) Changes in concerns of first-time mothers after one week at home. *J.O.G.N. Nursing, 10,* 391.

What Are the Special Concerns of Multiparas?

Postpartal teaching primarily focuses on the primipara, but Moss (1981) chose to investigate concerns of the multipara. She found the multipara is interested in growth and development and behavior. She is also concerned with family relationships and how the new baby will be accepted by the other children in the family. The nurse should assess each mother's needs individually and have these areas serve as the basis for each individual teaching plan.

Reference

Moss, J. (1981). Concerns of multiparas on the third postpartum day. *J.O.G.N. Nursing, 10,* 421.

Motherhood—A Time of Crisis?

Motherhood is identified by some as a time of developmental crises in a woman's life. A small sample of 6 women was used by Sheehan (1981) to assess women's adaptation to motherhood 6 weeks' postpartum. Specifically, the study attempted to identify variables that enable women to adjust successfully to motherhood in the 6 weeks following childbirth. The results substantiated the theory that the maternal adjustment period during the first 6 weeks after delivery constitutes a potential crisis in women's lives. The physical demands, their perception of the role transition, and identity reformation make women vulnerable to self-conflict and insecurity at this time. In order to facilitate maternal adjustment, health professionals should be prepared to educate young women on childcare and mothering.

Reference

Sheehan, F. (1981). Assessing postpartum adjustment. *J.O.G.N. Nursing, 10*(1), 19.

Does the Birth of a Baby Alter a Couple's Sexuality?

Difficulties can arise in the sexual adjustment of a marital relationship after the birth of a child. A study to find out how couples adjust sexually to changes that occur during the postpartal period was conducted on 42 couples following the birth of their first child (Hames, 1980). The questionnaire, administered to both husband and wife, included questions about breast change, vaginal bleeding, and sexual activity as they occurred in the first 4 to 6 weeks' postpartum.

Over 50 percent of the males and females felt that breast changes and vaginal bleeding did not inhibit their normal sexual activity. Most of the husbands and wives indicated they had adequate information regarding these areas but would have liked additional information in related areas. The study also showed that most of the subjects in both groups rated their knowledge in the three areas as having increased since the birth of the baby. It seems apparent that if health care providers are made aware of the informational needs of the postpartal couple they can provide information and advice that is specifically geared for each particular couple so that sexual harmony can be preserved.

Reference

Hames, C. T. (1980). Sexual needs and interests of postpartum couples. *J.O.G.N. Nursing, 9*(5), 313.

will be returning to school or taking a full-time job, who will care for the baby during these times?

Very young girls enjoy having you look at their baby with them and point out features or care points with them. They have none of the experience of older women with babies; they need a lot of help to determine what is "normal" and what is not.

Unwed women need visitors during the postpartal period. If the father of the child wants to visit and hold his newborn, he should be allowed this privilege; his self-esteem is important too. If the father of the child is not going to visit the mother, then another person, either the woman's mother or father or some other person who is important to her should be allowed to come instead.

Investigate the availability of a strong support person. If a woman does not seem to have such a person, help her make contact with a health care center (a well-child conference, a community health nurse, a pediatrician, a community clinic) so she has a resource person to call on when she has questions about baby care in the first few days or weeks of her baby's life.

The Unwed Father

Many an unwed father serves as a support person in labor and delivery for the child's mother. He enjoys holding and feeding and getting acquainted with his newborn in the postpartal period. He plans on visiting as much as a married father would during this time.

Other fathers are not interested in talking with the child's mother or even in holding the infant, but do want to see the child at least once. Their self-esteem is raised by knowing that they have had a healthy child. Some unwed fathers need the assurance that although they will not help raise the newborn, they have, nevertheless, fathered a healthy child.

The Mother Who Chooses Not to Keep Her Child

It is difficult for many nurses to accept the fact that some children are not wanted. The availability of birth control information and the increasing number of abortions that are being performed have reduced the number of these children. Nonetheless, some children are still unwanted.

There are many reasons for a child being born in this circumstance. A mother may be unmar-

ried or her marriage may be failing, and she does not want to raise a child alone. A woman may feel her family is already complete. The child may have been wanted if it had been a girl, or if it had been a boy. A woman may feel too old to have more children, or she expected to finish school first, or she would like to follow a career—the reasons are endless.

During pregnancy, most women decide whether or not they will keep their child. During labor, they express confidence in their decision, but with the birth of the child, they often find that their resolve wavers. A woman who was certain she was going to surrender her child for adoption may begin to feel she would prefer to change her mind. A woman who was certain she was going to keep her child becomes aware of the responsibility involved and decides that the best course for the child will be adoption. In either event, a mother's feelings become confused.

The wait in the delivery room for completion of perineal repair and preparations for transfer of the baby to a nursery is unusually long for a woman who chooses not to keep her child. She is usually alone, with no husband, no father of the child, to accompany her to the delivery room.

It is always a question whether a mother who has chosen adoption should see her child after delivery. There is a saying that if she holds the newborn once, she will never be able to go through with her original choice. Any decision to surrender a child that can be changed this easily has never been firm and probably would have changed in any event.

Every mother has a right to see, hold, and feed her child if she wishes. The mother who is not going to keep her child may find a great source of pride in her ability to produce a healthy child. The realization that he is well may give her a foundation to build a sounder future. It may make her feel truly a whole woman for the first time.

Do not attempt to persuade a woman to keep her child or to place her child for adoption while she is in the delivery room. She is extremely vulnerable to suggestion at this time, and such decisions are too long-range, too important to be made at such an emotional moment. Her earlier conclusion that she would not be able to be a good mother to the child may be a sounder one.

During the taking-in phase of the puerperium be especially careful that you do not influence the mother's decision making. Women enjoy having decisions made for them during this time and may ask you what you think is best.

It is not uncommon for mothers who surrender their infants for adoption to experience grief reactions like those of mothers whose children have died. If a mother decides to surrender her child for adoption, be certain that she is referred to an official adoption agency. An official agency gives the mother the best assurance that the parents chosen for her child will be the right parents. This assurance will help to relieve any misgivings or guilt the mother has about surrendering the child and should reduce the moments of doubt that can come in future years: Is my child well cared for? Is he getting everything I could have given him?

Some mothers do not openly voice a wish to give up their child, but they do show you by their actions that they feel little attachment to the child. The average mother approaches her newborn tentatively; this mother makes contact even more slowly. By the third or fourth postpartal day she is still barely touching the child and asking few questions about newborn care. She needs concrete help.

The hospital social service department can be of assistance in discussing and helping to plan the child's future. A married couple, as well as a single woman, may place an infant for adoption. More probably, family counseling is the mother's and family's needs.

The foundation of a firm mother-child relationship is laid in the first days of the infant's life. The mother who seems incapable of beginning to build this foundation should be able to rely on the professional nurse to recognize her problem and to offer her an avenue to a solution.

It is a fallacy to assume that everything will work out once the mother and infant get home. The number of battered children seen in hospital emergency rooms is the proof of the harm that can follow when assessment to detect this is inadequate in the first few days of life.

Sibling Visitation

Whether a child grows up feeling loved or not is partially dependent on how older siblings react to having a new family member. Waiting at home separated from their mother, listening only to telephone reports of what a new brother or sister looks like, is very difficult for children. They may picture the new baby as much older than he or she actually is. "He is eating well" may produce an image of a child sitting at a table using a fork and spoon. "He is sleeping well" may make them envision a child in a regular bed. "He weighs 7 pounds" is meaningless information. A chance to visit the hospital and see the new baby and mother reduces feelings that their mother cares more about the new baby than about them (their mother, after all, *is* spending her days with the

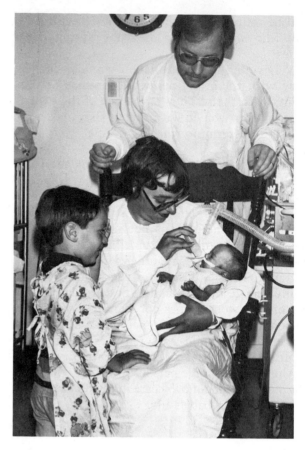

Figure 27-6 *Sibling visiting helps to make the new baby real. Here a brother visits with his parents even though the new baby is ill and needs supplemental oxygen. Note the mother's "en face" position. (Courtesy of the Department of Medical Photography, Children's Hospital, Buffalo, N.Y.)*

baby and not with them) and provides a true image of the new family member.

Children should be free of contagious diseases (upper respiratory disease, recent exposure to chickenpox) when they visit. They should be allowed to actually hold or touch the newborn (Figure 27-6).

Separation from children is often as painful for a mother as for the children. Sibling visitation usually goes a long way toward preventing postpartal depression by relieving some of the impact of separation. A mother needs to be cautioned that preschoolers' opinions of a new brother or sister may not be complimentary. This baby with little hair is not their idea of a "pretty baby." If they thought the new baby would be big enough to play with them, they may not feel he is a "big baby." Seeing the baby, however, even if his or her appearance is not what they expected, is helpful in terms of establishing strong relationships and is a practice to be encouraged in postpartal units.

Diagnosis: Parenting, Alterations in: Actual or Potential

Defining Characteristics: Actual and Potential

Lack of parental attachment behaviors

Inappropriate visual, tactile, auditory stimulation

Negative identification of infant/child's characteristics

Negative attachment of meanings to infant/child's characteristics

Constant verbalization of disappointment in infant/child's gender or physical characteristics.

Verbalization of resentment toward infant/child

Verbalization of role inadequacy

Inattention to infant/child's needs

Verbal disgust at infant/child's body functions

Noncompliance with health appointments for self and/or infant/child

Inappropriate or inconsistent discipline practices

Frequent accidents

Frequent illness

Growth and development lag in the child

History of child abuse or abandonment by primary caretaker

Verbalization of desire to have child call parent by first name versus traditional cultural tendencies

Infant/child receives care from multiple caretakers without consideration of his needs

Compulsive seeking of role approval from others

Actual

Abandonment

Runaway

Verbalization of inability to control child

Evidence of physical and psychological trauma

Utilizing Nursing Process

The puerperium is an important time in a woman's life: It is her first experience with mothering her new child, as well as her support person's first experience with fathering. The novelty of that experience is unchanged by whether the newborn is actually the second, third, or fourth child. In order that nursing care be comprehensive during this important time, nursing process should be incorporated.

Assessment

Assessment of a woman's psychological adjustment should begin with her reaction at birth (she is happy the baby is a girl or faintly disappointed; happy to be through with the pregnancy or still longing to be back in it) and continue with every contact with her in the next few days. Assess the extent and quality of her interaction with the child (does she hold and talk to her newborn?) and her overall mood (do you observe her crying? staring into space? not talking?) and her ability to "move out" and begin self- and infant care. Observe how she prepares for visitors. If a woman feels good about herself, even though she is exhausted from childbirth, she will "primp" for visitors. A woman who is depressed has no energy to do things such as wash her hair or ready herself for visitors.

Analysis

Nursing diagnoses during the postpartal period are usually either concerned with a woman's ability to accept and bond with a new child ("Potential for interference with bonding related to disappointment in the sex of the child" or a well diagnosis of "Family with adequate bonding related to acceptance of life stage") or related to her mood and acceptance of this life stage ("Fear related to lack of preparation for child care" or a well diagnosis of "Family with well-formed future plans related to acceptance of life change"). The North American Nursing Diagnosis Association accepted one diagnosis specific to parenting: "Parenting, alterations in." The defining characteristics of this diagnosis are shown in the box above. Many families do not remain in the hospital for an extended period following childbirth (often only 24 hours, and in alternative birth centers for as short a time as 4 hours) so goals for care must be short-term in order to be evaluated within the time of the patient contact.

Planning

When planning for care in the postpartal period, try to arrange procedures so there is optimal time for a woman to spend with her child and optimal time for adequate rest to relieve exhaustion. With exhaustion relieved, coping ability improves so the woman can then aid in planning for self-care.

Implementation

Implementations during this period are geared toward increasing a woman's self-esteem and allowing her to view herself as a new mother and the infant as part of her family. Do not be as quick to teach new mothers as to explore with them what they already know about childcare and what they think would be a sensible solution to a problem.

Teaching only solves an immediate problem; helping a mother to learn good problem-solving techniques allows her to solve the many problems in childrearing to come.

Evaluation

Evaluation of a mother's psychological adjustment to the postpartal period is important: If she fails to make an adequate adjustment, she will have difficulty integrating the infant into the family. The child's mental health, self-esteem, and ability to form a sense of trust will be affected. Because of the short contact time with families in the immediate postpartal period, evaluation must be continued at well-child evaluations during the first year.

Nursing Care Planning

Christine McFadden is a 15-year-old (gravida 1, para 1) you care for on her first postpartal day. The following is a nursing care plan you devise in relation to psychosocial aspects of the period.

Assessment

Patient states, "I look terrible! I'm so pale. And my hair is terrible."

Spent morning washing hair and redoing nail polish removed for cesarean birth delivery; talking on telephone to friends. Was reluctant to interrupt self-care to feed baby at both 10 and 2 o'clock feedings. Stated baby would have to wait for nail polish to dry even though baby was crying. Allowed maternal grandmother to feed child.

Analysis

Potential for interference with bonding related to inability to accept life change.

Locus of Decision Making. Shared.

Goal. Patient will achieve a balance in self- and infant care by 7 days postpartum.

Criteria. Patient will voice need to temporarily put infant's needs ahead of her own.

Nursing Orders

1. Encourage patient to do self-care in between times her infant needs her care.
2. Support interest in self (self-care is important for adolescent identity).
3. Review newborn needs and inability of infant to delay needs.

4. Explore future childcare plans for child's safety.

Mary Kraft is a 23-year-old woman you care for on the first day postpartum.

Assessment

Twice during the morning, patient was observed sitting on side of her bed crying. Stated, "I don't know why I'm doing this. I've never been happier." Husband scolded her for acting so inappropriately.

Analysis

Postpartal depression related to normal psychological change of period.

Locus of Decision Making. Patient.

Goal. Patient to maintain self-esteem despite seemingly inappropriate emotions.

Criteria. Patient to voice understanding of why depression occurs.

Nursing Orders

1. Review with patient that postpartal depression is common.
2. Explore if there are factors that are a concern or worry to her.
3. Assure her that postpartal depression runs a short, natural course and will pass.

Questions for Review

Multiple Choice

1. Mrs. Wells is a 27-year-old woman (gravida 1, para 1) who asks you immediately after delivery if she should request rooming-in with her infant. Your best response would be
   a. This puts too much responsibility on a first-time mother.
   b. It depends on whether she will breast-feed or not.
   c. Rooming-in allows increased maternal-newborn contact.
   d. Resting for the first 3 days postpartum will be better for her.

2. When you care for Mrs. Wells on the second day postpartum, you notice that she does not kiss her child during the time she holds him. The basis for this cool reaction probably is
   a. She is disappointed in the child's appearance or sex.
   b. She has difficulty accepting her role change.
   c. She is reacting normally to accepting a new child.
   d. Her cultural orientation does not include kissing children.

3. Which of the following actions would lead you to assess that Mrs. Wells is entering the taking-hold phase of the postpartal period?
   a. She sits and rocks her infant for long intervals.
   b. She is eager to talk about her delivery experience.
   c. She has not asked for anything for pain all day.
   d. She did her perineal care independently.

4. Mrs. Jones is a woman who states she did not plan her pregnancy and it took a long time in pregnancy for her to get used to having a baby. Which action below would make you believe *most* that she is now accepting the child well?
   a. She states she has named the child after a well-loved friend.
   b. She turns her face to meet the infant's eyes when she holds her.

   c. She comments that her baby has the most hair in the nursery.
   d. She asks you to use her camera to take a photo of the child.

5. On the third day postpartum, you discover Mrs. Wells sitting by her bed crying. She states nothing is wrong; she just "feels sad." Your best response to her would be
   a. "I'll keep confidential any problem you want to discuss with me."
   b. "You have a beautiful baby boy; you shouldn't feel sad about that."
   c. "Do you wish you'd had a girl instead of a boy?"
   d. "Feeling sad when you know you shouldn't must be very confusing."

6. Which action below would lead you to believe Mrs. Wells is still in the taking-in phase of the postpartal period?
   a. She spent the majority of her day talking about labor.
   b. She states she is "starving" and cannot get enough to eat.
   c. She walked to take a shower and wash her hair.
   d. She was interested in learning how to give her infant a bath.

Discussion

1. What is the advantage of asking a woman to fill out a standardized form such as the neonatal-perception inventory to evaluate her relationship with her newborn rather than just observing her?

2. Suppose two women, one a primipara and one a grand multipara, are hospitalized in the same room postpartally. What differences might you anticipate observing in their interaction with their newborns?

3. Women who plan to have a home birth often do so to preserve family integrity. Why might a home birth interfere with the "taking-in" phase of the puerperium?

Suggested Readings

Ball, J. (1982). Stress and the postnatal care of women. *Nursing Times, 78*, 1904.

Becker, C. (1980). The postpartum period: What is reality? *Canadian Nurse, 76*, 24.

Broussard, E. R., & Sturgeon, M. S. (1970). Maternal perception of the neonate as related to development. *Child Psychiatry and Human Development, 1*, 16.

Dunn, D. M., et al. (1981). Interaction of mothers with their newborns in the first half-hour of life. *Journal of Advances in Nursing, 6*, 27.

Freeman, M. H. (1979). Giving family life a good start in the hospital. *M.C.N., 4*, 51.

Furr, P. A., et al. (1982). A nurse-midwifery approach to early mother-infant acquaintance. *Journal of Nurse Midwifery, 27*, 10.

Gruis, M. (1977). Beyond maternity: Postpartum concerns of mothers. *M.C.N., 2*, 182.

Inglis, T. (1980). Postpartal sexuality. *J.O.G.N. Nursing, 9*, 298.

Klaus, M. H., & Kennell, J. H. (1982). *Maternal-infant Bonding*. St. Louis: Mosby.

Kyndely, K. (1978). The sexuality of women in pregnancy and postpartum. *J.O.G.N. Nursing, 7*, 28.

Martell, L. K., & Mitchell, S. K. (1984). Rubin's "puerperal change" reconsidered. *J.O.G.N. Nursing, 13*, 145.

Mercer, R. T. (1981). The nurse and maternal tasks of early postpartum. *M.C.N., 6*, 341.

Newton, L. D. (1983). Helping parents cope with infant crying. *J.O.G.N. Nursing, 12*, 199.

Pellegrom, P., et al. (1980). Primigravidas' perceptions of early postpartum. *Pediatric Nursing, 6,* 25.

Perry, S. E. (1983). Parents' perceptions of their newborn following structured interactions. *Nursing Research, 32,* 208.

Petrick, J. M. (1984). Postpartum depression: Identification of high-risk mothers. *J.O.G.N. Nursing, 13,* 37.

Pitt, B. (1973). Maternity blues. *British Journal of Psychiatry, 122,* 431.

Rubin, R. (1977). Binding-in in the postpartum period. *Maternal Child Nursing Journal, 6,* 67.

Sheehan, F. (1981). Assessing postpartum adjustment: A pilot study. *J.O.G.N. Nursing, 10,* 19.

Sholder, D. A. (1981). Portrait of a newborn: Preconceived ideas that 10 primigravidas have of their newborn's appearance. *J.O.G.N. Nursing, 10,* 98.

Skerrett, K., et al. (1983). Infant anxiety. *Maternal Child Nursing Journal, 13,* 51.

Tentoni, S. C., et al. (1980). Culturally induced postpartum depression: A theoretical position. *J.O.G.N. Nursing, 9,* 246.

Thomas, S. (1981). Maternal counselling: First steps in motherhood. *Nursing Mirror, 153,* 48.

Walz, B. L., et al. (1983). Maternal tasks of taking in a second child in the postpartal period. *Maternal Child Nursing Journal 12,* 185.

Wheeler, L. A. (1979). Sexuality during pregnancy and the postpartum. *Perinatal Press, 3,* 131.

Wieser, M. A., & Castaglia, P. T. (1984). Assessing early father-infant attachment. *M.C.N., 9,* 104.

28

Physiology of the Postpartal Period

OBJECTIVES

Following mastery of the contents of this chapter, you should be able to

1. Describe the process of uterine involution.
2. Describe the systemic physiologic changes that occur in the postpartal woman.
3. Describe the progressive changes that occur during the postpartal period.
4. Analyze the effects of the physiologic changes on a woman and her sexual partner.
5. Synthesize the local and systemic physiologic changes of the postpartal period with nursing process in order to achieve quality maternal-newborn nursing care.

THE POSTPARTAL PERIOD (the period of the puerperium) extends to the sixth week following birth of an infant. The period includes a wide range of physiologic changes that are both retrogressive in nature (the involution of the uterus and vagina) and some that are progressive in nature (the production of milk for lactation and the restoration of the normal menstrual cycle). Protecting the health of a woman as these changes occur helps preserve future childbearing function and her physical well-being, which is important for care of her new child. Because a mother's health needs as much protection during this stage as during pregnancy, this period is popularly termed the *fourth trimester* of pregnancy. Both the retrogressive and progressive changes that occur are discussed below.

Involution

Involution is the process whereby the reproductive organs return to their nonpregnant state.

Uterus

Involution of the uterus involves two main processes. First the area where the placenta was implanted is sealed off, and bleeding is therefore prevented. Second, the organ is reduced to its approximate pregestational size.

The sealing of the placental site is accomplished by rapid contraction of the uterus immediately following the delivery of the placenta. This contraction pinches the blood vessels entering the 7-cm-wide area left denuded by the placenta and controls bleeding. With time, thrombi form within the uterus sinuses and permanently seal the area. Eventually, endometrial tissue undermines the site and obliterates the organized thrombi, completely covering and healing the area. This process leaves no scar tissue within the uterus and thus does not compromise future implantation sites.

The same contraction process reduces the bulk of the uterus. Freed of the placenta and the membranes, the walls of the uterus thicken and contract, reducing the uterus from the size of a container large enough to hold a 7-pound fetus to the size of a grapefruit. Uterine contraction can be compared to a rubber band that has been stretched for many months and now is regaining its normal contour. None of the rubber band is destroyed; the shape is simply altered. A small number of cells of the uterine wall are broken down by an autolytic process into their protein components, and these components are then absorbed by the bloodstream and excreted by the body in urine. However, the main mechanism that reduces the bulk of the uterus is contraction. This is the reason the postpartal period, like pregnancy, is not a period of illness, of necrosing cells being evacuated, but primarily a period of healthy change.

With involution, the uterus will never completely return to its virginal state, but the reduction in its size is dramatic. Immediately after delivery the uterus weighs about 1,000 gm. At the end of the first week, it weighs 500 gm. By the time involution is complete (6 weeks), it will weigh approximately 50 gm (a prepregnant weight).

In the first minutes following delivery of the placenta, as contraction takes place, the fundus of the uterus may be palpated through the abdominal wall halfway between the umbilicus and the symphysis pubis. By an hour after delivery it has risen to the level of the umbilicus, where it remains for approximately the next 24 hours. From then on it will decrease a fingerbreath (F) (1 cm) a day in size. Thus, on the first postpartal day the fundus of the uterus will be palpable one fingerbreadth below the umbilicus; on the second, two fingerbreadths below the umbilicus; and so on. This movement can be recorded as 1 cm below the umbilicus, 2 cm below it, and so forth.

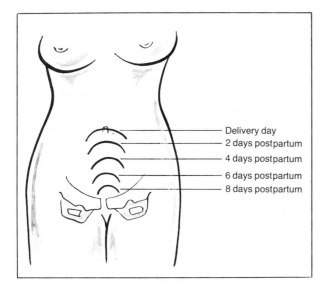

Figure 28-1 *Uterine involution. The uterus decreases in size at a predictable rate during the postpartal period. After 10 days, it recedes under the pubic bone and is no longer palpable.*

In the average woman the uterus will have contracted so much by the ninth or tenth day and be so far withdrawn into the pelvis that it can no longer be detected by abdominal palpation (Figure 28-1). Because oxytocin is released with breast-feeding, the uterus of the breast-feeding mother may contract even more quickly.

On palpation, the fundus can usually be felt in the midline of the abdomen, although occasionally it is found slightly to the right because the bulk of the sigmoid colon forced it to the right during pregnancy and it tends to remain in that position. Measurements of the height of the fundus should be made shortly after a woman's bladder has been emptied, because a full bladder will keep the uterus from contracting, push it upward due to the laxness of the uterine ligaments, and give a false reading.

Uterine involution may be retarded if any condition such as multiple gestation or hydramnios, exhaustion from prolonged labor or difficult delivery, grand multiparity, or physiologic effects of excessive analgesia is present. Contraction may be difficult in the presence of retained placenta or membranes or a full bladder. Involution will occur most dependably in a woman who is well nourished and ambulated early following birth (gravity may play a role).

An estimation of the consistency of the postpartal uterus is as important as measurement of its height. A well-contracted fundus feels firm. It can be compared with a grapefruit not only in size but also in tenseness, or consistency. Whenever the fundus feels soft or flabby, it is not as contracted as it should be, despite its position in the abdomen.

The first hour postpartum is potentially the most dangerous time for a newly delivered woman. If the uterus should become relaxed during this time (*uterine atony*) so the placental site is no longer well sealed, the woman will lose blood very rapidly because no permanent thrombi have yet formed at the placental site. Hemorrhage is the commonest cause of maternal morbidity and mortality in childbirth: This is a critical point at which it may occur.

In some women the contraction of the uterus after delivery causes cramps similar to those accompanying a menstrual period. These are termed *afterpains*. They occur more frequently in multiparas than primiparas and in mothers who have delivered large babies or had an overdistended uterus for any other reason. They are noticed most intensely with breast-feeding as the infant's sucking causes a release of oxytocin from the posterior pituitary, which increases contractions and thus the uncomfortable sensation in the mother's abdomen.

Abdominal Wall

The abdominal wall and the ligaments that support the uterus are obviously stretched during pregnancy and usually require the full 6 weeks of the puerperium to return to their former state. If a woman does postpartal exercises such as head raising or sit-ups, this tone returns more dependably.

Lochia

The separation of the placenta and membranes occurs in the spongy layer or outer portion of the decidua basalis. By the second day following delivery the layer of decidua remaining under the placental site (an area 7 cm wide) and throughout the uterus differentiates into two distinct layers. The inner layer attached to the muscular wall of the uterus will remain and serve as the foundation from which a new layer of endometrium will be formed. The layer adjacent to the uterine cavity will become necrotic and will be cast off as a uterine discharge similar to a menstrual flow. This uterine flow, consisting of blood, fragments of decidua, white blood cells, mucus, and some bacteria, is known as *lochia*.

The portion of the uterus where the placenta was not attached will be fully cleansed by this sloughing process and will be in a reproductive

Table 28-1 Characteristics of Lochia

Type of Lochia	Color	Duration	Composition
Lochia rubra	Red	1–3 days	Blood, fragments of decidua and mucus
Lochia serosa	Pink or brown-tinged	3–10 days	Blood, mucus, and invading leukocytes
Lochia alba	White	10–14 days (May last for 6 weeks)	Largely mucus; leukocyte count high

state in about 3 weeks. The placental implantation site will take approximately 6 weeks (the entire postpartal period) to be cleansed and healed.

For the first 3 days after delivery, the lochia discharge consists almost entirely of blood, with only small particles of decidua and mucus. Because of its red color, it is termed *lochia rubra*. As the amount of blood involved in the cast-off tissue decreases (about the fourth day), and leukocytes begin to invade the area as they do any healing surface, the flow becomes pink or brownish in color (*lochia serosa*). On about the tenth day, the amount of the flow decreases and becomes colorless or white (*lochia alba*). Lochia alba is present in most women until the third week following delivery, although it is not unusual for a lochia flow to last the entire 6 weeks of the puerperium. Characteristics of lochia are summarized in Table 28-1. There are several rules for judging whether lochia flow is or is not normal. These are shown in the Nursing Care Highlight on page 619.

Cervix

Immediately following delivery, the cervix is soft and malleable. Both the internal os and the external os are well open. Like contraction of the fundus of the uterus, retraction of the cervix begins at once. By the end of 7 days the external os is narrowed to the size of a pencil opening, and the cervix feels firm and nongravid again.

In contrast to the process of involution in the fundus, in which the changes consist primarily of old cells being returned to their former position by contraction, the process in the cervix does involve the formation of new muscle cells. Like the fundus, the cervix does not return exactly to its virginal state. The internal os will close as before, but, assuming that the delivery was vaginal, the external os will usually remain slightly open and appear slit-like or stellate (star-shaped) where it was round before. Finding this pattern on pelvic examination suggests that childbearing has taken place.

Vagina

Following a vaginal delivery the vagina is soft, few rugae are present, and its diameter is considerably greater than in a nonpregnant woman. The hymen is permanently torn and heals with small, separate tags of tissue. It takes the entire postpartal period for the vagina to involute (as in the uterus, by contraction) until it gradually returns approximately to its nonpregnant state. Thickening of the walls also appears to depend on renewed estrogen stimulation from the ovaries; a woman who is breast-feeding and in whom ovulation is delayed may continue to have thin-walled or fragile vaginal cells, which cause slight vaginal bleeding on sexual coitus until about 6 weeks' time. Like the cervix, the vaginal outlet will remain slightly more distended than before; if a woman practices Kegal's exercises, the strength and tone of the vagina will increase more rapidly. This effort may be important for both the woman's and her partner's sexual enjoyment.

Perineum

The perineum is put under a great deal of pressure during delivery, to which it responds by the development of edema and generalized tenderness following delivery. Portions may show ecchymosis from the rupture of surface capillaries. The labia majora and labia minora typically remain atrophic and softened in a woman as another indication that she has borne a child.

Systemic Changes

During pregnancy, the blood volume of the body increases 30 to 50 percent. The tendency of the body to retain water in interstitial tissue is also increased. Beginning with the second day of the puerperium, diuresis and diaphoresis (noticeable soon after delivery) combine to rid the body of these sources of excess fluid. Pregnancy hormones decrease as the placenta is no longer pres-

— *Nursing Care Highlight* —

Normal Characteristics of Lochia

Characteristic	*Description*
Amount	Lochia should approximate a menstrual flow in amount. Like the amount of menstrual flow, this amount will vary from woman to woman. Two women in adjoining beds may be having very different quantities of lochia discharge, yet each may be normal for that woman. Mothers who breast-feed tend to have less lochial discharge than those who do not, since the natural release of oxytocin during breast-feeding strengthens uterine contractions. Conservation of fluid for lactation may also be a factor. Lochial flow increases on exertion, especially the first few times a woman is out of bed, but decreases again with rest. A woman should be warned of this possibility or she may become unnecessarily alarmed by a sudden, heavy flow. The increase in amount that occurs with ambulation, however, is the result of vaginal discharge of pooled lochia, not a true increase in amount. Lochia amount truly does increase on strenuous exercise such as lifting a heavy weight or walking upstairs. Saturating a perineal pad in less than 45 minutes is considered an abnormally heavy flow.
Consistency	Lochia should contain no large clots. Clots may indicate that a portion of the placenta has been retained and is preventing closure of the maternal uterine blood sinuses. In any event, clotting denotes poor uterine contraction, which needs to be corrected.
Pattern	The pattern of lochia (rubra to serosa to alba) should not reverse. A red flow after lochia serosa or alba usually indicates that placental fragments have been retained or that uterine contraction is decreasing and new bleeding is beginning.
Odor	Lochia should not have an offensive odor. Lochia has the same odor as menstrual blood (sometimes compared with the odor of marigolds). An offensive odor usually indicates that the uterus has become infected. Immediate intervention is needed to halt postpartal infection.
Absence	Lochia should never be absent. Absence of lochia, like presence of an offensive odor, may indicate postpartal infection. Lochia may be scant in amount following cesarean deliveries, but it is never altogether absent.

ent. The level of chorionic gonadotropin in urine is almost negligible by 24 hours. By 1 week progestin, estrone, and estradiol are at prepregnancy levels. Estrol may be elevated for an additional week before it reaches prepregnancy levels.

Urinary System

During a vaginal delivery, the fetal head exerts a great deal of pressure on the bladder and urethra as it passes on the bladder's underside. This pressure may leave the bladder with a transient loss of tone and such edema surrounding the urethra that voiding is difficult. Thus, even though a bladder fills rapidly and becomes distended, a woman may have no sensation of having to void. The woman who has had a spinal anesthetic or a general anesthetic for delivery can feel no sensation in the bladder area until the anesthetic has worn off.

To prevent permanent damage to the bladder from overdistention, check a woman's abdomen frequently in the immediate postpartal period to see whether bladder distention is developing. A full bladder is felt as a hard or firm area just above the symphysis pubis. On percussion (placing one finger flat on the woman's abdomen over the bladder and tapping it with the middle finger of the other hand) a full bladder sounds resonant or echoing in contrast to the dull, thudding sound of nonfluid-filled tissue. Pressure on this area may make a woman feel as if she has to void, but she is then unable to do so. As the bladder fills it displaces the uterus; uterine position is thus a good gauge of whether the bladder is full or empty. If the uterus is becoming uncontracted and flabby and is being pushed to the side, the usual cause is an over-filled bladder. The hydronephrosis or increased size of ureters that occurred during pregnancy remains present for about 4 weeks' postpartum. The increased size of these organs enhances the possibility of urinary stasis and urine infection in the postpartal period.

During pregnancy, as much as 2,000 to 3,000 ml of excessive fluid accumulates in the body. An extensive diuresis begins to take place almost immediately following delivery so the body can get rid of the fluid—a response that increases the daily output of a postpartal woman greatly. Urinary volume may easily rise from a normal level of 1,500 ml to as much as 3,000 ml during the second to fifth day after delivery. This marked increase in urine production causes the bladder to fill rapidly.

In the postpartal period, urine tends to contain more nitrogen than normal. This development is probably due in part to a woman's increased muscle activity during labor and in part to the breakdown of protein that occurs during involution in a portion of the uterine muscle. Levels of lactose in the urine may be the same as during pregnancy. If any urine testing for sugar is done either during pregnancy or in the postpartum period, therefore, agents such as Clinistix or Tes-Tape that test only the glucose, not the lactose, component of sugar should be used.

Diaphoresis

Diaphoresis (excessive sweating) is another way by which the body rids itself of extra fluid. This response is most noticeable in the woman immediately following delivery.

Weight Loss

The rapid diuresis and diaphoresis during the second to fifth day postpartum will ordinarily result in a weight loss of an additional 5 pounds (2–4 kg) over the 12 or so pounds (5.8 kg) that the woman lost at delivery. Little loss occurs after 6 weeks. The weight she reaches at that time will be her baseline postpartal weight.

Circulatory Changes

The diuresis evident between the second and fifth days postpartum plus the blood loss at delivery acts to reduce the added blood volume the woman accumulated during pregnancy. This reduction occurs so rapidly that by the first or second week postpartum the blood volume has returned to its normal level before pregnancy.

Usual blood loss is 250 to 300 ml at delivery; 500 to 1,000 ml with a cesarean birth. A 4-point drop in hematocrit will occur with each 250 ml of blood lost. If the average woman enters labor with a Hct of 37 percent, therefore, it will be about 33 percent on the first postpartal day. If a woman was anemic during pregnancy, she can expect to continue to be anemic postpartum, although her hematocrit reading (proportion of red cells to proportion of circulating blood) may rise as extra fluid is lost. On the third day postpartum, a hemoglobin assessment is usually done to test for the presence of anemia, either from the pregnancy or from blood lost at delivery. If the hemoglobin is below 10 gm per 100 ml, supplementary iron is usually prescribed. As excess fluid is excreted, the hematocrit will gradually rise from hemoconcentration to prepregnancy levels by 6 weeks.

Women generally continue to have the same high level of plasma fibrinogen during the first postpartal weeks as they did during pregnancy. This is a protective measure against hemorrhage but unfortunately also increases the risk of thrombophlebitis formation. Leukocytes also increase in the blood. The white cell count may be as high as 30,000 mm^3 (mainly granulocytes), particularly if a woman had a long or difficult labor. This, too, is part of the body's defense system, acting against infection and as an aid to healing.

Take note of the laboratory reports on a postpartal woman and make certain that any abnormal finding, such as low hemoglobin, is brought to the attention of the physician or nurse-midwife. The woman's new responsibility at home will tax her energies enough. She does not need the additional burden of an undetected low hemoglobin level to increase her fatigue.

Any varicosities will recede but will rarely return to a completely prepregnant appearance. Although vascular blemishes such as spider angina fade slightly, they also invariably remain.

Gastrointestinal System

Digestion and absorption begin to be active again in the gastrointestinal system soon after delivery. A woman feels almost immediately hungry from the glucose used during labor and thirsty from the long period of restricted fluid plus the beginning diaphoresis. Unless she has the aftereffects of general anesthesia, she can eat without difficulty from nausea or vomiting during this time.

Hemorrhoids (distended rectal veins) that have been pushed out of the rectum due to the effort of pelvic stage pushing are often present. Bowel sounds are active but passage of stool through the bowel may be slow due to the still-present effect of relaxin on the bowel; bowel evacuation is difficult due to pain of episiotomy sutures or hemorrhoids.

Integument

Following delivery, the stretch marks on the abdomen (striae gravidarum) still appear reddened and may be even more prominent than during pregnancy when they were tightly stretched. A Caucasian woman can be assured that these will fade to a pale white; and they will be revealed as only slightly darker pigment in a black woman over the next 3 to 6 months. Excessive pigment on the face and neck (chloasma) and on the abdomen (linea nigra) will be barely undetectable in 6 weeks' time. Any diastasis recti (overstretching of the abdominal musculature) will always be present as a slightly indented, bluish-tinged area in the abdominal midline. Abdominal exercises are necessary to tighten muscle tone. Otherwise the muscle will remain protuberant and soft.

Systemic Exhaustion

As soon as delivery is completed, a woman experiences a sense of complete exhaustion. During the later months of pregnancy, worried that she might sleep through labor and have the baby at home, she might not have slept soundly. No position in bed was comfortable because of the fetus's activity or the presence of back or leg pain. All during labor she ate nothing and worked very hard, with little or no sleep.

She now has sleep hunger, which makes it difficult for her to cope with new experiences and to handle stressful situations. Her need for sleep probably adds to the development of postpartal depression. Protecting time for sleep can aid greatly in helping a woman get back to her normal energy level (Figure 28-2).

Vital Signs

Vital signs reflect the internal changes that are happening.

Temperature

Temperature is always taken orally during the puerperium because of the danger of vaginal contamination and the discomfort involved in rectal intrusion.

A woman may show a slight increase in temperature the first 24 hours of the puerperium because of the period of hydration she underwent during labor. If she receives adequate fluid during the first 24 hours, the temperature will be reduced and should be normal thereafter. As stated previously, most women are thirsty immediately after delivery and so are eager to drink. Drinking a large quantity of fluid is not a problem unless the woman is nauseated from a delivery anesthetic.

Any woman whose oral temperature rises above 38°C (100.4°F), excluding the first 24-hour period, is considered by criteria of the Joint Commission on Maternal Welfare to be febrile, and a postpartal infection should be suspected.

Occasionally, on the third or fourth day postpartum when milk "comes in," a woman's temperature rises for a period of hours because of the increased vascular activity involved in engorgement. This response is sometimes referred to as *milk fever*. However, if the elevation in temperature lasts more than a few hours, infection is a much more likely cause. Infection is a major cause of postpartal mortality and morbidity. Any rise in maternal temperature must be considered serious and suspect until proven otherwise.

Pulse

The pulse rate during the postpartal period is generally slightly lower than normal, between 60 to 70 beats. The decline is due to the increased amount of blood that returns to the circulatory system following delivery of the placenta. This increased volume raises blood pressure. The slowing of the heart is a compensatory mechanism to decrease the pressure in the circulatory system. As diuresis diminishes, the blood volume and blood pressure drop, and the pulse rate increases accordingly. By the end of the first week, the pulse rate has returned to normal.

Pulse rate should be evaluated carefully in the postpartal period. A rapid and thready pulse, for example, is a possible sign of hemorrhage. Be certain that you are comparing a woman's pulse rate

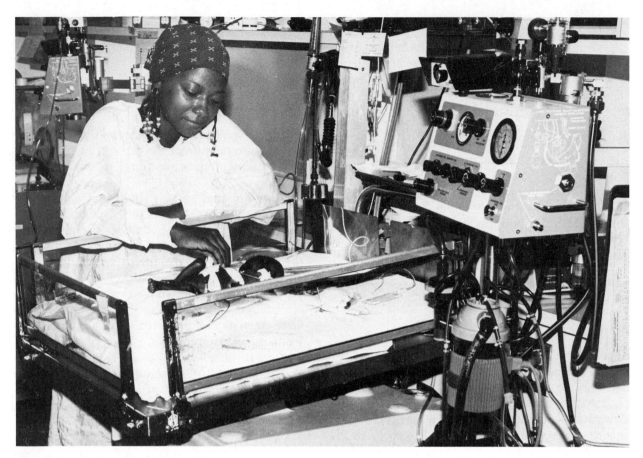

Figure 28-2 *Helping a woman balance rest and exercise so she can both over-come exhaustion and prevent circulatory complications is a major nursing responsibility during this time. Here a mother visits with her ill newborn. (Courtesy of the Department of Medical Photography, Children's Hospital, Buffalo, N.Y.)*

with the normal range in the postpartal period, not with the normal pulse rates in the general population; otherwise, you may misinterpret the finding.

Blood Pressure

Blood pressure should also be monitored during the postpartal period because of the information it gives about the presence of bleeding. A blood pressure reading should be compared with a woman's predelivery level rather than standard blood pressures, since blood pressure varies with the age of the woman.

If the reading is above 140 mm Hg systolic or 90 mm diastolic, postpartal pregnancy-induced hypertension, an unusual but serious complication of the puerperium, may be developing (see Chapter 39). Oxytocics are drugs frequently administered during the postpartal period to achieve uterine contraction. These drugs cause contrac-

tion of all smooth muscle, which means they constrict blood vessels and consequently increase blood pressure. Always take a blood pressure reading prior to administration of one of these agents; if it is over 140/90, omit the drug to prevent hypertension and possible cerebrovascular accident.

Progressive Changes

Two physiologic changes during the puerperium involve progressive changes, or the building of new tissue. For this reason, strict dieting that limits cell-building ability is contraindicated in the first 6 weeks following childbirth.

Lactation

The formation of breast milk (lactation) is initiated in a mother whether or not she plans to breast-feed. Early in pregnancy, the increased estrogen level produced by the placenta stimulates the growth of milk glands and of breast size from accumulated fluid and extra adipose tissue. For the first 2 days postpartum the average woman notices little change in her breasts from their pregnancy state. Midway through pregnancy, she started to secrete colostrum, the thin, watery prelactation secretion. She continues to excrete this fluid the first 2 days postpartum. On the third day, her breasts tend to become full and feel tense or tender as milk forms within breast ducts.

Breast milk forms as a result of the fall in estrogen and progesterone levels that follows delivery of the placenta (which causes an increase in prolactin and stimulates milk production). When the production of milk begins, a great deal of distention tends to occur in the milk ducts. A woman experiences this distention as a feeling of heat or throbbing breast pain. Breast tissue may appear reddened, its appearance simulating that of an acute inflammatory or infectious process. The distention is not limited to the milk ducts but occurs in the surrounding tissue as well, since blood and lymph enter the area to contribute fluid to the formation of milk. The feeling of tension in the breasts on the third or fourth day postpartum

is termed *engorgement*, and, although painful, is a welcome sign that breast milk production is starting. Whether milk production continues or not is dependent on the infant sucking at the breasts and the ability of milk to come forward in the breasts (a *let-down reflex*). Care of breasts postpartum and breast-feeding are discussed in Chapter 33.

Return of Menstrual Flow

With the delivery of the placenta, the production of placental estrogen and progesterone is no longer available to a woman; this decrease in hormones causes a rise in the production of FSH and therefore, with only a slight delay, the return of ovulation. This will initiate prepregnancy menstrual cycles.

If a woman is not breast-feeding, she can expect her menstrual flow to return within 8 to 12 weeks after delivery. If she is breast-feeding, menstrual flow may not return for 3 or 4 months, or, in some women, for the entire lactation period. However, the absence of a menstrual flow does not guarantee that a woman will not conceive during this time. She may be ovulating, with the absence of menstruation being the body's way of conserving fluid for lactation.

Utilizing Nursing Process

Being certain that a woman's body returns to its prepregnant state after birth is important in guarding the health of the woman and ultimately her family. Because of the importance of this time in a woman's life, care should be undertaken with a nursing process base to ensure its safety and comprehensiveness.

Assessment

Important assessments to be made in the postpartum period are uterine involution and breast health preparatory to breast-feeding. A woman is at great risk for hemorrhage in the postpartal period so assessments done during this time are some of the most critical assessments made in nursing. It is easy to discount the importance of these assessments because the overall context of the postpartal period is such a well period.

Analysis

The North America Nursing Diagnosis Association accepted no diagnoses specific to the postpartal period. Commonly used diagnoses are "Fatigue related to physiologic changes of childbirth," "Fear related to ability to breast-feed," or a wellness diagnosis of "Health maintenance needs

related to physiologic changes of pregnancy." Be certain that goals established during this time are realistic in light of a woman's changed life pattern. Although it is only 24 hours since she entered a hospital or birthing center, she leaves the facility a different woman from the one she was when she entered it.

Planning

Women should be able to monitor their own health during the postpartal period following adequate instruction. Planning, then, should include time for instruction. This effort becomes more and more important the earlier women are discharged from health care facilities.

Implementation

All implementations in the postpartal period should be family-centered so the beginning family is drawn as close together as possible during this important period of parent-child bonding.

Evaluation

Evaluation in the postpartal period is a double-edged process because it involves not only being certain that a woman is safe but that she is aware of how to maintain her health after she returns home from a health care facility. The ultimate proof of her well-being may not be fully evaluated until she attempts a future pregnancy.

Nursing Care Planning

Angie Baco, 42 years old (gravida 7, para 7) is a patient you care for on a postpartum unit.

Assessment

Patient has acute afterpains; states she feels "as if my stomach is falling out" when she ambulates; perineal suture line painful. Suture line intact, no erythema, no separation. Voiding in large amounts (over 100 ml).

Abdominal muscles soft. Fundus ½ F under umbilicus. Large amount of lochia rubra (2 pads every 2½ hours).

Analysis

Health maintenance need related to physiologic change of period.

Locus of Decision Making. Patient.

Goal. Patient to experience normal uterine involution by end of postpartal period.

Criteria. Fundus decreases at rate of 1 cm per day.

Nursing Orders

1. Relieve afterpain discomfort by appropriate analgesic (Tylenol gr. 10 every 4 hours ordered by M.D.).
2. Check uterine contraction and lochia flow q2h.
3. Check vital signs q2h until lochia flow is less.
4. Teach and help practice abdominal strengthening exercises starting 2nd PP day.
5. Teach monitoring of self-health by day of discharge.

Questions for Review

Multiple Choice

1. Mrs. Allis is a woman you care for during the postpartal period. During the first hour postpartum, Mrs. Allis seems to want to do nothing but sleep. This attitude probably reflects
   a. disappointment in her newborn.
   b. reluctance to begin her mothering role.
   c. exhaustion from delivery.
   d. lack of knowledge that she can be ambulatory.

2. Mrs. Allis has difficulty voiding following delivery. You would explain the reason for this as
   a. The bladder fills slowly following childbirth.
   b. She is not trying hard enough.
   c. She must have a cervical tear, reducing bladder sensation.
   d. Perineal edema makes voiding difficult.

3. You check Mrs. Allis's fundal height every 15 minutes during the first hour postpartum. The height of her fundus during this hour should be
   a. two fingerbreadths under the umbilicus.
   b. one fingerbreadth under the umbilicus.
   c. at the umbilicus.
   d. two fingerbreadths above the symphysis pubis.

4. You can expect Mrs. Allis's lochial discharge to change from rubra to serosa on which day postpartum?
   a. The first day.
   b. The third day.
   c. The seventh day.
   d. The tenth day.

5. Mrs. Allis tells you that her room is too warm because she has been perspiring excessively since delivery. Your best advice for her would be
   a. "You should try to get a cooler room."
   b. "Breast-feeding would decrease the problem."
   c. "I'll take your temperature before you feed your baby."
   d. "You should maintain a good fluid intake."

6. On the second postpartal day, Mrs. Allis gets out of bed to walk to the nursery and she notices a very heavy vaginal discharge. Which assessment factor below would help you decide the flow is within normal limits?
   a. The flow contains no clots over 3 cm.
   b. The flow is less than 200 ml.
   c. Her uterus is soft to your touch.
   d. The color of the flow is red.

Discussion

1. Uterine involution may be delayed under particular circumstances. What are these circumstances?
2. An important physiologic change following delivery is the reduction in body fluid. What are the measures you would use to assess that this is occurring?
3. Being able to identify normal lochia discharge protects women against developing infection. What are the parameters of a normal lochia flow?

Suggested Readings

Becker, C. (1980). The postpartal period: What is reality? *Canadian Nurse, 76,* 24.

Ezrati, J. B., et al. (1979). Puerperal mastitis: Cause, prevention and management. *Journal of Nurse Midwifery, 24,* 3.

Inglis, T. (1980). Postpartal sexuality. *J.O.G.N. Nursing, 9,* 298.

Kelley, M., et al. (1982). Hypertension in pregnancy: Labor, delivery and postpartum. *American Journal of Nursing, 82,* 813.

Leander, K., et al. (1980). Making love after birth. *Birth and Family Journal, 7,* 181.

Schrag, K. (1979). Maintenance of pelvic floor integrity during childbirth. *Journal of Nurse Midwifery, 24,* 26.

Schwalb, R. B., et al. (1984). Preventing infection during pregnancy—and after. *R.N., 47,* 44.

Scupholme, A. (1982). Puerperal inversion of the uterus: A case report. *Journal of Nurse Midwifery, 27,* 37.

Turton, P. (1980). Sleep and comfort during pregnancy and after birth. *Nursing (Oxford), 1,* 863.

Walker, S. (1980). Postpartum family planning. *Nursing Mirror, 153,* xxii.

Wallace, J. P. (1979). Exercise during pregnancy and postpartum. *Female Patient, 4,* 78.

29

The Postpartal Experience: Nursing Implementations

OBJECTIVES

Following mastery of the contents of this chapter, you should be able to

1. Assess a postpartal woman for both infant and self-care.
2. State a nursing diagnosis related to the problems of the postpartal period.
3. Plan nursing implementations related to care of the postpartal family.
4. Initiate implementations of safe care with a woman and her support person during the postpartal period.
5. Evaluate goal outcomes in both the immediate and late postpartal period.
6. Analyze the ability of nursing care to promote family-child bonding.
7. Synthesize knowledge of postpartal care with nursing process to achieve quality maternal-newborn nursing care.

NURSING IMPLEMENTATIONS in the postpartal period are always concerned with at least two major goals: aiding the physiologic changes of the period to occur as spontaneously as possible, and helping strengthen mother-child or parent-child bonding. Implementations can be divided into immediate and long-term care periods.

Immediate Postpartal Care

During the first 4 hours after delivery, a woman's care must be completed with extreme conscientiousness: At this time the uterus is prone to hemorrhage until myometrial vessels have healed closed. One of the worries with a couple delivering at home is that they will not appreciate how dangerous a time this is for the mother; with attention focused on the newborn, not on the woman, postpartal hemorrhage may occur.

Provision of Rest

After delivery a woman is a paradox. She is excited. She has a baby, a happening almost imposs-ible to believe, and she wants to hold and be with this new person in her life. She wants to talk to her support person about the experience, their child, and their future. At the same time she is exhausted and will instantly fall asleep.

This first wish of hers, to have time with her expanded family, should be granted in the birthing room immediately after the baby's birth. If the father did not watch the birth for some reason, time should be allowed for mother, father, and baby to be together as soon as possible. An old policy of sending the child immediately to a nursery ("infection control," "routine," just "the way things are done here") causes this first moment when the family would have a chance to be together to be forever lost. Rules of this nature should be revised: Lost with that moment is a long-to-be-remembered time of pride, fulfillment, and family sharing.

Following a first get-acquainted meeting with the infant, a woman should be encouraged to sleep to counteract the deficit she is experiencing from sleep lost during labor. All the procedures that must be carried out with the newly delivered mother (blood pressure, pulse, checking of fundal height, and perineal inspection) should be done swiftly and gently, to allow her as much sleep as possible. If she has discomfort from hemorrhoids, perineal stitches, or afterpains, she needs the cause of the discomfort addressed so that she can sleep.

Some women experience a shaking chill immediately after delivery or within a half hour of birth. This is probably due in part to a combination of the exhaustion and the exhilaration they are feeling. In part, it may also be an effect of the pressure changes in the abdomen that occur with reduction in the bulk of the uterus, or of temperature readjustment following the excessive sweating of labor. In any event, shaking chills at this point are common and a woman needs to be reassured that she does not have a developing cold or infection.

Covering a woman with a warm blanket, offering her a warm drink if she is not nauseated from an anesthetic, and assuring her that the occurrence is normal are usually enough to make the chill transient and allow her to fall into a sound, much-needed sleep. Most women will then sleep for at least an hour.

Although she may choose any position to sleep in, a woman may enjoy being able to sleep on her stomach (as she has not been able to do during pregnancy). A woman who has had a general anesthetic will sleep soundly for an hour or more. Because her gag reflex will not be functional until the bulk of the effect of the anesthetic is "blown off," she should be positioned on her side or on her abdomen so saliva will drain from her mouth and she will not aspirate.

Be certain that a woman who had spinal anesthesia (a subarachnoid or saddleblock regional block) remains flat with no more than one pillow for the entire first 8 hours. Sitting up following spinal anesthesia causes tension on the meninges and "spinal headache," an intense, annoying type of headache that leaves her incapacitated for up to a week at a time she wants to feel her best and be able to care for her new child.

There are many things that generally need to be taught in the postpartal period about self-care and baby care. During the first hour, however, learning these steps is not as important as sleep. Sleep hunger blocks out the ability to learn effectively, and teaching done at this time will probably have to be repeated later when the mother is more rested.

Promotion of Uterine Involution

For the first hour after delivery, the height of the fundus is at the umbilicus or even slightly above it. The height of the fundus and its consistency should both be determined by palpation at least every 15 minutes during this time. If a woman did not receive an oxytocic agent following delivery to help her uterus contract, someone should sit with one hand resting on the woman's abdomen, ready to assist the fundus to contract if it should become soft or relaxed during this important first hour. If the uterus is not contracted well when you first palpate it, because the uterus is a sensitive organ, gentle palpation or massage of the fundus usually causes it to contract immediately and become firm to the touch. Massage is a gentle rotating motion of the hand. It is good practice always to place one hand just above the symphysis pubis before massaging with the other hand in order to give adequate support to the uterus and avoid its inversion. Massage should never be hard or forceful, lest it be painful to the mother and cause the uterus to expend excess energy. A uterus that contracts too forcefully can become fatigued and subsequently unable to maintain contraction; the result will be uterine hemorrhage.

If massage does not seem to be effective in causing the uterus to contract, there may be a clot in the cavity of the uterus. The clot may be expressed from the uterus by gentle pressure on the fundus, but only after the uterus has been massaged. If the uterus is totally relaxed, the pressure may cause inversion, an extremely serious complication that leads to rapid hemorrhage and may necessitate an emergency hysterectomy to save

the woman's life. Another reason that the uterus may not be well contracted is because a rapidly filling bladder is preventing contraction.

Checking for uterine contraction is a painless procedure for the woman, takes only a moment of your time, and is of prime importance in determining whether the uterus is involuting properly.

Lochia Assessment

A woman can expect to have lochia following childbirth for 2 to 6 weeks. Characteristics of normal lochia and the change in pattern from red to pink to white are described in Table 28-1.

During the first hour postpartum, when the fundus is checked for contraction every 15 minutes, the mother's perineal pad should be removed and the character, amount, and color of the lochia discharge evaluated. In the first hour the lochia rubra may contain small clots. The amount of lochia should be evaluated in terms of the amount the woman has during a normal menstrual flow. Ask how often during a normal menstrual flow she changes pads or tampons.

Be certain that when you turn a woman to inspect her perineum, you check under her buttocks in order not to miss bleeding that may be pooling below her. If you observe a constant trickle of vaginal flow or a woman is soaking through a pad every 15 minutes, she is losing more than the average amount of blood. She needs to be checked by a physician or nurse-midwife to be certain that there is no cervical or vaginal tear present.

Perineal Assessment

At the time that lochia is evaluated the perineum should be inspected. Are any hematomas (bloodfilled, protruding spheres) forming because surface capillaries were broken? If she had an episiotomy, do the stitches in the suture line appear secure? Applying an ice bag or cold pack to the suture line during the first hour reduces edema, which allows you to observe the area more easily as well as reducing pain and promoting healing and comfort. Be certain not to place ice or plastic directly on the perineum: Wrap it first in a towel or disposable pad in order to decrease the chance of a thermal injury (easy to cause because the perineum has decreased sensation due to edema).

Vital Signs

Assessment of vital signs may supply the evidence that a woman is bleeding more profusely than desired because of the correlation between changing blood pressure (decreasing) and pulse (increasing) recordings with bleeding. During the first hour postpartum, both pulse and blood pressure should be taken and evaluated every 15 minutes. Remember that a pulse rate is normally slightly lower in the postpartal period (often 60–70 rather than 70–80 beats per minute).

Promotion of Elimination

Since the diuresis of the postpartal period begins almost immediately after delivery, a woman's filling bladder will quickly put pressure on the uterus and may interfere with effective uterine contraction. An overdistended bladder may cause damage to bladder function as well.

Offer a bedpan at the end of the first hour. Many women will have enough residual effect of epidural, spinal, or pudendal anesthesia at this time so that voiding is painless (later, when the anesthesia has worn off, the acid urine against episiotomy sutures may sting). Other women have too much perineal edema to be able to void this early.

If a woman's bladder is distended but she cannot void at the end of the first hour, she will need to be catheterized. Most women, however, do not have this much filling at this time. They must void within 4 to 8 hours after birth, however, because bladder distention will surely have occurred by that time.

Promotion of Breast-Feeding

For the first 2 days postpartum, women generally notice little change in breast tissue except perhaps a slight tingling sensation. Palpate a woman's breasts at the end of the first hour postpartum as a baseline determination for softness against which later assessments can be compared. During this time breast tissue should feel soft; it may feel slightly tender to the woman.

Suppression of Lactation

If a woman is not going to breast-feed, some intervention to stop the formation of breast milk is helpful in order to increase her comfort on the third or fourth day postpartum, when engorgement takes place.

Breast milk forms in mammary glands stimulated by the pituitary hormone prolactin. Administering either an estrogen or an androgen or both in combination to a woman soon after delivery will prevent prolactin from being produced. In the past, chlorotrianisene (TACE), a synthetic estrogen, was often prescribed orally for this purpose. Deladumone, which contains testosterone enanthate and estradiol valerate in combination, is an example of a commonly used androgen-containing drug. This was administered as a one-time injection immediately following delivery.

To be effective, these lactation-suppressing agents must be started immediately after delivery, or in the first hour postpartum. They are extremely effective in suppressing lactation but do have some side effects. Estrogen compounds should be used with caution in women susceptible to thrombophlebitis (presence of varicosities or family or past history of thrombophlebitis) as estrogen leads to increased blood clotting. Androgen compounds are likely to retard menstruation, so a woman who has received one of these drugs should be informed that her first menstrual flow may be delayed more than the normal 6 to 8 weeks after delivery.

A newer approach to lactation suppression is the oral administration of Parlodel. This compound directly decreases prolactin levels as its mode of action. Parlodel has the side effect of causing gastrointestinal pain so it should be given with meals in order to reduce this effect.

Promotion of Mother-Child (Parent-Child) Interaction

As soon as a mother wakes from her hour or two of needed sleep, she should have her baby brought into her room. If a woman did not have the opportunity to see her newborn in the delivery room because of a general anesthetic, she particularly needs to see her infant as soon as she wakes from anesthesia. Having to wait until all babies are brought to mothers is unreasonable. While she waits, she imagines there is something wrong with her baby or thinks "Why can't I see him?" "What is wrong with the people in this health care facility that they cannot appreciate my need to see him?!".

Listen to what women say about their newborns in this immediate postpartal period. Do they make positive statements ("I'm glad he's a boy") or negative ones ("I really hoped it would be a girl")? Do you hear, "She's cute" or "She looks like a circus clown with no hair"? First impressions may not be lasting ones; however, unless negative comments are identified so that extra discussion can revolve around, for example, what it feels like to have four boys, a woman will be discharged with her needs unmet. At home, away from health personnel who are attuned to how disappointment can interfere with mother-child interaction, she may have great difficulty adjusting to and relating to her new child.

Most women appreciate a bath at the end of their initial rest period (Figure 29-1). They enjoy

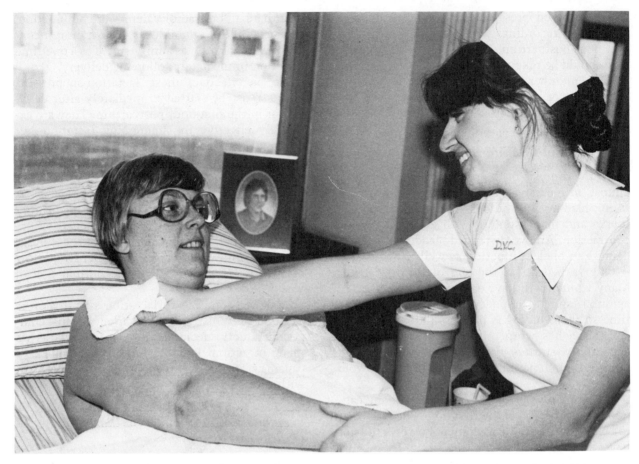

Figure 29-1 *A woman appreciates a bedbath following labor and delivery; this is also an excellent time for reviewing the events of labor.*

being administered to early in their taking-in phase and talking to a nurse about their labor and delivery experience. They enjoy having a nurse with them to serve as a sounding board, a point of reality to use to secure wandering thoughts such as, "I can't believe it's really over. I can't believe the baby's really born."

Following a bath and perineal care a woman can be transferred from a birthing or recovery room to a postpartal room. The most dangerous hour for her in childbearing is past.

A timetable for nursing interventions in the first hour postpartum is shown in the box on page 631.

Continued Implementations

Before World War II, most women stayed in a hospital for 10 to 14 days following childbirth; they expected to rest with little exertion for the first month at home. Changes in postpartal care took place during the war: With nursing care in short supply, women had to do more self-care and be-

gan to stay only 3 or 4 days. Today, with many women giving birth without the use of anesthetics, hospital stays are routinely becoming as short as 24 hours. Women delivering in alternative birth centers remain at the center only 4 to 8 hours (see the Nursing Research Highlight on page 631).

When hospital stays were long, the nursing role during this time centered around administering care. Now that health care stays are so much shorter, nursing care centers around *teaching* care. A woman must know how to care for herself to prevent introducing infection to her as-yet-unhealed uterus or suture line. She must be aware of danger signs and know whom to call if she notices any of them. She must understand safe baby care. Every contact with a woman includes some teaching information, therefore, in order to squeeze it all in. At the same time, learning does not take place if a learner is overwhelmed and hurried. Common sense is necessary to determine when it is a time to teach and when it is a time to observe or listen. Observation of mother-child or parent-child interaction and evaluation of the

Timetable for Nursing Interventions, First Hour Postpartum

Intervention	Timing
Evaluate fundal height and consistency.	q15 min
Evaluate color and amount of lochia.	q15 min
Assess perineum for hematoma or stressed suture line.	q15 min
Take pulse and blood pressure.	q 15 min
Check to see if lactation suppressant is desired.	During first hour
Assess bladder distention.	At end of hour
Ask woman to void.	At end of hour
Assess breasts.	At end of hour
Give bath, first perineal care.	At end of hour
Observe mother-child (parent-child) interaction.	At each encounter

woman's support system at home are the basis for much of the teaching.

Promotion of Involution

Following the first hour after delivery, the uterus may be evaluated for height and consistency less frequently: every hour for the next 8 hours, then once each nursing shift. If a woman is going home before 3 days, she should be taught to make this assessment herself. Always stress that she put one hand on the lower uterine segment for support before she massages the fundus. By the ninth or tenth day postpartum the uterus will have become so small that she will no longer be able to palpate it above the symphysis pubis.

Afterpains

Uterine contractions may cause uterine cramps similar to those accompanying menstrual flows in some women. They are particularly likely to occur in multiparas or women who have had large babies. They almost always occur with breast-

Nursing Research Highlight

Early Postpartal Discharge— A Viable Alternative?

As an alternative to home delivery a program was developed and established in a large tertiary care center to discharge low-risk mothers and babies 12 hours postpartum (Scupholme, 1981). A collaborative effort between the hospital-based nurse-midwifery service, obstetricians, pediatricians, and nurses from the medical center and the public health department, the program was offered to prenatal patients who attended the public health clinics or the prenatal clinic at the University of Miami Jackson Memorial Medical Center. Thirty-five mothers and babies completed the program. Home visits were made each day for 2 to 3 days and a clinic visit was scheduled at 7 to 10 days for the infant. Results from the pilot study indicate that early postpartal discharge with home visits is not only possible and well accepted by families, but also a safe and cost-effective alternative to the traditional hospital stay for families who want to return home as soon as possible after delivery.

Reference

Scupholme, A. (1981). Postpartum early discharge: An inner city experience. *Journal of Nurse Midwifery,* 26(6), 19.

feeding because the oxytocin released from the pituitary with breast-feeding increases the firmness of uterine contractions.

Women need to understand that this discomfort is normal and rarely lasts more than 3 days. If necessary, ibuprofen (Motrin), an analgesic that reduces inflammation and is specific for relief of afterpains, or a common analgesic such as acetaminophen (Tylenol) can be taken for relief. As with any abdominal pain, heat should never be placed on the abdomen. It may cause relaxation of the uterus and consequent uterine bleeding.

Muscular Aches

Many women feel sore and aching after labor and delivery because of the excessive energy they used for pushing during the pelvic division of labor. They say they feel as if they have "run for miles," an estimate that is actually comparable to the energy expended. A woman may need a mild analgesic for such pain. A backrub is effective for relieving aching shoulders or back. Assess carefully a woman who states she has pain on standing. *Luke's sign* (pain in the calf of the leg on standing or a position that dorsiflexes the foot)—like Homans' sign—suggests thrombophlebitis.

Lochia Assessment

Women should be encouraged to change perineal pads frequently as they begin self-care. Lochia is an excellent medium for bacterial growth, and constantly wet pads against a suture line slow healing. This is not often a problem for a woman while she is at a health care facility, but a woman who is trying to save money may try to conserve on the number of pads she uses at home. Be certain she knows not to use tampons until she returns for her postpartal checkup: She is high-risk for toxic shock syndrome until the uterus lining is completely healed. Be certain that the woman who will be discharged early knows the criteria against which to judge the type and amount of lochia (see the Nursing Care Highlight on page 619).

While she is at a health care facility, you need to inspect a woman's lochia discharge once every hour for the first 8 hours (following the important first hour), then every 8 hours. Make certain she understands that she must wash her hands after handling pads and must use only her own individual care equipment so that she does not contract or spread infection. Demonstrate good role modeling yourself in terms of hand washing and equipment use.

Perineal Care

Assessment

A woman who is going to be discharged early and who has perineal stitches should be taught to lie on her back and view her perineum with a hand-held mirror. Once a day for the next 7 days she should inspect for redness or sloughing of sutures or formation of pus at the suture line.

While she is in the health care agency you should check her perineum once every 8 hours, examining for any sign of infection or poor healing at a suture line. Ice to the perineum after the first hour is no longer therapeutic, and healing after the first hour takes place faster if blood is encouraged to enter the area through the use of heat, not cold application.

Many physicians and nurse-midwives order a soothing cream or anesthetic spray to be applied to the suture line. A cortisone-base cream, which helps to decrease inflammation in the area and therefore to decrease tension, is also helpful. Witch hazel preparations, because of their cooling effect, are a mainstay for relief of hemorrhoidal discomfort.

Cleanliness

In addition to measures to assess and alleviate perineal discomfort, every woman needs attention to perineal cleanliness in the postpartal period. Because the vagina lies in close proximity to the rectum, there is always a danger that bacteria will spread from the rectum to the vagina and cause infection. Lochia allowed to dry and harden on the vulva and perineum furnishes a bed for bacterial growth. Perineal care is thus necessary to prevent infection, but it also promotes healing and provides comfort.

Perineal care should be undertaken as a part of the daily bath and after each voiding or bowel movement—or as often as a woman wishes for comfort. If she is on bed rest during her first hours after delivery, you will need to provide perineal care for her. As soon as a woman is ambulatory, she can be instructed to carry it out herself.

Perineal care formerly was a sterile procedure, involving sterile gloves, sterile water, and sterile compresses—a complicated business for women to undertake. Most agencies now require only *clean* technique so women can carry it out after a minimum of instruction.

Agencies differ as to the type of cleansing that is done and the articles and solutions used. The solutions may range from warm tap water, which is poured over the vulva from a pitcher or spray can, to soap and water or a mild antiseptic solution applied to the perineum by gauze sponges or disposable washclothes. Cotton balls should not be used for cleaning the perineum if a woman had pubic hair shaved or has an episiotomy: They stick to the stubble of shaved pubic hair or the suture line and leave particles behind to invite lochia buildup.

Before beginning perineal care, wash your own hands. More postpartal infection is probably caused and spread by the unclean hands of caregivers than by unclean equipment. With a woman lying in a supine position in bed, remove the perineal pad from the front to back; the direction is important in preventing the portion of the pad that has touched the rectal area from sliding forward to the vaginal opening. A plastic-covered pad should be placed under the woman's buttocks to protect the bed during the procedure.

If actual washing is to be done, use a clean gauze square or a clean portion of the washcloth for each stroke, always washing from front to back, from the pubis toward the rectum. Rinse the area in the same manner and dry.

Be certain that none of the solution enters the vagina, since it might be a source of contamination. The labia normally have a tendency to close and cover the vaginal opening, which will prevent solution from entering if you do not separate them. If the solution is to be poured or sprayed and the woman is lying on her back, the flow will naturally be from front to back because of gravity. Again, the labia should not be separated or the solution will enter the vagina.

The entire perineum is tender, so your touch must be gentle or you will cause pain. Inspect the perineum to detect any stitches that are pulling out or any area that appears inflamed or exceptionally tense (beginning signs of suture-line infection or hematoma formation). It may be advantageous to have a woman turn on her side in a Sims' position, so that you fully view the episiotomy area; in some women better cleaning of the episiotomy area can be done in this position also.

If any cream for the episiotomy area has been ordered, it should be applied after the area has been dried (to apply it, use a clean gauze square or a fingercot). In unwrapping a new perineal pad to apply it, be careful that you do not grasp the portion of the pad that will touch the perineum; hold it by the bottom side or the ends. In applying the pad, first pin the front side and then the back, so that if it pulls with pinning, a clean part of the pad will lie over bacteria-prone areas, and the part that touched the rectal area will not lie over the vagina. Whether you are unpinning or pinning a perineal pad, the rule is the same: *front first*.

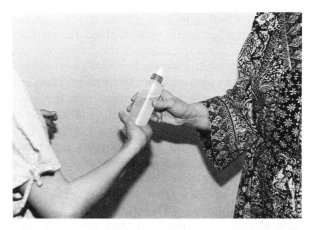

Figure 29-2 *A "peri" bottle used for perineal care.*

Self-Care

As soon as a woman is allowed to get up to go to the bathroom (if she delivered without an anesthetic, about 1 hour after delivery), she should be instructed in how to carry out her own perineal care.

The bathroom of a birthing room or a postpartal room should have a stand or shelf close to the toilet where a woman can place the equipment she needs for care: the spray bottle (a *peri* bottle, Figure 29-2), sponges to dry, her clean pad, and so forth. She needs instructions on how to remove the soiled perineal pad, where to dispose of it, and how to apply a clean pad. She needs to be told always to work from front to back and to be reminded of the importance of using any cream or medication that has been prescribed (some women believe that applying the cream or spray will sting and omit it). She should be cautioned not to flush the toilet until she is standing upright; otherwise, the flushing water may spray the perineum.

A woman usually prefers to do her own perineal care. If she is given a clear explanation as to why it is important to do it carefully, she usually does it well. However, self-care does not free you from your responsibility of checking a woman's perineum and ascertaining whether or not the suture line is healing and the lochia flow is normal as long as she remains in the health care agency. By continuing with these assessments, you remain a woman's first line of defense against postpartal complications.

Episiotomy Care

Episiotomy, the incision of the perineum made during the second stage of labor to avoid laceration of the perineum, is a frequently used obstetric procedure. You can expect many postpartal mothers to have perineal stitches at an episiotomy site. This area is usually 1 or 2 inches long, but if a laceration was involved, the stitches may extend from the vagina back to the rectum. Rarely, they extend forward toward the urethra.

It is easy to inspect an episiotomy incision and think that because of its minimal size it should not cause much discomfort to the mother. However, the perineum is an extremely tender area, and the muscles of the area are involved in many activities (sitting, walking, stooping, squatting, bending, urinating, defecating). Thus, an incision in this area causes a great deal of discomfort.

Most women are not forewarned about the tugging sharpness perineal stitches cause. Women expect the pain of labor to be excruciating and are usually pleasantly surprised to find that it is not nearly as bad as they feared. They usually do not expect, however, to have this unexplained pulling pain in the postpartal period. They are distracted by it when they want to pay attention to you talking about baby care. It interferes with their rest and sleep, with eating, and with being able to sit and hold the baby comfortably.

Do not underestimate the physical discomfort experienced by women following episiotomy and make every effort to alleviate this discomfort. Despite the greater frankness today, many women are embarrassed to discuss pain in this part of their body even with nurses. Unless you are alert and observant enough to mention the problem, some women may prefer to put up with the discomfort rather than to point it out themselves.

A woman needs an explanation that this discomfort is normal and fortunately does not usually last more than 5 or 6 days, since the perineal area heals rapidly. A woman may worry about additional discomfort when, as she supposes, the episiotomy sutures are removed. Explain to her that episiotomy sutures do not need to be removed; they are made of an absorbable material and are absorbed within 10 days.

Comfort

Most women who have an episiotomy require an oral or injected analgesic to relieve their perineal discomfort. Be certain a woman understands how to use any cream or suture-line spray ordered for her. Some women doubt the efficiency of suture-line medications or worry that applying the cream will hurt more than not applying it, so do not use these helpful aids unless urged to give them a trial.

Most physicians and nurse-midwives order a potent analgesic such as meperidine (Demerol) or codeine for the first 24 hours, then a milder type such as acetaminophen (Tylenol) for the remainder of the first week. Acetylsalicylic acid (aspirin) is not used routinely with pain during the postpartal period because it interferes with blood clotting and may make a woman more prone to hemorrhage from the denuded placental site.

Exercises. Some women find that carrying out a perineal exercise three or four times a day greatly relieves their discomfort. The exercise consists in contracting and relaxing the muscles of the perineum five times in succession as if trying to stop a voiding (Kegal's exercises). This effort improves circulation to the area and so helps decrease edema. It is only one of a number of postpartal exercises that can help a woman regain her prepregnant muscle tone and form. Others will be discussed later.

Because a normal sitting position stretches the perineal muscles, a woman needs to learn to sit a little differently until the perineum is healed. Before attempting to sit, she should squeeze her buttocks together and sit with them in that position. This seems like a small matter, but it can be most helpful to a mother who is listening to tips on breast-feeding or infant bathing and wants to pay attention to you and not be distracted by the physical discomfort of sitting.

Heat. Exposing the perineum to dry heat in the form of a perineal heat lamp or moist heat by a sitz bath are other ways of increasing circulation to the perineum and thereby reducing edema, promoting healing, and providing comfort.

Heat Lamp. For a heat lamp treatment, a woman lies in a supine position in bed with her legs flexed and spread to expose the perineum. Cleanse her perineum to prevent lochia from drying due to the heat. A heat lamp is then placed on a clean sheet on her bed. It is positioned between her legs, about 12 to 18 inches from the perineum. She should then be covered loosely by a drawsheet or bath blanket during the procedure so that she will not remain exposed.

The heat lamp should be left in place for 20 minutes and then removed. If it is left in place any longer, a woman will feel discomfort because of her position or a heat burn of the healing tissue may occur. The therapy is no longer effective after that time anyway, because heat causes vasoconstriction rather than vasodilatation after 20 minutes. After the procedure, which may be repeated three or four times a day, the washable parts of the lamp should be wiped with an appropriate antiseptic solution before it is returned to a storage area or used with another patient (in order to prevent the possible spread of infection).

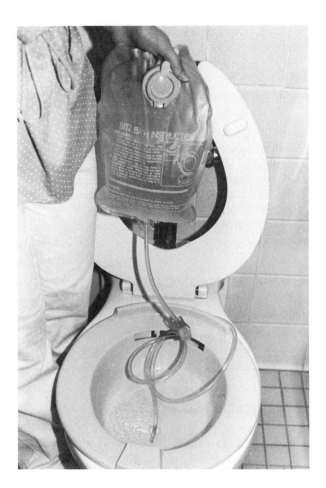

Figure 29-3 *A sitz bath being set up on a toilet.*

SITZ BATH. A sitz bath is a small portable basin that fits on a toilet seat with water constantly swirling in it (Figure 29-3). The movement of water is soothing to healing tissue, decreases inflammation by vasodilatation to the area, and therefore is effective in reducing discomfort and promoting healing.

Be certain that the water in the sitz bath is not too hot before you help a woman to use it. The woman herself will not be sensitive to the temperature because healing surfaces are not good indicators of heat and cold. This caution applies particularly to a woman who is using an analgesic cream or spray on the perineum or has a great deal of generalized perineal edema. Both these situations make her very prone to burns from scalding water unless you act to protect her.

Like a heat lamp treatment, a sitz bath should not last more than 20 minutes but may be repeated three or four times a day. Because of the soothing effect of the warm water and the sitting position, a woman may feel extremely tired and unsteady on her feet after using a sitz bath and may need help in getting back to bed. Procedure for a sitz bath is shown in the box on page 636.

IRRIGATION. A new method of bringing moist heat to the perineum is by a plastic spraying device that fits under a toilet rim and connects by a tubing to a warm water faucet. When the faucet is turned on, water jets out of the irrigating device and sprays the perineum. An advantage of this type of apparatus is that it does not have the potential for harboring bacteria as does a sitz bath.

K-Pads. K-pads are yet another means of bringing soothing warmth to the perineal area. These are rubber pads similar in appearance to hot-water bottles except that they are long and narrow, shaped to conform to the perineal area. The pad is attached to a pump that circulates warm water in much the same way as water circulates in a hypothermia blanket or alternating mattress. You must be familiar with the instructions that come with the pump before you attempt to use it or the temperature of the circulating water can become too hot (the set temperature can be locked in place with a key). To prevent chafing, the rubber pad should be covered by gauze or linen before being placed on the perineum. As with other heat treatments, 20 minutes achieves the desired effect, and the treatments should then be discontinued. Few hospitals have enough K-pads for each woman to have her own; therefore, the pad should be washed with an antiseptic solution after each use and before another patient uses it, as with all other postpartal equipment.

Breast Care

Assessment

The initiation of lactation is discussed on page 622. Early breast assessment and techniques to suppress lactation are discussed on page 629.

Relief of Discomfort

If a woman is breast-feeding, the sucking of the infant is the main treatment for relief of the tenderness and soreness of primary engorgement. (The techniques of breast-feeding are discussed in Chapter 33.) In addition, a woman needs a firm, supporting bra to eliminate a tugging sensation and possibly synthetic oxytocin (Syntocinon) nasal spray just prior to breast-feeding. The nasal spray is absorbed across the mucous membrane of the nose and helps bring milk forward in the breast ducts, thus reducing engorgement. A woman may find the application of hot or cold compresses or standing under a hot shower beneficial. An analgesic is usually also helpful. A woman who is breast-feeding needs reassurance that primary engorgement is a normal finding 3 or

Procedure 29-1

Sitz Baths

Purpose: To aid healing of the perineum through application of moist heat.

Procedure	*Principle*
1. Wash your hands; identify patient; explain procedure.	1. Prevent spread of microorganisms; ensure patient safety and cooperation.
2. Assess patient condition; analyze appropriateness of procedure; plan modifications as necessary.	2. A sitz bath can make a woman feel lightheaded; assess whether she is capable of ambulation.
3. Implement procedure by assembling equipment: a sitz bath, clean towel, and clean perineal pad.	3. Organization of equipment increases efficiency of procedure.
4. Place sitz bath on toilet seat; fill collecting bag with warm water, hang overhead so a steady stream of water will flow into basin through tubing.	4. Warm, flowing water increases circulation to perineum and so reduces inflammation and aids healing.
5. Assist woman to walk to bathroom; help her remove perineal pad and sit in bath. Instruct her in use of clamp on tubing to allow water to continue to flow.	
6. Provide privacy; be certain woman is not chilled; review call bell system for her.	6. Provide for safety and modesty.
7. After twenty minutes, assist woman to pat perineum dry and apply clean pad; assist her to return to room.	7. After twenty minutes, heat is no longer therapeutic as vasoconstriction occurs.
8. Evaluate effectiveness, cost, comfort, and safety of procedure. Plan health teaching such as advantage of continuing sitz baths after return home.	8. Health teaching is an independent nursing action always included in care.
9. Record on chart that sitz bath was taken, condition of perineum, and patient condition.	9. Document patient care and patient status.

4 days after delivery, so that she does not view it as a result of something she is doing wrong with breast-feeding. Engorgement with breast-feeding lasts about 24 hours.

A woman who is not breast-feeding experiences similar discomfort. However, when little or no milk is moved from the breasts, the accumulation inhibits further milk formation, and so engorgement will subside in about 2 days. Hot or cold compresses applied to the breasts three or four times a day during the period of engorgement, or an analgesic, provide relief. There are old wives' tales that restriction of fluid, tight binding, and pumping milk from the breasts aid in relieving discomfort. None of these methods is truly effective, and all are to some degree harmful and so should be avoided.

Hygiene

Further breast care during the postpartal period is directed toward cleanliness and support. These needs are basically the same whether or not a woman is breast-feeding.

Cleanliness. A woman should wash her breasts daily at the time of her bath or shower. If she is breast-feeding, she should not use soap on her breasts, since soap tends to dry and crack nipples and may lead to fissures and possible breast abscess. It is not necessary for women to wash their breasts more often than once daily even if they are breast-feeding. Excessive washing means unnecessary manipulation, making the process of breast-feeding more complicated than it should be.

To wash her breasts, a woman should never use cleaning products like those that come individually wrapped in foil packets. These products invariably have an alcohol base and are extremely drying to nipples.

Support. A woman should wear a bra for breast support for at least the first week after delivery. Breast-feeding women need breast support throughout the period of lactation. As lactation begins, the breasts increase in weight and feel heavy. Good support offers a degree of relief from the resultant pulling sensation and prevents unnecessary strain on the supporting muscles of the breasts, preserving muscle tone. Good support also positions the breasts in good alignment and diminishes the amount of engorgement caused by blocked milk ducts. A bra used during this time should give both support and uplift for best alignment. If a woman has not packed one in her suitcase, she can usually arrange to have one brought from home. Support can be provided by a breast binder (a straight binder brought around the chest and pinned from the bottom up to ensure uplift). A binder rarely gives the uplift of a good bra, however, and if engorgement is marked, it becomes very tight, and eventually wrinkled and uncomfortable.

A woman who has a considerable discharge of colostrum or milk from her breasts (breast-feeding or not) should insert clean gauze squares in her bra to absorb the moisture. These should be changed as often as necessary to keep the nipples dry. If nipples remain wet for any length of time, fissures may form and lead to infection.

Self-Examination

All woman should know how to examine their breasts in order that they can check them routinely for signs of breast carcinoma. This procedure can be taught during pregnancy, but many women are not interested in hearing about cancer prevention measures at that time—the possibility of their developing cancer seems far removed from what they are doing during pregnancy: creating life. In the postpartal period they are very conscious that they must remain well in order to raise this new child to maturity. They are receptive to having you review with them or teach them for the first time the technique of self-examination.

A day after a woman's menstrual period is the best time of the month for breast self-examination. During a menstrual period or just prior to it, breasts may be tender and the examination uncomfortable. A woman who is breast-feeding may not have a menstrual flow for 3 or 4 months. She should pick a day, say the first day of every month, to do the examination until menstrual flow "markers" return.

The technique of breast self-examination is discussed in Chapter 18. Caution women that they have a rim of supportive tissue in the lower half of each breast so they do not think they are feeling something abnormal when they discover it. If they are very slim, they may be able to palpate ribs through the breast tissue. This also is a normal finding. A breast-feeding woman will, of course, have a milk discharge when she squeezes her nipples. She may occasionally discover a distended milk gland that feels very much like a cyst or tumor. She should not worry about such lumps unless they persist beyond two breast-feedings.

Remind women that if they do find a lump or have nipple discharge in their breast by self-examination they should telephone their doctor about the finding but should not worry. Most lumps found in breasts are benign. Many women do not examine their breasts because they are afraid they will find something; other women find something but are then afraid to tell anyone about it. Breast carcinoma discovered early and treated promptly (often without removal of more than the local lesion) has an excellent cure rate. "Ostrich philosophy"—what you don't know won't hurt you—leaves a woman with little chance of cure and recovery.

Bladder Assessment

Many women need help to accomplish voiding in the first few hours after delivery. Like all patients, they have difficulty using bedpans. The position of the bedpan makes their perineal stitches hurt and, combined with the awkwardness involved, renders voiding impossible. Better results are obtained by helping the mother up to a bedside commode or to a nearby bathroom. You can be of further assistance by providing privacy (but remaining in close proximity since a woman may become dizzy if just getting out of bed), running water at the sink, or offering the woman a drink of water. Pouring warm tap water over the vulva, if that is consistent with the agency's policy of perineal care, may also help.

If these methods do not induce a woman to void, the physician may order a medication such as bethanechol chloride (Urecholine) to aid bladder contraction and emptying. If the medication does not help, the physician will usually order catheterization.

Because the perineum is usually edematous following delivery, the vulva in postpartal women appears out of proportion, and it is usually difficult to locate the urinary urethra for catheterization. Be certain that in catheterization you do not invade the vagina by mistake and by so doing carry contamination to the denuded uterus. Catheterization procedure is reviewed in the box below.

Occasionally, because of poor tone, the bladder in some women retains large amounts of residual urine following voidings. This urine harbors bacteria, which may cause bladder infection. Also, permanent loss of bladder tone can result if the distended condition is allowed to persist for any length of time.

The first voiding after delivery should be measured to detect urinary retention. Measurement of voidings can be accomplished by having a

---

Procedure 29-2

Female Urinary Catheterization

Purpose: To remove urine from the bladder by means of a catheter using sterile technique.

Procedure

1. Wash your hands, identify patient; explain procedure.
2. Assess patient condition; analyze appropriateness of procedure; plan modifications as necessary.
3. Implement procedure by assembling equipment: a good light source and a sterile catheterization tray, or separate component parts: sterile cotton balls, sterile basin, specimen container, gloves, drape, lubricant.
4. Provide privacy by bed curtains or closed room door. Cover patient with bath blanket or draw sheet to use as a drape to protect modesty. Position her in a dorsal recumbent position; place tray of equipment on bed between her legs.

5. Open the catheterization tray or set up a sterile field. Put on sterile gloves. Open sterile lubricant and drop a spot of it on a section of the tray so the catheter can be dipped into it using only one hand later.
6. Slide a sterile towel or drape under the woman's buttocks by asking her to lift her buttocks.

7. Place left hand on anterior surface of labia and gently spread them with your fingers so urinary meatus is evident. Do not allow labia to close over meatus again until catheter is inserted.
8. With sterile right hand, dip a cotton ball in antiseptic solution, wipe front to back down right side of urinary meatus; discard the cotton ball on rim of tray. Use a second cotton ball to wash left side of meatus, a third cotton ball to wash the center of meatus.

Principle

1. Prevent spread of microorganisms; ensure patient safety and cooperation.
2. Use the smallest size catheter (10F or 14F) practical to prevent trauma to the urethra.
3. Strict sterile procedure must be used to reduce the possibility of introducing urinary tract infection. A good light source is crucial to locate urinary meatus.

4. Catheterization requires exposure of the perineum. Proper draping not only protects against undue exposure but prevents chilling. For many women, the loss of modesty involved in catheterization is more uncomfortable than physical pain. Relaxation of the sphincter is important for catheter insertion and privacy aids relaxation.
5. Sequence of gloving varies depending on whether the tray is commercially prepared or you are organizing your own tray.

6. If the woman is unable to cooperate, you may need an assistant not only to help you place the drape but to support her legs in a knee-raised position.
7. The left hand is now contaminated and must not be returned to the sterile tray or catheter.

8. Always stroke front to back to avoid carrying microorganisms from the vagina or rectum forward to the meatus. The outer inch of a sterile field is considered contaminated so may be used for disposal of contaminated articles.

9. Use two cotton balls to dry meatus, stroking gently and carefully front to back. Pick up catheter about 3 inches from tip and lubricate it by touching tip to lubricant; place distal end in sterile basin.

10. Identify urinary meatus. Ask the woman to take a deep breath while you gently insert catheter into meatus about 2 inches. Do not force the catheter if you meet resistance. Do not allow tip of catheter to touch any surface but the meatus or you must discard it and use a new sterile one.

11. If the catheter is in the bladder, urine will immediately flow into the sterile basin. If urine does not return, advance catheter another inch.

12. If a urine specimen is desired, allow at least 5 ml of urine to flow into sterile specimen container from catheter. Allow remainder to flow into collecting basin. Once catheter is in place, secure it in place by left hand to free right hand to arrange basin and specimen container.

13. Following removal of the desired amount of urine, remove catheter gently but quickly; dry the perineum well.

14. Position patient comfortably if in bed or help to return to bed if procedure was done in a treatment room. Evaluate effectiveness, cost, comfort, and safety of procedure. Plan health teaching as needed, such as the fact that the next time she voids she may feel slight pain.

15. Record on chart that catheterization was accomplished, amount of urine obtained, whether a specimen was sent for analysis, and any abnormalities observed in procedure or urine.

9. If an iodine solution was used for disinfection, it is difficult to visualize meatus unless the solution is wiped away. Wiping away also prevents introduction of disinfectant to urethra. Addition of lubricant reduces trauma to urethra and facilitates insertion of catheter.

10. A distraction technique of this kind aids sphincter relaxation and reduces resistance to catheter insertion. The secret of successful catheterization is to be certain that you have identified urinary meatus and not a dimpling under the clitoris or the vaginal opening. In actual practice, perineal anatomy is not as obvious as it is in an anatomical drawing.

11. Urine return depends on the length of the individual urethra and the amount of urine in the bladder.

12. As a rule, do not initially remove more than 750 ml of urine from the bladder except under special circumstances; if a bladder is completely distended, removing all urine might cause such a loss of bladder tone that it will not respond to filling afterward. Such a shift in intra-abdominal pressure could also shift blood from the central circulation to the abdominal vessels so that the person grows dizzy from lack of cerebral perfusion.

13. Continued perineal moisture can lead to excoriation.

14. Health teaching is an independent nursing action always included as a part of care.

15. Document nursing care and patient status.

MODIFICATION OF PROCEDURE

Commercial catheterization kits are supplied with tweezers. These may be used to grasp the cotton balls for cleansing and drying the urinary meatus. The advantage of tweezers is that your glove is absolutely sterile when you pick up the catheter; a disadvantage is that they decrease your ability to determine how much pressure against the perineum you are using and may cause pain. You can keep the catheter tip sterile by grasping it 3 inches from the tip, or the length of the urinary urethra, making use of the tweezers optional.

woman void into a commode or into a urine collector placed in the toilet. Whether or not the bladder is emptying may also be judged by fundal height and position (a full bladder pushes the fundus up or to the side) or by palpating or percussing bladder prominence in the lower abdomen. If a woman is voiding less than 100 ml at a time or has a displaced uterus or a palpable bladder, the physician may order catheterizaiton for residual urine following a voiding. Be certain you know before catheterization how much residual there must be before you leave the catheter in place. As a rule, if the residual urine is over 150 ml, the catheter is left in place for 12 to 24 hours to give the bladder time to regain its normal tone and to begin to function efficiently.

Here is an example of why professional judgment is necessary in nursing. A woman may report that she is out of bed and using the bathroom to void. Only a person with knowledge of the extent of the diuresis being accomplished and the amount that should be voided during this time is able to estimate whether bladder function is adequate.

Fortunately, for most women who must be catheterized, the procedure need be done only once following delivery. After another 6 to 8 hours have passed and the bladder has filled again, some of the perineal edema has subsided, the bladder has achieved better tone, and a woman is able to void by herself if helped to the bathroom.

Catheterization in the postpartal period should not be used indiscriminately. On the other hand, it should be done before a woman's bladder is decompensated or the uterus is displaced and uncontracted and bleeding results.

Diaphoresis and Comfort

Newly delivered women often complain that their hospital or birthing center room is being kept too warm and to prove it they point out how heavily they are perspiring. Postpartal rooms often are kept warm so newborns will be comfortable in them, but the profuse perspiration normally comes more from the body's attempt to regulate fluid than from the heat.

A woman needs to be reassured that sweating not only is a normal postpartal event but is helping to bring her body back to its prepregnant state. She should be cautioned against becoming chilled during this time and perhaps contracting an upper respiratory infection. If she has soaking sweats, particularly at night, she usually prefers a hospital gown to one of her own. She needs frequent gown changes to be comfortable.

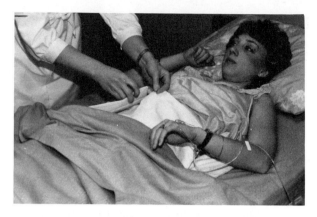

Figure 29-4 *If applying a binder postpartum, apply it from the top down to help contract the uterus.*

Abdominal Wall Assessment

Following childbirth, the abdominal wall and the uterine ligaments are stretched. The abdomen pouches forward. A woman may feel fat and unattractive. Wearing an abdominal binder or a girdle may make her more comfortable during the first few weeks postpartum but does not aid—and may actually hinder—the strengthening of the tone of the abdominal wall. If a scultetus or velco binder is applied for comfort in the postpartal period, it should always be applied from the top down, so that it pushes the uterus down, not up, and uterine contraction is not hampered (Figure 29-4).

A woman can best help her abdominal wall to return to good tone by good body mechanics and posture, adequate rest, and prescribed exercises.

Constipation

Many women have difficulty moving their bowels during the first week of the puerperium, and in most instances this inability worries them more than is necessary. If they have had an enema with labor, there is little solid waste in their intestine to be evacuated for the first 2 or 3 days. Constipation tends to occur because of the relaxed condition of the abdominal wall and the intestine, which is no longer pushed by the bulky uterus. For a bowel movement, the abdominal wall must exert pressure and, in this relaxed state, the pressure is not strong enough to be effective. Also, if hemorrhoids or perineal stitches are present, a woman may decline to try to move her bowels until she becomes constipated for fear of pain.

To prevent constipation, many physicians order a stool softener for their postpartal patients beginning with the first day after delivery. If a woman has not moved her bowels by the third day, a mild laxative or cathartic may be ordered for her. There is a danger in giving cathartics before the third day; the increase in intestinal activity may also cause increased activity in the uterus and lead to insufficient contraction.

Early ambulation, a good diet with adequate roughage, and an adequate fluid intake all aid in preventing the problem of constipation.

Hemorrhoids

The pressure of the fetal head on the rectal veins during delivery tends to aggravate or produce hemorrhoids. Some women find that the discomfort from distended hemorrhoidal tissue is their chief discomfort in the first few days following delivery. The discomfort can be relieved by sitz baths, anesthetic sprays, witch hazel, or astringent preparations or suppositories such as hydrocortisone acetate (Anusol-HC). A gentle manual replacement of hemorrhoidal tissue may be attempted. Assuming a Sims' position several times a day aids in good venous return of the rectal area and also reduces discomfort. Increased fluid and the administration of a stool softener prevents the irritation of hemorrhoids by hard stool.

Postpartal Exercises

Exercises to strengthen the abdominal and pelvic muscles may be started with the physician's or nurse-midwife's consent as early as the first day after delivery. A woman begins with easy exercises and gradually progresses to more difficult ones. She should continue these exercises until the end of the puerperium if she is to derive maximum benefit. Common abdominal and perineal strengthening exercises are shown in the box on page 642.

Involution

All during the postpartal period, lying on the abdomen gives support to abdominal muscles and aids involution, since it tips the uterus into its natural forward position. Most women welcome being able to lie on their abdomens after so many months when they could not lie this way and are anxious to assume this position. If it puts too much pressure on sore breasts, a small pillow under the stomach usually solves the problem.

A *knee-chest position is dangerous for a woman to assume until at least the third week*

postpartum. In a knee-chest position, the vagina tends to open. Because the cervical os remains open to some extent until the third week, there is a danger that air will enter the vagina and the open cervix, penetrate the open blood sinuses inside the uterus, enter the circulatory system, and cause an air embolism.

It is therefore good practice for a woman to avoid this position until she returns for a postpartal examination and is assured her cervix has closed properly. Women who have used a knee-chest position during pregnancy to relieve the pressure of hemorrhoids need to be instructed that a modified Sims position, such as they used for a rest position during pregnancy, is better for them now.

Bathing

Because of increased perspiration, most women enjoy a daily shower or bath. The first time a woman is allowed up to take a shower or tub bath she should have someone accompany her. Warm water tends to make many people light-headed and they become unsteady on their feet as they return to bed.

Formerly, women were not allowed to take tub baths following delivery for fear bacteria from the bath water would enter the vagina and cause infection. There appears to be little evidence that this is a real danger. The sitz bath has long been used for postpartal women, and this is no less a bath than a regular tub bath. Some women feel that baths are the only way of getting really clean, and the warm water in contact with the perineum gives them the secondary benefit of a sitz bath, namely, relief from perineal discomfort.

Weight Loss

The rapid diuresis and diaphoresis during the second to fifth day postpartum will ordinarily result in a weight loss of an additional 5 pounds over the 12 or so pounds that the woman lost at delivery.

A woman often feels thirsty during this period of rapid fluid loss and wants additional fluid. It seems a paradox that while the body is ridding itself of unwanted fluid it should also demand fluid. Part of this contradiction stems from a woman's having very little to drink during a part of her labor. She may say immediately following delivery, "I don't think I'll ever get enough to drink again." Part of the need for fluid stems from the increased amount of nitrogen being released from catabolized uterine cells. A woman needs to

Muscle Strengthening Exercises

Exercise	*Description*
Abdominal breathing	Abdominal breathing may be started on the first day postpartum, since it is a relatively easy exercise. Lying flat on her back, a woman should breathe slowly and deeply in and out five times, using her abdominal muscles. If she used this method of breathing as a labor exercise, she will be very familiar with it and will do it well. A woman who has never used it before needs some coaching to be certain she is using abdominal, not chest, muscles.
Chin-to-chest	The chin-to-chest exercise is excellent for the second day. Lying on her back with no pillow, a woman raises her head and bends her chin forward on her chest without moving any other part of her body (Figure 29-5). She should start this gradually, repeating it no more than five times the first time and then increasing it to 10 to 15 times in succession. The exercise can be done three or four times a day. She will feel her abdominal muscles pull and tighten if she is doing it correctly.
Perineal contraction	If a woman is not already using this exercise as a means of alleviating perineal discomfort, it is a good one to add on the third day. She should tighten and relax her perineal muscles five times in succession as if she were trying to stop voiding (Kegal's exercises). She will feel her perineal muscles working if she is doing it correctly.
Arm raising	Arm raising helps both the breasts and the abdomen return to good tone and is a good exercise to add on the fourth day. Lying on her back, arms at her sides, a woman moves arms out from her sides until they are perpendicular to her body. She then raises them over her body until her hands touch and lowers them slowly to her sides. She should rest a moment, then repeat the exercise five times.
Leg raising	Leg raising is a good exercise to add next. To do this the woman lies supine; she raises one leg upward and then very slowly lowers it again. She repeats this with the second leg (Figure 29-6). She should feel her abdominal muscles tense as she lowers her leg.
Sit-ups	It is well to wait until the tenth or twelfth day after delivery before attempting sit-ups. Lying flat on her back, a woman folds her arms across her chest and raises herself to a sitting position, keeping her knees outstretched and unbent. This exercise expends a great deal of effort and tires a postpartal woman easily. She should be cautioned to begin it very gradually and work up slowly to doing it 10 times in a row.

increase her fluid intake in order to rid her body of these wastes.

Some women need to be urged to drink adequate fluid in the first few days postpartum because they are restricting fluid in the hope of preventing their breasts from becoming engorged.

Other mothers are beginning diets that they hope will bring their bodies more quickly back to their nonpregnant, slim state. As mentioned previously, fluid restriction does little to thwart breast engorgement, and unless a woman is extremely obese, this is not a good time for dieting. The

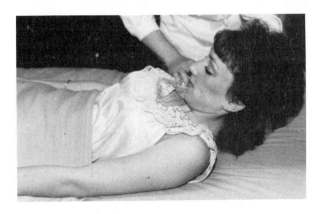

Figure 29-5 *Chin-to-chest is a good beginning postpartal exercise to strengthen abdominal muscles. From a supine position, a woman raises her chin and touches it to her chest.*

postpartal period is a time of rebuilding and readjusting, for which a woman needs both ample nourishment and adequate fluid intake. She should drink three to four 8-ounce glasses of fluid a day.

Nutrition

Postpartal nutrition should include a diet of between 2,500 and 2,600 calories daily and should be high in protein and the vitamins and minerals needed for good tissue repair. It should have an adequate supply of roughage to help restore the peristaltic action of the bowel. A woman who is breast-feeding needs an additional 500 calories and an additional 500 ml of fluid (these may be from the same source) in her diet to encourage the production of high-quality breast milk. Most mothers are hungry during the immediate post-

Figure 29-6 *Leg raising is another good beginning postpartal exercise to strengthen abdominal muscles.*

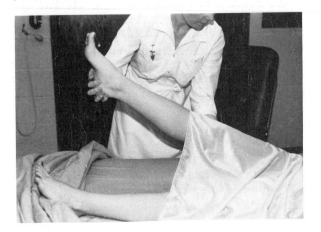

partal period and consume an adequate diet without urging.

On discharge a woman needs to be instructed to continue to eat a nutritious diet after she returns home. Some mothers become too fatigued during their first weeks at home to prepare adequate meals. Thus, neglecting to eat properly leads to more fatigue and so to an even less nutritious diet.

If a woman has any prenatal vitamins or supplementary iron preparations left over from pregnancy, she should, as a rule, continue to take them until her supply is used up. If she needs further supplements, her physician will order them for her either on discharge or when she returns for her postpartal checkup.

Rest

The importance of rest throughout the puerperium cannot be stressed too much. Throughout a woman's health care agency stay, time for naps (shoes off, feet up) should be provided. Discharge instructions should include a firm statement encouraging a woman to continue to get adequate rest when she is home. This will not be easy for her; she has a newborn who wakes at least twice a night, and relatives and friends come to see the baby during the day.

When families were closely knit and neighborhoods were smaller than they are today, every new mother had someone in her family or neighborhood to look after the baby while she napped. Today, a young couple is likely to live in an apartment building and may have no family or close friends nearby to call on. A single woman may have no nearby support people. If a woman has not thought through this problem before delivery, you can help her to look at her situation and see what is available. Perhaps a parent could come and stay for the first week. Perhaps the father of the newborn could take a week off from work or school to help out at home. Perhaps a friend at school or work could take part of the strain of the first week from the mother's shoulders. If none of these solutions seems appropriate, a woman might appreciate being given the name of a community service agency that supplies homemakers on a short-term basis; or you might make a referral to a community health agency, urging an early home visit.

A woman does not have an auspicious start for her role—being a mother instead of a daughter, a mother as well as a wife, a mother of three, not two—if she is so overcome by sleep hunger that her judgment and her common sense are blurred.

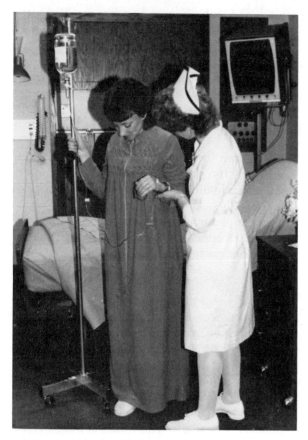

Figure 29-7 *Ambulating postpartally helps to prevent thrombophlebitis. Encourage this effort even if a woman has equipment attached such as intravenous therapy.*

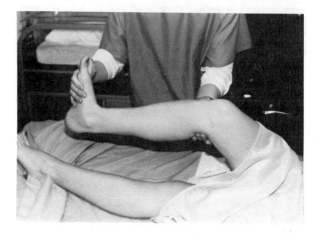

Figure 29-8 *Evoking Homans' sign (asking if a woman has pain in her calf on dorsiflexion of her foot) is a good test for the presence of thrombophlebitis.*

Early Ambulation

Getting a mother out of bed and assisting her to be ambulatory shortly after delivery seems inconsistent in the face of her exhaustion and need for rest. Those who ambulate quickly, however, in the fourth to eighth hour after delivery, have fewer bowel and bladder complications and fewer circulatory complications. They feel stronger and healthier by the end of their first week than do those who remain in bed during this time (Figure 29-7).

The first time a woman is out of bed after delivery she can expect to feel dizzy and wobbly. Before assisting her to ambulate, it is important that you be aware if she was given an anesthetic for delivery. A woman who has had a spinal anesthetic should remain flat in bed for at least 8 hours after delivery; earlier ambulation tends to cause spinal headaches, which are excruciating and difficult to relieve and often recur for days or weeks.

A woman should be allowed to dangle her legs on the edge of the bed for a few minutes the first time she is up. Then assist her as needed for the few steps to a chair or a nearby bathroom. Remain with her the first time she is up; some women are extremely unsteady on their feet and discover that a seemingly easy task like walking across the room becomes overwhelmingly difficult when one is exhausted.

Once a woman has been out of bed with your assistance, she may be up on her own as she wishes. She can begin to care for her own needs, including perineal care after instruction in good technique. However, it is important that she not be left with the impression during this time that because she is able to do these things she is now strictly on her own. She needs continued attention, to give her a feeling that people are concerned about her and enjoy caring for her. She needs professional attention to her physical wellbeing. She needs to be urged to rest every afternoon and to get a full night's sleep (some women who ambulate early will overdo).

A complication that may occur postpartally in women who do not ambulate early is thrombophlebitis of pelvic or leg veins. Homans' sign (pain in the calf on dorsiflexion of the foot) can be evoked by a simple test that reveals the presence of thrombophlebitis in leg veins. Simply flex the woman's leg, dorsiflex her foot, and ask if she feels pain in her calf (Figure 29-8). If there is pain in the calf of her leg, a thrombophlebitis is beginning. Do not massage the area: Massaging a thrombophlebitis may cause circulatory emboli.

This test should be done once each nursing shift or every 8 hours during the woman's health care agency stay. A timetable for continued nursing interventions during the postpartal period is given in Table 29-1.

Table 29-1 Timetable for Continued Nursing Interventions

Intervention	Timing 2 to 8 Hours Postpartum	Timing 1 to 4 Days Postpartum
Evaluate fundal height and consistency.	q1h	q8h
Evaluate color and amount of lochia.	q1h	q8h
Assess perineum for hematoma or stressed suture line.	q1h	q8h
Take pulse and blood pressure.	q2h	q4h
Assess bladder distention.	q2–4h	q4–8h
Take temperature.	q4h	q4h
Assess breasts.	q8h	q8h
Assess Homans' sign for thrombophlebitis.	q8h	q8h
Observe mother-child (parent-child) interaction.	At each encounter	At each encounter

Health Assessment

Careful health assessment is necessary during the puerperium in order that you can be aware of the psychological and physiologic state of the woman and to identify both actual and potential problems.

Health History

As with all health assessment, assessment during this time begins with history taking. Technical aspects of pregnancy, labor, and delivery can be learned from a woman's chart. The majority of this information is best obtained from the woman herself, however, as this questioning supplies not only information on events of her pregnancy or labor but on her emotions and impressions about them as well.

Family Profile. You need to know a woman's age, marital status, number of siblings, type of housing and community setting, occupation and education level, husband's occupation and education, and socioeconomic level. This information is necessary to evaluate the impact of this new child on the woman and her family. It lays a foundation for teaching of self- and child care (you cannot tell a mother who lives in a third-floor apartment not to walk up stairs, and a woman who must economize on money may not be able to purchase enough baby bottles to use a terminal sterilization technique). Knowing a woman's occupation and education is important in allowing you to plan teaching that is specific to her knowledge level and needs.

Pregnancy History. Information you need to know is para and gravida (and the reason for any discrepancy), expected pregnancy due date, nutrition during pregnancy, whether the pregnancy was planned or not, contraceptive use before pregnancy, her reaction at quickening, problems such as spotting or hypertension of pregnancy. This information helps you to evaluate a woman's potential for bonding (complications during pregnancy may greatly interfere).

Labor and Delivery History. The length of labor; position of fetus; type of delivery; any analgesic and anesthesia used; problems during labor such as fetal distress, hypotension syndrome, and presence of perineal sutures are all important data to gather. This information helps you to plan what procedures will be necessary in the postpartal period for care.

Infant Data. The sex, weight of infant, difficulty at birth or during labor, plans to breast-feed or formula feed, and any congenital anomalies present are facts needed. This information helps you to plan care for the infant and promote bonding with the parents.

Postpartal Course. Ask about general health, activity level since delivery, and a description of lochia, presence of pain of the perineum or abdomen or breasts, success with infant feeding, and response of herself and her support person to parenting.

Physical Assessment

A woman had a complete physical examination done in early labor. During the immediate postpartal period, therefore, she does not need all of this procedure repeated. She does need crucial assessments that examine particular aspects of health, however—an estimation of nutritional and fluid state, energy level, presence or absence of pain, breast health, fundal height and consistency, lochia amount and character, perineal integrity and circulatory adequacy. Be certain to provide privacy for physical assessment during this period. A frequent complaint of women dur-

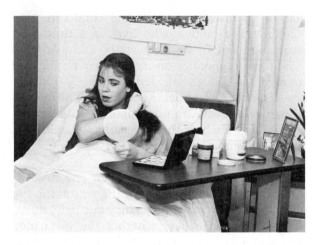

Figure 29-9 *Assess the degree of interest a postpartal woman takes in herself to help assess her mood and whether she has entered a stage of taking-hold. (Courtesy Department of Medical Photography, Millard Filmore Hospital, Buffalo, N.Y.)*

ing this time is a feeling that modesty is a forgotten concept on a maternity service.

General Appearance. A woman's general appearance in the postpartal period reveals a great deal about her energy level, her self-esteem, and whether she is moving into a taking-hold phase of recovery or not (see page 605). Before an assessment, ask her to void so she has an empty bladder. Observe the energy level she uses to do this task (quickly reaching for her robe and walking to the bathroom or listlessly and slowly going through the motions). Observe for a cringing expression or hand pressure against her abdomen that suggests pain on movement. Observe whether she has combed her hair or applied makeup or whether she is wearing her own clothing or an agency gown (Figure 29-9). Many women choose to sleep in an agency gown to prevent lochia stains on their own clothing, but a woman who is pleased with herself and her pregnancy and delivery experience usually changes to her own clothing and fusses with her appearance within an hour after delivery. A woman who is extremely exhausted or depressed does not. A woman whose labor progressed very rapidly and so came to the health care agency as an emergency admission may not have a comb or brush or her own clothing with her.

Hair. Ask a woman to lie supine in bed. Palpate her hair to determine its quality. Assess it for cleanliness or oil that suggests a lack of washing. A woman who had a good pregnancy diet has firm, lustrous hair; when a diet was deficient in nutrients, hair becomes listless and stringy. A

woman who feels good about herself following delivery wants to shower almost immediately because she is so diaphoretic. She invariably washes her hair also (she was so fatigued the last week of pregnancy she may not have washed it during that time). A mother who does not wash her hair may be depressed (although do not discount common sense problems such as lack of shampoo or being accustomed to having a hairdresser).

Many women begin to lose a quantity of hair in the postpartal period. While a woman's metabolism was elevated during pregnancy, hair growth was very rapid. She has many hairs reaching maturity at the same time and, as her body returns to a normal metabolism level, this hair is lost. You may need to assure her that this loss is not a sign of illness but just another aspect of returning to being not pregnant.

Face. Assess a woman's face for evidence of edema. This is most apparent early in the morning because she has had her head level during the night. Edema is manifested as puffy eyelids or a prominent fold of tissue inferior to the lower eyelid. It is normally negligible but will be very evident in a woman who had hypertension of pregnancy and so was accumulating excessive fluid. It will become evident in a woman who is developing hypertension of pregnancy in the postpartal period.

Eyes. Place your finger on a woman's lower eyelid and gently pull it downward to inspect the color of the inner conjunctiva. Normally this should appear pink and moist. The conjunctiva of a woman who is anemic from poor pregnancy nutrition or excessive blood loss at delivery will be very pale-colored. If a woman is dehydrated, the area will appear dry. Make a note to check the hematocrit determination of any woman with pale conjunctivae. Use common sense in assessing extremely fair-skinned or darkly pigmented individuals. The conjunctiva always appears lightly shaded in fair-skinned women. Dark-skinned women may have ruddy conjunctiva in the face of anemia.

Breasts. A woman should wear a bra in the postpartal period in order to offer support to breast tissue as increased accumulation of fluid preparatory to breast-feeding occurs. This precaution prevents undue stretching of ligaments and the occurrence of pendulous breasts later in life; and it also offers a great deal of comfort. Assess whether a bra is being used and whether it is an adequate, comfortable size. Properly fitted, the straps should not leave erythemic marks on the shoulders or the bottom part should not be pressing so firm against the breasts that reddened areas are left there. Breast tissue increases in size as breast milk forms; a bra that was adequate during pregnancy may no longer be adequate by the second or third postpartal day. Advise women to buy a nursing bra for the postpartal period that is one to two sizes larger than their pregnancy size in order to allow for this increase.

Ask a woman to remove her bra and cover her breasts with a towel or folded sheet to protect modesty; be certain during a breast examination that you observe the breast tissue as well as palpate it. Observe for size, shape, and color. Ask a woman to raise her hand over her head and tuck it under her head; this stretches and thins breast tissue. Palpate gently for firmness and warmth. The first and second day following delivery, breast tissue should feel soft; on the third day, as engorgement occurs, it becomes very firm and tense and may feel warm (described as *filling*). It may appear flushed. Occasionally, a firm nodule will be detected on palpation. This is usually only a temporary, "caked" milk duct or milk contained in a gland that is not flowing forward to the nipple. The location of the nodule should be noted, however, reported to the physician or nurse-midwife, and reassessed within 24 hours. Such caking of breast milk generally is relieved by the infant sucking. Any nodule needs reassessment, however, because a fibrocystic or malignant growth could be present unrelated to the pregnancy. Normal engorgement causes the entire breast to feel warm or appear reddened. If only one portion of a breast has these characteristics, mastitis, inflammation, or possibly infection of glands or milk ducts could be present.

Note whether the nipple is normally erect and not inverted. Assess the nipple for a crack or fissure or presence of caked milk. Squeezing the nipple is not necessary as it is painful to sensitive nipples and unnecessary nipple manipulation increases the risk of mastitis. To see if a woman who is breast-feeding is excreting colostrum or milk, place your thumb and finger on the breast alveoli, press backward, and then bring your finger and thumb together. A drop of colostrum (clear, watery in appearance) will be expressed for the first 2 days' postpartum; breast milk (white with a bluish tinge) will be present on the third to fourth day. Do not do this assessment with a woman who is not planning on breast-feeding because expression of milk encourages formation of new milk, an action she wants to avoid. Wipe away any colostrum or milk expressed with a tissue so nipples are left dry (excess moisture can lead to fissuring and infection).

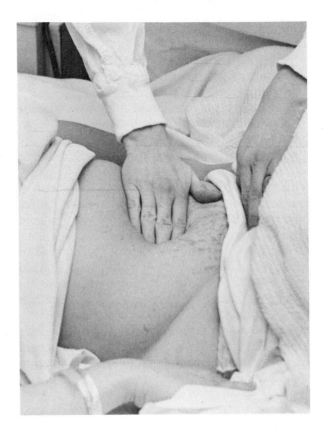

Figure 29-10 *To palpate the uterus, be certain to place one hand at the base of the uterus. This fundus is about four fingerbreadths below the umbilicus. Notice the striae gravidarum marks on the abdomen. (Courtesy of the Department of Medical Photography, Children's Hospital, Buffalo, N.Y.)*

Abdomen. Be certain the bed is flat for uterine assessment so the height of the uterus is not influenced by an elevated position. Observe a woman's abdomen for contour to detect distention and the appearance of striae or a diastasis. If a diastasis is present (a slightly indented, bluish-tinged groove in the midline of the abdomen), measure the width and length by fingerbreadths (F) (a fingerbreadth equals a centimeter). Palpate the fundus of the uterus by placing a hand on the base of the uterus just above the symphysis pubis and the other at the umbilicus. Press in and downward with the hand on the umbilicus until you "bump" against a firm, globular mass in the abdomen: the uterine fundus (Figure 29-10). Assess the fundus for consistency (firm, soft, or boggy), whether it is in the midline or not, and its height. Measure in fingerbreadths (2 F ↓ umbilicus, or centimeters beneath the umbilicus, etc.). Although this measurement seems less scientific than measuring the height of the uterus from the pubis, it is the most meaningful measurement because it is the gradual decline in size or distance from the umbilicus that is the meaningful relationship.

Never palpate a uterus without supporting the lower segment in order to prevent inversion (and in so doing cause a massage hemorrhage).

Palpating a fundus should not cause pain as long as the action is done gently. Pain on manipulation of the uterus suggests pelvic inflammatory disease. If the uterus is not firm (it should feel like a grapefruit) on palpating, massaging it gently with the examining hand generally causes it to contract and firm immediately. Possible causes of a failure to firm are extreme atony, retained placenta, or excessive blood loss. The woman's physician or nurse-midwife should be notified or an oxytocin administered if it has been ordered p.r.n. Placing the infant at breast will cause endogenous release of oxytocin and achieve the same effect.

Teach women to do self-assessment of their fundal height and consistency so if they return home following an hour or two of observation they can continue at home.

Perineum. To assess a woman's perineum, unfasten the anterior fastener of her perineal pad and remove it carefully, being certain it does not adhere to episiotomy stitches. Ask her to turn on her side into a Sims' position with her back toward you. Gently press on the upper buttock to lift it and inspect the perineum. Observe for ecchymosis, hematoma, and the condition and intactness of any episiotomy stitches. If a midline episiotomy was performed, which side the mother turns to does not make any difference. If a mediolateral incision is present, turning so the incision is on the bottom buttock often causes less pain and better visibility. An episiotomy incision is generally fused (edges sealed) by 24 hours following delivery; if it is a midline incision, it may be almost invisible, obscured by the perineal fold. Observe for erythema, intactness of stitches, edema, and any drainage or odor. If there is clotted lochia along the incision, the woman probably needs a review of postpartal perineal care.

Assess the rectal area for the presence of hemorrhoids. Count the number and appearance and note their size in centimeters.

Lochia. Inspect both the perineal pad and the perineum for lochia. Note the color, type (rubra, serosa, or alba), and presence of any clots; smell the pad for odor.

Lower Extremities. Assess the thigh for skin turgor by lifting a ridge of tissue and observing whether it falls readily back into place or not. Assess for edema at the ankle and over the tibia on the lower leg by observing for any indication of swelling and pressing into the tissue to detect pitting. Assess for any indication of thrombophlebitis by dorsiflexing the woman's ankle and asking her if she notices any pain in her calf on that motion (Homans' sign).

Laboratory Information

Women routinely have a hematocrit level done 24 hours after delivery to determine whether the blood loss at delivery left them anemic. This new determination should not be under 3 percent from the admission level. (Hemoglobin level should not be more than 2 mg decreased from admission.) Many physicians order a urinalysis done in the postpartal period. If a urinalysis is done during this time a clean-catch technique should be used, with a sterile cotton ball tucked in the vaginal introitus so lochia is not present in the specimen. Lochia changes the acidity, specific gravity, red blood cell count, and bacteria count of the specimen.

Preparation for Discharge

Childcare Instruction

Many women attend classes in newborn care during their pregnancies. They remember many points from these classes; but when they actually have a newborn, they become worried that they will not remember enough. Many mothers say childcare did not seem real during pregnancy. The postpartal period is therefore a time for teaching, reteaching, and offering anticipatory guidance to help in the new situations the family can expect when they go home.

During the taking-in phase of the puerperium, a woman may not show much interest in learning; she is more in need of the comfort of being taken care of. As she enters her taking-hold period, she grows increasingly receptive to advice and looks to you for the information she needs. Some nurses assume that multiparas will react negatively to child care suggestions. Multiparas are, after all, veterans of child care. If you listen carefully to the multipara, however, you will discover that a mother of three girls will feel insecure about the care of her new boy. A mother whose next youngest child is 5 years old admits

Nursing Research Highlight

Parity—Does It Make a Difference?

A belief held by health professionals and maternity patients is that childbirth becomes easier the second time around. A study by several researchers (Norr, Block, Charles, and Meyering, 1980) sought to determine the effects of parity on three areas: the pregnancy experience; the birth itself, including both obstetrical and psychosocial factors; and interactions with the baby during the immediate postpartum period. An interview and self-administered questionnaire completed on 249 women indicated that multiparas had more physical discomfort but fewer worries during pregnancy, and that they worried about labor more but prepared for birth less than did the primiparas. Multiparas re-

ceived less support during labor and also sought less contact with their babies during the hospital stay than the primiparas. Health professionals need to be aware that the benefits of parity are primarily limited to obstetrical factors and that multiparas basically are no better informed than primiparas. Therefore doctors, nurses, and childbirth educators should be more supportive and encourage others, especially husbands, to offer more attention.

Reference

Norr, K. L., Block, C. R., Charles, A. G., & Meyering, S. (1980). The second time around: Parity and birth experience. *J.O.G.N. Nursing, 90*(1), 30.

---

that in 5 years she has completely forgotten how small newborns are. She yearns to have a nurse who is comfortable with such small human beings reassure her that she is holding her new baby correctly and giving him the proper care. All mothers, whether primiparas or grand multiparas, therefore, need to be evaluated individually and helped at that point where you find they need guidance (see the Nursing Research Highlight above).

Group Classes

Providing group classes in bathing infants, preparing formula, breast-feeding techniques, problems of minimizing jealousy in older children, and maintaining health in the newborn and infant can be helpful to mothers and fathers as they can learn from other parents as well as from the instructor (Figure 29-11). Be certain that a time for questions and answers is allowed with such classes so that a mother can apply what she is being taught to her individual circumstances. Fathers should be able to attend the classes as well because many fathers give direct childcare for at least part of every day.

Individual Instruction

Every mother needs some individual instruction in how to care for her infant and how to care for herself after discharge. Rooming-in (see page

605) is an ideal setup for letting you observe and work with the mother and her baby. If a mother does not choose to keep the baby for the majority of the day, you should provide some time each day for her to handle her infant and ask any questions she has about childcare over and above time for feeding. How to bathe and feed the baby, how to care for the infant's cord and circumcision, a review of how much infants sleep during 24 hours, and how to fit a newborn into the family's

Figure 29-11 *Postpartal teaching can be done individually or here in a group of new mothers. (Courtesy of the Department of Medical Photography, Children's Hospital, Buffalo, N.Y.)*

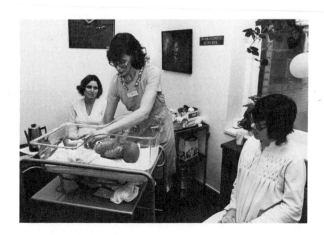

Postpartal Discharge Instructions

Area	Instructions
Work	All women should avoid heavy work (lifting or straining) for at least the first 3 weeks following birth. Women differ in their concept of heavy work, so it is a good idea to explore with the woman what she considers falls into this category. If she plans to do too much, you can perhaps help her to modify her definition of heavy work. It is usually advised that she does not return to an outside job for at least 3 weeks (better 6 weeks), not only for her own health but to enjoy the early weeks with her newborn.
Rest	A woman should plan at least one rest period a day and try to get a good night's sleep. She can rest during the day when her newborn is sleeping unless she has other children or an aged parent to care for. If she has other dependents, explore with her the possibility of a neighbor, another family member, or a person from a community health agency coming in to relieve her.
Exercise	A woman should limit the number of stairs she climbs to one flight a day for the first week at home. Beginning the second week, if her lochial discharge is normal, she may start to expand this activity. This limitation will involve some planning on her part, especially if her washing machine is in the basement and she must wash diapers every day, or if she must go up and down stairs to check on the baby. It is probably better to arrange for a place for the baby to sleep downstairs as well as upstairs, so the newborn has to be taken upstairs only at bedtime. She should continue with muscle strengthening exercises such as sit-ups and leg raising.
Hygiene	A woman may take either tub baths or showers. She should continue to apply any cream or ointment ordered for the perineal area and remember to continue to cleanse her perineum from front to back. Any perineal stitches will be absorbed within 10 days. She should not take vaginal douches until she returns for her postpartal checkup.
Coitus	Coitus is safe as soon as a woman's lochia has turned to alba and, if she has an episiotomy, it is healed (about the third week after delivery). Vaginal cells may not be as thick as formerly because prepregnancy hormone balance has not yet completely returned. Use of a contraceptive foam or lubricating jelly will aid comfort.
Contraception	A woman should begin a contraceptive measure with the initiation of coitus (if she desires contraception). If she wants an IUD, it may be fitted immediately following delivery or at her first postpartal checkup. A diaphragm must be refitted at a 6-week checkup. Oral contraceptives are begun about 2 to 3 weeks' postdelivery. Until she returns for this checkup, the woman and her sexual partner can use an over-the-counter spermicidal jelly combined with a condom in order to provide a high level of protection.

Follow-up

A woman should notify her physician or nurse-midwife if she notices an increase, not a decrease, in lochial discharge, or if lochia serosa or lochia alba becomes lochia rubra. Delayed postpartal hemorrhage can occur in women who become extremely fatigued. Getting adequate rest during the first weeks at home will do much to prevent this complication.

Four to 6 weeks after birth, a woman should return to her physician or nurse-midwife for an examination. This visit is important to ensure that involution is complete and reproductive life planning, if desired, can be further discussed.

pattern of living are topics that mothers like to have discussed. As with formal classes, the father should be included in these sessions. The problems that arise with newborn care are by their nature family problems, and every effort should be made by nursing personnel to help both parents prepare to deal with them. (Home care of the newborn is discussed in Chapter 34.)

Discharge Planning

Before a mother is discharged, she will be given instructions by her physician or nurse-midwife concerning her care at home. These instructions differ in some aspects among different health care providers but have common points that are summarized in the box on page 650.

Prior to discharge from the health care agency, a woman must be aware that she herself must return for an examination 4 to 6 weeks after delivery and she must make an appointment to take her baby to a pediatrician, family physician, or well-child clinic for an examination at 2 to 4 weeks.

It is important that discharge instructions be written for the family. The business of getting ready to go home, dressing the baby in new clothes for the first time, and experiencing the thrill of realizing the baby is really theirs to take home is so exciting that your oral instructions may go unheard (Figure 29-12). On the other hand, a mother should not simply be handed a list of instructions. All instructions should be reviewed with her to make certain that she understands them.

The health agency should have on its staff a community liaison person, ideally a nurse, to telephone mothers who are discharged within 24 hours to help them assess their own health and that of the baby and to answer questions from those women who lose their instructions or are

unable to interpret them after they have returned home. It is comforting to have a familiar person one trusts to turn to in the first few days a new baby is at home.

Making a telephone call to a mother 24 hours after discharge from a health care facility (particularly if she was discharged within 24 hours of birth) is a helpful way of evaluating if she is able to continue self-evaluation and infant care after discharge and integrate the new infant into the family.

Figure 29-12 *Parents dress new twins to take them home. In the exciting minutes of discharge, instructions are easily forgotten unless they are written. (Courtesy of the Department of Medical Photography, Millard Filmore Hospital, Buffalo, N.Y.)*

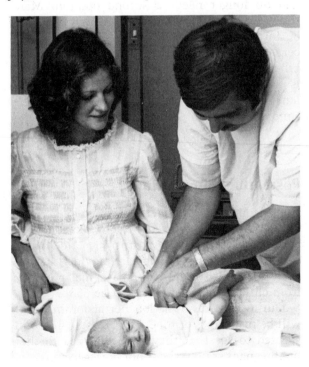

Twenty-Four Hour Discharge Assessment

Mother's Health

General energy level.

Is she resting every afternoon?

Presence of any pain?

Type and kind of lochia?

Is she eating well?

Does she have any difficulty with urinary or bowel elimination?

Infant's Health

What is his feeding pattern?

Has his cord fallen off yet?

What type of cord care is the mother giving?

Any problems with bowel or urine elimination?

What is his or her sleeping pattern?

If circumsized, what is the circumcision appearance?

Family's Health

Does she have help with household chores or infant care?

How does she feel about her new life role?

How does the father feel about his new role?

Are there problems with infant fitting in?

What do siblings think about or how do they act toward new infant?

Future Family Health

Does she have an appointment for a return health visit for herself?

Does she have an appointment for a return health visit for the infant?

Does she have any questions regarding sexuality or contraception?

In order for such a call to be maximally helpful, it is important that it be made fairly close to the day of discharge. If not, a woman generally solves any problems that she has—for better or worse—and no longer needs a second opinion. Many times such a call reveals concerns that could not be anticipated before discharge. Often these concerns can be managed by telephone advice. In other instances, a referral to a community agency is made following the contact as a means of problem solving. Major areas to be assessed at this time are shown in the box above.

Postpartal Examination

Every woman should have a checkup by her physician or nurse-midwife at 4 to 6 weeks following delivery (the end of the postpartal period) to assure herself and her health care provider that she is in good health and has no residual problems from childbearing (see box on page 653).

During this examination her abdominal wall will be inspected for tone. Her breasts will be inspected to see that they have returned to their nonpregnant state if she is not breast-feeding, and to see that they are unfissured and free of complications in the breast-feeding mother. Most important, a thorough internal examination is performed to see that involution is complete, that the ligaments and the pelvic muscle supports have returned to good functional alignment, and that any lacerations sustained during birth have healed.

If a woman does not have an adequate rubella antibody titer and anticipates further pregnancies, she may receive a rubella immunization (she could have this immediately following delivery). If she has hemorrhoids or varicosities as a result of the pregnancy, her physician will discuss with her whether further management of these conditions is necessary. You should discuss breast self-examination with her, as well as the necessity for a Pap smear every 3 years and a pelvic examination every year as a means of detecting cervical and uterine cancer. The postpartal examination should also be a time for a woman to discuss with you any problems she had with childbearing and any she now has with childrearing, since these are a continuum. Moreover, it should be a time to discuss a form of reproductive life planning if that is the family's wish and it was not discussed in the immediate postpartal period.

Six-Week Physical Assessment

Interview	*Areas of Assessment*
History	Assess chief concern, family profile (support system, bonding, self-esteem, family integrity), interval history, and review of systems (urinary system for pain, frequency, or stress incontinence along with gastrointestinal tract and reproductive tract in particular). Assess maternal intake. Some new mothers are too fatigued to eat well so they eat mainly carbohydrate foods or at least not a balanced diet.

Physical Examination	*Expected Findings*
General appearance	Alert; positive mood. If not, mother is probably still extremely fatigued.
Weight	Achieved prepregnant weight. If not, this will be her baseline postpregnant weight.
Hair	Healthy, firm hair. Excess loss of hair from early postpartal period has halted.
Eyes	Pink and moist conjunctivae. If pallor persists, diet may be inadequate due to fatigue.
Breasts	

Nursing mothers	Full and firm to palpation; blue veins prominent under skin; only slightly tender. No palpable nodules or lumps.
	    If erythematous or tender, mastitis may be present. If fissures on nipples are present, the mother may need to expose her nipples to air or apply additional cream.
	    An occasional filled milk gland may present as lump; reexamine following breast-feeding.

Nonnursing mothers	Return to prepregnant size. No palpable nodules or lumps.
Abdomen	Striae less prominent; linea nigra fading, muscle tone improving. No distended bowel from constipation. No distended bladder from retention. No history of pain, frequency, or blood on urination. (If no muscle tone is present, mother needs to increase abdominal exercises. For constipation, increase fluid and fiber. Urinary symptoms probably reflect a urinary infection that needs specific treatment.)
Perineum and uterus	No lochia; cervix closed; uterus has returned to prepregnant size. Pap test is normal. Ask her to bear down and observe for uterine prolapse, rectocele, or cystocele. If involution is not complete, reason for subinvolution must be investigated.
Lower extremities	Varicosities are barely noticeable.
Rectum	Hemorrhoids have receded to prepregnant size or are no longer observable.

Laboratory Report	
Laboratory values	Hct:37%; Hgb:11–12 mg/100 ml. If these are low, reassess diet. Possible iron supplement may be needed. Rubella antibody titer: 1:8. If low, additional immunization is needed.

Utilizing Nursing Process

Because the period of the puerperium is a time of both ending and beginning—the ending of the pregnancy and the beginning of a new life—careful nursing planning is necessary to help a woman learn safe self-care and to help the family incorporate the newborn with confidence. It is a time of letting go of health care personnel who have guided the couple through pregnancy—difficult to do until self-care can be accomplished at a safe level.

Assessment

Assessment of a woman during the puerperium is done by health interview, physical examination, and analysis of laboratory data. Most women do not realize that their uterine *fundus* will be palpable following delivery (or even what that *is*). They thought of labor and delivery as the time of danger, so they are perplexed by the number of assessments by health care personnel during this time. Most women can be taught to make self-assessments, particularly concerning fundal height and consistency and lochia flow (and need this assessment ability to return home safely).

Analysis

The North American Nursing Diagnosis Association accepted no diagnoses that are specific to the puerperium. A number of diagnoses are applicable to this time, however. "Discomfort, pain, related to perineal sutures," "Self esteem, altered, related to disappointment in sex of child," and "Potential for blood loss related to subinvolution" are examples of diagnostic statements applicable to this period.

When helping set goals for the postpartal period, be certain that a couple is thinking about activities and influences that will occur at home as well as in the health care agency. Setting a goal that can be achieved while a mother is isolated from her family influences but not after she returns home is not realistic (a goal to rest, for example, may be easy to accomplish in a hospital; very difficult to accomplish at home).

Planning

Couples having their first child have reactions that must be similar to those experienced by explorers of the New World. They are venturing on a journey that is totally new for them—and they are not at all certain that they will make a success of it. An important part of planning should be to make flexible plans (because a couple does not know yet if the child will sleep deeply or fitfully, is hungry at long or short intervals, or how terribly tired they can grow waking at least twice a night for a new infant). Brainstorming—practicing to produce at least three different methods of reaching any one goal—is excellent practice for parenting.

Implementation

Teaching and role modeling are important implementations for the postpartal period. Be certain in describing or demonstrating infant care that you stress the many different ways to do any task; the couple will need to take your suggestions or techniques and modify them to their own life style and infant's personality.

Evaluation

Evaluation of the postpartal couple should reveal a woman prepared to begin care for herself and her child, hopefully backed up by a meaningful support person. As women are discharged earlier and earlier from health care facilities following birth, follow-up evaluation must be done by a telephone call or at a postpartal return visit and well-child care visit. Evaluation that reveals a goal not met will be followed by reassessment and more analysis and planning, as the postpartal period is a time that positively or negatively influences the mental and physical health of both a woman and child for the remainder of their lives.

Nursing Care Planning

Mary Kraft is a 23-year-old woman you care for on a postpartal service.

Problem Area. Sleep needs.

Assessment

Patient states she is too tired to hold baby to feed him. Sleeping between procedures or meals.

Analysis

Exhaustion related to stress of labor and delivery.

Locus of Decision Making. Patient.

Goal. Patient to obtain adequate rest during hospital stay.

Criteria. Patient states she feels rested and is able to problem solve adequately.

Nursing Orders
1. Encourage bedtime by 10 P.M.
2. Allow to sleep through night uninterrupted except for breast-feeding.
3. Stress resting with feet and legs up for at least an hour every afternoon.
4. Promote a habit of resting during day while infant sleeps.
5. Assess support structure to allow her relief from housework at home.

Problem Area. Postpartal involution.

Assessment
Uterus at 2F ↓ U; firm and midline. Lochia rubra and mod. amt. No foul odor. No afterpains.

Analysis
Involution adequate related to healthy postpartal course.

Goal. Involution to be complete by 6 weeks.

Criteria. Uterus continues to remain firm and decrease 1 F per day. Lochia remains equal in amt. to menstrual flow with no large clots.

Nursing Orders
1. Assess uterine height and consistency q15 min for 1st hour; q8h thereafter.
2. Assess lochia for amt., type, description, and odor q15 min for 1st hour, then q8h.
3. Teach self fundal assessment in preparation for early discharge.

Problem Area. Perineal healing.

Assessment
Has "pulling" pain from episiotomy sutures. Dislikes heat lamp treatment. Refusing to use it. Perineal sutures are intact, no erythema, no separation. Doing own perineal care; dried lochia present on suture site.

Analysis
Potential for infection related to episiotomy site.

Goal. Patient will accomplish normal perineal healing.

Criteria. Patient's perineum will be free of pain and erythema by third postpartal day.

Nursing Orders
1. Ask M.D. for sitz bath order in place of heat lamp.
2. Review perineal care to be done 1× daily and after voiding or defecation so suture line remains cleaner.
3. Teach Kegal's exercises to encourage healing.

Problem Area. Bowel elimination.

Assessment
Patient has had no bowel movement as yet. Has hemorrhoids that are painful on movement or touch.

Analysis
Potential for interference with elimination related to painful hemorrhoids and lax abdominal muscles.

Goal. Patient will resume normal bowel elimination within 3 days.

Criteria. Patient will have bowel movements without bleeding or excessive pain qod.

Nursing Orders
1. Encourage oral fluid (at least 1,000 ml per day).
2. Ask M.D. for order for stool softener.
3. Teach chin and leg raising to strengthen abdominal muscles.

Problem Area. Readiness for discharge.

Assessment
Patient states she understands perineal care and does not want to stay away from home one minute longer than necessary. Her husband will stay home from work for 1 week. A neighbor and her mother are both available as support persons to answer questions on self- or child care as needed.

Analysis
Patient prepared for early hospital discharge.

Goal. Patient will return home at 24 hours postpartum.

Criteria. Postpartal course is without complication.

Nursing Orders
1. Ask for final questions regarding care.
2. Give self-care booklet for reference.
3. Remind of necessity for 4-week postpartal visit.
4. Remind of nursing liason number to call if questions regarding self-care arise.
5. Review physician's instructions on rest, exercise, douching, sexual coitus, and provide with written list of these if not given by M.D.

Questions for Review

Multiple Choice

1. Mrs. Malinowski is a woman you care for on the second day postpartum. She is reluctant to begin sitz baths. A health teaching point you would want to make with her would be that
   a. sitz baths cause perineal vasoconstriction and decrease bleeding.
   b. the longer a sitz bath is continued the more therapeutic it becomes.
   c. sitz baths increase the blood supply to the perineal area.
   d. sitz baths may lead to increased postpartal infection.

2. Mrs. Malinowski asks you about perineal care. Advice you would give her includes
   a. not using soap on her perineum.
   b. washing her perineum with her daily shower.
   c. using an alcohol wipe to wash her suture line.
   d. avoiding washing lochia from the suture line.

3. Which fact would you ask Mrs. Malinowski to report to you?
   a. absence of lochia
   b. red-colored lochia for the full first 24 hours
   c. lochia that has the odor of menstrual blood
   d. absence of fever on the second day

4. Mrs. Malinowski is concerned that her abdomen is extremely lax. Which exercise would you suggest she start on the second day postpartum to tighten these muscles?
   a. sit-ups
   b. pelvic rocking
   c. Kegal's exercises
   d. chin-to-chest

5. When doing a health assessment, which fundal finding would you expect to be present on the second postpartal day?
   a. fundus height 4 cm below umbilicus and midline
   b. fundus two fingerbreadths above symphysis pubis and hard
   c. fundus 4 cm above symphysis pubis and firm
   d. fundus two fingerbreadths below umbilicus and firm

6. In palpating for fundal height, which technique is preferable?
   a. Place one hand at base of uterus; one on the fundus.
   b. Place one hand on fundus, one on perineum.
   c. Rest both hands on the fundus.
   d. Palpate the fundus with only fingertip pressure.

7. Mrs. Malinowski has painful hemorrhoids. A rest position you would suggest for her the second day postpartum is
   a. supine with uterus pressed to the side.
   b. a Sims' position.
   c. a knee-chest position.
   d. Trendelenburg's position.

8. Mrs. Malinowski has varicosities. Following her last pregnancy she had a mild thrombophlebitis. Which of the following procedures would you question before carrying out for her?
   a. administering Tylenol for afterpains
   b. encouraging her to begin perineal exercises
   c. administering diethylstilbestrol as a milk suppressant
   d. encouraging her to drink all the fluid on her tray

9. Which assessment would you use to diagnose for thrombophlebitis?
   a. Ask her if she has pain in her groin on bending her knee.
   b. Ask her if she has pain on uterine massage.
   c. Ask if she has pain in her calf on dorsiflexion of her foot.
   d. Ask her to report any pain on hyperextension of her foot.

10. Mrs. Malinowski still feels exhausted on the second postpartal day. Your best advice for her would be
    a. not even to try to get out of bed for another 2 days.
    b. to walk with you the length of her room.
    c. to walk the length of the hallway to regain her strength.
    d. not to elevate her feet when she rests in a chair.

Discussion

1. Women differ in the amount of activity they engage in following childbirth. What are some factors that would make a difference in level of activity?
2. Many women remain in a health care facility only 24 hours following delivery. What is important health-teaching information prior to discharge for such a woman?
3. Assessing a woman for bladder filling postpartally is a major nursing responsibility. What measures would you use to do this?

Suggested Readings

Avery, M. D., et al. (1982). An early postpartum hospital discharge program: Implementation and evaluation. *J.O.G.N. Nursing, 11,* 233.

Ball, J. (1982). Stress and the postnatal care of women. *Nursing Times, 78,* 1904.

Brandon, S. (1983). Depression after childbirth. *Health Visitor, 56,* 13.

Bull, M. J. (1981). Change in concerns of first-time mothers after one week at home. *J.O.G.N. Nursing, 10,* 391.

Carr, K. C., et al. (1982). Early postpartum discharge. *J.O.G.N. Nursing, 11,* 29.

Cranley, M. S., et al. (1983). Women's perceptions of vaginal and cesarean deliveries. *Nursing Research, 32,* 10.

Foster, R. S. (1980). How to encourage breast self-examination. *Female Patient, 5,* 36.

Fraleigh, D. (1984). Combined mother-baby care. *Canadian Nurse, 80,* 25.

Gorrie, T. M. (1979). A postpartum evaluation tool. *J.O.G.N. Nursing, 8,* 41.

Horn, B. M. (1981). Cultural concepts and postpartum care. *Health Care, 2,* 516.

Ketter, D. E., et al. (1983). In hospital exercises for the postpartal woman. *M.C.N., 8,* 120.

Laryea, M. (1981). The post-natal period: A time of change. *Nursing (Oxford), 1,* 939.

Malinowski, J. (1978). Bladder assessment in the postpartum patient. *J.O.G.N. Nursing, 7,* 14.

Mansell, K. A. (1984). Mother-baby units: The concept works. *M.C.N., 9,* 132.

Moss, J. R. (1981). Concerns of multiparas on the third postpartum day. *J.O.G.N. Nursing, 10,* 421.

Myneck, A. (1981). Instituting a postpartum self-medication program. *M.C.N., 6,* 422.

Nelms, B. C. (1983). Attachment versus spoiling. *Pediatric Nursing, 9,* 49.

Oakley, A. (1981). Adjustment of women to motherhood. *Nursing (Oxford), 1,* 899.

Palkovitz, R. (1982). Fathers' birth attendance, early extended contact and father-infant interaction at five months' postpartum. *Birth, 9,* 173.

Paukert, S. (1982). Maternal-infant attachment in a traditional hospital setting. *J.O.G.N. Nursing, 11,* 23.

Petrowski, D. D. (1981). Effectiveness of prenatal and postnatal instruction in postpartum care. *J.O.G.N. Nursing, 10,* 386.

Strelnick, E. G. (1982). Postpartum care: An opportunity to reinforce breast self-examination. *M.C.N., 7,* 249.

Trevathan, W. R. (1983). Maternal "en face" orientation during the first hour after birth. *American Journal of Orthopsychiatry, 53,* 92.

Wallace, J. P. (1979). Exercise during pregnancy and postpartum. *Female Patient, 4,* 78.

Weaver, R. H., et al. (1983). An exploration of paternal-fetal attachment behavior. *Nursing Research, 32,* 68.

VII

The Newborn

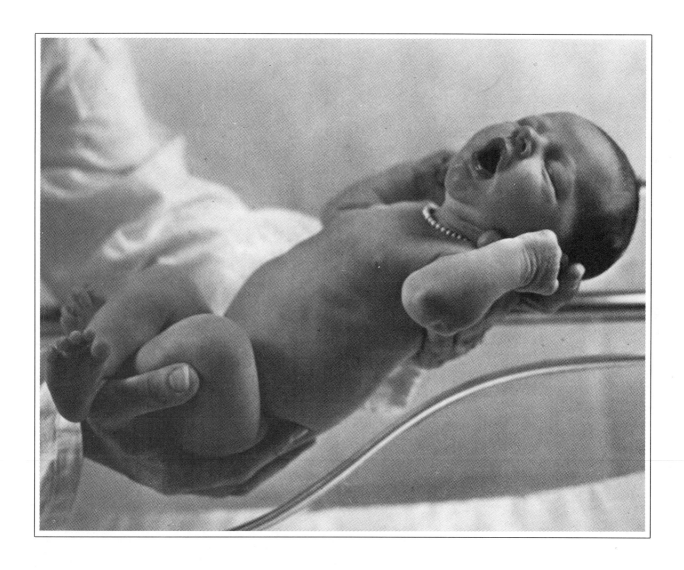

30

Personality Development in the Newborn

OBJECTIVES

Following mastery of the contents of this chapter, you should be able to

1. Describe tasks necessary for a newborn to complete to adjust to an extrauterine environment.
2. Describe the development of bonding and temperament in a newborn.
3. Assess the degree of bonding that is evident in an infant-parent relationship.
4. State a nursing diagnosis related to personality development in the newborn.
5. Plan nursing interventions to assist infants develop a sense of trust.
6. Implement nursing care to promote bonding and personality development through such techniques as sensory stimulation.
7. Evaluate goal outcomes related to personality development.
8. Analyze ways that nursing care can foster the development of a sense of trust.
9. Synthesize knowledge of personality development in the newborn with nursing process to achieve quality maternal-newborn nursing care.

INFANTS ARE NOT, as some parents assume, passive, parasitic creatures who take and take and never give back. They are alert, participating individuals who are interested in interacting with people around them, particularly the person who gives them primary care (Figure 30-1).

Infants are people-oriented—how much so can be demonstrated by their reaction to people versus objects. A baby will recognize his primary caregiver's face by 4 months of age but will not recognize his bottle until he is 5 months old. He will cry at 4 months if a person who was playing with him leaves him, but not until 5 months will he cry when a toy is taken away from him.

The classic experiments of the Harlows (Harlow and Zimmerman, 1970) with newborn monkeys demonstrated how baby monkeys yearn for something more from a mother than physical nourishment. The experimenters fed one group of newborn monkeys from a bottle attached to a wire mesh "mother." A second group was fed from a bottle attached to a soft terrycloth "mother." When the monkeys were frightened, all of them clung to the terrycloth "mother," even those who had not been fed by "her."

A human baby demonstrates this same behavior, enjoying being cuddled, held tightly, and mothered. She reciprocates very soon by cooing and smiling in response to her mother's face.

Newborn Tasks

A newborn has certain developmental tasks that he or she must master to mature and adjust to the environment. Duvall (1971) has isolated a number of these. The infant has to

1. Achieve physiologic equilibrium following birth. This involves learning to sleep and be active at appropriate times, so that the newborn receives enough nourishment and has enough exercise to remain physiologically sound.
2. Learn to take foods satisfactorily; sucking is not as instinctive for some infants as others. Developing a taste for new textures and foods is more difficult for some infants than for others.
3. Achieve controlled elimination and not be frightened by own body urges.
4. Learn to manage own body. This involves developing coordination, the ability to move about, assurance, and competence.
5. Learn to adjust to other people.
6. Learn systems of communication. This involves both verbal and nonverbal learning.
7. Learn to express and control feelings.
8. Lay the foundations of self-awareness. This involves seeing oneself as a separate entity and finding personal fulfillment both with and without others.
9. Learn to love and be loved.

The greatest task of a new mother is to conceive of her newborn as an individual with separate needs and to rely on what the infant's behavior tells her (to be able to interpret cues). By 2 months of age, most infants can indicate by their cry whether they are feeling cold, hungry, wet, or lonesome. Since the mother spends a great deal of time with the infant in these first months, she has an opportunity to recognize these nonverbal cues and to be aware of individual needs.

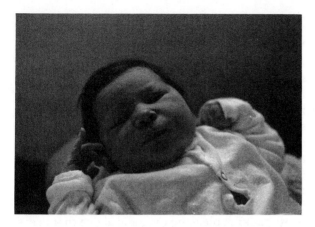

Figure 30-1 *Personality is apparent in a newborn from the start. Note the alert, searching interest.*

Developmental Task: Trust Versus Distrust

A developmental task is one that is best achieved at a particular time in life so that the individual can proceed to the next step of maturity.

Erikson (1963) proposes that the personality developmental task of the infant period is to form a sense of trust. When the infant is hungry, the mother feeds and makes her comfortable again; she is wet, and the mother changes her and makes her comfortable again; she is cold, and the mother holds and warms her and makes her comfortable again. By this process, infants learn to trust that when they have a need, or are in distress, a person will come to take care of them.

A synonym for *trust* in this connotation might be *love*. By the way that the infant is handled, fed, talked to, and held, he learns to love and be loved. The infant who has a variety of caregivers, who sometimes is fed on a rigid schedule and sometimes when he is hungry, who sometimes is treated roughly and sometimes gently, has difficulty learning to trust anyone. If a person cannot trust people, he cannot enjoy deeply satisfying interactions with people. If he cannot trust others, he has difficulty trusting himself or feeling self-esteem. Children who are raised by multiple caretakers may have difficulty establishing close relationships as adults.

The importance of establishing this ability to love or trust early becomes evident when development is thought of sequentially. If the first developmental step is inadequate, this inadequacy will pervade all future steps. The end results will be an adult who is unable to form deep relationships with others. Such adults are unable to instill a sense of trust in their own children, and thus the inadequacy is perpetuated from generation to generation.

How does a mother encourage a sense of trust in her infant? Trust arises out of a sense of confidence that one knows what is coming next. This does not mean that a mother should set up a rigid schedule of care for her child. It does imply that she should establish *some* schedule: breakfast, bath, playtime, nap, lunch, walk outside, quiet playtime, dinner, story, bedtime, for example. This gentle rhythm of care gives the infant a sense of being able to predict what is going to happen, to feel that life has some consistency. All little children thrive on routine: the same story read over and over again, the same bedtime routine over and over, the same spoon every day for lunch. The newborn period is not too early for children to learn family traditions that will help them to feel secure in their world as they grow. Some mothers have difficulty seeing this as important. They are so tired of work routines that they want to raise their child as a "free spirit." Do not discourage this philosophy altogether. However, it may be helpful to suggest a few modifications to try to instill a little order into the infant's life.

As important as a rhythm of care is that the care is given largely by one person. This person can be the mother, a grandmother, a conscientious baby-sitter, a foster mother, the father, or anyone who can give consistent care. A mother who is going to work during the first year of her baby's life should try to arrange for one person to care for her child or a day care center where one person will give consistent care. She should discuss her method of child care with baby-sitters, so that changes in baby-sitters do not disrupt the routine of care.

The person who gives an infant constant care must actively interact with the child in order to provide a sense of trust. Passively caring for an infant, never talking to her or stroking her while feeding and changing, is the same as not being with her at all. Some mothers feel self-conscious talking to a baby who does not talk back. Or they think such interaction can wait until the child is older. The rule that parents should not talk baby talk to the baby is a good one, because children will not learn the correct pronunciation of words from baby talk. Be sure, however, that a mother is not interpreting the rule as "don't talk to babies."

Pointing out to a mother the importance of interacting with her child helps her to include this form of stimulation as she cares for the baby's physical needs.

Rooming-in helps a mother to feel secure about

caring for her baby before she is discharged from the hospital. Looking at the baby with her, pointing out that such things as the faint red marks over the eyebrows are normal in newborns, or that the irregular manner that newborns use to breathe is normal, helps her begin to interact with the baby. Even if a mother does not choose rooming-in, she needs to have extra time with her baby. She needs to do more for him during her hospital stay than just feed him and then quickly return him to the nursery again.

If a woman is going to have a short hospital stay or delivers at an alternate birth center, she should spend as much time as possible with her baby during this time. Unfortunately, she may be so exhausted following delivery or still be in a taking-in phase of recovery from childbirth that she is not able to use the time with her baby effectively. Try to identify a support person in her family or among her friends whom she will be able to use when she is at home to answer the questions about her baby that would have been answered by nurses if she had stayed in the hospital longer.

Sensory Stimulation

Because small infants react strongly to sensory stimuli, the sensory stimulation the mother intends to give her baby is a good area to explore.

Hearing

An infant appears to enjoy soft, musical sounds or soft, cooing voices; he or she starts at the sound of harsh, raucous rattles or loud bangs. A mother should choose first toys in terms of the sounds they make. They should not be chosen because they appeal to her, but according to their suitability for an infant who is just being introduced into the modern world of high-intensity sound.

Sight

Babies appear to enjoy watching their mothers' faces more than any toy. A mother should make a point of initiating eye-to-eye contact with her newborn right from the beginning. Most mothers are aware that infants also enjoy mobiles. Occasionally, a mother overdoes the amount of visual stimulation she gives her child. He has so many patterns around him, so many dangling objects over his head as he lies in his crib, that he must feel overwhelmed. Again, mothers should consider how all these trappings appear from the child's view.

Taste

Mealtime every day is a time for fostering trust. Feedings should be at the infant's pace, and the amounts should fit her needs, not the mother's idea of what she should eat. Again, she should not be overwhelmed by too many stimuli. New foods should be introduced one at a time, so that the child can accustom herself to a new taste before another new one is introduced. The temperature of formula or food should be neither too hot nor too cold. An infant should be held while she is fed, so that she feels secure; she should have adequate sucking pleasure over and above that necessary for feeding.

Touch

An infant needs to be touched, to experience skin-to-skin contact. His clothes should feel comfortable: soft rather than rough; dry rather than wet diapers. He needs to be handled with assurance and gentleness. Some mothers handle their sons roughly, trying not to make them "sissies." Such mothers need reminding that right now their sons are babies; later on, they will have time enough to become men.

It is interesting to explore with new mothers how much they appreciate the benefits or meaning of touch. Sometimes one observes a mother at a social gathering who brings her baby in an infant carrier, leaves him there all during the visit, and takes him out to the car in the carrier when she leaves. The mother has avoided touching by always interposing a plastic barrier between her and her child. Such a mother is not necessarily cold or distant. Probably, no nurse ever took the time to talk to her about the psychological aspects of infant care.

Infant Development

Most mothers ask a number of questions relating to a baby's development: When will he be able to sit up? When will she be able to turn over? When can I expect him to begin to talk? It is good for a mother not to expect these milestones of development to occur before they normally do or she will fear that her infant is retarded. Furthermore, it is dangerous when she believes that certain capabilities develop later than they actually do. If she thinks her child is too young to move to the edge of a bed, she may leave him or her there unattended, setting the scene for a fall.

You should be familar with the developmental milestones of infancy in order to be able to answer the mother's questions intelligently. Be sure that mothers understand that babies all proceed through developmental stages, but at different rates. The fact that an older child walked at 12 months does not mean a new brother or sister will walk this early. Some babies walk as late as 22 months and are still within the normal limits of development. An older child may not have turned over until 4 months old; the new baby may flip over at 3 months. The ages at which milestones are established are averages only.

A guide such as the developmental screening items devised by Provence (1968) is a helpful reference to use in discussing development in the first 24 months of life. This is shown in Table 30-1.

Temperament

Temperament is not a characteristic that arises during childhood or in adult life. Infants are born with temperament, which can be defined as characteristic reaction patterns to situations. It is important to explore this concept with new mothers. Awareness that infants are not all alike, that some adapt quickly to new situations, others adapt slowly, some react intensely, some passively, helps the new mother to understand her child better, to learn more quickly the cues her child is giving her, and therefore to deal with him or her more constructively (Figure 30-2).

Thomas et al. (1971) have identified nine different reaction patterns in infants.

Activity Level

Some infants have a high level of motor activity and are rarely quiet. They wiggle and squirm in their crib as early as 2 weeks of age. The mother puts such a child to sleep in one end of the crib and finds her in another corner of the crib an hour later. The child will not stay seated in her bathtub. She refuses to be controlled by a playpen. She is constantly "on the go." Other babies move very little, stay where they are placed, appear to take in their environment in a quieter, more docile way. Both patterns are normal; they merely reflect extremes of the scale of motor activity, which is one characteristic of temperament.

Rhythmicity

Some infants manifest a regular rhythm in their physiologic functions. They tend to awake at the same time each morning. They appear hungry at regular 4-hour periods. They nap the same time every day, have a bowel movement the same time every day. They are predictable, easy-to-care-for infants in that the mother learns early what to expect from them. On the other end of the scale are infants with an irregular rhythmicity. They rarely awake at the same time 2 days in a row. They may go a long time without eating one day and the next day appear hungry almost immediately after a feeding. Such a child is difficult to care for because the mother cannot easily plan a schedule for him. She must constantly adapt her daily schedule to the infant's.

Approach

Approach refers to the child's response on initial contact with a new stimulus. Some infants approach new situations in an unruffled manner. They smile and "talk" to strangers, and will accept new food without any spitting out or fussing. They explore new toys without apprehension. Other infants demonstrate withdrawal rather than approach. They cry at the sight of strangers, new toys, new foods, the first time a tub bath is introduced. They are difficult children to take on vacation because they react so fearfully to new situations.

Adaptability

Adaptability is the infant's ability to change his reaction to stimuli over a period of time. The infant who is adaptable changes his first reaction to situations without exhibiting extreme distress. The first time he was placed in a bathtub he protested loudly, but by the third time he is happily sitting in it splashing (Figure 30-3). This contrasts with the infant who cries for months whenever he is put into the bathtub or who cannot seem to accustom himself to a new bed, a new playpen, or a new caregiver.

Intensity of Reaction

Some infants react to situations with their whole being. They cry loudly when their diapers are wet, when they are hungry, when their mother leaves them. Others rarely fuss over irritations such as wet diapers. They wait for their mother to prepare food, and they have a mild or low-intensity reaction to stress.

Distractibility

An infant who is easily distracted is easily managed. A pacifier diverts and calms her. If she is crying over the loss of a toy, she can be ap-

Table 30-1 Items for Developmental Screening, Ages 1 to 24 Months

Age (Months)	Posturing and Gross Motor Development	Grasping Patterns	Play and Use of Toys	Speech	Reactions to Others and Staff
1	Asymmetrical postures predominant	Hands fisted or partially open Grasps voluntarily when toy is placed *in* hand	Follows visually Holds rattle briefly (not reflexively)	Makes small throaty noises Vocalizes responsively to people (musical cooing)	Looks at face of adult Smiles responsively
3	Lifts head high in prone position Rolls prone to supine				Follows moving person visually Distinguishes mother from others
5	No head lag when pulled to sit Rolls supine to prone	Grasps toy when held *near* hand Palmarwise grasp of block	Shows interest in playthings Shows displeasure at loss of toy	Vocalizes spontaneously to self and to toys Localizes sounds	*Initiates* contact by smiling or vocalizing Plays with own foot
7	Sits with trunk erect with support Sits alone	Transfers object from hand to hand Grasps block with thumb and index	Looks briefly for toy that disappears	Vocalizes "da, ba, ha"	Reacts to strangers Pushes away examiner's hand
9	Belly crawl Creeps on all fours		Plays with two toys simultaneously	Vocalizes "dada, mama" (*non*specific)	Plays pat-a-cake, so-big, bye-bye
11	Pulls to a stand	Grasps pellets with pincer grasp (index and thumb)	Shows preference for one toy over another	Vocalizes "mama, dada" (specific)	Cooperates in dressing (e.g., pushes arm with sleeve)
13	Walks a few steps alone		Enjoys "putting in and taking out" games	Two words (besides *mama, dada*)	Finger-feeds Rolls ball to adult with pleasure
15	Walks well alone Starts and stops with control			Uses 1–6 words, including names Uses jargon	Hugs and gives kiss to parent
18	Climbs into adult chair		Piles 3–4 blocks Looks at picture book Explores drawers and cabinets	Names one or two common objects	Identifies parts of own body (e.g., eye, nose)
21	Squats and returns to standing position Runs well		Pushes small cars, etc., about	Combines 2–3 words spontaneously Vocabulary of 20–50 words	Feeds self with spoon
24	Walks up and down stairs alone		Beginning fantasy play: takes care of doll or teddy bear; "goes to store"; etc.	Begins to use pronouns, *I, you, me* Uses three-word sentences	Imitates parents in domestic activities (dusts, sweeps, puts on father's hat, etc.)

Source: Provence, S. (1968). Developmental history. In R. Cooke & S. Levin (Eds.). *The biologic basis of pediatric practice* (Vol. 2, p. 1738). New York: McGraw-Hill. Copyright © 1968 by McGraw-Hill Book Company. Used with permission.

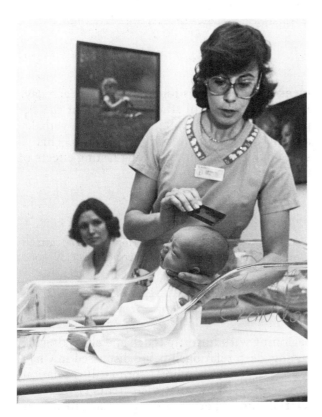

Figure 30-2 *Classes on newborn care can help a mother realize the individual characteristics of her child. Here a nurse styles a newborn's hair. (Courtesy of the Department of Medical Photography, Children's Hospital, Buffalo, N.Y.)*

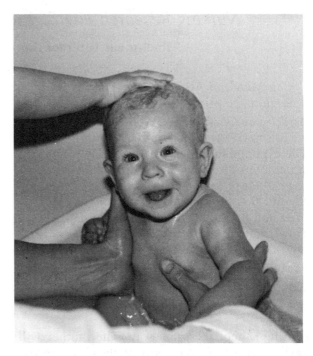

Figure 30-3 *Temperament makes infants respond to new experiences in different ways. Here an infant demonstrates good adaptability to a new situation, a tub bath.*

peased by the offer of a new one. Other infants are nondistractible. No offer will distract them from the object they want. The mother of such an infant may describe her as "bullheaded" or unwilling to compromise.

Attention Span and Persistence

Attention span in infants is variable. One infant will play in a playpen by himself with one toy for an hour; another will spend no more than a minute or two with each toy. Degree of persistence is also variable. Some infants will keep trying to perform an activity even when they fail time after time; others stop trying after one unsuccessful attempt.

Threshold of Responsiveness

Threshold of responsiveness is the intensity level of stimulation that is necessary to evoke a response. Infants with a low threshold of responsiveness need very little stimulation to evoke a reaction. Infants with a high threshold level do not react to mild stimuli; they need intense stimu-

lation before they demonstrate a change in behavior.

Mood Quality

The infant who is "always happy, always laughing" can be categorized as having a positive mood quality. The infant whose mother describes him as "always fussy, always cranky" has a negative mood quality. Obviously, the baby's mood pattern can make a major difference in the mother's enjoyment of the baby, and a mother who has fun with her baby is bound to spend more time with him or her than one whose baby reacts negatively.

Infants who have a normal activity level, a regular rhythmicity, who approach and adapt easily, who have a long attention span, high level of persistence, and a positive mood quality are "ideal" babies to care for. Much harder for new mothers to learn to care for are the highly active infants, especially if they demonstrate irregular physiologic rhythms, withdraw rather than approach, and are nonadaptable.

It is good to talk to a mother about her child's reaction patterns, since these patterns tend to persist, and the way the child will react in the future depends a great deal on present performance. The child who withdraws rather than approaches in breast-feeding may approach toilet training or

Nursing Research Highlight

Attachment Intervention

Can Maternal Attachment Be Enhanced by Prenatal Intervention?

Attachment intervention is a term used by Carter-Jessop (1981) in her study of ten primiparas. The experimental group in this study received attachment intervention during the last trimester of their pregnancies. This process involved encouraging the mothers to feel for the babies' parts and to check the fetal position daily. These mothers were also encouraged to notice how they could affect fetal activity. They were instructed to gently rub and stroke their abdomens over the babies for short periods each day. Results of this small study revealed that the experimental mothers were happier, more verbal, and more comfortable with their babies. This study did not examine the long-lasting effects of this process.

Reference

Carter-Jessop, L. (1981). Promoting maternal attachment through prenatal intervention. *M.C.N.*, 6(2), 107.

---

starting school the same way. The mother will have to focus more on preparing the child for new activities than will the mother whose child approaches new situations easily. The mother who is aware that her baby shies away from new experiences, such as baths and new foods, will take it in her stride when she is slow in adapting to nursery school at age 4, knowing that this is her child's way.

It was in the natural course of events to notice such reaction patterns in children when extended families were common. Grandmothers, with their more objective view, observed and reported consistent nonadaptability or withdrawal patterns that busy mothers, involved in everyday care, did not have time to notice. Mothers are likely to remain unaware of these patterns unless nurses bring them to their attention before they take their babies home. Nurses who do so are giving good anticipatory guidance. If a new mother has difficulties with her baby, she is likely to assume that it is her fault. If she is aware of temperamental differences in infants, some of the burden of guilt will be lifted. She will be able to accept her infant as being hard to manage. Understanding—which is the beginning of acceptance and respect for a child as an individual—is essential for successful childrearing.

Bonding

Bonding is the initial psychosocial reaction that takes place between parents and a child in which parents "claim" or identify with the infant as "their" infant; in other words, they match the visual image they carried with them during pregnancy with a particular child. Steps of bonding, beginning with fingertip touch and climaxing in a lasting, deep relationship, are discussed in Chapter 30. Although bonding is primarily a relationship influenced by what the parents bring to the relationship (whether they are ready to be parents, whether they have a capacity to love, their goals and expectations of the child, unusual happenings during pregnancy such as a move or loss of a job that interfered with the process), the infant also contributes to whether bonding will occur readily or with difficulty. These are important contributions: Where some of the problems of poor bonding that occur from the parents' standpoint can be solved, those that stem from the infant are much more difficult to solve. He or she cannot change to accommodate or become the parents' idealized child. (See the Nursing Research Highlight above.)

Major among the factors that contribute to poor bonding is an infant being of a different sex than was expected. Spend time talking to parents about whether they had a preference for one sex or the other. Help them to find positive things about having a child of the opposite sex than they desired (bedroom space will be easier, the father will enjoy having a son to role model for, etc.). Point out positive attributes about the child as you give care (hair is curly, her disposition is good).

Sex Stereotyping

In previous generations, boys and girls were raised very differently, not only in the way they were handled, but in the types of toys and clothing purchased for them as well. This early indoctrination contributed to sexual stereotypes such as women being less assertive and men having the power and decision-making ability. Stereotypic qualities such as these put women at a disadvantage; if women were more assertive, perhaps situations such as wife abuse would be less frequent.

Helping new parents to limit sex stereotyping (choosing pink for girls, blue for boys, baseball bats for boys, dolls for girls, etc.) from the first days of their child's life is an action that can help promote sexual equality for the next generation.

Utilizing Nursing Process

Many mothers have not thought ahead to what their newborn is going to be like (he or she was only a vague, hard-to-visualize being all during pregnancy); they are surprised to hear that their infant is an individual and has a unique personality from the start. Some mothers know so little about newborns they believe they are born with their eyes closed like kittens or at least without vision (and therefore have not done much planning about infant stimulation during pregnancy). In order that they can fully appreciate their child's needs and individuality, interventions should be planned and comprehensive.

Assessment

Assess a mother's interactions with her new child at each contact with her; include not only the length of time she spends with the child but the quality of the relationship (Does she hold the baby? Talk to him? Does she only observe her from across the room?). Assess her general knowledge of newborns because, as a rule, the more she knows, the easier it will be for her to begin interaction. Encourage her to keep her infant with her for the majority of the day so she has time to get acquainted and begin to appreciate individual differences in her child.

Analysis

The North American Nursing Diagnosis Association accepted one diagnosis specific for newborns:

"Parenting, alterations in: actual or potential." The defining characteristics of this diagnosis are shown in the box on page 611. A well diagnosis such as "Bonding well established, related to well newborn" may be appropriate. Help mothers to set realistic goals for their interventions with newborns based on the newborns' capabilities.

Planning

As a lot of helping a mother learn more about her infant's personality is teaching her about normal newborns, planning includes finding ways that time for individual teaching can be incorporated into a day.

Implementation

During procedures such as teaching breast- or formula feeding, make a point of stressing that all procedures will need to be modified after the mother returns home, based on the individual preferences of her newborn. Be certain you role model good infant care (holding infants warmly, not clinically), as an unsure mother watches you very carefully for guidance.

Evaluation

Evaluation should include whether the infant's individual characteristics can be identified and whether nursing care has been modified enough to accommodate the characteristics of an individual child.

Nursing Care Planning

John Kraft is a 1-day-old baby you care for.

Assessment

Mother states: "I thought he'd be bigger. He felt a lot bigger inside me." Father concerned because he heard a nurse say the baby has "downy hair." As Mrs. Kraft has a sister with Down's syndrome, he wondered if someone was trying to tell him his son has Down's syndrome, and he asked how soon someone will be able to test him for IQ.

Analysis

Potential for interference with bonding related to parental concern over infant's health.

Locus of Decision Making. Parents.

Goal. Parents to accept newborn as well baby by 1 week of age.

Criteria. Parents hold baby warmly and voice positive comments about his progress.

Nursing Orders

1. Ask M.D. to confirm that child does not have Down's syndrome.
2. Demonstrate newborn's alert behaviors such as following finger, listening to voice.
3. Review parents' information base about normal newborns.
4. Encourage parents to voice any other concerns they have so these can be relieved and allow parent-child bonding to be optimal.

Questions for Review

Multiple Choice

1. Mrs. Valandos is a 22-year-old mother who feels badly that she is not as assertive a person as she would like to be. What advice would you give her to help her newborn daughter be more secure and confident?

   a. "Don't hurry to meet her needs so she learns to express herself."

   b. "Expose your daughter to new faces at least once a week."

   c. "Provide a consistent, stable environment for her."

   d. "Allow her to cry for 15 minutes each time before picking her up."

2. Mrs. Valandos asks you when she can expect her infant to return her smile. Based on normal development, your best answer would be

   a. 1–2 weeks.

   b. 4–6 weeks.

   c. 8–12 weeks.

   d. 12–16 weeks.

3. Mr. Valandos asks you about the best newborn toy. Based on newborn abilities, which of the following would you suggest?

   a. blocks for stacking

   b. a mobile to hang over her crib

   c. colored marbles to fit into a bottle

   d. a box that makes a piercing sound when opened

4. Mrs. Valandos will need childcare 2 days a week in order to return to work. Which suggestion below would you make to her concerning this?

   a. Using family members would be an ideal choice.

   b. She should employ one person consistently.

   c. A day care center with varied caregivers is stimulating.

   d. An older woman will supply the mothering she is unable to give.

5. The developmental task of the first year is to form a sense of trust. This task consists of learning

   a. to love and be loved.

   b. what kind of person you are.

   c. to reason objectively.

   d. where you fit into the world.

6. Bonding is the process that lays the basis for a sense of trust. Which comment by Mrs. Valandos would best make you believe she is bonding well?

   a. She spends her time observing her baby in the nursery.

   b. She holds her infant to bottle-feed her.

   c. She bought an expensive going-home dress for her.

   d. She is concerned that the baby's hair will not be curly.

Discussion

1. Suppose parents have a first child with an easy temperament and a second child with a difficult temperament. What problems can you anticipate they will have raising the second child? What suggestions could you make to them?

2. Encouraging the formation of a sense of trust in an infant is a parenting responsibility. What suggestions could you make to new parents about this?

3. Based on the developmental changes in the first 3 months of life, what safety points would you want to be certain a mother was planning to provide?

Suggested Readings

Carey, W. (1970). A simplified method for measuring infant temperament. *Journal of Pediatrics, 77,* 188.

Dunn, D. M., et al. (1981). Interaction of mothers with their newborns in the first half hour of life. *Journal of Advances in Nursing, 6,* 27.

Duvall, E. M. (1971). *Family development* (4th ed.). Philadelphia: Lippincott.

Erikson, E. (1963). *Childhood and society* (2nd ed.). New York: Norton.

Fraleigh, D. (1984). Combined mother-baby care. *Canadian Nurse, 80,* 25.

Furr, P. A., et al. (1982). A nurse-midwifery approach to early mother-infant acquaintance. *Journal of Nurse Midwifery, 27,* 10.

Harlow, H. F., & Zimmerman, R. (1970). Affectional responses in the infant monkey. In P. Mussen, J. Conger, & J. Kagan (Eds.). *Readings in child development and personality* (2nd ed.). New York: Harper & Row.

Klaus, M. H., et al. (1970). Human maternal behavior at the first contact with her young. *Pediatrics, 46,* 187.

Klaus, M. H., & Kennell, J. H. (1970). Mothers separated from their newborn infants. *Pediatric Clinics of North America, 17,* 1015.

Mansell, K. A. (1984). Mother-baby units: The concept works. *M.C.N., 9,* 132.

Newton, L. D. (1983). Helping parents cope with infant crying. *J.O.G.N. Nursing, 12,* 199.

Oliver, C. M., et al. (1978). Gentle birth: Its safety and its effect on neonatal behavior. *J.O.G.N. Nursing, 7,* 35.

Perry, S. E. (1983). Parents' perceptions of their newborn following structured interactions. *Nursing Research, 32,* 208.

Provence, S. (1968). Developmental history. In R. Cooke and S. Levin (Eds.). *The biologic basis of pediatric practice* (Vol. 2). New York: McGraw-Hill.

Sholder, D. A. (1981). Portrait of a newborn: Preconceived ideas that ten primigravidas have of their newborn's appearance. *J.O.G.N. Nursing, 10,* 98.

Skerrett, K., et al. (1983). Infant anxiety. *Maternal Child Nursing Journal, 12,* 51.

Thomas, A., et al. (1971). *Behavioral individuality in early childhood.* New York: New York University Press.

31

Physiologic Development in the Newborn

OBJECTIVES

Following mastery of the contents of this chapter, you should be able to

1. Describe normal height and weight parameters in the newborn.
2. Describe body system changes that occur as an adjustment to extrauterine life.
3. Describe neurologic function and reflexes of a newborn.
4. Describe the normal appearance of a newborn.
5. Analyze nursing measures that help the newborn adjust to extrauterine life.
6. Synthesize knowledge of newborn physiology with nursing process to achieve quality maternal-newborn nursing care.

NEWBORNS UNDERGO many profound physiologic changes at the moment of birth and probably psychological changes as well. They are released from a warm, snug, darkened, liquid-filled environment in which all their basic needs are met. Suddenly they are in a chilly, glaring, unbounded, gravity-based, outside world.

Within minutes of being plunged into this strange environment, a newborn's body must initiate respirations and accommodate the circulatory system to extrauterine oxygenation. Within 24 hours neurologic, renal, endocrine, gastrointestinal, and metabolic functions must be operating competently in order for life to be sustained.

How well a newborn can achieve these major adjustments will depend on his or her genetic endowment, the competency of the intrauterine environment, the concern and management received during the labor and delivery period, and the concern and management received as a neonate or during the *neonatal period* (the time from birth through the first 28 days of life). Nursing has a major contribution to make at all these stages.

Two thirds of infant deaths occur in the neonatal period. Over half occur in the first 24 hours after birth—an indication of how hazardous a time this is for the infant and the close observation for indications of distress needed at this time.

A Newborn Profile

It is not unusual to hear the comment that "all newborns are alike" from people viewing a nursery full of babies. In actuality, every child is born with individual physical and personality characteristics that make him or her unique right from the start.

Some infants are born stocky and short, some large and bony, some thin and rangy. Some have a temperament that causes them to feed greedily, protest procedures loudly, and perhaps respond to their mother's inexperienced handling with restlessness and spitting up. Other infants appear to protest little, to sleep soundly, to accept passively this new step in life. As you gain experience in working with newborns, it becomes easier to differentiate infants who are merely demonstrating the extremes of normal newborn characteristics from those whose behavior or appearance indicates a need for more skilled care than is available in normal nursery surroundings.

Weight

The birth weight of newborn infants differs, depending on the racial, nutritional, intrauterine, and genetic factors that were present during conception and pregnancy. The weight in relation to the gestation age should be plotted on a standard neonatal graph like the one shown in Figure 31-1, so that it can be interpreted meaningfully. Plotting in this manner helps to identify infants at risk and to separate those who are small for their gestation age (children who have suffered intrauterine growth retardation) from low-birth-weight infants (infants who are a good weight for their gestation age, formerly termed *premature*). These first measurements also serve to establish a baseline for future measurements.

A reason for plotting weight, height, and head circumference is to point out disproportionate measurements (see Appendix H). All three of these measurements should fall close to the same percentile for the same child. An infant who falls within the fiftieth percentile for height and weight and whose head circumference is in the ninetieth percentile may have abnormal head growth. A newborn who is in the fiftieth percentile for weight and head circumference but in the third percentile for height may have a growth problem such as achondroplastic dwarfism.

As a rule of thumb, Caucasian newborns generally weigh approximately a half pound more than children of other races (probably because of better nutrition in the mother during pregnancy). Sec-

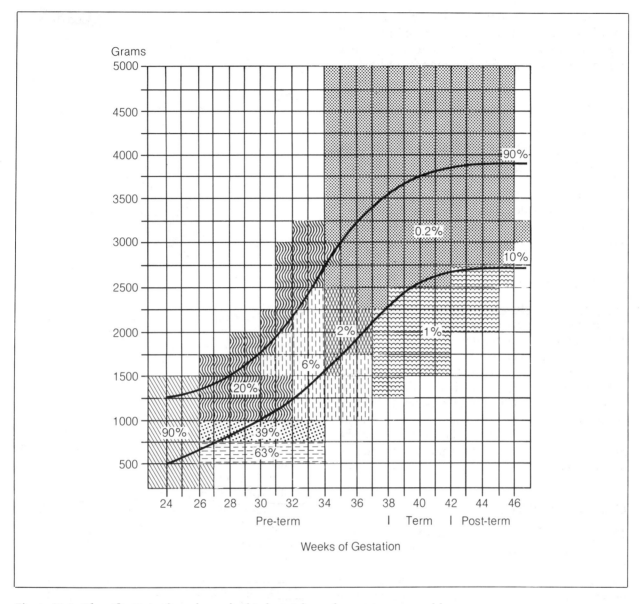

Figure 31-1 *Classification of newborns by birth weight and gestation age and by neonatal mortality risk. From Koops, B. L., Morgan, L. J., & Battaglia, F. C. (1982). Neonatal mortality risk in relation to birth weight and gestational age: An update.* Journal of Pediatrics, *101, 969.*

ond children generally weigh more than first-borns; weight continues to increase with each succeeding child in a family.

The average birth weight (the fiftieth percentile) for a white mature female newborn is 3.4 kg (7.5 pounds) and for a white mature male newborn, 3.5 kg (7.7 pounds). The arbitrary lower limit of normal is 2.5 kg (5.5 pounds). Under this weight the child is termed a low-birth-weight infant and is given high-risk priority. Birth weight exceeding 4.7 kg (10 pounds) is unusual, but weights as high as 7.7 kg (17 pounds) have been documented. When an infant over 4.7 kg is born, a maternal illness such as diabetes mellitus must be suspected.

The newborn loses 5 to 10 percent of birth weight (6 to 10 ounces) during the first few days after birth. This weight loss occurs because the infant is no longer under the influence of maternal hormones (which are salt- and fluid-retaining); he or she voids and passes stools; and intake until about the third day of life is limited by the relatively low caloric content of colostrum, the fluid preceding breast milk (or feeding of glucose water if bottle-fed). The infant may also have difficulty in establishing sucking.

Following this initial loss of weight, the newborn has one day of stable weight and then will begin to gain about 2 pounds a month (6 to 8 ounces weekly) for the first 6 months of life.

Length

The average birth length (the fiftieth percentile) of a white mature infant female is 53 cm (20.9 inches). For white mature males it is 54 cm (21.3 inches). The lower limit of normal length is arbitrarily set at 46 cm (18 inches). Below this limit the child is considered to be preterm. Babies with a length as great as 57.5 cm (23 inches) have been reported.

Head Circumference

The head circumference is 34 to 35 cm (13.5 to 14.0 inches) in a mature newborn. A mature newborn with a head circumference greater than 37 cm or less than 33 cm (14.8 or 13.2 inches) should be carefully investigated for neurologic damage, although occasionally a newborn will fall within these limits and still be perfectly normal. Head circumference is measured with a tape measure drawn across the center of the forehead and the most prominent portion of the posterior head (the occiput) (Figure 31-2).

Chest Circumference

The chest circumference in a newborn is about 2 cm (¾ to 1 inch) less than head circumference. It is measured at the level of the nipples. If a large amount of breast tissue or edema of the breasts is present, this measurement will not be accurate until the initial edema has subsided.

Vital Signs

Temperature

The temperature of newborns is about 37.2°C (99°F) at the moment of birth because they have been confined in an internal body organ. Their temperature falls almost immediately to below normal because of (a) heat loss, and (b) immature temperature-regulating mechanisms. The 21° to 22°C (68° to 72°F) temperature of delivery rooms can add to this. Newborns lose heat by four separate mechanisms: convection, conduction, radiation, and evaporation.

Convection is the flow of heat from the body surface to cooler surrounding air. The effectiveness of convection depends on the velocity of the

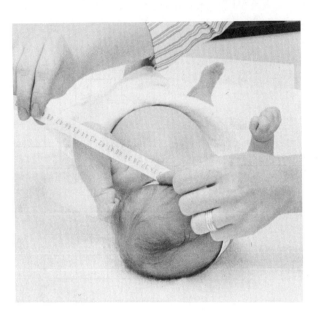

Figure 31-2 *Head circumference is measured between points just above the eyebrows to the protuberant point of the occiput. (Courtesy of the Department of Medical Photography, Children's Hospital, Buffalo, N.Y.)*

flow (a current of air cools faster than nonmoving air). Being certain that there are no drafts from windows or air conditioners reduces convection heat loss.

Conduction is the transfer of body heat to a cooler solid object in contact with the baby. If the baby were laid on a cold counter, for example, or on the cold base of a warming unit, he or she would quickly lose heat to the colder metal surface.

Radiation is the transfer of body heat to a cooler solid object *not* in contact with the baby. A baby can lose heat by radiation to cold objects such as a cold window surface or an air conditioner across the room.

Evaporation is loss of heat through conversion of a liquid to a vapor. Newborns are wet; they lose a great deal of heat as the amniotic fluid on their skin evaporates. To prevent this rapid loss of heat, they should be dried immediately. Remember to dry their faces; the head is a large surface area in an infant. Covering their wet hair with a cap reduces evaporation and radiation cooling.

A newborn not only can lose heat easily by the above means but has difficulty conserving heat under any circumstances. Insulation, an efficient means of conserving heat in adults, is not effective in newborns as they have little subcutaneous fat to provide insulation. Shivering, a means of increasing metabolism and thereby providing heat, is rarely seen in newborns.

Newborns can conserve heat by constricting

blood vessels. Brown fat, a special tissue found in mature newborns, apparently helps to conserve or produce body heat. Brown fat is found in greatest proportion in the intrascapular region, the thorax, and the perirenal area. It is thought to aid in the control of temperature in the neonate in much the same way it does in the hibernating animal. In later life it may influence the proportion of body fat retained.

Because newborns have difficulty conserving body heat, exposure to cold can be extremely detrimental at this time of life.

Infants exposed to cool air will kick and cry to increase their metabolic rate to produce more heat. This reaction, however, also increases their respiratory rate; an immature infant with poor lung development will have trouble making such an adjustment. An infant who cannot increase his respiratory rate in response to increased needs will be unable to deliver sufficient oxygen to his system. The resultant anaerobic catabolism of body cells releases acid. Every newborn is born slightly acidotic, and any new buildup of acid may lead to severe, life-threatening acidosis. The infant also becomes fatigued, and additional strain is thus placed on an already stressed cardiovascular system.

Drying and wrapping newborns and placing them in warmed cribs or drying them and placing them under a radiant heat source are the best mechanical measures to help conserve heat (Figure 31-3). All infant care should be done speedily to avoid exposing the infant unnecessarily. Any procedure during which the infant must be uncovered (e.g., resuscitation, circumcision) should be done under a radiant heat source to prevent damaging heat loss. If chilling is prevented, a newborn's temperature stabilizes at 37°C (98.6°F) within 4 hours after birth.

A few newborns run a transient fever between the second and fourth days of life; the temperature may rise as high as 40°C (104°F). The infant's skin will be dry, the fontanelles may be sunken, and urinary output may be decreased. This reaction tends to occur in infants who do not suck well or who for other reasons receive a lower-than-normal fluid intake during the first few days of life. The lowered intake, along with normal water loss, leads to a physiologic fever. The condition can be relieved by increasing the amount of formula or giving water between breast-feedings. If oral intake is a problem, intravenous fluid may be given. With the increase in fluid, the dehydration and symptomatic fever disappear.

A newborn who has a bacterial infection may, in contrast to an adult, run a subnormal temperature. Therefore, when a neonate's temperature does not stabilize shortly after birth, the cause should be investigated so that corrective measures can be taken.

Pulse

The heart rate in utero averages 120 to 160 beats per minute. Immediately after birth, as a newborn struggles to initiate respirations, the heart rate may be as rapid as 180 beats per minute. Within an hour after birth, as the infant settles down to sleep, the heart rate falls to an average of 120 to 140 beats per minute, where it stabilizes.

The heart rate of a neonate is often irregular because of immaturity of the cardiac regulatory center in the medulla. Transient murmurs may be due to the incomplete closure of fetal circulation shunts. During crying, the rate may rise again to 180 beats per minute.

The femoral pulses can be felt readily in a newborn, but the radial and temporal pulses are more difficult to palpate with any degree of accuracy. Thus, a newborn's heart rate should always be determined by listening for an apical heartbeat for a full minute. It is important that the femoral pulses be palpated, since their absence suggests possible coarctation (narrowing) of the aorta.

Respiration

The respiratory rate of a newborn in the first few minutes of life may be as high as 80 respirations

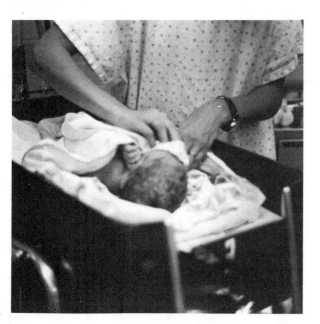

Figure 31-3 *Drying and wrapping a newborn reduces the amount of heat lost as it protects against evaporation.*

per minute. As respiratory activity is established and maintained, the rate settles to an average of 30 to 50 per minute when the child is at rest. Respiratory depth, rate, and rhythm are likely to be irregular, and short periods of apnea (without cyanosis) that may occur are normal. Respiration can be observed most easily by watching the movement of the abdomen, since breathing primarily involves the use of the diaphragm and abdominal muscles.

Coughing and sneezing reflexes are present at birth to clear the airway. Neonates are nose-breathers and show signs of acute distress if the nostrils become obstructed. Short periods of crying increase the depth of respiration and aid in aerating deep portions of the lungs and so are beneficial to the newborn. Long periods of crying exhaust the cardiovascular system and have no purpose. This is an important fact for the mother to know.

Blood Pressure

The blood pressure of a newborn is approximately 80/46 mm Hg at birth. By the tenth day it rises to about 100/50 mm Hg. Blood pressure is not routinely measured in newborns unless certain cardiac anomalies are suspected. The blood pressure readings in the newborn are somewhat inaccurate. The cuff width used must be no more than two thirds the length of the upper arm or thigh for any degree of accuracy to be achieved. The blood pressure tends to increase with crying (and a newborn cries when disturbed and manipulated by such procedures as taking blood pressure).

A flush method may be used to take blood pressures in infants: Apply a blood pressure cuff to the child's upper arm or the thigh. Wrap the portion of the extremity distal to the cuff with an Ace bandage. Inflate the blood pressure cuff to about 200 mm Hg of pressure; remove the Ace bandage. The skin distal to the cuff will appear pale. Release pressure in the cuff slowly until the distal portion of the extremity flushes (becomes pink). Read the manometer at this point. Flush pressure is about halfway between systolic and diastolic blood pressure. If the newborn's blood pressure is 80/40, for example, the flush pressure will be about 60 (Figure 31-4). Table 31-1 shows normal flush readings.

Newer ultrasonic or Doppler methods of taking blood pressure are effective with newborns and more accurate than traditional measuring. A Doppler technique bounces high frequency sound waves off body parts; the rate and pitch at which they return depend on the density of the body part

Figure 31-4 *Technique for measuring flush blood pressure. A. A blood pressure cuff is applied. The distal extremity is wrapped snugly with an Ace bandage. B. The blood pressure cuff is inflated; the Ace bandage is removed. C. As pressure in the cuff is released, the pressure at which the distal extremity "flushes" or pinkens is the flush blood pressure. (Courtesy of the Department of Medical Illustration, State University of New York at Buffalo.)*

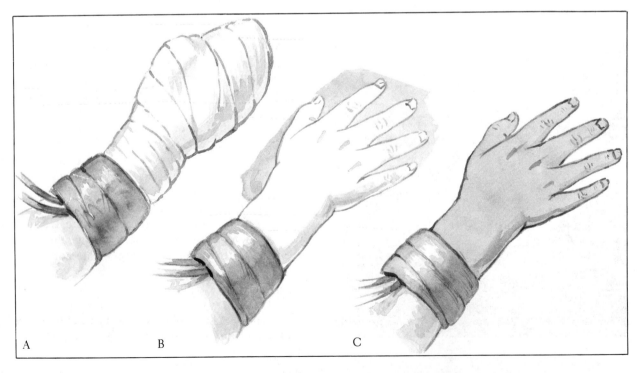

A   B   C

Table 31-1 Flush Blood Pressure in Infant Arm

| Age | Blood Pressure (mm Hg) | |
	Average	Range
1–7 days	41	22–66
1–3 months	67	48–90
4–6 months	73	42–100
7–9 months	76	52–96
10–12 months	76	62–94

Source: From Moss, A. J. (1978). Indirect methods of blood pressure measurement. *Pediatr. Clin. North Am., 25,* 3.

that is struck. If a Doppler lead is placed over an artery, either the movement of the blood (pulse wave) or the tension of the blood (blood pressure) can be interpreted as a digital readout or a monitor print. Electronic blood pressure recording is not used with well newborns but is helpful when an almost continuous assessment is necessary in high-risk infants.

Cardiovascular System

Changes in the cardiovascular system are necessary at birth because the blood was formerly oxygenated by the placenta and now must be oxygenated by the lungs. When the cord is clamped, a newborn is forced to take in oxygen through the lungs. As the lungs are inflated for the first time, pressure in the chest in general and particularly in the artery leading to the lungs (pulmonary artery) is greatly decreased. This decrease in pressure in the pulmonary artery plays a role in causing the ductus arteriosus to close. As pressure increases in the left side of the heart from increased blood volume, the foramen ovale closes because of the pressure against the lip of the structure. Since the remaining fetal circulatory structures—the umbilical vein, two umbilical arteries, and the ductus venosus—are no longer receiving blood, the blood within them clots, and the vessels atrophy.

Figure 31-5 shows the respiratory and cardiovascular changes at birth. These changes in the cardiovascular system begin to occur with the first breath. Table 31-2 shows the timetable of obliteration of fetal cardiovascular structures.

Total Blood Volume

As the uterus contracts after the birth of the baby, an additional 50 to 125 ml of blood is pushed into the umbilical cord and into the newborn's circulation. The cord pulsates. If the cord is cut before

the pulsating ceases, the newborn will not receive this additional blood.

On balance, additional blood appears to be helpful to most newborns. It increases the infant's store of hemoglobin for the months ahead when iron intake will be low because of a diet that is predominantly milk. However, the additional blood may be harmful to infants who are Rh-sensitized, since it loads them with even more maternal antibodies. Further, because infants are already polycythemic, the additional blood may lead to pulmonary edema from an overload of circulating blood. Finally, pulmonary rales and transient cyanosis appear to be associated with late clamping of the cord in some infants.

The peripheral circulation of a newborn remains sluggish for at least the first 24 hours. It is not uncommon to observe cyanosis in the feet and hands and for the feet to feel cold to the touch for this period of time (acrocyanosis).

Blood Values

A newborn's blood volume is 80 to 110 ml per kilogram of weight, or about 300 ml. The oxygen dissociation curve of fetal blood is shifted to the left (the quantity of oxygen bound to hemoglobin and partial pressure of oxygen is greater in fetal blood than after birth).

Because of the nature of fetal circulation, a baby is born with a high erythrocyte count, around 6 million per cubic millimeter. A newborn's hemoglobin level averages 17 to 18 gm per 100 ml of blood. Hematocrit is between 45 to 50 percent. Capillary heel pricks may reveal a high Hct or hemoglobin because of sluggish peripheral circulation. Warming the extremity before the blood drawing improves the accuracy of this value by increasing circulation movement.

Once proper lung oxygenation is established, the need for the high erythrocyte count diminishes. Therefore, within a matter of days, the erythrocyte count begins to fall. A bilirubin level at birth is 1 to 4 mg per 100 ml. Any increase over this amount reflects the rate of red cell breakdown.

The decrease in red blood cells reaches its lowest level at 3 months of age (the life span of red blood cells), when the hemoglobin level may be as low as 11 or 12 gm per 100 ml of blood, the total red cell count as low as 3 to 4 million per cubic millimeter. Although this is a normal decrease, an iron supplement should be added early to an infant's diet to keep the decline at a minimum.

A newborn has an equally high white blood count at birth, about 15,000 to 45,000 cells per cubic millimeter. Polymorphonuclear cells (neutrophils) account for a large part of this leukocy-

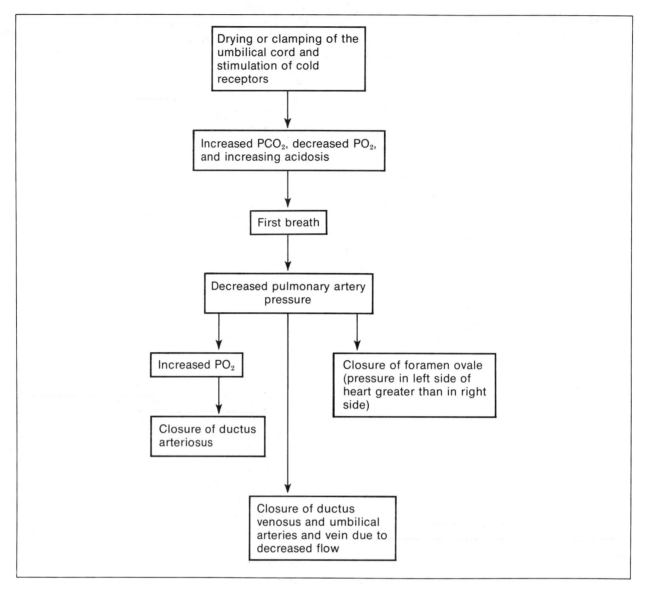

Figure 31-5 *Circulatory events at birth.*

tosis, but by the end of the first month, lymphocytes become the predominant type. It should be remembered that this leukocytosis is a response to the trauma of birth and is nonpathogenic; an increased white cell count should not be taken as evidence of infection. On the other hand, although the high white cell count makes infection difficult to prove in a newborn, infection must not be dismissed as a possibility if other signs of infection (e.g., pallor, respiratory difficulty, or cyanosis) are present.

Blood values in the newborn are summarized in Appendix G.

Blood Coagulation

The majority of newborns are born with a prolonged coagulation or prothrombin time because their blood levels of vitamin K are lower than normal. Vitamin K is synthesized through the action of intestinal flora and is necessary for the formation of Factor VII (proconvertin), Factor IX (plasma thromboplastin component), and Factor X (Stuart-Prower factor). A newborn intestine is sterile at birth unless membranes were ruptured more than 24 hours before delivery. Flora must therefore accumulate before vitamin K can be synthesized. Because almost all newborns have poor blood coagulation, vitamin K (AquaMEPHYTON) is given routinely to newborns in most hospital delivery rooms.

Respiratory System

The first breath of an infant is initiated by a combination of cold receptors, a lowered PO_2 (PO_2 falls from 80 to as low as 15 mm Hg), and an

Table 31-2 Changes in the Cardiovascular System at Birth

Structure	Approximate Time of Obliteration	Structure Remaining
Foramen ovale	1 year (probe patent)	Fossa ovalis
Ductus arteriosus	1 month	Ligamentum arteriosum
Ductus venosus	2 months	Ligamentum venosum
Umbilical arteries	2–3 months	Lateral umbilical ligament Interior iliac artery
Umbilical vein	2–3 months	Ligamentum teres (round ligament of liver)

Source: Adapted from Moore, M. L. (1972). *The newborn and the nurse.* Philadelphia: Saunders.

increased PCO_2 (PCO_2 rises as high as 70 mm Hg). A first breath requires a tremendous amount of energy to pull in. A pressure of about 40 to 70 cm H_2O is required. The presence of lung fluid is a mechanism that makes the first breath easier than if dry alveolar walls had to be pulled apart to inflate alveoli. Lung fluid is quickly absorbed by lung blood vessels and lymphatics.

Breaths following the first one are easier, requiring only about 6 to 8 cm H_2O pressure. Within 10 minutes of birth, an infant has established a good residual volume. By 10 to 12 hours of age, vital capacity is established at infant proportions. The heart in a newborn takes up proportionately more space than in an adult so the amount of lung expansion space available is proportionately limited.

An infant who is delivered by cesarean section does not have as much lung fluid expelled at birth as a baby delivered vaginally. He or she is therefore likely to have more difficulty with establishing effective respiration (excessive fluid blocks air exchange space). Infants who are immature and whose alveoli collapse each time they exhale (lack of pulmonary surfactant) have trouble in establishing effective residual capacity and so establishing effective respirations. If alveoli do not open well, an infant's cardiac system is compromised as closure of the foramen ovale and ductus arteriosus depends on free blood flow through the pulmonary artery and good oxygenation of blood. An infant who has difficulty establishing respiration at birth should be examined closely in the

postpartal period for a cardiac murmur or indication that he or she still has patent cardiac structures that did not close.

Gastrointestinal System

Although the gastrointestinal tract is usually sterile at birth, bacteria may be cultured from the intestinal tract in most babies within 5 hours after birth; at 24 hours of life they can be cultured from all babies. Bacteria enter the tract via the infant's mouth. Some mouth bacteria are airborne; others may come from vaginal secretions at the time of birth, from hospital bedding, and from contact at the breast. Accumulation of bacteria in the gastrointestinal tract is necessary for digestion as well as for the synthesis of vitamin K. Since milk, the infant's main diet for the first year, is low in vitamin K, this intestinal synthesis is necessary.

Although a newborn stomach holds 60 to 90 ml, a newborn has limited ability to digest fat and starch because the pancreatic enzymes lipase and amylase are deficient for the first few months of life. He regurgitates easily because of an immature cardiac valve. Immature liver functions may lead to lowered glucose and protein serum levels.

Stools

The first stool of the newborn is usually passed within 24 hours after birth and consists of meconium, a sticky, tar-like, blackish green, odorless material formed from mucus, vernix, lanugo, hormones, and carbohydrates that have accumulated during intrauterine life. An infant who does not pass a meconium stool by 24 hours after birth should be examined for the possibility of meconium ileus, imperforate anus, or bowel obstruction (see Chapter 46).

About the second or third day of life, in response to the feeding pattern, the newborn stool changes in color and consistency, becoming green and loose. This is termed a *transitional stool,* which may resemble diarrhea to the untrained eye. By the fourth day of life, breast-fed infants pass three or four light yellow stools per day. These are sweet-smelling, because breast milk is high in lactic acid, which reduces the amount of putrefactive organisms in the stool. An infant who receives formula usually passes two to three bright yellow stools a day. These have a slightly more noticeable odor than do breast-fed babies' stools.

When solid foods are introduced into the infant's diet, the stools again change, gradually becoming like the brown, odorous stools of adults.

An infant placed under phototherapy lights to be treated for jaundice will have bright green stools because of increased bilirubin excretion.

Make a habit of inspecting newborn stools and recording their color, consistency (soft, hard), and size (small, medium, large). If mucus is mixed with the stool, milk allergy or some other irritant factor should be suspected. Newborns with obstruction of the bile ducts will have clay-colored (gray) stools because the bile pigments do not enter the intestinal tract. If the stools remain black or tarry, intestinal bleeding should be suspected. Blood-flecked stools usually indicate an anal fissure. Occasionally, a newborn swallows some maternal blood during delivery and will either vomit fresh blood immediately after birth or pass a tarry stool in two or more days. Maternal blood may be differentiated from fetal blood by a dip stick Apt test.

Urinary System

The newborn should void within 24 hours after birth. The first voiding may be pink or dusky because of uric acid crystals that were formed in the bladder in utero. An infant who is not fed for 12 to 16 hours after birth may take a little longer to void, but the 24-hour cutoff point is a good rule of thumb. Infants who do not void within this time should be examined. Possible causes are urethral stenosis and absent kidneys or ureters.

The presence of obstruction in the urinary tract can be tested by observing the force of the urinary stream in both male and female infants. Male newborns should void forcefully, so that urine forms a small projected arc. Female newborns should void with enough force so that the urine forms a stream, and voiding is not just continuous dribbling. Urine that is projected farther than normal may also be a sign of urethral obstruction. A normal urine stream is evidence that there is no major constriction of the urinary tract and is an indication of good kidney function.

The kidneys of newborns do not concentrate urine well, and thus the urine is usually light in color and odorless. The infant is about 6 weeks of age before much control over reabsorption of fluid in tubules is evident.

A single voiding in a newborn is only about 15 ml so is easy to miss in a thick diaper; specific gravity is 1.008 to 1.010. The daily urinary output for the first one or two days is about 30 to 60 ml total. By one week, total volume has risen to about 300 ml. A small amount of protein may be present in voidings the first few days of life until kidney glomeruli more fully mature.

Autoimmune System

The newborn infant has difficulty forming antibodies against invading antigens until reaching 2 months of age. This is the reason immunizations against childhood diseases are not given to babies less than 2 months old. However, the infant at birth has antibodies (IgG) from the mother that have crossed the placenta—in most instances antibodies against poliomyelitis, measles, diphtheria, pertussis, rubella, and tetanus. There is little natural immunity transmitted against varicella (chickenpox) or herpes simplex. Hospital personnel with herpes simplex eruptions (cold sores) should not care for newborns. Herpes simplex II virus becomes systemic in the newborn, a rapidly fatal form of the disease.

Neuromuscular System

Mature newborns demonstrate general neuromuscular function by moving extremities and attempting to control head movement. Limpness or total absence of a muscular response to manipulation is never normal and suggests narcosis, shock, or cerebral injury. A newborn occasionally makes twitching or flailing movements of extremities in the absence of a stimulus because of the immaturity of the nervous system.

Reflexes

A multitude of reflexes are present and can be tested in a newborn infant. Those that can be elicited with consistency by using simple maneuvers are discussed briefly.

Blink Reflex

A blink reflex in a newborn serves the same purpose as it does in an adult, that is, to protect the eye from any object coming near it by rapid eyelid closure. It may be elicited by shining a strong light such as a flashlight or otoscope light on the eye. It can rarely be elicited by a sudden movement toward the eye.

Rooting Reflex

If a newborn's cheek is brushed or stroked near the corner of the mouth, the child will turn the head in that direction. This reflex serves to help the baby find food. As the mother holds the child and allows her breast to brush the baby's cheek, the baby will turn toward the breast. The reflex disappears about the sixth week of life. At about this time, the eyes focus steadily and a food source can be seen. Thus the reflex is no longer needed.

Sucking Reflex

When an infant's lips are touched, the baby makes a sucking motion. Thus, as the lips touch the mother's breast or a bottle, the baby sucks and so takes in food. The sucking reflex begins to diminish at about 6 months of age. It disappears immediately if it is never stimulated—for example, in a newborn with a tracheoesophageal fistula who is not allowed to take oral fluids. It can be maintained in such an infant by offering the child a pacifier after the fistula has been corrected by surgery and until oral feedings can be given normally.

Swallowing Reflex

The swallowing reflex in the newborn and in the adult is the same phenomenon. Food that reaches the posterior portion of the tongue will be automatically swallowed. (Gag, cough, and sneeze reflexes are also present in order to maintain a clear airway in the event that normal swallowing does not keep the pharynx free of obstructing mucus.)

Extrusion Reflex

If any substance is placed on the anterior portion of an infant's tongue, the baby will extrude it. This is a protective reflex to prevent the swallowing of inedible substances. The reflex disappears at about 4 months of age. Until then an infant may seem to be spitting out or refusing solid food placed in his mouth.

Palmar Grasp Reflex

When an object is placed in a newborn's palm, the child will grasp it by closing his fingers on it (Figure 31-6). Mature newborns grasp so strongly that they can actually be raised from a supine position and be suspended momentarily from an examiner's fingers. The reflex disappears at about age 6 weeks to 3 months. A baby begins to grasp meaningfully at about 3 months of age.

Plantar Grasp Reflex

When an object touches the sole of a newborn's foot at the base of the toes, the toes grasp in the same manner as the fingers do. The reflex disappears at about 8 to 9 months of age in preparation for walking, although it may be present in sleep for a longer period of time.

Step (Walk)-in-Place Reflex

When newborns are held in a vertical position and their feet touch a hard surface, they will take

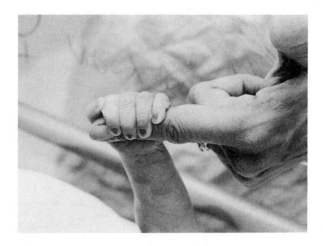

Figure 31-6 *Palmar grasp reflex. (Courtesy of the Department of Medical Photography, Children's Hospital, Buffalo, N.Y.)*

a few quick alternating steps (Figure 31-7). This reflex disappears by 3 months of age. By 4 months of age, the baby can bear a good portion of weight unhindered by this reflex.

Placing Reflex

The placing reflex is similar to the step-in-place reflex, except it is elicited by touching the anterior surface of a newborn's leg against the edge of a bassinet or table. A newborn will make a few quick lifting motions as if to step on the table.

Tonic Neck Reflex

When infants lie on their backs, their heads usually turn to one side or the other. The arm and the leg on the side to which the head turns ex-

Figure 31-7 *Step-in-place reflex. (Courtesy of the Department of Medical Photography, Children's Hospital, Buffalo, N.Y.)*

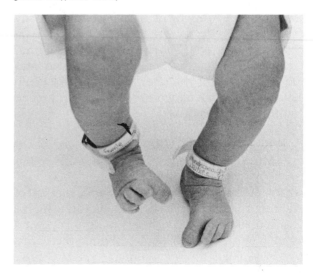

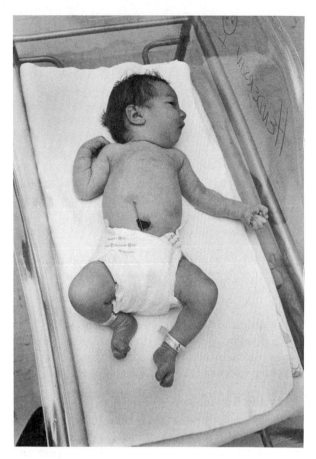

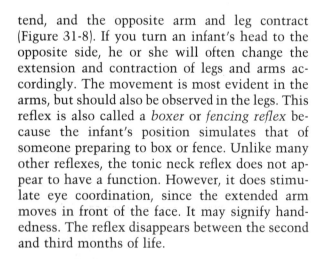

Figure 31-8 *Tonic neck reflex. (Courtesy of the Department of Medical Photography, Children's Hospital, Buffalo, N.Y.)*

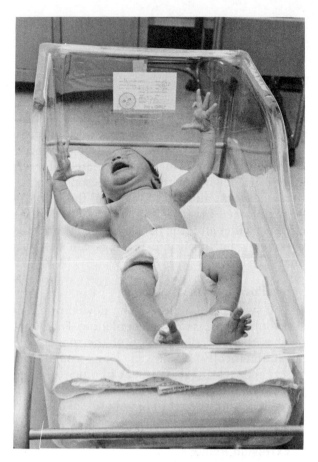

Figure 31-9 *Moro reflex. (Courtesy of the Department of Medical Photography, Children's Hospital, Buffalo, N.Y.)*

tend, and the opposite arm and leg contract (Figure 31-8). If you turn an infant's head to the opposite side, he or she will often change the extension and contraction of legs and arms accordingly. The movement is most evident in the arms, but should also be observed in the legs. This reflex is also called a *boxer* or *fencing reflex* because the infant's position simulates that of someone preparing to box or fence. Unlike many other reflexes, the tonic neck reflex does not appear to have a function. However, it does stimulate eye coordination, since the extended arm moves in front of the face. It may signify handedness. The reflex disappears between the second and third months of life.

Moro Reflex

A Moro (startle) reflex (Figure 31-9) can be initiated by startling the infant by a loud noise or by jarring the bassinet. The most accurate method of eliciting the reflex is to hold infants in a supine position and allow their heads to drop backward an inch or so. They abduct and extend their arms and legs. Their fingers assume a typical C posi-

tion. They then bring their arms into an embrace position and pull up their legs against their abdomen (adduction). The reflex simulates the action of someone trying to ward off an attacker, then covering up to protect himself. The reflex is strong for the first 8 weeks of life. It fades by the end of the fourth or fifth month, when the infant can roll away from danger.

Babinski's Reflex

When the side of the sole of a newborn's foot is stroked in an inverted J curve from the heel upward, the newborn fans his or her toes (positive Babinski sign) in contrast to the adult, who flexes the toes. This reaction occurs because of the immature stage of nervous system development. It remains positive (toes fan) until at least 3 months of age, when it is supplanted by the down-going or flexing adult response.

Magnet Reflex

If pressure is applied to the soles of the feet of an infant lying in a supine position, he or she pushes back against the pressure. This and the

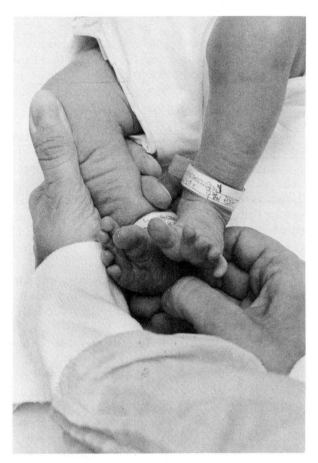

Figure 31-10 *Crossed extension reflex. When the sole of the foot is irritated, the newborn makes an attempt to push away the irritating object. (Courtesy of the Department of Medical Photography, Children's Hospital, Buffalo, N.Y.)*

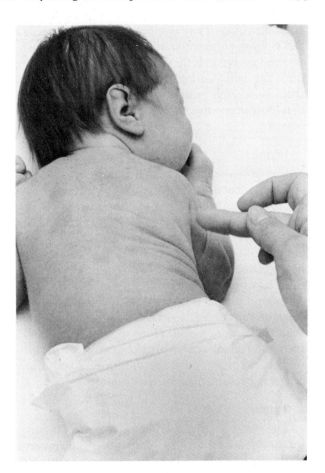

Figure 31-11 *Trunk incurvation reflex. When the paravertebral area is irritated, the newborn flexes his or her trunk. (Courtesy of the Department of Medical Photography, Children's Hospital, Buffalo, N.Y.)*

two following reflexes are tests of spinal cord integrity.

Crossed Extension Reflex

If one leg of a newborn lying supine is extended and the sole of that foot is irritated by being rubbed with a sharp object such as a thumbnail, the newborn will raise the other leg and extend it as if trying to push away the hand irritating the first leg (Figure 31-10).

Trunk Incurvation Reflex

When newborns lie in a prone position and are touched along the paravertebral area by a probing finger, they will flex their trunk and swing their pelvis toward the touch (Figure 31-11). This is an easy reflex to elicit and is another test of spinal cord integrity.

Landau Reflex

When a newborn is held in a prone position with a hand underneath supporting the trunk, he or she should demonstrate some muscle tone. While babies may not be able to lift their head or arch their back (as they will at 3 months of age), neither should they sag into an inverted U position. The latter response indicates extremely poor muscle tone, and such an infant needs referral for further investigation as to its cause.

Special Senses

Recent investigation reveals that special senses are much better developed than was previously believed.

Hearing

A newborn can hear as soon as amniotic fluid drains from or is absorbed from the middle ear by way of the eustachian tube—within hours after birth. Newborns appear to have difficulty locating sound (or at least may not turn toward a sound). Perhaps they must learn to interpret small differences between sounds arriving at their two ears at different times. They respond to a sound such as a bell ringing a short distance from their ear by generalized activity. If they are actively crying at the time the bell is rung, they will stop crying and seem to attend. Similarly, they calm in response to a soothing or motherly voice and startle at loud noises.

Vision

Newborns see as soon as they are born and possibly have been "seeing" in utero for months. As the uterus and the abdominal wall stretch at the end of pregnancy, the fetus may be able to distinguish shadowy light and dark images. Newborns demonstrate sight at birth by blinking at a strong light (blink reflex) or following a bright light or toy a short distance with their eyes. Because they cannot follow past the midline of vision, they lose track of objects easily, so it is sometimes reported that they cannot see. They focus best at 9–12 inches on black and white objects; at 3 months they can follow past the midline. A pupillary reflex is present from birth.

Touch

The sense of touch is well developed at birth. Infants demonstrate this ability by quieting at a soothing touch and by the presence of sucking and rooting reflexes, which are elicited by touch. They react to painful stimuli.

Taste

Taste buds are developed and functioning before birth to such an extent that a newborn has discriminatory ability. A fetus in utero will swallow amniotic fluid more rapidly than usual if glucose is added to sweeten its taste; the swallowing will decrease in amount if a bitter flavor is added. A newborn will turn away from a bitter taste such as salt but will readily accept the sweet taste of milk or glucose water.

Smell

The sense of smell is present in a newborn as soon as the nose is clear of mucus and amniotic fluid. Newborns turn toward their mothers' breast partly out of recognition of the smell of breast milk and partly as a manifestation of the rooting reflex.

Appearance of the Newborn

Skin

Inspection of the skin of a newborn reveals many findings that are characteristic of the newborn period.

Color

Most mature newborns have a ruddy complexion because of the increased concentration of red blood cells in blood vessels and the decrease in the amount of subcutaneous fat, which makes the blood vessels more visible.

Cyanosis. The infant's lips, hands, and feet are very likely to appear cyanotic from immature peripheral circulation. Acrocyanosis is so prominent in some infants that a line seems to be drawn across the wrist or ankle, with pink skin on one side and blue on the other, as if some stricture were cutting off circulation. This is a normal phenomenon in the first 24 to 48 hours after birth.

Generalized mottling of the skin is common. Generalized cyanosis, however, is always a cause for concern, since it usually indicates an underlying disease state.

It is important to observe an infant in both a quiet and a crying state. A newborn with atelectasis may be cyanotic when quiet and grow pink when crying and aerating a larger number of alveoli. Infants with congenital heart disease, on the other hand, usually demonstrate the opposite pattern. Such an infant has normal color when quiet but becomes cyanotic when the activity of crying demands better oxygen transport than the damaged heart is able to supply.

Newborns are nose-breathers. Any infant whose posterior nares are obstructed by membrane or bone (bilateral choanal atresia) will be cyanotic, the degree of cyanosis depending on the extent of obstruction. You can help diagnose the cause of this form of cyanosis by holding a wisp of cotton in front of one of the nares (after compressing the opposite naris and closing the infant's mouth) and observing the cotton for movement on inspiration and expiration. Obstruction can also be detected by an infant's discomfort or by holding a stethoscope diaphragm next to the nares and listening for the sound of moving air.

Mucus obstructing the respiratory tract will cause sudden cyanosis and apnea in a newborn who had previously had a good color. Suctioning the mucus relieves the condition. Suctioning may be performed through the mouth if there appears to be a large amount of mucus at the back of the throat, but the nose should be suctioned as well because in the infant this is the chief conduit for air.

Cyanosis may result because of damage to the infant's central nervous system at birth. However, if such damage is the cause, the infant usually has other manifestations of damage as well: a very rigid or floppy muscle tone, a poor Apgar score, absence of a strong Moro reflex, or perhaps a high-pitched cry.

Pallor. Pallor in newborns is usually the result of anemia. Anemia may be due to the following: excessive blood loss at the time the cord was cut; inadequate flow of blood from the cord into the infant at birth; fetal-maternal transfusion; low iron stores caused by poor maternal nutrition during pregnancy; or blood incompatibility in which a large number of red blood cells were hemolyzed in utero. It may be the result of internal bleeding (the baby should be watched closely for signs of blood in stools or vomitus). Infants with central nervous system damage may appear pale as well as cyanotic. A gray color in newborns is generally indicative of infection. Twins may be born with a twin transfusion phenomenon, in which one twin is larger and has good color and the smaller twin has pallor.

Jaundice. Jaundice appears in about 50 percent of all newborns as a normal process of the breakdown of fetal red blood cells (physiologic jaundice). The infant's skin and sclera of the eyes become yellow in color.

A fetus has a high red blood cell count to provide for more efficient oxygen and carbon dioxide transport while in utero. As red blood cells are destroyed (the high hemoglobin level immediately begins to be reduced), heme and globin are released. Globin is a protein component that is reused by the body and so is not a factor in the developing jaundice. Heme is further broken down into iron (which is also reused and so is not involved in the jaundice) and protoporphyrin. Protoporphyrin is further broken down into indirect bilirubin. Indirect bilirubin is fat-soluble and cannot be excreted by the kidneys in this state. It is therefore converted by the liver enzyme glucuronyl transferase into direct bilirubin, which is water-soluble, is incorporated into stool, and excreted in feces. In many newborn infants, liver function is so immature that the conversion to direct bilirubin cannot be made, and it therefore remains bilirubin in the indirect form. When the level of indirect bilirubin rises above 7 mg per 100 ml, bilirubin permeates tissue outside the circulatory system, and the infant begins to appear jaundiced. As long as the bilirubin remains in the circulatory system, the red of the red blood cells obscures its color.

If the level of indirect bilirubin rises above 10 to 12 mg per 100 ml, treatment should be considered. It is important that the level not rise above 20 mg per 100 ml. At this point, bilirubin interferes with the chemical synthesis of brain cells and causes permanent cell damage, a condition termed *kernicterus*, which will leave permanent neurologic effects and possibly will cause mental retardation. If treatment for physiologic jaundice in newborns is necessary, early feeding (to speed passage of feces through the intestine and prevent reabsorption of bilirubin from the bowel) and phototherapy (exposure of the infant to light to initiate maturation of liver enzymes) are the means generally instituted (see Chapter 47).

Some breast-fed babies have more difficulty in converting indirect bilirubin to direct bilirubin than do formula-fed babies because breast milk contains pregnanediol (a metabolite of progesterone), which depresses the action of glucuronyl transferase. Although stopping nursing in the first week of life must never be a decision taken lightly, if the level of indirect bilirubin rises above 10 mg per 100 ml, breast-feeding is usually halted for 1 to 2 days until the level falls again. If the mother expresses her milk manually for the few days that she is not breast-feeding, so that her milk supply does not decline, high indirect bilirubin is not a contraindication to breast-feeding.

Physiologic jaundice generally occurs on the second or third day of life. Jaundice occurring in an infant under 24 hours old is usually a result of a blood incompatibility reaction. The old rule that jaundice is serious in an infant under 24 hours of age but not in one over 24 hours is not an adequate assessment standard. No matter what the cause of jaundice, the level of indirect bilirubin must not be allowed to rise to damaging heights if the well-being and mental capabilities of the child are to be protected. Jaundice can be assessed grossly by inspection. Discoloration from jaundice begins in the head and is evident in the trunk and lower extremities only when it is extensive (Figure 31-12).

Many hospital laboratories do not report indirect bilirubin levels; they report only the total bilirubin and the direct bilirubin level. To reveal the indirect level, you subtract the direct level from the total level report.

Harlequin Sign. Occasionally, because of immature circulation, an infant who has been lying on his side will appear red on the dependent side of the body and pale on the upper side, as if a line had been drawn down the center of his body. This is a transient phenomenon and, although startling, of no clinical significance. The odd coloring fades immediately if the position is changed or the baby kicks or cries vigorously.

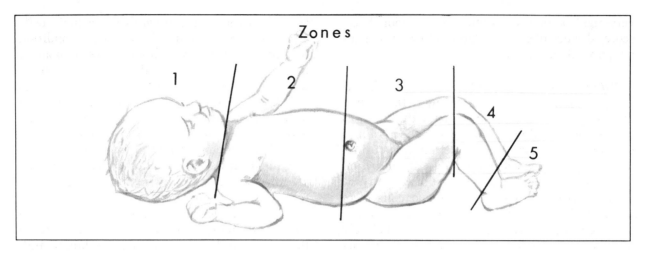

Figure 31-12 *Jaundice may be estimated to some degree by the zone on the child that it has reached. The indirect bilirubin level of zone 1 is 4 to 8 mg/100 ml; of zone 2, 5 to 12 mg/100 ml; of zone 3, 8 to 16 mg/100 ml; of zone 4, 11 to 18 mg/100 ml; of zone 5, 15 mg/100 ml. Based on data from Kramer, L. I. (1969). Advancement of dermal icterus in the jaundiced newborn. American Journal of Diseases of Children, 118, 454.*

Birthmarks

A number of commonly occurring birthmarks can be identified in newborns.

Hemangiomas. The hemangiomas are vascular tumors of the skin. Three separate types are found.

Nevus flammeus (Figure 31-13) is a macular purple or dark-red lesion (sometimes termed *port-wine stain* because of its deep color) that is present at birth. The lesions generally appear on the

Figure 31-13 *Nevus flammeus (port-wine stain) formed of a plexus of newly formed capillaries in the papillary layer of the corium. It is deep red to purple, does not blanch on pressure, and does not fade with age. (Reproduced with permission of Mead Johnson & Company, Evansville, Ind.)*

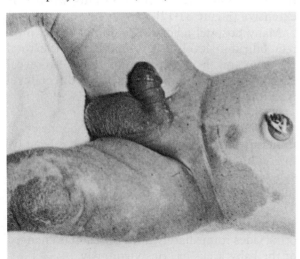

face, although they are often found on the thighs as well. Lesions above the bridge of the nose tend to fade; the others are less likely to. Because they are level with the skin surface (macular), they can be covered by a cosmetic preparation later in life or can be removed surgically.

Nevus flammeus lesions also occur as a lighter, pink patch at the nape of the neck (termed a *stork's beak mark*) (Figure 31-14). These lighter nevus flammeus lesions do not fade either but are covered by the hairline and so are of no consequence. They occur more often in girls than boys.

Strawberry hemangiomas are elevated areas formed by immature capillaries and endothelial cells (Figure 31-15). Most are present at birth, although they may appear up to 2 weeks following birth. Formation is associated with the high estro-

Figure 31-14 *Stork's beak mark, commonly occurring on nape of neck. It blanches on pressure; although it does not fade, it is covered by hair. (Reproduced with permission of Mead Johnson & Company, Evansville, Ind.)*

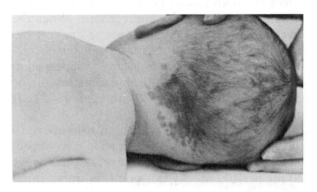

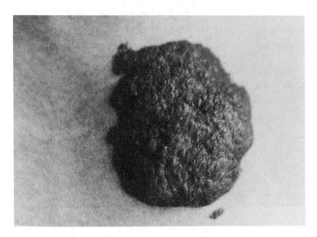

Figure 31-15 *Strawberry hemangiomas consist of dilated capillaries in entire dermal and subdermal layers. They continue to enlarge after birth but usually disappear by age 10 years. (Reproduced with permission of Mead Johnson & Company, Evansville, Ind.)*

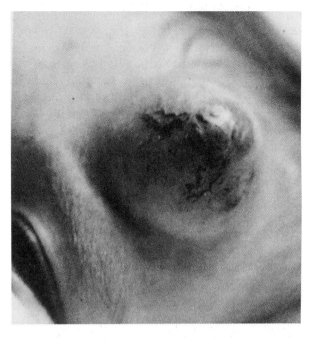

Figure 31-16 *Cavernous hemangiomas consist of a communicating network of venules in subcutaneous tissue and do not fade with age. (Reproduced with permission of Mead Johnson & Company, Evansville, Ind.)*

gen levels of pregnancy. They may continue to enlarge from their original size up to 1 year of age. After the first year they tend to be absorbed and shrink in size. By the time the child is 7 years old, 50 to 75 percent of these lesions have disappeared. A child may be 10 years old before the absorption is complete. Application of cortisone ointment may speed their disappearance by interfering with the binding of estrogen to its receptor sites.

It is important for a mother to understand that the mark may grow; otherwise, she may confuse it with cancer (a skin lesion increasing in size is one of the seven danger signals of cancer). She should also understand that the mark will disappear. This second concept keeps her from thinking of her child as imperfect or disfigured. Surgery to remove them may lead to secondary infection, leaving scarring and permanent disfigurement.

Cavernous hemangiomas (Figure 31-16) are formed of dilated vascular spaces. They are usually raised and resemble a strawberry hemangioma in appearance. They do not disappear. They can be removed surgically. Cavernous hemangiomas may bleed internally, leading to hyperbilirubinemia or anemia. Children who have one obvious skin lesion may have additional lesions on internal organs. Blows to the abdomen such as occur in childhood games, therefore, can cause bleeding from internal hemangiomas.

It is important to learn to differentiate the various types of hemangiomas so that you neither give false reassurances to parents nor worry them unnecessarily about these lesions.

Mongolian Spots. Mongolian spots are slate-gray patches seen across the sacrum or buttocks

and consist of a collection of pigment cells (melanocytes). They tend to occur in children of Asian, southern European, or African extraction. They disappear by school age without treatment. The mother should be told that they are not bruises, since she may be concerned that her baby has a "weak back" or has sustained a birth injury.

Vernix Caseosa

Vernix caseosa, the white cream-cheese-like substance that serves as a skin lubricant, is usually noticeable on a newborn's skin, at least in the skin folds, for the first 2 or 3 days of life. The color of the vernix should be carefully noted, since it takes on the color of the amniotic fluid. If it is yellow, the amniotic fluid was yellow from bilirubin; if it is green, meconium in the amniotic fluid is indicated. In most instances, the color of the amniotic fluid is noted in the labor room or delivery room. However, if the membranes ruptured while the mother was at home, so that the color of the amniotic fluid was not observed, the color of the vernix may provide this information. It is important information to have because the color of the amniotic fluid may suggest the presence of erythroblastosis neonatorum or fetal distress (see Chapter 47).

Vernix caseosa is gradually absorbed by the newborn's skin, and part of it is washed away with each bath. Whether it should be washed away or not is controversial. Although it protects delicate skin from abrasions, it may be a breeding ground for bacteria. For cosmetic reasons, mothers usually prefer that it be washed off, particularly if it is blood-stained from the delivery. Harsh rubbing should never be employed, however, because the newborn's skin is tender, and breaks in the skin from too vigorous attempts to remove the vernix may open portals of entry for bacteria.

Lanugo

Lanugo is the fine downy hair that covers a newborn's shoulders, back, and upper arms. The immature child (37 to 39 weeks' gestation age) has more lanugo than the mature infant; postmature infants rarely have lanugo. Most mothers are familiar with lanugo, but occasionally a mother may worry because her small baby girl has thick, almost gorilla-like hair on her arms. Lanugo is rubbed away by the friction of bedding and clothes against the newborn's skin. By age 2 weeks it has disappeared, never to return.

Desquamation

Within 24 hours of birth, the skin of most newborns has become extremely dry. The dryness is particularly evident on the palms of the hands and the soles of the feet. It may result in areas of peeling similar to those following a sunburn. This is normal and needs no treatment. If a mother wishes, she may apply some hand or body lotion to lubricate the dry areas.

Infants who are postmature or have suffered intrauterine malnutrition have extremely dry skin with a leathery appearance and cracking in the skin folds. This should be differentiated from normal desquamation.

Milia

Newborn sebaceous glands are immature. At least one pinpoint white papule (a plugged or unopened sebaceous gland) can be found on the cheek or across the bridge of the nose of every newborn. Such lesions, termed *milia* (Figure 31-17), disappear by 2 to 4 weeks of age as the sebaceous glands mature and drain. Mothers need to be told that the lesions are not acne or some other skin disease but are normal in newborns.

Erythema Toxicum

In 30 to 70 percent of normal mature infants, a newborn rash, erythema toxicum, is observed (Figure 31-18). It usually appears in the first to fourth day of life but may appear in infants up to 2 weeks of age. It begins with a papule, increases in severity to become erythema by the second day, then disappears by the third day. It is sometimes

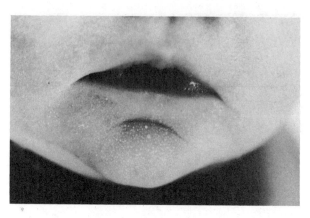

Figure 31-17 *Milia are unopened sebaceous glands frequently found on the nose, chin, or cheeks of a newborn. They disappear spontaneously in a few weeks' time. (Reproduced with permission of Mead Johnson & Company, Evansville, Ind.)*

called *flea-bite rash* because the lesions are so minuscule. One of the chief characteristics of the rash is its lack of pattern. It occurs sporadically and unpredictably as to time and place on skin surfaces. It may last a matter of hours rather than days. It is probably a response to irritation of the infant's skin by sheets and clothes. It needs no treatment.

Forceps Marks

If forceps were used for delivery, there may be a circular or linear contusion matching the rim of the blade of the forceps on the infant's cheek (Figure 31-19). This mark disappears in 2 to 3 days along with the edema that accompanies it. The mark is the result of normal forceps usage and

Figure 31-18 *Erythema toxicum is found on almost all newborns. The reddish rash consists of sporadic pinpoint papules on an erythematous base. It fades spontaneously in a few days. (Reproduced with permission of Mead Johnson & Company, Evansville, Ind.)*

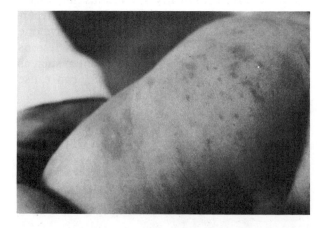

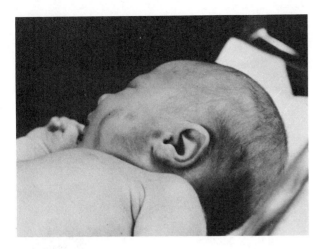

Figure 31-19 *Forceps marks are commonly found in infants delivered by forceps. Such marks are transient and disappear in a day or two. (Reproduced with permission of Mead Johnson & Company, Evansville, Ind.)*

does not denote unskilled or too vigorous application of forceps.

Skin Turgor

Newborn skin should feel resilient if the underlying tissue is well hydrated. If a fold of the skin is grasped between the thumb and fingers, it should feel elastic. When it is released, it should fall back to form a smooth surface. If severe dehydration is present, the skin will not smooth out again but will remain as an elevated ridge. This is seen in infants who suffered malnutrition in utero, who have taken no fluid for a long time after birth, or who have certain metabolic disorders such as adrenogenital syndrome.

Head

A newborn's head is disproportionately large, about one fourth of the total length; in an adult, the head is one eighth of total height. The forehead of the newborn is large and prominent. The chin appears to be receding, and it quivers easily if the infant is startled or cries.

Fontanelles

The fontanelles are the spaces or openings where the skull bones join. The anterior fontanelle is at the junction of the two parietal bones and the two fused frontal bones. It is diamond-shaped and measures 2 to 3 cm (0.8 to 1.2 inches) in width and 3 to 4 cm (1.2 to 1.6 inches) in length. The posterior fontanelle is at the junction of the parietal bones and the occipital bone. It is

triangular and measures about 1 cm (0.4 inch) in length.

The anterior fontanelle will be felt as a soft spot. It should not appear indented (a sign of dehydration) or bulging (a sign of increased intracranial pressure). The fontanelle may bulge if the newborn strains to pass a stool or cries vigorously, and with vigorous crying, a pulse may sometimes be seen in the fontanelle. The posterior fontanelle is so small in some newborns that it is not readily felt. The anterior fontanelle normally closes at 12 to 18 months of age. The posterior fontanelle closes by the end of the second month.

Sutures

The skull sutures, the separating lines of the skull, may override at birth because of the extreme pressure exerted by passage through the birth canal. Overriding is a normal, transient phenomenon. When the sagittal suture between the parietal bones overrides, the fontanelles will be less perceptible than usual. Suture lines should never appear separated in newborns. Separation denotes increased intracranial pressure from either abnormal brain formation, abnormal accumulation of cerebrospinal fluid in the cranium (hydrocephalus), or an accumulation of blood from a birth injury such as subdural hemorrhage.

Molding

The part of the infant's head (usually the vertex) that engages the cervix is molded to fit the cervix contours and appears prominent and asymmetrical; it may be so extreme in the baby of a primiparous woman that it looks like a dunce cap (Figure 31-20). This is a normal finding, although worrisome to mothers. The head is restored to its normal shape within a few days of birth.

Caput Succedaneum

Caput succedaneum (Figure 31-21A) is edema of the scalp at the presenting part of the head. It may involve wide areas of the head or may be the size of a goose egg. The edema will gradually be absorbed and disappear about the third day of life. It needs no treatment.

Cephalhematoma

A cephalhematoma is a collection of blood between the periosteum of the skull bone and the bone itself caused by rupture of a periosteum capillary due to the pressure of birth (Figure 31-21B). The blood loss is negligible, but the swelling is generally severe and is well outlined as an egg. It may be discolored (black and blue) because of the presence of coagulated blood. A caput suc-

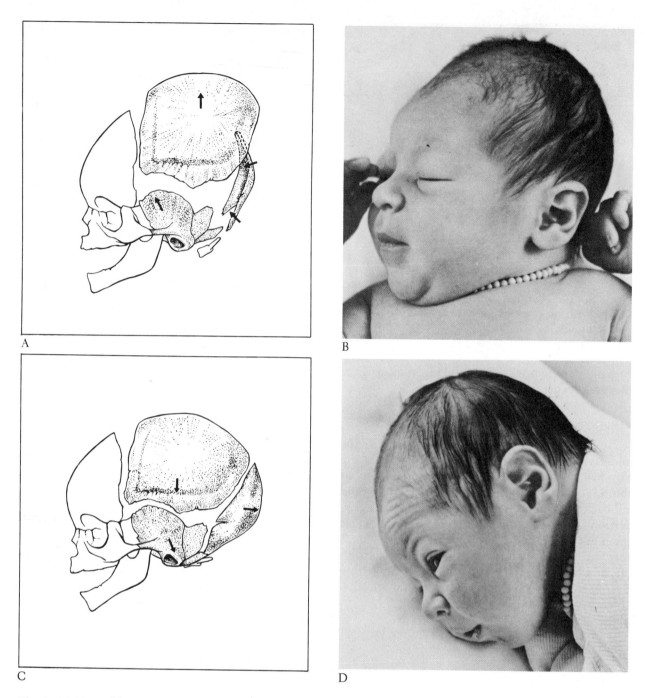

Figure 31-20 *Molding. (A, B) The infant head molds to fit the birth canal more easily. On palpation, the skull sutures will be felt to be overriding. (C, D) The head shape returns to normal within 1 week. (Reproduced with permission of Mead Johnson & Company, Evansville, Ind.)*

cedaneum may involve both hemispheres of the head, but a cephalhematoma is confined to an individual bone, so that the associated swelling stops at the bone's suture line.

It takes weeks for a cephalhematoma to be absorbed. It might appear that the blood could be aspirated to relieve the condition. However, this procedure would introduce the risk of infection, an unnecessary intrusion since the condition will subside by itself. As the blood captured in the space is broken down, a great deal of indirect bilirubin may be released, leading to jaundice.

Craniotabes

Craniotabes is a localized softening of the cranial bones. The bone is so soft it can be indented by the pressure of an examining finger. The bone returns to its normal contour when the pressure is removed. The condition corrects itself without treatment after a matter of months.

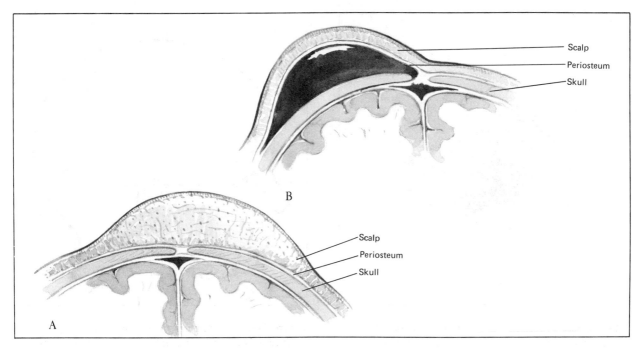

Figure 31-21 *A. Caput succedaneum. From pressure of the birth canal, an edematous area is present beneath the scalp. Note how it crosses the midline of the skull. B. Cephalhematoma. A small capillary beneath the periosteum of the skull bone has ruptured, and blood has collected under the periosteum of the bone. Note how the swelling now stops at the midline. Since the blood is contained under the periosteum, it is necessarily stopped by a suture line. (Courtesy of the Department of Medical Illustration, State University of New York at Buffalo.)*

Craniotabes is probably due to pressure of the fetal skull against the mother's pelvic bone in utero. It is more common in firstborn infants than in infants born later because of the lower position of the head in the pelvis the last 2 weeks of pregnancy in primiparous women. It is an example of a condition that is normal in a newborn but is pathological if found in an older child (probably the result of faulty metabolism or kidney dysfunction).

Eyes

Almost without exception the irises of the eyes of newborns are gray or blue. They do not assume their permanent color until the child is about 3 months of age.

The eyes should appear clear, without redness or a purulent discharge. Occasionally, a purulent discharge for the first 24 hours of life is seen if silver nitrate drops were administered in the delivery room to prevent ophthalmia neonatorum (gonorrheal conjunctivitis). The use of an antibiotic ointment such as erythromycin in place of silver nitrate prevents this reaction.

With few exceptions, newborns cry tearlessly because the lacrimal ducts are not fully mature at birth.

Sometimes a small subconjunctival hemorrhage results from pressure during delivery that causes rupture of a small capillary. This appears as a red spot on the sclera, usually on the inner aspect of the eye, or as a red ring around the cornea. The bleeding is slight and needs no treatment. It will be absorbed in two to three weeks, with no evidence that it ever existed. However, the baby's mother should be assured that the hemorrhage is unimportant. Otherwise, she may assume that the baby is bleeding from within the eye and that vision will be impaired.

Edema is often present around the orbit or on the eyelids. It will remain for the first two or three days until the newborn's kidneys are capable of evacuating fluid efficiently.

The cornea of the eye should be round and proportionate in size to that of an adult eye. A cornea that is larger than usual may be the result of congenital glaucoma. An irregularly shaped pupil, such as one with a keyhole shape (a portion of the iris is missing), is termed a *coloboma*. This may be an isolated finding but must be further investigated because the retina and the child's eyesight may be involved (Figure 31-22).

The pupil should be observed for any whiteness or opacities, which indicate congenital cataract. This should be especially watched for in

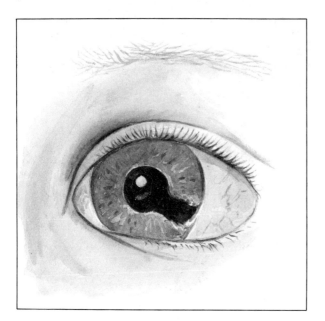

Figure 31-22 *Coloboma. The inferior portion of the iris is incompletely formed, leaving a "keyhole" pupil. (Courtesy of the Department of Medical Illustration, State University of New York at Buffalo.)*

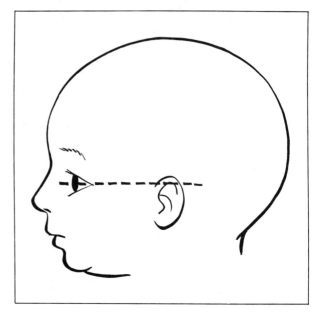

Figure 31-23 *Estimating height of the ears. If a line is drawn from the inner and outer canthus of the eye, it touches the pinna of the ear if the ears are normally set. This is an important determination to make, since low-set ears may be indicative of chromosomal abnormalities.*

infants whose mother had a history of rubella during pregnancy or if cytomegalic inclusion disease or galactosemia is suspected.

Ears

The newborn's external ear is still not as completely formed as it will be eventually, and the pinna tends to bend easily. When putting an infant on his or her side after feeding, be sure that you place the ear in good alignment. If you allow an infant to sleep on an ear in a deformed position, it tends to assume that position permanently.

The level of the top part of the external ear should be on a line drawn from the inner canthus to the outer canthus of the eye and back across the side of the head (Figure 31-23). Ears that are set lower than this are found in infants with certain chromosomal abnormalities, particularly trisomy 18 and 13, syndromes in which low-set ears and other physical defects are coupled with mental retardation (Chapter 6).

Small tags of skin are sometimes found just in front of the ear. Although they may be associated with chromosomal abnormalities, they are generally isolated findings and are of no consequence. They can be removed by ligation when the child is a few months of age. Directly in front of the ear is a common place for a dermal sinus to be present. The area should be inspected for a pinpoint-

size opening. The sinus is usually small and can be removed without consequence when a child is near school age.

Nose

A newborn's nose may appear large for the face. As the child grows, the rest of the face will grow more than the nose, and the discrepancy will disappear. One or two milia are usually present on the tip or bridge of the nose.

Mouth

A newborn's mouth should open evenly when the baby cries. If one side of the mouth moves more than the other, cranial nerve injury may be indicated. A newborn's tongue appears large and prominent in the mouth. Since the tongue is short, the frenulum membrane is attached close to the tip of the tongue, creating the impression in some mothers that the infant is "tongue-tied." At one time it was almost routine to snip a newborn's frenulum membrane to lengthen it. Now this procedure is regarded as harmful, since it leaves a portal of entry for infection, risks hemorrhage because of the low level of vitamin K in most newborns, and causes feeding difficulties by making the tongue sore and irritated.

The palate of the newborn should be intact. Occasionally, one or two small, round, glistening, well-circumscribed cysts (Epstein's pearls) are present on the palate, a result of the extra load of calcium that is deposited in utero. They are of no significance and need no treatment since they disappear spontaneously in a week's time. The mother may be concerned about them, mistaking them for thrush. Thrush, a *Candida* infection, usually appears on the tongue and sides of the cheeks as white or gray patches.

All newborns have some mucus in their mouths. If babies are placed on their side, the mucus drains from their mouths and gives them no distress. If their mouths are filled with so much mucus that they seem to be blowing bubbles, they may have a tracheoesophageal fistula. This must be determined before a child is fed; otherwise formula can be aspirated into the lungs from the inadequately formed esophagus.

It is unusual for the newborn to have teeth, but sometimes one or two will have erupted. Any teeth present must be evaluated for stability. If they are loose, they should be extracted, lest they be aspirated with a feeding. Small white epithelial pearls (inclusion cysts) may be present on the gum margins.

Neck

The neck of a newborn is short and often chubby. It is creased with skin folds. The head should rotate freely on the neck. It should flex forward and back. If there is rigidity of the neck, congenital torticollis from injury to the sternocleidomastoid muscle during birth should be considered. In infants whose membranes were ruptured more than 24 hours prior to birth nuchal rigidity suggests meningitis.

The neck is not strong enough to support the total weight of the head, but in a sitting position the infant should make a momentary effort at head control. When lying prone, newborns can raise their heads slightly, usually enough to lift them out of mucus or spit-up formula. If they are pulled to a sitting position from a supine position, their heads will lag behind considerably; however, again, they should make some effort to control and steady their heads as they reach the sitting position.

The trachea may be prominent on the front of the neck. The thymus gland may be enlarged because of the rapid growth of glandular tissue in comparison with other body tissues. The thymus gland triples in size by 3 years of age; it remains at that size until the child is about 10 years old.

After that, its size begins to decrease. Although the thymus may appear to be bulging in the newborn, it is rarely a cause of respiratory difficulty as was previously believed.

Chest

The chest in some infants looks small because the infant's head is so large in proportion. Not until the child is 2 years of age does the chest measurement exceed that of the head.

In both female and male infants, the breasts may be engorged. Occasionally, the breasts of newborn babies secrete a thin, watery fluid popularly termed *witch's milk*. Engorgement occurs in utero as a result of the influence of the mother's hormones. As soon as they are cleared from the infant's system, the engorgement and any fluid present subsides (about a week). Fluid should never be expressed from infant breasts. The manipulation may introduce bacteria and lead to mastitis.

The clavicles should be straight. A lump on one or the other may indicate that a fracture occurred during delivery and calcium is now being deposited at that point.

Overall, the appearance of the chest should be symmetrical. Respirations are normally rapid (30 to 50 per minute) but not distressed.

Retraction (the chest wall drawn in with inspiration) should not be present. A retracting infant is using such strong force to pull air into the respiratory tract that he or she sucks in the anterior chest muscles. Retraction is shown in Figure 31-24.

Abdomen

The contour of the newborn abdomen is slightly protuberant. A scaphoid or sunken appearance may be indicative of missing abdominal contents.

For the first hour after birth, the umbilical cord appears as a white, gelatinous structure marked with the red and blue streaks of the umbilical vein and arteries. The vein and arteries should be counted when the cord is first cut in the delivery room to be certain they are present. In 0.5 percent of deliveries (3.5 percent of twin deliveries), there is only a single umbilical artery, and in a third of such infants this single artery is associated with a congenital heart anomaly. Since the anomaly may not be readily apparent, any child with a single umbilical artery needs close observation and assessment until all anomalies are ruled out.

After the first hour of life, the cord begins to dry up, shrink, and become discolored like the

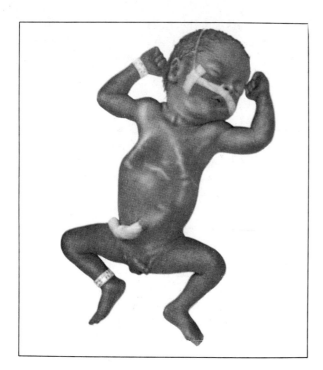

figure 31-24 *Sternal retraction in a newborn. Retraction indicates labored and difficult breathing. (From Clinical Education Aid, No. 5, Ross Laboratories, Columbus, Ohio, 1960.)*

dead end of a vine. By the second or third day it has turned black. It sloughs by the sixth to tenth day, leaving a granulating area a few centimeters across that heals during the following week.

There should be no bleeding at the cord site. Bleeding suggests that the cord clamp has been loosened or the cord has been tugged loose by the friction of the bedclothes. The base of the cord should appear dry. A moist or odorous cord suggests infection. If present, infection should receive immediate treatment or it may enter the newborn's bloodstream and cause septicemia. Moistness at the base of the cord may also indicate a patent urachus (connection between the bladder and the umbilicus) with urine draining at the cord site.

The base of the cord should also be inspected to be certain there is no defect in the abdominal wall (umbilical hernia). If there is a fascial (abdominal wall) defect less than 2 cm wide, it will generally close by itself by school age; a defect more than 2 cm wide will probably require surgical correction. Taping or putting buttons or coins on the abdomen is an old time remedy and does not help such defects to close. Heavy taping may in fact worsen the condition by preventing the development of good muscle tone in the abdominal wall. The tape also tends to keep the cord moist and make infection more likely than when the cord is dry.

Anogenital Area

The anus of the newborn must be inspected to be certain that it is patent and not covered by a membrane (imperforate anus). This condition is best determined by inserting a rectal thermometer into the rectum for the length of the bulb or by inserting the tip of a lubricated little finger. The time after birth that the infant first passes meconium should be noted. If a baby does not do so in the first 24 hours, the suspicion of imperforate anus or meconium ileus is aroused.

Male Genitalia

The scrotum in most male infants is edematous. It may be deeply pigmented in black or dark-skinned infants. Rugae should be evident in the mature infant.

Both testes should be present in the scrotum. Male infants who do not have one or both testes in the scrotum (cryptorchidism) need further referral to establish the extent of the problem. It could be due to agenesis (absence of an organ), ectopic testes (the testes cannot enter the scrotum because the opening to the scrotal sac is closed), or undescended testes (the vas deferens or artery is too short to allow them to descend). Infants with agenesis of the testes are usually referred for investigation of other anomalies. Since the testes arise from the same germ tissue as the kidney, agenesis of the testes may indicate agenesis of a kidney also.

The penis of newborns is usually small. It should be inspected to see that the urethral opening is at the tip of the glans, not on the dorsal surface (epispadias) or the ventral surface (hypospadias).

The prepuce (foreskin) of the penis should be examined to be certain it is not stenosed. In most newborns it slides back poorly from the meatal opening. Although today most male infants are circumcised, the necessity for this operation can be questioned. It is rare to find an infant who physically requires it (with a foreskin so constricting that it interferes with voiding or circulation), and surgery this early in life poses the risk of hemorrhage and infection. Circumcision should not be done if hypospadias or epispadias is present; the plastic surgeon may want to use the foreskin as tissue in the repair of these conditions.

Female Genitalia

The vulva in female newborns may be swollen because of the action of maternal hormones. In some infants a mucous vaginal secretion is present, which is sometimes blood-tinged. Again, this is due to the action of maternal hormones, and the discharge will disappear as soon as the infant's system has cleared the hormones. The discharge should not be mistaken for an infection or taken as an indication that a trauma has occurred.

Back

A newborn should be turned to a prone position and the back observed to determine whether or not the spine is straight. The spine appears flat in the lumbar and sacral areas; the curves seen in the adult appear only when a child is able to sit and walk. The base of the spine should be inspected carefully to be certain no dermal sinus is present there. This looks like a pinpoint opening in the skin.

A newborn normally assumes the position maintained in utero, in which, typically, the back is rounded and the arms and legs are flexed on the abdomen and chest. A child who was born in a frank breech position will tend to straighten the legs at the knee and bring them up next to the face. The position of a baby delivered by a face presentation sometimes simulates opisthotonos because the curve of the back is deeply concave.

Extremities

The arms and legs of a newborn are short. The hands are plump and clenched into fists. Newborn fingernails are soft and smooth and are usually long enough to extend over the fingertips.

The arms and legs should move symmetrically (unless an infant is demonstrating a tonic neck reflex). An arm that hangs limp and unmoving suggests injury to the clavicle or the brachial or cervical plexus or fracture of a long bone, all of which are possible birth injuries.

The legs are bowed as well as short. The sole of the foot appears to be flat because of an extra pad of fat in the longitudinal arch. In the mature infant there are many crisscrossed lines on the sole of the foot. Absence of such marks usually indicates immaturity.

The feet of many newborns turn in (varus deviation) because of intrauterine position. This simple deviation needs no correction if the feet can be brought to the midline position by easy manipulation; when the infant begins to bear weight, they will align themselves. If a foot does not align readily or will not turn to a definite midline position, a talipes deformity (clubfoot) may be present. The condition needs investigation, since con-

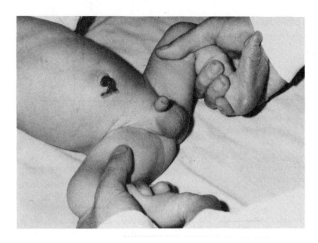

Figure 31-25 *Hip abduction. In a newborn, both hips should abduct so completely they lie almost flat against the mattress (180 degrees). (Reproduced with permission of Mead Johnson & Company, Evansville, Ind.)*

genital problems of this kind are best treated in the newborn period.

With the newborn in a supine position, both legs can be flexed and abducted to such an extent that they touch or nearly touch the surface of the bed (Figure 31-25). If the hip joint seems to lock short of this distance (160 to 170 degrees) hip subluxation (a shallow and poorly formed acetabulum) is suggested; a click heard as the femur head strikes the acetabulum is another indication of this. Subluxated hip may be bilateral but is usually unilateral. It is important that hip subluxation be discovered as early as possible, since correction, as in correction of talipes deformities, is most successful if initiated early.

When lying on the abdomen, newborns are capable of bringing their arms and legs underneath them and raising their stomach off the bed enough for a hand to be slipped underneath. This ability helps to prevent pressure or rubbing at the cord site because in this position the cord site does not actually touch the bedding. The immature infant does not have this ability, and thus its presence or absence is an indication of maturity.

Physiologic Adjustment to Extrauterine Life

All infants seem to move through a period of irregular adjustment in the first 6 hours of life before their body systems stabilize. This has been described as a transition period. The first phase lasts about half an hour. During this time the

Table 31-3 Periods of Reactivity: Normal Adjustment to Extrauterine Life

Assessment	First Period (First 15 to 30 Minutes)	Second Period (30 Minutes to 120 Minutes)	Third Period (2 Hours to 6 Hours)
Color	Acrocyanosis	Color stabilizing; pink all over	Quick color changes occur with movement or crying
Temperature	Baby's temperature begins to fall from intrauterine temp. of 100.6°F	Temperature stabilizes at about 99°F	Temperature increases to 99.8°F
Heart rate	Rapid, as much as 180 per minute while crying	Slowing to between 120 and 140 per minute	Wide swings in rate with activity
Respirations	Irregular; 30–90 per minute while crying; some nasal flaring, occasional retraction may be present	Slows to 30–50 per minute; barreling of chest occurs	Respirations become irregular again with activity
Activity	Alert; watching	Sleeps	Awakes
Ability to respond to stimulation	Reacts vigorously	Difficult to rouse	Becoming responsive again
Mucus	Visible in mouth	Small amount present while sleeping	Mouth full of mucus causing gagging
Bowel sounds	Able to be heard after first 15 minutes	Present	Often has first meconium stool

Source: Desmond, M. N., et al. (1963). The clinical behavior of the newly born: The term baby. *Journal of Pediatrics, 62,* 307.

baby is alert and exhibits exploring, searching activity, often making sucking sounds. Heartbeat and respiratory rate are rapid. This is called the *first period of reactivity.*

Next comes a quiet, resting period. Heartbeat and respiratory rate slow; the infant generally sleeps for about 90 minutes.

The third period, between 2 and 6 hours of life, is the *second period of reactivity.* The infant wakes, often gagging and choking on mucus that has accumulated in the mouth. He or she is again alert and responsive and interested in the surroundings.

These three periods are summarized in Table 31-3. Infants who are ill or who had difficulty at birth do not pass through these typical stages; they may never have periods of alertness or periods of quiet. Their vital signs may not fall and rise again, but remain rapid; their temperature may remain subnormal. Exhibition of this typical pattern, therefore, is an indication that the infant is well and adjusting well to extrauterine life.

Utilizing Nursing Process

Although the average newborn infant adjusts to extrauterine life with amazing ease, because so many physiologic changes are necessary for this to be accomplished, nursing care during the period must be designed by use of the nursing process.

Assessment

Assessment of a newborn consists of observation of the total infant for normal physiologic functioning. This is done immediately at birth and is continued at every contact with the infant. Teach mothers to make assessments concerning their infant's temperature and respiratory rate so that they continue to monitor their infant's health at home.

Analysis

A nursing diagnosis during the first few days of life might be a well diagnosis such as "Physiologic adjustment to extrauterine life within normal parameters." If a minor deviation from the normal is present, it may be one such as "Anxiety related to hemangioma on left thigh" or "Anxiety related to coloring from physiologic jaundice." Be certain that goals established during this time are realistic in terms of the short time an infant will remain in a health care facility.

Planning

Planning nursing care during this period must be done so that the newborn teaching necessary can be scheduled in between time for adequate rest for the mother so the mother not only knows enough about her newborn to care for him or her at home but has the energy to be able to carry out the needed care.

Implementation

A major phase of implementation in the newborn period is role modeling to help a new mother grow confident with her newborn. Be aware how carefully mothers observe you for guidance in child care. Preserving newborn warmth and energy is important to all interventions.

Evaluation

Evaluation should reveal that a mother is able to give beginning newborn care with a degree of confidence. Be certain that women have made arrangements for continued health supervision for their newborns so evaluation can be continued and the family's long-term health needs met.

Questions for Review

Multiple Choice

1. Baby Swensen is a 7 pound, 6 ounce male infant. In assessing his weight in the newborn period, what would you accept as a normal newborn weight loss?
   a. 1–2 percent of birth weight
   b. 5–10 percent of birth weight
   c. 10–15 percent of birth weight
   d. 15–20 percent of birth weight

2. A major adaptation that a newborn makes at birth is closure of fetal circulatory shunts. The shunt that must close between the aorta and pulmonary artery is the
   a. foremen ovale.
   b. ductus arteriosus.
   c. venous artery.
   d. duct of Heim.

3. Baby Swensen has a very prominent elevation on his left parietal area. Which finding below would assure you that the elevation is a caput succedaneum, not a cephalhematoma?
   a. No ecchymosis is present.
   b. The area does not feel warm.
   c. The area crosses a suture line.
   d. The area is soft and yielding.

4. In order to assess gastrointestinal function, you observe the time of the first meconium stool. The time you use as a marker of a normal time interval is
   a. 2 hours following birth.
   b. 2 hours after the first feeding.
   c. 12 hours following birth.
   d. 24 hours following birth.

5. The reason lung expansion is so difficult in a newborn and first breath is such a stress is that
   a. alveoli are filled with amniotic fluid.
   b. alveoli cells do not soften until exposed to oxygen.

   c. the chest cartilage is noncompliant.
   d. the alveoli are collapsed at birth.

6. The most accurate method of eliciting a Moro reflex in Baby Swensen would be to
   a. startle him with a loud noise.
   b. raise his head and drop it backward.
   c. jiggle his bassinet.
   d. raise his hands over his head

7. Baby Swensen has a strawberry hemangioma birthmark on his left thigh. You would want to tell his mother concerning this mark that
   a. it may continue to grow during the first year.
   b. it is a permanent birthmark.
   c. it may become cancerous later in life.
   d. it will fade by 3 months' time.

8. Baby Swensen has thick vernix caseosa in his skin folds. The purpose of this substance is to
   a. initiate vitamin D utilization.
   b. absorb bilirubin from skin cells.
   c. promote circulatory vasodilatation.
   d. moisten and lubricate the skin.

9. At birth, Baby Swensen is given vitamin K. The reason for this treatment is
   a. vitamin K will aid respiratory function.
   b. his liver is too immature to produce vitamin K until 6 days of age.
   c. vitamin K helps prevent retinal infections.
   d. he has no intestinal flora to synthesize vitamin K at birth.

10. On the second day of life, Baby Swensen's indirect bilirubin level is rising rapidly. Indirect bilirubin in the newborn occurs from
    a. breakdown of vitamin K by the liver.
    b. release of sequestered red blood cells from the pancreas.
    c. trapped cord blood being evacuated.
    d. destruction of red blood cells by hemolysis.

Discussion

1. Assessing vital signs in a newborn is part of an initial first assessment. What are normal findings for vital signs?
2. Some newborn reflexes are helpful to use in showing a mother how alert her newborn is. What reflexes would you elicit to do this?

3. Parents often inspect a newborn carefully for skin lesions or birthmarks. How would you explain the cause and course of a mongolian spot, a strawberry hemangioma, and milia to new parents?

Suggested Readings

Adams, M. E. (1981). Neonatal abilities: Pictures in nursing. *Nursing (Oxford), 1,* 913.

Barnett, M. M., et al. (1982). Infant outcome in relation to second stage labor pushing method. *Birth, 9,* 221.

Coles, E. R. (1983). Babies' sleeping habits. *Midwife Health Visitor and Community Nurse, 19,* 322.

Davidson, S., et al. (1981). Appearance, behavior and capabilities: Teaching new parents infant ABCs. *Canadian Nurse, 77,* 37.

Davis, V. (1980). The structure and function of brown adipose tissue in the neonate. *J.O.G.N. Nursing, 9,* 368.

Desmond, M. N., et al. (1963). The clinical behavior of the newly born: The term baby. *Journal of Pediatrics, 62,* 307.

Levy, H. L., et al. (1982). The current practice of newborn screening. *Hospital Practice, 17,* 89.

Ludington-Hoe, S. M. (1983). What can newborns really see? *American Journal of Nursing, 83,* 1286.

Sahu, S. (1984). Birthweight, gestational age and neonatal risks. *Perinatology/Neonatology, 8,* 28.

Moore, M. L. (1972). *The Newborn and the Nurse.* Philadelphia: Saunders.

Scharping, E. M. (1983). Physiological measurements of the neonate: Methods of accurately measuring vital signs are constantly being refined. *M.C.N., 8,* 70.

Schiffman, R. F. (1983). Temperature monitoring in the neonate: A comparison of axillary and rectal temperatures. *Nursing Research, 32,* 208.

Starr, T. (1984). The baby at birth. *Nursing (Oxford), 2,* 608.

32

Health Assessment of the Newborn

OBJECTIVES

Following mastery of the material in this chapter, you should be able to

1. Describe history taking pertinent to newborn health.
2. Describe techniques of physical examination used with newborns.
3. Describe the components of a comprehensive health assessment of the newborn.
4. Analyze ways that health assessment can be incorporated into health teaching for the new family.
5. Synthesize knowledge of newborn health with nursing process to achieve quality maternal-newborn nursing care.

NEWBORN ASSESSMENT is an important role of the maternal-newborn nurse. You use such assessment skills doing initial delivery room or birthing room examinations, initial nursery admission examinations, or discharge examinations. A community health nurse or a nurse in a pediatrician's office might visit a new mother in her home before her baby's first visit to a health care agency. You might also use the skills of newborn health assessment doing monthly well-child assessments in a physician's office or child care clinic.

Health assessment of a newborn involves three phases: assessment of the pregnancy, labor, and delivery by reference to the records and by history taking; physical assessment of the infant; and assessment of the parent-newborn interaction.

All three phases are equally important. The 9 months the infant spent in utero and the circumstances of delivery can have as much effect on the baby's health as anything that comes after birth. Infants, in order to thrive, need not only to be physically healthy but to have someone to take good care of them and interact with them. The three phases in newborn assessment overlap and intertwine.

History Taking

Some information on the pregnancy and delivery can be obtained from the health care facility charts of a mother and infant. Part of it must be gained from interviewing the mother.

For a pregnancy history, you need to know the para and gravida of the mother, the date of her last menstrual period, and the predicted date of confinement. Double-check the date of confinement by Nägele's rule. Is there any suspicion the infant is immature or postmature by these dates?

When did the mother go for medical supervision during the present pregnancy? Did she keep appointments? What was her nutritional state and her general health during the pregnancy? Did the milestones of pregnancy occur on schedule (e.g., cessation of nausea and vomiting by 4 months, quickening of the fetus at 4½ to 5 months)? Were there any complications during pregnancy such as spotting or beginning hypertension? Did the mother take vitamins, iron, and folic acid during the pregnancy? Did she take any other medication? Were there any injuries such as falls or car accidents? Were any X-ray films made? Does she have any chronic illness such as heart or kidney disease?

If you have access to a mother's health care facility admission record, examine it to determine whether she entered the facility in good health. Was her blood pressure within normal limits? Did she have any signs of infection that could spread to the newborn and impair the newborn's health?

Examine the mother's labor and delivery room record for the length and type of her labor, the type of delivery, kind of analgesia or anesthetic used, problems in delivering the child or the placenta. Examine the infant's birth record for presentation, position, time the membranes ruptured, whether or not aseptic technique was broken during delivery, fetal heart rate during labor and delivery, time in which breathing was established after birth, weight (plotted on a neonatal estimation of gestation age chart—see Figure 31-1), and Apgar score. Check to be certain eye prophylaxis was done and vitamin K was administered (see Chapter 34).

Following examination of the birth record, an infant's nursery chart should be studied for further points of history. The time the infant first passed a stool and first voided will be important in assessing the functioning of the intestinal and urinary systems. A child's response to feeding and tolerance of feedings provide a clue not only to the state of health of the gastrointestinal system but also to the baby's overall maturity and well-being.

If you do not have a mother's chart, ask her to tell you about her pregnancy, labor, and delivery and the condition of the infant at birth. Ask specifically if the infant cried right away; if there was any cyanosis or jaundice (ask "turn blue or yellow?" with most women); if any special equipment was used with the baby. A mother has a keen interest in the baby at that time and so is generally an excellent informant on his or her condition immediately after birth.

What was the outcome of previous pregnancies? Are all previous children healthy? Were there any complications at delivery or in the newborn period with these children? Are there any familial diseases?

Physical Assessment of the Newborn

In the physical assessment of adults and older children, the sequence of assessment is usually overall inspection, then detailed assessment of body parts from head to toe, including certain neurologic components. Many examiners find it more satisfactory to examine infants under 1 year of age by beginning with an overall inspection and then assessing body parts, proceeding from *toe to head*, finishing with the neurologic evaluation. This method has the advantage of a gentle and untraumatic beginning and postpones the parts of the examination that are certain to upset the infant and cause crying, particularly examination of the mouth and throat. Because it is necessary for an infant to be relaxed and not crying while the chest and abdomen are examined, many examiners start with these body parts after the initial inspection and then proceed from the feet upward. Since it is unrealistic to expect the infant to cooperate in any way during the assessment, this third method appears to have the most merit and is the order of assessment presented here.

Inspection

Body proportion is an important observation to make before the newborn is disturbed. Are the infant's proportions typical newborn proportions? Is the head about one fourth of overall height? Is the head circumference slightly larger than the chest circumference? Are the legs and arms short in proportion to the trunk? Although the arms appear to be short, fingertips should reach to midthigh. Does the child have gross anomalies? What position does the baby assume? Is it consistent with the delivery presentation? With the gestation age? Breech-born babies ordinarily assume their delivery position, possibly with legs extended. Vertex-born babies are typically slightly flexed. Browborn babies often arch their backs. Immature babies do not flex well (they frogleg).

Are the arms and legs positioned symmetrically (as they should be unless the infant is exhibiting a tonic neck reflex)? (See page 681.)

If lying in a prone position, does the baby exhibit good muscle tone by pulling his knees well under himself and raising his abdomen off the bedding? Does he make sucking movements with his lips? Are his respirations easy or labored? Is the chest retracting while at rest? (Occasional retractions—inward movement of the sternum with inspiration—in a mature infant are normal; persistent retraction is a sign of respiratory distress.) What is his color? Ruddy? Pale? Cyanotic? Jaundiced?

All of these observations are important to make initially since they become increasingly difficult to make once an infant has become upset.

Assessment of the Chest

Examination of the chest follows the general procedure of all examination: inspection, palpation, percussion, and auscultation (see Chapter 18). Note the size and contour of the chest. It should appear to be almost as large in the anteroposterior diameter as in width. Inspect the respiratory movements. Healthy findings are easy respirations at a rate between 30 to 50 per minute if quiet, 50 to 80 if crying. If retractions are present, are they intercostal or subcostal? Are they constant or occasional? Is the chest symmetrical? (An enlarged heart may make the left side of the chest appear larger; a diaphragmatic hernia in the right side of the chest may make that side appear larger.) What is the respiratory rate? Do both sides of the chest move with respirations? Is the number of ribs even on each side? Are the clavicles straight?

Inspect the breasts for inflammation (possible infection), presence of breast tissue (the presence of palpable breast tissue is a sign of maturity), drainage, and the presence of supernumerary nipples (usually found below and in line with the normal nipples). Note whether or not the point of maximum impulse of the heart is visible on inspection, as is normal in newborns.

Begin palpating the chest in a systematic order from the top down or from side to side. Do the ribs feel smooth? Examine the clavicles for intactness. A crepitant feeling denotes fracture. A bony prominence on the clavicle may mean that the clavicle was fractured at delivery and callus formation is beginning. Palpate the anterior chest to ascertain the point of maximum intensity of the heartbeat. Can you feel a thrill radiating from that point (thrills suggest heart disease)? Palpate the breast tissue for engorgement; estimate the size of engorgement in centimeters. Palpate the supraclavicular and the axillary lymph nodes for any enlargement (should not be present).

Chest percussion in a newborn does not always produce meaningful findings, although total lack of resonance on one side of the chest in comparison with the other side might suggest that primary atelectasis or a diaphragmatic hernia is occluding chest space. You should be able to locate the left lateral aspect of the heart by percussion. Lung tissue sounds resonant; as your finger moves over the heart, the sound dulls.

Auscultate heart sounds. Begin at the point of maximum intensity (the heart apex). What is the heart rate? How about the rhythm (listen long enough to be certain that you have heard the rhythm through both inhalation and exhalation)—is it even? Are the sounds clear and distinct? Are there any extra sounds? Do you hear a murmur? Do you hear a splitting of the heart sounds? Is it a fixed or a changing split? The first heart sound is caused by closure of the tricuspid and mitral valves; the second sound, by closure of the pulmonary and aortic valves. Splitting (the sound of *l-lub* instead of *lub*; *d-dub* instead of *dub*) implies that a valve is closing after its mate, not at the same time. (Physiologic splitting of the second heart sound widens on inspiration; pathologic splitting caused by delayed closure of the pulmonary valve is fixed—that is, it does not change with inspiration or expiration.)

Auscultate at "listening posts" for the sounds of the different valves—that is, at the fourth or fifth left interspace of the ribs for the mitral valve, the second interspace at the left of the sternum for the pulmonary valve, the second interspace on the right of the sternum for the aortic valve, and at the junction of the sternum and xiphoid for the tricuspid valve. Auscultate below the left axilla for radiating sounds. Listening posts for heart sounds are shown in Figure 32-1.

After you have a good mental picture of the heart sounds, auscultate the chest for breath sounds. Listen to the anterior upper left chest, anterior upper right chest, lower left chest, middle and lower right chest (everyone has two lung lobes on the left side, three lobes or spots to listen to on the right side).

Because the newborn's alveoli open slowly over the first 24 to 48 hours to full capacity and the baby invariably has mucus in the back of the throat, listening to lung sounds often reveals the sounds of rhonchi and perhaps transient other findings. Adventitious chest sounds are summarized in Table 32-1.

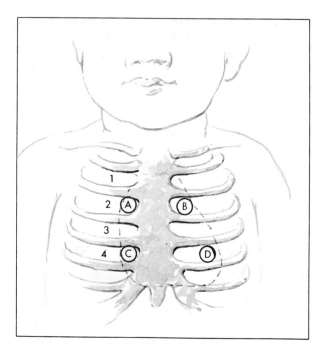

Figure 32-1 *Listening posts for heart sounds. Heart valves are not at these points, but these are the points to which the sounds radiate best. A = aortic valve, B = pulmonary valve, C = tricuspid valve, D = mitral valve. (Courtesy of the Department of Medical Illustration, State University of New York at Buffalo.)*

Lastly, turn the baby on his or her abdomen and listen in the four posterior chest quadrants for radiating heart sounds and for breath sounds.

Assessment of the Abdomen

Assessment of the abdomen proceeds from inspection to auscultation, palpation, and percussion. Inspect the skin carefully for color and the presence of superficial veins (superficial veins are generally present in a newborn). Inspect the umbilical area to determine whether the cord is free from drainage. Inspect the cord clamp to be certain it is secure. A newborn's abdomen should appear slightly protuberant. A depressed abdomen suggests missing organs.

It is good practice to auscultate the abdomen before palpating or percussing it; abdominal pressure will shift intestinal contents and lessen the already low intensity of bowel sounds. These are tinkling sounds, and if they are not present, bowel obstruction is suggested. You have to listen for at least a minute to detect bowel sounds, since they occur at a rate of perhaps only two to five per minute.

Begin palpation by testing the skin of the abdomen for turgor. Grasp the skin between your

Table 32-1 Adventitious Chest Sounds in Newborns

Term	Source of Sound	Description	Importance
Rhonchi	Air passing through mucus in a major air passage	A coarse, snoring sound	Little importance in newborns as mucus in the back of the throat causes transmitted sound
Rales	Air passing through fluid in alveoli	Simulates the crackle of cellophane	Should be investigated. Can be the sound of unabsorbed lung fluid; also can be a sign of pneumonia
Stridor	Air being pulled through a narrowed airway, often caused by immature trachea cartilage	A high crowing (rooster-like) sound heard on inspiration	Should be investigated. May be beginning sign of tracheal obstruction
Wheezing	Air being pushed through narrowed bronchioles	A whistling heard on expiration	Should be investigated. May be a beginning sign of obstruction
Grunting	Air being pushed through a partially closed epiglottis	A "grunt" heard on expiration	Should be investigated. Infants with respiratory distress syndrome (hyaline membrane disease) typically grunt to maintain pressure in alveoli
Absent or diminished breath sounds	If air is not entering a lung or lobe of a lung on one side, breath sounds are absent or quieter on that side	Soft, difficult-to-hear breath sounds	Should be investigated. Suggests lack of aeration such as occurs with atelectasis

thumb and index finger to raise it, then release it and note whether or not it returns to its former position. With good hydration, the crease disappears immediately; if the raised portion of skin remains raised, poor turgor or poor hydration is indicated.

First palpate the abdomen superficially, then deeply. Follow a systematic order so that no quadrant is inadvertently overlooked. Begin in any quadrant and palpate clockwise back to the first quadrant. The edge of the liver is usually palpable in newborns at 1 to 2 cm below the right costal margin. The edge of the spleen may be palpable 1 to 2 cm below the left costal margin. To detect the liver and spleen, be certain you palpate from the lower to the upper quadrants so that your fingertips bump against their lower edges. Otherwise, your fingers will be on top of the organs and you will not detect their presence.

No areas of weakness or hernias of muscle should be discernible on palpation; no tenderness should be present. Tenderness is difficult to determine in a newborn, but if it is extreme, the infant will cry or thrash about or possibly tense abdominal muscles to protect the abdomen as you palpate it.

Attempt to identify the presence of kidneys by pressing deeply. The right kidney can usually be palpated (at least its lower pole), since it is lower than the left kidney; the latter is more difficult to locate because the intestine is bulkier on the left side, and the left kidney is higher in the retroperitoneal space. Nonetheless, you should try to locate it; the child's voiding only demonstrates that there is at least one kidney, not that there are two. Attempt to evaluate kidney size. Are the kidneys normal in size (about the size of a walnut)? If a kidney is enlarged, a polycystic kidney or pooling of urine from a ureteral obstruction is suggested. Be certain your fingernails are clipped close to your fingertips before you undertake kidney palpation. Otherwise, you will cut the baby's abdominal skin as you press in deeply enough to locate kidneys.

Palpate the umbilical ring. Is it open or closed? If open, how wide is the opening? A fascial ring more than 2 cm in diameter is generally accepted as wider than one that will close spontaneously.

Last, percuss the abdomen to determine resonance and to confirm the location of the inferior margin of the liver and spleen and the superior margin of the bladder.

Elicit an abdominal reflex. Stroking each quadrant of the abdomen will cause the umbilicus to move or "wink" in that direction. This superficial abdominal reflex is a test of spinal nerves T-8 through T-10. The reflex may not be demonstrable in newborns until the tenth day of life.

Assessment of the Lower Extremities

Begin with the feet and inspect one foot at a time. Inspect for color. Separate the toes and count them. Watch for webbing (syndactyly), extra toes (polydactyly), or unusual spacing of toes, particularly between the big toes and the others (a finding in certain chromosomal disorders, although also a normal finding in some families). Test to see whether the toenails become blanched and refill after pressure.

Observe the foot for position. Feet tend to turn in (varus deviation) because of intrauterine position, and they tend to turn out (valgus deviation) in infants who consistently sleep in a prone position. Check to see that the foot aligns with the ankle. Put the ankle through a range of motion to evaluate whether or not the heel cord is unusually tight. Check for ankle clonus by supporting the lower leg in the left hand and dorsiflexing the foot sharply two or three times by pressure on the sole of the foot. Following the dorsiflexion, one or two continued movements are normal; rapid alternating contraction and relaxation (clonus) is abnormal (suggests neurologic involvement).

The skin of the legs should be inspected for color and tested for warmth. The skin of the thigh should be tested for turgor. Align the legs and examine for an abnormal degree of bowing (tibial torsion). Flex and extend the knee joint. Check the muscle tone of the lower extremities by extending them, then releasing them and observing the action. The mature newborn will immediately flex them again, but the immature infant will not make a motion this strong.

Inspect the posterior thighs for asymmetrical skin folds as are seen in hip dysplasia. Check further for hip dysplasia by turning the infant to a supine position, flexing the hips and knees and attempting to abduct the hips (Figure 31-25). With good joint function, the hips should abduct 160 to 170 degrees. The presence of hip dysplasia is further supported by feeling the joint slip in your hands or hearing a click as the head of the femur strikes the ridge of the acetabulum.

The thighs should flex on the abdomen with the knee in a flexed position. Inability of the infant to extend his leg from this position is a sign of meningitis (Kernig's sign), which is rare in a newborn but possible when the membranes ruptured early.

Palpate the inguinal area in both male and female infants for unusual masses that would sug-

gest hernia or enlarged lymph nodes. Palpate the femoral pulses (at the inguinal ligament) and compare their strength (should be present and equal).

Assessment of the Genitalia and Rectum

The foreskin of the uncircumcised male infant should be retracted to visualize the urethral opening. Normally, the foreskin retracts far enough for you to locate the meatus; it does not retract over the entire glans.

A few adhesions of the prepuce may be present in newborns but are of no consequence unless they cause obstruction of the urinary meatus.

The urinary meatus should be inspected for appearance and to determine that it is located at the end of the penis (ruling out epispadias or hypospadias). If the opening is round rather than slit-like, scar tissue formation from infection should be suspected.

The scrotum should be inspected for normal asymmetry (the left side is invariably slightly larger). The testes should be palpated to be certain they are descended. Make a practice of pressing your left hand against the inguinal ring before palpating for the testes, so that they do not slip upward out of the scrotal sac as you palpate (Figure 32-2). Note whether or not rugae are present on the scrotum (rugae are a sign of maturity).

The cremasteric reflex is elicited by stroking the internal side of the thigh. As the skin is stroked, the testis on that side moves perceptibly upward. This is a test of the integrity of spinal

Figure 32-2 *Procedure for blocking the inguinal canal when examining the scrotal contents. From Alexander, M., & Brown, M. S. (1978). Pediatric physical diagnosis for nurses. New York: McGraw-Hill.*

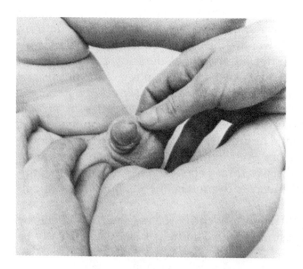

nerves T-8 through T-10. The response may be absent in newborns less than about 10 days old.

Inspect the genitalia of the female newborn for gross structures: labia majora and minora (often enlarged from maternal hormone influence), clitoris (also often enlarged), and the urethral and vaginal openings. In most newborns, vulvar edema is so severe that locating the urethral and vaginal openings is difficult. Vaginal secretions are present in most newborn females, and they are sometimes blood-tinged, again, from maternal hormone effect.

In both sexes, it is important to observe the stream of urine. It should be forceful and especially in males should curve upward in an arc. Observation of a urine stream is usually possible during the course of physical assessment, since the infant voids with crying; further, the abdomen is chilled, contracting the bladder slightly.

A rectal examination, done by inserting your little finger (encased in a fingercot) into the child's rectum, should be a part of newborn assessment. Patency of the rectum and anus is thus determined.

Assessment of the Upper Extremities

Observe the infant for the position of the arms, which should be held flexed at the elbow. The hands are held clenched. Inspect the skin for color, warmth, and turgor. Test the upper extremities for muscle tone by unflexing the arms for approximately 5 seconds. When you release an arm, it should return immediately to its flexed position. Hold the arms down by the sides and note their length. The fingertips should cover the proximal thigh. Unusually short arms may signify achondroplastic dwarfism.

Examine the fingernails for color and blanching and refilling of the nails. Separate the fingers and count them. Observe for webbing between fingers. Observe for unusual curvature of the little finger and inspect the palm for a simian crease (a single palmar crease in contrast to the three creases normally seen in a palm). Both simian creases and inward-curved little fingers are signs of Down's syndrome, although curved fingers and simian creases may also occur normally. Test the wrist for range of motion. It should rotate laterally and medially and flex and extend. Palpate the radial pulses and estimate for symmetrical strength. Palpate the long bones for possible fracture.

A scarf sign is a test for movement of the shoulder and an indication of muscle tone and therefore of muscle maturity. With the infant lying on the back and with the chin in the midline, an arm is brought across the chest toward the opposite shoulder and thus up against the chin in the manner of a scarf. In the mature newborn, the hand should reach to the acromion process but no farther. If the hand goes past the acromion process, muscle tone may be lax, indicating immaturity. This is shown in Figure 32-7D, page 711.

Assessment of the Neck

Inspect the neck for good body alignment. Does the infant hold the head straight, or is it tipped to one side, as happens with torticollis (a torn sternocleidomastoid muscle)?

Observe the infant in a prone position. Does she make an attempt to lift her head? Pull the infant to a sitting position from a supine position and observe for head control. A newborn will have complete head lag until she reaches the sitting position, when she will make a momentary attempt at head support. After this momentary effort, her head will fall forward in a lax manner.

Palpate the sides of the neck for the posterior and anterior cervical, submental, postauricular, and occipital lymph nodes (Figure 32-3). Palpate the sternocleidomastoid muscle for masses (a hematoma forming from birth injury). Palpate the trachea to be certain that it is in the midline and that the thyroid gland on its lateral aspects is not enlarged.

Turn the infant's head from side to side. Extend it and flex it. Observe for crying or signs of pain when you flex the neck (a test for meningeal irritation). Inspect the anterior neck closely for a dermal sinus, since this is a common opening point for such sinuses.

Assessment of the Head

Observe the head and face for symmetry. Observe the infant while crying or smiling to see whether both sides of the mouth move in the same direction. Observe the distance between the eyes to detect hypotelorism or hypertelorism (narrowly or widely set eyes).

Inspect the head for molding and the presence of caput succedaneum or cephalhematoma. With the infant in a sitting position, locate and palpate the fontanelles for size and tension. Tension of the fontanelles is deceptive if an infant's head is lowered. Palpate the suture lines for overriding or wide spacing. Feel the hair for texture. Well-nourished newborns have full-bodied hair; poorly nourished or immature infants have stringy, lifeless hair.

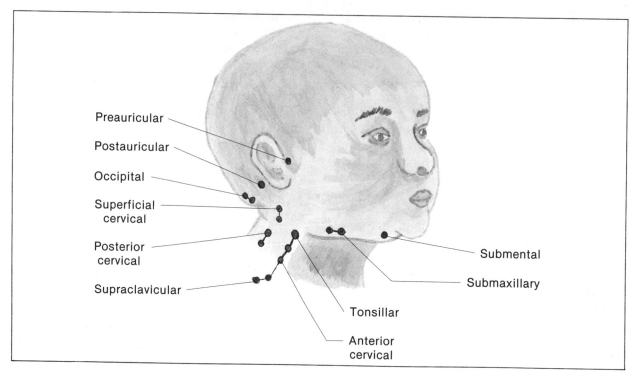

Figure 32-3 *Lymph nodes of the head and neck.*

Assessment of the Eyes

With the infant in a supine position, lift the head. This maneuver usually causes the baby to open his eyes. Observe the eyes for periorbital edema (indicated by a bulging of the eye globe) or a sunken appearance (a sign of dehydration). Note any subconjunctival hemorrhage (small innocent hemorrhagic areas on the eye sclera). Check for the presence of strabismus by observing whether or not a light shined into the eyes strikes the same place on both corneas (Figure 32-4). Transitory strabismus is common in newborns. Test for a blink reflex by shining a light on the eye (a blink reflex is not readily elicited in a newborn by an object moving toward the eye).

Test for pupillary constriction by shining an otoscope light first in one eye and then in the other. Bring the light downward from the forehead or in from the side of the eye, so that the pupil must make an immediate adjustment to the sudden bright light; if you bring the light gradually toward the eye, pupillary constriction will occur so gradually that it is easy to miss. Note whether the corneas are the same size and color. Look for haziness (possible cataract) or an irregular shape such as a coloboma (keyhole pupil) (see Figure 31-22).

Test for a red reflex by bringing an otoscope light up to about 6 inches from the eye. The retina will be visualized as a red disk. Such visualization demonstrates that the cornea, the lens, and the liquid of the eye are clear enough to be seen through and is a gross indication that the retina is intact. The retina and the red reflex are better revealed by use of the ophthalmoscope head of the otoscope.

Figure 32-4 *Hirschbrung's test. When a light is shined into a newborn's eyes, the light reflex should strike the pupils at the same point if they are in good alignment.*

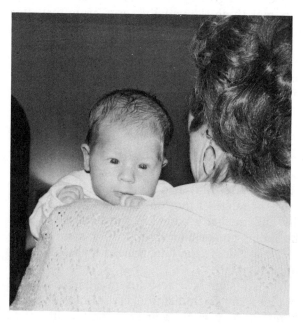

Assessment of the Ears

Inspect the outer ear for size, shape, and position (the upper portion of the pinna should be on a line drawn backward from the lateral canthus of the eye) (see Figure 31-23). Inspect the skin immediately in front of the ear for a dermal sinus.

Visualizing the tympanic membrane in a newborn is difficult and generally is not attempted because amniotic fluid and flecks of vernix fill the canal and obliterate the drum and its accompanying landmarks.

It is good practice to test the newborn's hearing by ringing a bell held about 6 inches from each ear. If he or she is crying, the infant who can hear will stop momentarily; if quiet, a newborn will blink the eyes, appear to attend to the sound, and may startle. This method of testing is not highly accurate. A negative response should be noted, however, and the child should be retested at a later time. In many health care facilities all newborns are tested by a standardized response to sound before discharge.

Assessment of the Nose

Inspect the nose for general appearance. Is it unusually broad? Is any ecchymosis present? Are the nares flaring as in an infant with respiratory distress? Shine the otoscope light into the nose to note whether the septum is straight and to attempt to view the turbinates (the cartilage processes on the sides).

Test for choanal atresia by closing the newborn's mouth and compressing one naris at a time with your fingers. Note any discomfort or distress.

Assessment of the Mouth and Throat

Inspect the lips for symmetry. Note any tendency toward a cleft. Introduce a tongue blade into the mouth and inspect the gums for the presence of teeth or a cleft. Look at the tongue and buccal membrane for evidence of thrush (rare under 4 or 5 days of age). Thrush, a monilian infection, appears as white patches on the tongue or mucus membrane. Note the movement of the tongue. Does the infant hold it in the midline or does it deviate to one side?

Inspect the palate for intactness or an unusually high arch; the latter is associated with chromosomal abnormalities. Note any Epstein's pearls (calcium deposits) on the palate or inclusion cysts on the gums (normal).

Introduce the tongue blade farther into the mouth. Using a good light source, gag the newborn by pressing on the base of the tongue with the tongue blade. Note whether the gag reflex is present. Observe in the fleeting instant that the posterior pharynx is visible whether or not the uvula is in the midline and the posterior wall of the pharynx is free of a pharyngeal cyst.

Because newborns have a large quantity of mucus in the back of their throats, turn them on their stomachs or turn their heads to the side following elicitation of a gag reflex so mucus can drain.

Assessment of the Back

Because you want to leave a newborn in a prone position for a few minutes after eliciting the gag reflex, to be certain he or she is not choking on secretions, this is a good time to examine the back.

Lanugo is usually evident across the shoulders of newborns. The spine, particularly in the sacral area, should be inspected carefully for any tuft of hair or indentation that would reveal spina bifida occulta (see Chapter 46).

Inspect the scapulae for symmetry. Inspect the coccygeal area for a pilodermal sinus.

Assessment of the Neurologic Function

Stroke the back to calm or quiet a newborn before attempting to elicit any reflexes.

These reflexes should be elicited: rooting, sucking, palmar grasp, plantar grasp, step-in-place, placing, trunk incurvation, magnet, crossed extension, Landau, Babinski, tonic neck, and Moro. The techniques for eliciting these reflexes are discussed in the preceding chapter.

Two deep tendon reflexes should be included in the examination: the patellar and the biceps. A patellar reflex can be elicited in a newborn by tapping the patellar tendon with the tip of a finger; in older children or adults a percussion hammer is needed to demonstrate this reflex. The lower leg will move perceptibly if the child has a mature reflex. A biceps reflex is difficult to elicit in a newborn. To demonstrate this reflex, place the thumb of your left hand on the tendon of the biceps muscle on the inner surface of the elbow. Tap the thumb as it rests on the tendon. You are more likely to feel the tendon contract than to observe movement. A biceps reflex is a test for spinal nerves C-5 and C-6; a patellar reflex is a test for spinal nerves L-2 through L-4.

Table 32-2 Clinical Criteria for Gestational Assessment

	Gestation Age (Weeks)		
Finding	*0–36*	*37–38*	*39 and Over*
Sole creases	Anterior transverse crease only	Occasional creases in anterior two-thirds	Sole covered with creases
Breast nodule diameter	2 mm	4 mm	7 mm
Scalp hair	Fine and fuzzy	Fine and fuzzy	Coarse and silky
Earlobe	Pliable; no cartilage	Some cartilage	Stiffened by thick cartilage
Testes and scrotum	Testes in lower canal; scrotum small; few rugae	Intermediate	Testes pendulous; scrotum full; extensive rugae

Source: Usher, R., et al. (1966). Judgment of fetal age. *Pediatric Clinics of North America, 13,* 835.

Assessment of the Infant's Cry

Assessing a newborn's health is a complex task because of the multitude of normal variations present and because many subtle changes occur as newborns recover from the birth process and establish respirations and other body functions.

If the child did not cry during the physical assessment, irritate the soles of the feet or pinch a leg. Evaluate the sound of the cry for loudness and pitch. A brain-injured newborn has a high, shrill cry; an immature infant has a weak cry; a child with laryngeal stridor has a hoarse cry.

Measurements

Securing accurate measurements of the head, chest, abdominal circumferences, and length is part of a newborn assessment. It is good to leave these measurements to the last so that the newborn is not tired out by them before the neurologic assessment. The measurements must be plotted on a growth chart such as that shown in Appendix F in order to be interpreted meaningfully.

Assessment of Gestation Age

The best way of judging whether a newborn is a term infant is not by the due date but by the specific findings of the physical assessment.

There are many indexes of maturity. Usher (1966) has proposed the five criteria given in Table 32-2 as a basis for evaluating gestational maturity. These are easy, quick criteria to use for assessment of all newborns.

Dubowitz Maturity Scale

Dubowitz (1970) has devised a gestational rating scale whereby newborns can be observed and tested and rated as to maturity level based on much more extensive criteria.

All newborns that appear to be immature by Usher's criteria or who are light in weight at birth or early by date should be assessed by means of the more definitive criteria. Although completing a Dubowitz assessment takes practice, it is a tool that can be used successfully by nurses. Alone in a small community hospital nursery, debating whether the infant just delivered needs immediate medical intervention or can wait until morning for care, the nurse who can do a Dubowitz examination and report a standardized gestation age report may make the difference in the physician's actions.

The Dubowitz scale has been modified by Ballard (1977) to an assessment that can be completed in 3 to 4 minutes. The assessment consists of two portions (Figures 32-5 and 32-6). The first is a series of observations about such things as skin texture and color, lanugo, foot creases, and genital, ear, and breast maturity. The body part is inspected and given a score of 0 to 5 as described in Figure 32-5. This observation scoring should be done as soon as possible after birth as skin assessment becomes much less reliable after 24 hours.

To complete the second half of the examination, you observe or position the baby as shown in Figure 32-6. Again, the child is given numerical scores from 0 to 5. Examples of reflexes or tests of maturity are shown in Figure 32-7.

To establish the child's gestation age, the total score obtained (on both sections) is compared to

	0	1	2	3	4	5
SKIN	gelatinous red, transparent	smooth pink, visible veins	superficial peeling &/or rash, few veins	cracking pale area, rare veins	parchment, deep cracking, no vessels	leathery, cracked, wrinkled
LANUGO	none	abundant	thinning	bald areas	mostly bald	
PLANTAR CREASES	no crease	faint red marks	anterior transverse crease only	creases ant. 2/3	creases cover entire sole	
BREAST	barely percept.	flat areola, no bud	stippled areola, 1–2 mm bud	raised areola, 3–4 mm bud	full areola, 5–10 mm bud	
EAR	pinna flat, stays folded	sl. curved pinna, soft with slow recoil	well-curv. pinna, soft but ready recoil	formed & firm with instant recoil	thick cartilage, ear stiff	
GENITALS Male	scrotum empty, no rugae		testes descending, few rugae	testes down, good rugae	testes pendulous, deep rugae	
GENITALS Female	prominent clitoris & labia minora		majora & minora equally prominent	majora large, minora small	clitoris & minora completely covered	

Figure 32-5 *Physical maturity assessment criteria. From Ballard, J. L., et al. (1977). A simplified assessment of gestational age. Pediatric Research, 11, 374.*

the rating scale in Figure 32-8. As can be seen by this scale, an infant with a total score of 5 is at 26 weeks' gestation age; a total score of 10 reveals a gestation age of about 28 weeks; a score of 40 total points is found in infants at term or 40 weeks' gestation.

Using such a standard method of rating maturity is helpful in detecting infants who are small for gestation age (they are light in weight but the neuromuscular and physical observation scales will be adequate for their weeks in utero) and those who are immature because of a miscalculated due date. An infant who is found to be at a lower gestation age than was predicted by the mother's calculation of due date needs careful observation in the neonatal period and should not be admitted to routine nursery care.

Brazelton Neonatal Behavioral Assessment Scale

The Brazelton Neonatal Behavioral Assessment Scale is a rating scale devised by Brazelton (1973) to evaluate the newborn's behavioral capacity or ability to respond to set stimuli. Six major categories of behavior—habituation, orientation, motor maturity, variation, self-quieting ability, and social behavior—are assessed. These terms are defined in Table 32-3.

It is important that one have a wealth of experience with newborns before utilizing a Brazelton Neonatal Behavioral Assessment Scale. Perform-

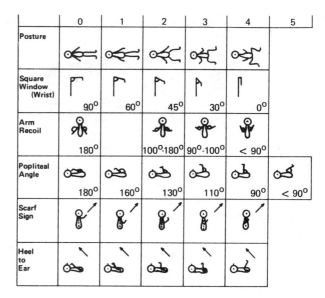

Figure 32-6 *Neuromuscular maturity assessment criteria. Posture: With infant supine and quiet, score as follows: arms and legs extended = 0; slight or moderate flexion of hips and knees = 1; moderate to strong flexion of hips and knees = 2; legs flexed and abducted, arms slightly flexed = 3; full flexion of arms and legs = 4. Square window: Flex hand at the wrist. Exert pressure sufficient to get as much flexion as possible. The angle between hypothenar eminence and anterior aspect of forearm is measured and scored. Do not rotate wrist. Arm recoil: With infant supine, fully flex forearm for 5 seconds, then fully extend by pulling the hands and release. Score as follows: remain extended or random movements = 0; incomplete or partial flexion = 2; brisk return to full flexion = 4. Popliteal angle: With infant supine and pelvis flat on examining surface, flex leg on thigh and fully flex thigh with one hand. With the other hand extend leg and score the angle attained according to the chart. Scarf sign: With infant supine, draw infant's hand across the neck and as far across the opposite shoulder as possible. Assistance to elbow is permissible by lifting it across the body. Score according to location of the elbow: elbow reaches opposite anterior axillary line = 0; elbow between opposite anterior axillary line and midline of thorax = 1; elbow at midline of thorax = 3; elbow does not reach midline of thorax = 4. Heel to ear: With infant supine, hold infant's foot with one hand and move it as near to the head as possible without forcing it. Keep pelvis flat on examining surface. From Ballard, J. L., et al. (1977). A simplified assessment of gestational age. Pediatric Research, 11, 374.*

ing an assessment by use of the scale requires training in the different techniques so that it is used consistently from one individual to another.

There are 27 behavioral items (Table 32-4) that are evaluated on a score of 1 to 9 and 20 elicited responses or reflexes scored on a 3 point scale. An "average" baby scores about the midpoint on each

Premature Infant

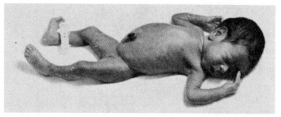

Full-term Infant

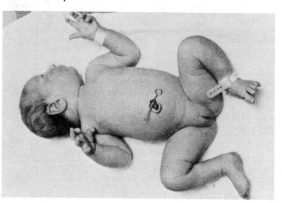

RESTING POSTURE   *The premature infant is characterized by very little, if any, flexion in the upper extremities and only partial flexion of the lower extremities. The full-term infant exhibits flexion in all four extremities.*

A

Premature Infant, 28–32 Weeks

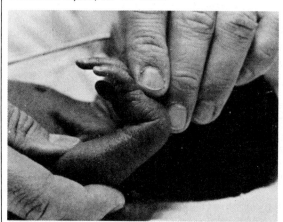

Full-term Infant

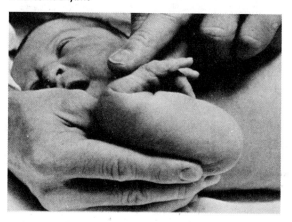

WRIST FLEXION   *The wrist is flexed, applying enough pressure to get the hand as close to the forearm as possible. The angle between the hypothenar eminence and the ventral aspect of the forearm is measured. (Care must be taken not to rotate the infant's wrist.) The premature infant at 28–32 weeks' gestation will exhibit a 90° angle. With the full-term infant it is possible to flex the hand onto the arm.*

B

Figure 32-7 *Examples of reflexes or tests used to judge gestation age. A. Posture. B. Square window. C. Recoil of extremities. D. Scarf sign. E. Heel to ear. F. Plantar creases. G. Breast tissue. H. Ear. I. Male genitals. J. Female genitals. From Sullivan, R., et al. (1979). Determining a newborn's gestational age. M.C.N., 4, 38. Original source: R. L. Schreiner (Ed.). (1978).* Care of the newborn. *Indianapolis: Indiana University Press.*

Flex Extremities and Hold

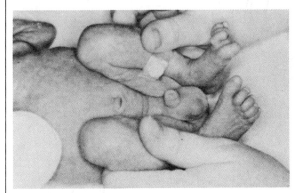

Extend

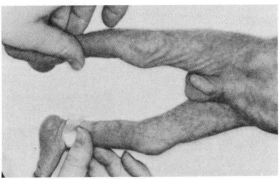

RECOIL OF EXTREMITIES   *Place the infant supine. To test recoil of the legs (1) flex the legs and knees fully and hold for five seconds, (2) extend by pulling on the feet, (3) release. To test the arms, flex forearms and follow same procedure. In the premature infant response is minimal or absent; in the full-term infant extremities return briskly to full flexion.*

C

Response in Premature Infant

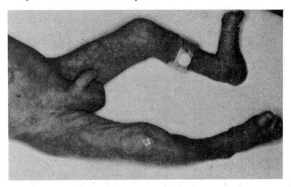

Response in Full-term Infant

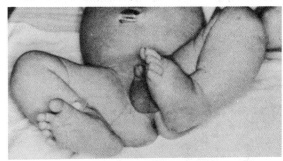

Premature Infant

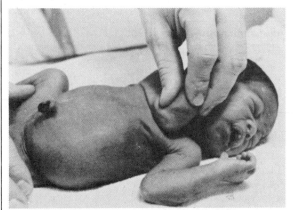

SCARF SIGN   *Hold the baby supine, take his hand, and try to place it around his neck and above the opposite shoulder as far posteriorly as possible. Assist this maneuver by lifting the elbow across the body. See how far across the chest the elbow will go. In the premature infant the elbow will reach near or across the midline. In the full-term infant the elbow will not reach the midline.*

D

Full-term Infant

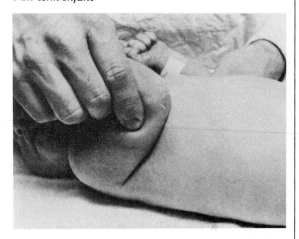

Figure 32-7 (continued)

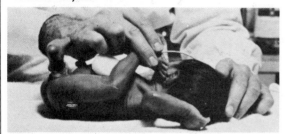

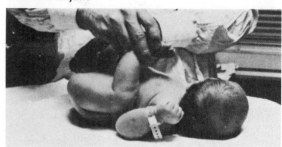

Premature Infant   *Full-term Infant*

HEEL TO EAR   *With the baby supine and his hips positioned flat on the bed, draw the baby's foot as near to his ear as it will go without forcing it. Observe the distance between the foot and head as well as the degree of extension at the knee. In the premature infant very little resistance will be met. In the full-term infant there will be marked resistance; it will be impossible to draw the baby's foot to his ear.*

E

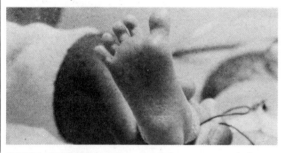

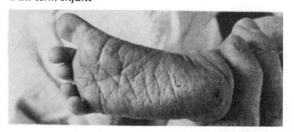

Premature Infant   *Full-term Infant*

SOLE CREASES   *The sole of the premature infant has very few or no creases. With the increasing gestation age, the number and depth of sole creases multiply, so that the full-term baby has creases involving the heel. (Wrinkles that occur after 24 hours of age can sometimes be confused with true creases.)*

F

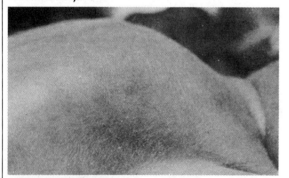

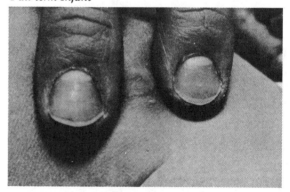

Premature Infant   *Full-term Infant*

NIPPLES AND BREAST   *In infants younger than 34 weeks' gestation the areola and nipple are barely visible. After 34 weeks the areola becomes raised. Also, the infant of less than 36 weeks' gestation has no breast tissue. Breast tissue arises with increasing gestation age due to maternal hormonal stimulation. Thus, an infant of 39–40 weeks will have 5–6 mm of breast tissue, and this amount will increase with age.*

G

Figure 32-7 (continued)

valuable for helping everyone involved in the infant's care come to know him or her as an individual and be more able to meet newborn needs.

Assessment of the Parent-Newborn Interaction

The manner in which new parents handle their infant is the result of several factors: their expectations of a newborn baby, their familiarity with newborns, perception of themselves as parents, and the events occurring during pregnancy. To assure yourself that parents and the child will be able to establish a good relationship, you need to observe the parents handling the child and to discuss with them the significant events of pregnancy and plans for the child.

It is helpful to know whether or not the pregnancy was planned. If it was not, how did they feel when the mother first suspected that she was pregnant? When pregnancy was confirmed? At quickening? During labor? At delivery? When they first saw or held the child?

Most women can name a point in pregnancy when they knew they wanted the baby. Such a point may not have been reached during pregnancy; it may not have been reached until delivery or until the woman first fed the baby. Some mothers are unable to say that they know they want a child until he or she has been home for a number of weeks.

In the hospital, it is important to ask the mother to try to identify this point. If she cannot do so by the time she leaves the hospital, she is still within the normal time period of response. The physician who will be caring for the infant or the community health nurse who will be visiting the child should be informed, however, that maternal-child interaction is still incomplete, so that they can be alert to the need for counseling if interaction does not improve in the coming months.

Chapter 29 describes the pattern of initial maternal contact. Be certain that you handle the newborn with the mother present; seeing you in action may speed up the process of learning how to handle her baby. Performing a physical assessment at the mother's bedside (Figure 32-9) gives her an opportunity to watch skilled newborn handling and to ask questions about her newborn. Further, as you note your findings on the newborn's reflexes, vaginal discharge, caput succedaneum, and so on, you can immediately assure the mother that these are normal newborn findings.

Utilizing Nursing Process

Health assessment of an infant at birth is an important responsibility so that any deviation from the normal can be identified and early therapy begun. In order to be well done, assessment should be structured to use nursing process.

Assessment

Assessment of an infant's health at birth includes history (gained from the pregnancy record), physical examination, laboratory reports such as hematocrit and blood type, and also an assessment of the parent-child interaction and beginning of bonding: Whether this occurs will influence a baby's life strongly. In addition to these formal inspection and examination times, be alert to appearance and activity every time you give care. Newborns have a disadvantage over older persons in that they are unable to detail their concerns. Your observation and inspection, then, must be more detailed in order to compensate.

Analysis

A nursing diagnosis used with a newborn is most often a well diagnosis such as "Stability of body systems related to adequate adjustment to ex-trauterine environment." Some diagnoses will be concerned with minor deviations from the normal, such as "Mother's concern related to strawberry hemangioma on infant's left arm" or "Fear of mother related to uneven respiratory rate of newborn." One goal established should relate to how the family plans to ensure comprehensive health follow-up for the child.

Planning

The initial newborn assessment is done immediately after birth. If performed in a delivery room, which is cool, a radiant warmer should be used to prevent the child from chilling. Plan for later assessments to be done at a time when a child is not hungry, which lessens the baby's distress. Planning to do a health assessment in the mother's postpartal room so she can observe the full inspection and ask any questions she has about her new child promotes mother-child bonding.

Implementations

All implementation of health assessment of newborns must be done with respect for conservation of the infant's heat and energy. Be certain to use aseptic technique with instruments so an infection is not accidentally spread from one infant to another. Be careful that any blood taken for laboratory determinations is not delayed in transit to the laboratory; newborns do not have enough blood for extra samples to be taken due to simple carelessness.

Evaluation

The final evaluation of whether a newborn is totally well or not must be delayed until later in the first year of life. A health assessment in the first few days of life, however, should be able to determine whether it is safe for the infant to be discharged without immediate care interventions.

Nursing Care Planning

The following is a health assessment made on Baby Kraft (John Joseph) on his first day of life.

Assessment

Examination done at mother's bedside; mother asked questions about meaning of rash.

Well-proportioned, black male newborn.
Wgt: 6 lb. 5 oz.—10% (AGA). Hgt: 19½ inches—25%. Head circumference: 34 cm—25%.
Head: Molding at vertex still prominent; ant. font.: 3 × 4 cm and soft; post. font.: pinpoint. Edematous raised area on right parietal 3 cm diameter, no discoloration.
Hair: Mature in thickness and character.
Eyes: Small subconjunctival hemorrhage right eye. Extraocular muscles grossly intact. Follow both sides to midline. Edema on eyelids present; mild inflammatory response on conjunctiva present.
Ears: Normal alignment; apparent patent canal meatus; firm cartilage, no discharge. Pinpoint dermal sinus in front of right ear, not inflamed, no discharge.
Nose: Midline septum, no discharge, patent.
Mouth: Midline uvula, palate intact, no teeth; 2 epithelial cysts on soft palate; gag reflex intact.
Neck: Midline trachea, no dermal sinuses, supple, no nodes palpable. Clavicles intact.
Heart: Rate 130, normal tones, no murmur heard.
Lungs: Air exchange all lobes, rate 30; rhonchi heard in both upper lobes.
Chest: Symmetrical, no retractions, breast tissue palpable 2 cm; no discharge.
Abdomen: Soft, no masses. Liver palpable 1 cm, spleen not palpable, 2 kidneys palpable.
Genitalia: Urinary meatus present; left testis not palpable; scant rugae on left scrotum.

Extremities: Full range of motion; hips abduct to 180 degrees.
Back: No dimples, hair tufts visible.
Skin: Slate gray 2 × 3 cm macular area in sacral area; scattered pinpoint papules on erythematous base on abdomen, back, arms, and legs.

Analysis

Newborn male with stability of major body systems related to adequate adjustment to extrauterine life; left testis not palpable. Caput succedaneum, mongolian spot, and erythema toxicum present.

Locus of Decision Making. Parents.

Goal. Infant will continue transition to extrauterine life without complication.

Criteria.
1. Testicular abnormality to be confirmed or ruled out by M.D.
2. If testicular abnormality is confirmed, plan of care to be outlined for parents before discharge.

Nursing Orders
1. Parents not told of undescended testis—wait for M.D. confirmation to avoid unnecessary concern.
2. Discuss mongolian spot, caput, and newborn rash with mother and assure her these are normal.
3. Notify private pediatrician of testicular abnormality. Parents want early discharge, 24–48 hours if possible.

Questions for Review

Multiple Choice

1. You are planning a health assessment on Baby Christus. In reviewing his mother's hospital record, which finding would be most important for you to locate?

   a. if his position in utero was posterior or anterior
   b. if he breathed spontaneously or not at birth
   c. if his mother used prepared childbirth exercises
   d. if he was a planned pregnancy or not

2. Baby Christus weighed 7 pounds, 3 ounces at birth. Based on this birth weight, which procedure below would be necessary for you to do?
   a. Plot his weight on a gestation age graph.
   b. Arrange for additional blood work for cholesterol level.
   c. Turn off the radiant heat warmer for physical assessment.
   d. Ask for additional consent to examine him.

3. On inspection, you note that Baby Christus has a normal newborn head proportion. This is
   a. one-half his total length.
   b. one-fourth his total length.
   c. one-sixth his total length.
   d. one-eighth his total length.

4. You assess Baby Christus' respiratory rate. In a newborn, you would recognize this as typically
   a. 12–16/minute.
   b. 16–20/minute.
   c. 20–30/minute.
   d. 30–50/minute.

5. On inspecting Baby Christus' abdomen, which finding would you note as abnormal?
   a. abdomen slightly protuberant (rounded)
   b. liver palpable 2 cm under the right costal margin
   c. bowel sounds present at 2 to 3 per minute
   d. clear drainage at the base of the umbilical cord

6. You assess Baby Christus for possible congenital hip dysplasia. The finding that would suggest this problem is
   a. inability of the right hip to externally rotate.
   b. crying on straightening of the right leg.
   c. continual drawing of his legs under him while prone.
   d. inward rotation of his right foot.

7. If Baby Christus is a term infant, you would expect to find what pattern of sole creases?
   a. creases covering one fourth of the foot
   b. longitudinal but not horizontal creases
   c. creases on three fourths of the foot
   d. heel but not anterior creases

8. You inspect genitalia. Which procedure below would you *not* include in your assessment?
   a. Palpate if testes are descended into the scrotal sac.
   b. Inspect the genital area for irritated skin.
   c. Inspect if the urethra opening appears circular.
   d. Retract the foreskin over the glans to assess for secretions.

9. Baby Christus is a well newborn. On examining his eyes, which finding below would you expect to discover?
   a. He follows your finger a full 180°.
   b. He has a white rather than a red reflex.
   c. He follows a light to the midline.
   d. He produces tears when he cries.

10. You elicit a gag reflex on Baby Christus to inspect his throat. Following this, which would be your best action?
    a. Sit him up abruptly.
    b. Turn his head to the side.
    c. Leave the tongue blade in his mouth for a count of 10.
    d. Speak to him calmly and reassuringly until he stops crying.

Discussion

1. It is important when doing physical assessment of newborns to prevent them from becoming chilled during the process. How would you control this in a birthing room? In a hospital nursery?
2. Performing a newborn assessment by a mother's bedside helps her get acquainted with her infant. What findings in a newborn would be most important to discuss with her?
3. Rating a newborn as to gestational age is only learned with practice. Describe how you would perform this using Usher's and Ballard's criteria.

Suggested Readings

Adams, M. E. (1981). Neonatal abilities . . . pictures in nursing. *Nursing (Oxford)*, 1, 913.

Ballard, J. L., et al. (1977). A simplified assessment of gestational age. *Pediatric Research*, 11, 374.

Barnett, M. M., et al. (1982). Infant outcome in relation to second stage labor pushing method. *Birth*, 9, 221.

Barrie, H. (1981). Examination of the newborn. *Midwife Health Visitor and Community Nurse*, 17, 422.

Brazelton, T. B. (1973). Neonatal Behavioral Assessment Scale. *Clinics in Developmental Medicine*, Vol. 50. Philadelphia: Lippincott.

Brodish, M. S. (1981). Perinatal assessment. *J.O.G.N. Nursing*, 10, 42.

Buckner, E. B. (1983). Use of Brazelton neonatal behavioral assessment in planning care for parents and newborns. *J.O.G.N. Nursing*, 12, 26.

Dubowitz, L., et al. (1970). Clinical assessment of gestational age in the newborn infant. *Journal of Pediatrics*, 77, 1.

Dunn, D. M., et al. (1981). Interaction of mothers with their newborns in the first half-hour of life. *Journal of Advances in Nursing*, 6, 27.

Evans, M. L. (1983). Tips for taking a child's blood pressure quickly. *Nursing 83*, 13, 61.

Garn, S. M., et al. (1981). Effect of maternal cigarette smoking on Apgar scores. *American Journal of Diseases of Children*, 135, 503.

Labson, L. (1983). The newborn: Quick postdelivery check. *Patient Care*, 17, 16.

Labson, L. H. (1983). Newborn exam: Evaluation in the nursery. *Patient Care, 17,* 95.

Levy, H. L., et al. (1982). The current practice of newborn screening. *Hospital Practice, 17,* 89.

Ludington-Hoe, S. M. (1983). What can newborns really see? *American Journal of Nursing, 83,* 1286.

Magowan, M., et al. (1980). The effect of an antibiotic spray on umbilical cord separation time. *Nursing Times, 76,* 184.

Maisels, M. J., & Conrad, S. (1982). Transcutaneous bilirubin measurements in full-term infants. *Pediatrics, 70,* 464.

Nelson, K. B., & Ellenberg, J. H. (1981). Apgar scores as predictors of chronic neurologic disability. *Pediatrics, 68,* 36.

Ostler, C. W. (1979). Initial feeding time of newborn infants: Effects upon first meconium passage and serum indirect bilirubin levels. *Issues in Health Care of Women, 1,* 1.

Parker, S., et al. (1981). Newborn behavioral assessment: Research, prediction, and clinical uses . . . the Brazelton Neonatal Behavioral Assessment Scale. *Children Today, 10,* 2.

Phibbs, R. H. (1980). The birth was normal . . . but is the baby? *Birth and Family Journal, 7,* 215.

Plante, D., et al. (1984). Expanding the nurse's role through formal assessment of the neonate. *J.O.G.N. Nursing, 13,* 25.

Scharping, E. M. (1983). Physiological measurements of the neonate: Methods of accurately measuring vital signs are constantly being refined. *M.C.N., 8,* 70.

Schiffman, R. F. (1982). Temperature monitoring in the neonate: A comparison of axillary and rectal temperatures. *Nursing Research, 31,* 274.

Usher, R., et al. (1966). Judgment of fetal age. *Pediatric Clinics of North America, 13,* 835.

Wilson, L. J. (1984). How to give baby's first physical. *R.N., 47,* 44.

33

Nutritional Needs of the Newborn

OBJECTIVES

Following mastery of the contents of this chapter, you should be able to

1. Describe normal newborn nutritional requirements.
2. Assess a newborn as to whether he or she is receiving adequate nutrition.
3. State a nursing diagnosis related to newborn nutrition.
4. Plan with a mother a method of infant feeding that will be satisfying for both her and the infant.
5. Implement feeding procedures with newborn infants.
6. Evalute goal outcomes in relation to both mother and infant satisfaction.
7. Analyze ways that nurses can help mothers problem solve feeding difficulties.
8. Synthesize knowledge of normal newborn nutrition with nursing process to achieve quality maternal-newborn nursing care.

BECAUSE PROPER NUTRITION is essential for optimal growth and development, knowledge of good infant nutrition is a fundamental requirement for persons involved in the health supervision of newborns. In no other area of nutrition, with the possible exception of weight control or diabetes, is the nurse asked more questions than she is asked about the process of infant feeding.

Nutritional Allowances for the Newborn

Although breast-feeding is for many reasons the method of choice for feeding human infants, a mother should be urged to choose for herself the method of infant feeding, breast or bottle, that will be most satisfying and convenient for her. No matter which method she chooses, the end result must meet the nutritional and psychological needs of her infant.

Nutrition is extremely important in the early months of life, because brain growth is proceeding at a rapid rate during this time. Infants in whom kwashiorkor (a protein depletion disease) develops when they are 3 to 6 months old may fail to reach their full intellectual or psychological development. Mental retardation has been observed in infant rats when their caloric intake is inadequate. Rats, piglets, and puppies fed a diet adequate in calories but deficient in protein show signs of degenerative changes in nerve cells.

As important in terms of growth is the maternal stimulation or love the infant receives. This is directly related to feeding, since the mother is close to her infant during feeding time and the baby will be particularly sensitive to her demonstration of affection or to her lack of warmth. An infant who does not experience a warm relationship with his or her mother may fail to thrive as surely as one denied sufficient protein or calories. (See the Nursing Research Highlight on page 723.)

Caloric Requirement

Growth in the neonatal period and early infancy is more rapid than at any other period of life. Therefore, the caloric requirements exceed those at any other age. A newborn and an infant up to 2 months of age require 120 calories per kilogram of body weight (50 to 55 calories per pound) every 24 hours to provide an adequate amount of food for maintenance and allow for growth as well. After 2 months of age, the amount gradually declines until the requirement at 1 year is down to 100 calories per kilogram, or 45 calories per pound per day. In adults, the requirement is 42 calories per kilogram, or 20 calories per pound per day.

The actual caloric requirement, of course, depends on the activity of the baby and the rate of growth. An active infant, one who cries frequently and squirms constantly, will need more calories than one who is more passive and is content to spend long hours playing quietly or just studying the environment.

A large number of mothers tend to feed their babies more calories than they physiologically need (especially extra quantities of milk), believing that a chubby-cheeked baby with fat legs is a healthy one. This is not necessarily the case; an overweight baby is more likely to become an overweight adult than one whose weight is within the usual range during the first year of life. The fat cells in the overweight infant appear to increase in size and remain large, so that such a baby tends to be obese ever afterward. Unusually rapid weight gain in the early months of life of a term infant is related to obesity and overweight in later childhood (Eid, 1970).

A formula should contain about 9 to 12 percent of the calories as protein and 45 to 55 percent of

===== *Nursing Research Highlight* =====

Will Early Bonding Affect Nutritional Intake?

A study of 85 full-term normal infants was conducted to determine the relationship between early bonding in the immediate postdelivery period and initial infant feeding patterns in bottle-fed newborns (Brodish, 1982). Analysis of the data showed that a significant effect of bonding was increased benefit to infant status. This was demonstrated by improved nutritional intake and less weight loss.

Reference

Brodish, M. (1982). Relationship of early bonding to initial infant feeding patterns in bottle-fed newborns. *J.O.G.N. Nursing, 11,* 248.

---

the calories as lactose carbohydrate. The balance should be fat, of which about 10 percent (4 percent of the calories) should be linoleic acid.

Protein Requirement

Because of the extremely rapid growth during infancy and because protein is necessary for the formation of new cells and the maturation and maintenance of existing cells, protein requirements are high during the newborn and infancy period. The nutritional allowance of protein for the first 2 months of life is 2.2 gm per kilogram of body weight; for ages 2 to 6 months it is 2.0 gm per kilogram; for ages 6 months to 1 year it is 1.8 gm per kilogram. Both human milk and cow's milk provide all the essential amino acids. Histidine, an amino acid that appears to be essential for infant growth but is not necessary for adult growth, is found in both forms of milk.

Cow's milk contains about 16 percent of its calories as protein; human milk, about 8 percent. Thus the milk in a formula containing cow's milk must be diluted. Undiluted cow's milk creates such a rich solute load (the amount of urea and electrolytes that must be excreted in the urine) that newborn kidneys are overwhelmed. The protein in cow's milk differs from that in human milk in composition as well as in amount. The main protein in human milk is lactalbumin; the main protein in cow's milk is casein. The curd tension in milk is related to the amount of casein present. Thus, the curd in cow's milk is large, tough, and difficult to digest; in human milk, the curd is softer and easier to digest.

Fat Requirement

Linoleic acid is an essential fatty acid necessary for growth and skin integrity in infants. It is found in both human and cow's milk, but human milk contains about three times as much. Infants fed on skimmed milk for long periods of time (when other sources of food are not being offered) may become deficient in linoleic acid. Therefore feeding skimmed milk is not the answer to controlling obesity in young infants. In addition, skimmed milk does not contain sufficient calories (only about half as many).

Carbohydrate Requirement

Lactose, the disaccharide found in human milk, appears to be the most easily digested of the carbohydrates. It improves calcium absorption and aids in nitrogen retention, both of which are positive factors. When included in a formula, it produces stools most like those of a breast-fed baby, in which gram-positive rather than gram-negative bacteria predominate, another positive factor. An adequate carbohydrate level in a formula allows protein to be used for building new cells rather than for calories, encouraging normal water balance, and preventing abnormal metabolism of fat.

Cow's milk contains about 29 percent of its calories as carbohydrate; human milk, 37 percent. Cow's milk formulas need added carbohydrate to bring their carbohydrate content up to that of human milk.

Fluid Requirement

Maintaining a sufficient fluid intake in newborns is important because their metabolic rate is high and metabolism requires water. An adult uses 25 to 30 calories per kilogram of body weight in 24 hours for metabolism. In the same period, a newborn utilizes 45 to 50 calories per kilogram. This high rate of metabolism requires a large amount of water. In addition, the surface area of the newborn is large in relation to body mass. Thus, a baby loses a larger amount of water by evaporation than does an adult.

Water is distributed differently in the newborn than in the adult. In an adult, about 20 percent of body weight is extracellular fluid; in a newborn, 30 to 35 percent of body weight is extracellular fluid. Consequently, loss of fluid or inadequate fluid intake, which depletes the extracellular water supply, can affect as much as 35 percent of the newborn's fluid component. Because the kidneys of a newborn are not yet capable of fully concentrating urine, the newborn cannot conserve body water by this mechanism and must have an adequate fluid intake to prevent dehydration.

The fluid requirement for a newborn is 160 to 200 ml per kilogram (2.5 to 3.0 ounces per pound) per 24 hours.

Mineral Requirement

Calcium

Calcium is an important mineral because of its contribution to bone growth. Calcium levels tend to fall after birth, and phosphate levels tend to rise. Since milk is high in calcium, tetany from a low calcium level seldom occurs in infants who suck well, whether taking human milk or cow's milk formula. Both milks contain more calcium than phosphorus, but the ratio is higher in human milk than in cow's milk (2:1 versus 1.2:1.0).

Iron

The infant of a mother who had an adequate iron intake during pregnancy will be born with iron stores that, theoretically, will last for the first 3 months of life, until he or she begins to produce adult hemoglobin. Because not all mothers' diets are iron-rich during pregnancy (and socioeconomic level is not a good criterion for judging the quality of a diet), the American Academy of Pediatrics (1976) recommends that an iron supplement be given to formula-fed infants for the entire first year of life.

Fluoride

Fluoride is essential for building sound teeth and for resistance to tooth decay. When an infant's teeth are first forming during pregnancy, it is important for mothers to drink fluoridated water. The lactating mother should continue drinking fluoridated water (although fluoride does not pass in great amounts in breast milk), and formulas should be prepared with fluoridated water. This is an essential point to remember, because a mother may think she is helping her child by using bottled "natural" water in the formula rather than the chlorinated (but fluoridated) water from a tap.

If a mother is breast-feeding or a source of fluoridated water is not available (the family drinks well or spring water or bottled water, or the tap water is not fluoridated), it is recommended that a fluoride supplement be given: 0.25 mg daily (Fomon, 1979).

Vitamin Requirement

Vitamin additives are necessary for the bottle-fed infant.

Formerly, vitamin C was introduced by adding orange juice to the diet and vitamin D by adding cod liver oil. Orange juice causes colic or skin rashes in some infants, and it is a rare infant who takes cod liver oil well. Therefore, as with iron, the American Academy of Pediatrics recommends supplemental multi-vitamins (A, C, and D) for the entire first year of life. Infants taking commercially prepared formulas do not need additional vitamins because such formulas already contain them.

Breast-Feeding

All women should be asked during pregnancy if they have thought yet about whether they plan to breast-feed or formula-feed their newborn.

Mothers who expect to breast-feed can practice a few simple techniques toward the end of pregnancy to improve milk production and ease of feeding. Nipple rolling—that is, holding the nipple between the thumb and finger and rolling it gently to cause it to protrude—done two or three times a day, is helpful in releasing adhesions at the base of the nipple and in making it more protuberant.

Practicing breast massage to move the milk forward in the milk ducts (manual expression of milk) is helpful. This allows a woman who may feel diffident about handling her breasts to grow accustomed to it and will enable her to assist with milk production in the first few days after birth. Manual expression consists of supporting the breast firmly, then placing the thumbs on the areolar margin and pushing inward and backward toward the chest wall until secretion begins to flow (Figure 33-1). During the last months of pregnancy and immediately following birth, the fluid obtained will be colostrum. By the third day of infant life, milk will be obtained.

A woman should avoid using any soap on her breasts during pregnancy because soap tends to dry and crack nipples. The use of creams or lo-

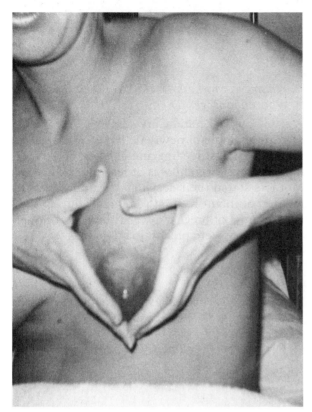

Figure 33-1 *Manual expression of milk. The breast is supported firmly and the thumbs are pushed back firmly until breast milk begins to flow. From Murdaugh, Sr. A., & Miller, L. E. Helping the breast-feeding mother.* American Journal of Nursing, 72, 1420.

tions other than lanolin or A&D ointment does not help in any way and may overstimulate the nipples because of too much handling, leading to nipple fissures and soreness.

Physiology of Breast-Feeding

Milk is formed in the acinar or alveolar cells of the mammary glands. (Internal breast anatomy is shown graphically in Figure 8-14.) Colostrum, a thin, watery, high-protein fluid, has been secreted by these cells since the fourth month of pregnancy. With the delivery of the placenta, the level of progesterone in the mother's body falls dramatically, stimulating the production of prolactin, an anterior pituitary hormone. Prolactin acts on the acinar cells of the mammary glands to stimulate the production of milk. Moreover, when an infant sucks at the breast, nerve impulses travel from the nipple to the hypothalamus to stimulate the production of prolactin-releasing factor. This factor then passes to the pituitary and stimulates further active production of prolactin. Other anterior pituitary hormones such as ACTH, TSH, and growth hormone probably also play a role in growth of the mammary glands and their ability to secrete milk.

Milk flows from alveolar cells through small tubules to reservoirs for milk, *lactiferous sinuses,* behind the nipple. This constantly forming milk is termed *foremilk.* Its availability depends very little on the infant's sucking at the breast. Foremilk is produced in all mothers 3 to 4 days after delivery.

A second result of an infant's sucking at the breast is release of oxytocin from the posterior pituitary. Oxytocin causes smooth muscle to contract so it stimulates the uterus to contract, and the breast-feeding mother will feel a small tugging or cramping in her lower pelvis during the first few days of breast-feeding. Oxytocin causes the collecting sinuses of the mammary glands to contract too, forcing milk forward through the nipple and making it readily available for the baby. This action is termed the *let-down reflex.* In addition, new milk, termed *hind milk,* is formed after the let-down reflex. Hind milk tends to be higher in fat than foremilk and is the milk that will make the breast-fed infant grow most rapidly.

Colostrum

Colostrum is composed of protein, sugar, fat, water, minerals, vitamins, and maternal antibodies. It is high in protein and fairly low in sugar and fat. Its low fat content makes it easy to digest.

Physiologic Advantages of Breast-Feeding

The advantages and disadvantages of breast-feeding are a popular subject. Everyone seems to feel compelled to take a position on one side or the other.

The easiest way for a woman to decide whether to breast-feed is to ask herself what would please her most and make her most comfortable. If she is comfortable and pleased with what she is doing, her infant will be comfortable and pleased, will enjoy being fed, and will thrive. The choice is that simple. (See the Nursing Research Highlight on page 726.)

Advantages for the Mother

There are a number of physiologic benefits to the woman from breast-feeding.

1. The incidence of breast cancer in women who breast-feed appears to be lower than in those who do not. In a study in Boston (Moore, 1967), mothers who breast-fed for more than 3 months had a significantly lower incidence of

Nursing Research Highlight

Breast-Feeding

Inconsistencies in Nurses' Knowledge About Breast-Feeding

Hayes (1981) studied 203 nurses involved in supporting and counseling breast-feeding mothers during a hospital stay. Inconsistencies among the majority of nurses in their ability to support breast-feeding women and understand the mechanisms of successful breast-feeding were demonstrated. It was concluded from this study that nursing school does not necessarily prepare a nurse with adequate information to counsel mothers on breast-feeding. Before attempting to teach a new mother, a nurse must be sure that her suggestions are based on adequate knowledge.

Reference

Hayes, B. (1981). Inconsistencies among nurses in breastfeeding knowledge and counseling. *J.O.G.N. Nursing, 11,* 430.

When Do Mothers Decide to Breast-Feed and Who Encourages Them?

A study by Beske and Garvis (1982) used a convenience sample of newly delivered primiparas who were breast-feeding and had just delivered infants whose weight was at least 5.5 pounds. Mothers stated their decisions regarding the method of infant feeding were made during the first months of pregnancy, and the baby's father and the baby were predominant sources of encouragement.

Reference

Beske, E., & Garvis, M. (1982). Important factors in breast feeding success. *M.C.N., 7,* 174.

---

breast cancer than did those who did not breast-feed or who breast-fed for less than 3 months.

2. The release of oxytocin from the posterior pituitary aids uterine involution.
3. Women in whom varicosities develop during pregnancy are prone to thrombophlebitis following delivery. If such women breast-feed and thus are not given estrogen to suppress lactation, they are not subjected to the increased risk of thromboembolic complications with administration of this drug.

Many mothers feel that breast-feeding will give them the best chance of forming a true symbiotic bond with their child. This is not necessarily true. A mother who holds her baby to bottle-feed can form this bond equally well. Many mothers feel that breast-feeding is a foolproof contraceptive technique. Again, they are incorrect. Among mothers who breast-feed, 50 percent start ovulating by the fourth week postpartum (Cronin, 1968).

Some mothers are reluctant to breast-feed because they fear it will tie them down to have to be available to feed the baby every 3 or 4 hours. In reality, their situation is no different from that of the mother who is bottle-feeding; she also has to be available every 4 hours. Both breast-feeding and bottle-feeding mothers should have time away from their babies occasionally. Both can prepare bottles of formula for the baby-sitter or father to use while they are away.

Advantages for the Baby

Breast-feeding has certain physiologic advantages for the baby. Breast milk contains secretory immunoglobin A (IgA), which binds large molecules of foreign proteins including viruses and bacteria and keeps them from being absorbed through the gastrointestinal tract into the infant. *Lactoferrin* is an iron-binding protein present that binds iron in such a way that pathogenic bacteria that require iron for growth cannot utilize it. This decreases the growth of such bacteria. *Lysozyme* is an enzyme present that apparently actively destroys bacteria by lysing (dissolving) their cell membranes. It may increase the effectiveness of antibodies. Leukocytes are present in breast milk and provide protection against infectious invaders. Macrophages in breast milk are responsible for producing *interferon*, which interferes with virus growth. The *bifidus factor* is a specific growth-promoting factor present that the bacteria *Lactobacillus bifidus* needs in order to grow. The presence of *Lactobacillus bifidus* interferes with colonization of the gastrointestinal tract by pathogenic bacteria.

In addition to these anti-infection properties,

breast milk contains the ideal electrolyte and mineral composition for human infant growth. Breast milk is higher in lactose than is cow's milk. Lactose is a readily digested sugar that provides ready glucose for rapid brain growth. The ratio of cysteine to methionine (two amino acids) in breast milk also appears to favor rapid brain growth in early months. Although the protein content of breast milk is less than that of cow's milk, it is more readily digested by the infant and therefore the infant may actually receive more. Breast milk contains nitrogen in compounds other than protein and so the infant receives cell-building materials from sources other than just protein. Breast milk contains more linoleic acid, an essential amino acid for skin integrity, than does cow's milk. It contains less sodium, potassium, calcium, and phosphorus than do many formulas. These lower levels are enough to supply infant needs, and they spare the infant's kidneys from having to process a high renal solute load of unused nutrients. Breast milk also has a better balance of trace elements such as zinc than do formulas.

Babies on breast milk appear to have less difficulty with regulation of calcium-phosphorus levels than those who are bottle-fed. Cow's milk formulas contain a high level of phosphorus. As the phosphorus level in the infant's bloodstream rises, the calcium level falls because of the inverse relationship between phosphorus and calcium. Decreased calcium levels in the newborn lead to tetany. The increased concentration of fatty acid in commercial formulas may bind calcium in the gastrointestinal tract and further increase the danger of tetany.

There is a great deal of discussion about the benefits of breast-feeding from the standpoint of the formation of the dental arch. Babies suck differently from a breast than from a bottle (Figure 33-2). Infants pull their tongue backward as they suck from a breast; they thrust it forward to suck from a rubber nipple. Tongue thrusting may lead to malformation of the dental arch.

Mothers who have a familial history of allergy are usually encouraged to breast-feed and thus eliminate the possibility of exposing the infant to cow's milk protein, which is allergenic this early in life.

Beginning Breast-Feeding

Breast-feeding should begin as soon after delivery as possible. Ideally, the first breast-feeding should begin immediately while the mother is still in a birthing room and the infant is in the first reactivity period. The release of oxytocin from breast-feeding at this time not only gets the production of milk off to an early start but stimulates uterine contraction as well. If the mother is fatigued—and it is a rare mother who is not—adding this new skill of child care at this point may only convince her that breast-feeding is not for her, however, so when to initiate breast-feeding should be individually considered.

The infant should be fed by 4 to 8 hours after delivery if not fed at birth, provided color, respirations, and temperature are normal. It is important that infants grasp the areola of the nipple, as well as the nipple itself, when they suck. This gives them an effective sucking action and helps to empty the collecting sinuses completely. To prevent nipples from becoming sore and cracked, an infant should be fed for only 5 minutes at each breast at each feeding the first day. The time at each breast is increased 1 minute per day until, by the sixth day, a baby is nursing for 10 minutes at each breast at each feeding. This schedule also keeps the infant from becoming fatigued. At each feeding, the infant should be placed first at the breast he or she fed at last in the previous feeding. Thus each breast is completely emptied at every other feeding.

Milk forms to the extent that it is used. If the breasts are completely emptied, they completely fill again. If half-emptied, they only half-fill, and after a time, milk production will be insufficient for proper nourishment.

As important as making certain that infants are grasping the areola of the breast is helping them to break away from the suction of the breast when they are through feeding. This can be done by inserting a finger in the corner of the mouth or by pulling the chin down (see Figure 33-3). Otherwise they may pull too hard on the nipple and cause cracking or soreness.

Breast-feeding is, in more simple cultures, the method of feeding babies that is used by all mothers; the technique is learned early. In the United States most mothers must be shown the technique because they have had few, if any, opportunities to observe the process. One of the first things a mother needs to learn to do before she will be a successful breast-feeder is relax. If she is tense and anxious, she will not achieve a good let-down reflex, and her infant will have difficulty getting adequate milk. She will become more tense and anxious because her infant does not seem content, the infant will have more difficulty, and shortly she will stop breast-feeding.

Relaxing is not easy when you are a new mother because perineal stitches hurt (and never underestimate the sharpness and the pain of

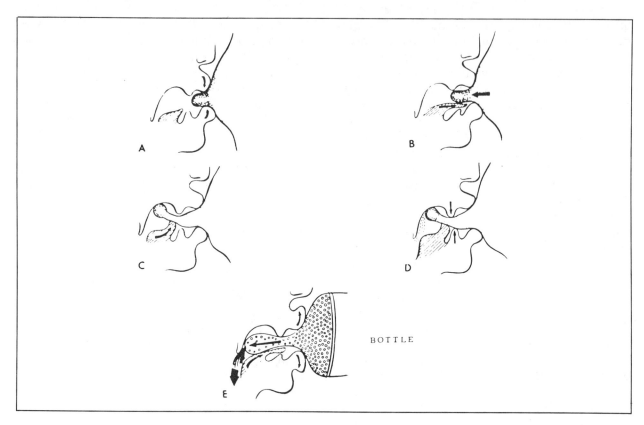

Figure 33-2 *Sucking mechanism at the breast (A–D) and bottle (E). A. The lips of the infant clamp in a C shape at the concave junction of nipple and areola, fitting like a glove. The cheek muscles contract. B. The tongue thrusts forward to grasp nipple and areola. C. The nipple is brought against the hard palate as the tongue pulls backward, bringing the areola into the mouth. Negative pressure is created by action of tongue and cheeks against the nipple, and the result is a true sucking motion. D. The gums compress the areola, squeezing milk into the back of the throat. Milk flows against the hard palate from the high-pressure system of the breast to the area of negative pressure at the back of the throat. E. In contrast, the large rubber nipple of a bottle strikes the soft palate (causing gagging) and interferes with the action of the tongue. The tongue moves forward against the gum to control the overflow of milk into the esophagus. From Applebaum, R. M. (1970). The modern management of successful breast feeding. Pediatric Clinics of North America, 17, 203.*

stitches) and the baby is so small and looks so helpless and dependent.

Lying on her side with a pillow under her head is a good position for the mother to assume when she is first attempting breast-feeding (Figure 33-4). It is comfortable for her and allows the infant to rest on the bed, also a comfortable position. Figures 33-5 and 33-6 show alternative positions for breast-feeding. The mother should wash her hands before breast-feeding as she would if she were bottle-feeding, to be sure they are free of pathogens picked up from handling perineal pads. She need not wash her breasts before feeding unless she notices a lot of caked colostrum on the nipple.

If a mother brushes the infant's cheek with her nipple, the baby will turn toward the breast (rooting reflex). Be careful that *you* do not initiate a rooting reflex by trying to press the baby's face against the mother's breast and causing the child to turn *away* from the mother. Such a move may make her think her baby does not like breast-feeding.

If a mother has large breasts, the infant may have trouble breathing while nursing because breast tissue is pressing against his nose. A mother may prevent this by grasping the areolar margin between her thumb and forefinger, holding the bulk of the breast supported. The nipple is thus made more protuberant as well.

The breasts will secrete only colostrum the first 1 to 2 days. On the third or fourth day, milk

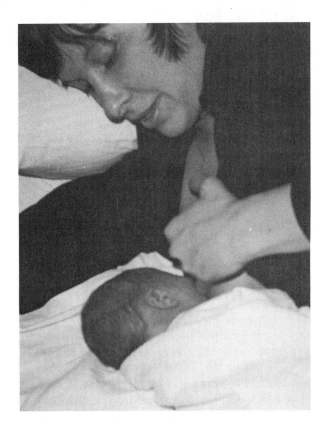

Figure 33-3 *Pressing a finger against the corner of the baby's jaw to release suction. From Murdaugh, Sr. A., & Miller, L. E. (1972). Helping the breast-feeding mother. American Journal of Nursing, 72, 1420.*

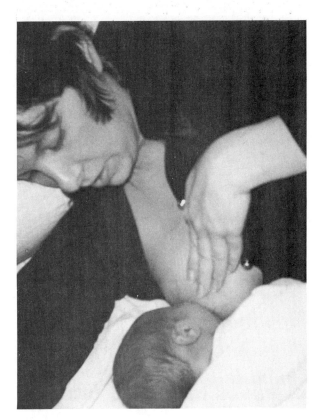

Figure 33-4 *Side-lying position for breast-feeding. Notice how the mother holds the bulk of breast tissue away from the infant's nose. From Murdaugh, Sr. A., & Miller, L. E. (1972). Helping the breast-feeding mother. American Journal of Nursing, 72, 1420.*

will form. The infant should be put to the breast and encouraged to suck during the first 2 days since the stimulation of sucking aids the formation of breast milk. Breast milk looks like skimmed milk; it is thin and almost blue-tinged in color. Many mothers need assurance that the

Figure 33-5 *Reversing the baby's position to ease sore nipples. From Murdaugh, Sr. A., & Miller, L. E. (1972). Helping the breast-feeding mother. American Journal of Nursing, 72, 1420.*

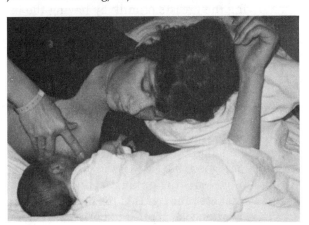

color and consistency are normal for breast milk. Otherwise, they think their milk is not nutritious enough for their infants.

Babies should be fed as often as hungry the first few days of life, because they are receiving only colostrum and so need the nutrients and fluid obtained by frequent sucking. Further, the more often the breasts are emptied, the more efficiently they will fill and continue to maintain a good supply of milk. A baby may need to be fed as often as every 2 or 3 hours for the first few days.

A newborn being breast-fed will often drop off to sleep during the first few feedings, as bottle-fed infants do. In order for milk production to be effectively stimulated, and to ensure an adequate fluid intake, the infant should be kept awake and urged to suck. The mother can prevent this falling asleep by waking a baby up well before feeding by handling him and stroking his back, changing his position during feeding, or rubbing his arms and chest. Tickling the bottom of a baby's feet wakes him up effectively, but most mothers are unwilling to cause their newborns discomfort in order to keep them awake. This may be the first sign that the mother is transferring the protectiveness she

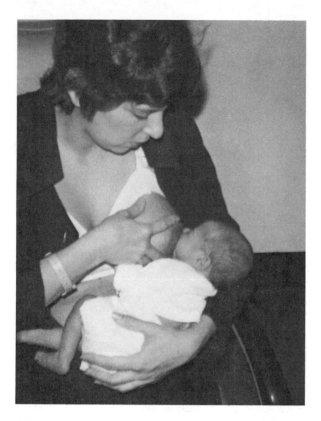

Figure 33-6 *Sitting position for breast-feeding. From Murdaugh, Sr. A., & Miller, L. E. (1972). Helping the breast-feeding mother.* American Journal of Nursing, *72, 1420.*

felt all during pregnancy toward her own body to that of her newborn and is therefore a positive rather than a negative reaction.

If an infant seems to tire easily or is too affected by the delivery anesthetic to suck vigorously, the mother can massage her breasts to increase the flow of milk while the infant sucks. This is the same breast massage she practiced during pregnancy. If the infant is sucking strongly and effectively, and sucking is well paced, she should not attempt breast massage. Massage will increase the flow of milk to such an extent that the infant will begin to choke or aspirate.

If an infant is not sucking well at all, the mother can use breast massage following the first feedings to empty her breasts manually. This will ensure good milk production for the time when the infant is ready to suck.

An infant who is taking in little breast milk because of poor sucking or insufficient nipple projection, which makes it difficult to grasp the nipple and suck effectively, needs some fluid supplementation. Many people believe that additional fluid should not be given in a bottle, since the infant may become accustomed to a bottle rather than to the breast. They recommend that

the extra fluid be given by spoon or medicine dropper. However, the infant needs this additional fluid only for the first 3 or 4 days of life. After that, the mother's breast milk has formed, the infant is free of effects of anesthesia, and he or she will obtain adequate fluid without supplementation. Further, the danger of aspiration rises with medicine-dropper, spoon, or cup feedings. Finally, some mothers are ready to stop breast-feeding at the slightest sign of trouble, and having to give supplementary feedings by medicine dropper may precipitate their rejection of breast-feeding. Thus, the advantages of giving supplemental fluid by bottle seem to outweigh its disadvantages.

Common Problems with Breast-Feeding

The common problems that arise with breast-feeding, if handled intelligently by the health care personnel advising the mother, will pass and be as nothing to her. Handled wrongly, or overemphasized, they may so complicate breast-feeding that a mother is discouraged from continuing it. It is bizarre that complications should deter a mother from using the most natural and least complicated of all infant feeding methods.

Engorgement

On the third or fourth day, when breast milk comes in, a mother may notice swelling, hardness, tenderness, and perhaps heat in her breasts. The skin may appear red, tense, and shiny. This is engorgement and is caused by vascular and lymphatic congestion arising from an increase in the blood and lymph supply to the breasts. An infant has difficulty sucking on engorged breasts because the areola is too hard to grasp (Figure 33-7). The mother has difficulty with nursing because her breasts are extremely painful, and the baby's sucking accentuates the discomfort.

The primary method of relief for engorgement is emptying the breasts of milk by having the infant suck more often than previously, or at least continuing to suck as much as before. Unfortunately, the breasts are so sore that it is difficult for a mother to continue to breast-feed unless she is given something to alleviate the pain. An analgesic may be necessary, but some mothers find that ice packs applied for 20 minutes at a time give relief. Others find that warm packs applied for a comparable length of time afford the most relief. In addition, good breast support from a firm-fitting bra prevents the pulling feeling.

If an infant cannot grasp the nipple to suck strongly, warm packs applied to both breasts for a

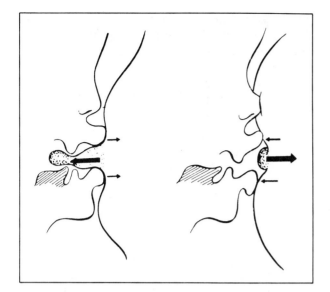

Figure 33-7 *The relationship of breast engorgement and sore nipples. Left, when an infant sucks at a normal breast, his lips compress the areola and fit neatly against the concave nipple-areola junction. He also has room to breathe. Right, if the breast is engorged, the nipple-areola junction becomes convex. The infant attempts to suck the inverted nipple, causing soreness and damaging the nipple epithelium. Furthermore, normal breathing space does not exist. Preventing engorgement will prevent sore nipples by allowing the infant a proper grasp. From Applebaum, R. M. (1970). The modern management of successful breast feeding.* Pediatric Clinics of North America, 17, 203.

few minutes before feeding will often facilitate drainage and promote softness so that the infant can suck. Synthetic oxytocin (Syntocinon) nasal spray used for a few minutes prior to feeding may also be effective. Syntocinon is absorbed across the nasal mucosa and acts to contract milk ducts and bring milk forward. Manual expression or the use of a hand breast pump to complete emptying of the breasts after the baby has nursed is helpful in maintaining or promoting a good milk supply during the period of engorgement.

Engorgement is a transient problem. Unfortunately, it occurs just as the mother feels she is becoming skilled at breast-feeding. Suddenly her breasts are swollen, hot, and painful. She may worry that she has an infection or that the baby is not getting enough milk.

Mothers need to be assured that engorgement not only is normal but is to be welcomed because it means that breast cells are actively working to form milk. Mothers also should be told that engorgement is only temporary and will begin to subside 24 hours after it becomes apparent.

Sore Nipples

Sore nipples may result from improper sucking, that is, from the infant's not grasping the areola as well as the nipple; from forcefully pulling the infant from the breast; from the infant's sucking too long a time at a breast because the mother did not place the infant on the same breast where he or she nursed last at the previous feeding; or from the nipple's remaining wet from leaking of milk.

Nipples feel sore because they are cracked or fissured. Healing a fissure here is the same as healing irritated skin anywhere else on the body. Exposing the nipples to air by leaving the bra unsnapped for 10 to 15 minutes after feeding is often sufficient to clear up the problem. A mother should avoid using the plastic liners that come with nursing bras, so that air is always circulating around her breasts. Application of a lanolin-based cream following air exposure may toughen the nipple and prevent further irritation.

If normal air-drying is not effective, simultaneous exposure to a 20-watt bulb in a gooseneck lamp two or three times a day may be helpful. The light should be 12 to 18 inches away from the breasts to prevent burns, and it should be left in place about 10 minutes.

Sore nipples, like engorgement, are not a contraindication to breast-feeding. They are enough to discourage a mother, however, if she does not realize that they are a temporary result of adjustment to nursing, both hers and her baby's. Using a plastic breast shield to protect a nipple during feeding may help. If nipples are so sore that she cannot nurse, the baby should be given supplemental formula for a day or two, and the breast milk should be expelled manually until the nipples have had a chance to heal. Do not use a hand pump with sore nipples, or fissures will worsen.

If the baby's sucking patterns are corrected, and if the mother uses air exposure following feedings and returns to nursing again by gradually increasing the time the baby sucks at each feeding, the problem of sore nipples is unlikely to become acute again.

Assessing Amount of Milk Taken

Many mothers who are breast-feeding wonder whether the infant is getting enough to eat. They watch a woman bottle-feeding and listen to her report, "She took 3 ounces this feeding," and wish they could tell as surely that their infant is getting an adequate intake.

They can be assured that the ultimate test of whether a baby, either breast-fed or bottle-fed, is getting enough to eat is whether he or she seems content between feedings and is gaining weight, not the actual amount taken. Although the bottle-feeding mother measures the amount of formula as a way of determining this criterion in the early weeks, very soon she too is using the alternative criterion: Her baby is happy and growing larger.

At one time breast-fed babies were weighed before each feeding and then again after each feeding. The difference in weight gave a gross estimate of the amount of breast milk they had taken. If a mother is particularly worried that her infant is not getting anything to eat, the baby can be weighed for a few feedings to assure her that the infant is taking in milk. This practice should not be routine, however. It is better to help the mother begin to use the criteria she will use at home. That way she will develop confidence in her judgment to evaluate her child's health, a role that will be hers for the next 18 years.

Advice on Going Home

Some mothers do well with breast-feeding while they are in the hospital but after going home grow discouraged with the process and stop.

A mother must regard breast-feeding time as a time in which she is devoting herself only to feeding the baby. If she approaches it with an attitude such as "I'll get this over as quickly as possible so I can get to something else," her let-down reflex will be affected, and she will discover that she no longer has adequate milk. If milk remains in her breasts, either because it did not move forward as it should have (weak let-down reflex) or because the infant sucked poorly or not at all, the tension created inhibits subsequent milk production.

Mothers who do not remember to begin nursing the baby at the breast finished on the last time may find their milk supply decreasing. It is easy to remember this in the hospital, but the many distractions at home may make the sequence hard to keep in mind. Pinning a safety pin to the bra strap on the correct side is a useful aid to memory.

Another problem of mothers after they return home is fatigue. A mother needs to realize that she cannot expect to feed a baby, by any method, attend many social functions, and be a perfect housekeeper and gourmet cook. Adequate rest periods during the day are essential. Sitting relaxed in a comfortable chair with her feet elevated, feeding her baby and enjoying it, is an excellent way to rest.

A mother must take in adequate fluid to maintain an adequate milk supply. In the hospital fluid intake is supervised by health care personnel.

When she is at home and involved in other things, she may neglect to take adequate fluids. Sometimes a mother will deliberately limit fluid intake after she returns home in the hope of shedding the pounds she put on during pregnancy.

Mothers who are breast-feeding should drink at least four 8-ounce glasses of fluid a day; many women need to drink six glasses. A daily diet plan for a lactating mother compared with her intake during and before pregnancy is given in Table 33-1.

At one time mothers were given a list of foods not to eat while they were breast-feeding because it was thought they caused diarrhea, constipation, or colic in infants. Today there are no rules other than to use common sense. A mother can eat anything during lactation that agrees with her and is taken in moderation. She should not eat foods to which she is allergic or that cause gastrointestinal upsets. But then such foods should be avoided whether or not she is lactating.

Many mothers stop breast-feeding after they return home because they have no one to talk to about their problems or to give them support. A nurse who works as a hospital-community liaison person receives countless calls from breast-feeding mothers asking for support or advice. The community health nurse is another person to whom mothers turn for help.

Mothers should be made aware of the La Leche League, an international organization of breast-feeding mothers that has chapters in most major cities. In addition to sponsoring classes on breast-feeding, a helpful service the league offers is its hot line, through which a breast-feeding mother who is discouraged or is having difficulty can contact a member and ask for advice. *The Womanly Art of Breastfeeding*, published by the La Leche League (1971), is a comprehensive and readable book for mothers.

Drugs and Breast Milk

For years people talked about a placental "barrier," which theoretically protected the fetus from drugs taken by the mother. A similar protection was postulated for breast milk. Today it can be shown that the fetus is very susceptible to drugs ingested by the mother. The same is true of breast-fed infants. Almost any drug may cross into the acinar cells and be secreted with breast milk.

Drugs that should be avoided by breast-feeding mothers because of their harmful effect on an infant are shown in Table 33-2.

The rule that a mother followed all during pregnancy, that she should take no drug unless pre-

Table 33-1 Quantities of Food Necessary During Pregnancy and Lactation

Food Group	Active Nonpregnant Woman	Pregnant Woman	Lactating Woman
Meat	2 servings of meat, fowl, or fish daily; 3–5 eggs per week	3 servings of meat, fowl, or fish daily; 1 egg per day	3–4 servings of meat, fowl, or fish daily; 1 egg per day
Vegetables			
Dark green or deep yellow	1 serving (at least 3 times per week)	2 servings per day	2 servings per day
Other vegetables	2 or more servings per day	1 serving per day	1 serving per day
Fruits			
Citrus, melon, strawberry, tomato	1 serving per day	1 or more servings per day	2 or more servings per day
Other fruits	1 serving per day	1 serving per day	2 servings per day
Bread and cereals	4 or more servings per day	4 servings per day	4 servings per day
Milk	1 pint (two 8-oz glasses) per day	1 quart (four 8-oz glasses) per day	Four–six 8-oz glasses per day
Additional fluid	As desired	At least two glasses per day	At least two glasses per day

scribed or approved by her physician, continues to apply during lactation.

Prolonged Jaundice in Breast-Fed Infants

Physiologic jaundice may persist for a longer time in breast-fed than in bottle-fed infants because pregnanediol (a breakdown product of progesterone) in breast milk depresses the action of glycuronyl transferase enzyme. Discontinuing breast-feeding for a day or two usually corrects this problem, causing the indirect level of bilirubin to drop and the jaundice to clear. The mother should pump her breasts manually during this time to protect her supply of breast milk. Prolonged jaundice is not a reason to discontinue breast-feeding permanently.

If the jaundice progresses, a mother should be referred to a health care facility. She may be reporting a rise in direct bilirubin level caused by obstruction of the bile ducts.

The Working Mother

Many women return to work while continuing to breast-feed by bringing the infant with them to their work setting; others express additional breast milk at the end of feedings, freeze or store this in the refrigerator, and have it ready and convenient for the baby's caregiver to administer by bottle. Still others provide supplementary feedings for the infant by commercial formula. Breast-feeding can be done in public places without undue exposure if the mother wears a smock-type or a button-type blouse that she lifts or unfastens only as much as necessary; covering any bared breast with a shawl or towel assures modesty. In some work settings, employers have strong feelings about breast-feeding and women need to review with an employer the best way to allow them to continue breast-feeding, perhaps by use of a private office or screened area.

Supplemental Feedings

A breast-feeding mother may leave her child during the day or evening in the care of a baby-sitter, just as a bottle-feeding mother may. She needs to express breast milk manually and leave it bottled in the refrigerator or prepare a single bottle of formula for the time she is away. If she chooses to use formula, one of the commercial formulas is

Table 33-2 Drug Excretion in Breast Milk and Effect on the Infant

Drug	Excreted	Implications
Analgesics		
Acetaminophen (Datril, Tylenol)	Yes	No significant effect on infant from therapeutic doses.
Acetylsalicylic acid (aspirin)*	Yes	Tendency toward bleeding noted; if given to nursing mother, should be given after nursing; check infant for adequate sources of vitamin K.
Codeine	Yes	No significant effect on infant reported from therapeutic doses.
Heroin†	Yes	Controversial reports as to the long-term effect on infant; usually goes through withdrawal depending on maternal dose.
Meperidine hydrochloride (Demerol)	Yes	No significant effect on infant from therapeutic doses.
Methadone*	Yes	Controversial as to whether user should breast-feed; if she does, the daily dose should be given after the feeding, and the next feeding should be by bottle.
Morphine	Yes	No significant effects on infant from therapeutic doses.
Pentazocine (Talwin)	No	
Phenylbutazone* (Azolid, Butazolidin)	Yes	Drug should be used judiciously; manufacturer states that it is excreted in cord blood and breast milk; infant should be monitored; may increase kernicterus—highly protein-bound.
Propoxyphene hydrochloride (Darvon)	Yes	No significant effect on infant from therapeutic doses.
Anticoagulants		Differing opinions as to whether mother on anticoagulants should nurse; all agree that if she does, infant should be monitored with the mother.
Bishydroxycoumarin* (Dicumarol)	Yes	May cause hypoprothrombinemia in infant; monitor infant.
Ethyl biscoumacetate* (Pelentan, Tromexan)	Yes	No significant effect on infant from therapeutic doses, but monitor infant; do not use if infant suffered any birth injury such as cephalhematoma, or forceps damage resulting in vascular injury.
Heparin	No	
Phenindione† (Dindevan, Hedulin)	Yes	May cause hypoprothrombinemia; one incident of massive hematoma in infant whose mother received it.
Warfarin sodium* (Coumadin)	Yes	May cause hypoprothrombinemia; monitor infant.
Anticonvulsants		
Phenytoin* (Dilantin)	Yes	Methemoglobulinemia in breast-fed infant; enzyme induction may occur.
Primidone† (Mysoline)	Yes	Manufacturer recommends breast-feeding be avoided, since substantial amounts found in breast milk; drowsiness may occur in newborn.
Antidiabetics		
Chlorpropamide (Diabinese)	Yes	No significant effect on infant from therapeutic doses.
Insulin	Yes	Destroyed in the infant's GI tract.
Tolbutamide (Dolipol, Mobenol, Orinase, Tolbutol)	Yes	No significant effects on infant from therapeutic doses.

Table 33-2 (continued)

Drug	Excreted	Implications
Antidiabetics (continued)		
Tolazamide (Tolinase)	?	Has not been completely evaluated; 6.7 times more potent than tolbutamide.
Antihistamines		
Chlorpheniramine maleate (Chlor-Trimeton)	Yes	May cause drowsiness in the infant.
Diphenhydramine (Benadryl, Benhydril)	Yes	No adverse effects on infant from therapeutic doses.
Promethazine hydrochloride (Phenergan)	Yes	No significant effects on infant from therapeutic doses.
Trimeprazine tartrate (Temaril)	Yes	No significant effects on infant from therapeutic doses.
Anticholinergics		
Atropine sulfate†	Yes	May inhibit lactation and may cause atropine intoxication in infant; although documentation scarce, best avoided until further research available.
Scopolamine	Yes	No significant effects on infant from therapeutic doses.
Antihypertensives—Diuretics		
Acetazolamide* (Diamox)	Yes	Infant may develop idiosyncratic reaction to this sulfonamide diuretic.
Furosemide (Lasix)	No	Women ill enough to receive Lasix should not breastfeed.
Hexamethonium	Yes	Rarely used drug; very toxic.
Reserpine† (Serpasil)	Yes	May cause nasal stuffiness, drowsiness, and diarrhea in infant, galactorrhea in mother.
Spironolactone (Aldactone)	No	Watch for potassium deficiency and dehydration in mother.
Thiazides†	Yes	Manufacturer suggests avoiding; watch fluid, electrolyte balance.
Anti-infectives		With all anti-infectives that cross into breast milk, the possibility of sensitization of the infant must be considered.
Amantadine hydrochloride† (Symmetrel)	Yes	May cause skin rash and vomiting; manufacturer suggests avoiding.
Aminoglycosides*	Yes	Should be reserved for severe infection; avoid in high G-6-PD-deficient populations, as hemolysis may occur.
Ampicillin	Yes	No significant effects on infant from therapeutic doses.
Chloramphenicol* (Chloromycetin)	Yes	May affect infant's bone marrow; avoid use, particularly during the first 2 weeks of life.
Erythromycin* (E-Mycin, Erythrocin, Ilosone, Ilotycin)	Yes	Appears in breast milk in concentrations higher than that of maternal plasma; sensitization possible; estolate form (Ilosone) may cause jaundice.
Isoniazid†	Yes	If possible, avoid use during lactation; if given, infant must be monitored for toxicity.
Mandelic acid†	Yes	Probably best avoided during lactation; for this urinary antiseptic to be effective, urine must be strongly acid and fluids must be limited.
Metronidazole† (Flagyl)	Yes	No adverse oral or GI effects noted in infants, but some authors feel that because of possible carcinogenicity it would be best to avoid, as long-term effects are not known.

Table 33-2 (continued)

Drug	Excreted	Implications
Anti-infectives (continued)		
Nalidixic acid† (NegGram)	Yes	Hemolytic anemia, especially in G-6-PD populations.
Nouobiocin†	Yes	May cause kernicterus in large doses.
Penicillin	Yes	Possibility of sensitization; may alter intestinal flora of infant.
Quinine	Not in clinically significant amounts	In very high maternal doses, thrombocytopenia in infants.
Sulfonamides*	Yes	Avoid in high G-6-PD populations; high doses for long-term use is questionable; may cause kernicterus; avoid in the first 2 weeks of life.
Tetracyclines†	Yes	Slows bone growth and deposits in bones and teeth.
Cancer-Chemotherapeutic Agents†		Breast-feeding is generally considered ill-advised in patients receiving chemotherapy.
Hormones Estrogen, progestogen, androgens†	Yes	Breast-feeding not indicated if mother is on oral contraceptives; may alter the composition of breast milk (decreasing the amounts of protein, fats, and minerals); long-term effects on infants have not been adequately determined.
Corticosteroids†	Yes	Should be avoided by the nursing mother, as they may interfere with normal function and cause growth suppression.
Laxatives Aloe*	Yes	Conflicting evidence regarding catharsis in infants; avoid in high doses.
Cascara†	Yes	Thought to cause diarrhea in infants.
Danthron† (Dorbane, Dorbantyl, Doxan, Doxidan)	Yes	Conflicting reports regarding the cathartic effect of these drugs; probably best avoided.
Dioctyl sodium sulfosuccinate (Colace)	No	No reports of having caused any problems in the infant.
Milk of magnesia	No	No adverse reactions noted.
Phenolphthalein (Evac-U-Lax, Ex-Lax, other nonprescription drugs)	Yes	No significant effects noted in usual doses.
Psyllium hydrophilic mucilloid (Metamucil)	Yes	No adverse reactions noted.
Senna compounds*	Yes	Controversial reports with moderate doses; high doses may cause diarrhea in infants.
Muscle Relaxants Carisoprodol† (Rela, Soma)	Yes	According to manufacturer, two to four times more concentrated in breast milk than in maternal blood plasma; infant may experience CNS depression and GI upset.
Methocarbamol (Robaxin)	Yes	No significant effects on infant from therapeutic doses.
Oxytocics Ergot preparations†	Yes	May suppress lactation by blocking the release of prolactin; symptoms in the infant may include vomiting, diarrhea, cardiovascular changes.

Table 33-2 (continued)

Drug	Excreted	Implications
Oxytocics (continued)		
Oxytocin	Yes	Oxytocin nasal spray used prior to breast-feeding appears to increase the volume of milk produced; may be used for hemorrhaging mothers; very short half-life.
Psychotropics—Psychotherapeutics		
Butyrophenones, haloperidol* (Haldol)	Unknown	Manufacturer recommends that benefits must outweigh risk in the use of these drugs, since their safe use in pregnancy and lactation has not been established.
Chlordiazepoxide* (Librium)	Yes	No significant effects on infant from therapeutic doses; some authors suggest using caution.
Diazepam* (Valium)	Yes	May cause weight loss, lethargy, jaundice in the infant; some authors feel that breast-feeding should be discontinued if high doses are given to mother.
Imipramine* (Tofranil)	Yes	Safe use during lactation has not been established.
Lithium carbonate† (Lithonate, Lithane)	Yes	May alter electrolyte balance; most authors state that indications for its use should be unequivocal; long-term effect on infant unknown; best avoided until further evidence available.
Phenothiazines* (Compazine, Thorazine, etc.)	Yes	All phenothiazines are excreted in breast milk, and except for reported jaundice in the infant and galactorrhea, no other effects are known at this time.
Sedatives—Hypnotics		
Barbiturates†	Yes	May increase the activity of hepatic drug metabolizing enzymes; high single dose may cause more drowsiness than small, multiple doses.
Bromides† (ingredient in many nonprescription sleeping medications)	Yes	May cause rash and drowsiness in infant; difficulty in feeding, lethargy, hypotonia or hypertonia.
Chloral hydrate (Noctec, Somnos)	Yes	Drowsiness in infant.
Chloroform†	Yes	Anesthetic effect in infant.
Glutethimide* (Doriden)	Yes	May cause drowsiness in infant; one author suggests avoiding during lactation; manufacturer suggests caution during lactation.
Meprobamate† (Equanil, Miltown)	Yes	Very high level in milk (two to four times maternal plasma); alternate drug advised; if given, infant should be monitored for signs of meprobamate toxicity.
Thyroid and Antithyroid Preparations		
Carbimazole† (Neo-Mercazole)	Yes	May cause goiter in infant.
Methimazole† (Tapazole)	Yes	Manufacturer recommends that user not breast-feed.
Thiouracil† (+ derivatives)	Yes	Excreted in high levels (3 to 12 times maternal plasma levels); may cause goiter or agranulocytosis.
Thyroid	Yes	No significant effects on infant with therapeutic doses
Thyroxine sodium† (Choloxin)	Yes	Manufacturer states that use in pregnancy and lactation is contraindicated.
Iodides		
¹³¹I† (radioactive)	Yes	All radioactive agents should be avoided in the breast-feeding mother.

Table 33-2 (continued)

Drug	Excreted	Implications
Iodides (continued)		
Iodides† (contained in many nonprescription cough preparations)	Yes	Infant's thyroid functioning may be affected; avoid taking large or frequent doses of iodide-containing cough preparations; may have thyrotropic effect on infant or cause rash.
Vitamins, Minerals, Food Products Vitamins		
B_1 (thiamine)	Yes	Mothers with severe deficiency (beriberi) should not nurse because of excretion of toxic substances, sodium pyruvate and methylglyoxal, which have caused infant death.
B_6 (pyridoxine)	Yes	Some authors report that it successfully suppressed lactation in doses of 150–200 mg po tid.
B_{12} (cyanocobalamin)	Yes	No effect with therapeutic doses.
D (calciferol)	Yes	High doses may cause hypercalcemia in infant.
K	Yes	No significant effects on infant with therapeutic doses.
Caffeine* (many nonprescription drugs contain caffeine: Awake, 100 mg; No-Doz, 100 mg; Sta-Alert, 100 mg; Vivarin, 200 mg; and coffee and tea, 100–150 mg per cup)	Yes	Unless large amount ingested, no significant effect on infant; ingestion of large quantities of tea or coffee can cause irritability and poor sleeping patterns in infants.
Carrots	Yes	In large quantity, may cause yellow discoloration of skin.
Egg protein	Yes	Allergic sensitization possible.
Fava bean	Yes	In G-6-PD-deficient infants, hemolysis has occurred.
Fluoride (toothpaste, water supply, tablets)	Yes	Not significant in usual quantities; excess may affect tooth enamel; La Leche League advises either *not* breast-feeding or to stop taking fluoride tablets; may cause GI upsets, rash in infants.
Vaccines–Immunosuppressives DPT	Yes	Probably no immunity transfer to baby.
Poliovirus	Yes	If infant is immunized after 6 weeks, probably negligible effect on antibody titer.
Rh_0 (D) immune globulin (human) (Gamulin Rh, RhoGAM)	No	
Rubella	No	Probably no transfer of live virus to infant.
Other Alcohol (ethyl alcohol)	Yes	No significant effect in moderate amount; prolonged ingestion of large amounts may intoxicate infant; large doses may also inhibit the milk ejection reflex, whereas small amount of alcohol prior to nursing may enhance the milk let-down.
Clomiphene citrate (Clomid)	Unknown	May suppress lactation.
Dihydrotachysterol* (DHT)	Yes	May cause hypercalcemia in infant (osteoporosis, bone dysgenesis).
L-dopa	Unknown	May suppress lactation by inhibiting prolactin secretion.
Lead†	Unknown	Caution against the use of lead acetate ointment in breast creams, as it may lead to encephalitis.

Table 33-2 (continued)

Drug	Excreted	Implications
Other (continued)		
Marijuana†	Yes	May interfere with DNA and RNA formation.
Mercury†	Yes	In cases of mercury contamination in the environment, watch infant for CNS symptoms and mercury intoxication.
Nicotine*	Yes	Probably very little effect on infant with moderate use (20 cigarettes per day or less); may decrease milk production; one recorded case of nicotine intoxication in infant (restlessness, vomiting, diarrhea, insomnia, circulatory disruptions)—mother smoked 20 cigarettes per day; infants of smoking mothers absorb smoke through GI tract, respiratory tract, and skin.

* Use with caution in nursing mother.
† Avoid drug whenever possible.

Source: Dickason, E. J., et al. (1978). *Maternal and infant drugs and nursing intervention.* New York: Mc-Graw-Hill. Copyright © 1978 McGraw-Hill Book Company. Used with the permission of McGraw-Hill Book Company.

best, because these formulas so closely resemble breast milk. Buying the prepackaged and prepared type is the most convenient; the mother need only take a bottle of it down from a shelf, and it is ready. If cost is a problem, the powdered type is probably the next best solution. The powder can be stored for long periods, and one bottle at a time can be prepared.

The mother may notice breast discomfort if she is away from her baby at feeding time. After breast-feeding has been established, missing one feeding will not affect the production of milk enough to make a difference at the next feeding. Thus, there is no need for her to express milk manually to safeguard a milk supply, although she may prefer to do so to reduce the tension and discomfort that she feels.

Burping the Breast-Fed Baby

Some infants seem to swallow very little air when they breast-feed; others swallow a great deal. As a rule, it is helpful to bubble the baby after he or she has emptied the first breast and again after the total feeding.

Weaning

Mothers who breast-feed do so for varying lengths of time. Some breast-feed for 1, 2, or 3 months, then wean the child from breast to bottle. Other mothers breast-feed until the child is 6 to 12 months of age and then wean directly to a small cup or glass.

Discontinuing breast-feeding should be done gradually to prevent engorgement and pain in the breasts. A woman should first omit one breast-feeding a day, substituting a bottle-feeding or milk from a glass or cup. Then she should omit two breast-feedings, then three, and so on, until the child is feeding entirely from a bottle, glass, or cup. If the breasts are not emptied, the resulting pressure leads to milk suppression and natural, gradual discontinuance of breast milk secretion.

Common problems mothers may experience with breast-feedings are summarized in Table 33-3.

Formula-Feeding

There is little controversy over the proposition that breast-feeding is the best method of feeding human infants—except when a mother does not want to breast-feed. A mother (or her support person) who feels that breasts are "dirty", that breast-feeding is a form of promiscuity, or who is uncomfortable with the thought of exposing her body in this way, cannot hold a baby warmly and gently and cannot enjoy feeding her infant. Mothers who plan to return to work or who have older children to watch may choose not to breast-feed. Mothers who develop a breast abscess may be advised not to breast-feed. Formulas that closely resemble human milk and are safe for infant feeding are available for the infant who will be bottle-fed.

Table 33-3 Common Problems of Breast-Feeding

Problem	Cause	Nursing Interventions
Engorgement.	Lymphatic filling as milk production begins.	Engorgement subsides best if infant can be encouraged to suck normally; warm packs to breasts prior to feeding may help soften breast tissue; oxytocin nasal spray prior to feeding may aid the let-down reflex.
Sore nipples.	Infant not gripping entire areola. Nipple kept wet.	Help infant to grasp nipple correctly; expose nipple to air between feedings; lanolin cream afterward to help harden nipple; possible heat lamp treatments.
Mother worried about amount of milk being taken.	Mother cannot see the amount taken.	Assure mother that the best way to judge amount taken is to note if infant is gaining weight and appears content between feedings.
Infant does not suck well.	Possible effect of anesthesia. Infant brought to mother when not hungry. Infant exhausted by crying from hunger.	Adjust feeding pattern to child's need; assure mother that effect of anesthesia is temporary.
Mother reports infant's stools are loose and thin.	Stools are normally looser and lighter in color than in formula-fed babies.	Examine stool; assure and explain normal stool pattern.
Mother tired.	Exhaustion is a common postpartal finding due to psychosocial and physiologic adjustments of time.	Help mother to plan rest times; assess diet and fluid intake.

Commercial Formulas

Commercial formulas are designed to simulate breast milk as closely as possible in terms of protein, carbohydrate, fat, mineral, and vitamin content. Commercial formulas contain 20 calories per ounce when diluted according to directions. Common brands are shown in Table 33-4.

There are four separate forms of commercial formulas available: a powder that the mother combines with water; a condensed liquid type that she dilutes with an equal amount of water; a ready-to-pour type, which requires no dilution; and individually prepackaged and prepared bottles of formula (Figure 33-8).

The powder is the least expensive type but the most difficult for the mother to prepare. It does not dissolve well and must be beaten with a hand beater to remove lumps. The prepackaged type has the advantage of never needing refrigeration or preparation (take off a bottle cap and it is ready), but it is the most expensive. The ready-to-pour type is convenient but also expensive. Many mothers are not aware of the existence of the liquid condensed type and need to be informed that it is available and is convenient and economical. The cost is as much as 50¢ to $2 a day less than that of the ready-to-pour or prepackaged types, which amounts to a savings of $15 to $60 a month.

Commercial formulas may be purchased with added iron, so that additional iron supplementation is not necessary. As indicated, they also contain added sufficient vitamins.

You should be familiar with all four types of commercial formula in order to discuss their advantages and disadvantages with mothers. Cost should not be the only basis for a choice. Acceptance by the infant and convenience for the mother are also important factors to consider.

Calculation of a Formula

The calculation of a newborn formula is not, and should not be, a complicated procedure. There are only a few rules of thumb to learn.

1. The total fluid used for 24 hours must be sufficient to meet the child's fluid needs; 2.5 to

3.0 ounces of fluid per pound of body weight per day (160 to 200 ml per kilogram) is needed.
2. The protein requirement is 1 gm per pound of body weight per day (2.2 gm per kilogram).
3. The number of calories required per day is 50 to 55 per pound of body weight (100 to 120 per kilogram).

If an infant is going to be discharged on a commercial formula, total fluid is all that needs to be calculated. The 7-pound infant needs 17.5 to 21.0 ounces (7 × 2.5 to 3.0 ounces) of formula per day. As commercial formula contains 20 calories per ounce, this supplies 350 to 420 calories per day, which can be divided into six feedings of 3.0 to 3.5 ounces each. The 9-pound infant needs 22.5 to 27.0 ounces of fluid per day, which supplies 450 to 540 calories.

A rule of thumb to determine how much an infant usually takes at a feeding is to add 2 or 3 to the infant's age in months. A newborn (0 age) takes 2 to 3 ounces each feeding; a 3-month-old infant, 5 to 6 ounces; and a 6-month-old infant, 8 ounces per feeding. As infants change from six to five feedings a day (at about 4 months of age), they begin to take more at each feeding to keep their total intake the same.

You should be able to calculate formulas and, using the minimum requirements of fluid and calories per day, evaluate the adequacy of an infant's intake.

Prepared Formulas

Mothers today almost all use commercial formulas. The rare woman who is not going to use a commercially prepared formula must prepare one herself, with milk, added carbohydrate, and water. Babies cannot digest cow's milk for at least 4 months and it should not be used before then (and preferably not until the infant is 1 year of age).

Types of Milk

Evaporated Milk. Evaporated milk is whole milk from which 60 percent of the water has been removed. Because the solution is concentrated, its caloric content and its protein content are almost twice as high as those of whole milk (44 calories, usually considered as 40 calories for calculation, and 2 gm protein per ounce). Evaporated milk is sterile, and it is inexpensive. It has other advantages: It can be stored without refrigeration as long as the can is unopened; it has a fine curd, both because it is homogenized and because the casein curd is reduced in size in the evaporating process. Before using evaporated milk you must first dilute it with at least an equal part of water

to restore the water removed in its processing. There is a possibility that evaporated milk may contain a fairly high lead content from leaching of the metal can into the milk during storage.

Condensed Milk. It is important for you to be able to differentiate condensed milk from evaporated milk. Some mothers use the terms interchangeably, but they are two different products and cannot be interchanged in formulas. Condensed milk is evaporated milk to which sugar has been added. It contains about 100 calories per ounce and is intended for use in rich desserts and puddings. It is too rich for infant feeding, and the additional sugar will usually cause intestinal upset and diarrhea. Make certain you know which product a mother is talking about when she tells you what milk she is using.

Skimmed Milk. Skimmed milk is milk from which the bulk of the fat has been removed. Whole milk has about 3.5 gm of fat per 100 ml of milk; skimmed milk has 0.2 to 1.0 gm; 2 percent skimmed milk has 2 gm per 100 ml of milk. Thus the caloric content is reduced from the 20 calories per ounce of whole milk to 10 to 12 calories. Skimmed milk is not appropriate for continuous long-term feeding in infants (as long as this is the only food source) because of its low caloric and low fat content.

Dried Milk. Dried milk is whole or skimmed milk from which the water has been completely evaporated. A fine curd is produced by the drying process. The powder can be stored for indefinite periods without refrigeration. Each brand has its own directions for reconstitution, and the mother should follow them accurately. The milk appears pale after reconstitution, and occasionally a mother will try to make it more nutritious by adding less water than specified. This will not result in a more nutritious mixture but in a stronger mixture that is less easy to digest and may be vomited.

Goat's Milk. In the United States, in contrast to some other countries, goat's milk is rarely used in preference to cow's milk, but in certain rural areas its use is widespread. The curd tension of goat's milk is lower than that of cow's milk, so an infant may do well on a goat's milk formula. Another advantage is that goats rarely contract tuberculosis; however, they are susceptible to brucellosis. Goat's milk is not recommended over a long period of time for infants because it is deficient in folic acid.

Table 33-4 Infant Formula Product Comparison with Breast Milk and Cow's Milk

| Formula | Nutrient source | | | Energy per oz | | Nutrients g/100 ml | | |
	Protein	Carbohydrate	Fat	kcal	kJ	Pro	Carbohydrate	Fat
Breast milk	Lactalbumin, casein	Lactose	High in olein, low in volatile fatty acids	22	92	1.1	6.8	4.5
Cow's milk	Lactalbumin, casein	Lactose	Milk fat	20	84	3.5	4.9	3.7
Well infant formulas								
Similac (Ross)	Nonfat cow's milk	Lactose	Soy oil, coconut oil	20	84	1.5	7.3	3.6
Enfamil (MJ)	Nonfat cow's milk	Lactose	Soy oil, coconut oil	20	84	1.5	7.0	3.7
Premature								
Similac Low Birth Weight (Ross)	Nonfat cow's milk	Lactose, poly-cose	Soy oil, coconut oil, MCT oil	24	100	2.2	8.5	4.5
Enfamil Premature (MJ)	Demineralized whey, nonfat cow's milk	Glucose polymers, lactose	Corn oil, MCT oil, coconut oil	24	100	2.4	8.9	4.1
Increased energy/oz								
Similac 24 with Iron (Ross)	Nonfat cow's milk	Lactose	Soy oil, coconut oil	24	100	2.2	8.5	4.3
Similac 27	Cow's milk	Lactose	Coconut oil, soy oil,	27	113	2.5	9.5	4.8
Enfamil 24 with Iron (MJ)	Nonfat cow's milk	Lactose	Soy oil, coconut oil	24	100	1.8	8.3	4.5
Decreased energy/oz								
Similac 13 with Iron (Ross)	Cow's milk	Lactose	Coconut oil, soy oil	13.2	55.2	1.1	4.6	2.3
Enfamil 13 (MJ)	Nonfat cow's milk	Lactose	Soy oil, coconut oil	13.2	55.2	1.0	4.5	2.4
Electrodialyzed								
SMA (Wyeth)	Nonfat cow's milk, demineralized whey	Lactose	Oleo, coconut oil	20	84	1.5	7.2	3.6
PM 60/40 (Ross)	Nonfat cow's milk, demineralized whey	Lactose	Safflower oil, soybean oil	20	84	1.6	7.6	3.5
Soy protein-lactose free								
Isomil (Ross)	Soy protein isolate	Corn syrup, sucrose	Coconut oil, soy oil	20	84	2.0	6.8	3.6
Prosobee (MJ)	Soy protein isolate, supplement with L-methionine	Corn syrup solids	Soy oil, coconut oil	20	84	2.0	6.9	3.6

Table 33-4 (continued)

Minerals

Mg/100 ml Iron	meq/L Ca^{2+}	p^{2+}	Ha^+	K^+	Cl^-	Osmolality mosmol/kg H_2O	Renal solute load mosmol/L	Considerations
0.1–0.15	17	8	7	13	11	300	75	
0.05	59	60	22	35	28	288	23	Cow's milk alone is not suitable for an infant formula. Evaporated milk is diluted 1 part evaporated milk, 2 parts water, with 5% corn syrup added.
— c̄ iron 1.2	26	23	11	20	15	290	108	Formulas used for normal infant feeding. Formula with iron recommended. (Some infants do not tolerate iron-fortified formulas. With usage they may become colicky and/or constipated.)
— c̄ iron 1.2	28	27	12	18	15	290	110	
0.3	36	33	16	26	24	290	154	Formulas modified to meet the increased growth needs of the premature infant.
0.12	48	28	14	23	19	300	220	
0.15	36	33	14	27	21	360	150	Formulas used for infants with a limited intake or infants recovering from illness with increased energy needs.
Tr.	40	36	17	32	22	420	171	
1.52	33	33	15	21	18	355	130	
0.7	20	18	10	15	12	190	84	Formulas used with infants who have not been fed enterally for several days/weeks. Also, used when a conservative initial formula is needed for newborns during first 24–48-hour period.
0.10	18	18	8	12	10	182	70	
1.26	22	20	6.5	14.4	10.4	300	91	Formulas provide a lower renal solute load and lower amounts of sodium and potassium. (Whey is demineralized by electrophoresis.) Protein and mineral content is comparable to breast milk. Formulas are used with infants who have impaired renal or cardiovascular function and infants with diabetes insipidus.
0.26	20	12	7	15	7	260	92	
1.2	35	24	13	18	15	250	126	Formulas used for infants with milk sensitivity or lactose or sucrose intolerance, and for infants with galactosemia.
1.3	32	32	18.7	18	16	160	127	Other soy-based formulas are Neomul-soy and CHO-Free (Syntex).

Table 33-4 (continued)

Formula	Nutrient source			Energy per oz		Nutrients g/100 ml		
	Protein	Carbohydrate	Fat	kcal	kJ	Pro	Carbohydrate	Fat
Hydrolyzed protein								
Nutramigen (MJ)	Casein hydrolysate	Sucrose, modified tapioca starch	Corn oil	20	84	2.2	8.8	2.6
Pregestimil (MJ)	Casein hydrolysate, L-trytophan, L-cystine, L-tyrosine	Corn syrup solids, modified tapioca starch	Corn oil MCT	20	84	1.9	9.1	2.7
High protein–lower fat								
Probana (MJ)	Whole nonfat cow's milk, banana powder, casein hydrolysate	Dextrose, banana powder, lactose	Milk fat, corn oil	20	84	4.2	7.9	2.2
Altered fat–lactose free								
Portagen (MJ)	Sodium caseinate	Corn syrup solids, sucrose	MCT oil (88%), corn oil (12%)	20	84	2.4	7.8	3.2
Inborn errors of metabolism								
Lofenalac (MJ)	Casein hydrolysate (most phenylalanine removed), fortified with tyrosine, tryptophan, histidine, methionine	Corn syrup solids, modified tapioca starch	Corn oil	20	84	2.2	8.8	2.7
Phenyl-free (MJ)	Amino acids	Sucrose, corn syrup solids, modified tapioca starch	Corn oil	25	105	3.8	6.2	0.64
Carbohydrate-free								
CHO-Free (Syntex)	Soy protein isolate		Soy oil	20	84	1.8	6.4 c̄ added CHO	3.5
Transition formula								
Advance (Ross)	Cow milk, soy protein	Corn syrup	Soy oil, corn oil	20	84	2.0	5.5	2.7

Table 33-4 (continued)

Minerals

Mg/100 ml	meq/L					*Osmolality* mosmol/kg H₂O	*Renal solute load* mosmol/L	
Iron	*Ca²⁺*	*p²⁺*	*Ha⁺*	*K⁺*	*Cl⁻*			*Considerations*
1.27	32	28	14	17	13	443	130	Formulas used for infants sensitive to intact protein, and infants recovering from prolonged diarrhea. These formulas avoid possible GI absorption of intact protein because the protein is hydrolyzed. The formulas contain a high percentage of free amino acids, and the remainder of the protein is in the peptide form.
1.27	32	25	14	18	16	338	125	
0.15	58	53	27	31	21	592	250	Formula high in protein (24% of calories), and lower in fat. Formula is used for infants with poor absorption (celiac disease, acute diarrhea).
1.88	32	28	14	22	16	236	150	Formula high in MCT oil which is more readily hydrolyzed and absorbed. The formula is used with infants who have a defect in the hydrolysis of fat, (C.F., pancreatic insufficiency, chronic liver disease, biliary atresia, or obstruction), a defect in absorption (sprue, idopathic steatorrhea, resection of intestine, blind-loop syndrome), a defective lipoprotein-lipase system (hyperchylomicronemia) or faulty chylomicron formula (β-lipoproteinemia), or defects in fat transportation (intestinal lymphatic obstruction, lymphangiectasia, chylothorax, chyluria, chylous ascites exudative enteropathy).
1.3	32	28	13.9	17.4	13.3	454	130	Formula used for infants and children with phenylketonuria. Initially to meet phenylalanine needs, whole milk or formula is added.
2.3	57	55.2	20.7	34.1	26.8	920	170	Formula used for older children with phenylketonuria. The formula contains no phenylalanine.
1.04	41.6	40.3	15.8	23	14.4	480 c̄ added dextrose	125	Formula used for infants with carbohydrate intolerances. Carbohydrate of choice can be added (i.e., polycose, dextrose) slowly to provide 6.4% of total energy.
1.2	26	23	13	22	16	210	131	Formula used as a transition between infant formula and cow's milk

Source: Howard, R. B., & Herbold, N. H. (1982). *Nutrition in Critical Care.* New York: McGraw-Hill.

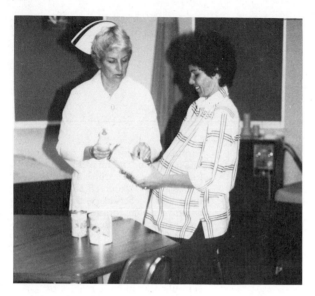

Figure 33-8 *Choosing which type of formula to use can be confusing. Here a nurse reviews options with a woman during pregnancy.*

Types of Carbohydrate

Commercial formulas are self-contained and need no added carbohydrate. A whole- or evaporated-milk formula will need additional carbohydrate. Sugar additives all contain 120 calories per ounce. Sugar may be added in the form of Dextri-Maltose, Karo syrup, or sucrose (table sugar).

Dextri-Maltose. Dextri-Maltose is a commercial preparation that consists of maltose and dextrin, carbohydrates that are easily broken down into monosaccharides. It is frequently recommended for infant formulas. Because the powder is light and fluffy in texture, 4 tablespoons are required to make an ounce (120 calories).

Karo Syrup. Karo syrup (a corn syrup) is easily digested and is inexpensive. It is important to remember that because Karo syrup is thick and heavy only 2 tablespoons are required to make an ounce (120 calories). A mother may switch from one to another of these carbohydrates (a neighbor suggests that Karo is less expensive, or the mother is out of Dextri-Maltose and uses the Karo she has on hand). When she switches to Karo, she must remember to add only half as much Karo as she did Dextri-Maltose.

If a baby who is on an evaporated-milk formula has diarrhea, it is a good idea to explore with the mother the amount of corn syrup being used.

Sucrose. Sucrose is table sugar, and it may be used in formulas. Since it tends to taste very sweet, however, and is difficult to dissolve, it is

not used often. Two tablespoons contain 120 calories.

Caution mothers not to use honey in formulas. This has been associated with the development of *Clostridium botulinum* in infants.

Calculation of Prepared Formulas

In addition to a familiarity with fluid, caloric, and protein requirements, a few additional rules of thumb are necessary to know for calculating adequate prepared infant formulas.

1. Carbohydrate must be added to bring the caloric content of home-prepared formulas up to an adequate level for infant growth.
2. Evaporated milk is the milk of choice for prepared formulas and is prescribed (undiluted) in the proportion of 1 ounce to 1 pound of body weight (30 ml per 2.2 kg).
3. A formula that meets the preceding requirements (sufficient milk, carbohydrate, total fluid, and calories) will be adequate in minerals, but iron and possibly fluoride, as well as vitamin C, must be added.

Following these principles, a discharge formula for a 7-pound newborn whose mother will be using evaporated milk would be as follows:

Total amount of fluid required:
$$7 \times 3 \text{ ounces} = 21 \text{ ounces}$$
Total amount of calories required:
$$7 \times 50\text{--}55 = 350\text{--}385 \text{ calories}$$
Total amount of evaporated milk needed:
$$7 \times 1 \text{ ounce} = 7 \text{ ounces}$$

The amount of evaporated milk needed (7 ounces) will provide 280 calories (7×40 calories). The mother will need to add 2 tablespoons (1 ounce) of corn syrup or 4 tablespoons of Dextri-Maltose (1 ounce) to make 120 additional calories and bring the total caloric value up to 400 calories. The total fluid needed is 21 ounces, so the mother will need to add about 14 ounces of water. The formula, then, contains 7 ounces of evaporated milk, 14 ounces of water, and 2 tablespoons of corn syrup or 4 tablespoons of Dextri-Maltose. This formula provides approximately 20 calories per ounce.

The formula could be divided into six feedings of 3.5 ounces each.

A discharge formula for a 9-pound infant would be the following:

Total fluid required:
$$9 \times 3 \text{ ounces} = 27 \text{ ounces}$$
Total calories required:
$$9 \times 50\text{--}55 \text{ calories} = 450\text{--}495 \text{ calories}$$
Total evaporated milk needed:
$$9 \times 1 \text{ ounce} = 9 \text{ ounces}$$

The amount of evaporated milk needed (9 ounces) will provide 360 calories (9 × 40 calories). The mother will need to add 2 tablespoons of corn syrup (1 ounce) or 4 tablespoons Dextri-Maltose (1 ounce) to make 120 additional calories and bring the total calories up to 480. The total fluid need is 27 ounces, so the mother will need to add 18 ounces of water. The formula, then, is 9 ounces of evaporated milk, 18 ounces of water, and 2 tablespoons of corn syrup (or 4 tablespoons of Dextri-Maltose). The formula could be divided into six feedings of 4.5 ounces each. It provides approximately 18 to 19 calories per ounce.

Supplies for Formula-Feeding

Bottles

To prepare a full day's formula, a mother needs eight bottles. Only six are actually required for 24 hours, but the two additional bottles will take care of the first two feedings on the next day, giving her a chance to prepare formula for that day a little ahead of time. She may select a type of bottle from any of those available, all of which have advantages and disadvantages. If she is going to sterilize the formula, she should be guided into buying glass rather than plastic bottles, since plastic eventually deteriorates from being exposed to high heat. A newer form of bottle is available that is actually an empty shell into which a disposable plastic bag is inserted. The advantages of these bottles are that only the nipples and bottle caps need be washed and that many babies feeding from them suck less air, reducing the chance of colic. The disadvantages are that terminal sterilization cannot be used and that the mother must continue to purchase the disposable liners.

Nipples

The nipple of the bottle should be firm enough so that the infant will suck on it vigorously. A soft, flabby nipple allows a baby to suck in milk too rapidly and does not fulfill the need for sucking. Nipples come in two forms: the crosscut nipple (which has a slit across the top) and the standard single-hole nipple. A mother has to decide after experimentation which is best for her baby. She should buy single-hole nipples first; if they are not satisfactory, she can enlarge the hole by pressing a red-hot needle into the hole, or she can purchase crosscut nipples. If an infant finishes a feeding in 20 minutes, the nipple hole is probably adequate as is.

A way to judge a nipple's adequacy is to hold the bottle of milk with nipple attached upside down. The milk should drop through the nipple at a rate of about one drop a second.

Many mothers are too eager to enlarge nipple holes, so that "the baby doesn't tire" or because "the baby works so hard at sucking that he perspires." Babies do perspire when they suck, but sucking is a pleasurable and needed activity for them.

Bottle Caps

A bottle cap is necessary after preparation of the formula to keep the nipple clean until it is used. If the mother is feeding the baby outdoors or anywhere there are flies about, she should cover the nipple with a bottle cap while she stops feeding to bubble the baby.

Preparation of Formula

Infant formulas must be prepared with careful attention to cleanliness and accuracy. The American Academy of Pediatrics states that if a mother is using chlorinated water and pasteurized milk, proceeds with clean technique, then refrigerates the formula until it is ready to be used, she does not need to sterilize the formula. Sterilization is necessary, however, if any of these conditions cannot be met—that is, if the mother uses unchlorinated well or spring water, unpasteurized milk, or a technique that is not absolutely clean.

All mothers, whether or not they are going to sterilize, need to begin preparation of the formula with clean equipment. Bottles, nipples, and bottle caps need to be washed with warm, soapy water or detergent. Water should be squeezed through the nipple holes to be certain they are patent and not clogged with milk. The bottles, caps, and nipples should be rinsed well to remove all soap.

If the mother is not going to sterilize, but is using presterilized formula, she need only do the following to prepare a full day's supply of formula: wash off the top of the can with warm soapy water and rinse; open the can; pour the desired amount of formula and water into each clean bottle; put on the nipples, with care not to handle the nipple projection. Finally, she puts on the bottle caps and refrigerates the bottles.

Aseptic Method of Sterilization

In addition to thoroughly washed bottles, caps, and nipples, for aseptic sterilization, a mother needs the following: a large pan with a cover, a small pan with a cover, measuring cup (calibrated), measuring tablespoon, can opener, long-handled spoon, funnel (optional), tongs, teakettle or pan for boiling water, and a bowl or pitcher in which to mix ingredients.

The steps for preparing formula by the aseptic method are as follows:

1. Place all equipment except the nipples in the large covered pan and boil in water for 10 minutes.
2. Place the nipples in the small pan and boil them for 3 minutes. Boiling them too long makes the rubber soft and the nipples useless.
3. Boil the amount of water required for the formula in the teakettle or pan for 5 minutes.
4. Drain the water from the pan of equipment and let the pan stand for a minute until the equipment is cool enough to touch. Remove the measuring cup by the handle; do not touch the inside. From the teakettle, pour the correct amount of boiled water required for the formula into the measuring cup. Pour the water into the pitcher or bowl.
5. Measure the required amount of sugar or syrup into the boiled tablespoon. Add to the water in the bowl or pitcher, and stir until dissolved.
6. If evaporated milk or a commercial formula that requires dilution is going to be used, wash the top of the can with soap and water, rinse with water as hot as available. Open the can with the boiled can opener.
7. Pour the required amount of milk or commercial formula into the boiled measuring cup and pour into the pitcher along with the water-sugar mixture. Stir with the long-handled spoon.
8. Pour the formula into sterile bottles (may have to use boiled funnel), put on the nipples, touching only the edges, and cover with bottle caps.
9. Refrigerate the formula until needed.

Aseptic sterilization is the form to use with disposable bottles, since these cannot be sterilized by the other method. With disposable bottles, the following changes are made: In step 1, omit boiling the bottles, since they have been sterilized. In step 3, be sure to allow the water to cool for at least 15 minutes before proceeding, since formula that is too hot will melt some brands of disposable bottles.

Terminal Sterilization

Terminal sterilization is the safest, most efficient form of sterilization, since it eliminates any contamination of the bottles that may have occurred during preparation of the formula, and equipment does not have to be boiled separately. The disadvantage of terminal sterilization is the long cooling period required before the formula can be used (about 2 hours). Thus, the mother must prepare and sterilize formula at least 2 hours before she needs it. Further, some brands of disposable bottles cannot be terminally sterilized, because they will usually melt and leak if exposed to high heat. Terminal sterilization procedure is as follows:

1. Wash the bottles, nipples, and caps. Prepare the formula, using a clean (not sterilized) bowl, spoon, and can opener. Fill the bottles, and put on the nipples and caps. The caps should not be screwed absolutely tight or the pressure inside from the steam as they boil will break the bottles. A good idea is to tighten the caps to the limit and then loosen them half a turn.
2. Place the bottles in a bottle sterilizer or a large Dutch oven. The rack on the bottom of the sterilizer or pan must be in place; the heat will make the bottles crack if they rest directly on the pan bottom. A high Dutch oven (covered) can be used for sterilizing as long as it is high enough for the bottles to stand upright in it. To protect the bottles from cracking, either a metal pie pan punched with holes (to simulate a rack) or a dishcloth should be placed on the bottom of the pan. Fill the sterilizer up to the line marked on the sterilizer, or up to the shoulders of the bottles, place on the stove to boil, and boil for 25 minutes after boiling starts, determined by listening to the sound of the boiling water and the gentle jiggling of the bottles. The lid should not be lifted to check for boiling, since pressure in the bottles from steam will force milk up into the nipples and clog the holes.
3. After 25 minutes, turn off the stove and move the sterilizer to a cool burner. Do not lift the lid until the sides are cool enough to be touched with bare hands. If the lid is lifted before that, milk will be forced up into the nipples and will clog them. The sterilizer takes about 2 hours to cool. When it is cool enough to touch, remove the bottles, tighten the caps, and refrigerate the bottles.

Preparing Individual Bottles

Many women today do not prepare a whole day's formula at one time but make up individual bottles as needed. Mothers who are breast-feeding and using supplemental bottles do the same thing.

If the mother is using ready-to-pour formula, she merely cleans the bottle, nipple, and cap, pours the desired amount of formula into the bottle, and puts on the nipple and cap. If she is using a condensed formula that needs to be diluted, she adds the correct amount of formula and an equal amount of water.

Techniques of Bottle-Feeding

To warm or not to warm formula is up to the mother, since studies have shown that infants who are fed cooled formula directly from the refrigerator thrive as well as infants who are fed warmed formula. Most mothers feel uncomfortable giving cool formula, however, and choose to warm it. The bottle can be removed from the refrigerator about an hour before feeding time and allowed to come up to room temperature gradually. Or it can be put into a pan of hot water or warmed up in a pan of water on the stove.

Heating it on the stove is the quickest method, and if the baby is hungry and crying, this is often the method chosen. A mother should be certain she does not allow the pan to boil dry or the bottle of milk will burst (this happens to every mother at least once, usually with the last bottle of formula on hand). She also must be sure to check the temperature of the formula by allowing a drop or two to fall onto the inside of her wrist, so that it will not burn the baby's mouth. She should not heat disposable bottles on the stove; they tend to melt and then leak during feeding. Heating bottles in a microwave oven is potentially dangerous, because in such ovens the milk in the center of the bottle becomes hotter than that near the plastic or glass side of the bottle. An infant can burn his tongue from the hot milk at the center.

Once a bottle has been used, any contents remaining should be thrown away. It should never be stored and reused. In sucking, an infant exchanges a small amount of saliva for milk. Because milk is a good growth medium for bacteria and the baby's mouth harbors many bacteria, the bacteria content in reused formula is likely to be high.

Feeding an infant is a skill that, like all skills, has to be learned. A mother needs a comfortable chair (and so does a nurse who feeds babies) and adequate time (at least half an hour) to enjoy the process of feeding and not to rush the baby. The baby is held with the head slightly elevated, to reduce the danger of aspiration and retention of bubbles. The mother should be sure that the nipple is filled with milk as the baby sucks, and he is sucking milk, not air. You can tell that a baby is sucking effectively if small bubbles rise in the bottle with sucking (Figure 33-9).

Babies in the early weeks should be bubbled after every ounce of fluid taken. A mother may place the baby over her shoulder and gently pat or

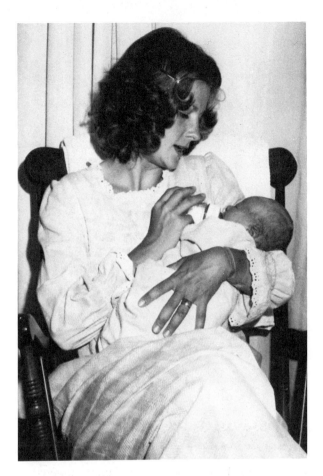

Figure 33-9 *Urge women who will be formula feeding to make themselves comfortable and spend time in interaction with the infant. (Courtesy of the Department of Medical Photography, Millard Filmore Hospital, Buffalo, N.Y.)*

stroke the back. This position is not always satisfactory for small infants, since their head control is poor, and the mother may not be able to support the baby's head and pat the back at the same time.

Holding the baby in a sitting position on her lap, leaning him or her forward against one hand, with the index finger and thumb supporting the head, is the best position to use for bubbling because it provides head support and yet leaves the other hand free to pat the baby's back (Figure 33-10). Mothers usually have to be shown this method. It does not seem as natural as putting the baby against the shoulder.

Some nurses are taught to feed babies by holding them in a supine position on their knees, not cradled in their arms in a motherly fashion. Theoretically, this position gives you a better view of the infant's face, so that you will see any signs of distress in the infant immediately. It also keeps the infant away from your clothes and hair, which

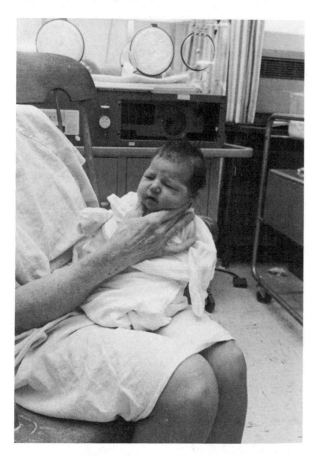

Figure 33-10 *A sitting position for burping a new-born. The infants head is well supported by the anterior hand. (Courtesy of the Department of Medical Photography, Children's Hospital, Buffalo, N.Y.)*

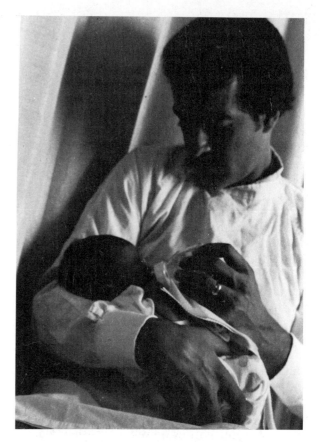

Figure 33-11 *Fathers enjoy (and need) interaction with their newborns. Here a father gives a supplemental glucose feeding to his newborn.*

are possible sources of infection. In practice, you can see the infant's face as clearly in the latter, motherly position as in the former one. Your gown should be clean, and in a newborn nursery, your hair should be short or controlled.

It is foolish to try to teach mothers to hold their babies warmly and comfortably if they are watching nurses holding and feeding infants in a cold, "clinical" manner.

Mothers need to be reminded not to prop up bottles. A mother whose infant spits up following feedings may feel that propping will relieve spitting up because it will reduce the amount of handling involved. Others prop up bottles because it allows them to feed the baby and do something else at the same time, such as preparing dinner. Babies who spit up actually need to be held more than babies who do not, because they are in greater danger of aspiration. Mothers might have to shift their usual dinner time to some other hour to coincide with their newborn's stomach clock. This is not an easy adjustment to make because husbands and older children have stomach clocks as well. Many a father enjoys feeding

the baby while his wife prepares dinner or simply relaxes (Figure 33-11). A mother who appreciates what it means to her baby to be held and made to feel secure will more readily make sitting down for feedings a top priority and will prop up very few bottles.

A mother should be cautioned that her infant may not eat well the first day home from the hospital because of the change in environment and the increase in activity and stimulation; for the same reason, the baby might not eat well when traveling. However, some infants eat as if they are starved on their first day home, probably because of the increase in activity. Common problems with formula-feeding are summarized in Table 33-5.

Introducing Solid Foods

The time to introduce solids to an infant's diet depends on a variety of factors: the baby's temperament and ability to accept new experiences, the mother's readiness to introduce solids (most

Table 33-5 Common Problems of Formula-Feeding

Problem	Cause	Nursing Interventions
Infant sucks for a few minutes, then stops and cries.	Either nipple is blocked and infant is unable to get milk or flow is too fast and baby has choking sensation.	Show mother how to test flow of milk from the nipple (hold bottle upside down); milk should flow from nipple at rate of about 1 drop per second.
Infant does not "bubble" well after feeding.	Some infants swallow little air with feeding. Mother may be handling infant too tentatively.	Observe baby feeding and mother's technique of handling; rubbing a newborn's back may be more effective than patting it.
Mother reports loose stools.	Bowel movements from formula-fed infants are not quite as loose as those from a breast-fed infant but so different from adult stools that a mother may be concerned.	Examine stool; assure and explain normal stool pattern.
Mother tired.	Exhaustion is a common postpartal finding due to psychosocial and physiologic adjustments of time.	Help mother to plan rest times; assess diet intake.

mothers are too eager to do so), the degree of development of the musculature of the jaw that enables the baby to bite, the maturity of digestive enzymes, and the fading of the extrusion reflex.

In order to digest the complex structure of solid food, the infant needs salivary enzymes. These are not present until 2 to 3 months of age. The extrusion reflex lasts until 3 or 4 months of age.

Biting is an accomplishment that becomes possible at about 6 months of age.

Nutritionally, an infant does not appear to need solid food until 5 or 6 months of age, as long as he or she is breast-feeding and receives a daily supplement of fluoride or is taking an iron-fortified commercial formula and receives a daily supplement of fluoride.

Utilizing Nursing Process

Infant nutrition is an important area of child care because it strongly influences a child's continued growth and development. Planning of good nutrition involves use of nursing process.

Assessment

Assessment of infant nutrition begins in pregnancy with assessment of the mother's (and father's) attitudes and choices about infant feeding. It is well accepted that breast-feeding is the preferred method of newborn nutrition; however, if a particular mother does not choose to breast-feed, she should not be made to feel guilty for her choice. In the same situation and with her same values, you would undoubtedly make the same decision.

Once infant feeding begins, teach a mother to assess whether the amount the infant is receiving is adequate—not by how long the baby takes to empty a breast or a bottle but by whether he or she is growing and happy and alert.

Analysis

The North American Nursing Diagnosis Association accepted three diagnoses specific to nutrition: Nutrition, alteration in, less than body requirements; nutrition, alteration in, more than body requirements; and nutrition, potential for more than body requirements. Although the characteristics that define these diagnoses pertain mainly to adults, one of them for a potential alteration is: Reported use of solid food as major food source before 5 months of age.

Planning

If a mother knows during pregnancy that she will breast-feed, she can begin gentle nipple rolling exercises to toughen nipples. The mother does not need to do this precaution, however: She can change her mind and still breast-feed even if she omitted this step. A mother who plans on formula feeding needs to think through how she will purchase formula and what supplies in terms of bottles and such she will need. Just as you need to help mothers plan on how to initiate a method of feeding, you often need to plan with them *not* to introduce solid food too early. Otherwise many mothers introduce solid food as early as 1 month of age; this premature arrangement may result in the baby not receiving enough milk for growth.

Implementation

A major phase of implementation in infant nutrition is supporting a mother's choice for the type of feeding she has chosen and helping her learn to trust her judgment as to when her infant is full and content. Help mothers to make both types of infant feeding as "natural" as possible by being certain they are comfortable during feeding and eliminating any extra procedures such as weighing the baby or excessive washing of breast tissue.

Evaluation

Evaluation should include not only whether an infant is thriving on the nutrition pattern chosen but whether the parents are satisfied with the method and find it an enjoyable time to be with their newborn.

Nursing Care Planning

Baby Kraft (John Joseph) is a 1-day-old newborn you care for.

Assessment

Mother states, "I thought breast-feeding would be hard. It's easier than it looks."

Infant breast-feeding q2h; 6 minutes each breast. Sucks eagerly; content between feedings. Voidings qs; meconium stool ×1. Skin turgor good, mucous membranes moist.

Weight: Birth weight minus 2 oz.

Analysis

Nutrition by breast-feeding established well at day 1 level.

Locus of Decision Making. Parent.

Goal. Breast milk to be entire nutritional pattern for 6 months.

Criteria.

1. Breast-feeding to be viewed as an enjoyable experience by parents.
2. Mother is knowledgeable of breast-feeding technique by discharge (24–48 hours).
3. Mother to use hospital liaison nurse as reference person for breast-feeding concerns when at home (no community or family support person identified).

Nursing Orders

1. Review physiology of engorgement with mother as she will be at home by third day postpartum when this occurs.
2. Review care of engorgement (warm compresses prior to feeding; encourage infant to suck).
3. Review practice of checking with M.D. before

beginning any medication while breast-feeding.
4. Review need for rest and adequate fluid intake while at home.
5. Review availability of hospital liaison nurse for consultation while at home.

Baby Collins (no name yet) is a 2-day-old infant you care for.

Assessment

Mother (19 years old) asking to feed baby but unable to hold her for entire feeding because of "pain from c-birth incision."

Grew concerned when baby spit up some mucus; asked when she will be old enough to feed by spoon.

Infant taking about 2 oz 20 cal/oz formula q4h. Sucks readily; voiding qs; meconium stool ×2. Skin turgor good; mucous membranes moist.

Weight: Birth weight minus 3 oz.

Analysis

Nutrition adequate for day 2 of life.

Locus of Decision Making. Shared.

Goal. Commercial formula to be entire nutrition for 6 months.

Criteria.

1. Mother to view formula feeding as enjoyable experience.
2. Mother to increase feeding time as physical condition improves.
3. Maternal grandmother to serve as resource person at home for nutritional problems.

Nursing Orders

1. Observe mother-infant interaction at each contact.
2. Encourage mother to feed infant so she grows accustomed to spitting up and handling infant.
3. Review adequacy of formula for infant and why there is no need for solid food.
4. Review feeding technique (hold, milk in nipple, burping, etc.)

Questions for Review

Multiple Choice

1. Mrs. Green is a primigravida you care for; she intends to breast-feed. She asks you how soon she can breast-feed following delivery. Your best answer would be
   a. immediately after birth.
   b. after the infant is allowed to rest first.
   c. the infant will be given a first feeding of formula.
   d. her infant will be given water for the first 24 hours.

2. On the first day postpartum, Mrs. Green is concerned that her milk has not yet "come in." You would explain to her that
   a. most mothers *do* have milk by 1 day postpartum.
   b. she will not have breast milk until 7 days postpartum.
   c. her infant must not be sucking well or she would have milk by now.
   d. breast milk normally comes in on the third to fourth postpartum day.

3. In planning nutrition for infants, you should be aware that a newborn's calorie requirement per pound each 24 hours is
   a. 50–55 calories.
   b. 100–120 calories.
   c. 150–170 calories.
   d. 200–225 calories.

4. In order to evaluate nutrition adequacy, you should be aware that breast milk contains an average of how many calories?
   a. 12 calories/oz
   b. 20 calories/oz
   c. 24 calories/oz
   d. 30 calories/oz

5. Mrs. Green points out to you that her infant has loose, yellow stools. Although the infant is healthy in every other way, she is concerned this means he is allergic to her breast milk. You would explain to her that
   a. she might try burping the infant more frequently.
   b. the stools of breast-fed infants are normally loose.
   c. she might consider changing to a soy-bean formula.
   d. her child may need to be investigated for bile duct disease.

6. Mrs. Green lives on a farm and, after breast-feeding for 3 months, plans to begin her infant on goat's milk. Your best response to her would be that

   a. goat's milk is superior in nutrition to cow's milk.
   b. human infants are unable to digest goat's milk.
   c. the infant will not drink goat's milk after breast milk.
   d. goat's milk will need to be supplemented with folic acid.

7. Mrs. Green asks you when she can begin to introduce solid food. Your best response to her would be
   a. as soon as her infant begins to act hungry at bedtime.
   b. infants do not need solid food until 5 to 6 months of age.
   c. she should delay solid food until the infant is 1 year of age.
   d. infants do well with solid food by 2 months' time.

8. On the fourth day postpartum, Mrs. Green develops breast engorgement. Which of the following measures would you recommend to her as a means of alleviating this problem?
   a. Discontinue breast-feeding for 24 hours.
   b. Decrease her fluid intake to below 500 ml per 24 hours.
   c. Encourage her to continue regular breast-feeding.
   d. Have her apply lanolin cream to each breast.

9. Mrs. Green is concerned that the infant is sucking too long at each breast. She asks how long her baby should nurse at each breast after she is home. Your best answer would be
   a. no longer than 3 minutes.
   b. the average baby empties a breast in 10 minutes.
   c. at least a half hour at each breast to ensure emptying.
   d. forty-five minutes is an average time interval.

Discussion

1. Choosing a commercial formula is difficult today because of the many brands and types available. What type would you recommend for a woman who must economize? For a woman who is more concerned with convenience than cost?
2. Many women stop breast-feeding after they leave the hospital because they do not believe they can return to work and continue breast-feeding. What are suggestions you could make to help a woman integrate breast-feeding and return to work?
3. Engorgement with breast-feeding causes pain. What are suggestions you could make to lessen this discomfort?

Suggested Readings

American Academy of Pediatrics. (1976). Committee on Nutrition: Iron supplementation for infants. *Pediatrics, 58,* 765.

American Academy of Pediatrics. (1978). Committee on Nutrition: Breast-feeding. *Pediatrics, 62,* 591.

American Academy of Pediatrics. (1980). Committee on Nutrition: On the feeding of supplemental foods to infants. *Pediatrics, 65,* 1178.

Appel, J. A., & King, J. C. (1979). Energy needs during pregnancy and lactation. *Nutrition and Health Promotion, 1,* 7.

Applebaum, R. M. (1970). The modern management of successful breast feeding. *Pediatric Clinics of North America, 17,* 203.

Bragdon, D. B. (1983). A basis for the nursing management of feeding the premature infant. *J.O.G.N. Nursing, 12,* 51s.

Bromberger, P. L. (1982). Premature infant's nutritional needs. *Perinatology/Neonatology, 6,* 79.

Catz, C., & Giacoia, G. (1972). Drugs and breast milk. *Pediatric Clinics of North America, 19,* 151.

Cronin, T. J. (1968). Influence of lactation upon ovulation. *Lancet, 2,* 422.

Eid, E. E. (1970). Follow-up study of physical growth of children who had excessive weight gain in the first 6 months of life. *British Medical Journal, 2,* 74.

Fisher, C. (1984). The initiation of breast-feeding. *Midwives Chronicle, 97,* 39.

Fomon, S. J., et al. (1979). Recommendations for feeding normal infants. *Pediatrics, 63,* 52.

Frantz, K. B., et al. (1979). Breastfeeding works for cesareans, too. *R.N., 42,* 38.

Houston, M. J. (1984). Supporting breast feeding at home. *Midwives Chronicle, 97,* 42.

La Leche League International. (1971). *The womanly art of breastfeeding* (13th ed.). Dansville, Ill.: Interstate Printers & Publishers.

Leonard, L. G. (1982). Breastfeeding twins: Maternal-infant nutrition. *J.O.G.N. Nursing, 11,* 148.

MacDonald, J. (1983). The working mother and her breast-feeding infant. *Canadian Nurse, 79,* 21.

Martinez, G. A., et al. (1981). Milk feeding patterns in the United States during the first 12 months of life. *Pediatrics, 68,* 863.

Moore, F. D., et al. (1967). Carcinoma of the breast. *New England Journal of Medicine, 277,* 293.

Mullett, S. E. (1982). A practitioner comments on research findings: Helping mothers breastfeed. *M.C.N., 7,* 178.

Riordan, J., & Countryman, B. A. (1980). Basics of breastfeeding: The anatomy and psychophysiology of lactation. *J.O.G.N. Nursing, 9,* 210.

Rogan, W. J., et al. (1980). Pollutants in breast milk. *New England Journal of Medicine, 302,* 1450.

Sterk, M. B. (1983). Understanding parenteral nutrition: A basis for neonatal nursing care. *J.O.G.N. Nursing, 12,* 45s.

VanPoppel-Ray, D., & Jenaway-Estok, P. (1984). Infant feeding choice and the adolescent mother. *J.O.G.N. Nursing, 13,* 115.

34

Newborn Care: Nursing Implementations

OBJECTIVES

Following mastery of the contents of this chapter, you should be able to

1. Assess a newborn's immediate needs and care.
2. State a nursing diagnosis related to an immediate newborn need.
3. Plan nursing care that is individualized for an infant during the first few days of life.
4. Implement techniques of newborn care such as bathing, temperature assessment, and umbilical cord care.
5. Evaluate goal criteria as to whether care is specific for newborn needs.
6. Analyze ways that newborn care can be individualized to meet specific infant needs.
7. Synthesize knowledge of newborn care with nursing process to achieve quality maternal-newborn nursing care.

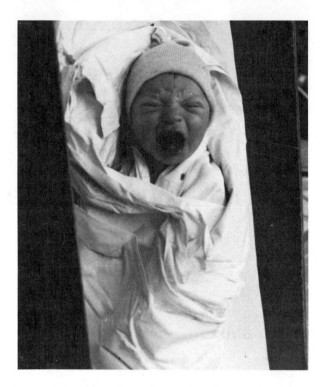

Figure 34-1 *A newborn wrapped and capped to conserve body heat.*

NURSING CARE of the newborn is a continuation of the care the fetus received during pregnancy and during labor and delivery.

Care at Birth

An island for newborn care should be provided in the delivery room or birthing room apart from the equipment needed for the mother's care. A radiant heat table or a warm bassinet, a warm soft blanket, and equipment for oxygen administration, resuscitation, suction, eye care, identification, and weighing the newborn must be provided.

In most health care facilities, the delivering physician or nurse-midwife hands the newborn to the nurse moments after birth to begin care. You should wash your hands thoroughly with an appropriate antiseptic solution; then, holding a warm sterile blanket, grasp the infant through the blanket by placing one hand under the back and the other around a leg. Newborns are slippery because they are wet from amniotic fluid and vernix caseosa.

Rub infants dry so that no body heat is lost by evaporation. Then swaddle them loosely with the blanket so that respiratory effort is not compromised, and lay them on their side in a warmed bassinet or unwrapped on a radiant heat table. Placing a cap on the head helps conserve heat (Figure 34-1). The bassinet should be tipped to a 30-degree Trendelenburg's position to allow mucus or fluid to drain from the mouth. The tilt should not be exaggerated or the infant's abdominal contents will be pressed against the diaphragm, interfering with lung expansion.

Evaluation of Respirations

Good respiratory function obviously has the highest priority. A Silverman and Andersen index (1956) can be used to estimate degrees of respiratory distress in infants. A newborn is observed once and scored on the items listed in Table 34-1. As shown, each item is given a value of 0, 1, or 2. These values are then added. A total score of 0 indicates no respiratory distress. Scores of 4 to 6 indicate moderate distress. Scores of 7 to 10 indicate severe distress. Note that this index's scores are opposite those of the Apgar. In an Apgar score, a value of 7 to 10 denotes a well infant. On a Silverman and Andersen score, a value of 7 to 10 denotes a seriously distressed infant.

Table 34-1 Evaluation of Respiratory Status

Feature Observed	Score		
	0	1	2
Chest movement	Synchronized respirations	Lag on inspiration	Seesaw respirations
Intercostal retraction	None	Just visible	Marked
Xiphoid retraction	None	Just visible	Marked
Nares dilatation	None	Minimal	Marked
Expiratory grunt	None	Audible by stethoscope only	Audible by unaided ear

Source: Silverman W. A., & Andersen, D. H. (1956). A controlled clinical trial of effects of water mist on obstructive respiratory signs, death rate and necroscopy findings among premature infants. *Pediatrics, 17,* 1. Copyright American Academy of Pediatrics 1956.

Suctioning

Mucus should be suctioned from a newborn's mouth by a bulb syringe as soon as the head is delivered. As soon as an infant is born, he or she should be held for a few seconds with the head slightly lowered for further drainage of secretions. Mucus must be removed from the mouth and pharynx before the first breath to prevent aspiration of the secretions. If an infant continues to have an accumulation of mucus in the mouth or nose following these first steps, you may need to suction further when the baby is placed in the bassinet (Figure 34-2). Use a bulb syringe or a soft small (No. 10 or 12) catheter. With a De Lee glass trap between the catheter and the suction tubing, the mucus obtained can be observed for color, consistency, and the presence of any blood. Vigorous suctioning should never be employed. It irritates the mucous membrane and leaves portals of entry for infection. Brisk suctioning has also been associated with bradycardia in newborns. If a bulb syringe is used, the bulb should be decompressed before being inserted in the infant's mouth or the force of decompression will force the secretions back into the pharynx or bronchi. When an infant is born with meconium-stained amniotic fluid, it is important that the infant be not only suctioned but intubated so that deep tracheal suction can be accomplished before the first breath. This action

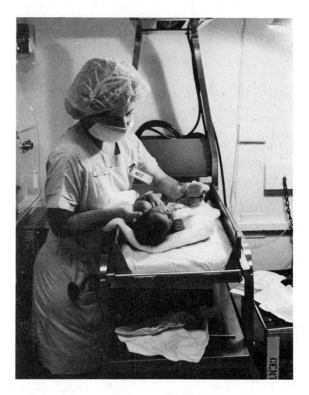

Figure 34-2 *Suctioning the newborn. A newborn is suctioned by means of a bulb syringe to remove mucus from the mouth. The head-down-and-to-the-side position facilitates drainage. Care is given with the infant under a radiant heat source. From Roberts, J. E. (1973). Suctioning the newborn.* American Journal of Nursing, 73, 63.

prevents meconium, which is very irritating to lung tissue, from being drawn into the lungs with the first breath.

Recording First Cry

A crying infant is a breathing infant because the sound of crying is made by a current of air passing over the larynx. The more lusty the cry, the more assurance there is that the newborn is breathing deeply and forcefully. Vigorous crying also helps to "blow off" the extra carbon dioxide that makes all newborns slightly acidotic and thus helps to correct this condition. Although gentleness is necessary to make an infant's transition from intrauterine life to extrauterine life as untraumatic as possible, most people believe you should not be so motherly in handling a newborn in the delivery room that you rock or jiggle the baby to completely stop this initial crying.

It is important to note what time after birth the child first gasped and cried and whether or not he or she was able to maintain respirations unaided. The newborn who does not breathe spontaneously, or who takes a few quick gasping breaths but is unable to maintain respirations, needs resuscitation as an emergency measure (see Chapter 47).

Control of Body Temperature

As discussed in Chapter 31, newborns have difficulty in regulating body temperature. They tend to become chilled in the delivery room because they are wet and the temperature of the room is low. Nursing care should be accomplished as quickly as possible, with minimum exposure of a child to chilling. Any extensive procedures such as circumcision or resuscitation should be done under a radiant heat source to reduce heat loss. There is no need for the infant to be removed immediately from a birthing or delivery room in order to prevent chilling. This is an important time for parents to have an opportunity to begin interaction. Newborns are very alert (first period of activity) and respond well to their parents' first tentative touches or interaction with them. Although the temperature of newborns who are dried and wrapped and held by their parents in the delivery room apparently falls slightly lower than that of infants placed in heated cribs, their rectal temperature does not fall below safe limits (Phillips, 1974).

Apgar Scoring

At 1 minute and 5 minutes after birth, the newborn must be observed and rated according to an Apgar score (Apgar, 1958). As shown in Table 34-2, heart rate, respiratory effort, muscle tone, reflex irritability, and color are rated 0, 1, or 2; all five scores are then added. An infant whose total score is under 4 is in serious danger and needs resuscitation. A score of 4 to 6 means that the condition is "guarded" and a baby may need clearing of the airway and supplementary oxygen. A score of 7 to 10 is considered a good Apgar rating, indicating that the infant scored as high as do 70 to 90 percent of infants at 1 and 5 minutes after birth (10 is the highest score possible). The Apgar score standardizes infant evaluation and serves as a baseline for future evaluations. There is a high correlation between low 5-minute Apgar scores and mortality and morbidity, particularly neurologic morbidity.

An Apgar rating is most accurate when it is done by a nurse. (Obstetricians tend to rate high; pediatricians tend to rate low.) For this reason you should be very familiar with how the rating is carried out. The following points should be considered in obtaining an Apgar rating.

Table 34-2 Apgar Scoring Chart

Sign	Score		
	0	*1*	*2*
Heart rate	Absent	Slow (below 100)	Over 100
Respiratory effort	Absent	Slow, irregular; weak cry	Good; strong cry
Muscle tone	Flaccid	Some flexion of extremities	Well flexed
Reflex irritability			
Response to catheter in nostril or	No response	Grimace	Cough or sneeze
slap to sole of foot	No response	Grimace	Cry and withdrawal of foot
Color	Blue, pale	Body pink, extremities blue	Completely pink

Source: Apgar, V., et al. (1958). Evaluation of the newborn infant—second report. *Journal of the American Medical Association, 168,* 1985. Copyright © 1958, American Medical Association.

Heart Rate

Auscultating the newborn chest with a stethoscope is the best way of determining heart rate. However, heart rate may also be obtained by observing and counting the pulsations of the cord at the abdomen if the cord is still uncut at 1 minute after birth. The newborn's heart rate ranges between 150 and 180 beats per minute immediately after birth as he or she struggles to begin respirations.

Respiratory Effort

A mature newborn usually cries spontaneously at about 30 seconds after birth. By 1 minute he or she is maintaining regular, although rapid, respirations. Difficulty might be anticipated in a newborn whose mother received large amounts of analgesics or a general anesthetic during labor or delivery.

Muscle Tone

Mature newborns hold the extremities tightly flexed, simulating their intrauterine position.

They should resist any effort to extend their extremities.

Reflex Irritability

One of two possible cues is used to evaluate reflex irritability, *either* the newborn's response to a suction catheter in the nostrils *or* the response to having the soles of the feet slapped. A baby whose mother was heavily sedated will tend to have a low score in this category.

Color

All infants appear cyanotic at the moment of birth. They grow pink with or shortly after the first breath. The color of newborns thus corresponds to how well they are breathing. Acrocyanosis (cyanosis of the hands and feet) is so common in newborns that a score of 1 in this category can be thought of as normal.

Care of the Umbilical Cord

The umbilical cord pulsates for a moment after the infant is born as a last flow of blood passes from the placenta into the infant. Two Kelly clamps are applied to the cord about 8 inches from the infant's abdomen, and the cord is cut between the clamps. It is then clamped again by a cord clamp, such as a Hazeltine or a Kane clamp, or tied with cord string or umbilical tape before the Kelly clamp is released. If a string is used, it should be tied in a square knot gently but firmly, so that the hands do not slip and tear the cord in the process of tying. The Kelly clamp on the maternal end of the cord should not be released following cord cutting; otherwise, blood still remaining in the placenta will leak out. This loss is not important since the mother's circulation does not connect to the placenta. It is messy, however, and that is why the clamp is left in place.

Inspect the infant's cord to be certain it is clamped or tied securely. If the clamp loosens before thrombosis obliterates the umbilical vessels, hemorrhage will result. As previously mentioned, the number of cord vessels should be counted and noted while the infant is in the delivery or birthing room. Cords begin to dry almost immediately, and by the time of the infant's first thorough physical examination in the nursery, the vessels will be obscured.

Care of the Eyes

Although the practice may shortly become obsolete (it is in Europe), every state requires that newborns receive prophylactic treatment against gonorrheal conjunctivitis of the newborn. Such infections are acquired from the mother as the infant passes through the birth canal. Silver nitrate is the drug that was exclusively used for prophylaxis in the past; today tetracycline and erythromycin ointments are becoming more commonly used. Silver nitrate comes prepared in wax ampules that are opened by puncturing one end with a pin supplied by the manufacturer. The face of the newborn should be dried first with a soft gauze square, so that the skin is not slippery. It is difficult to open a newborn's eyes. The best procedure is to shade the eyes from the overhead light and open one eye at a time by pressure on the lower and upper lids. Two drops of a 1% solution of silver nitrate are dropped one drop at a time into the conjunctival sac of each eye. Be careful not to drop any on the infant's cheek, since it may stain the skin a brown color. This is a transient phenomenon, but it causes needless worry to the parents. Do not drop the solution directly on the eye cornea or it will cause excessive pain. Silver nitrate should *not* be washed away with saline after instillation. A drawback of silver nitrate therapy is that a chemical conjunctivitis, characterized by inflammation, edema, and a purulent discharge, will result from instillation. Chemical conjunctivitis is confusing in the newborn period because it simulates an infectious process and makes the diagnosis of a true infection difficult. Antibiotic ointments eliminate the conjunctivitis and are easy to instill (simply squeeze a line of ointment along the lower conjunctival sac from the inner canthus outward).

Prophylaxis against gonorrheal conjunctivitis was first proposed by Credé, a German gynecologist, in 1884. For this reason, it is often referred to as the Credé treatment and may be listed that way on a health care facility form. Penicillin ophthalmic ointment or drops may be used for eye prophylaxis. This is effective against most gonorrheal strains, but its use is generally discouraged because of the dangers of introducing penicillin sensitivity at an early age.

Babies born outside hospitals (in taxicabs, for example) must have the prophylactic treatment administered on admission to the hospital; it is also required in babies born at home. Because it is a birth routine it is easy to forget in infants who are born elsewhere in these ways.

Vitamin K Administration

All newborns should receive an injection of 1 mg of water-soluble vitamin K (AquaMEPHYTON)

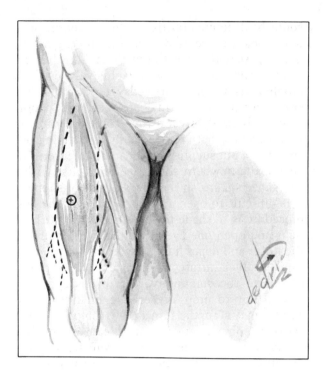

Figure 34-3 *Preferred site for intramuscular injection in a newborn: lateral aspect of the anterior thigh. (Courtesy of the Department of Medical Illustration, State University of New York at Buffalo.)*

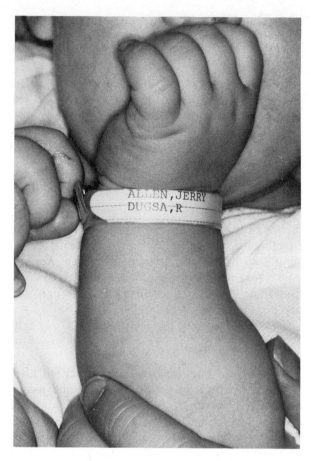

Figure 34-4 *A newborn identification band in place. Note how the wrist is almost the size of the hand in a newborn.*

in the delivery room. Higher doses may lead to hyperbilirubinemia and should not be given. Vitamin K is administered intramuscularly, usually into the lateral anterior thigh, the preferred site for all injections in the newborn (Figure 34-3).

Identification

Some form of identification must be attached to all newborns before they are removed from the delivery or birthing room. One traditional form is a plastic bracelet or bead necklace with permanent locks that need to be cut to be removed (Figure 34-4). A number that corresponds to the mother's hospital number, the mother's full name, and date and time of birth, and the sex of the baby compose the information necessary for identification. If the identification band is attached to a newborn's arm or leg, two bands should be used. A newborn's wrist and hand, as well as ankle and foot, are not very different in width, so bands tend to slide off with very little movement.

Following the attachment of the identification bands, the infant's footprints may be taken (Figure 34-5) and thereafter kept with the baby's chart for permanent identification. Although the value of foot-printing is being questioned, care should be taken in securing them since they will

Figure 34-5 *Newborn footprints. (Courtesy of the Department of Medical Photography, Children's Hospital, Buffalo, N.Y.)*

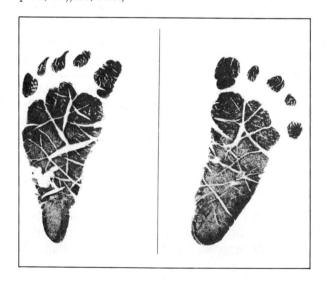

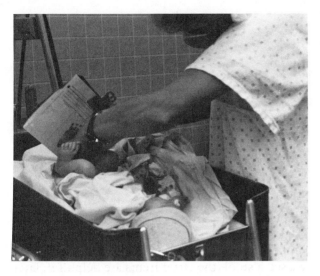

Figure 34-6 *Footprinting a newborn for identification.*

be part of the permanent record (Figure 34-6). Gleason (1969) suggests the following procedure for obtaining accurate and identifiable prints.

1. Proper equipment must be used, including a disposable footprinter ink plate and high-gloss paper.
2. As soon as the infant is wrapped in a warm blanket, his or her foot should be wiped clean. Vernix caseosa is thus prevented from drying on it and it is easier to clean when the actual footprinting is done.
3. After respiratory and circulatory functions have been established, but before the baby is taken from the delivery room, the foot should be cleansed gently but thoroughly. Scrubbing too vigorously makes a newborn's skin peel. The foot should be dried. Flex the baby's knee so that the knee is close to the abdomen, and grasp the ankle between your thumb and middle finger. Next, press your index finger on the upper surface of the foot just behind the newborn's toes to prevent the toes from curling. Press the footprinter gently against the sole of the foot.
4. The footprint paper, attached to a hard surface such as a clipboard, should be pressed gently against the inked foot. The heel should be pressed on the chart first, then the foot "walked" onto the chart with a heel-to-toe motion. The foot should not be rolled back and forth in the hope of making a better print; the result will only be a blurry print.
5. Any excess ink should be wiped from the infant's foot. The baby should then be well swaddled to prevent chilling. The mother's index fingerprint or thumbprint is commonly

placed on the same paper, along with the mother's and child's number.

If footprinting is required, it should be done in the same way on babies who are born outside the hospital when they are admitted to the newborn nursery for follow-up care.

Measurements

The newborn should be weighed nude and without a blanket in the delivery or birthing room. Height and head, chest, and abdominal circumferences should be measured in the newborn or transitional nursery. Doing these measurements while the infant is still damp, only exposes a newborn unnecessarily to chilling.

Assessment

A newborn is given a preliminary physical examination immediately following birth to detect such grossly observable conditions as meningocele, cleft lip and palate, hydrocephalus, birthmarks, imperforate anus, tracheoesophageal atresia, and bowel obstruction. This assessment may be the responsibility of the delivering physician, the anesthesiologist, a pediatrician, or nurse. The health assessment must be done rapidly, so that the newborn is not exposed for a long period of time, yet it must not be done so swiftly that important findings are overlooked.

The immediate birth appraisal should include auscultation of the chest for heart and respiratory sounds (perhaps already done as a part of Apgar scoring). Van Leeuwen and Glenn (1968) suggest a number of procedures that can be performed to rule out the common birth anomalies. These procedures and their screening importance are shown in Table 34-3.

A thorough generalized inspection and tentative gestation age determination should be included in the immediate birth appraisal in addition to the procedures that have been described.

Mother-Child Interaction

As mentioned in Chapter 24, the mother or parents should be allowed some time to be with a child before the child is removed to a nursery (unless the baby is in distress). Except for the few moments allowed for inspection of fingers, toes, and sex, the infant should be kept wrapped during the visit to prevent chilling and compromise of respiratory function. If a mother wishes to begin breast-feeding immediately following birth, she may do so.

Table 34-3 Congenital Anomaly Appraisal

Procedure	Abnormalities Considered
Inquire for hydramnios.	Presence of hydramnios suggests congenital gastrointestinal or genitourinary obstruction or extreme prematurity.
Appearance of abdomen.	Distended abdomen suggests ascites or tumor. Empty abdomen suggests diaphragmatic hernia.
Passage of nasogastric tube (No. 8 feeding catheter).	Failure to pass nasogastric tube through nares on either side establishes choanal atresia. Failure to pass it into the stomach confirms presence of esophageal atresia.
Aspiration of stomach with recording of color and amount of fluid.	With excess of 20 ml of fluid, or yellow fluid, duodenal or ileal atresia is suspected.
Insertion of rectal catheter.	Failure to obtain meconium suggests imperforate anus or higher obstruction.
Counting of umbilical arteries.	The presence of one artery suggests possible congenital urinary anomalies or chromosomal trisomy (if other portions of examination are consistent).

Source: Van Leeuwen, G., & Glenn, L. (1968). Screening for hidden congenital anomalies. *Pediatrics, 41,* 147. Copyright American Academy of Pediatrics 1968.

Birth Registration

The physician or nurse-midwife who delivered the infant must be certain a birth registration is filed with the Bureau of Vital Statistics of the state in which the infant is born. The infant's name, the parents' names, and the date and place of the birth must be recorded. Official birth information is important in proving eligibility for school and later for voting, passports, Social Security benefits, and so on.

Record Keeping

Be certain the birth record lists the following: the time of birth; the time the infant breathed; whether respirations were spontaneous; the child's Apgar score at 1 and 5 minutes of life; whether eye prophylaxis was given; whether vitamin K was administered; the general condition of

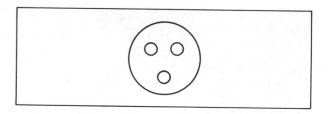

Figure 34-7 *A chart abbreviation for a three-vessel cord.*

the infant; the number of vessels in the umbilical cord; whether cultures were taken (they are taken if at some point sterile delivery technique was broken); and whether the infant (a) voided and (b) passed a stool (the latter items are helpful if, later on, the diagnosis of bowel obstruction or absence of a kidney is considered). Many people record a three vessel cord with the symbol in Figure 34-7. Don't mistake this drawing as a smiling face or assume it is not important.

Gentleness in Care

The philosophy of caring health care providers has always been that newborns should be handled as gently at birth as they are at any other time. The image of the obstetrician holding the newborn up by his heels and spanking him to make him breathe has existed only in Hollywood movies. It has long been accepted that holding a baby by the feet and letting the back extend fully is probably painful after the months in a flexed position in utero; a measure such as spanking is not as effective in helping a newborn to breathe as is gentle stimulation such as rubbing the back.

Leboyer, a French obstetrician (see Chapter 26), has stressed in recent years that gentleness at birth should be a prime priority of care. In addition to the accepted measures mentioned, he advises dimming the delivery room lights to reduce the pain of sudden exposure to light and immersing the newborn in a tub of warm water shortly after birth.

Gentleness at birth must extend to nursing interventions in order for the concept to be complete in all situations, whether specific Leboyer interventions are carried out or not.

Continuing Care

General Principles

A newborn should be kept in either a birthing room or a careful-watch nursery (Figure 34-8) for optimal safety for the first few hours of life. This

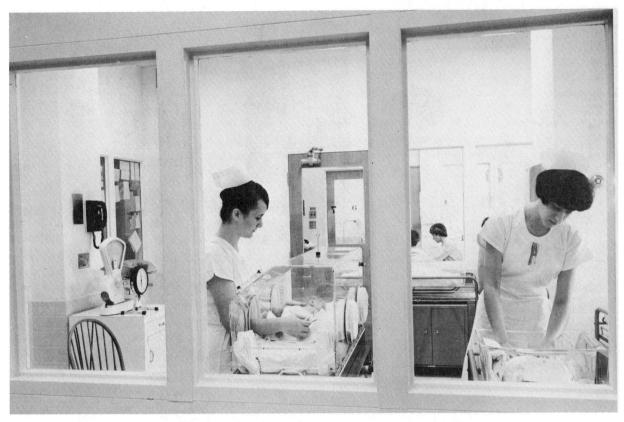

Figure 34-8 *An observation nursery. Following delivery, newborns need at least an hour of "careful watch" care either in a birthing room or in a special nursery before they are transferred to a regular nursery or the mother's rooming-in unit. (Courtesy of the Department of Medical Photography, Children's Hospital, Buffalo, N.Y.)*

nursery functions as a recovery room and provides a space where intensive care can be given during the first crucial period of life.

Following careful-watch time, whether a central care system or a rooming-in system is used, certain general principles always apply:

1. Infants should be housed in close proximity to the postpartal unit. The nurseries and the postpartal unit should, in fact, be a continuous service, so that the mother and child are thought of as one unit.
2. Each infant should have his or her own bassinet (Figure 34-9). Compartments in the bassinet should hold a supply of diapers, shirts, gowns, and individual equipment for bathing and temperature taking. The sharing of equipment leads to the spread of infection.
3. The temperature of the baby's environment should be about 75°F (24°C). When procedures that require undressing the infant for an extended period of time are being done (e.g., circumcision), a radiant heat source should be used.

4. Areas where babies are housed should be well lighted for the easy detection of jaundice and cyanosis. Nonglossy white or pale beige walls are best.
5. An oxygen source and emergency call lights should be readily accessible.
6. Personnel, parents, or siblings caring for newborns should wash their hands and arms to the elbows thoroughly with an antiseptic solution before handling infants. Personnel should wear cover gowns or nursery uniforms.
7. Personnel with infections (herpes simplex, sore throats, upper respiratory infections, skin lesions, or gastrointestinal upsets) should be excluded from caring for mothers and infants until the condition is completely cleared. Babies should be excluded from the rooms of mothers with any of these infections. A Polaroid photograph can be taken or the baby can be carried to the door of the mother's room, however, and shown to her, so that she can follow progress. If the infant is breast-fed, milk should be manually expressed during the time the infant is excluded in order to maintain the

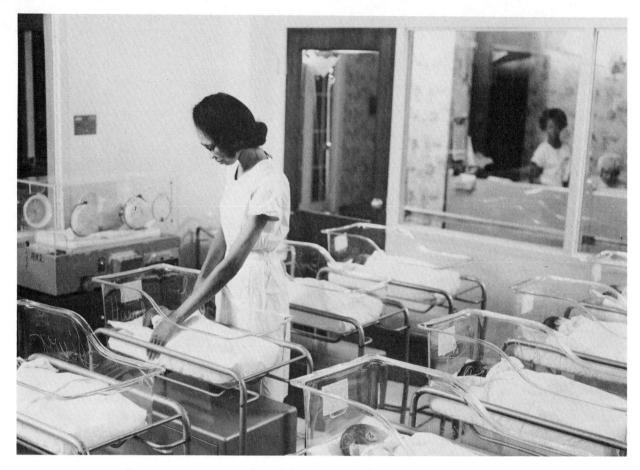

Figure 34-9 *A newborn nursery. Each infant has a self-contained unit for care. (Courtesy of the Department of Medical Photography, Children's Hospital, Buffalo, N.Y.)*

milk supply and allow for breast-feeding as soon as it is safe.

8. The number of babies housed together in a nursery should not exceed 16. Then, if an infection occurs, it will spread to no more than 16 babies. It is best if nurseries are limited to six newborns and are used on a rotating basis, so that each one can be cleaned between each group of six babies.

9. Any baby born outside the hospital or under circumstances conducive to infection (e.g., rupture of the membranes more than 24 hours before birth) should be admitted to a special isolation nursery or a closed Isolette for at least 24 hours until negative cultures show that he is free of infection. Any newborn in whom symptoms of infection develop (skin lesions, fever, and so on) should be removed from a central nursery and placed in an isolation nursery to prevent the spread of infection to other babies. There is no reason for a mother not to visit a baby housed in isolation care. She may, in fact, have more need to hold her baby than the average mother, because she has an extra reason to be worried that something is wrong with her child. However, as staff members do, she must use isolation techniques at these visits.

Admission to the Nursery

When the newborn arrives at the recovery nursery, the cord should be checked for any possibility of bleeding, and any antibiotic ointment or triple dye required by agency policy should be applied. The infant's measurements—height, weight, and head circumference—should be taken and recorded. Color and respirations should be noted. Be sure that the infant's identification band or necklace is in place. The baby should be reswaddled in a warm blanket and placed in a bassinet or in the mother's arms, or placed nude except for a diaper in a heated Isolette. An infant should be laid on his or her side.

During the first hour of life newborns should be observed closely for changes in color or respiratory effort. Leaving them on their side allows mucus to drain from their mouth. Some physicians prefer newborns to rest with the foot of the bassinet elevated at a 15- to 20-degree angle. This position obviously aids the drainage of mucus, but it may also unnecessarily increase intracranial pressure.

At the end of the first hour of life, a newborn's temperature should be taken. If it is subnormal and the baby is in a bassinet, he or she should be placed in an Isolette for additional heat. If the baby's temperature is normal, he or she can be bathed quickly to remove excess vernix caseosa and any blood, then dressed in a shirt and diaper, reswaddled in a snug blanket or sheet (to give the baby a feeling of the tight confines of the uterus he or she is used to), and placed in a bassinet or returned to the mother's side. If the mother is going to keep her baby with her during this time, she needs close observation. She is more tired than she realizes and may fall asleep easily.

When newborns awake or are awakened from their first period of sleep, they usually appear hyperreactive to stimuli. Their cries will be vigorous and their reflexes active. Mucus may have been pooling in their mouths during sleep; now, with activity, they gag and choke. This may be the body's way of ensuring good circulation and lung expansion during this time. In any event, an infant's temperament should not be judged by these actions. They are not necessarily typical of what behavior will be thereafter.

Occasionally, a child remains groggy when awakened. Extremities are floppy and head control lags behind normal. Such babies are probably still affected by analgesia or anesthesia; however, they may be demonstrating the first signs of increased intracranial pressure or infection. In either event, such babies should be watched closely for respiratory difficulty. Either they are candidates for a special care nursery or they will need to remain in the admitting nursery longer than the average child, until the grogginess passes.

Newborn Assessment

Following an hour of undisturbed rest, the newborn should have a thorough physical assessment, the details of which are discussed in Chapter 32. In addition, he should have a heel-stick hematocrit or hemoglobin determination and a Dextrostix test for hypoglycemia. Both hematocrit and Dextrostix determinations require a minimum of blood and can be obtained by nurses.

Newborn anemia is difficult to detect by clinical observation. Anemia may have been caused by hypovolemia due to bleeding from placenta previa or abruptio placentae, or perhaps from a cesarean birth that involved incision into the placenta. As dangerous to the newborn as anemia is the presence of an excess of red cells (polycythemia), probably caused by excessive flow of blood into the infant from the umbilical cord.

Heel-stick hematocrits reveal both of these conditions, and treatment can be instituted. The mean hematocrit at 1 hour of life is about 62 percent. If the hematocrit is below 40 percent, the infant will probably be transfused with fresh whole blood. Newborns with a hematocrit over 75 percent will probably have a modified exchange transfusion with low-hematocrit blood to reduce the hematocrit value.

If the Dextrostix reading is less than 45 mg per 100 ml of blood, the physician will probably order 10% dextrose in water or infant formula given orally immediately. Treating hypoglycemia is important, because excessive hypoglycemia leads to brain damage. If an infant is showing the symptoms of hypoglycemia (see Chapter 47), intravenous glucose will be administered.

Mother-Child Interaction

If a mother was not awake for the delivery, the baby should be taken to her room for at least a short visiting period as soon as she is awake and the baby's first hour of rest is over. The mother who delivered under a general anesthetic has a harder time believing that the pregnancy is over and that her child has been born than does the mother who was wide awake during delivery. Making her wait to see her baby until the first routine feeding time, which may be as late as 12 hours after birth, is unfair to her and may harm her relationship with the baby.

First Feeding

A mature newborn who will be breast-fed may be breast-fed immediately after birth. A baby who will be formula-fed receives a first feeding at 6 to 12 hours of age. This is a test feeding, to be certain that the infant can swallow without gagging and aspirating and to rule out the presence of a tracheoesophageal fistula connecting the esophagus and trachea and causing the infant to aspirate the feeding.

A first feeding is traditionally given by the nursery nurse, but there is no reason why the mother cannot give this feeding if a nurse remains in attendance. One approach to first feedings is to take the newborn to the mother for a visiting period and then bring the baby back to the nursery for her first feeding. This method serves several purposes. It allows the mother some time with her infant, assures you that the infant swallows properly, and protects the mother from possibly having to see her baby choking and spitting, which is frightening to a first-time mother, who wants and needs to do everything perfectly.

A first feeding consists of about an ounce of sterile water. Glucose water, which used to be the traditional first feeding fluid, if aspirated, has proved to be almost as irritating to the lungs as aspirated formula. Some physicians prefer that a baby who will be breast-fed also be given a test feeding of sterile water. This feeding can follow the initial delivery room breast-feeding experience because babies do not obtain much fluid at this first feeding, since only colostrum is present in the mother's breast. It is mainly a time to give both mother and baby practice in being together and getting used to each other, which is important to the success of breast-feeding.

Following an initial feeding of water, the formula-fed infant will be fed about every 4 hours. The next three or four feedings will be glucose water (Figure 34-10), and then formula-feeding will be started. Breast-fed infants do best on a de-

mand schedule or when fed as often as every 2 hours for the first few days of life. They may receive supplemental glucose water after each feeding for the first 2 or 3 days to prevent hypoglycemia. Infant feeding is discussed in detail in Chapter 33.

Daily Care

The routines of a newborn's daily care may be carried out largely by the nursery staff or by the parents, depending on the policy of the particular health care agency and the wishes of the parents.

Temperature

During the first day of life, a newborn's temperature is usually taken every 4 hours. Thereafter, unless the temperature is elevated or subnormal, or the infant appears to be in distress, once a day is often enough for temperature to be recorded during a health care facility stay. It is better to take axillary temperatures in the newborn

Figure 34-10 *A newborn receives a bottle feeding. Notice the motherly position the nurse uses to feed him. (Courtesy of the Department of Medical Photography, Children's Hospital, Buffalo, N.Y.)*

Figure 34-11 *Taking an axillary temperature. Notice how the infant's arm is held snugly against the thermometer tip. An immature infant, he has an indwelling gavage tube and cardiac monitor leads in place. (Courtesy of the Department of Medical Photography, Children's Hospital, Buffalo, N.Y.)*

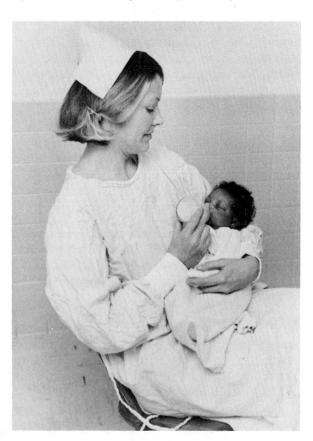

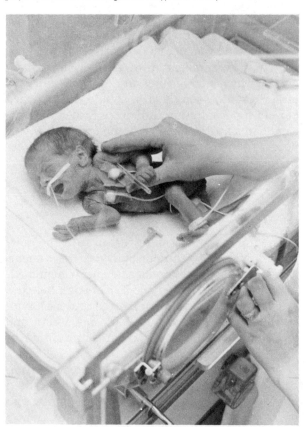

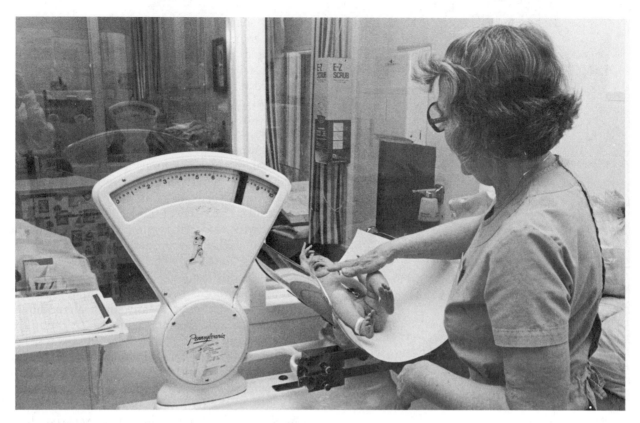

Figure 34-12 *Weighing a newborn. Notice the protective hand held over the infant. (Courtesy of the Department of Medical Photography, Children's Hospital, Buffalo, N.Y.)*

period to avoid injury to the rectal mucosa. If an axillary temperature is being recorded, the thermometer must be held firmly in the axilla with the child's arm pressed against it for 5 minutes (Figure 34-11).

Electronic thermometers are ideal for use with newborn infants since they register the temperature almost instantaneously and minimize the amount of manipulation necessary.

Weight

A newborn should be weighed on the delivery or birthing room scale at birth and on the nursery scale when admitted to the nursery (to establish a baseline weight against which all others will be compared). Thereafter, he or she should be weighed nude once a day at approximately the same time every day. More frequent weighing subjects the infant to unnecessary manipulation. The weight each day should be compared with the preceding day's weight to be certain that the infant is not losing more than the normal physiologic weight loss (5 to 10 percent of birth weight). Too often, the daily weighing of newborns is regarded as busywork by nurses rather than the health assessment tool that it is. The

first indication that newborns have an inborn error of metabolism, such as adrenogenital syndrome (salt-dumping type), or that dehydration is occurring, may be an abnormal loss of weight. Weighing the baby every day is only half the task. Comparing a day's weight to the weight of the day before and interpreting the two figures meaningfully is a nursing assessment.

An individual scale liner should be used with each baby to prevent the spread of infection from infant to infant. A baby should never be left alone on a scale and should be protected by a sheltering hand during the weighing procedure (Figure 34-12). Even a newborn can twist and turn enough to fall from a scale if left alone.

Bathing

In most hospitals a newborn is bathed once a day, although the routine may vary to include a full bath one day and a partial one the next. Bathing may be done by you in the nursery or by you or one of the parents at the mother's bedside. The room should be warm (about 75°F, 24°C) to prevent chilling during bath time. Bathwater should be around 98° to 100°F (37° to 38°C), a temperature that feels pleasantly warm to the elbows or

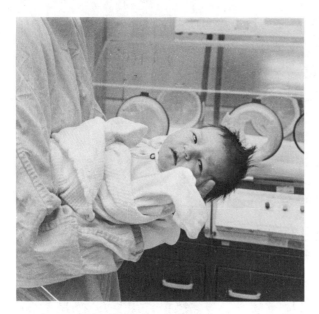

Figure 34-13 *A football hold. Such a position supports the infant's head and back and leaves the nurse's or mother's other hand free for assembling or using equipment. (Courtesy of the Department of Medical Photography, Children's Hospital, Buffalo, N.Y.)*

wrist. The soap used should be mild and without a hexachlorophene base. Bathing should take place prior to, not after, a feeding, to prevent spitting up or vomiting and possible aspiration.

The equipment for the bath consists of a basin of water, soap, a washcloth and towel, a comb, and clean diaper and shirt. It should be assembled beforehand, so the baby is not left exposed while the bather goes for more equipment.

Until a newborn's cord falls off, at about the seventh to tenth day of life, he or she should be sponge-bathed, not immersed in a tub. It is best if a bath proceeds from the cleanest to the most soiled areas of the body, that is, from the eyes and face to the trunk and extremities and last to the diaper area. The eyes should be wiped with clear water, and a clean portion of the washcloth should be used for each eye to prevent spread of any infection present to the other eye. The face should also be washed in clear water to avoid skin irritation by soap, but soap may be used on the rest of the body.

Hair is washed daily with the bath. The easiest way to wash a newborn's hair is first to soap it with the baby lying in the bassinet, then hold the infant in one arm over the basin of water as you would a football (Figure 34-13), and then splash water from the basin against the head to rinse the hair. Dry the hair well to prevent chilling.

Each portion of the baby's body should be washed, and each portion should be rinsed, so that no soap is left on the skin (soap is drying and newborns are prone to desquamation), and then dried. The skin around the cord should be washed, with care taken not to soak the cord. A wet cord remains in place longer than a dry one and furnishes a breeding ground for bacteria. Particular care should be given to the creases of skin, where milk tends to collect if the child spits up after feedings.

In male infants, the foreskin of the uncircumcised penis generally does not retract. It should not be forced back or constriction of the penis may result. The vulva of female infants should be washed with the bath, wiping from front to back to prevent rectal contamination of the vagina or urethra.

Most health agencies do not apply powder or lotion to newborns because some infants are allergic to these products. Many adult talcum powders contain zinc stearate, which is irritating to the respiratory tract; they should always be avoided. If the newborn's skin seems extremely dry, so dry it is cracking and portals for infection are becoming apparent, a lubricant such as Nivea oil added to the bathwater or applied directly to the baby's skin should relieve the excessive dryness. Because vernix caseosa may serve a protective function, some people recommend that newborn babies not be bathed, except for the washing away of meconium from the rectal area or bloodstreaked vernix from the face.

Diaper-Area Care

With each change of diapers, the baby's diaper area should be washed with clear water and dried. This prevents the ammonia in urine from irritating the infant's skin and causing diaper rash. Following the cleaning, an ointment such as Vaseline or A&D may be applied to the buttocks. The ointment keeps ammonia away from the skin and also facilitates the removal of meconium, which is very sticky and tarry in consistency. Be certain the diaper is folded below the level of the umbilical cord so that when the diaper becomes wet, the cord does not become wet also.

Rest

The newborn should be allowed to sleep with a minimum of disturbance between feedings. A newborn may sleep as much as 20 out of 24 hours, although the time varies widely depending on the activity or temperament of the infant. The infant should be positioned on alternate sides following feedings, to keep respiratory secretions or mucus from collecting or pooling in one lung or the other and to prevent flattening of one side of his head.

Healthy newborns have enough head control to move their head up out of spit-up milk on a sheet, so they may safely sleep on their stomach; some infants are unable to sleep in *any other* position. In infants who sleep constantly on the abdomen, however, a valgus deviation of the foot may develop. For this reason, changing the infant's sleeping position, from side to side and occasionally onto the abdomen, seems to have merit.

Identification

The identification bands of infants should be checked to see that they are in place during baths and before a child is removed from the bassinet or Isolette or from the nursery for any reason. When a baby is taken to a mother for feeding, the number on his or her band should be checked with hers before being handed to her or left with her. On discharge, it is extremely important that the number of the baby's band be checked to see that it corresponds with the number of the mother. Otherwise, a baby could be accidentally discharged with the wrong mother.

Continuing Parent-Child Relationship

Every attempt should be made during an infant's hospital stay to promote a good parent-child relationship. A mother should be encouraged to hold and get acquainted with her infant not only at feeding time but at other times as well. Encourage her to think of the infant as an individual, not just an extension of herself. Encourage her to talk to her baby. She will be surprised how intently the infant listens to the sound of her voice and how he responds to her—how from the very beginning he seems to be saying that he is a new, wholly unique person and that his mother should listen and pay attention to his needs. When a father visits, he may need some encouragement to hold his child if he feels self-conscious. Siblings need an opportunity to interact with the new baby as well (Figure 34-14).

A mother should have infant care demonstrated to her (Figure 34-15), and before discharge she should have a chance to care for her baby enough to be comfortable handling her. She should spend some time just watching her sleep, to become accustomed to the sucking and twitching movements that are characteristic of sleeping infants. She should feed and bubble her baby often enough to have confidence in the feeding method she has chosen and not to be upset if no bubble is forthcoming or the infant spits up at the end of the feeding. She should have an opportunity to change diapers enough so that she can grow skilled at it (handling and folding diapers to the

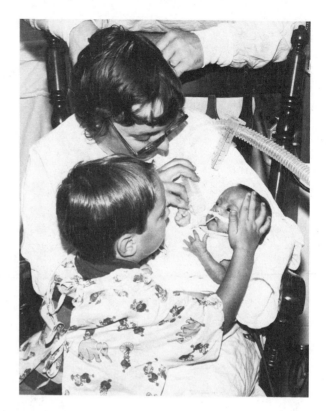

Figure 34-14 *Sibling visitation allows an older child to gain a realistic view of the new baby. Here a 3-year-old sees a new brother for the first time. (Courtesy of the Department of Medical Photography, Children's Hospital, Buffalo, N.Y.)*

correct size is difficult at first). She also needs to change diapers to observe bowel movements. Many new mothers assume that a newborn's stools will be brown and firm and are surprised at their black or yellow color and loose consistency. A new mother needs the opportunity to be surprised at these things while she is in the hospital, where there are knowledgeable people around her, rather than at home, where she might become alarmed.

Phenylketonuria Testing

Every infant, by state law, must be screened for phenylketonuria by a blood test before being discharged from the hospital. This is a simple test requiring three drops of blood from the heel of the baby dropped onto a special piece of filter paper. The baby must have been on formula or breast-fed for two days (must have had an intake of phenylalanine, an essential amino acid found in milk) before the test will be accurate. Be certain you check that the infant has received adequate milk before taking the blood sample. Otherwise, the results may be false-negative (a child with phenylketonuria will test as if normal). Many institu-

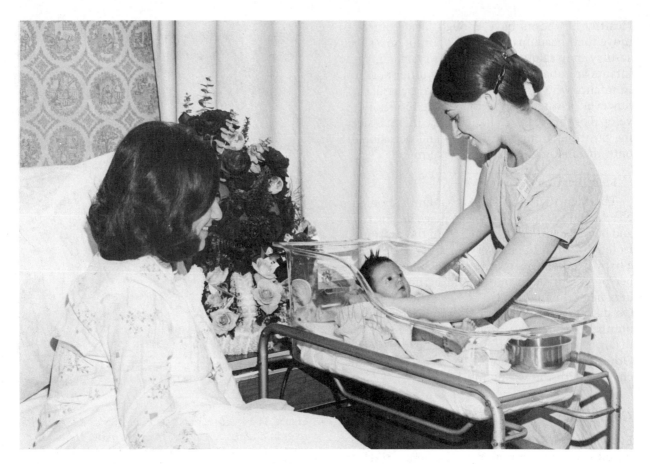

Figure 34-15 *In a rooming-in unit, a mother has her child with her for a greater part of the day, and mother-child interaction is thus increased. Here, the nurse is demonstrating a newborn bath by the mother's bedside. (Courtesy of the Department of Medical Photography, Children's Hospital, Buffalo, N.Y.)*

tions are beginning other metabolic tests at birth (such as screening for hypothyroidism) that need filter paper blood tests taken also. If the baby is discharged before the third day of life, the mother must be made aware that they were not done so she will remind her primary health care provider to obtain the blood sample at a first health supervision visit. Blood sampling of this nature is done best by a spring-activated lancet rather than a regular lancet so the skin incision is made so quickly that it is painless.

Record Keeping

A daily log of the baby's progress during the first days of life should be kept, including the number of voidings; the number, consistency, and color of bowel movements; the infant's color and degree of activity; the condition of the cord and skin; and the general feeding adaptation of the infant.

In hospitals where patient charts are put on microfilm after a period of time, special provision should be made to preserve the footprint record, if it is required for identification.

Discharge of the Newborn

Before a newborn is discharged, a thorough physical assessment should be performed. Its purpose is to determine whether or not some congenital defect or birth injury is present that has not been detected up to this point and to discover any condition that may have developed in the preceding three or four days.

Be certain that the mother has thought through child care at home. Try to anticipate problems she may have, so that they can be averted or solved. An important aspect to discuss with a mother who is not going to breast-feed is what she will use to feed the baby for the next 24 hours until she has had time to prepare formula. Most hospitals supply or sell a discharge formula kit to mothers to tide them over until they can prepare formula at home.

Be sure the mother has chosen when and where she is to take her newborn for health supervision. The identification bands should be checked one final time with her identification band before the infant is discharged to her.

Care of the Newborn at Home

The day a newborn comes home from a hospital or alternate birth center is an important day in the life of most families. Taking a long-wished-for baby home after a normal pregnancy and delivery is a time of happiness. Parents are strongly aware of their responsibility for the new child or perhaps frightened because they feel unable to cope with their new life situation.

Talking with a mother about her plans for home care of her child will help her make more realistic plans.

Housing

The physical environment of the home to which the child will be discharged is a good subject to explore with parents. Is it an apartment or a house? How many flights of stairs will the mother have to climb when she takes the baby home? When she takes the baby out in a carriage? To go back and forth to the baby's room? How many other people live in the home? Are there grandparents who will visit or help care for the child? Does the mother have anyone to turn to if she has questions about the baby? If she is unmarried, is she returning to her famly's home or her own apartment? Will the baby be sleeping in a room by himself or with older children? Will the mother be the primary caregiver to the child?

Does she have a bed for the baby? Is there a refrigerator in which formula can be stored? Is there adequate heat? An infant needs a temperature of 70° to 75° during the day and 60° to 65°F at night. Are the windows draft-free? Are they screened to keep out insects? Is there a danger that rats might attack the baby?

Does the mother or do the parents have a source of income? If not, what sort of referral should be made so that money can be provided to care for this child?

These are not prying questions but are a means of ascertaining whether the home that will receive the child is adequate and safe for him. All the good prenatal and postnatal care is wasted if an infant contracts pneumonia the first week home because no one at the hospital took the time to ask the right questions about the home environment.

Daily Care

Infants thrive on a gentle rhythm of care, a sense of being able to anticipate what is to come next. Most mothers have questions to ask concerning the kinds of care a newborn baby needs and how the care should be scheduled.

Every mother should decide what is the best daily at-home routine for her and her child. There are no fixed rules of infant schedules. There is no set time an infant must be bathed every day. There is not even a rule that he or she must have a bath every day. There is no rule that all infants must be in bed for the night by 8 o'clock. If the father works evenings, it may be important for the family to have the baby awake at midnight when he comes home from work, so that he has some time to spend with the baby.

Your aim in helping a mother plan her schedule of care is to arrive at one that (a) offers a degree of consistency (a mother cannot expect an infant to stay awake until midnight five nights a week, then go to sleep at 7 o'clock the next two nights); (b) appears to satisfy the infant; and (c) satisfies the parents, giving them a sense of well-being, a sense of contentment with their child.

Help the mother to realize that her infant is a real person with individual needs. Although physically part of the mother and father, the baby is still an individual in his or her own right. A schedule should respect that individuality. Some parents have difficulty with newborns because they do not appreciate this simple fact. They may be upset when they find their baby wants to be fed at 6 o'clock at night, just when they usually have their dinner; that he has needs he insists be met on his terms. They are surprised to find their infant is a real person who coos and "talks" and smiles at them, having assumed that he was going to be passive in his relationship to them for a long time.

Babies enjoy the gentle motion of a rocking chair. Mothers need to include a rocking chair in their budget as part of basic baby equipment (as should hospitals as part of basic nursery equipment).

As the mother cares for the baby, urge her to "discuss" things with her baby. It does not matter whether she talks about day-to-day happenings or about all her future hopes and aspirations for her child. The important thing is that she begin communicating with her child and establish a closeness that can continue all the years of the child's growing up. Talking to a baby is also necessary for speech development.

Bathing

Most mothers today are overly concerned with the technique of bathing their newborns, as if it were a complicated procedure that must be done just one way. In reality, there are only a few simple guidelines to follow in giving a baby a bath. In warm weather it is refreshing for the infant to have a daily bath. It is not necessary to bathe the baby if the house is chilly or if the mother feels that she is too tired or that she would not enjoy it. Washing the infant's face and neck (to wash away milk spills) and the diaper area (to avoid rash from ammonia irritation) is sufficient in lieu of a bath in these instances. In some infants, however, the hair needs to be washed as frequently as every other day in order to keep dry, scaling patches (cradle cap, or seborrheic dermatitis) from forming. Bath time should be fun for both mother and baby. It is a good time for mother-child interaction and is perhaps the first project they accomplish together.

The major piece of equipment needed for bathing babies at home is a baby bathtub placed on a table or counter of comfortable height so the mother does not have to stretch or bend. If the mother does not own a baby bathtub, there is really nothing wrong with bathing an infant in the kitchen sink. As soon as the baby begins to have good back support (at 5 or 6 months), he or she can be bathed in the family bathtub. Until this time, the baby is too slippery to be held firmly in an adult tub by a mother who has to stretch to reach him at all.

Water for bathing should be pleasantly warm. There is no need for the mother to take the temperature of the water, but she should feel it with her wrist or elbow to judge that it is pleasantly warm.

Additional bath articles she will require are a towel and washcloth, clean from the laundry basket or linen closet (there is no need to buy high-priced infant towels); hand soap (whatever type the rest of the family uses, but one cake should be used just for the baby); and a comb or hairbrush. No lotion or oil is necessary for routine use on babies. If the infant's skin appears dry, the mother may use a mild hand lotion or baby oil on the dry areas if she wishes. If the baby tends to have diaper rash, she may routinely use an ointment such as A&D on the diaper area after the bath and after each diaper change. Powders, like oils, are unnecessary. They create a pleasant "baby"

smell, however, so many mothers enjoy using them; but if powder is used too liberally, the infant will inhale it.

Babies should have only sponge baths until the cord comes off, at about the seventh to tenth day of life. Mothers need to be reminded that the fontanelles can be washed. Otherwise, they will wash around them.

When the baby is ready for a tub bath, the mother should place him on a soft towel on the tabletop and wash his eyes first, using clear water and different portions of the washcloth for each eye, to prevent the spread of any infection present to the other eye. Next, the face is washed in clear water. The hair is lathered, and then the infant is held over the bathtub in a football position (see Figure 34-13) and the soap is washed away.

The easiest way to complete the bath after the hair is washed is to lay the infant on his back on the tabletop and lather his front, then turn him on his abdomen and lather his back. Then pick him up and, slowly and gradually, holding his back supported, lower him into the bathwater to rinse him off.

Some babies take readily to bathing and enjoy it from the start. Others are furious at being exposed to this new sensation and take a month or more before they begin to smile and splash as they are washed. It helps to accustom these "slow-to-adapt" infants to bathing if the mother uses a gentle, soothing touch and speaks calmly. If the infant reacts strongly to being submerged in water, the mother can continue to give sponge baths for a longer time than usual. The guideline on bathing is that infants *may* be submerged once the cord comes off, not that the infant *must* be submerged once the cord is off.

Cord Care

It is important to remind the mother to keep the cord dry until it falls off. She should fold diapers down in front so that a wet diaper will not touch the cord area. If the mother uses plastic pants on the baby, she should be certain that these are folded down below the cord as well.

The use of creams, lotions, and oils on the cord should be avoided since they tend to slow drying of the cord and invite infection. Some physicians like the mother to dab rubbing alcohol onto the cord once or twice a day to hasten drying; others prefer that the cord be left strictly alone.

After the cord falls off, a small, pink granulating area about a quarter of an inch in diameter may remain. This should also be left clean and dry until it has healed (about 24 to 48 more hours). If it remains as long as a week, it may require cautery with silver nitrate to speed healing.

Clothing

A mother invariably dresses her infant too warmly. She should use only enough clothing to keep him or her comfortably warm. The less clothing the baby wears, the easier dressing is and the greater the baby's freedom to move and exercise. A mother can judge how much clothing is enough by how much she needs to put on herself. If she needs a sweater, her infant does also; if she is warm, her infant does not need a sweater. On very hot days, just a diaper will be enough clothing. The mother has to learn to trust her own judgment and not be swayed by friends who constantly tell her to put more clothing on the infant.

Selecting a Layette

Women may have questions as to buying clothing for a newborn. In selecting clothes several principles should be kept in mind:

1. Clothes should be easy to launder. Since newborns spit up and wet through several layers of clothing, all their clothes have to be changed after a feeding. Everyday clothes should be simple, with no trimming to irritate sensitive skin or complicate laundering. The woman will probably want to choose one dress-up outfit, but even this should be easy to launder.
2. Clothes should be easy to put on the baby. Shirts that open in the front and are fastened by ties or snaps are easier to put on newborns than those that slip over the head. Plastic pants that snap at the sides go on more easily than those with elastic tops.
3. Clothes should be large enough to allow for growth. A baby will outgrow a 3-month or even a 6-month size before it is worn out. Size 12 months, although large for a newborn, allows for growth.

Diapers. The selection of diapers involves a major decision; the child will wear diapers long after he has outgrown his baby clothes. The choices available are cloth diapers, disposable diapers, or a diaper service. The woman's choice will be based on the experiences of her friends and neighbors and the washing facilities she has available. If she has no washing machine, she will find a diaper service or disposable diapers more convenient than a daily trip to the laundromat.

At first thought it seems as if a diaper service or buying disposable diapers is expensive. This makes purchasing cloth diapers seem a preferable choice. However, when the costs of water, bleach, softener, soap, wear and tear on a washing machine, and replacing worn-out diapers are added in, the expense is probably comparable. Mothers often use a cloth diaper to cover their shoulder while burping the baby, so they may want to buy some even if they are not going to be using them as diapers.

Basic Layette. A basic layette for a newborn usually consists of

6 shirts
6 nightgowns or kimonos
6 receiving blankets
1 bunting or heavy blanket
6 diaper pads or plastic pants
1 sweater, cap, and bootie set
1 outfit for dress-up
1 rubber sheet to protect the mattress
3 or 4 dozen diapers (or about 10 disposable diapers per day)
4 rustproof diaper pins to use with cloth diapers.

Special sheets are not necessary; nor are special towels and washcloths as long as freshly laundered ones are used for the baby. Additional purchases might include a baby bathtub, additional basic clothing, baby lotion, oil, or powder, as preferred, and a diaper pail if cloth diapers are to be used. If a decision is to bottle-feed, the woman will need to purchase equipment for this as well. Both breast-feeding and bottle-feeding are discussed in Chapter 33.

Circumcision

Most male infants today are circumcised (have the foreskin of the penis removed surgically). There is little medical reason for the procedure as only a few men have such a tight prepuce that it interferes with voiding. Although enlightened parents are no longer asking to have this done, many still do because uncircumcised males have to include cleaning under the foreskin as part of routine bathing in order to avoid infection from accumulated secretions whereas circumcised males do not. Another reason for having the procedure done is that, since most boys are circumcised, being circumcised makes a boy appear like his classmates in school. Jewish males, of course, undergo circumcision as an important religious ceremony.

At one time, circumcision was completed immediately following birth. This policy had some disadvantages: The infant probably has a prolonged clotting time at birth (lowered amount of vitamin K), and he is exposed unnecessarily to the cold of the delivery room. It also prevents the parents from enjoying the wide awake phase of the infant at birth.

If circumcision is to be done, it is probably best performed during the first or second day of life. It is unfair to mothers to have the procedure done the day of discharge from a hospital (this does happen at alternative birth centers because of the short stay). Infants may bleed following the circumcision, and this timing puts the responsibility for observing bleeding on the new mother rather than on experienced nursing personnel.

Circumcision is theoretically a painless procedure although local anesthesia may be injected to ensure this. A few infants appear to be fussy for the first hour following the procedure as if they are uncomfortable. For the procedure, the infant is immobilized, either by restraining hands or by a special restraining board. The penile area is prepared and draped (Figure 34-16). A specially designed clamp is fitted over the end of the penis, stretching the foreskin taut (Figure 34-17). The stretching inhibits sensory conduction to the foreskin. Under sterile conditions, the skin is then quickly cut with a sharp scalpel and removed. The area is covered by sterile petrolatum gauze to keep the diaper from rubbing against it. The infant should be checked for bleeding at the circumcision site every 15 minutes for the first hour, then every 30 minutes for the next 4 hours. At every diaper change, a notation as to the state of healing should be recorded. The petrolatum gauze should remain in place for 24 hours unless

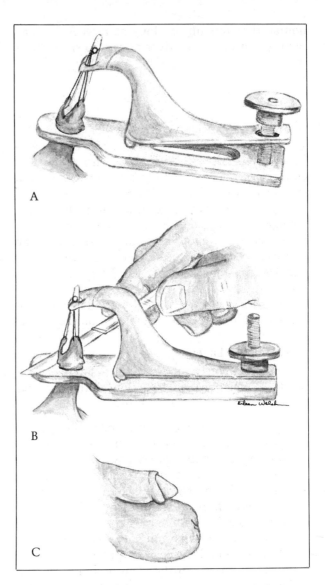

Figure 34-17 *Newborn circumcision. A. Foreskin clamped. B. Foreskin being cut. C. Circumcised infant penis.*

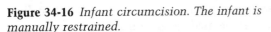

Figure 34-16 *Infant circumcision. The infant is manually restrained.*

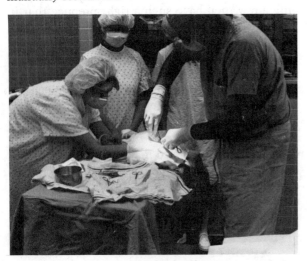

it is soiled by stool. After 24 hours, application of a petroleum jelly (Vaseline) to the site seems comforting for another 48 hours until healing is complete. Keeping the diaper pinned firmly helps to reduce bleeding and prevents the diaper from rubbing against the site.

Circumcision sites appear red and sore but should never have a strong odor or a discharge. A thin yellow exudate forms over the healing surface within 24 hours of the procedure (similar to a scab). Do not confuse this with an infectious exudate or attempt to wash it away.

At discharge, the circumcised infant seems most comfortable if the healing site is kept covered by an ointment such as Vaseline for 4 to 5 days. This prevents the diaper from touching and clinging to the healing tissue and causing bleeding with diaper changes. The mother should observe the site daily and report to her physician any redness, foul odor, or discharge that suggests infection.

Health Problems in the Newborn

Mothers who have private physicians call them for advice on health problems in their newborns. Mothers who do not have private physicians are urged to phone either the agency where they delivered, or a community health nurse or the agency which will provide well child care if they are concerned about some aspect of care. A high proportion of newborn problems can be managed successfully by advice given on the telephone by a nurse in consultation with a physician.

Many child care problems that arise with newborns are simply the result of a mother's misinterpretation of the child's reactions or are problems of the child's adjustment to a new world and new stimuli, which takes a little time. Mothers ask questions about cord care, bathing, and feeding, and they often call about the common illnesses of infancy.

Constipation

Constipation is rare in breast-fed infants because their stools tend to be loose. Rarely, constipation may occur with bottle-fed infants if the diet is too deficient in fluid. Some infants on iron-fortified commercial formula tend toward constipation. The problem can be corrected by adding more fluid or carbohydrate to the diet. Some babies need a formula change because they have grown since the formula was prescribed and now have a greater fluid requirement. Offering a bottle of water with a teaspoon of Karo syrup added may be helpful.

Some mothers misinterpret the normal pushing movements of a newborn as constipation—infants do make faces, get red in the face, and make small grunting noises when passing stools. As long as the stool is not hard and no fresh blood is on the stool (as might occur with a rectal fissure), this is not constipation but an example of a new mother's misinterpreting her infant's behavior.

If the infant is constipated, and the problem persists beyond a few months of age, the addition of bulky foods such as fruits or vegetables generally relieves it. One half to 1 ounce of prune juice daily may be given as a temporary measure. It is better not to give prune juice over a long period of time (mothers often believe that if a little is good for the baby, a lot will be even better), since too much of it will cause diarrhea.

All infants with a history of constipation for more than a week should be examined for an anal fissure or a tight anal sphincter. Softening the hard stools by means of an oral stool softener, therefore alleviating the pain of defecation, often solves the problem and helps an anal fissure to heal. If the infant has an unusually tight anal sphincter, the mother will be given instructions to dilate the sphincter two or three times daily until it stretches sufficiently to eliminate the obstipation. Hirschsprung's disease (congenital aganglionic megacolon) may be manifested early in life as constipation. If no stool is found on rectal examination of a constipated infant, congenital aganglionic megacolon is suggested.

Loose Stools

Many new mothers report loose stools in their infants as a problem because they are unfamiliar with the consistency of the normal newborn's stools. Every mother needs to handle and care for her newborn enough in the health care agency before discharge to be familiar with what a newborn's stools are like before she goes home.

When talking to a mother about the problem of loose stools, you need to investigate the duration of the condition, the number of stools per day, their color and consistency, and the presence of any mucus or blood. Is there associated fever, cramping, vomiting? Does the infant continue to eat well? Does the infant appear well? Is the infant thriving?

The infant of a mother who is mixing formula inaccurately, adding too much sugar, or not diluting formula properly will have loose stools. Correcting the problem, of course, is simply a matter of correcting the error in formula preparation. Occasionally, loose stools begin with the introduction of solid food. In this instance, food sensitivity is suggested. Ask exactly what foods the baby is being fed. Malabsorption syndrome may be the cause, since it may manifest itself first by loose stools.

As previously mentioned, stools of breast-fed infants are usually softer than those of formula-fed infants. Further, a laxative taken by the mother while breast-feeding may cause the infant to have loose stools.

Infants who have loose stools and associated symptoms (fever, cramping, vomiting, loss of appetite, loss of weight) should be seen by a physician. Dehydration occurs rapidly in a small infant who is not eating and is losing body water in loose stools.

Colic

Colic is paroxysmal abdominal pain. It generally occurs in infants under 3 months of age who are formula fed. The discomfort appears abruptly. The infant cries loudly and pulls his legs up against his abdomen. His face is red and flushed, his fists clench, and his abdomen is tense. If offered a bottle, the infant will suck vigorously for a few minutes as if he were starved, then stop when another wave of intestinal pain overwhelms him.

The cause of colic is unclear. It may occur in susceptible infants from overfeeding, from swallowing too much air while feeding, or from being on a formula too high in carbohydrate. Its occurrence is associated with a tense and unsure mother. Women who fear that their infants will have congenital abnormalities tend to have infants with colic more than do women who do not have this concern.

Colic should not be dismissed lightly as an unimportant disease of infancy. It is a major problem for the mother because it is so frightening. The infant appears to be in acute pain and distress. Since colic persists for hours and usually in the middle of the night, neither mother nor child gets adequate rest. This is a bad beginning to a mother-child relationship, which needs to be strong and binding for the mother to enjoy mothering and for the infant to thrive in her care. Prevention of colic or the relieving of colic may do as much for the future mental health of the child as it does for his temporary pain and discomfort.

A thorough history should be taken on infants with the symptoms of colic, since intestinal obstruction or infection may mimic an attack of colic and will be misinterpreted by the casual interviewer. Ask how long the problem has been going on and about the frequency and time of attacks (colic usually occurs at bedtime). Ask for a description of what happens just prior to the attack and what the attack of colic is like. Ask for associated symptoms. It is important to know the number of bowel movements associated with the condition, since bowel movements are not abnormal with colic. Constipated stools or narrowed "ribbon" stools suggest other complicating problems. Ask about the family medical history. Allergy to milk may simulate colic.

The mother of a baby with colic should be asked the type of formula the infant is being fed and how she is preparing it. Explore with her how she is feeding the baby and whether she is bubbling her adequately. While feeding the baby, the mother should hold her in as upright a position as possible, so that air bubbles can rise. Both bottle-fed and breast-fed babies should be bubbled thoroughly after feeding. After feeding, many babies with colic are more comfortable sleeping on their abdomen than on their side or back. A towel rolled under the abdomen for a little extra pressure is often helpful.

A mother may feel uneasy placing a baby under 3 months of age on her stomach to sleep. This creates no problem in a well newborn (and a baby with true colic is a well baby), who will have no difficulty in lifting her head to clear the airway. Some persons recommend placing a hot-water bottle under the infant's stomach, but this should be discouraged as a common practice; a basic rule in dealing with any abdominal discomfort is to avoid heat because the pain may be symptomatic of appendicitis. Such a diagnosis is highly unlikely in an infant, but the mother will remember that a hot-water bottle was recommended for her infant's abdominal pain and may use one with an older child whose pain may be due to appendicitis.

Changing to a commercially prepared formula from an evaporated milk formula may alleviate colic. Changing the type of bottle to one with a disposable bag that collapses as the baby sucks and reduces the amount of air swallowed may be helpful.

Occasionally, a colicky baby needs sedation to relieve his pain and to give him and his mother some rest. It is important to think of colic as a problem for two people, the infant and the mother, or a vicious circle begins. The infant cries and the mother becomes tense and unsure of herself. The colic worsens because the infant senses her tenseness. He cries more, the mother becomes even more unsure, and so on.

Colic almost magically disappears at 3 months of age. If the mother can be supported until this milestone arrives, she will discover that despite the colic her infant has grown during this time. *Support* is the prime word in colic. Three months of living with a fussy, crying, unappeasable infant seem like 3 years.

Sleeping Patterns

Mothers who call about their infant's sleeping patterns may be concerned because they think the baby is sleeping too much or because he appears to be sleeping too little.

A baby sleeps an average of 16 hours out of every 24 in his first week home and sleeps an average of 4 hours at a time. By 4 months of age he sleeps an average of 15 hours out of 24 hours and 8 hours at a time (through the night).

Mothers try various devices to induce a baby to sleep through the night much earlier than at 4 months of age. One approach is introducing solids (particularly cereal) early, in the first weeks of life, on the theory that the cereal's bulk will fill up the infant's stomach for the night, and therefore he will not wake up crying to be fed. Actually, there is no correlation between the age at which solid food is introduced and the baby's capability for sustained sleep. A baby wakes every 4, 5, 6, or 8 hours for feeding because of physiologic need for fluid. It is, of course, exhausting for mothers who are already tired from the experience of labor and delivery to have to wake at night and feed a newborn. It is a rare husband who can feed a newborn at night without waking his wife to ask her whether he is doing everything correctly. Thus, having a husband say he will take over at night may not really help.

Be certain that a mother who is troubled about her baby's waking at night is describing a newborn who is healthy in every way: taking a sufficient amount of formula or spending enough time at the breast every day, sleeping well during the day, having normal bowel movements, and being normally active. You should have a total picture before blindly assuring a mother of anything. But once you are satisfied that the mother is simply describing a normal baby waking at night for a feeding, assure her that he is normal and that there is no reason to try to eliminate this feeding. Knowing that her baby is not sick, that you are concerned with her problem and willing to listen to her, and that every other mother of a newborn is also up at night does not solve her difficulty, but it is a help. Being assured that a baby's behavior is normal is always welcome news to parents.

Crying

Many new mothers are not prepared for the amount of time a newborn spends in crying. Whenever the mother saw the baby while at the health care agency, she was sleeping. She woke her up to feed her, and she immediately went back to sleep. It is not uncommon to hear a mother say on leaving the hospital with a newborn, "I'm sure she's going to be a good baby. I've never heard her cry."

Brazelton (1962) reports that infants cry an average of 2¼ hours out of every 24 for the first 7 weeks of life. The incidence of crying seems to peak at age 6 or 7 weeks and then taper off.

Almost all infants have a period during the day when they are wide awake and invariably fussy.

Each new mother needs to recognize this period as normal and not concern herself that her child is ill because once a day he seems out of sorts. She might use this fussy time for bathing him or playing with him, arranging her schedule to cope with his wakefulness. The most typical time for wakefulness to occur is between 6:00 and 11:00 P.M., which unfortunately is a time when the mother is tired and least able to tolerate crying.

Spitting Up

Almost all babies do some spitting up, formula-fed more than breast-fed babies. A mother who does not handle her infant very much while at an alternative birth center or hospital may, in the first week home, interpret spitting up as vomiting or a sign of infection.

Ask a mother to describe carefully what she means by spitting up. How long has the baby been doing it? How frequently does he do it? What is the appearance of the spit-up milk? Almost all milk that is spit up smells sour, but it should not contain blood or bile. What is the intensity of the spitting? Does the baby spit out forcefully, or is the mother just describing a mouthful of milk rolling down his chin? Are there any associated symptoms (diarrhea, abdominal cramps, fever, cough, cold, inactivity)? What has she tried as a remedy?

If the mother describes associated symptoms, the child should be seen by a physician, because she is describing an ill child. If he is spitting up so forcefully that the milk is projected 3 or 4 feet away, she may be describing beginning pyloric stenosis (obstruction of the pyloric opening from the stomach). This requires medical or surgical intervention.

If she is describing an infant who two or three times a day (or sometimes after every feeding) spits up or allows a mouthful of milk to roll down his chin, she is describing the normal spitting up of early infancy.

Ask her to describe how she bubbles the baby; thorough bubbling often reduces spitting up. Changing formulas (which she will probably suggest as a solution) generally has little effect. Spitting up decreases in amount as the baby better coordinates his swallowing and digestive processes and possibly because as he grows older he is more often in an upright position, and gravity corrects the problem.

Colds

Upper respiratory infections are infrequent in children under 1 month of age. A mother sometimes reports that her newborn has a stuffy nose, or makes "snoring noises" in his sleep, or sneezes occasionally. Most newborns continue to have some mucus in the upper respiratory tract and posterior pharynx for about two weeks after birth, and it is this, not a cold, that causes the snoring noise. Infants also breathe irregularly for about the first month. A new mother who did not room in with her child at the hospital may wake at night, notice this breathing pattern, and become alarmed that her child is in respiratory distress.

Ask a mother about the exact duration, nature, frequency, and intensity of the symptoms she is reporting. Is she describing normal newborn breathing? A head cold with rhinitis? A cold in which bronchial and lung areas are involved? Ask for associated symptoms such as fever, vomiting, and diarrhea. Ask what action she has taken to relieve the symptoms. Ask for a careful description of what sound the baby is making. Stridor is a harsh, vibrating, high-pitched, shrill, or crowing noise that is marked on inspiration. It is a sign of respiratory obstruction.

If a mother is describing normal newborn breathing, she needs to be reassured about its normality. If there is no fever (ask her if she has actually taken the baby's temperature or is judging fever by touch), but the baby has symptoms of congestion and rhinitis, the physician may wish her to purchase a nasal syringe and gently suction secretions from the infant's nose, particularly before feeding. Infants cannot suck and breathe at the same time. An infant with a stuffy nose will constantly stop sucking to breathe. He becomes fatigued, his intake falls, dehydration may occur, and a simple cold becomes complex.

Most physicians prefer to examine a young infant with upper respiratory symptoms to be certain his lungs are clear. If the infant has a fever, he should be examined to determine the reason for the fever.

Skin Problems

Diaper Dermatitis

Some newborns have such sensitive skin that diaper rash is a problem from the first few days of life. Diaper rashes have a variety of causes; most commonly irritation from feces, urine, or laundry products creates the problem.

Feces Irritation. In an infant who does not have her diapers changed as frequently as she might, so that feces remain in contact with the skin, dermatitis from fecal contact may result, with the rash involving the perianal area. More

frequent changing of diapers and screening the skin from fecal material with an ointment such as Vaseline or A&D Ointment is the solution to the problem.

Urine Irritation. After a time, the urine in urine-soaked diapers breaks down into ammonia, a chemical that is extremely irritating to infant skin. Ammoniacal dermatitis is usually a problem of the second half of the first year of life, when the infant is producing a larger quantity of urine than he did initially, but in some infants it is a problem from the first week on. Again, frequent diaper changing and application of Vaseline or A&D Ointment may be the answer. Some infants may have to sleep without diapers at night in order to relieve the problem. Some need to have plastic pants removed to decrease irritation. Disposable diapers may cause the difficulty; often changing the brand of diapers helps.

Rinsing cloth diapers in a final rinse of methylbenzethonium chloride (Diaparene) helps to discourage the breakdown of urine. Exposing the infant's diaper area two or three times a day to a low-wattage light bulb may also be beneficial. However, when using this heat source, the parents must make sure that the light bulb is at least 12 inches away so it does not touch the infant's buttocks or clothes or the sheets, since they may become dangerously hot. Caution them not to face a male infant toward the light or his urine stream might shatter the bulb.

Irritation from Laundry Products. Any time the entire diaper area is erythematous and irritated, so that the outline of the diaper appears on the skin, the products the family is using to wash diapers are suspect as the cause of the irritation. Parents should rinse diapers well, removing all soap and fabric softener. If they are washing diapers at a laundromat, paying for an extra rinse cycle may be a problem. If the family adds up the cost of washing diapers, buying soap and softener, and rinsing adequately, they may find that disposable diapers or diapers from a diaper service are actually more economical.

Miliaria

Miliaria (prickly heat) rash occurs most often in warm weather or on babies who are overdressed or sleep in overheated rooms. Clusters of pinpoint-sized, reddened papules with occasional vesicles and pustules and surrounded by erythema usually first appear on the neck. They may spread upward to around the ears and onto the face or down onto the trunk.

Bathing the infant twice a day during hot weater, particularly if a small amount of baking soda is added to the bathwater, is helpful in clearing up the rash. Eliminating sweating by reducing the amount of clothes on the infant or lowering the room temperature will bring about almost immediate improvement and prevent further eruption.

Seborrheic Dermatitis (Cradle Cap)

Cradle cap is a common scalp condition of early infancy characterized by dirty-looking, adherent, yellow, crusting patches. The skin beneath the patches may be slightly erythematous. Cradle cap can be largely prevented by frequent shampoos (every other day). The patches may be removed by oiling the scalp with mineral oil or Vaseline at night. This softens the crusts, which can then be removed by shampooing the next morning.

Infection

Oral Candidiasis

Oral candidiasis (thrush) is a *Candida* infection in which numerous small white and gray patches are present on the tongue and buccal membrane. During delivery, the baby contracts the infection from *Candida* organisms in the mother's vagina. Milk curds remaining on the tongue after feeding simulate thrush. Milk curds can be scraped away, but thrush cannot. Infants with thrush need to be referred to a physician, since a prescription antifungal agent (usually nystatin) is necessary for treatment.

Candidiasis

Candidiasis is a *Candida* infection of the diaper area. The anal mucosa and perianal skin appear macerated, and raw red areas spread from the anus outward. The irritation does not respond to the usual measures. The infant should be seen by a physician, since, again, nystatin is necessary for treatment.

Impetigo

Although it is almost impossible to judge the nature of skin lesions from a telephone account, ask a mother to describe minutely the lesion that concerns her. It may be impetigo, a skin infection most often caused by a streptococcus. The lesions begin as pustules that rupture into thick, honey-colored crusts. Because impetigo is ordinarily due to a streptococcal infection, it must be treated systemically with an antibiotic, usually penicil-

lin, so the infant should be referred to a physician for care.

Health Maintenance at Home

There is no need for parents to continue to weigh an infant while at home. This practice may only cause worry, since an infant's weight gains fluctuate. Parents should learn to judge an infant's state of health in terms not of increases in weight but of overall appearance, eagerness to eat, general activity, and disposition.

A mother should be shown in the health care facility how to take the infant's temperature rectally. Then, if she suspects a fever, she can take the temperature before calling her physician for advice. This is best done in infants if the infant is positioned prone over the mother's knee (Figure 34-18).

Parents should know before they leave a birth setting what kind of follow-up care their child is going to have. Pediatricians or general practitioners will visit women while they are hospitalized, discuss their philosophy of child care, and give a woman an appointment for a visit to the office in about 4 weeks. If parents choose a well-child conference, health maintenance organization, or pediatric clinic for care, they should be given the telephone number of the agency, so that they can call for an appointment for the child.

It is important that parents understand the necessity for follow-up care for a baby. A mother is conscientious throughout pregnancy because she wants to bring a well child into the world. She now needs to begin a health care program that will keep her child well.

Recommendations for preventive health care for the first 5 years of life are presented in Table 34-4. This is a guide for the care of well children who receive competent parenting, who have not manifested any important health problems, and who are growing and developing satisfactorily. Children with special problems would need more frequent care or different patterns of care.

Newborn Safety

Accidents are the leading cause of death from age 1 month through 24 years and are second only to acute infections as a cause of acute morbidity and as a reason for visits to the physician throughout childhood.

Most accidents in infancy occur because parents either underestimate or overestimate the child's ability. Helping parents to get to know the

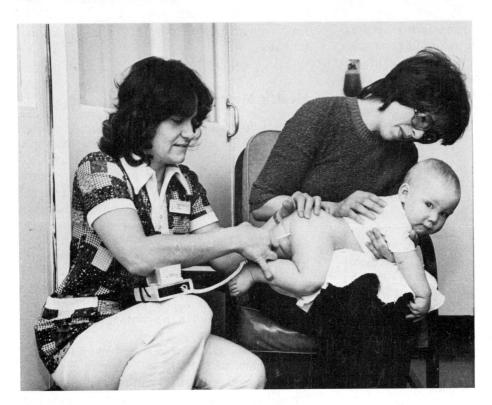

Figure 34-18 *Taking a rectal temperature on an infant. Notice how the nurse's hand restrains the infant. (Courtesy of the Department of Medical Photography, Children's Hospital, Buffalo, N.Y.)*

newborn in the hospital, therefore, is important not only in terms of getting a parent-child relationship off to a good start but also for the child's future safety.

Prevention of Aspiration

The leading type of fatal accident in the newborn period is aspiration. Explore with the mother who will bottle-feed her baby whether she intends to prop bottles up or hold her baby for feeding. Some mothers prop up an evening bottle in the baby's bed; others prop a bottle up at dinnertime or when they are with older children. Others prop bottles up all the time. All of these mothers are propping bottles up because they do not appreciate what being held and rocked and made to feel secure means to a small infant. Furthermore, they are overestimating the infant's ability to push away the bottle, sit up or turn his head to the side, and cough, or clear his airway if milk should flow too rapidly into his mouth and he begins to aspirate it.

If mothers must prop up bottles—and it is unrealistic to think you can persuade all mothers not to do so—be certain a mother understands she must never leave her infant alone with a propped bottle. An infant farther away than arm's

reach feeding from a propped-up bottle is an accident waiting to happen.

When final night bottles are propped up, milk is left in contact with the teeth for hours. This leads to a high incidence of decay of deciduous teeth (bedtime-bottle syndrome). If deciduous teeth become so decayed or abscessed that they have to be removed, eruption of the permanent teeth may be adversely affected, since the space for this eruption is not adequate. Exposure to infection is an additional hazard if tooth extraction is necessary.

In other instances of aspiration, the mother has underestimated her baby's ability to grasp and place objects in her mouth. A newborn's grasp and sucking reflexes give her this ability automatically, so from day 1, the mother must be certain that nothing comes within her baby's reach that should not be in her mouth. She should make certain that toys have no small parts that will snap off. She must keep any object painted with lead-base paint out of her reach. Rattles should be checked to make sure that whatever makes the noise cannot come out. The baby's clothes should have no buttons on the front that the child can pull off. Diaper pins should be closed and put well out of the newborn's reach while the mother changes diapers. Even a newborn can wiggle to a

Table 34-4 Recommendations for Preventive Health Care, by Age

Health Supervision Procedure	2–4 Weeks	Months								5–6 Years
		2	4	6	9–12	15	16–19	23–25	35–37	
History	x	x	x	x	x	x	x	x	x	x
Measurements										
Height and weight	x	x	x	x	x	x	x	x	x	x
Head circumference	x	x		x		x		x		
Blood pressure									x	x
Sensory screening										
Sight	x	x		x					x or	x
Hearing				x					x or	x
Developmental appraisal	x	x	x	x	x	x	x	x	x	x
Physical examination	x	x	x	x	x	x	x	x	x	x
Immunizations										
DPT†		x	x	x		x				x
Oral polio		x	x	x*		x				x
Combination measles and mumps						x				
Laboratory procedures										
Tuberculin test					x or	x			x	
Hematocrit or hemoglobin					x				x or	x
Urinalysis									x	
Urine culture (girls only)									x	x
Discussion and counseling	x	x	x	x	x	x	x	x	x	x
Dental screening	x	x	x	x	x	x	x	x	x	x
Initial dental examination								x or	x	

* Optional.
† In some agencies pertussis vaccine is no longer routine.

new position to touch an attractive object. The safe distance for objects in relation to the baby rapidly expands from an arm's reach to yards away. In a very short time, safety will require objects to be locked in cupboards.

Prevention of Falls

Falls are a second major cause of infant accidents. A mother underestimates her infant's ability to turn over or crawl. No infant, beginning at birth, should ever be left on a surface unattended. Normal newborn wiggling can easily bring a baby to the edge of a bed or tabletop and over the edge. You will note that many mothers in rooming-in units leave a newborn infant lying on the bed while they answer the telephone or go to the bathroom. They will justify this carelessness by saying that babies do not turn over until they are 3 months old. These mothers are revealing how little they know about a newborn's capabilities or about newborn safety.

Car Safety

Car accidents are a safety problem all during childhood. Infants who are laid on a car seat unprotected by any kind of restraint are at great risk if an accident should occur. The car stops suddenly, and the infant is thrown to the floor, or out of the car, or through the windshield. Infants standing on car seats are in equal danger. Many mothers do not think of an infant car seat as being an essential piece of equipment for a baby. They envision buying one "later on, when the baby sits up." If they are going to be transporting the infant in the car, however, this could be the most important piece of baby equipment they will buy.

Infant car seats are important pieces of equipment for a family to purchase because a parent holding a baby cannot hold onto him in a crash (centrifugal force causes the infant to weigh as much as 450 lbs). The infant hits the dashboard with the force of a fall from a three-story building (even in a car moving as slowly as 30 mph). If the adult holding the infant does not have a seat belt attached, the adult can be thrown into the infant and actually kill him or her.

In January of 1981, a federal safety standard took effect that requires infant car seats to meet additional standards for testing. It is advisable for parents to check that the seat they are purchasing (or borrowing) was built after this date. A local health department or local Red Cross should have a list of all the different car seats available and their comparable features and costs.

For a 17 to 20-pound baby, the best type of seat is an "infant-only" seat. It faces the back of the car, is fairly light-weight, and can double as a household seat. The ideal type should have a five-point harness with broad straps that spread the force of a collision over the chest and hips and a shield that will cushion the head (Figure 34-19).

Other seats (convertible ones) support babies up to 18 to 20 pounds in a backward position; these can then be turned to face forward for children up to 40 to 43 pounds. These convertible seats are larger and heavier than infant-only seats. They may be too large for some small cars. They are more expensive but would be the only seat parents need to buy. Some seats use only a lap belt to secure the seat to the car seat; others have a "top tether" or additional strap to secure the seat as well. In order for a seat to be safe and meet federal standards for infant safety, a parent must use the top tether straps on those seats supplied with them. If this seems inconvenient, they

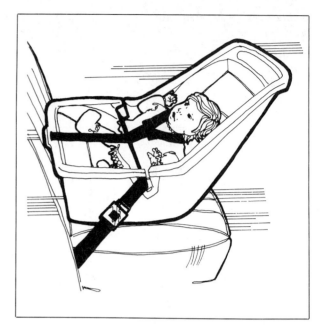

Figure 34-19 *An infant car seat. (Gerber products.)*

should buy a brand of seat that does not require this extra strap.

To place an infant in the seat, a parent should dress her in clothing with legs, as the harness crotch strap must pass between the baby's legs for a snug and correct fit. Teach not to use a sack sleeper or papoose bunting or wrap the baby in a bulky blanket. In order to support the baby's head, the parent probably needs to use a rolled receiving blanket or towel or diaper on each side of the head. To provide extra warmth, they can cut holes in a blanket for the harness and crotch straps. Put the blanket in the seat; pull the seat straps through the blanket holes. Place the baby in the seat, buckle her in, then fold the blanket over the baby for warmth. Drape a second blanket over the seat as needed.

A parent should keep the baby in a backward position until he is able to sit up without support, is restless and struggles to sit up, or weighs at least 17 pounds. Caution parents that plastic car seats grow very warm in a car on a hot day and to test the surface before placing the infant on it. Parents should try out the seat in their car to be certain that seat belts reach around the seat and the car seat is wide enough to support the depth of the infant seat before they pay for it. If finances are a problem, parents should check with their local hospital or Red Cross to see if they have a loan program for car seats. Urge parents to always use the seat even on short trips and to use a seatbelt for themselves at the same time. A common argument is that safety seats are too bothersome to use and too expensive to buy. You can compare this cost to paying insurance premiums to protect health (no one likes that either but they do it).

Common mistakes that parents often make with car seats, the avoidance of which should be stressed in teaching, are:

Not using the harness.
Not placing an infant seat facing backward.
Not attaching the top tether when required.
Not securing the seat belt to attach the seat.
Wrapping the infant in a blanket so the strap doesn't fit securely.

Other Safety Measures

Mothers with older children may need to be reminded that children under 5 years of age, as a group, are not responsible enough or knowledgeable enough about newborns to look after their safety. Some preschoolers are so jealous of a new baby that they will harm a baby if left alone with him or her.

Explore the plans for the infant's sleeping space with the mother. Make sure the baby is not going to sleep in the same bed with parents. The danger of accidental suffocation by bedding or by the pressure of a 150-pound adult is too great. Caution mothers not to use pillows in cribs or bassinets for the same reason.

The Role of Stress in Accidents

Time spent talking to parents about accident prevention is always time well spent because what you are actually doing is helping parents to know their child better. Anticipatory guidance in this area is not always successful in preventing accidents, however. In some instances a parent may believe that none of these things will happen to her child. In others, stress factors may be operating; these have been shown to play as great a role in accidents as do unsafe conditions. Meyer, et al. (1963) have identified a number of factors associated with accidental injury in children by com-

Table 34-5 Factors Associated with Accidental Injuries

Family Factor	Percentage in Which Factor Was Present	
	Accident Group	*Comparison Group*
Parents unresponsive to child's needs	87	3
Maternal health incapacity	54	2
Disruptive supervisory shift	52	0
Family separated or unstable	44	5
Other family life stress	35	1
Instability in community	16	2

Source: Meyer, R. J., et al. (1963). Accidental injury to the preschool child. *Journal of Pediatrics, 63,* 95.

paring the incidence of certain family life events in the families of over 100 preschool children injured seriously enough to require hospitalization with their incidence in a matched control group. The results of the study are shown in Table 34-5.

Parents in families in which one of these stress factors is operating are particularly in need of accident prevention counseling. If you have conducted a careful admission interview with the mother and have spent time getting acquainted with both parents on the labor or postpartal unit, you will be aware of many such factors. If a family appears to have so many life contingencies bearing in on it at this time that parents do not seem capable of beginning good infant care, or if a family needs extra guidance for any reason, a referral to a community health agency should be made. The agency will arrange for a community health nurse to visit the home to provide guidance and help and to suggest further referral if necesary.

Utilizing Nursing Process

Nursing care for the newborn is important care because an infant is unable to have full input in planning. In order that care be individualized, it must be done by using nursing process.

Assessment

Be certain in assessing newborns that you fully unwrap them so you can observe the infants fully. Be certain that you do not begin to consider newborn assessment procedures such as temperature

taking as "routine." Include assessment of a mother's ability to care for the infant: This ability will ultimately influence the infant's growth and development.

Analysis

The North American Nursing Diagnosis Association approved no diagnosis specifically relating to newborn care. Many diagnoses are applicable to this time period, however. "Fear related to uncertainty of newborn care" or a well diagnosis of "Adequate adaptation to new mothering role related to acceptance of new life style" are commonly used. Because of the early discharge of many infants, be certain that care goals established during this time are realistic for the short time frame available.

Planning

Based on assessment of a mother's knowledge and capabilities, plan health teaching that is important for her to have before she can care for a newborn independently. If a mother will be staying at the health care facility only a few hours, you need to limit this information to only those few items that are vital for safe infant care in order to prevent overwhelming the woman with instructions.

Help a mother plan newborn care that will allow the infant to fit into her family life style without a great deal of change in the family pattern. On the other hand, help her to appreciate that, because her new infant is a unique individual, some modification will need to be made in order to include him and make him feel secure in the pattern.

Implementation

A great deal of implementation in the area of newborn care involves role modeling as a new mother is unsure of herself and looks to you for guidance and demonstration.

Evaluation

Evaluation is a double process: evaluating how the infant responds to procedures and how well parents are able to initiate them.

Nursing Care Planning

Baby Kraft (John Joseph) is a 1-day-old infant you care for immediately after birth.

Problem Area. Extrauterine adjustment.

Assessment

Mother states, "He's beautiful." Father present at delivery, pleased with child's sex.

Birth from LOA position; breathed at 30 seconds. Apgars: 8 and 9. No anesthesia, no forceps.

Catheter inserted through left naris, esophagus, and into stomach; 15 ml stomach contents removed. No gross anomalies, no hydramnios, 3-vessel cord.

Weight 6 lbs. 5 oz.

Analysis

Adequate adjustment to extrauterine life related to well newborn.

Locus of Decision Making. Parents.

Goal. Patient to make physiologic adjustment to extrauterine life within normal parameters.

Criteria. Patient to establish respiratory and cardiovascular extrauterine changes within 1 hour of birth.

Nursing Orders

1. Infant to remain in birthing room for 1 hour postpartum, then transfer to rooming in, 2nd floor.
2. Footprinting, ID identification done; review with parents.
3. Administer vitamin K 1 ml to left thigh.

4. Erythromycin ointment to both eyes following initial parent-child interaction.
5. Initial breast-feeding in birthing room.
6. Encourage mother to hold to maintain temperature.

Problem Area. Circumcision.

Assessment

Permission for procedure signed by both parents. Want it done immediately because of early discharge.

Circumcision done in birthing room by Dr. Collins. Slight bleeding from surgery site: Vaseline gauze applied. Baseline pulse: 140, regular. Vitamin K administered prior to procedure.

Analysis

Potential for blood loss related to circumcision.

Goal. Patient to have minimum blood loss and no infection at site.

Criteria. Bleeding is confined to staining; no erythema at site develops or systemic temperature elevation develops.

Nursing Orders

1. Vaseline gauze for 24 hours; then Vaseline as needed.
2. Check vital signs q15min for 1 hour, then 30 min for 4 hours.
3. Keep diaper snug for pressure; position on side to decrease irritation
4. Show site to mother and review care and possible symptoms of infection.

Quesions for Review

Multiple Choice

1. Baby Green is a newborn you care for and record the Apgar score for at birth. A normal 1-minute Apgar score is
   a. 1–2.
   b. 5–9.
   c. 7–10.
   d. 12–15.

2. On an Apgar evaluation, reflex irritability is tested by
   a. raising the infant's head and letting it fall back.
   b. slapping the sole of a foot and observing the response.
   c. dorsiflexing the foot against pressure resistance.
   d. tightly flexing the infant's trunk and then releasing it.

3. You teach Mrs. Green to care for her infant's cord. Instructions you would give her are to
   a. keep it dry.
   b. wash it with soap and water.
   c. apply Vaseline to it daily.
   d. cover it with dry gauze.

4. Phenylketonuria testing is done by a blood sample. This blood specimen should be taken
   a. within an hour after birth.
   b. at 24 hours after birth.
   c. on the third or fourth day following birth.
   d. at 2 weeks or the first well-child visit.

5. Baby Green will be formula-fed. You anticipate his first infant feeding will be
   a. glucose water.
   b. sterile water.
   c. dilute formula.
   d. normal saline.

6. You take Baby Green's temperature daily. The best way to do this daily is
   a. orally.
   b. by axillary method.
   c. rectally.
   d. abdominally.

7. When you teach Mrs. Green about formula feeding, what liquid would you suggest she feed the baby at bedtime?
   a. orange juice
   b. formula
   c. normal saline
   d. water

8. Mrs. Green asks what will be the safest way to transport her infant in the car to take him home. You would recommend
   a. holding the infant on her lap.
   b. using an infant seat that faces backward.
   c. using an infant seat that faces forward.
   d. placing the infant in a bassinet in the backseat.

Discussion

1. Determining an Apgar score can be a nursing responsibility. What observations would you complete and rate for this score?
2. A mother asks you why you are giving her infant an injection in the delivery room. How would you explain the purpose of vitamin K to a new mother?
3. Deciding whether to have an infant circumcised or not is a decision new parents must make. What are the pros and cons of circumcision?

Suggested Readings

Apgar, V., et al. (1958). Evaluation of the newborn infant—second report. *Journal of the American Medical Association, 168,* 1985.

Brazelton, T. B. (1962). Crying in infancy. *Pediatrics, 29,* 578.

Bryant, B. G. (1984). Unit dose erythromycin ophthalmic ointment for neonatal ocular prophylaxis. *J.O.G.N. Nursing, 13,* 83.

Buckner, E. B. (1983). Use of Brazelton neonatal behavioral assessment in planning care for parents and newborns. *J.O.G.N. Nursing, 12,* 26.

Carey, W., & McDevitt, S. (1978). Revision of the infant temperament questionnaire. *Pediatrics, 61,* 735.

Christophersen, E. R., & Sullivan, M. A. (1982). Increasing the protection of newborn infants in cars. *Pediatrics, 70,* 21.

Coles, E. R. (1983). Babies' sleeping habits. *Midwife Health Visitor and Community Nurse, 19,* 322.

Davidson, S., et al. (1981). Appearance, behavior and capabilities: Teaching new parents infant ABCs. *Canadian Nurse, 11,* 37.

Davies, A. (1980). Hypothermia: The invisible baby killer. *Nursing Mirror, 151,* 34.

Denson, S. E. (1980). Routine care of the normal neonate. *Issues in Health Care of Women, 2,* 91.

Dowham, M. A. P., et al. (1981). The risks of overheating in young babies. *Health Visitor, 54,* 325.

Dunn, D. M., et al. (1981). Interaction of mothers with their newborns in the first half-hour of life. *Journal of Advances in Nursing, 6,* 271.

Evans, M. L. (1983). Tips for taking a child's blood pressure quickly. *Nursing 83, 13,* 61.

Fraleigh, D. (1984). Combined mother-baby care. *Canadian Nurse, 80,* 25.

Furr, P. A., et al. (1982). A nurse-midwifery approach to early mother-infant acquaintance. *Journal of Nurse Midwifery, 27,* 10.

Gleason, D. (1969). Footprinting for identification of infants. *Pediatrics, 44,* 302.

Goebel, J. B., et al. (1984). Infant car seat usage: Effectiveness of a postpartal educational program. *J.O.G.N. Nursing, 13,* 33.

Gray, M. (1980). Neonatal resuscitation. *Journal of Emergency Nursing, 6,* 29.

Kavanagh, C. A., & Banco, L. (1982). The infant walker—a previously unrecognized health hazard. *American Journal of Diseases of Children, 136,* 205.

Labson, L. (1983). The newborn: Quick postdelivery check. *Patient Care, 17,* 16.

Lauri, S. (1981). The public health nurse as a guide in infant child-care and education. *Journal of Advances in Nursing, 6,* 297.

Mason, T. N. (1982). A hand ventilation technique for neonates. *M.C.N., 7,* 366.

Meyer, R. J., et al. (1963). Accidental injury to the preschool child. *Journal of Pediatrics, 63,* 95.

Perry, S. E. (1983). Parents' perceptions of their newborn following structured interactions. *Nursing Research, 32,* 208.

Phillips, C. R. (1974). Neonatal heat loss in heated cribs vs mother's arms. *J.O.G.N. Nursing, 3,* 11.

Romanko, M. V., & Brost, B. A. (1982). Swaddling: An effective invention for pacifying infants. *Pediatric Nursing, 8,* 259.

Scanlon, J. W. (1980). Routine neonatal procedures: Risk/benefit calculations and informed consent. *Birth and Family Journal, 7,* 219.

Silverman, W. A., & Andersen, D. H. (1956). A controlled clinical trial of effects of water mist on obstructive respiratory signs, death rate, and necropsy findings among premature infants. *Pediatrics, 17,* 1.

Snyder, D. M. (1980). Future directions in the care of the full-term infant. *Birth and Family Journal, 7,* 264.

Styles, W. (1981). Common problems and their management: Significant symptoms and possible causes in the first 18 months. *Nursing (Horsham), 1,* 968.

Van Leeuwen, G., & Glenn, L. (1968). Screening for hidden congenital anomalies. *Pediatrics, 41,* 147.

Wayland, J. R., et al. (1983). Newborn circumcision: Father's involvement. *R.N., 46,* 42.

Zukowsky, K., et al. (1982). Maintaining the infant's skin integrity. *Critical Care Nurse, 2,* 53.

VIII

High-Risk Pregnancy

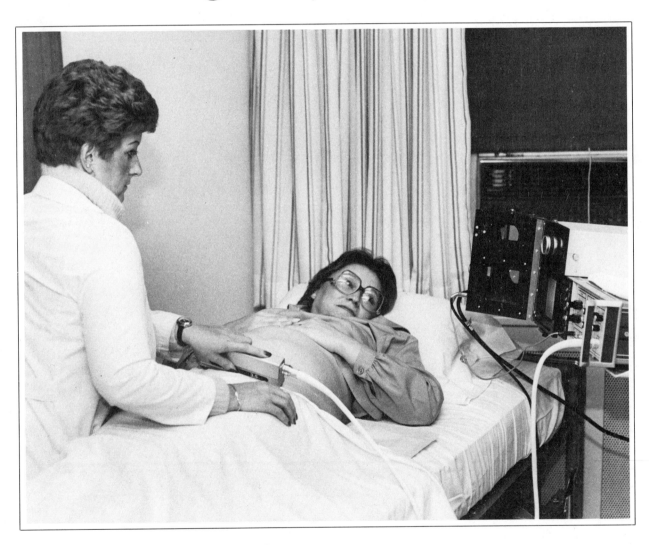

35

Identifying the High-Risk Mother

OBJECTIVES

Following mastery of the contents of this chapter, you should be able to

1. Define the term *maternal high risk*.
2. Describe common psychological, social, and biophysical situations that lead to high-risk categorization.
3. Describe common emotions such as depression, guilt, or fear that may occur in a high-risk pregnancy.
4. Analyze the problems that may occur with a high-risk pregnancy in regard to acceptance of the pregnancy.
5. Synthesize the knowledge of high-risk pregnancy with nursing process to achieve quality maternal-newborn nursing care.

A HIGH-RISK INFANT is one who is born with less ability or chance to survive or a greater chance to be left with a permanent handicap, either psychosocial or physiologic, than the average child. A *high-risk pregnancy* is one in which some maternal factor, either psychosocial or physiologic, is apt to result in the birth of a high-risk infant or in some way harm the woman herself.

Some women enter pregnancy with a chronic illness that, superimposed on the pregnancy, makes it high-risk. Other women enter pregnancy in good health but then develop a complication of pregnancy that causes it to become high-risk. Other women's particular circumstances—poverty, lack of support people, poor coping mechanisms, genetic inheritance, past history of pregnancy complications—cause the pregnancy to be categorized as high-risk.

In most instances, no single factor causes a pregnancy to be classified this way. The pregnancy of a woman who is a known diabetic, for example, is automatically termed one with greater-than-normal risk. The fetus growing in utero in an environment in which hyperglycemia is the rule runs increased danger. During the pregnancy, the woman, worrying that something will happen to her baby, fails to begin the "pregnancy work" that she must do so that bonding can take place. At birth, the child is in double jeopardy. Not only may the baby be born with a handicap

but he or she is high-risk for poor maternal-child attachment as well.

Another example is a teenage girl who delivers a low-birth-weight infant. The infant, again, has a double problem. Not only are the baby's physical systems immature, but the immaturity of the mother and her inability to give him care compound the problem.

Remembering that the term *high risk* rarely refers to just one causative factor helps you plan nursing care. Because high-risk factors are often compounded, nursing care must be multidimensional in scope if it is going to be effective.

Table 35-1 lists common psychological, social, and physical factors that, when present, can cause a pregnancy to be categorized as high-risk. Categorizing these risks as minimal, moderate, or extensive differs with each woman because of her individual coping mechanisms and level of support. A woman living in a poverty environment, for example, isolated on a mountain top would be extremely high-risk for a poor nutritional intake during pregnancy; a woman with a similar income who could depend on a nutritional program and counseling from a community health nurse might be only minimal-risk.

Defining the Concept of High-Risk

The circumstances that can cause a pregnancy to be high-risk are endless when the concept is broadened to include psychosocial aspects.

A high-risk classification system such as Goodwin's Antepartum Fetal Risk Score (see Table 18-11) should be used routinely with all pregnant women to attempt to identify early in pregnancy those who have a physiologic interference. Rose's criteria of factors that interfere with mothering attachment (see Table 13-1) should also be used at antenatal visits to try to identify psychosocial reasons for special care during pregnancy.

Accepting the Pregnancy

The first psychological task a mother has to complete with any pregnancy is accepting the pregnancy. She must get used to the idea that a new cycle of life is beginning. This is difficult when there is a possibility that the pregnancy will not come to term. Many people feel, superstitiously, that if they plan on something, something will go wrong. If they do not plan, and proceed as if nothing is happening, everything will then go all right.

Table 35-1 Factors that Categorize a Pregnancy as High-Risk

Prepregnancy	Pregnancy	Labor and Delivery
Psychological	*Psychological*	*Psychological*
History of drug dependence (including alcohol)	Loss of support person	Frightened by labor and delivery experience
History of abusive behavior	Illness in a family member	Lack of participation due to anesthesia
History of tolerating battering	Decrease in self-esteem	Separation of infant at birth
Cigarette smoker	Drug abuse (including alcohol and cigarette smoking)	Lack of preparation for labor
History of mental illness	Poor acceptance of pregnancy	Delivery of infant who is disappointing in some way (sex, appearance, congenital anomalies)
History of poor coping mechanisms		Illness in newborn
Mental retardation		
Social	*Social*	*Social*
Occupation involving handling of toxic substances (including radiation and anesthesia gases)	Refusal of or neglected prenatal care	Lack of support person
Environmental contaminants at home	Exposure to environmental teratogens	Inadequate home for infant care
Isolated	Disruptive family incident	Unplanned for cesarean birth
Lower economic level	Decreased economic support	Lack of access to continued health care
Poor access to transportation for emergency care		Lack of access to emergency personnel or equipment
High altitude		
Highly mobile life style		
Poor housing		
Lack of support people		
Physical	*Physical*	*Physical*
Visual or hearing impaired	Subject to trauma	Hemorrhage
Pelvic inadequacy or malshape	Fluid or electrolyte imbalance	Infection
Uterine incompetency, position, or structure	Intake of teratogen such as a drug	Fluid and electrolyte imbalance
Secondary major illness (heart disease, diabetes mellitus, kidney disease, hypertension, chronic infection such as tuberculosis, hemopoietic or blood disorder, malignancy)	Multiple gestation	Dystocia
	A bleeding disruption	Precipitous delivery
	Poor placental formation or position	Lacerations of cervix or vagina
	Gestational diabetes	Celphalopelvic disproportion
	Nutritional deficiency of iron, folic acid, or protein	Induced labor
Poor gynecologic or obstetric history	Poor weight gain	Internal fetal monitoring
History of previous poor pregnancy outcome (spontaneous abortion; stillbirth)	Pregnancy-induced hypertension	Anesthesia, analgesia
	Infection	Forceps delivery (other than outlet)
History of child with congenital anomalies	Amniotic fluid abnormality	Retained placenta
Obesity	Postmaturity	Cesarean birth
Pelvic inflammatory disease	Conception under 1 year from last pregnancy	
History of inherited disorder		
Small stature		
Potential of blood incompatibility		
Younger than 18 years or older than 35 years		

This is similar to the philosophy of the ancient Greeks, who believed that gods were basically vengeful, spiteful beings. Lullabies originated, in fact, to keep away the evil god Lilith: It was believed that singing certain songs over babies kept Lilith from knowing a baby was in the house.

This philosophy is healthy in that it protects the woman from being hurt, and if this is the third or fourth or fifth pregnancy that has not come to term, she needs something of this nature to get her through the experience. It is unhealthy, however, in terms of mother-child bonding. It never lets the work of accepting the pregnancy—or accepting the child—begin.

During her current pregnancy visit, ask a woman with a history of high-risk pregnancies, "Are you starting to feel pregnant yet? Have you made any plans for the baby yet? Have you thought about where this baby is going to sleep yet?" to find out where she is in terms of accepting the pregnancy.

You cannot force her to think about being pregnant. She needs the protection of not thinking for her own mental health. You can, however, document how far along she is in the process of accepting the pregnancy. Then at the birth of her child the extra help she requires to interact effectively with her child will be recognized and can be given.

Accepting the Child

The second psychological step which must be taken in all pregnancies is accepting the child, a change from "I'm pregnant" to "I'm having a baby." This step too is difficult to take when the pregnancy is high-risk and the outcome is guarded. How much a woman wants a child can be measured by the amount of strain, inconvenience, medical visits, laboratory tests, and added expense she is willing to undergo to continue a pregnancy.

Women need support from health personnel during procedures such as nonstress tests or amniocentesis when they are called for. Some need support when, despite all they have endured, the pregnancy ends without a viable child or with a very damaged one. At some point, in this event, the physician, who has also invested energy in this pregnancy, and the woman's family support people, who have been with her through the experience, leave. The only person left standing at the end of the bed is you. Knowing what to say, or *not* say, at such a time begins with an appreciation of what high-risk pregnancies mean to women.

Identifying Coping Abilities

The ability to cope with a stressful situation depends on a woman's perception of the event, the support people available, and her ability to cope successfully with stress in the past.

Perception of the Event

It is difficult to predict high-risk situations in terms of psychosocial criteria because what is a crisis for one person in this area may not be for another; what one person can cope with easily, another finds overwhelming.

The multiple factors in high-risk pregnancy often make it difficult for a person to perceive clearly the extent of the problem. A woman might be able to cope with being hospitalized during the last half of pregnancy (because of pregnancy-induced hypertension, for example) if she were married and had a supportive husband. Being single and still in school makes the forced hospitalization not only financially disabling but career defeating as well.

Timing has a great deal to do with perception of the event. At first, when a physician tells the woman that something is going wrong with a pregnancy, because she cannot see inside herself, she cannot believe that anything is the matter. It is often hard to talk to people during this time of initial diagnosis about the problem because they have not yet admitted there is one. Time, however, forces a woman to accept what is happening. Weeks are passing, but her abdomen is not growing any larger (or her blood pressure is not getting any better and other signs are appearing).

At health care contacts, it is a good habit to explore with women during pregnancy what they know about their situation. At some point, when they have internalized the fact that they have a problem, they are ready to talk about it and what it means to them. It may be 4 or 5 weeks from the time they were first told about their situation before they are able to perceive it as what it is and not what they would like it to be.

In order for women to understand what is happening to them, they must have explanations that are at their level of comprehension. The average woman knows very little about the way babies grow in utero. She accepts on faith the concepts that a fetus can live surrounded by fluid without drowning, that enough nutrients will cross the placenta to sustain him, that labor will not harm him. When something is interfering with these processes she does not understand its importance because she never understood the basic process.

Serving as a factual source of information for mothers with high-risk pregnancies is an important role. The physician with whom you work will undoubtedly reserve the right to tell the woman what her diagnosis is. Check with her that she understood the explanation. Nothing is worse than having a test for fetal well-being done and then waiting days for the results. Check that she was called and told the results. Caution women not to get information on prognosis from their friends at the supermarket; it is invariably wrong because the circumstances their friends are relating were so different. Caution them not to read medical books from the library; new discoveries make statements about prognosis inaccurate very quickly. Advise them to use their physician as their source of medical information. If they are reluctant to ask the physician questions because they are afraid of taking up too much of his or her time, ask the questions for them. People cannot begin to deal with problems until they are aware that they have them. They cannot appreciate the extent of a problem until they understand it.

Women with physical interferences during pregnancy may be referred to specialty clinics or obstetrical specialists for care during their pregnancy. They may be hospitalized for care in specialized units some distance from their home and their support people. Communicating with these new caregivers may be difficult for the woman. Asking questions of specialists may be harder for her than asking questions of her family doctor. Working in high-risk areas, remember how new and strange everything seemed to you your first day there. Women coming for care are rarely comfortable with these strange new settings. Finding a nurse they can talk to, who will intercede for them with people who intimidate them by their importance, is their chief hope when they walk in the door. It is the thing that will keep this experience in perspective for them.

Support People

Someone who is an excellent support person for the tasks of everyday living and who is adequate during a normal pregnancy may be no help at all when a complication of pregnancy occurs. Some women, therefore, have their usual support people cut off from them during a high-risk pregnancy. In many instances they are able to reach out to secondary support people such as members of their church or a community group. Others are left with no one to fill the gap. They do not recognize unless it is pointed out to them that health care personnel are willing and able to serve as support people to them.

Ask at prenatal visits, "How is this affecting everyone at home?" You may discover a woman in the midst of many people but very much alone.

Coping Success

Ways of coping with situations in the past may not seem relevant or meaningful now because this stress seems so different, so much more serious than anything that happened in the past. Comments such as "We've come through worse things" or "We've had trouble before" are good to hear. They show that the woman is relying on past performance to sustain her in the present crisis.

Immobilizing Reactions to High-Risk Pregnancy

How women react to being told that something about the pregnancy is not going as hoped varies with the individual person and how much she wants the pregnancy or the child. A number of emotions are generally present, however.

Fear

Although the possibility exists that any woman might die with a pregnancy, it is a light, barely perceived fear for the majority of women, something that flickers once through their mind the day they are diagnosed as pregnant and again when they begin labor.

For a woman with a high-risk pregnancy, fear of dying may remain very real all during pregnancy. The woman with a small pelvis may fear being mutilated at birth or bleeding to death; the woman with hypertension may worry that her cerebral arteries will burst from pressure and leave her dead or paralyzed. Women worry that the child is dying inside them. A child who is part of them, dying inside them, is the same as dying themselves.

Living with fear of this nature for 9 months is defeating (Figure 35-1). A woman cannot make plans—to move or not to move, to go back to school or not—because 9 months from now she may be dead. She cannot begin to bond with her child. She feels that she will never mother this child because she will die.

She needs reassurance at every step of the way that her condition is not this serious (providing that is true information). At delivery, relief that she is all right, that she has survived the pregnancy intact, may be her chief feeling. She may

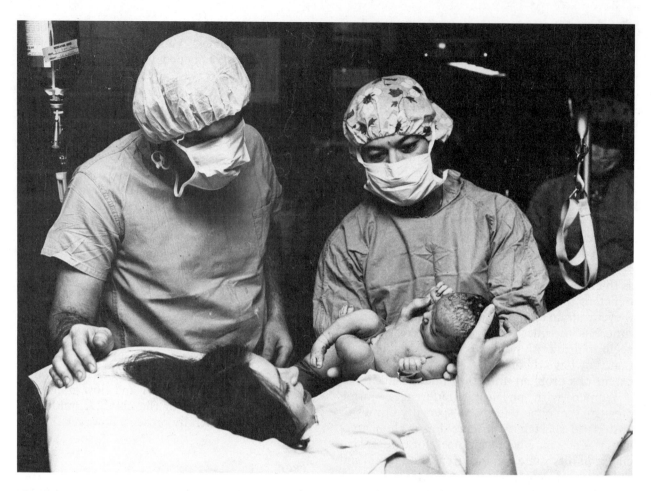

Figure 35-1 *A mother and father meet one of two new twins. This moment may seem a long way off for the woman with a high-risk pregnancy. (Courtesy Department of Medical Photography, Children's Hospital, Buffalo, N.Y.)*

not be ready to care for her child until the realization that she is really safe has been worked through.

Guilt

Most women accept the responsibility of eating better, not taking medications, and getting more rest as the price to pay for having children. They feel rewarded for their efforts when they see a perfect baby. If something is going wrong with the pregnancy, they search their minds to discover what it was they did or did not do that caused it. Even if what is happening has no documented cause—pregnancy-induced hypertension, for example—they often feel as if they are at fault. If only they were a better person, if only they had not insisted on buying expensive furniture, playing baseball the Sunday before, this would not be happening. It is punishment for their greed, their lack of charity, their selfishness.

A woman who believes she caused the mishap is having difficulty perceiving the event clearly.

She cannot use her support people because she feels they no longer respect her or care about her (she imagines they hold her as responsible as she holds herself). She has trouble relating the way she dealt with past events to the present because she wishes she had done things differently in the past.

Guilt, therefore, is a destructive emotion during pregnancy. It puts a woman in the worst possible position to cope with what is happening to her. Guilt can never be totally eliminated from her mind, but making certain that she knows the cause of the problem (or that no cause is known) is a help. If the cause *is* unknown—premature labor, for example—it is good to list things that are *not* the cause: running upstairs, picking up a 2-year-old, eating a rich meal. If the woman did do something in pregnancy that is hurting the fetus—smoke heavily, drink heavily, use a street drug—assuring her that people understand she did not mean to hurt the child (or did not realize that she was hurting the child) is a help.

At birth, a woman who feels guilt about what

she has done or imagines she has done may have difficulty beginning interaction with her child. She needs some time first to see that the infant responds to her and does not dislike her before she can give herself freely to the relationship.

Depression

Chronic depression is a numbing state. It blocks out all emotions so that nothing can be felt. If a woman cannot feel, she cannot adapt to her pregnancy or to bonding with her child.

In order to protect themselves from feeling the full shock of learning that their child will be born malformed or has died, women may begin a pattern of *anticipatory grief* after they are first told that something is wrong with the pregnancy. At one time, this reaction was encouraged. People pictured a woman as letting herself down through the stages of grief easily and gently rather than being assaulted with the full blow all at once. It seemed therapeutic. What happened, however, when the child was born normal or did not die? A woman had already mourned for the child, who was already dead in her mind. She could not revive her feelings to reestablish an effective relationship with the child.

Children who cannot be loved because they have already been mourned as dead are termed *vulnerable children* (Green & Solnit, 1964). They tend to have behavior problems as they grow older (they demand to be noticed and loved, to be counted among the living).

Based on a philosophy that preventing anticipatory grief is therapeutic for maternal-child bonding, therefore, the approach to telling high-risk women that their pregnancy is threatened has changed. In the past, a woman who had bleeding at 3 months' gestation, for instance, was told that bleeding at that point generally meant pregnancy loss. The chance was good that painless bleeding would go on to cramping and loss of the child; better to get prepared for that. Today, with the same symptoms, a woman is told that bleeding all by itself is not a meaningful happening. There is no reason to think yet that the pregnancy is lost.

This change in philosophy does not mean that the woman is not told the basic truth. It means that she is told an optimistic truth: "You have symptoms of pregnancy-induced hypertension, but with rest, we feel sure we can keep them under control and get you the baby you want," not "You have pregnancy-induced hypertension, so prepare for the worst."

It is important that all health personnel in contact with the woman understand the philosoph-ical difference in those two pieces of information. Nothing is worse than being told two stories, or feeling that one is being told less than the truth. A woman must have confidence in health care providers during pregnancy: She is laying her life in their hands.

Signs of Grieving

The grieving or mourning process affects everyone a little differently, but there are enough common signs of grief so that it is possible to identify the woman who is undergoing chronic grief or has begun to grieve for the fetus inside her.

Denial. The first step in grief is denial. Denial is a temporary pain reliever and a necessary step on the way to acceptance and the beginning of grief. Although a woman had just been told that the fetus has not grown since the last prenatal visit a month ago, she may want to talk instead about the new color the examining room has been painted. She may want to talk about her sister's children, who are all small. Hiding the knowledge of what is happening or rationalizing the cause reduces the pain of the knowledge.

Anger. The second step in grief is often anger. A change from thinking, "Surely not me" to "It's not fair that this is happening to me." When a woman is angry about what is happening inside her, she may project her anger inappropriately at people or things. She is angry at the bus she rode to the office; angry at the receptionist for asking her her name; angry at you for tightening a blood pressure cuff too tightly. It is difficult to respond to this kind of anger because it erupts so suddenly and so unfairly. Your first reaction is likely to be anger in return. After all, you applied the blood pressure cuff as you usually do and you are not responsible that the receptionist did not remember the woman's name or the bus was late. A more therapeutic reaction is to accept the anger for what it is—a stage of grief—and respond accordingly: "I'm sorry the cuff felt uncomfortable, but you seem angry about more than the blood pressure. Would it help to talk to me about it?"

Bargaining. Bargaining is a stage of grief in which a woman tries to "trade off" what is happening to her for something more acceptable. She might say, "If I ever make it through this pregnancy, I'm going to go to nursing school and do things for other people the way you do" (i.e., if God will only let her have a perfect baby, she will spend the rest of her life doing good). A mother may feel very betrayed if after this type of bargaining, the pregnancy is lost.

Depression. The fourth stage of grief is a change from "It's not fair that this is happening to me" to "Yes, it is happening to me." Crying is the most common sign that this stage has been reached. The woman may ask more questions about the problem than she did previously. She may want to talk more about her hopes and expectations of this pregnancy or child than she did before. She may seem upset by laboratory reports when before she accepted them calmly even though they were equally ominous. On the surface, it seems as if she has taken a step backward. She was managing so well; now she seems so out of control. In reality, this is the first time she has allowed herself to really feel what is happening to her, the first time the laboratory report seemed to be about her.

Acceptance. The final stage of grief is acceptance, a change to "not only is this thing happening to me, but I can live with the fact that it is happening to me." Following this, the woman puts herself back together again and goes on with life. It may be as long as 6 weeks after the first time she was told that something was wrong before she reaches this stage. If the pregnancy is lost, a woman needs to have a return appointment to the health care setting about this time for an evaluation of whether she has worked through a grief process to this stage.

If the pregnancy is threatened but not lost, you do not like to see a woman reach this stage. If she completes mourning for a child who is still alive, the mother-child bonding will be inadequate.

Lowered Self-Esteem

For generations, fertility and the ability to bear and raise children were regarded as a woman's chief functions. Even today, if a woman has difficulty fulfilling these, she may feel that she is less than other women despite any other achievement she has made. During pregnancy, all women need to be reminded of all the other things they are besides being pregnant so that if a pregnancy is lost, or the outcome of the pregnancy is not perfect, they still retain their self-esteem. Low self-esteem will not allow maternal-child bonding to happen. The woman needs time at birth to get acquainted with her newborn before she can believe that a child would like her and respond to her.

The High-Risk Father

Many women have a hard time understanding what is happening when there is an interference with normal pregnancy. Fathers, who often know less about normal pregnancy than women, understand even less. They receive most of their reports secondhand—not from the physician or you but from their wife or sexual partner. They may feel reluctant to call and ask questions, to admit that they do not know something. Their perception of the event is likely to be distorted, therefore. A father may tell a woman that she misunderstood or did not listen well to the explanation; thus, because he does not understand, he lowers her self-esteem further.

Fathers are generally left feeling extremely helpless in their one-person-removed position. They want a child and yet have no control over the pregnancy's outcome. In addition, by wanting this pregnancy, they may have caused the person they love most to be hurt.

Their emotions during the pregnancy, like the woman's, range through fear, depression, guilt, and anger. They need careful explanations of what is going on in order to control these feelings. They cannot be support people with overwhelming guilt and doubt about what it is they are expected to be supportive of.

Including the father of the infant in health visits and counseling not only allows him to be a better support person but also provides the mother with the support she needs during a high-risk pregnancy.

Suggested Readings

Adamsons, K. (1979). Centralizing care of high-risk OB patients. *Perinatology/Neonatology, 3*, 14.

Becker, C. H. (1982). Comprehensive assessment of the healthy gravida. *J.O.G.N. Nursing, 11*, 375.

Gillespie, S. A. (1980). Childbirth in the 80s: What are the options? *Issues in Health Care of Women, 2*, 11.

Green, M., & Solnit, A. (1964). Reactions to the threatened loss of a child: A vulnerable child syndrome. *Pediatrics, 34*, 58.

Howley, C. (1981). The older primipara: Implications for nurses. *J.O.G.N. Nursing, 10*, 182.

Ishida, Y. (1980). How to deal with grief in childbirth. *Female Patient, 5*, 74.

Labson, L. H. (1981a). High-risk pregnancy: Trimester 1: Assessing risk and options. *Patient Care, 15,* 76.

Labson, L. H. (1981b). Taking the high-risk pregnancy to term. Trimesters 2 and 3. *Patient Care, 15,* 132.

Morrison, J. C., et al. (1981). Management of the pregnancy patient with cardiovascular disease. *Journal of Cardiovascular and Pulmonary Technology, 9,* 17.

Raphael-Leff, J. (1984). Varying needs . . . women vary greatly in their response to birth. *Nursing Mirror, 158,* v.

Rusinski, P. S. (1981). The employed pregnant worker: The risks of physical exertion. *Occupational Health Nursing, 29,* 19.

Sammons, L. N. (1981). Battered and pregnant. *M.C.N., 6,* 246.

Seller, M. J. (1982). Preconception care and neural tube defects. *Midwife Health Visitor and Community Nurse, 18,* 470.

Sweeney, P. J. (1983). Genital herpes and pregnancy. *Perinatal Press, 7,* 19.

Tipping, V. G. (1981). The vulnerability of a primipara during the antepartal period. *Maternal Child Nursing Journal, 10,* 61.

Tull, M. W., et al. (1981). Effects of caffeine on pregnancy and lactation. *Pediatric Nursing, 7,* 51.

Wheeler, L., et al. (1981). Pregnancy-induced hypertension. *J.O.G.N. Nursing, 10,* 212.

Williamson, S. (1981). Problems associated with long-term hospitalization of antenatal patients. *Midwives Chronicle, 94,* 160.

36

The Woman with Preexisting Illness

OBJECTIVES

Following mastery of the contents of this chapter, you should be able to

1. Describe common illnesses such as heart disease, diabetes mellitus, renal and blood disorders that can cause complications when they exist with pregnancy.
2. Assess a woman with a preexisting illness during pregnancy.
3. State a nursing diagnosis regarding the effect of a preexisting illness on pregnancy.
4. Plan implementations that will help ensure a safe pregnancy outcome when a preexisting illness occurs with pregnancy.
5. Implement care to help ensure a safe psychological and physiologic pregnancy outcome for a woman with a preexisting illness during pregnancy.
6. Evaluate goal criteria regarding pregnancy outcome when a preexisting illness is present.
7. Analyze ways that nurses can be instrumental in aiding a safe pregnancy outcome for women with preexisting illness.
8. Synthesize knowledge of preexisting illnesses and nursing process to achieve quality maternal-newborn nursing care.

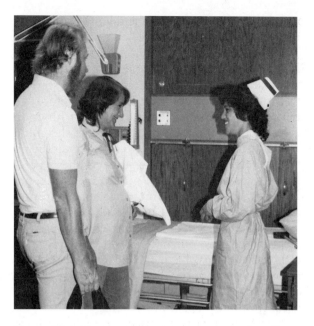

Figure 36-1 *Pregnancy is a crisis situation for all women. It can be an extreme crisis when a woman enters pregnancy with a preexisting illness. Here a woman is admitted to the hospital for fetal assessment.*

If every pregnancy is considered a crisis situation in itself—and it is—it is obvious that the advent of a complication such as an accompanying disease can place a very severe burden on a woman and her family (Figure 36-1). Any woman benefits from the support and the skill of a professional nurse who helps her work through the tasks of pregnancy, accepting it and preparing to become a mother. The support and skill of a professional nurse are essential to a woman who, in addition to the usual tasks of pregnancy, must question whether or not she and her baby will be all right.

THE LEADING CAUSES of maternal death during pregnancy are hemorrhage, infection, hypertension of pregnancy, anesthesia complications, ectopic pregnancy, heart disease, and thromboembolism.

When a woman enters pregnancy with a chronic condition such as heart disease or kidney disease, the course of a normal pregnancy imposed on these disease conditions can cause complications either of the disease process or with the pregnancy and fetal health. In addition, interferences with the safe outcome of the pregnancy may leave a woman less equipped to function as a mother or to undergo a future pregnancy.

Cardiovascular Disease and Pregnancy

As more and more congenital heart anomalies are corrected in early infancy and rheumatic fever is being more actively prevented and treated so that cardiac damage is reduced, the number of women of childbearing age with a heart disease is diminishing. Heart disease is still a continuing problem in pregnancy (affecting about 1% of pregnancies), however, because improved management during pregnancy has enabled women with heart disease—who, in the past, never would have dared to try—to attempt pregnancy. A woman with heart disease needs a team approach to care during pregnancy, one that combines the talents of an internist, obstetrician, and nurse.

A woman should visit her obstetrician or family physician before conception, so that a health care team can become familiar with her state of health when she is not pregnant and therefore can make baseline evaluations of her heart function and anticipate the individual problems she could expect during pregnancy. A woman should begin prenatal care as soon as she suspects she is pregnant (1 week after the first missed menstrual period), so that close watch on her general condition and circulatory system can be maintained.

The two most frequent heart conditions that affect pregnancy outcome are rheumatic fever with valvular involvement and uncorrected coarctation of the aorta. Heart disease that occurs specifically with the pregnancy (peripartal heart disease) can also occur but is rare.

Pregnancy taxes the circulatory system of every woman even without cardiac disease because during pregnancy the cardiac volume and cardiac output increase about 30 (perhaps as much as 50) percent. Most of this increase occurs in the first 6 months of pregnancy, and then this greater blood volume continues to be maintained for the remainder of pregnancy.

Because of the increased blood flow past valves, heart murmurs are heard in many women during pregnancy. These are functional (innocent) murmurs, which are transient and will disappear following the pregnancy. Heart palpitations on sudden exertion are also normal in pregnancy. Neither of these symptoms is a sign of heart disease, but merely of normal physiologic adjustment to pregnancy.

Effect of Heart Disease

The dangers of pregnancy in a woman with heart disease occur mainly because of the increased circulatory volume. The most dangerous time for her is the twenty-eighth to thirty-second weeks when the blood volume first reaches its highest level. A woman's heart may become so overwhelmed by this increased blood volume that her cardiac output falls to the point that vital organs (including the placenta) are no longer perfused adequately with arterial blood, and their oxygen and nutritional requirements are thus not met. Cardiac failure will affect fetal growth if maternal blood pressure is not sufficient to provide an adequate supply of blood to the placenta. The infants of women with severe heart disease tend to have low birth weights because not enough nutrients are available due to poor placenta perfusion; this poor perfusion level may lead to severe fetal dis-

tress if blood flow is not adequate for carbon dioxide exchange and the environment of the fetus becomes acidotic. Premature labor may occur with cardiac disease, which exposes an infant to the hazards of immaturity at birth. An infant may do poorly during labor (evidenced by late deceleration patterns on a fetal heart monitor) if cardiac decompensation has reached a point of placental incompetency. Heart failure can be divided into that which primarily affects the right heart and that which primarily affects the left heart.

Left-Sided Heart Failure

Left sided heart failure occurs with mitral stenosis and mitral insufficiency (the most common cardiac sequelae of rheumatic heart disease) and aortic coarctation. It occurs when the left ventricular output is less than the total volume of blood received by the left atrium from the pulmonary circulation. This imbalance puts back pressure on the pulmonary circulation, causing it to become distended and systemic blood pressure to fall. With pulmonary vein distention, the pulmonary vascular bed also engorges. When this vessel pressure reaches a point of about 25 mm Hg, fluid passes from the pulmonary capillary membranes into the interstitial spaces surrounding the alveoli and then into the alveoli themselves (pulmonary edema). This occurrence interferes with oxygen–carbon dioxide exchange as the fluid coats the exchange space. If pulmonary capillaries rupture under the pressure, small amounts of blood will leak into the alveoli. This situation will be manifested by a productive cough of blood-speckled sputum.

As the oxygen saturation of the blood decreases, chemoreceptors stimulate the respiratory center to increase the respiratory rate. At first this is noticeable only on exertion, then finally with rest also. As the systemic fall in blood pressure registers on the pressoreceptors in the aorta, a woman's heart rate increases and peripheral vasoconstriction occurs in attempts to increase the systemic blood pressure. As the fall in blood pressure is registered with the renal angiotension system, both sodium and water retention occur (an attempt to raise blood pressure through increased blood volume). The increased blood volume from fluid retention compromises circulation still further. As the oxygen saturation level falls still further from this, body cells receive little oxygen and a woman experiences increased fatigue and weakness and dizziness (specifically from lack of oxygen in brain cells).

As pulmonary edema becomes severe, a woman will be unable to sleep in any position but one with her chest and head elevated (orthopnea).

Elevating her chest allows fluid to settle to the bottom of her lungs and frees up oxygen exchange space. She may also notice paroxysmal nocturnal dyspnea or suddenly waking at night very short of breath. This phenomenon occurs because heart action is more effective with her at rest. With the more effective heart action, interstitial fluid is returned to the circulation during the first half of the night; this overburdens the circulation, causing increased left-side failure and increased pulmonary edema during the later half.

Right-Sided Heart Failure

Congenital heart defects such as pulmonary stenosis and ventricular septal defect (VSD) may result in right-sided heart failure. Right-sided failure occurs when the output of the right ventricle is less than the blood volume the heart receives at the right atrium from the vena cava or venous circulation. This condition results in congestion of the systemic venous circulation and decreased cardiac output to the lungs.

With right-sided failure, the right ventricle cannot pump all the blood forward: Blood pools in the right ventricle, then the right atrium, then the vena cava. Blood pressure falls in the aorta because less blood is reaching it; pressure becomes very high in the vena cava with jugular and portal venous distention. Both the liver and spleen become distended. Distention of abdominal vessels leads to exudate of fluid from the vessels into the peritoneal cavity (ascites). Fluid moves systemically into interstitial spaces (peripheral edema). Liver enlargement can cause extreme dyspnea in a pregnant woman as the pressure of the enlarged liver will be against the diaphragm as it is pressed upward by the enlarged uterus.

Classification of Heart Disease

The determination of whether a woman with heart disease can complete a pregnancy successfully depends on the type and extent of her disease. As a rule, a woman with artificial but well-functioning heart valves can be expected to complete a pregnancy without difficulty as long as she has consistent prenatal and postpartal care. The occasional woman with a pacemaker implant can also expect to complete pregnancy successfully. In order to predict pregnancy outcome, heart disease in pregnancy is separated into four categories based on the criteria originated by the New York State Heart Association, as shown in Table 36-1. A woman with class I or II heart disease by this table can expect to experience a normal pregnancy and delivery. Women with class III can complete a pregnancy if they abide by almost

Table 36-1 Classification of Heart Disease

Class	Description
I	Patients have no limitation of physical activity. Ordinary physical activity causes no discomfort. They do not have symptoms of cardiac insufficiency and do not have anginal pain.
II	Patients have slight limitation of physical activity. Ordinary physical activity causes excessive fatigue, palpitation, and dyspnea or anginal pain.
III	Patients have a moderate to marked limitation of physical activity. During less than ordinary activity they experience excessive fatigue, palpitation, dyspnea, or anginal pain.
IV	Patients are unable to carry on any physical activity without experiencing discomfort. Even at rest they will experience symptoms of cardiac insufficiency or anginal pain.

Source: The Criteria Committee of the New York State Heart Association. (1979). *Nomenclature and criteria for diagnosis of diseases of the heart and blood vessels* (8th ed.). Boston: Little, Brown.

complete bedrest. Women with class IV heart disease are poor candidates for pregnancy: They are in cardiac failure even when at rest and free of pregnancy.

Assessment

Assessment of a woman with heart disease begins with a thorough health history so you are aware of her prepregnancy heart status. Ask about her level of normal exercise performance (what level can she do before growing short of breath and what physical symptoms does she experience, such as cyanosis of the lips or nailbeds). Ask if she normally has a cough and edema. Every woman with heart disease should report coughing during pregnancy and should be seen even if she assumes it is just a simple upper respiratory infection because pulmonary edema from heart failure may first be manifested as a cough.

Evaluation of edema in women with heart disease must never be taken lightly. You have to ask yourself whether the edema is the normal edema of pregnancy (innocent), the beginning of pregnancy-induced hypertension (serious), or the edema of heart failure (serious). The normal edema of pregnancy involves only the feet and ankles. Edema of either pregnancy-induced hypertension or heart failure may *begin* as ankle edema. (As an extra aid, remember that edema of pregnancy-induced hypertension usually begins after the twenty-fourth week.) If the edema is a sign of heart failure, other symptoms will probably also be present: irregular pulse, rapid or difficult respirations, and perhaps chest pain on exertion. Be certain to record a baseline blood pressure, pulse, and respiratory rate in either a sitting or lying position early in pregnancy and then at future health visits always take these in the same position for the most accurate comparison. Assessing for nailbed filling (should be under 5 seconds) and jugular venous distention is helpful throughout pregnancy. If a woman's heart disease involves right-sided failure, assessment of liver size at visits is helpful. This becomes difficult and probably inaccurate late in pregnancy as the enlarged uterus presses the liver upward.

For additional cardiac status assessment, a woman may have an ECG or chest X-ray or echocardiogram done at periodic points in the pregnancy. Assure her that an ECG merely measures cardiac electrical discharge and does not harm the fetus in any way. Echocardiography uses sonography and is also not harmful to the fetus. Chest X-ray is safe as long as she is offered a lead apron to cover her abdomen during the exposure. An ECG may become inaccurate late in pregnancy as the enlarged uterus presses upward on the diaphragm and displaces the heart laterally.

Analysis

A nursing diagnosis for a woman with heart disease usually concerns her body's inability to circulate blood adequately. As therapy may include complete bedrest, it may regard her concern (or the family's concern) over this step. Be certain that goals established for her are realistic to her circumstance. Not all women with heart disease will be able to complete a pregnancy successfully; some infants of women with severe involvement will be born with the effects of placental insufficiency: neurologic involvement or mental retardation.

Planning and Implementations

A woman with heart disease needs to take measures during pregnancy to rest and strengthen her heart action. Many nursing interventions are concerned with helping her to achieve this goal.

Rest. A woman with heart disease needs more rest during pregnancy than the average woman to lessen the strain of the increased burden on her heart. Remember that at the point that cardiac output is not enough to meet systemic body demands, peripheral vasoconstriction occurs. As the uterus is a peripheral organ, this causes uterine/placental constriction. A rest program must be carefully designed, therefore, so the woman stops exercising *before* this point is reached. Exactly how much rest she is to have should be carefully detailed. She may need to discontinue work early in pregnancy rather than work until midpregnancy or the end of pregnancy as the average woman usually plans to do. Exactly what type of work she will be allowed to do should be covered as well. Allowing "normally heavy" housework may mean nothing more strenuous than dusting to some women. To others, it may mean washing windows, turning mattresses, and shoveling snow. Make certain that a woman's definition of "heavy work" is the same as your's and the physician's.

Many women need two rest periods a day (fully resting, not getting up frequently to answer the door or telephone) and a full night's sleep at night (not tossing and turning because of excess noise or heat in the room). Many physicians prefer that women with heart disease remain on complete bed rest after the thirtieth week of pregnancy. The purpose of this measure is to ensure that the pregnancy will be carried to term, or at least past the thirty-sixth week, so that the likelihood of fetal maturity increases. Rest should be in the left lateral recumbent position to prevent hypotension and increased heart effort.

Nutrition. A woman with heart disease may need closer supervision of her nutrition during pregnancy than does the average woman. She must gain enough weight to ensure a healthy pregnancy and a healthy baby, but not so much that she gains excess weight. Excess weight gain causes her to have unnecessary additional cells to supply with nutrients. This may overburden her heart and circulatory system.

Be certain that the woman is taking an iron supplement so that she does not become anemic. Anemia requires the body to circulate blood more vigorously in order to distribute oxygen to all body cells—difficult if her heart is already taxed. If a woman was following a sodium-restricted diet prior to pregnancy, these limitations may be continued during pregnancy. As sodium is necessary for fluid volume, however, and allowing a woman's body to retain enough blood volume to supply blood to the placenta is important, a woman's sodium intake is usually *limited*, not severely restricted, during pregnancy. Furosemide (Lasix) may be taken during pregnancy to reduce peripheral edema.

Medication. A woman who needed digitalis for heart action before pregnancy will continue to require it during pregnancy. A woman who was not digitalis-dependent before pregnancy may need such therapy prescribed as pregnancy advances and her cardiac output has to be increased or strengthened (the action of a digitalis preparation is to slow and strengthen myocardial contraction). Help her understand that this need does not mean her degree of heart function is becoming less; it is caused by the increased circulatory strain of pregnancy. She should continue to think of herself as a fully functioning person. Although digitalis preparations cross the placenta, they do not appear to be teratogenic.

A woman who was taking penicillin prophylactically following rheumatic fever in order to prevent a recurrence (often taken for 10 years following rheumatic fever, or at least until age 18) should continue to take this during pregnancy because penicillin is not known to be a fetal teratogen. Close to delivery, some physicians begin women with valvular or congenital heart disease on a course of prophylactic penicillin. This treatment is because the postpartal period always involves some mild invasion of bacteria from the denuded placental site on the uterus (which is why lochia is always considered potentially contaminated). As these invading bacteria may be streptococci, the bacteria often responsible for subacute bacterial endocarditis, a course of penicillin at this time and through the postpartal period offers her needed protection.

It is often difficult to keep healthy women from taking over-the-counter medicines during pregnancy. It is sometimes as difficult to encourage women who need medicine during pregnancy to take it. They must understand that there are valid exceptions to the rule of "no medicine during pregnancy" so they continue to take necessary heart medication.

Avoidance of Infection. A systemic infection almost automatically increases body temperature, causing a woman to have to expend more energy and increase her cardiac output. This insult may be too much for a woman with heart disease to withstand. Caution women to avoid visiting or being visited by people with infection. She should alert health care personnel at the first indication of an upper respiratory tract or urinary tract infection (be certain she knows the symptoms) so antibiotic therapy, if warranted, can be started early in the course of the infection.

Reduction of Psychological Stress. Reducing psychological stress in a high-risk pregnancy

is a worthy goal but often unattainable: The reason for the worry and stress *is* the high-risk pregnancy. Factors outside the pregnancy, however, such as financial responsibilities or lack of support persons, should be reduced to the minimum possible. Provide extra time at prenatal visits for discussing any problems a woman is developing. Be certain that the woman understands that the purpose of any fetal assessment test, such as a nonstress test, is prophylactic; this assurance will lessen unnecessary worry.

A woman with heart disease needs a great deal of support during pregnancy. She is worried, not only for the fetus, but also—realistically—for herself. In many instances, a well-meaning physician, family member, or friend had told her long ago that she would never be able to have children. Much as she would like to believe the obstetrician who is telling her now that she can, the old prediction keeps running through her mind. If she feels that the pregnancy will never reach a safe conclusion, it is hard for her to follow instructions; everything seems more or less in vain. She is unable to begin pregnancy bonding. She needs the frequent reinforcement of being told that everything is going well. Reinforce teaching points and positive aspects of the pregnancy for support people as they can reinfect the woman with their concern and worry.

It helps some women to look at the pregnancy one day at a time rather than at the entire pregnancy. Today, everything is going well. Let's do everything that is necessary today. Tomorrow we will think about what needs to be done then.

Delivery. Many women with heart disease should not push with contractions; pushing requires more effort than they should expend. The anesthetic of choice for delivery in women with heart disease is therefore often an epidural or a caudal anesthetic, which blocks out both pain and the urge to push, making labor and delivery effort-free as well as pain-free. If an epidural anesthetic is used, low forceps will be used for delivery. A woman may be disappointed that her delivery is not more "natural"; help her to remember that her ultimate goal is a healthy newborn and these are the measures that can achieve that hope for her.

Monitor both fetal heart beat and uterine contractions continuously during labor; late decelerations on fetal monitoring and ineffective uterine contractions may occur from poor uterine perfusion. Assess the mother's blood pressure, pulse, and respirations frequently. Rapidly increasing pulse rate (over 100) is a good indication that her heart is pumping ineffectively and therefore has

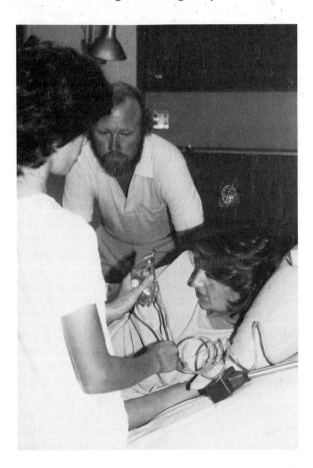

Figure 36-2 *A woman with heart disease may need oxygen administered during labor to supply oxygen to the fetus.*

increased its rate in an effort to compensate. Assess her level of fatigue by her ability to turn in bed; fatigue indicates poor heart compensation. Be certain she remains in a side-lying position to reduce the possibility of supine hypotension syndrome. If she has some pulmonary edema it may be necessary for her to have her chest and head elevated (semi-Fowler's position) in order to breathe adequately; she may need oxygen administrated to maintain adequate placental exchange (Figure 36-2).

If she has a congenital heart defect or valvular disease, she may be begun on penicillin prophylactically during labor if this treatment was not already begun during pregnancy. If an intravenous line is begun, regulate the rate carefully to avoid adding extra fluid to an already overworked circulatory system.

The Postpartal Period. The period immediately following delivery may be the most critical time for a woman with heart disease. With delivery of the placenta, the blood that supplied the placenta is now released into the general circulation, and the blood volume increases between 20 to 40 percent. During pregnancy, the rise in blood volume occurred over a 6-month period. Following delivery, it takes place within 5 minutes, so the heart must make a rapid and a major adjustment. In order to prevent a sudden distention of the abdominal veins following delivery of the placenta, a physician may (or may ask you to) apply pressure to the woman's abdomen and then gradually release it so blood theoretically enters her circulation more slowly.

Despite the extra workload on her heart, a woman should be ambulated early to avoid the formation of emboli; she may need to wear elastic stockings to increase venous return. If she was not already begun on prophylactic antibiotics previously, she will be started on them immediately postpartally to discourage subacute bacterial endocarditis due to a mild postpartal infection. In the postpartal period ergot compounds to encourage uterine involution must be used with caution as they tend to increase blood pressure. Estrogen compounds to decrease lactation should also be used cautiously; they may lead to thromboembolus.

A woman with heart disease is very interested in close inspection of her baby in the delivery room. She needs more assurance than "You have a beautiful baby." She needs to know that her infant does not appear to have a heart defect. Be sure to point out that acrocyanosis is normal, so that she does not interpret her baby's severe peripheral cyanosis as cardiac inadequacy.

A woman with heart disease can breast-feed without difficulty as a rule, although she needs individual assessment before beginning. Do not start postpartal exercises to improve abdominal tone until her physician approves them, though Kegal's exercises are acceptable for perineal strengthening. Suggest a stool softener if it has not been prescribed to prevent her from straining with bowel movements. The woman needs contraceptive information so that she delays a second pregnancy at least a year. If she chooses sterilization as her contraceptive method, this procedure is generally delayed rather than done in the postpartal period to allow for better circulatory stabilization.

A woman may require a longer-than-usual hospital stay in order that her cardiac condition can be stabilized. Be certain the woman has thought through what help she will need at home so she can continue periods of adequate rest. Be certain she has a return appointment for a postpartal checkup for both her gynecologic health and cardiac status.

Peripartal Heart Disease

An extremely rare condition, peripartal heart disease, originates late in pregnancy in women with no history of previous heart disease; it is apparently due to the effect of the pregnancy on the circulatory system. Since it occurs most often in women from low socioeconomic areas, the possibility of accompanying protein malnutrition is suggested; it may also occur in women with hypertension of pregnancy. Late in pregnancy, the woman develops signs of myocardial failure (shortness of breath, chest pain, edema). Her heart begins to increase in size (cardiomegaly). Activity must be sharply reduced. Many women need diuretic and digitalis therapy. Low-dose heparin may be administered to decrease the risk of thromboembolism.

If the cardiomegaly persists past the postpartal period, it is generally suggested that she not attempt any further pregnancies.

Mitral Stenosis

Mitral stenosis is the heart defect most likely to occur with rheumatic fever. During pregnancy, the normally occurring increase in heart rate and cardiac output forces an increased flow of blood through the stenosed valve. There is pressure in the left atrium due to the inability of the valve to handle the increased flow. Pulmonary veins become distended. Pressure on lung capillaries causes a transexudate of fluid into lung or pulmonary edema.

Management is aimed toward decreasing the flow of blood through the mitral valve. A woman may be placed on oral diuretics to limit plasma volume. Digitalis therapy will reduce the heart rate. If she is taking a diuretic for an extended time, the woman will probably be placed on a potassium supplement as well so she does not become potassium-depleted. Prophylactic penicillin will reduce the possibility of subacute bacterial endocarditis due to the stasis of blood flow at the damaged valve. A woman whose symptoms are becoming so severe that it is evident her heart is failing can undergo cardiac surgery to repair the valve during pregnancy. With this insult to her body and the long period of anesthesia, the fetal risk from the procedure is obviously high.

Pulmonary Artery Hypertension

The maternal risk during pregnancy is very high (about 50 percent) if pulmonary artery hypertension exists (Burrow & Ferris, 1982). A woman might have this condition due to a mitral stenosis or a congenital heart defect such as Eisenmenger's syndrome. Death may occur from congestive heart failure at the time of delivery or early in the postpartal period because of the increased blood flow following the delivery of the placenta. Since it tends to decrease vascular resistance in the lungs, oxygen inhalation should be used during labor and delivery. Anesthesia that causes hypertension should be avoided (the heart cannot make this adjustment; it is already overtaxed). Blood loss at delivery must be replaced, but very cautiously lest rapid intravenous administration tax the mother's circulatory system further. Following delivery, she may be started on heparin anticoagulant therapy to reduce the chance of pulmonary vascular thrombosis from the relative stasis in the pulmonary artery.

Artificial Valve Prosthesis

Once women with a heart valve prosthesis were told they should not become pregnant. Today, caring for a woman with a valve prosthesis during pregnancy would not be unusual. Many women with valve prostheses take oral anticoagulants to prevent the formation of clots at the valve site. This kind of medication may increase the risk of congenital anomalies in infants, however. Women may therefore be placed on heparin therapy to reduce this risk prepregnancy (heparin does not cross the placenta). Subclinical bleeding from an anticoagulant may cause placental dislodgment, so a woman must be observed closely for signs of premature separation of the placenta. If coagulation therapy other than heparin is continued, anticoagulant therapy may be discontinued about 2 weeks prior to delivery to reduce the level in the fetus at birth and prevent the baby being born with a coagulation defect. Regional block anesthesia into the spinal cord is generally not used at delivery because of the danger of bleeding into the spinal cord from surrounding vessels if some difficulty with coagulation still exists. Important goals of care with the woman with heart disease are shown in the Nursing Care Highlight on page 806.

Anemia and Pregnancy

Because the blood plasma volume expands during pregnancy slightly ahead of the red cell count, most women have a pseudoanemia of early pregnancy. This condition is normal and should not be confused with the true anemia that can occur as a complication of pregnancy. Anemia during

Nursing Care Highlight

The Woman with Heart Disease

Goal of Care	Implementations
Assess baseline cardiac function	Assess blood pressure, pulse, and respiratory rate.
	Schedule echocardiography or ECG as indicated.
	Assess exercise tolerance by history.
	Assess presence of edema.
Conserve energy	Plan and urge additional rest periods a day.
	Help her plan for sufficient sleep at night.
	Clarify with her what housework or other activities she will be able to continue during pregnancy.
Maintain nutrition	Be certain the woman is taking her iron supplement.
	Urge her to prepare meals early in the day when she is not fatigued.

pregnancy limits oxygen exchange at the placental site because of the reduced amount of hemoglobin present.

Iron Deficiency Anemia

Many women enter pregnancy with an iron deficiency anemia resulting from poor diet, heavy menstrual periods, or unwise weight-reducing programs. When the hemoglobin level is below 11 gm (hematocrit under 35%), iron deficiency is suspected. Women may have erythrocyte indexes done to determine the cause of the low hematocrit level. Iron deficiency anemia is characteristically a microcytic (small-sized red blood cell), hypochromic (less hemoglobin than the average red cell) anemia: When iron is not available for incorporation into red blood cells, they are not as large or as rich in hemoglobin as normally. Mean corpuscular volume (MCV, or the size of the average erythrocyte) and mean corpuscular hemoglobin (MCH, or the amount of hemoglobin in the average erythrocyte) will both be low.

All women should take an iron supplement during pregnancy as prophylactic therapy against iron deficiency anemia; those with iron deficiency anemia will receive therapeutic levels of medication.

Be certain to ask a woman at prenatal visits whether she is taking her iron supplement. Women do not appreciate the value of iron; it is an over-the-counter medication and therefore it does not seem as urgent or important to take as a prescription drug. Some women who find that iron compounds tend to constipate them stop taking their iron supplement after a few weeks. If this is a problem, a stool softener such as dioctyl sodium sulfosuccinate (Colace) may be prescribed with the iron compound. Aside from limiting the amount of oxygen available for fetal exchange (oxygen is carried in combination with hemoglobin; a decreased hemoglobin amount decreases oxygen transportation), the woman will feel chronically tired if she has iron deficiency anemia. Nine months of pregnancy with iron deficiency anemia makes a pregnancy something to be endured, not a beginning step to firm mother-child bonding (Figure 36-3).

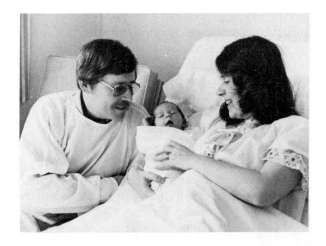

Figure 36-3 *A mother and father share time together after birth of their child. For the woman with a preexisting illness, this moment seems far away during pregnancy. (Courtesy of the Department of Medical Photography, Children's Hospital, Buffalo, N.Y.)*

Folic Acid Deficiency

Megaloblastic anemia due to low levels of vitamin B_{12} or folic acid may occur during pregnancy. Folic acid deficiency has serious effects on fetal development and may be responsible for early abortion or abruptio placentae (premature separation of the placenta). For this reason, all women should receive a folic acid supplement during pregnancy. Routine vitamin preparations prescribed during pregnancy contain folic acid. Over-the-counter nonpregnancy multivitamin preparations generally do not. Ask at prenatal visits whether a woman is taking her prescribed vitamin source. In order to save money, she may not have had the prescription filled and may be using an over-the-counter, less expensive type, not aware of the difference.

If there are small children in the house, caution the woman that she must regard iron compounds and pregnancy vitamins as medicine and keep them away from small hands. Both iron compounds and pregnancy-prescribed vitamins, because of the folic acid content, are dangerous if ingested by young children.

The term *megaloblastic anemia* implies that the red blood cells are enlarged. Thus the MCV with folic acid deficiency is elevated, in contrast to the lowered level seen with iron deficiency anemia. These large cells are not functional, however, so poor placental oxygen exchange occurs.

Sickle Cell Anemia

Sickle cell anemia is a recessively inherited hemolytic anemia. Approximately 1 in every 12 black Americans has sickle cell *trait*—that is, carries a recessive gene for S hemoglobin but is asymptomatic; 1 in every 576 black women theoretically has the disease (Ship-Horowitz, 1984). The sickle cell *trait* does not appear to influence the course of pregnancy in terms of pregnancy-induced hypertension, prematurity, abortion, or perinatal mortality. Such women should take the regular iron and folic acid supplement during pregnancy. There may be an increased incidence of asymptomatic bacteriuria, however, if the trait is present resulting in an increased incidence of pyelonephritis. Clean-catch urines should be collected periodically during pregnancy to attempt to detect developing bacteriuria while it is still asymptomatic.

Pregnancy can be a severe complication for a woman with sickle cell *disease*. With the disease, the majority of red blood cells are irregular or sickle-shaped. They do not carry as much hemoglobin as normally shaped red blood cells. When oxygen tension is reduced, as happens at high altitudes, or blood becomes more viscid than usual (dehydration), the cells tend to clump because of the irregular shape. This clumping results in infarcts and blockage of vessels. The cells will then hemolyze. At any time in life, sickle cell anemia is a threat to life if vital blood vessels such as those to the liver, the kidneys, the heart, the lungs, or the brain are blocked. In pregnancy, blockage to the placental circulation will lead to direct fetal compromise and fetal death. Early in pregnancy when a woman may be nauseated, her fluid intake may be decreased and dehydration is a real possibility. Pooling of blood in the lower extremities because of uterine pressure may take place as pregnancy advances, leading to increased sickling of blood cells. If a woman develops an infection that raises her temperature and causes her to perspire more than normally or she contracts a respiratory infection that compromises air exchange so that her PO_2 is lowered, she will be hospitalized for observation until it is established that she is not beginning a sickle cell crisis and hemolysis of crowded cells has not started. All during pregnancy, ask about her diet (she must include enough fluid—at least four glasses daily) and whether she is sitting for long periods during the day. She needs always to rest with her legs elevated when sitting in a chair; lying on her side in a modified Sims' position encourages return venous flow from the lower extremities.

A woman with sickle cells disease may normally have a hemoglobin level of 6 to 8 mg per 100 ml, and this is the level she will maintain during pregnancy unless it is corrected. Hemolysis in a sickle cell crisis may occur so rapidly that her hemoglobin level falls to 5 to 6 mg per 100 ml in a few hours. There is an accompanying rise in her indirect bilirubin level because she cannot conjugate the bilirubin released from red blood cells being so quickly destroyed. Following a crisis, she may have jaundiced sclerae.

Interventions in sickle cell crisis include replacing sickled cells with normal cells by exchange transfusion (this can be done prophylactically during pregnancy and just prior to labor), administering oxygen as needed, and increasing the fluid volume of the circulatory system to lower viscosity. An exchange transfusion serves a secondary purpose of removing a quantity of the increased bilirubin level as well as restoring hemoglobin level. Women with sickle cell disease are not given an iron supplement during pregnancy as a rule. The cells cannot incorporate the added iron as can normal cells, and there may therefore be an excessive buildup from a supplement. They do need a folic acid supplement be-

---

Nursing Care Highlight

**Signs and Symptoms of
Urinary Tract Infection**

Pain on urination
Frequency of urination
Hematuria

Bacterial count over 100,000 colonies/ml in a
   clean-catch specimen
Lumbar pain and tenderness

---

cause of the overproduction of marrow trying to counteract hemolysis. If these women do not have adequate folic acid, they may develop megaloblastic anemia following a crisis.

When the fetus is mature, delivery must be individualized. The woman must be kept well hydrated in labor. For delivery, she generally receives nerve block anesthesia rather than a general anesthetic to avoid the possibility of anoxia.

Women generally are interested in determining at birth whether their child has inherited the disease. As the disorder is recessively inherited, with one of the parents having the disease and the other free of the disease, the chances that the child will inherit the disease are zero. If one parent has the disease and the partner has the trait, the chances that the child will be born with the disease are 50 percent (see Chapter 6).

Symptoms of sickle cell disease do not become clinically apparent in the child until the hemoglobin converts to a largely adult pattern (in 3 to 6 months). Fetal hemoglobin is composed of two alpha and two gamma chains; adult hemoglobin is composed of two alpha and two beta chains. Since the sickle cell trait is carried on the beta chain, it will not be manifested until the chain appears. Electrophoresis of red blood cells at birth, however, will reveal the manifestation of the disease on the few beta chains present (infants have about 15 percent adult hemoglobin at birth).

A woman with sickle cell disease needs to be seen frequently during the antepartal period. In underdeveloped countries the maternal mortality in women with sickle cell disease is about 18 percent. One third to one half of all pregnancies end in abortion, stillbirth, or neonatal death.

Urinary Tract Disorders and Pregnancy

As adequate kidney function is important for a successful pregnancy outcome, any condition that interferes with kidney or urinary function is potentially serious.

Urinary Tract Infection

Urinary tract infection occurs in 1 to 2 percent of pregnancies. Many nonpregnant women have asymptomatic bacteriuria. In a pregnant woman, because of the stasis of urine in the dilated ureters, asymptomatic infections are greatly increased in importance because they can flame into pyelonephritis. The organism most commonly responsible for urinary tract infection is *Escherichia coli* from an ascending infection. A urinary tract infection can also occur as a descending infection or begin in the kidneys from the filtration of organisms present from other body infections.

With pyelonephritis a woman notices pain in the lumbar region (usually on the right side) that radiates downward. The area is tender to palpation. She may have accompanying nausea and vomiting, malaise, pain, and frequency of urination (see the box above). Her temperature may be elevated only slightly or may be as high as 103 to 104°F (39–40°C). The infection usually occurs on the right side because the uterus is pushed to that side by the large bulk of the intestine on the left side. The greater compression on the right ureter creates greater stasis on that side.

A clean-catch urine should be obtained for a culture and a sensitivity test (see Procedure 18-1). The sensitivity test report will determine which antibiotic will be prescribed. Ampicillin is effective against most organisms causing urinary tract infection and is a safe antibiotic for pregnancy. Nitrofurantoin (Furadantin) is also frequently ordered. The sulfonamides are used early in pregnancy but not near term: They interfere with protein binding of bilirubin; this could lead to hyperbilirubinemia in the newborn. Similarly, tetracyclines are contraindicated in pregnancy; they cause retardation of bone growth and staining of the fetal teeth.

A woman needs to take additional fluid to flush out the infection from the pelvis of the kidney. Never tell her to "push fluids" or "drink lots of water." Tell her a specific amount to drink every day (up to 3 or 4 liters per 24 hours), to make certain that her fluid intake will be sufficiently increased.

A woman can promote urine drainage by assuming a knee-chest position for 15 minutes morning and evening. In this position the weight of the uterus is shifted forward, freeing the ureter for drainage. Women should assume a knee-chest position for about 15 minutes twice a day during pregnancy not only as prophylaxis against urinary tract infection but against the development of hemorrhoids and varicosities.

Be certain to ask a woman about any associated symptoms, such as frequency of urination, when she is describing back pain during pregnancy so that you do not interpret this symptom of developing urinary tract infection as normal backache. An increased incidence of premature labor and fetal loss is associated with pyelonephritis.

If a woman has one urinary tract infection during pregnancy, the chance that she will develop another late in pregnancy is high. She may therefore be kept on prophylactic antibiotics throughout the remainder of the pregnancy. Ask a woman at prenatal visits whether she is continuing to take this type of prophylactic medicine. While women have pain and symptoms of urinary frequency, they take medication very well. When they no longer have any clinical evidence that they are sick, their compliance rate begins to fall dramatically. The woman may need to post a chart on her refrigerator door or in her bathroom to remind herself to take this kind of medication (Figure 36-4). Leaving the medicine on a counter to remind herself to take it is not a good habit to develop. Shortly she will have a new baby in the house. Encourage her to keep medicine out of sight and reach so as to get into the habit of childproofing even at this early stage.

Chronic Renal Disease

In previous years, children with chronic renal disease did not reach childbearing age or were advised not to have children because of the high risk during pregnancy. Today, women with chronic renal disease are having children. Children have been born to women who have even had renal transplants.

Pregnancy increases the work load on the kidneys because a woman's kidneys must excrete waste products not only for herself but for the fetus for 9 months. Many women with renal dis-

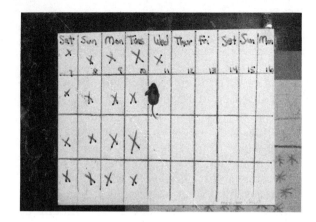

Figure 36-4 *A reminder sheet for medication compliance. Few women remember to take medicine without one; a refrigerator magnet marks the time for the next dose.*

ease take corticosteroids (Prednisone) at a maintenance level, and they should continue to do so throughout pregnancy. Although reports of animal studies have demonstrated an increased incidence of cleft palate from the taking of corticosteroids during pregnancy, this side effect does not appear to happen in humans.

It is difficult to interpret kidney function tests during pregnancy. Many women spill a trace of glucose and protein during pregnancy because of increased glomerular permeability. If a woman is told about this possibility, she will understand that it is an expected change of pregnancy, not a forecast of diminishing kidney function. Many women with renal disease have an elevated blood pressure; a woman's blood pressure level during pregnancy must be compared both to her prepregnancy and to normal levels in order to be meaningful.

Because the glomerular filtration rate increases during pregnancy, normally a woman is able to clear waste products for both herself and the fetus from her body with such efficiency that her serum creatinine and blood urea nitrogen (BUN) levels are actually slightly below normal during pregnancy. Normal blood creatinine is 0.7 mg per 100 ml; during pregnancy it is about 0.5 mg per 100 ml. BUN is normally 13 mg per 100 ml; during pregnancy it is about 9 mg per 100 ml. Women with kidney disease who normally have an elevated blood creatinine level over 1.7 gm per 100 ml or a BUN over 30 mg per 100 ml probably should not undertake a pregnancy: The increased strain on already damaged kidneys may lead to kidney failure.

Toward the end of pregnancy, fetal well-being may normally be evaluated by urinary estriol determinations. These findings can be erroneous, however, in women with renal disease because estriol is low if the woman is taking prednisone and because of the overall decreased output. They must always be interpreted in light of a woman's kidney-diseased state, not compared to normal values.

Infants of women with chronic renal disease tend to have intrauterine growth retardation. If a woman is taking steroids, her baby may be hyperglycemic at birth because of the suppression of insulin activity by corticosteroids at birth.

Women with kidney transplants should be considered individually in terms of their ability to carry a pregnancy to term before a pregnancy is initiated. Criteria that should be evaluated are a woman's general health and the time since the transplant (preferably more than 2 years), whether she has proteinuria, signs of graft rejection, hypertension, her level of serum creatinine, and whether she is taking medication to reduce graft rejection. If her drug usage is limited to Prednisone and azathioprine (an antimetabolite, but no reports of fetal compromise have been made with this), pregnancy may be possible for her.

Women with renal disease need a great deal of support during pregnancy. They are aware that kidneys are vital for life and that the stress of pregnancy on damaged kidneys may cause them to fail. They are aware that they are risking not only the life of the growing child inside them but their own.

They need extra time with their infant at birth for bonding as they may have had difficulty beginning bonding during pregnancy. They need extra assurance that the baby is well.

Reproductive Tract Disorders and Pregnancy

Reproductive tract disorders during pregnancy are always potentially serious because many of these disorders can cause interference with fetal growth.

Vulvitis

Vulvitis is inflammation of the vulva. It generally occurs not as a disease condition in itself, but as a result of a vaginitis that is creating excess vaginal discharge; the constant moisture against the vulva leads to inflammation and discomfort. Vulvitis also may occur as an allergy or sensitivity to a feminine hygiene or contraceptive product, pediculosis or scabies, poor hygiene, the presence

of stress incontinence, or a sexually transmitted disease (herpes may be vulvar). Chickenpox (varicella) may present with vulvar lesions. A high incidence is found in women with diabetes mellitus and those taking ovulation suppressants (oral contraceptives) because of the high incidence of vaginitis in such women.

Vulvitis is manifested as itching or pain; the area appears swollen and reddened. Urination may cause intense burning from the acid urine

Table 36-2 Comfort Measures for Vulvitis

Measure	Rationale
1. Wash vulva BID with mild, nonperfumed soap and water; pat dry front to back.	Removing secretions decreases irritation. Washing front to back prevents spread of rectal contamination forward.
2. Apply cornstarch for comfort.	Talc should be used sparingly as it may be associated with ovarian cancer.
3. Sitz baths or warm moist compresses TID for comfort.	Warm moist heat is soothing in removing edema and keeping the area free of irritating discharge.
4. Follow instructions concerning a vaginal infection.	Only when the vaginal discharge is eliminated will the vulvitis clear.
5. Avoid bubble bath, feminine hygiene sprays.	Products may cause local irritation; bubble bath may contribute to urinary tract infections.
6. Take acetaminophen (Tylenol) q4h for comfort.	Itching is a minimal pain sensation so analgesics reduce itching as well as pain.
7. Do not scratch the area. Apply a cold compress to decrease the sensation of pruritus.	Scratching leaves abrasions that may be secondarily infected.
8. Use an anesthetic spray or hydrocortisone cream only as prescribed.	Some absorption occurs with topical application so toxic systemic symptoms can occur.
9. Wear cotton underwear. Sleep without underwear.	Nylon or silk underwear does not allow evaporation and keeps perineum moist.

reduces discomfort. Applying an ointment such as A&D Ointment also reduces discomfort, but moist lesions appear to take longer to heal than dry ones. Ointments, therefore, prolong the active period of the lesion.

After an active infection has receded, it is recommended that the woman discard any product such as an ointment or dusting powder she used: The herpesvirus can survive for a considerable length of time outside the body and use of the product again could reactivate an infection. A new drug, acyclovir (Zovirax), is available as a topical ointment. It destroys the virus by interfering with DNA reproduction. Be certain when applying it that you use a finger cot to prevent possible spread of virus or absorption of the drug by your finger. Acyclovir should not be used by pregnant women, as it has not been proven safe for the fetus.

A herpes infection is dangerous during pregnancy. The primary form can lead to spontaneous abortion; if lesions are present in the vagina at birth, the virus can be spread to the newborn. Herpes infections in newborns involve a lethal systemic infection (discussed in Chapter 47). Because there is an association with cervical cancer, any woman who has a genital herpes infection should conscientiously have a Pap test yearly for the remainder of her life. The use of a condom appears to prevent the spread of herpes between sexual partners.

Gonorrhea

Gonorrhea is caused by the gram-negative coccus *Neisseria gonorrhoeae*; there are over a million cases of the infection reported yearly. Women are rarely aware that they have active gonorrhea because in women, the disease is asymptomatic. Their male partners usually have symptoms of burning on urination, frequency, and a purulent penile discharge.

Gonorrhea is potentially serious. It can lead to severe pelvic inflammatory disease with resulting infertility; if a woman has active gonorrhea at the time of delivery, the newborn may contract the organism, causing blindness from ophthalmia neonatorum (discussed in Chapter 47).

In early pregnancy, at the time of the Pap test, most physicians also take a routine culture for gonorrhea or draw blood for gonorrheal antibodies. If a culture is positive, the woman is treated with large doses of penicillin (penicillin G procaine, 4.8 million units intramuscularly, in two sites on one visit), plus probenecid, 1 gm orally one-half hour before the injection of penicillin. Probenecid delays urinary excretion of penicillin and maintains high blood levels of penicillin for a sustained time. Women who are sensitive to penicillin may be treated with erythromycin.

Condyloma Acuminata

Condyloma acuminata is a fibrous tissue overgrowth on the external vulva covered by thick epithelium. It tends to occur in women who have a chronic vaginitis and long-term vulvar irritation. Caused by the epidermatrophic virus that causes common warts (verrucae), these lesions tend to occur on the vestibule and labial folds. They can, however, be located at any point on the vulva or intravaginally. At first they appear as discrete papillary structures, which then spread and enlarge and coalesce to form large cauliflower-like lesions. They may become secondarily ulcerated and infected; when this occurs, a foul vulvar odor may develop. Because the disorder is transmitted by a virus, it is a sexually transmitted disease.

Therapy for such lesions is aimed at dissolving the lesions and also ending any secondary infection present. Twenty percent solution of podophyllin in tincture of benzoin may be effective in first blanching the lesions and then causing them to slough away in 2 to 3 days' time. Trichloroacetic acid (Negatol) may also be effective for this purpose. Large lesions may be removed by cryocautery or knife excision. With cryocautery, edema at the site is evident immediately; lesions become gangrenous and sloughing occurs in 7 days. Healing will be complete in 4 to 6 weeks with only slight depigmentation at the site. Sitz baths and a lidocaine cream may be soothing during the healing period. Unless they are bothersome, lesions may be left in place during pregnancy and removed during the postpartal period. Their presence appears to have no effect on the fetus. A chronic vaginitis, if present, should be treated to prevent recurrence of the condylomata.

Respiratory Disorders and Pregnancy

Chronic respiratory disorders can worsen during pregnancy. The rising uterus compresses lung space at a time when increased lung function is needed to provide adequate oxygen exchange for the fetus as well as for the woman.

Upper Respiratory Tract Infection

Upper respiratory tract infection (common cold) tends to occur with heightened severity during pregnancy. With pregnancy there is normally some degree of nasal congestion. With even a minor cold, therefore, a woman finds it difficult to breathe. Women should be cautioned that, unless they have a fever with a cold, taking aspirin or acetaminophen (Tylenol) is unnecessary and they should be very cautious about taking aspirin within 2 weeks of their delivery date (could cause a blood coagulation problem in the infant). Because common colds are invariably caused by a virus, antibiotic therapy is ineffective except to prevent a secondary infection.

Influenza

Influenza is caused by a virus that has been isolated and identified as type A and type B. It spreads in epidemic form and is accompanied by high fever, extreme prostration, aching pains in the back and extremities, and generally a sore, raw throat. There is some correlation between influenza outbreaks and congenital anomalies in newborns. During the famous Asian flu epidemic of the 1950s (caused by a variant of type A virus), premature labor and abortion rates increased. Influenza is treated with an antipyretic to control fever and perhaps a prophylactic antibiotic to prevent a secondary infection.

Pneumonia

Pneumonia is caused by a bacterial or viral invasion of lung tissue. Following the invasion, an acute inflammatory response with exudate of red blood cells, fibrin, and polymorphonuclear leukocytes into the alveoli occurs. This process poses a serious complication of pregnancy because as fluid collects in alveolar spaces oxygen/carbon dioxide exchange becomes limited. Extreme collection of fluid will limit the oxygen available to the fetus. The woman will be placed on an appropriate antibiotic. There is a tendency for women with pneumonia late in pregnancy to begin premature labor. During labor oxygen should be administered so that the fetus has adequate resources during contractions.

Asthma

Asthma is paroxysmal wheezing and dyspnea in response to an inhaled allergen. About 1 percent of all pregnant women have asthma. Most people who are susceptible to allergens in this way are said to be *atopic* individuals; they have a predisposition to allergy over and above others. Inhalation of the allergen results in an immediate histamine release from IgE immunoglobulin interaction, which stimulates constriction of the bronchial smooth muscle, marked mucosal swelling, and the production of thick bronchial secretions. These three processes reduce the lumen of air passages markedly. A woman has difficulty with air exchange; on exhalation, she makes a high-pitched whistling sound (bronchial wheezing) caused by air being pushed past narrow, fluid-filled bronchial spaces. Asthma has the potential for reducing the oxygen supply to the fetus because of this poor respiratory exchange pattern.

Many women find that their asthma is improved during pregnancy because of high circulating levels of corticosteroids. A woman should check with her physician concerning the safety of the medications she routinely takes for this disorder *before pregnancy* to be certain she can safely continue them during pregnancy and during breast-feeding. Many women with asthma take a corticosteroid routinely; this medication can be continued during pregnancy. Saturated solution of potassium iodide (SSKI) taken as a cough medication is harmful during pregnancy because it can lead to suppression of fetal thyroid function.

Pulmonary Tuberculosis

Tuberculosis is a disease that should have been eradicated in view of the effective treatment now available. However, in some highly populated areas, spread still occurs and its incidence is actually increasing. Worldwide, it is still one of the leading causes of death.

With tuberculosis, lung tissue is invaded by *Mycobacterium tuberculosis*, an acid-fast bacillus. Inflammation begins at the point of bacillus contact (termed a *Ghon complex*). Macrophages surround the bacillus; but rather than actually killing it, they only remain surrounding the invasion site (now termed a *tubercle*). Sensitized T lymphocytes group in the area and fibrosis, calcification, and a final ring of collagenous scar tissue develops, encircling the tubercle, effectively sealing off the organisms from the body and any further invasion or spread. The presence of the sensitized T lymphocytes will cause a positive tine or PPD (purified protein derivative) test for the rest of the individual's life.

In high-risk areas for tuberculosis, women should be skin-tested with a tine or PPD method at their first prenatal visit. A chest X-ray film can then be taken of women who show positive reactions to skin testing. Women need to be cautioned that a positive reaction does not necessarily mean that they have the disease; it can also mean that they have at some time been exposed to it and so have antibodies in their system. A chest X-ray film confirms the diagnosis.

A woman with tuberculosis shows symptoms of a chronic cough, weight loss, hemoptysis, night sweats, a low-grade fever, and chronic fatigue.

Women with active tuberculosis should be treated during pregnancy. Isoniazid (INH), ethambutol hydrochloride, rifampin, streptomycin, and para-aminosalicylic acid (PAS) may all be given without apparent teratogenic effects. Isoniazid may cause hepatitis-like symptoms of nausea, anorexia, malaise, fever, and enlarged liver in the mother. It may also result in a peripheral neuritis if a woman does not take supplemental pyridoxine as well. Ethambutol may cause optic nerve involvement (optic atrophy and loss of green color recognition) in the mother. To detect this problem, a woman can be tested monthly by the color code on a Snellen eye chart.

A woman who has had tuberculosis is usually advised to wait a full year, perhaps 2 years, before attempting to conceive after her tuberculosis becomes inactive because tuberculosis lesions never actually disappear but are only "closed off" by calcium deposits in the lung and therefore made inactive. A woman who has active tuberculosis, or has had it recently, must be especially careful to maintain an adequate level of calcium during pregnancy in order to ensure that tuberculosis pockets form or are not broken down. Recent inactive tuberculosis can become active during pregnancy, because pressure on the diaphragm from below changes the shape of the lung, and a sealed pocket may be broken in this process. Pushing during labor may increase intrapulmonary pressure and cause the same phenomenon. Recently inactive tuberculosis may become active during the postpartal period, as the lung suddenly returns to its more vertical prepregnant position and breaks open calcium deposits.

A woman with a recent history of tuberculosis should have at least three negative sputum cultures before she holds or cares for her infant. If these are negative, there is no need to isolate the infant from the mother; she can even breast-feed. If there is active tuberculosis in the home, the infant is generally sent home on prophylactic isoniazid or given a BCG vaccine (Calmette-Guerin bacillus vaccine) to prevent the newborn from contracting the disease.

Collagen Disorders and Pregnancy

A number of collagen disorders have a high incidence in young adult women.

Juvenile Rheumatoid Arthritis

Juvenile rheumatoid arthritis, a disease of connective tissue with joint inflammation and contracture, occurs for unknown reasons but is probably the result of an autoimmune or infectious response. IgG and IgM antibodies known as the *rheumatoid factor* have been found in the serum of almost all persons with rheumatoid arthritis. The disease can increase in severity with emotional or physical stress.

The disease pathology is synovial membrane destruction. Inflammation with effusion, swelling, erythema, and painful motion of the joints occurs. Over a period of time formation of granulation tissue fills the joint space, resulting in permanent disfigurement and loss of joint motion.

Women with juvenile rheumatoid arthritis frequently take corticosteroids and salicylate therapy to prevent joint pain and loss of mobility. Symptoms of the disease may improve during pregnancy because of the increased circulating level of corticosteroids in the maternal bloodstream during pregnancy. During the postpartal period, when a woman's corticosteroid levels fall to normal again, arthritis symptoms will probably recur.

Women who take large amounts of salicylates may have prolonged pregnancies (salicylate interferes with prostaglandin synthesis and so may delay the onset of labor contractions). An infant may have a bleeding defect due to a high salicylate level. For this reason a woman is asked to decrease her intake of salicylates about 2 weeks before term.

She should continue to take corticosteroids during pregnancy if they are necessary to control her symptoms. Despite reports that exposure to corticosteroids during pregnancy leads to increased congenital anomalies in animals, humans do not seem to be affected. Since urinary estriol levels may be decreased in a woman taking prednisone, levels must be evaluated in light of the prednisone therapy. The fetal adrenal output is apparently suppressed and less estrogen is formed.

A woman should not take phenylbutazone or indomethacin to reduce inflammation during pregnancy. These two drugs are known teratogens.

Systemic Lupus Erythematosus

Systemic lupus erythematosus (SLE) is a multisystem chronic disease of connective tissue that can occur in women of childbearing age (its highest incidence is in women 20 to 40 years of age). With onset of the illness, widespread degeneration of connective tissue, especially of the heart, the kidneys, the blood vessels, spleen, skin, and retroperitoneal tissue, occurs. The most marked skin change is a characteristic erythematous butterfly-shaped rash on the face. Most serious of the kidney changes are fibrin deposits that plug and block the glomeruli, leading to necrosis and scarring. The thickening of collagen tissue in the blood vessels causes vessel obstruction. This process is life-threatening to a woman when blood flow to vital organs is compromised and to the fetus when blood flow to the placenta is obstructed. A woman may take a corticosteroid and salicylate to reduce symptoms of joint pain and inflammation.

The naturally increased circulation of corticosteroids during pregnancy may lessen symptoms in some women. In others, the chief complication of the disorder—acute nephritis with glomeruli destruction—may occur during pregnancy.

With nephritis, a woman's blood pressure will rise. She will have hematuria and decreased urine output. Proteinuria and edema may begin. It is difficult to differentiate these symptoms from those of pregnancy-induced hypertension except that with the latter there is no hematuria.

Infants of women with systemic lupus erythematosus tend to be small for gestational age due to the decreased blood flow to the placenta. The incidence of abortion and premature birth rises. During the postpartal period there may be an acute exacerbation of symptoms in a woman as corticosteroid levels again fall to normal.

Gastrointestinal Diseases and Pregnancy

The gastrointestinal disorders that young adult women tend to be most prone to are hiatal hernia, peptic ulcer, cholecystitis, and appendicitis.

Hiatal Hernia

Hiatal hernia is a condition in which a portion of the stomach extends and protrudes up through the diaphragm into the chest cavity. Although the condition can be constantly present, it most often occurs only sporadically following increased peristaltic action. Hiatal hernia may generate symptoms during pregnancy as the uterus pushes the stomach against the diaphragm and increases the hernia. With a hiatal hernia, a woman has symptoms of heartburn, gastric regurgitation, indigestion, and dysphagia (difficulty swallowing); heartburn is particularly extreme if she lies supine following a full meal. Heartburn that the woman cannot seem to relieve will become noticeable during pregnancy at about the twentieth week. The woman may lose weight because of her inability to eat. If the problem is extreme, she may have hematemesis (vomiting of blood).

That a hiatal hernia is present may be diagnosed by X-ray examination or direct endoscopy. A woman can be assured that the X-ray covers only her stomach and esophagus; it is safe during pregnancy. Direct endoscopy offers the advantage of bypassing X-ray, however. Symptoms can be relieved by small frequent feedings and antacid administration. Following pregnancy, as the uterine pressure is decreased, the symptoms become less noticeable or disappear.

Peptic Ulcer

Peptic ulcer occurs in about 15 percent of the U.S. population (Bullock, 1984). A peptic ulcer is an erosion of the lining of the stomach or duodenum (most often duodenum) that results from overproduction of acid-pepsin balance in the organ. Miniature vessels in the submucosal layer are destroyed; this action leads to necrosis of cells until a large ulceration occurs. A woman will notice sharp epigastric pain that may radiate to the back 90 minutes to 3 hours after eating; she often wakes at night with sharp pain. The pain is caused by irritation of exposed nerve surfaces to stomach acid; it can be immediately relieved by food or fluid ingestion. As the ulceration deepens, hemorrhage or rupture into the peritoneal space may occur. Peptic ulcers are diagnosed by an upper GI X-ray series or direct endoscopy. Direct endoscopy has an advantage during pregnancy in that it does not involve radiation.

Women with peptic ulcer need to continue their bland prepregnancy diet during pregnancy. They can expect symptoms to decrease during pregnancy because stomach acidity decreases during that time. They should be forewarned that, following pregnancy, symptoms will probably return to prepregnancy level; and they should maintain their diet in the postpartal period.

Cholecystitis and Cholelithiasis

Cholecystitis (gallbladder inflammation) and cholelithiasis (gallstone formation) are most frequently associated with women over 40, obesity, multiparity, and ingestion of a high-fat diet. Gallstones are most frequently formed from cholesterol. Hypercholesterolemia occurs during pregnancy; whether it leads to increased cholecystitis or cholelithiasis during pregnancy is questionable. Symptoms of both cholelithiasis and cholecystitis (constant aching and pressure in the right epigastrium, perhaps accompanied by jaundice) typically occur following a meal rich in fat. These conditions are diagnosed by X-ray and history. As therapy, a woman can eat a low-fat but not a fat-free diet during pregnancy because of the importance of linoleic acid for fetal growth.

Surgery for gallbladder involvement may be done during pregnancy if a woman's symptoms cannot be controlled by conservative dietary management for the remainder of the pregnancy. Obviously, major surgery during pregnancy that requires a general anesthetic carries some degree of risk to the fetus.

Appendicitis

Because appendicitis is a disease of young adults, it can occur in the young pregnant adult. Any woman with abdominal pain during pregnancy—a basic danger sign—should call the health care agency. Differentiating the cause of the pain (an acute abdomen) from a disorder that is special to the pregnancy (abruptio placentae, ectopic pregnancy) is often difficult.

Assessment

History taking is important. Appendicitis usually begins with a few hours of nausea (the woman skipped lunch because she just did not feel hungry). An hour or two of generalized abdominal discomfort follows. The woman may have vomiting during this time. Then comes the typical sharp, peristaltic, lower-right-quadrant pain of acute appendicitis.

This is different from the pain of an overstretched round ligament. Pain from the round ligament occurs with sudden motion and is only transient. It is also different from that of ectopic pregnancy; with ectopic pregnancy, although pain may be sharp and in a lower quadrant, there is no nausea and vomiting. In the nonpregnant woman the sharp, localized pain of appendicitis appears at McBurney's point (a point halfway between the umbilicus and the iliac crest on the lower right abdomen). If you press at that point, it is not so tender while you are pressing; releasing your hand abruptly, however, causes the abdominal contents to jiggle, and the jiggling of the inflamed appendix brings sharp pain (rebound tenderness). In a pregnant woman the appendix is often displaced upward in the abdomen, and the localized pain may be so high in the abdomen it resembles the pain of gallbladder disease. Blood work will reveal leukocytosis. Temperature may be elevated. There are typically ketones in the urine.

A woman should take nothing to eat and no laxatives while she is waiting to be seen by a physician, as increasing peristalsis by these actions tends to cause an inflamed appendix to rupture.

Planning and Implementation

If a woman is near term (past 36 weeks) and there is reason to believe that the fetus is mature, a cesarean birth may be chosen to deliver the baby and then the inflamed appendix is removed. If appendicitis occurs early in pregnancy, an abdominal incision to remove the inflamed appendix can usually be made without disturbing the pregnancy. As long as the anesthesiologist is aware that the woman is pregnant and carefully controls oxygen levels during anesthesia administration, the outcome of the pregnancy will be good.

If the appendix ruptures before surgery, the risk to both mother and fetus increases dramatically. With rupture, infected material is free in the peritoneum. It can spread by the fallopian tubes to the fetus. Generalized peritonitis is such an overwhelming infection it is difficult for a woman's body to combat it effectively and maintain the pregnancy too.

Viral Hepatitis

Hepatitis may occur from invasion of either the A or B virus. Hepatitis A is spread by contact with another person who has the infection or by ingestion of fecally contaminated water or shellfish; it can also be contracted by contamination from a syringe or needle. Hepatitis B virus (serum hepatitis) is spread by transfusion of contaminated blood or blood products; it can also be spread by semen, so it is considered a sexually transmitted disease. Hepatitis A has an incubation period of 2 to 6 weeks, hepatitis B of 6 weeks to 6 months. Both viruses lead to liver cell necrosis with scarring and inability to convert indirect to direct bilirubin or excrete direct bilurubin.

A woman will notice symptoms of nausea and vomiting. Her liver area may feel tender. Jaundice is a late symptom. On physical examination, her liver is found to be enlarged. Her bilirubin level will be elevated, as her liver is unable to complete bilirubin conversion; her liver transaminase value will be increased. Specific antibodies against the A or B virus can be detected in her blood serum. Urine will be dark yellow from excretion of bilirubin by this alternative route; stools will be light-colored from lack of bilirubin.

For therapy, the woman will be put on bed rest and is encouraged to eat a high caloric diet. Use enteric precautions (wear a cover gown, wash hands well on entering and leaving the room; wear gloves to handle articles contaminated with fecal material). If a woman has hepatitis B infection, use precautions with blood samples or blood-drawing equipment.

The danger of hepatitis during pregnancy is a

high incidence of abortion or premature labor. The fetus may contract the hepatitis B virus during the pregnancy or during delivery. Following delivery, the infant should be washed well to remove any maternal blood, and hepatitis B immune globulin (HBIG) administered. The infant needs to be observed carefully for symptoms of infection over the first few months of life. The mother will be advised not to breast-feed: hepatitis B antigens can be passed by breast milk.

Crohn's Disease

Crohn's disease is inflammation of the terminal ileus. The highest incidence is found in the Jewish race, with apparent family predisposition. It occurs most often between the ages of 15 and 20 years. The cause of Crohn's disease is unknown, but an autoimmune process may be responsible. The bowel develops shallow, longitudinal ulcers with areas of bowel stricture between them. Malabsorption, particularly of vitamin B_{12} (a substance whose absorption takes place almost entirely in the ileum) occurs. A woman will experience chronic diarrhea, weight loss, occult blood in stool, and nausea and vomiting. If extreme, obstruction and fistula formation with peritonitis can occur.

Crohn's disease obviously has the potential for interfering with fetal growth if malabsorption occurs. Therapy for the disorder is total rest for the gastrointestinal tract by administration of total parenteral nutrition. Although it is possible to sustain a pregnancy by this route, it is obviously not a desirable nutrition pattern.

Neurologic Conditions and Pregnancy

Neurologic conditions that affect the young adult, and therefore the pregnant young adult, are few in number.

Recurrent Convulsions

Recurrent convulsions (epilepsy) have a number of causes, such as head trauma or meningitis. The majority of instances of recurrent convulsions, however, occur for unknown reasons (idiopathic epilepsy).

Before convulsions could be as well controlled as they can be today, recurrent convulsions were so incapacitating that women who suffered from them were generally advised not to have children. Today, there is no contraindication to such a woman's having children as long as she is aware

that the medications she must take to control convulsions may increase the chance of anomalies in her infant.

In the early months of pregnancy, women with recurrent convulsions often need help with relief of nausea and vomiting. They must not become so nauseated that they are unable to take their seizure control medications. They have to understand that the rule against taking medication during pregnancy does not apply to their seizure control medications.

Many women wonder what a convulsion during pregnancy might do to their unborn child. Convulsions vary so much from person to person that it is impossible to answer the question without knowing the individual woman's seizure pattern. Petit mal convulsions (often just a rapid fluttering of the eyelids, a moment's staring into space) will have no effect on the fetus. Grand mal convulsions (sustained clonic-tonic full-body involvement), because of the anoxia that can occur from the spasm of chest muscles, could conceivably affect the fetus. Ordinarily, persons having grand mal convulsions do not need oxygen administered to them during a convulsion. In pregnancy, administering oxygen by mask is good prophylaxis to ensure adequate fetal oxygenation. If a convulsion should occur, the woman must be evaluated to be certain that it was from her underlying disease, not from pregnancy-induced hypertension.

Dilantin (phenytoin sodium), a drug frequently prescribed for the control of grand mal seizures, appears to be teratogenic, resulting in a Dilantin syndrome (mental retardation and a peculiar facial proportion, not unlike that of the fetal alcohol syndrome). Tridione, a drug often used to control petit mal seizures, is also a known teratogen. A woman with recurrent convulsions, therefore, is in a catch-22 position of having to take drugs to safeguard her own health, but by taking them she may not be safeguarding the health of the fetus.

Women who have taken Dilantin for years may have developed chronic hypertension as a drug side effect. A baseline blood pressure should be established early in pregnancy so that later changes can be interpreted in terms of an already elevated pressure.

Despite all the information at hand about diseases, the actual cause of convulsions is still unknown, and they continue to be regarded as a mysterious or "strange" disease. In the past, people with convulsions were thought to be possessed by devils; in witch-burning times, women with convulsions met death at the stake. In many people's minds, this is still a "dirty," or unclean, disorder. For this reason, many women with recurrent convulsions have low self-esteem. To counteract this, all through pregnancy, the woman requires encouragement and support for the things that she is doing right.

A woman should be told to alert hospital personnel at the time of delivery about her recurrent convulsions and to report the type of medication she is taking. An anesthesiologist needs to know about her tendency to convulsions before administering anesthesia; during the excitement phase of anesthesia, a convulsion may occur if protective measures have not been taken.

A woman will often worry that her child will have convulsions as he or she grows older. If her convulsions are the result of an acquired disorder—infection, such as meningitis, or head trauma—there is no basis for thinking they will be inherited: She can be assured that her child will have no more tendency toward convulsions than any other child. If the etiology of her convulsions is unknown (idiopathic epilepsy), the chances that her child will have them too are slightly higher than in the normal population. This prediction is only theoretical, however, and cannot be made without a thorough review of the onset and nature of a woman's disorder.

Be certain the woman has her newborn with her for long periods so you can point out to her that sudden jerking motions such as occur when a newborn is startled (a Moro reflex) or quivering of the jaw with prolonged crying are normal. She should not interpret these as seizure activity.

Endocrine Disorders and Pregnancy

As a normal effect of pregnancy, the thyroid gland enlarges (hypertrophies) slightly as a result of increased vascularity due to the heightened metabolic rate necessary to supply nutrients to both the maternal and fetal systems. A woman with preexisting thyroid difficulty may have difficulty making this pregnancy transition.

Hypothyroidism

Hypothyroidism is a rare condition in young adults; women with untreated hypothyroidism are often sterile (anovulatory). As their thyroid cannot increase function to maintain even normal limits (and during pregnancy, cannot increase to a pregnancy level) these women often have a history of early spontaneous abortion. A woman with hypothyroidism fatigues easily and tends to be obese; her skin is dry (myxedema) and she has little tolerance for cold. Most women with hy-

pothyroidism take thyroxin to supplement what their body cannot produce. A woman who is taking thyroxin for therapy needs to consult with her obstetrician and internist about becoming pregnant. She needs to go for early diagnosis and close follow-up as soon as she suspects she is pregnant (1 week past her missed menstrual period). As a rule, her dosage of thyroxin will be increased for the duration of the pregnancy in order to simulate the effect that would normally occur in pregnancy. Be certain that a woman realizes the importance of this increased dose and that the rule against taking medication during pregnancy does not apply to her.

Following the pregnancy, this dose is gradually returned to her prepregnancy level. Be certain a woman does not continue to take her pregnancy dosage (trying to be economical and use up her pills) or she will pass the line between normality and hyperthyroidism.

Hyperthyroidism

Hyperthyroidism causes symptoms of rapid heart rate, exophthalmia (protruding eyeglobes), heat intolerance, nervousness, heart palpitation, and weight loss. Hyperthyroidism is more apt to be seen in pregnancy than hypothyroidism. If undiagnosed, a woman tends to develop heart failure during pregnancy because her rapid heart rate cannot adjust to the volume overload. She is more prone to symptoms of hypertension of pregnancy and premature labor than the average woman. In nonpregnant women, hyperthyroidism may be diagnosed by a radioactive uptake of ^{131}I. This diagnostic procedure should not be used during pregnancy as the fetal thyroid will also incorporate this drug, resulting in possible destruction of the fetal thyroid.

Treatment for hyperthyroidism includes the administration of thioureas (methimazole or propylthiouracil) to reduce thyroid activity. These drugs are unfortunately teratogens in that they cross the placenta and lead to hypothyroidism and enlarged thyroid gland (a goiter) in the fetus. If this abnormal neck growth enlarges enough it can obstruct the airway and make resuscitation difficult in an infant at birth.

A woman must be regulated on the lowest doses of drugs possible and cautioned to keep a careful record of doses taken so she does not forget a dose or accidentally duplicate one.

Surgical treatment to reduce the functioning of the thyroid gland can be accomplished, but this action is generally not the treatment of choice due to the need for general anesthesia to accomplish it. Following a pregnancy, if a woman desires other children, the procedure might be done as an interpregnancy measure.

Diabetes Mellitus

Unlike most diseases, diabetes in pregnancy is increasing in frequency. Before insulin was produced synthetically (1921), women with diabetes either failed to survive to reach childbearing age, were infertile, or had spontaneous abortions early in pregnancy.

Now that diabetes can be well controlled, three new problems have developed: (a) how to bring a woman with diabetes through a pregnancy in good control, (b) how to protect her infant in utero from the adverse effects of the diabetes, and (c) how to care for the infant in the first 24-hour period after birth until the insulin-glucose regulatory mechanism stabilizes. Many women with diabetes cannot take birth control pills because progesterone interferes with insulin activity and therefore increases blood glucose levels. The estrogen in contraceptives has the potential for increasing lipids and cholesterol levels. In a woman with a potential for vessel complications, taking such a substance is a questionable practice. Intrauterine devices lead to a high incidence of pelvic inflammatory disease; as women with diabetes have difficulty fighting infections, these are not advised either. Reproductive planning, therefore, may be a fourth concern for a diabetic woman.

Complications from diabetes occur in about 1 in every 500 pregnancies. The perinatal infant mortality for pregnancies complicated by diabetes is between 10 and 30 percent, an inordinately high figure (Dansforth, 1982). When diabetic control is poor, a woman is more prone to pregnancy-induced hypertension, hydramnios, and infection (particularly monilial infection) than are other women. Infants of poorly controlled diabetic women tend to be large (over 9 pounds) because of overstimulation of pituitary growth hormone during intrauterine life and excessive subcutaneous fat deposits. A large-size infant may cause delivery problems due to cephalopelvic disproportion. There is a high incidence of congenital anomaly, abortion, and stillbirth in infants of women with uncontrolled diabetes; and at birth they are more prone to hypoglycemia, respiratory distress syndrome, hypocalcemia, and hyperbilirubinemia. The first 7 weeks of pregnancy are the most important time during pregnancy for the fetus; if a woman's serum glucose level can be kept from becoming hyperglycemic during this time, the chances of congenital anomaly are greatly lessened (Miller, N.E., 1983). Infants of severely involved women tend to have intrauterine growth retardation so are small and may do poorly with extrauterine adaptation.

The primary problem in any woman with diabetes is control of the balance between insulin and blood glucose in order to prevent acidosis. Acidosis is dangerous during pregnancy as it is a chief threat to the fetus.

When the insulin amount is insufficient, as with diabetes mellitus, glucose cannot be used by body cells. The cells register their glucose want and the liver quickly converts stored glycogen to glucose to increase the blood glucose level. Because of the insulin insufficiency present, the body cells still cannot use the glucose, and the blood glucose levels continue to rise (hyperglycemia).

When the level of blood sugar of a pregnant woman is 100 to 150 mg per 100 ml, the kidneys begin to excrete quantities of glucose in the urine in an attempt to lower the level (glycosuria). Because of the heavy osmotic action, the increased amount of glucose in the urine reduces fluid absorption in the kidney, and large quantities of fluid are lost in urine (polyuria).

Dehydration begins to occur; the blood becomes concentrated and the blood volume falls. Cells cannot receive adequate oxygen, and anaerobic metabolic reactions take place, causing large stores of lactic acid to pour out of muscle into the bloodstream. To try to replace glucose, fat is mobilized from fat stores, metabolized, and poured into the blood as ketone bodies. These two acid sources, ketone bodies and lactic acid, lower the pH of the blood. The woman is in metabolic acidosis.

As the body continues to attempt to find a source of energy for body cells, protein stores are next tapped. Protein catabolism reduces the supply of protein for body cells. Destroyed body cells result in the loss of potassium and sodium from the body.

Diabetes in poor control, therefore, interferes with the glucose, fat, and protein metabolism of the body. It creates an environment in which there is poor placental perfusion due to sluggish blood movement and, because of the acidosis, one that may be toxic to the fetus (the fetus cannot use oxygen when body cells are acidotic). Hydramnios occurs in at least 25 percent of diabetic women, probably due to hyperglycemia in the fetus, which causes a fluid shift to amniotic fluid. Amniocentesis may be done to decrease the level of amniotic fluid throughout pregnancy. This technique unfortunately exposes a woman to potential infection and premature labor.

All women experience a number of changes in

the glucose-insulin regulatory system during pregnancy. A woman appears to have a decreased insulin sensitivity or insulin resistance (that is, insulin does not seem normally effective during pregnancy), a phenomenon that is probably caused by the presence of the hormone human placental lactogen (chorionic somatomammotropin) and high levels of cortisol, progesterone, and catecholamines. Placental insulinase causes increased breakdown or degradation of insulin. In the kidneys, glomerular filtration of glucose is increased (the glomerular excretion threshold is lowered), causing minimal glycosuria. In the pancreas, the rate of insulin secretion is increased; systemically, the fasting blood sugar is lowered.

The resistance to or destruction of insulin, however, prevents the blood glucose in a normal pregnancy from falling to dangerous limits, despite the increased insulin secretion. The insulin resistance may cause difficulty for a pregnant woman with diabetes in that she must increase her insulin dosage beginning at about the twenty-fourth week of pregnancy in order to prevent hyperglycemia. With this high insulin intake, there is a danger that the continued use of glucose by the fetus could lead to hypoglycemia between meals; this problem is very apt to occur during the night. A low maternal level of glycogenic amino acids (used by the liver to produce glucose) can add to this complex. If this occurs, a woman may become ketoacidotic from breakdown of stored fat between meals, particularly during the second and third trimester of pregnancy. If a woman has preexisting nephropathy (revealed by proteinuria, decreased creatinine clearance, and hypertension), the risk of fetal growth retardation, asphyxia, stillbirth, and maternal pregnancy-induced hypertension rises markedly.

Classification of Diabetes Mellitus

The National Institutes of Health has classified diabetes according to Table 36-4. White (1978) has divided diabetes into various categories in order to predict pregnancy outcome (see Table 36-5). The pregnancy outcome becomes less successful with more diabetic involvement in the mother. In class A (gestational diabetes), fetal survival is high. Infants of mothers in classes D and E may have a perinatal mortality as high as 25 percent. Class F and class R women may have a perinatal mortality close to 100 percent. Women with diabetes mellitus this severe are generally advised not to become pregnant (Miller, N. E., 1983).

Both a woman with diabetes that occurs just during pregnancy (gestational diabetes) and one with overt diabetes need more frequent prenatal visits than the average woman. Those with overt diabetes are usually seen weekly (preferably in a high-risk diabetic center, where an internist, an obstetrician, a nurse, a diabetic educator, and a nutritionist work in combination). Women with gestational diabetes are usually briefly hospitalized early in pregnancy to see whether insulin will be necessary or whether diet management will be enough. Women with known diabetes may be regulated on insulin pump therapy just prior to pregnancy by a short hospital stay.

Table 36-4 Classification of Diabetes Mellitus

Type	Title	Description
Diabetes mellitus		
I	Insulin-dependent	Formerly juvenile-onset diabetes. Little or no insulin is manufactured by pancreas; occurs mainly in children.
II	Noninsulin-dependent	Formerly maturity-onset diabetes. Can be controlled by diet alone. Ketosis does not tend to occur.
Secondary		Occurs from a secondary disease such as pancreatic tumor or cystic fibrosis.
Impaired glucose tolerance		Formerly chemical or latent diabetes. Fasting plasma glucose level is slightly elevated but true diabetes cannot be said to be present.
Gestational diabetes		Diabetes that occurs for the first time during pregnancy and recedes at the end of pregnancy.

Source: National Diabetes Data Group. (1979). *Classification of diabetes mellitus and other categories of glucose intolerance.* Hyattsville, MD: National Institutes of Health.

Table 36-5 White's Classification of Diabetes Mellitus

Class	Description
A	Pregnant woman whose glucose tolerance test is only slightly abnormal. Dietary regulation is minimal; no insulin is required (gestational diabetes is included here).
B	Pregnant woman whose diabetes is of less than 10 years' duration or whose disease began at age 20 or older. There is no vascular involvement.
C	Pregnant woman whose diabetes began between ages 10 and 19 or whose disease has lasted from 10 to 19 years. There is minimal vascular involvement.
D	Pregnant woman whose diabetes has lasted 20 years or more or whose disease began before age 10. There is greater vascular involvement than in class C. D1 = Under age 10 at onset. D2 = Over 20 years' duration. D3 = Beginning retinopathy is present. D4 = Calcified vessels of legs are present. D5 = Hypertension is present.
E	Pregnant woman in whom calcification of the pelvic arteries has been demonstrated on X-ray. (Technique is not used during pregnancy because of teratogenic effect of X-ray.)
F	Pregnant woman whose diabetes has caused nephropathy.
H	Cardiopathy is present.
R	Pregnant woman with active retinitis proliferans.

Source: White, P. (1978). Classification of obstetric diabetes. *American Journal of Obstetrics and Gynecology, 135,* 229.

Assessment

All women who have a history of large babies (9 pounds or more), unexplained fetal loss, congenital anomalies in previous pregnancies, unexplained natal or neonatal loss, obesity, or a family history of diabetes (one close relation or two distant ones) should be screened for diabetes early in pregnancy by a glucose tolerance test and at every prenatal visit by glucose determination of a routine urine specimen.

A woman with diabetes should go to her obstetrician for care before she becomes pregnant; during this waiting period, her condition can be well regulated so she has no hyperglycemia during the early weeks of pregnancy when the ten-

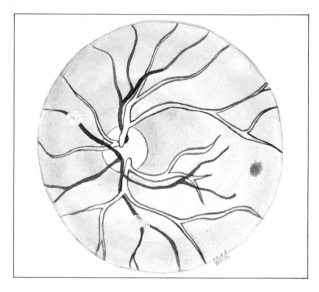

Figure 36-6 *The typical retina change in a woman with diabetes. The "cloud-like" lesion is caused by exudate from the blood vessel.*

dency for congenital anomalies is highest. The woman should use a basal body temperature graph to determine pregnancy at the earliest possible time. The best insulin control program for her during pregnancy can then be established. The measurement of glycosylated hemoglobin (Hgb A1) is a helpful measure of the degree of hyperglycemia present. As glucose circulates in the bloodstream, it binds to a portion of the total hemoglobin in the blood. This body process is glycosylatin. The amount of glucose that attaches to hemoglobin this way will be high if the hemoglobin has been exposed to a greater level of glucose than normally. Measuring glycosylated Hgb (Hgb A1 or Hgb A1c) reflects the average blood glucose level over the last 4 to 6 weeks (the time the red blood cells were picking up the glucose). The upper normal level of Hgb A1c is 6 percent and that of Hgb A1 is 8.2 to 9.5 percent. If a woman begins pregnancy with an elevated Hgb A1, her chance of delivering an infant with a congenital anomaly is increased (Kitzmiller, 1983).

Frequent ophthalmic examination (at least once each trimester) should be scheduled during pregnancy as background retinal changes such as increased exudate (Figure 36-6), dot hemorrhage, and macular edema proceed during pregnancy, and as this condition progresses it can lead to blindness. Laser therapy to halt these changes can be done during pregnancy without risk to the fetus.

Blood and Urine Glucose Monitoring. All women with diabetes can be taught to do blood glucose monitoring to determine if hyperglycemia or hypoglycemia exists rather than depend on urine testing. Blood glucose levels offer a more accurate picture of a woman's available glucose than urine testing. Blood testing also avoids the problem of overreading caused by pregnant women spilling lactose in the urine. A woman uses a Dextrostix technique (see Procedure 47-1), with one of her fingertips as the site of lancet puncture. If she uses a glucose meter with a digital readout, such as an Ames Glucometer, it is easier for her to assess the level than if she merely compares the color of the test strip to a color-coded chart. When she discovers hypoglycemia is present, she can correct this by taking a simple sugar such as a sugar cube, followed by a complex sugar such as a tablespoon of peanut butter if her next meal is over 30 minutes away.

In addition to blood monitoring, most women with diabetes test their urine daily for glucose and acetone. In the past insulin dosage was usually regulated to keep urine 1+ for glucose (negative for acetone) in order to prevent hypoglycemia, a condition that might be present but hidden if a woman's urine showed no glucose on repeated tests. Hyperglycemia may be the environmental influence that causes birth anomalies in the fetus, however, so an attempt is made today to keep a woman's state truly regulated during pregnancy, neither hyperglycemic nor hypoglycemic. Any finding of acetone should always be reported without fail. Acidosis during pregnancy must be prevented because maternal acidosis leads to fetal anoxia due to fetal inability to use oxygen when body cells are acidotic. The most frequent time during pregnancy for insulin coma (hyperinsulinism) is the second and third month; for diabetic coma (hypoinsulinism), the sixth month.

If urine is to be tested for glucose by a dipstick method during pregnancy, it should be done by a double void technique and by a method that measures only glucose, not all sugars: Late in pregnancy and during the postpartal period, lactose, the sugar of breast milk, may spill into the urine and cause a positive reaction if all sugars are measured. Benedict's solution and Clinitest methods measure all sugars. Clinistix and Tes-Tape, on the other hand, measure only glucose and are the preferred measurements during pregnancy. Many juvenile diabetic patients (Type I diabetes) are taught to use Clinitest tablets exclusively. Thus, during pregnancy, they not only have to change their insulin dosage (a change that brings a feeling of insecurity) but also must change the method of urine testing.

The glucose level in urine is not an accurate measure of actual blood sugar, even with a changed method of testing: Due to the decreased

Table 36-6 Diagnostic Criteria for Gestational Diabetes

Sample	Value
Fasting	105 mg per 100 ml
1 hour	190 mg per 100 ml
2 hour	165 mg per 100 ml
3 hour	145 mg per 100 ml

Source: National Diabetes Data Group. (1981). National Institutes of Health, Hyattsville, MD.

renal threshold, glucose may be spilled at unusually low glucose serum levels. Assessing a woman's blood glucose by blood monitoring is much more accurate. In addition to testing for glucose and for acetone, frequent urine cultures (one each trimester) are usually done to detect asymptomatic urinary tract infection.

Glucose Tolerance Tests. A 1-hour glucose tolerance test is the assessment most often chosen in early pregnancy to rule out diabetes. For the 1-hour test, a woman fasts overnight and reports to the health care agency early in the morning. A fasting blood glucose is drawn; she is given an oral 100-gram glucose load, and 1, 2, or 3 hours later, a venous blood sample is taken for blood glucose. Criteria for diagnosis of gestational diabetes (the point at which it is said to be present) is shown in Table 36-6.

Placental Function Tests

Because women with diabetes tend to have infants with an increased incidence of birth anomalies, a woman may have a serum test for alpha-feto-protein done at 15 to 17 weeks to check for spinal cord defects and an ultrasound examination done at 18 weeks' gestation for inspection of gross abnormalities.

To predict placental insufficiency, a woman may be asked to collect a 24-hour urine three times a week after the twenty-eighth to thirty-second week of pregnancy for estriol determination. A sudden drop in estriol in the urine or a low, flat curve may indicate that the pregnancy must be terminated as the fetus is no longer doing well in utero. It is important to begin these determinations as early as the twenty-eighth to thirty-second week of pregnancy in order to establish a baseline, since women with diabetes frequently have small placentas, and the amount of estriol secretion may be low-normal from the first test. A creatinine clearance test may also be ordered each trimester. A normal creatinine clearance suggests that the woman's vascular system is intact and uterine perfusion is probably adequate.

Placental functioning may also be established by means of a weekly nonstress test (see Chapter 15) if the woman is in good diabetes control, or by a daily nonstress test if her regulation is poor. Fetal stress tests are difficult procedures for a woman. Having to wait during each test to hear how the fetus is doing, and having to do this weekly, is something like having to take a final examination every week. The woman feels that it is somehow her fault, her doing, her failure (it is, after all, her diabetes) if the monitor equipment shows fetal distress. The failure may be absolute, for if the distress is acute, the fetus can no longer live in utero. If the gestation age is no more than 34 to 35 weeks, the chances of continuing life outside the uterus are also small.

These tests take 1 to 2 hours to complete. The time can be used to teach the woman controlled breathing or used as a short rehearsal time for actual labor. Thus a positive tone can be added to the test, which may counterbalance the tension the test evokes in some women. A father is often unable to take off time from work to come to the hospital and be with his wife or sexual partner once or twice a week while she is having these tests. The woman needs someone with her to give her emotional support. She needs health care personnel who will help her to minimize the feeling that she is all alone.

A woman may be asked to self-monitor fetal well-being by a count-to-ten test (see Chapter 15). Be certain she knows that fetal activity varies depending on her activity and meal patterns so she is not alarmed at discovering this herself.

Sonography to determine fetal growth, amniotic fluid volume, placental location, and the biparietal diameter may be taken at the twenty-eighth week and then again at the thirty-sixth to thirty-eighth weeks of pregnancy. With fetal growth retardation, there is often accompanying oligohydramnios. With poor disease control, there is hydramnios formation in as many as 25 percent of pregnancies (probably due to hyperglycemia in the fetus, which causes a fluid shift to amniotic fluid). Amniocentesis may be done to reduce fluid but this technique submits the fetus to possible infection and early labor. L/S ratio (see Chapter 15) by amniocentesis is undertaken by the thirty-sixth week of pregnancy to asssess fetal maturity. The L/S ratio in pregnancies complicated by diabetes tends to not show maturity as early as in other pregnancies because the synthesis of phosphatidyl glycerol, the compound that stabilizes surfactant, is delayed in a diabetes-complicated pregnancy. Although it is known

that administering corticosteroids to a mother during the last week of pregnancy can hurry lung maturity, corticosteroids may also impair fetal insulin release and perhaps fetal islet development. Therefore, with a fetus who already has a risk at birth from poor glucose control, this avenue is not usually attempted.

Implementations

The chief implementation for women with diabetes during pregnancy is teaching them to monitor their own health regarding such areas as nutrition and exercise.

Nutrition Management. Many women who are childbearing age and who have had diabetes since early childhood do not follow a strict diabetic diet, but eat sensibly and then cover any excess of food eaten with additional insulin. This type of regimen is apt to require excessive insulin during pregnancy. A woman is well advised, therefore, to alert her health care providers that she is anticipating a pregnancy and before she becomes pregnant begin to follow a more knowledgeable diabetic diet regimen that includes exchange lists.

She should wait to become pregnant until she has good disease control. She should be aware of sensible nutrition patterns such as including a complex carbohydrate in meals to delay absorption of glucose, adequate fat to delay gastric emptying and prevent hyperglycemia, a protein source to reduce the possibility of postabsorption hypoglycemia, and high fiber, also to delay absorption from the intestine. Women are extremely vulnerable to hypoglycemia at night due to the continuous fetal use of glucose during the time they sleep. Urge a woman to make her final snack of the day one of protein and complex carbohydrate, which will be slowly digested during the night.

Dietary control of maintaining an adequate glucose intake so that hypoglycemia does not occur due to a daily dose of insulin may be extremely difficult early in pregnancy because of nausea and vomiting. A 2,200-calorie diet (30–35 calories per kilogram ideal body weight), divided into three meals and three snacks is a usual regimen for a woman with diabetes during pregnancy. Keeping calories evenly distributed during the day helps to keep the blood glucose constant. Protein intake should be 1.3 to 1.7 gm per kilogram (125 gm protein), carbohydrate should be 200 to 500 gm, and fat 70 to 80 gm daily.

Even though a woman is overweight, she should not reduce her intake below 1,800 calories during pregnancy. A diet too low in carbohydrate causes breakdown of fat, which produces acidosis.

In a woman with diabetes, the weight of the infant is directly correlated with the weight the woman gained in pregnancy (which directly correlates with her disease control). She must thus be extremely diet-conscious in order to maintain good control and keep her weight gain to a suitable amount (about 25 pounds), in the hope of limiting the size of her infant and making a vaginal delivery possible. If she cannot eat due to vomiting or nausea early in pregnancy or heartburn in later pregnancy, she must telephone the health care agency. She may need temporary intravenous fluid supplementation during these times.

Insulin. Because of the change in body metabolism, a woman's insulin dosage will have to be changed during pregnancy. If she has been taking one particular kind of insulin and a specified dosage for a long time before the pregnancy, changing the type and dosage is frightening to her. She has no confidence in other types of insulin and other dosages. She needs to be informed that reregulation is a necessity for pregnancy because of the changes in her metabolism.

Early in pregnancy she may need less insulin because the fetus is taking so much glucose for rapid cell growth; later in pregnancy she will need an increased amount.

The dosage and type of insulin will be specific for each woman. The insulin is usually a short-acting type combined with an intermediate type. This is self-administered in combination one half hour before breakfast and again just before dinner in the evening.

Remind women of the time interval that insulin takes to reach its peak. An intermediate insulin given prebreakfast reaches its peak after lunch or late in the afternoon just before dinner. The regular insulin given prebreakfast reaches its peak just after breakfast. An intermediate insulin given in the evening reaches peak into the next day before breakfast; the evening regular insulin injection peaks after dinner or at bedtime. Knowing when insulin reaches its peak level makes blood glucose monitoring meaningful for women.

Be certain that women are using an insulin injection technique of stretching the skin taut and injecting at a 90° angle. As insulin is absorbed more slowly from the thigh than the upper arm, a woman should maintain a consistent, rotating injection routine. Insulin is adjusted to keep a fasting blood sugar within 60 to 120 mg per 100 ml and a 1 hour postprandial level between 110 to 170 mg per 100 ml. Oral hypoglycemia agents (aside from being controversial at present for any patient) are not used for regulation because, unlike insulin, they cross the placental barrier and are teratogenic.

Insulin Pump Therapy (Continuous Subcutaneous Insulin Infusion). Because no matter how carefully a woman maintains her diet and balances her exercise level, she will have some periods of relative hyperglycemia and hypoglycemia, the best solution that can be devised is to administer insulin by a continuous pump during pregnancy.

When pump therapy is begun, a woman is usually hospitalized for at least 3 days in order to ensure that she is familiar with the equipment and that the proposed insulin coverage is indeed adequate for her. An insulin pump is an automatic pump about the size of a transister radio; a syringe of regular insulin is placed in the pump chamber; a thin polyethylene tubing leads to the woman's abdomen where it is implanted into the subcutaneous tissue of her abdomen by a small-gauge needle (Figure 36-7). Throughout the day at a continuous rate, the pump edges the syringe barrel forward, infusing insulin continually into her subcutaneous tissue. Before a snack and before a meal, the woman manually presses a button on the pump and forces a bolus of insulin forward to increase her insulin amount for these large carbohydrate times. The site of the pump insertion is cleaned daily and covered with sterile gauze; the site is changed every 24–48 hours to ensure absorption is still optimum.

Restrictions with pump therapy include keeping it dry, so a woman must remove the pump

Figure 36-7 *Using an insulin pump during pregnancy is the best assurance that insulin levels will remain constant.*

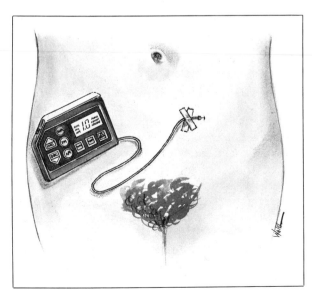

(not the syringe and tubing) while showering. She removes both the needle and pump to bathe or swim (caution her not to leave it disconnected for over an hour). She might prefer to wear clothing that hides the pump's outline (it can either be held against her abdomen by an over-shoulder sling or hung from a belt around her waist). In order to assess the pump's delivery of insulin, a woman must do blood glucose determinations throughout the day (4 times—fasting and 1 hour after each meal). When pump therapy first begins she must wake at night and do a 2 A.M. blood glucose as this is such a vulnerable time for hypoglycemia.

Exercise. When a woman begins to exercise during pregnancy, she may notice excessive glucose fluctuations. Women are urged, therefore, to begin a pregnancy exercise program prior to pregnancy, when glucose fluctuation can be evaluated and foods and snacks adjusted accordingly before a susceptible fetus is involved. When a woman whose diabetes is well controlled exercises, she lowers her blood glucose level because of uptake of glucose by the muscle. This effect lasts for at least 12 hours following exercise. If the arm in which she injects insulin is actively exercised, the effect will be greatly increased. To avoid the phenomenon, a woman should eat a snack of protein or complex carbohydrate before exercise and she should maintain a consistent exercise program (either aerobic or some other exercises every day or not at all, but not sporadically). In a woman who is in poor diabetic control, an exercise period will cause hyperglycemia and ketoacidosis as the liver both releases glucose and breaks down fatty acids to attempt to supply enough for the exercise (yet the body cannot use them because of inadequate insulin).

Timing for Delivery

Before women were managed with maximum control during pregnancy, the timing of the delivery was a chief concern. One of the most hazardous times for the infant is the thirty-sixth to fortieth weeks of pregnancy (the fetus is drawing large stores of maternal nutrients because of its large size). In the past many pregnancies were terminated early enough to prevent fetal loss from placental insufficiency due to poor perfusion during these susceptible weeks; caregivers could only hope that the termination was not so early that immaturity of the child would pose further complications.

Today, when accurate assessment of fetal age is available and the pregnancy can be maintained within safe limits for a longer period of time, the last weeks of pregnancy are not as hazardous and the chance the infant will be born immaturely is not as great. A woman may be hospitalized from the thirty-fourth or thirty-seventh week until delivery, however, as a "careful watch" time for her.

For many years, cesarean birth was almost routinely performed in pregnant diabetic women at about 37 weeks' gestation. Cesarean birth was chosen because it is very difficult to induce labor this early in pregnancy. The cervix is not yet ripe or responsive to labor contractions. Further, babies of diabetic women were invariably large, making vaginal delivery difficult. And finally, a fetus suffering placental dysfunction or insufficiency, which may occur with maternal diabetes, will not do well in labor and may actually be killed. Early cesarean deliveries, however, often resulted in immature infants who died in the neonatal period.

Today, with fetal heart monitoring equipment and the availability of tests for fetal maturity and well-being, the time for delivery is much more individualized. When it can be demonstrated that fetal lung tissue is still immature and the placenta is still adequate, delivery can be delayed. When placental function appears to be growing inadequate (and, it is hoped, fetal lung tissue will appear to be mature at the same time) delivery can be instituted.

As surfactant does not appear to form as early in these fetuses as in others (due to the decreased level of cortisone present because of high serum glucose levels), 2.5 : 1 rather than 2 : 1 is usually accepted as a mature L/S ratio. The presence of phosphatidyl glycerol ensures lung maturity.

Delivery should be vaginal if possible. Cesarean birth always presents a high risk for the fetus, and because of the difficulty of glucose-level regulation, the fetus of a diabetic mother is already under enough stress. Labor is induced by rupture of the membranes or an oxytocin infusion. Both maternal labor contractions and fetal heart sounds should be monitored continuously during labor, so that placental dysfunction can be detected if it does occur (Figure 36-8). An internal fetal monitor may be used with frequent scalp pH recordings. The woman's glucose level must be regulated during labor by an intravenous infusion of regular insulin, with blood glucose assay every hour. Regulating the glucose level carefully during labor reduces the possibility of rebound hypoglycemia in the newborn.

If a woman will be given a regional block anesthetic, be certain that a glucose solution is not used as a plasma volume expander (or its presence is accounted for by additional insulin administration).

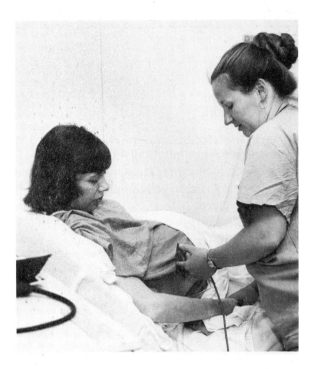

Figure 36-8 *Women with preexisting illness can expect to have the fetal heart rate monitored during labor. (Courtesy of the Department of Medical Photography, Children's Hospital, Buffalo, N.Y.)*

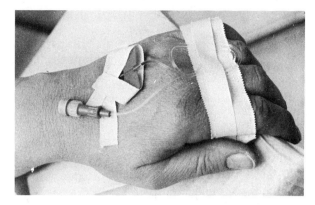

Figure 36-9 *A heparin trap. A heparin trap is an injection adaptor that fits into the distal end of scalp vein tubing; it is used to administer intermittent intravenous medications or withdraw blood.*

Postpartal Adjustment

During the postpartal period, a diabetic woman has to undergo another readjustment to insulin regulation. Often, she needs no insulin during the immediate postpartal period; she will then return to her prepregnant insulin requirements. Diabetic women may breast-feed, because although insulin passes into breast milk it is destroyed in the infant's stomach. A woman requires careful observation during the immediate postpartal period because, if hydramnios was present during pregnancy, she is at risk of hemorrhage from poor uterine contraction.

You will need to either monitor blood glucose levels or collect fractional urine specimens (all urine from 6 A.M. to 12 noon; all urine from 12 noon to 6 P.M., all urine from 6 P.M. to midnight) to be analyzed for glucose content. If many blood glucose measurements will be taken, suggest that a heparin trap be used (Figure 36-9) so the woman is not pricked over and over for blood samples. Blood drawing from a heparin trap is shown in Procedure 36-1, page 830.

Be certain a woman has contraceptive information as appropriate. Remind her that before she plans a second pregnancy, she will first need to be certain that her disease is stabilized and in good control (the first 7 weeks of pregnancy are the crucial fetal developmental times). Women can

be reassured that pregnancy does not appear to add to the long-term effects of diabetes so they feel free to plan another pregnancy at a later date. Goals of care for the woman with diabetes are summarized in the Nursing Care Highlight on page 831.

Gestational Diabetes

Between 2 to 3 percent of all women develop glucose intolerance during pregnancy, called *gestational diabetes*. It is unknown whether glucose intolerance results from inadequate insulin response to carbohydrate or from excessive resistance to insulin; a combination may occur. Once the phenomenon occurs, however, a woman will have a diabetic state for the remainder of pregnancy.

Most women with gestational diabetes are identified because they have a positive glucose urine test at a prenatal visit on a random specimen. A postprandial test or glucose tolerance test is then scheduled and the diagnosis is established. Be certain that a woman is provided some time to talk about what the diagnosis means to her before she leaves. Does anyone else in the family have diabetes? How does she perceive this person—as mainly ill or predominantly well? If there is an Aunt Sally in the family who can never come to dinner because she has to have all of her food specially prepared, who cannot drive her car because she is afraid she might faint, who cannot go on vacation because she does not want to be any distance from her doctor, what diabetes means to this woman during pregnancy is totally different from what it means if Aunt Sally holds a full-time job, volunteers in community or political activities, and—oh, by the way—has diabetes. In the latter instance the woman who is diagnosed as having diabetes during pregnancy has just been

Procedure 36-1

Blood Sampling from a Heparin Trap

Purpose: Remove blood for sampling without necessity of venipuncture.

Plan	*Principle*
1. Wash your hands; identify patient; explain procedure.	1. Prevent spread of microorganisms; ensure patient safety and cooperation.
2. Assess patient condition; analyze appropriateness of procedure; plan modifications as necessary.	2. Nursing care is always individualized based on patient need.
3. Implement procedure by assembling equipment: 1 syringe filled with 1 ml of dilute heparin; 2 empty syringes; 3 No. 25 needles, alcohol wipe.	3. Using small needles prevents tearing the rubber trap.
4. Wipe heparin trap with alcohol, insert empty syringe and needle and withdraw heparin solution until blood appears in syringe. Remove syringe.	4. If heparin solution entered blood sample, it would dilute the sample.
5. Rewipe trap; insert empty syringe and needle and withdraw blood sample. Withdraw syringe.	5. Amount of blood needed depends on laboratory requirements.
6. Rewipe trap; insert heparin filled syringe and inject solution to fill tubing. Withdraw syringe.	6. Heparin filled tubing will keep blood from coagulating in tubing and preserve patency of tubing.
7. Evaluate effectiveness, cost, comfort, and safety of procedure. Plan health teaching as needed, such as the purpose of blood assessments.	7. Health teaching is an independent nursing action always included in care.
8. Record timing and amount of blood sample; patient reaction to procedure.	8. Documentation of nursing care and patient status.

told that she has a disease that is a minor inconvenience; in the former she has been given a lifelong sentence of disability. Thinking that a baby who is not even born yet has made one this incapacitated is not a healthy beginning to maternal-child bonding.

Dietary management during pregnancy is generally all that is necessary for most women with gestational diabetes. A woman is placed on a controlled diabetic diet with the goal of preventing both fasting and postprandial hyperglycemia. If postprandial hyperglycemia persists despite the diet, the woman will be started on an insulin regimen. Insulin administration is used more and more often today to attempt to reduce macrosomia (overgrowth) in the fetus. With this additional measure, the woman should be able to complete a normal pregnancy without macrosomia and delivery problems in the fetus. The

symptoms of diabetes fade and disappear following delivery as her endogenous insulin again becomes more effective.

Women who develop this phenomenon during pregnancy need to be aware that they may develop diabetes later in life (as many as 20–50% will do so in the next 10–20 years) (Kitzmiller, 1983). A current ethical problem concerns the administration of insulin to women during pregnancy, as this may result in their forming antibodies to insulin and being unable to use it later in life when needed for long-term management.

Musculoskeletal Disorders

As pregnancy usually occurs in young women, musculoskeletal problems in pregnancy are few.

Nursing Care Highlight

The Woman with Diabetes

Goal	Implementations
Prevent congenital anomalies or macrosomia.	Urge woman with diabetes to prevent pregnancy until she has good disease control in order to prevent congenital anomalies in her infant: The first 7 weeks of pregnancy are the most critical time during which fetal anomalies tend to occur.
Maintain glucose/insulin balance.	Support the use of insulin pump therapy during pregnancy.
	Teach women to perform blood glucose monitoring.
	Support women's efforts to change urine testing method to Clinistix or Tes-Tape or Diastix.
	Teach women to maintain a fasting blood glucose between 60–120 mg/dl and a 1-hour postprandial level between 110–170 mg/dl. HgB A1 levels will remain level if occasional hyperglycemia occurs. Use this determination to reassure the woman that her effort at dietary control is worthwhile.
Maintain fetal well-being.	Support women during nonstress tests.
	Use testing times for "practice" sessions for true labor.
	Teach technique of self-monitoring by count-to-ten test.

Scoliosis and Pregnancy

Scoliosis is lateral curvature of the spine; it occurs most often in females about 12 years of age; if not corrected at this time, it continues to grow progressively worse until it causes cosmetic deformity and even interferes with respiration and heart action because of chest compression. Pelvic distortion that occurs in association with this can interfere with childbirth.

Girls with scoliosis may wear a Milwaukee brace during their adolescent years to maintain an erect posture (Figure 36-10). Obviously, such a brace cannot be continued during the last half of pregnancy; this may lead to such increased spinal displacement that a girl is medically advised to abort the pregnancy. Other girls have Harrington rods (stainless steel rods) implanted on both sides of their spinal vertebrae to strengthen and straighten their spine. If such rod implantations are in place prepregnancy, they do not interfere with the pregnancy; a woman will notice some back pain as does the average woman from tension on back muscles. If a woman's pelvis is distorted, a cesarean birth may need to be anticipated for a safe delivery. If a vaginal delivery is permitted, plot the course of labor on a Friedman graph so an unusually long first stage of labor suggesting cephalopelvic disproportion can be recognized.

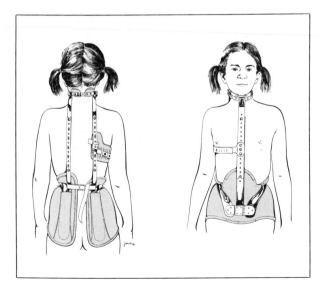

Figure 36-10 *A Milwaukee brace used for stabilization of the spinal column in scoliosis. (Courtesy W. P. Blount, M.D., Professor of Orthopedic Surgery, Milwaukee, Wisconsin.)*

Knee-Cartilage Disorders and Pregnancy

As many more adolescent girls and young adult women participate in sports today than ever before, an increasing number of women of childbearing age have weakened knee cartilage from having dislocated a knee joint during active sports play. During pregnancy, when all body cartilage softens, combined with the excessive abdominal weight the woman carries, the woman may dislocate her knee again.

Any woman who has had a previous knee injury of this type should have it reevaluated early in pregnancy. She may need to wear a knee support such as an Ace bandage or a knee immobilizer for the last 3 months of pregnancy in order to prevent the knee joint from separating again. Discuss with her the advantage of prevention: If the knee cartilage should not be able to sustain her added weight and dislocates again, she will surely fall. (She will then need to have a cast or knee immobilizer applied for about 6 weeks.) Preventing the dislocation prevents possible injury due to a fall and will allow her to be fully mobile at the time she has a new child to care for. She can be assured that a knee immobilizer in place at the time of delivery will not interfere with delivery; if a lithotomy position and stirrups are necessary, a modified stirrups position can be devised for her.

Drug Dependence and Pregnancy

Drug dependence is an increasing problem during pregnancy because it is a growing problem in women of childbearing age. A drug-dependent person craves a drug for either perceived psychological or physical well-being. The number of drugs that can lead to such a state can be categorized as stimulants, depressants, and psychedelics.

Stimulants include drugs such as amphetamines that give a feeling of increased productivity. They are termed *uppers* or *speed* by users. *Depressants* give a feeling of passive, calm well-being. Barbiturates, tranquilizers, narcotics, alcohol, and volatile solvents (airplane glue and gasoline) are examples. These are termed *downers* by users and may be alternated with uppers for increased effect. Sniffing gasoline during pregnancy is doubly dangerous, as this habit can lead to lead poisoning or neurologic damage in both mother and fetus.

Psychedelic drugs give a feeling of "spacing out" or being removed from reality. Drugs such as lysergic acid diethylamide (LSD), phencyclidine hydrochloride (PCP, or angel dust), mescaline or cannabis (marijuana) are termed *trippers* or *hallucinogens*.

The Drug-Dependent Woman

Typically, drug-abusing women are in the younger age group. They have less standardized life styles because they spend their money for drugs rather than for home furnishings. Settled-appearing women may be drug-dependent, however. Use of amphetamines (begun originally as an aid to dieting) is not confined to any one age group. The use of barbiturates and alcohol occurs at *any* age.

Occasional drug use is found in women from all social classes and education levels. Carr (1977) has identified three characteristics of the typical deeply involved drug-dependent woman. She is from a disrupted family background (many of these women leave home as adolescents, they have few meaningful support people and few skills or little education to use to support themselves). She has had negative sexual experiences (many drug-dependent women have been victims of incest or rape). She has low self-esteem. She uses drugs to ease psychological pain, fill a sense of emptiness, and promote social interaction.

A woman who is greatly dependent on drugs is apt to have difficulty following prenatal instructions. Although she means to eat well, if she is addicted to street drugs such as barbiturates or narcotics, she rarely has enough money for both drugs and food. Her nutrition during pregnancy is apt to be inadequate. Further, she is unlikely to have money for supplemental vitamins or iron preparations.

Abused drugs cross the placenta readily. As a result, the fetus of an addicted mother is exposed to the drug. If a woman uses a drug that she injects, she may well develop hepatitis unless her injection equipment is clean each time. Because a majority of women addicts become prostitutes to earn money for drugs, they are likely to contract sexually transmitted diseases, posing an additional threat to the fetus.

The drug-abusing woman may be reluctant to come for prenatal care, afraid that she will be "found out" and reported to legal authorities. She may not have the money to pay for prenatal services or transportation to and from a clinic. If she is using a drug that only sustains her for 4 hours, she cannot wait long at a health care facility to be seen for an appointment.

The infants of drug-abusing women tend to be small for gestation age and to have a higher-than-average incidence of congenital anomalies. They will have the same withdrawal symptoms after birth as the mother would if she abruptly stopped taking the drug.

Because the fetus is exposed to drugs that must be processed by the liver during pregnancy, his or her liver is forced to mature faster than normally. For this reason, newborns of drug-abusing women seem better able to cope with bilirubin at birth than other babies; hyperbilirubinemia is rarely a problem. Fetal lung tissue also appears to mature more rapidly than is normal. Thus even though the infant is born prematurely the chance of developing a condition such as respiratory distress syndrome is less than average.

If at all possible, the narcotic-dependent woman should be enrolled in a methadone maintenance program or a drug withdrawal program during pregnancy. Infants born of a woman on methadone do not escape withdrawal symptoms (some infants appear to have more severe reactions to methadone withdrawal than to heroin withdrawal), but because the woman is being provided drugs legally, the fetus is assured better nutrition, better care, and less exposure to pathogens such as the hepatitis virus. Drug withdrawal symptoms of the newborn are discussed in Chapter 47.

Drug-dependent women need your support during pregnancy. They are women of low self-esteem who need reassurance at prenatal visits that everything is going well with the pregnancy. They need anticipatory guidance throughout pregnancy because they may have no one to share their problems or worries with them or to answer questions about pregnancy for them. Pregnancy may become a stimulus for drug withdrawal so this year in their life can become a maturing and healthy one for them.

The Alcohol-Dependent Woman

Alcohol abuse is a problem for all age groups. Young women may use alcohol to supplement the effect of narcotics or barbiturates. Older women may use it exclusively because it is so readily available and legal and acceptable for their style of life.

Formerly it was believed that alcohol, per se, had no effect on a growing fetus. Any effect during pregnancy was from malnutrition because a woman spent her money on alcohol rather than food. Now it is evident that alcohol itself has an effect on the growing fetus. Infants of alcohol-dependent women tend to be small for gestation age and have mental retardation and an unusual facial appearance, including a prominent nose or bird-like face (fetal alcohol syndrome).

All women should be cautioned not to drink alcohol during pregnancy. Ask at prenatal visits, "What is your usual alcohol consumption?" A term such as *social drinker* is meaningless, and you need to ask a woman who uses it to define it. Some social drinkers drink a cocktail every 3 months; other social drinkers have 5 cocktails every day.

Most women who are alcohol-dependent are not aware of their dependency. The only reason they drink so much, they say, is that alcohol is forced on them at parties or that it is necessary as a part of their job to attend luncheons, receptions, and so forth. They are certain they can stop this very afternoon. When a reason for stopping such as pregnancy occurs, they are distressed to find that they cannot stop. They enjoy alcohol and depend on it to make them feel comfortable at social functions or under stress.

Withdrawing from using alcohol, if a woman is dependent, is as complicated as withdrawing from other drugs. Joining Alcoholics Anonymous is very helpful. A woman's support people may have to be involved in helping her avoid situations where she is most likely to feel the need for alcohol.

At a time in life when she needs to have high self-esteem (she is about to have a baby; that involves thousands of decision-making opportunities every day, and effective decision making requires high self-esteem) a woman discovers that she is not even independent enough to control what she drinks or does not drink in a day's time. She needs reassurance that the things she is doing right are right. Many women with a high alcohol consumption are vitamin B deficient because of the interaction between alcohol and the synthesis of vitamin B. They may need a vitamin B supplement during pregnancy in addition to other vitamins. Care of the infant with a fetal-alcohol syndrome is discussed in Chapter 47.

The Cigarette-Dependent Woman

Smoking is considered a form of drug ingestion because nicotine is absorbed in the process of smoking cigarettes. Infants of cigarette-smoking women tend to be small for gestation age. Furthermore, the incidence of prematurity in these infants is increased, probably because of constriction of uterine arteries due to the vasoconstriction action of nicotine. Prematurity may result from high carbon monoxide levels in the bloodstream.

Stopping smoking is very difficult; one can be as dependent on cigarettes as on any other drug. If a woman cannot stop, she should be urged to cut back the number of cigarettes smoked to 10 per day. All prenatal offices should have prominent *Please, No Smoking* signs.

Women who quit smoking often express strong desires for snack foods, to have "something in my mouth." Review with them at prenatal visits their nutritional intake for the last 24 hours to see whether, now that they are not smoking so much, they are taking in more carbohydrate-rich than protein-rich food. They will invariably gain more weight during pregnancy than might otherwise be expected, and they need assurance at prenatal visits that the extra weight gain is a compensation for stopping smoking, not the sudden weight gain of edema from pregnancy-induced hypertension.

Assure a woman that health personnel appreciate the problem she has in reducing smoking; it is preferable that she gain extra pounds for having stopped smoking than that she deliver a premature baby because of smoking.

Utilizing Nursing Process

Because a medical complication of pregnancy is such a potential threat to a pregnancy outcome, nursing care for a woman and her family must be based on nursing process so the woman can be provided with the best opportunity for a good pregnancy outcome.

Assessment

In order for assessment to be accurate when a woman has a preexisting illness, you must have both knowledge of normal pregnancy health and signs and symptoms of medical illnesses such as cardiac disease or diabetes mellitus that complicate pregnancy. Many of the assessments involve electronic monitoring such as fetal monitoring; other assessments depend on observation of more subjective findings such as the extent of edema or exhaustion. These assessments are best made by health care personnel who care for a woman consistently throughout the pregnancy.

In the absence of a consistent care provider, teach a woman to assess her health in relation to objective parameters. Teach her to report exhaustion, for example, in relation to daily activity. ("Two weeks ago, I could walk a block without being short of breath; today I could walk only half a block. The last time I was in for a checkup, edema did not occur until bedtime; now I notice it every afternoon by the time my child comes home from school.")

Analysis

The North American Nursing Diagnosis Association accepted no nursing diagnoses specific for complications of pregnancy, but many diagnoses related to the signs or symptoms of medical conditions are applicable to these situations. A diagnosis of this kind might be "Air exchange, ineffective, related to lung congestion," "Potential for circulatory inadequacy, related to documented heart disease," or "Potential for fetal macrosomia related to maternal diabetes mellitus." Be certain that goals established are realistic in light of the mother's health and the restrictions placed on her by her health. One family member with illness affects all family members; goals should speak to the entire family's health.

Planning

Planning with a woman with a preexisting medical condition must be done based on the pattern of her life before the pregnancy. Planning adequate rest during a normal pregnancy, for example, usually means planning for two rest periods a day. For a woman with cardiac disease, however, who took two rest periods a day before pregnancy, this would be ineffective planning. Remember that the additional medical supervision needed during pregnancy may involve increased expenses for the family; you may need to help the family plan on ways to meet these needs.

Implementation

A great deal of implementation for a woman with a preexisting medical illness is teaching her the new or additional measures that she needs to take during pregnancy in order to maintain her health so she can remain at home as long as possible and hospitalization can be kept to a minimum. Imaginative solutions to problems must be created or, after a time, a woman may not be able to adjust adequately to the changes she must make.

Evaluation

If evaluation of goals at health care visits reveals that a goal is not being met, new assessment and analysis and planning need to be done. In some instances, a goal is not met because a woman did not appreciate the need for an added pregnancy measure (she is so used to adjusting and compensating for her illness, she feels as if she can sense when she needs further restrictions). Evaluation may reveal that a woman needs more psychological support in order to continue to consistently follow a pregnancy routine. Nine months is a very long time to not know if restrictions or following a new regime is going to be successful or not.

Nursing Care Planning

Angie Baco, 42 years old, is a woman who develops gestational diabetes during her seventh pregnancy. The following is a nursing care plan you might devise for her at 20 weeks of pregnancy.

Problem Area. Regulation of insulin/glucose balance.

Assessment

States, "I feel dizzy all the time. I'm thirsty all the time. My diabetes has come back, hasn't it?" Patient had gestational diabetes treated by diet alone during last pregnancy 7 years ago. One-hour postprandial tolerance test done at 12 weeks of this pregnancy was normal. One-hour postprandial blood sugar done today is 200 mg/100 ml. (Normal is under 190 mg/100 ml.) Urine tests 2+ glucose, trace of acetone on random sample. SG = 1.020. Hydration adequate by skin turgor.

Analysis

Fear related to abnormal glucose/insulin regulation.

Locus of Decision Making. Shared.

Goal. Patient to learn self-care necessary to manage problem of gestational diabetes.

Criteria. One-hour postprandial glucose level to remain under 190 mg/100 ml.

Nursing Orders

1. Patient to test blood serum for glucose once daily at home. To keep a weekly chart and report a level over 120 mg/100 ml.
2. Patient to test urine for glucose and acetone by Tes-Tape four times daily; to keep weekly record.
3. Educate as to signs of hypoglycemia: weakness, dizziness, tachycardia.
4. Patient to ingest a diet of 2,200–2,400 cal/daily as three meals and three snacks.
5. Schedule for hospital admission for evaluation of diabetes and possible insulin therapy.
6. Arrangements must be made for 7-year-old child while mother is hospitalized. Husband to call when arrangements are complete.

Problem Area. Inadequate fetal growth.

Assessment

Uterine height equal to 4 months' gestation. Weight gain 1 lb since last visit (total weight gain is 18 lbs).

Analysis

Potential for inadequate fetal growth related to effect of gestational diabetes.

Goal. Fetal growth to proceed normally during pregnancy.

Criteria. Fundal height measurements to be adequate by McDonald's rule during pregnancy.

Nursing Orders

1. Measure fundal growth at each prenatal visit.
2. Patient to report for weekly health care visit.
3. Instruct in 24-hour collection procedure for estriol collection to begin at 30 weeks of pregnancy.
4. Teach techniques of fetal assessment tests such as nonstress test beginning at 28 weeks of pregnancy.
5. Teach technique of assessing fetal movements for self-monitoring.

Problem Area. Potential for monilial infection.

Assessment

Patient states she has extreme "itching" of vulva. Vulvar area reddened; linear abrasions from scratch marks present. Vaginal examination reveals white, plaque-like lesions that do not scrape away. M.D. confirmed vaginal monilia infection.

Analysis

Potential for monilia infection related to diabetes mellitus.

Goal. Patient to learn self-care to complete pregnancy without further monilia infection.

Criteria. Vagina to be free of plaques on examination for remainder of pregnancy.

Nursing Orders

1. Patient to insert Monostat vaginal suppository two times daily for 7 days.
2. Sexual partner to use nystatin ointment on glans of penis three times daily for 7 days.
3. Educate regarding cotton underpants during day; use no underwear at night.
4. Daily bath and dry well to keep perineal area dry and clean.

Questions for Review

Multiple Choice

1. Mrs. Soo is a woman who develops gestational diabetes. An assessment that you would want to make with Mrs. Soo at each prenatal visit is to
   a. test urine for sugar with a Clinitest technique.
   b. measure increase in abdominal diameter with a tape measure.
   c. test urine for glucose with a Tes-Tape technique.
   d. measure serum for insulin level by a fingerprick.

2. A nursing diagnosis that you might establish related to Mrs. Soo is
   a. potential for hydramnios related to glucose/insulin imbalance.
   b. potential for placenta previa related to diabetes mellitus.
   c. potential for cerebral vascular accident related to diabetes mellitus.
   d. potential for hypertension related to glucose/insulin imbalance.

3. Mrs. Soo is beginning on insulin pump therapy during pregnancy. The advantage of an insulin pump is that
   a. less total insulin will be needed daily.
   b. hypoglycemia during the night is less apt to occur.
   c. insulin administration will be more consistent.
   d. hyperglycemia can never occur.

4. You encourage Mrs. Soo to maintain an active exercise period during pregnancy. Prior to this exercise period, you would advise Mrs. Soo
   a. to inject a bolus of regular insulin.
   b. to eat a high carbohydrate snack.
   c. to eat a complex carbohydrate snack.
   d. to add a bolus of long-acting insulin.

5. The change in insulin during pregnancy that is most apt to occur is
   a. insulin is more effective than normally.
   b. insulin is not released because of pressure on the pancreas.
   c. insulin is not available because it is used by the fetus.
   d. insulin is less effective than normally.

6. Mrs. Cramer is a woman with asthma. Which variation in her disease is most apt to occur during pregnancy?
   a. The change in chest contour will increase her degree of involvement.
   b. The increased level of corticosteroids will decrease symptoms.
   c. Estrogen levels will dilate bronchioles and reduce symptoms.
   d. Symptoms of asthma increase due to increased progesterone levels.

7. What precaution would you advise Mrs. Cramer to take regarding her asthma?

a. continue all her medication for asthma throughout pregnancy
b. stop all medication 2 weeks before birth
c. stop all her asthma medication for pregnancy
d. consult her obstetrician as to the safety of her medications

8. Mrs. Talwin had pulmonary tuberculosis a year ago. During pregnancy, which instruction would you be certain to give her?
   a. maintain a high level of calcium intake
   b. avoid contracting an upper respiratory infection
   c. maintain a high vitamin C intake during pregnancy
   d. be prepared to have her child by cesarean birth

9. Following birth, which instruction would you give her?
   a. Her baby needs a diagnostic test (tine test) for tuberculosis at birth.
   b. Her baby should have a supplement of calcium for at least 3 months.
   c. Tuberculosis bacillus passes in breast milk so she should formula feed.
   d. She should have three negative sputum cultures before she nurses her baby.

10. Mrs. Ford has sickle cell anemia. At her 3-month visit, she tells you that her physician has suggested she have periodic exchange transfusions during pregnancy. Which rationale below explains the purpose for this?
    a. Exchange transfusions remove carbon dioxide from her blood.
    b. Her baby is developing sickle cell anemia.
    c. Exchange transfusion replaces sickled cells with normal ones.
    d. She is becoming jaundiced.

11. Mrs. Ford asks you if her infant will develop sickle cell disease. You would base your answer on which of the following?
    a. Sickle cell anemia is recessively inherited.
    b. Sickle cell anemia has no more than a polygenic inheritance pattern.
    c. Sickle cell anemia is dominantly inherited.
    d. Sickle cell anemia is not inherited; it occurs following a malaria infection.

Discussion

1. You meet a woman who has type I (juvenile) diabetes. She states she is nervous about changing her insulin dose during pregnancy. How would you explain to her the reason for this?

2. A woman with heart disease tells you she is having trouble getting enough rest daily because of two small children she must care for. What suggestions might you make to her?

3. Sexually transmitted diseases during pregnancy have the potential of being teratogenic. What questions would you want to include in a pregnancy history to help assess for these diseases?

Suggested Readings

Bali, C. (1983). Teaching intensive diabetic care in pregnancy. *Diabetes Education.* 9(Suppl), 38s.

Boxall, E. H. (1983). Hepatitis problems in the pregnant and nursing mother and the newborn. *Midwives Chronicle,* 96, 226.

Bullock, B. L., & Rosendahl, P. P. (1984). *Pathophysiology.* Boston: Little, Brown.

Burr, R. E. (1983). Continuous subcutaneous insulin infusion therapy associated with pregnancy. *Diabetes Education,* 9(Suppl), 30s.

Burrow, G. N., & Ferris, G. F. (1982). *Medical complications during pregnancy* (2nd ed.). Philadelphia: Saunders.

Carr, J. N. (1977). Psychological aspects of pregnancy, childbirth and parenting in drug dependent women. In J. L. Rementeria (Ed.), *Drug Abuse in Pregnancy and Neonatal Effects.* St. Louis: Mosby.

Ceresa, C. C., et al. (1983). Nutritional aspects of diabetes care and pregnancy. *Diabetes Education,* 9(Suppl), 21s.

Coustan, D. R. (1981). The pregnant patient with overt diabetes: Practical guide to management. *Perinatology/Neonatology,* 5, 27.

Dansforth, D. N. (Ed.). (1982). *Obstetrics and gynecology* (4th ed.). Philadelphia: Harper & Row.

Dewees, C. B. (1982). Hematologic disorders in pregnancy. *Nursing Clinics of North America,* 17, 57.

Fawcett, J. (1981). Needs of cesarean birth parents. *J.O.G.N. Nursing,* 10, 372.

Frankl, W. S. (1982). Cardiac disease and pregnancy: Better management, fewer surprises. *Consultant,* 22, 213.

Fredholm, N., et al. (1984). Insulin pumps. *American Journal of Nursing,* 84, 36.

Good-Anderson, B. (1983). Home blood glucose monitoring in the pregnant diabetic. *J.O.G.N. Nursing,* 12, 89.

Gould, S. F., et al. (1981). Obesity in pregnancy. *Perinatology/Neonatology,* 5, 49.

Guthrie, D. W., & Guthrie, R. A. (1982). *Nursing management of diabetes mellitus* (2nd ed.). St. Louis: Mosby.

Ho, E. (1984). Diabetes mellitus in pregnancy. *Nursing Mirror,* 158, 37.

Huff, T. A. (1981). Exercise planning for insulin-dependent diabetics. *Consultant,* 21, 71.

Iffy, L. (1981). When diabetes complicates . . . or results from . . . pregnancy. *Consultant,* 21, 61.

Jacobi, A. G. M. (1982). Obstetric anesthesia and the cardiac patient. *Perinatology/Neonatology,* 6, 51.

Jacobson, H. N. (1983). Prevention of prematurity. *Perinatology/Neonatology,* 7, 17.

Kitzmiller, J. L. (1983). Obstetrical care . . . for diabetic women. *Diabetes Education,* 9(Suppl), 41s.

Lalli, C. M., et al. (1981). Pregnancy and chronic obstructive lung disease. *Chest,* 80, 759.

McBride, A. B. (1982). Obesity of women during the childbearing years: Psychological and physiological aspects. *Nursing Clinics of North America,* 17, 217.

McKay, S. R. (1980). Smoking during the childbearing years. *M.C.N.,* 5, 46.

Miller, L. D. (1983). Eisenmenger's syndrome and the pregnant patient. *J.O.G.N. Nursing,* 12, 175.

Miller, N. E. (1983). Nutritional management of diabetes in pregnancy. *Perinatology/Neonatology,* 7, 37.

Nunez, L., et al. (1983). Pregnancy in 20 patients with bioprosthetic valve replacement. *Chest,* 84, 26.

Nyman, J. E. (1980). Thrombophlebitis in pregnancy. *American Journal of Nursing,* 80, 90.

Osborne, N. G., et al. (1984). Sexually transmitted diseases and pregnancy. *J.O.G.N. Nursing,* 13, 9.

Raphael-Leff, J. (1984). Varying needs . . . women vary greatly in their response to birth. *Nursing Mirror,* 158, v.

Reith, S. (1982). Pregnancy complicated by renal failure. *Nursing Times,* 78, 1753.

Richart, R. M. (1979). When a renal transplant patient becomes pregnant. *Contemporary OB/GYN,* 13, 153.

Roberts, J. M. (1979). When the hypertensive patient becomes pregnant. *Contemporary OB/GYN,* 13, 49.

Schuler, R. N. (1979). When a pregnant woman is diabetic: Antepartal care. *American Journal of Nursing,* 79, 448.

Schwalb, R. B., et al. (1984). Preventing infection during pregnancy—and after. *R.N.,* 47, 44.

Ship-Horowitz, T. (1984). Nursing care of the sickle cell anemic patient in labor. *J.O.G.N. Nursing,* 13, 381.

Ueland, K. (1979). What's the risk when the cardiac patient is pregnant? *Contemporary OB/GYN,* 13, 117.

Weil, S. G. (1981). The unspoken needs of families during high-risk pregnancies. *American Journal of Nursing,* 81, 2047.

White, P. (1978). Classification of obstetric diabetes. *American Journal of Obstetrics and Gynecology,* 130, 229.

37

Pregnancy at Age Extremes

OBJECTIVES

Following mastery of the contents of this chapter, you should be able to

1. Describe the special risks of pregnancy in an adolescent and a woman over age 35.
2. Describe pertinent assessments to make with a woman at an age extreme.
3. State a nursing diagnosis related to pregnancy at an age extreme.
4. Plan nursing care that considers the growth and development needs of the adolescent or the woman over age 35.
5. Describe implementations to protect the pregnancy of an adolescent or the woman over age 35.
6. Evaluate goal achievement in terms of both fetal outcome and maternal health and maturity.
7. Analyze the role of nursing care for a pregnant woman at an age extreme.
8. Synthesize knowledge of pregnancy age extremes with nursing process to achieve quality maternal-newborn nursing care.

ALTHOUGH THE AVERAGE WOMAN seen in a prenatal care setting is probably a married young adult who has planned her pregnancy, many women seen in care settings are at age extremes—adolescents who need special consideration because both physically and psychosocially they are immature, and women over age 35 who need yet other special considerations because their bodies may have passed a point of optimum childbearing and whose psychosocial adjustment to pregnancy at this time in life may be difficult. Care of women in these two age extremes is a concern because although the pregnancy rate is declining among the average population, it is increasing in women in these two age extremes.

Adolescent Pregnancy

Nine percent of the U.S. population consists of teenagers. The pregnancy rate is increasing in this age group due to a number of factors: the earlier age of menarche in girls today (many girls begin menstruating at 10 years of age, so are ovulating and able to conceive by 11 years of age); the increased awareness of coitus from the constant bombardment of the media; and a lack of knowledge (or inability to use) contraceptive information (see the Nursing Care Highlight on page 840).

At least half of all teenagers are sexually active (Green, 1983). At one time, this statistic on adolescent sexual activity was very skewed (60 percent of boys but only 20 percent of girls were sexually active). Today it represents an almost equal distribution (about 60 percent of boys; 45 percent of girls). This increased level of sexual activity in girls cannot help but lead to an increased pregnancy rate. The statistic also reflects a life style change among the girls who are pregnant. At one time, adolescent pregnancy occurred in a girl who was very active sexually (the 20 percent of girls who were involved with the 60 percent of sexually active boys). Today many adolescent girls who are pregnant are as sexually exclusive to one partner as are their older married counterparts.

Contraceptive measures that are effective with adolescents are discussed in Chapter 11. An inability to obtain adequate knowledge of contraceptive measures by the adolescent population is a problem that can be dealt with by the health care profession. Providing information, however, does not solve the entire problem: Part of the adolescent population's dilemma is a secondary lack of finances to secure protection such as ovulation suppressants or a diaphragm. A great deal of difficulty arises also from an adolescent egocentric phenomenon that makes girls believe that pregnancy could not happen to them (they are special). An often-not-recognized phenomenon is that many adolescent girls want pregnancy to happen because being pregnant frees them from an intolerable school or home situation and will give them someone to love either through a male who will then offer to marry them or a child who will love them. This phenomenon puts a tremendous responsibility on a newborn baby (to furnish love and change a girl's life); child abuse can occur when the newborn cannot meet these expectations.

The day of the sheltered "secret" home for unmarried pregnant girls, where they would stay for 9 months, deliver, place the child for adoption, and return home as if nothing had happened to them, is almost over. Something did happen, however much a girl and her family wanted to pretend it did not; the girl was left with the psychological scars of starting to love a kicking stranger inside her and then having to give the baby

Nursing Care Highlight

Adolescent Pregnancy

1. One million adolescents become pregnant each year; 30,000 of these girls are under age 15.
2. Births to adolescent girls represent one fifth of all U.S. births.
3. As many as 90 percent of adolescent mothers keep their babies.
4. The maternal death rate for women aged 15 to 19 years is 13 percent greater than for women in their early 20s.
5. Infants of adolescent mothers are two to three times more likely to die during the first year (largely due to immaturity).
6. Fewer than 50 percent of adolescent girls receive prenatal care before the sixth month of pregnancy.

Source: Green, K. W. (1983). Pregnancy in adolescence: Facts, risks, and special considerations. *Consultant, 23,* 187.

---

away, never to be mentioned again. Today, pregnant girls attend prenatal clinics or go to physicians' offices as most older women do. They deliver at community hospitals and the majority of them (as many as 90 percent) keep their babies. Few deliver in alternative birth centers as adolescent pregnancy is a high-risk status. A birthing room within a hospital is possible as long as there is no suspected cephalopelvic disproportion present. Home births for adolescents are not recommended because of the automatic high risk of cephalopelvic disproportion.

The Developmental Crises of Adolescence

As discussed in Chapter 7, pregnancy in an adolescent is particularly fraught with anxiety because the developmental tasks of pregnancy are superimposed on those of adolescence. Developmental tasks of adolescents are four-fold: to establish a sense of self-worth and a value system, to establish heterosexual relationships, to become emancipated from parents, and to choose a vocation. A girl who is in the process of separating from her parents may be devastated by the knowledge that in 9 months someone will be dependent on her. She may have decreased ability to separate from her parents because she needs their financial help more than ever before to obtain prenatal care and buy pregnancy vitamins. If she must depend on their health insurance, she may feel virtually "trapped" into dependence.

Help adolescents at health care visits to make their own health care decisions as much as possible so they can feel independent in the middle of dependency. Making such decisions as where she will hang her medication reminder sheet (on the refrigerator, her bathroom mirror, her school locker) is this type of decision: If it hangs in the kitchen, her mother will monitor it; in her bedroom or in her school locker, she alone will monitor it. She may not be able to choose when she comes for care (the only afternoon her mother has the car to drive her is Tuesday afternoons), but at a visit there are many things she can do to feel independent (weighing herself, holding a mirror to view the pelvic exam, being interviewed separately from her parent).

Parents may have difficulty allowing their daughter to participate in independent health care decisions and you may need to remind them that a pregnant woman of any age may sign permission for her own health care and her infant's health care.

Pregnancy may interfere with the development of a sense of intimacy and cause difficulty establishing future intimate relationships if a girl realizes that her present relationship has led to a situation detrimental to her. In order to prevent this blockage, help her view the pregnancy as a growth-producing experience. Almost everyone can point to a day in their life when they "grew up" (perhaps a day a parent became ill or they left home for college). This pregnancy experience can be her growing-up revelation, or a positive experience for her.

Establishing a value system or a sense of identity can be difficult if health care personnel treat a pregnant adolescent as though she were shameless and irresponsible. It is important that she think of herself as a worthwhile person or she may have trouble establishing a sound value system. In order to be able to make a sound vocational selection, she needs to be encouraged to continue high school even though pregnant so that she can both accomplish her chosen goals in life and support her future child.

Prenatal Care

Adolescents need prenatal care because pregnant teenagers have a high incidence of hypertension of pregnancy, iron deficiency anemia, and premature delivery. They tend to give birth to high-risk infants.

Unfortunately, many adolescents come late for prenatal care. As many as 50 percent do not present for care until they are 6 months' pregnant, well past a point of organogenesis and the main months when teratogenic effects could have occurred. About 14 percent of pregnant adolescents receive no prenatal care (Green, 1983).

Part of this lack of prenatal care occurs because a girl may deny that the pregnancy exists (if no one says that it is so, it is probably not so). Not going for prenatal care is also a way of protecting the pregnancy (if she does not tell anyone, no one can suggest that she have an abortion and end the pregnancy). After the sixth month, abortion is no longer a possibility so she can feel free to come for care without being subjected to this suggestion.

Other factors contributing to the lack of prenatal care are lack of knowledge of the importance of prenatal care and dependence on others for transportation. A girl may feel awkward in a prenatal setting (an adult setting) and frightened about her first pelvic examination. Every community should have a facility that is designed especially for adolescents, or all settings should be as accepting of adolescents as of older women so this last possible reason for poor prenatal care can be eliminated. Failure to design such facilities is a denial of adolescent pregnancy on the part of health care providers.

Health Assessment

The adolescent girl needs a detailed health history taken at her first prenatal visit. It is best to take this history without the girl's parents present. The girl needs practice in being responsible for her own health. Having to account for her health practices during the past month helps her to make this step. It also helps prevent her from fabricating the truth so that a parent does not become angry with her.

Ask at a prenatal visit why there was a delay, if one occurred, in seeking care. Acknowledge that "protecting" a pregnancy is a desirable characteristic, but a better method is to continue with prenatal care.

If a parent of a girl accompanies her, ask her separately if she has any concerns she would like to discuss. A young adolescent is very much still a daughter, and her mother is as concerned about her health during this pregnancy as she was at health visits during which the girl was being seen for a cold or a sports injury.

Fathers involved in pregnancies outside marriage are increasingly accompanying girls into physicians' offices to have the diagnosis established. Although the father has no legal right to participate in a girl's decision concerning pregnancy or abortion, or decisions about whether the child will be adopted or not at the pregnancy's end, he is not devoid of feelings for either the girl or the conceived child. A father may have wanted to marry the girl, even before a child was conceived. He may feel sorrow if he cannot provide adequately for the girl. If a complication occurs, he feels genuine grief in the same way the girl does. He needs compassionate understanding as much as the girl. The concept of the father as someone who irresponsibly used a girl is an old wives' tale and reveals a lack of understanding of human, especially adolescent, behavior.

Adolescents have a difficult time relating to authority figures. This process is made easier if a primary nursing pattern is established during the prenatal period.

Chief Concern

Elicit why a girl thinks she is pregnant (some girls present not with the acknowledgment that they are pregnant but concerns such as "weight gain" or "tired all the time"). Many girls depend on health care providers to think of pregnancy as a possible reason for their symptoms. This passivity is part of denial or pregnancy protection (if you discover the pregnancy, not her, it is less her "fault"; if you are not clever enough to discover she is pregnant, she may not be able to trust you with her secret). Think *adolescent pregnancy* when an adolescent presents with vague, hard-to-define symptoms. If you miss the importance of what she is saying when she is mentioning symptoms such as "tired" and "nauseated," she may ask if someone will feel her stomach. If you say no, there is no reason to do that for any of the symptoms she has mentioned, she may produce bigger symptoms, such as terrible stomach pain. Think *adolescent pregnancy* when you hear a "growing" history. This approach to history giving is potentially dangerous because if the symptoms she mentions are urinary tract problems or back pain, an unsuspecting physician might order an X-ray or intravenous pyelogram to aid in diagnosis.

Adolescents have not been exposed to many women who are pregnant; they may not be aware that symptoms such as urinary frequency, fatigue, and vaginal discharge are common to pregnancy. Asking what symptoms she has and following them with a short, reassuring statement that they are part of a normal pregnancy helps her to resist treating these symptoms with over-the-counter medications.

Many adolescents have irregular menstrual cycles; they may not know the date of their last menstrual flow. They have difficulty with such questions as, "Was your last menstrual flow normal?" (Their knowledge of "normal" is limited.) An adolescent may never weigh herself so be unaware of what her prepregnancy weight level was. Accept this lack of information as one of the problems of caring for an adolescent girl.

As pregnancy progresses, listen for signs of nest-building behavior during a pregnancy history. An adolescent girl may not have the financial resources of a more mature woman for buying clothing or a bed for the baby. She may reveal nest-building best by asking you an increased number of questions about newborns. Suggesting that she make one article of clothing for the baby or save her own money for one article is a way of actively involving her in the pregnancy and gives you a measure of nest-building potential (the girl who week after week spends the money on something else is probably not as involved in the pregnancy as the girl who puts even a dime away a week toward a pair of baby shoes).

Many adolescent girls come late to a health care facility for prenatal care because they had difficulty telling their parents about the pregnancy. Such a girl needs to be urged to tell someone what is happening. Role playing may be an effective technique for helping her. Most girls report on a second visit that their parents were not nearly as angry as they had anticipated. The parents knew that their daughter and her boyfriend were going steady and were being left unsupervised. Some parents react as if they had been waiting to hear this news, having accepted it as inevitable months before.

Family Profile

Adolescents may leave home if their family disapproves of their pregnancy. Others do not leave home, but separate themselves emotionally. Trying to manage by themselves leaves young girls with tremendous financial difficulties and few support people. Ask a girl at prenatal visits where she is living, what the source of her income is, and whom she would call if she suddenly became ill.

Asking about home life may reveal an incestuous relationship. If the girl is under legal age, incest is often considered as child abuse; be aware about its legal status in your state and make the necessary report.

Due to family relation problems, a girl may need help in making arrangements for the next few months. Will her parents allow her to live at home during the pregnancy? If not, is there a relative she may go to? Is there an institution such as a Salvation Army home for unwed mothers in the community that will shelter her during her pregnancy? What kind of financial support does she need? It is important that a girl continue in school if at all possible. A high-school education is necessary to obtain marketable skills. A girl will have little chance of supporting herself and her baby later on if she is not allowed to graduate from high school now.

Once she has the baby, returning to school will be difficult because she will have baby-sitter problems and because she may feel she is more mature than the other girls (or the other girls may make her feel this way). Any school that obtains federal money cannot discriminate against a student for a handicap. Many states interpret pregnancy as a handicapping condition, so in most states a girl cannot be forced to leave school (or even asked to go to an alternative school) because of pregnancy. You may need to be a girl's advocate with the Committee for the Handicapped regarding school placement. Ask at health assessments if she is continuing with school. Pregnancy is an egocentric time when outside interests do not always seem important. Help her to see that the 9 months of pregnancy will go faster if she is busy. Remaining in school and doing well in school is a way of keeping busy.

Past Health History

Many adolescents are very unaware of past illnesses they have had. If a girl does not know about illnesses such as measles or mumps, ask her permission to ask her parent or ask her to obtain this information by the next health visit. Ask specifically about sexually transmitted diseases and whether she thinks any sexual partner of hers has had one.

Ask if she was ever treated for a seizure disorder. Many children are put on long-term seizure medication such as phenobarbital for febrile seizures and then grow so used to taking it that they no longer think of it as medicine. The girl will need to be evaluated in terms of whether she still needs to continue the medication; all seizure medication has a potential teratogenic effect in pregnancy.

Gynecologic History

The average adolescent can describe her gynecologic history (when menstruation began, length of periods, and duration of menstrual cycles). Ask about dysmenorrhea, which is common in young adolescents. Having acute dysmenorrhea may make pregnancy a very desired state for her (no pain for 9 months).

Day History

Few adolescents are aware of how much information can be gained from a typical day history; they will not give good detail unless asked about specifics. Be certain a girl knows the purpose of a day history—so you can learn more about her as a whole—not to discover if she is doing things during the day she should not. Adolescents are very private people; to allow you to walk through their world for a day is a breech of philosophy.

Ask especially for nutritional practices, activity, use of drugs, and support people: These findings have direct influences on the outcome of the pregnancy.

Review of Systems

Finish a health history with a review of systems. Adolescents grow bored with this detailing of body systems. Be certain they view it as a "final mop-up" operation so they can see the end of question-asking is approaching.

Physical Examination

As a technique of physical assessment with teenagers, be certain to comment on findings as you proceed. "This is an accessory nipple. Did anyone ever tell you that before?" is the kind of comment that not only achieves assessment but makes a health examination a learning experience for a girl and relieves anxiety (adolescents tend to be very concerned about body appearance).

During pregnancy adolescents are prone to pregnancy-induced hypertension: be certain to obtain a baseline blood pressure determination at the first prenatal visit. Few adolescents have ever been told what their blood pressure measurement is, even if it has been taken, so they will not know their usual level. Adolescents are often active in a waiting room—walking to get a magazine, returning it, looking out the window—whereas older women tend to accept waiting by seating themselves. Be certain that a girl has 15 minutes of rest before you take a blood pressure or you will measure a false-high recording.

Use a Doppler technique to obtain fetal heart tones if possible; this "proof" helps the adolescent girl accept the pregnancy as real. Make a point of fundal height growth from visit to visit because this change also helps her to see the pregnancy is really happening. Adolescents tend to fail to bring urine specimens with them for their appointments and ask to void for you at the visit. If a girl cannot void, in order not to be criticized,

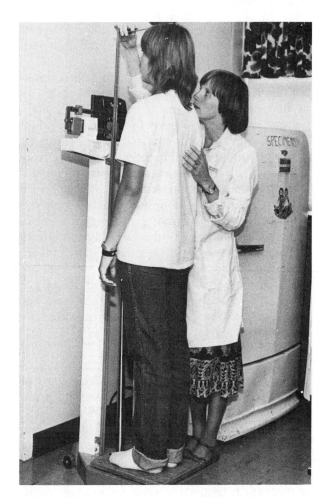

Figure 37-1 *Baseline weight and height measurements are important to an adolescent pregnancy.*

she may return a cupful of water to you as her specimen. If in doubt as to the substance you are testing, check the specific gravity. The specific gravity of water is 1.000. Urine specific gravity ranges from 1.003 to 1.030.

Many adolescents like to weigh themselves at prenatal visits. Weight gain in early pregnancy is one of the ways they have proof that they are pregnant. It is good practice to make a note of what type of clothing the girl is wearing the first time she is weighed (jeans, a halter top) so later weight determinations can be compared more accurately (Figure 37-1).

Prenatal Teaching

Adolescents are often unwilling to follow health care advice if it makes them different in any way from their peers. On the other hand, because adolescents often do not have well-established health practices, they are very "moldable" to well health practices. They need a great deal of health teaching during pregnancy because they do not know many of the common everyday measures of care that an older woman has gained through experience over the years.

Adolescent girls may respond to health teaching that is directed to their own health more than to that of the fetus inside them: "Eat a high-protein diet because protein makes your hair shiny (or prevents split fingernails)." "Taking the iron supplement should make you feel less tired." These are true statements and appeal to an adolescent's preoccupation with self. This type of health teaching is the only form to which the adolescent who is denying her pregnancy can respond. Be careful about overselling the effects of something in health teaching. Adolescents are suspicious of people in authority. If you are caught in a lie, their suspicions that adults are not to be trusted are confirmed, and they may not return to the office or clinic for further care.

Nutrition

Good nutrition is a major problem during an adolescent pregnancy. The girl's diet must not only be sufficient to maintain her own health and allow for growth of the fetus but provide for the needs of her own growing body. Protein, iron, folic acid, and vitamin A and C deficiencies may become acute. Besides eating larger amounts of food than an older woman, the pregnant adolescent must eat the proper foods and possibly abandon the food fads she has been following. Some girls are so peer-oriented that they balk at substituting a glass of orange juice for a cola beverage because no one else they know drinks juice. The best you will be able to accomplish is to secure her agreement to order a noncaffeine soft drink.

Many adolescent girls are very willing to eat a nutritious diet during pregnancy; they simply do not know what good nutrition is. Some girls have little choice in what foods are prepared at home. To change her dietary pattern you may have to talk to the person who cooks for her.

Remember that if a girl is attending school, she eats at least one meal away from home each day. If she travels by school bus, she may have to leave by 6:00 or 7:00 in the morning and need suggestions on how to construct a quick but healthy breakfast. If she leaves home this early she will have a long time interval until lunchtime. Suggest midmorning snacks that are not just empty calories. Be certain that nutrition education includes how to brown-bag or buy a nutritious cafeteria lunch (Type A school lunches are discussed in Chapter 20). Many adolescents eat at least one meal a week at a fast-food restaurant. Teach her to include some meat and to avoid cola beverages because of their caffeine content.

Adolescents are poor takers of medicine. They need frequent reminders that vitamin supplements during pregnancy not only have to be purchased but have to be swallowed as well. Be sure a girl has a medication reminder chart at home.

Weight Gain

Adolescents should gain the usual 11 to 13 kg (25 to 30 lbs) recommended for all pregnant women. You may need to remind some adolescents that it is good to gain weight during pregnancy, especially if they are attempting to hide the pregnancy by trying not to gain.

Activity and Rest

Assess a girl's level of sports activities and which ones should be discontinued during pregnancy (diving, gymnastics, touch football). Some girls play sports not for the exercise per se but for the feeling of "team," or companionship. You may need to suggest alternative activities for her (joining the drama club or a language club, inviting friends over once a week for Monopoly or trivia tournaments), or she will feel the loss of these activities very much.

Adolescent girls may not plan enough rest during pregnancy, especially if they are proceeding as if nothing is happening to them. Exploring their day with them and devising ways they could rest without compromising a busy social calendar is helpful.

Pregnancy Information

A young girl often has distorted concepts about her body. Despite all the health information given to children in school, it still is not uncommon to find an adolescent girl who thinks that her baby is growing in her stomach. Such a girl is unwilling to eat large meals during pregnancy (or eat at all) for fear of suffocating the fetus. All adolescent girls need education on the physiologic changes during pregnancy. They need information about labor and delivery to counteract scare stories from peers. This learning is a way that pregnancy will be a growth experience for them. At the end they will know a great deal more about their body and ability to monitor their own health.

Preparation for Childbirth

Adolescents have a strong need for peer companionship. When they become pregnant, they are cut off from many fellow adolescents. They are often "ripe," therefore, to join a class of adolescents in preparation for childbirth. They are excellent students because being a student is so age-appropriate for them. They have enough magical belief still operating that they are not skeptical about prepared childbirth. Believing that prepared childbirth will work for them is often a self-fulfilling prophecy.

During a course's review of reproductive anatomy, some adolescents who have just completed a biology course may show much more knowledge than do older women. Make a point of noticing this headstart; in other areas such as pregnancy care or "savvy" of childbearing, they will know less than other women.

Delivery Decisions

Pelvic measurements should be taken early and accurately in adolescent girls; cephalopelvic disproportion is a very real possibility due to the girl's incomplete pelvic growth. Most girls respond well to the news that their baby will have to be delivered by cesarean birth and many are frankly relieved. Surgery seems controlled and simple when compared with the agonies of labor that they imagine are in store. The decision on the method of delivery should be shared with the girl and her parents when it is reached by the health care team. It cannot be stressed enough that adolescents, for the most part, want to know the truth. They tend to regard the withholding of information, such as that their child must be delivered by surgery, not as a way of protecting them from worry but as an indication that they are being treated like children.

Plans for the Baby

An adolescent needs additional time at prenatal visits to talk to a good listener concerning her feelings about being pregnant. Scared? Bewildered? Numb? Happy? The plans for the baby should be discussed. Often the girl does not begin to make plans for the baby until very late in pregnancy. She should know the options available so that when she is ready to begin planning she knows the alternatives: keeping her baby or placing the baby in a temporary foster home or for adoption. She needs to make some plans for her life after the pregnancy. Will she continue in school? Try to get a job? Marry?

Complications of Pregnancy

Adolescent pregnancy has an increased incidence of pregnancy-induced hypertension, iron deficiency anemia, and cephalopelvic disproportion. Cephalopelvic disproportion leads to an increased incidence of cesarean births. An adolescent will probably have other children. Although it is not mandatory that all her children be delivered by cesarean birth, having one this way increases the chances for other cesarean births.

Pregnancy-Induced Hypertension

Adolescents are five times more prone to pregnancy-induced hypertension (PIH) than the average woman. Establishing a baseline blood pressure is a problem in adolescent girls because they have probably not had blood pressure taken since a preschool checkup as many as 10 years before. When caring for adolescent girls for any health assessment, make a point of telling them about blood pressure so they will be better health care consumers.

The best intervention for reducing blood pressure during pregnancy is bedrest, preferably in a left side-lying position. Bedrest is difficult for a teenager because she grows bored early and being confined to bed limits her interactions with peers and schooling. Remember many adolescents may rest better if they are lying on a living room couch or a sleeping bag on the kitchen floor where they can be aware of the household activity than in an upstairs bedroom where they have to get up time and again to see what is happening; it is also easier for a parent to enforce bedrest if a girl is within eyesight. If called too many times to a bedroom for small tasks, a mother tends to say, "Get up and get it yourself this time" and breaks the bedrest.

Girls on bedrest at home need activities to keep them busy. Possible chores include homework, obviously. Listening to the radio or a stereo can occupy hours. "Assignments" from the health care agency such as reading about good toys for newborns may be helpful to occupy time. A daily telephone call from the health care facility not only occupies time but shows concern and offers an opportunity to enforce health teaching points.

If a girl is going to be on bedrest for a portion of the pregnancy, she will need to make arrangements for continuing school. If the end of the pregnancy is near, she may be able to have a friend bring her homework assignments. If the bedrest period will be over 2 weeks, however, she will need to make arrangements for home tutoring. You may need to advocate for her with the school system for this service (remembering that only under a few circumstances can it be denied on the basis of pregnancy).

Be certain that a girl does not interpret being placed on bedrest as being *ill.* This feeling may cause her to limit her oral intake (sick people should eat cautiously). It may cause her to limit body hygiene (sick people can not be out of bed to bathe) and so she may develop a vaginal infection.

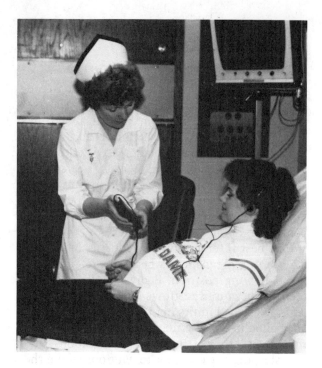

Figure 37-2 *Nurses on units where adolescents are hospitalized serve as adult role models. Here a nurse helps a pregnant adolescent adjust a stereo sound level.*

If the hypertension continues following a period of bedrest at home (or if the symptoms of PIH are acute when they are first discovered) the girl will be admitted to the hospital so bedrest can be better enforced. If you are caring for her during this period, establish a routine of bedrest so she knows exactly what you mean (does it mean strictly confined to bed or allowed to sit up part of the day in a lounge chair with legs elevated? Could she lie on a stretcher by the desk? Can she take a shower once a day? Use the bathroom?). Knowing what the exact rules are from the beginning prevents misunderstandings and hurt feelings (no-one-understands-me situations).

Help find activities that will occupy her. Many adolescents like listening to music; a hospital unit where many adolescents are hospitalized is well advised to buy headphones that fit common pieces of stereo equipment (Figure 37-2) so girls can listen to programs and still keep the noise level to an acceptable level (other women hospitalized on the unit with severe hypertension need quiet to avoid convulsions). If loud music is contraindicated for a girl because of the danger of convulsions, devise activities such as a board game (the girl pulls a card and moves a number of spaces only if she can answer a question such as "What would be a good newborn toy?") or flashcards with similar questions. Such an activity not

only passes time but playing it with staff members exposes the girl to good adult role models and helps to increase her knowledge of newborns or pregnancy.

Another method of controlling fluid accumulation is to reduce a girl's salt intake. Adolescents tend to eat high-salt foods such as potato chips, popcorn, and lunch meats (ham and bologna). Review with the girl how many of these she is eating and help her reduce by subsituting other snacks (unsalted popcorn, fruit).

Thrombophlebitis

Adolescents are at little risk for thrombophlebitis because their veins are so elastic that even with the pressure of the fetus pressing against the pelvic veins, they still achieve good vein flow. Caution girls not to sit with crossed legs and to rest with legs elevated for at least an hour a day, however, so subtle vein changes do not occur that will become extreme varicosities in a future pregnancy.

Iron Deficiency Anemia

Many adolescent girls are iron deficient because their low protein intake cannot balance the amount of iron lost with menstrual flows. A girl's deficiency is revealed by chronic fatigue, pale mucous membranes, and a hemoglobin under 11 gm per 100 ml. Iron deficiency anemia is associated with pica or the ingestion of inedible substances. Adolescent girls' cravings for ice cubes or candy bars may be a further result.

A pregnancy compounds iron deficiency anemia because a girl must supply enough iron for fetal growth and her increasing blood growth. All women—especially adolescents—should take an iron and folic acid supplement (folic acid is important for red blood cell growth) during pregnancy.

Unfortunately, of all age groups adolescents tend to have the poorest rate of medicine compliance. Help a girl plan a daily time for taking her nutrition supplement. If she has to hurry in the morning to get ready for school, she might do better to take the supplement with dinner or along with brushing her teeth at bedtime. Help her to make a medicine reminder chart. At first this seems "childish"; stress that in any busy day, no one has time to remember medicine without one; that you make them out for all women, not just adolescents. Review with her how many iron-rich foods she eats daily; an iron supplement is not a supplement until her diet is already strong in iron-rich foods.

After an adolescent begins on iron therapy,

blood can be drawn in another week for a reticulocyte count to prove that the iron supplement has been taken (as soon as the body has iron, it will begin forming immature red blood cells, or reticulocytes, very rapidly). If the reticulocyte count is not elevated, the girl probably did not take the supplement. Taking a stool swab and assessing it for the black tinge of an iron supplement is another method of evaluating medicine compliance.

Premature Labor

Review with adolescent girls the signs of labor contractions by the third month of pregnancy. Stress that labor contractions begin as only a sweeping contraction no more intense than menstrual cramps. Stress that any vaginal bleeding is suspicious until ruled otherwise. Adolescent girls have gained much of their knowledge of labor from television (where a woman suddenly announces she is in labor and within 15 minutes delivers a baby). They dismiss light contractions as being due to anything but labor. If contractions last for over 15 minutes and nothing appears to be happening, they assume that they are not in labor.

Hemorrhoids

Many adolescents develop hemorrhoids during pregnancy because of the disproportion of their body size to the fetus, which puts extra pressure on pelvic vessels and causes blood to pool in rectal veins. Remind a girl to rest with feet elevated for an hour a day and to sleep in a Sims' position at night to allow good rectal vein flow for this extended time. If hemorrhoids are severe, she may need a soothing cream such as Preparation H (an over-the-counter product). She needs instructions to replace protruding hemorrhoids after a bowel movement (many adolescents are very afraid to do this for fear of rupturing them). Assuming a knee-chest position for 15 minutes at the end of the day is often helpful. Assuring her that this is a pregnancy-related phenomenon that will fade following the pregnancy helps her deal with the problem as short-term.

Striae

Because an adolescent's skin is very elastic, she may not develop striae during pregnancy. Others may develop many striae across the sides of the abdomen because it has to stretch so far because of their small size. Applying cocoa butter or suntan lotion is probably not very effective in relieving these, but it is therapeutic in giving the girl some definite action to take to discourage them. She can be assured that following pregnancy, because she has such elastic skin, these marks will fade with little remaining streaking.

Chloasma

Excess pigment deposition of the face and neck appears as often in adolescents as in older women. Adolescents may be more conscious of this pigment, however, because, overall, they are more conscious and concerned about their facial appearance. Suggesting a cover makeup and reassurance of fading following pregnancy help.

Labor

Adolescent labor does not differ from labor in an older woman if no cephalopelvic disproportion is present. This problem may be suggested by lack of engagement at the beginning of labor, a prolonged first stage of labor, and, finally, poor fetal descent. Plotting labor on a Friedman graph is a good way to detect labor that is becoming abnormal at these points. Be certain that a girl has a support person with her so she can relax during labor and breathe effectively with contractions. If this person is also an adolescent, you may need to serve as the true support person or at least spend considerable time supporting him in order that he can effectively support the girl in labor. It is important that a first labor be a positive experience so the girl does not have to live in dread of a second pregnancy.

The Postpartal Period

Young adolescents are more prone to postpartal hemorrhage than the average woman because, if the girl's uterus is not yet fully developed, it is overdistended by pregnancy. An overdistended uterus does not contract readily in the postpartal period. The young adolescent may also have more frequent or deeper perineal and cervical lacerations because of the size of the infant in relation to her body. On the other hand, young adolescents are generally healthy and have supple body tissue so perineal stretching may occur very readily; if a laceration does occur, it heals readily without complication.

The immediate postpartal period may be an almost unreal time for the adolescent. Birth is a stress for all women and such a major crisis that it is difficult to integrate. It may be particularly difficult for an adolescent to deal with. The girl may block out the hours of labor as if they did not happen; if she was particularly frightened by labor, she may have been administered an amnesic or a narcotic so her memory of the labor hours is unclear. Urge her to talk about labor and delivery to make the happening real to her.

Infant Care

Many adolescents consider themselves to be very knowledgeable in child care because they have baby-sat for a neighbor child or a young brother or sister. They may be overwhelmed in the postpartal period to realize that when the baby is their own, childcare does not seem as simple because of the increased responsibility (when the child cries, they cannot merely hand him over to someone; at the end of 4 hours, when they are tired of caring for the baby, they cannot merely leave him and walk away). Even though you discussed this change with the girl during the pregnancy, these feelings are not real until the child is actually born. Spend time with the girl observing how she handles the infant; demonstrate a bath and changing the baby as appropriate. Model "mothering": She may not have had a good role model and will watch very carefully how you hold and care for the child.

Marriage

Many adolescent girls marry during pregnancy in order to legitimize the pregnancy. For some couples, who were going to be married eventually in any event, this happening is only fulfilling a natural conclusion of the relationship and is sound planning. For others, marriage only compounds their problems by removing them from their important support people. The majority of adolescent marriages entered into under these circumstances do not last over 3 years. Because pregnancy is a poor time for problem solving, many adolescents today are waiting until the pregnancy is over to make this type of life commitment. At the end of 9 months, if the father of the child is still supportive and interested in marriage, a girl might feel they have a chance of making a successful life together.

The Woman over 35

No woman over 35 likes to be referred to as elderly, but women over 35 who are pregnant for the first time are traditionally termed *elderly primiparas*. In the past, it has been assumed that a woman of this age was past the optimum age for childbearing so she would have a great many complications undertaking a pregnancy. In actual practice, there is little documentation that complications (with the exception of greater chromosomal abnormality) increase beyond this age.

A first pregnancy at this age has the potential, however, for being a high-risk pregnancy from several standpoints. A woman is more likely to have conditions such as hypertension, varicosities, or hemorrhoids prior to pregnancy than is a younger woman; these are conditions that, if they increase in severity during pregnancy, can lead to complication. If she has not thought through a pregnancy as a circumstance leading to a long-term commitment and not just a 9-month wait, she may have difficulty integrating the happening into her life.

Even if a woman has been waiting to become pregnant, she has a major role change to undertake because she is probably well established in a career, an accustomed routine at home, or in community groups—or all of these—and she needs to discuss how the pregnancy and childrearing are going to fit into her life. Although she may feel rich in the number of support people she perceives as being around her, she may have few "pregnancy support" people. Perhaps few friends her age are also having babies; some of the women she knows may even be close to becoming grandmothers. This lack leaves her without access to the daily "shop talk" of other pregnant women—someone to turn to, to ask whether the backache or urinary frequency she is experiencing is normal. The only things her friends may remember about pregnancy and labor are their highs and lows (many women that age delivered their children under general anesthesia and actually have little memory of labor).

The woman over 35, then, needs access to health care personnel who can supply her with factual information. She needs a sympathetic ear to listen to her while she works through this role change in her life (Figure 37-3). Because more women are choosing careers today, the number of women who established their career early in life and then begin their families past the age of 30 is also increasing. Nurses need to look directly at the needs of these women, not as a small, unusual section of women, but as representing a major portion of women they will care for.

Developmental Tasks and Pregnancy

The developmental crisis of the over-35 age group is developing a sense of generativity or community awareness. A woman in this age group who is pregnant may begin to feel torn during pregnancy: Half of her wants to continue with her community activities or career commitments and half of

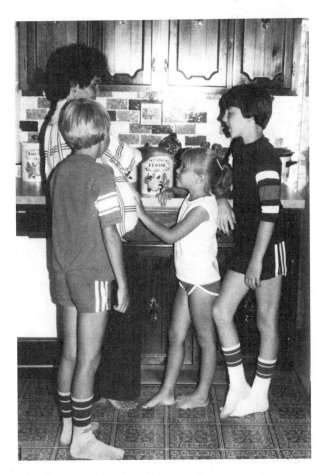

Figure 37-3 *One of the joys of having a child for a woman over 30 is sharing the event with older children.*

her wants to day dream or concentrate on the fetus inside her and her new life. You may need to help her balance her life so she can manage crossing two life spans this way.

Prenatal Care

Because the woman over 35 is more prone to complications of pregnancy she should begin prenatal care early in pregnancy. Unfortunately many women of this age come late for care because they are unable to believe they are pregnant (if they were not planning on being pregnant, they do not believe it; if they were planning on it, they do not believe they are lucky enough to be pregnant). Others mistakenly believe that their lack of menstruation is due to early menopause so they do not seek an early health care consultation.

Women may perform their own pregnancy tests at home to confirm for themselves that they are pregnant. They may then come late for pre-

natal care because they have no need to come early for pregnancy confirmation. Educate women that there are many other important reasons for early pregnancy care than pregnancy confirmation. Knowing that she is pregnant should be more reason for a woman to come for care, not less. As many women this age are employed, you may have to adjust the time for prenatal visits to conform to their work schedule so they continue to come for care regularly.

Most men in this age group were raised to believe that pregnancy was women's business, so they do not accompany their wives for prenatal visits. Urge them to attend with their wives for more active participation in the pregnancy.

Health Assessment

As the average woman is well and does not, unfortunately, go for a yearly physical as many men do, she may have had little experience with health care providers. As for the adolescent, pregnancy at this time of life can be a growth experience for the woman and can serve to acquaint her with a woman's health care facility that hopefully she will continue to attend for the rest of her life.

Chief Concern

Most women in the over-35 age group move confidently through their day, priding themselves on their independent life style and so may feel very foolish that months have passed before they have put together the obvious fact that they are pregnant. Explore with a woman exactly what symptoms she has: Some women mistake pregnancy for menopause, but others mistake menopause for pregnancy. The latter group need counseling on how to accept this phase of their life rather than pregnancy. If a woman did not realize that she was pregnant, she may have self-medicated. Ask if she has been taking any medication to relieve symptoms such as nausea or fatigue she reports.

Family Profile

Many women who are pregnant for the first time over age 35 are women who have recently changed their life pattern (recently married or have only recently become involved in a meaningful sexual relationship). Where a younger woman often waits a period of time after marrying to become pregnant, the over-35 aged woman may plan to become pregnant immediately as she senses her reproductive years are "running out." Because of this feeling of a ticking clock, she may find herself making many adjustments at once (not only adjusting to a new life partner, house or apartment, and perhaps a new community, but now a pregnancy).

Identify her source of income (her income may be large if she is a career woman and stopping work for the pregnancy may reduce her family income greatly); her support people (she may have more complications than the average woman so need more support); and how many people depend on her (children from a partner's former marriage, elderly parents, a workplace that "could not run without her," an elderly neighbor). Pregnancy causes her to turn inward and become dependent to some degree; her responsibilities to these people may make this phase of pregnancy difficult for her.

Past Medical History

Asking a woman about past illnesses not only reveals illnesses the woman has had but her previous relationship to the health care system. Some women were told when they were younger that they might have difficulty becoming pregnant because of endometriosis or because they had a benign ovarian tumor removed. They have a need to talk about how lucky they feel that was not true (and maybe how resentful they are about the time they have spent worrying about it for the past year).

Be certain to ask about kidney and heart disease, circulatory difficulties (particularly a history of thrombophlebitis), diabetes, tuberculosis, urinary infections, abdominal or gynecologic surgery.

Gynecologic History

Some women who delay childbearing until over 35 years of age have used a contraception method such as oral ovulation suppressants for years so the menstrual history they describe to you is strongly affected by this regulation (a "perfect" 28-day cycle). Ask what their cycle was before they began on oral contraceptives: This natural pattern may more truly reflect their menstrual health. If she was taking an oral contraceptive, ask when was the last time she took a pill (if she did not realize she was pregnant, she may have continued taking these into the pregnancy). Flag the chart of a woman who has recently had an IUD removed in order to become pregnant because with an IUD in place, a woman may have had heavy menstrual flows and be iron-deficient.

Ask specifically about whether a woman has ever had a sexually transmitted disease (include herpes in your questioning), frequent vaginal infections (many women on oral contraceptives have chronic occurrence), and if she has a history of endometriosis or pelvic inflammatory disease (adhesions could have formed that make her high risk for ectopic pregnancy). Many women with chronic monilial or trichomoniasis vaginal infections self-medicate with douches. Caution a woman not to continue this self-therapy but to telephone the health care facility for pregnancy instructions on care.

Day History

A day history is a good way to obtain information relating to nutrition, personal habits, sleep, and activity. Think as the woman describes this part of her history how you will need to modify nutrition and rest and sleep counseling based on her life style. Ask specifically about her job and estimate the amount of walking or back strain this entails. Ask about recent diet or exercise programs and if she belongs to a health club (saunas and hot tubs are contraindicated during pregnancy because of the possible hyperthermia). Identify personal habits such as cigarette smoking and alcohol consumption. A great many women in this age bracket smoke cigarettes; business women may drink alcohol daily while entertaining business contacts.

Assess for nest-building behavior. Some women who are good organizers do not buy baby clothing or furniture until close to term, planning to buy everything at once in tightly spaced, efficient trips. They make well-organized lists earlier on, however, of what they will buy; these lists are nest-building actions.

Review of Systems

A review of systems is usually a productive part of a health history in the woman over age 35 as reminders of health areas help her to recall problems she has had that did not come to her mind at first.

Physical Examination

A woman over age 35 needs a thorough physical examination at her first prenatal visit to establish her general health and in particular to identify any circulatory disturbances. Inspect her lower extremities well for varicosities. Be certain to test a urine sample for specific gravity as well as glucose and protein to better assess kidney function.

Assess for fetal heart sounds and fetal movement at prenatal visits as a hydatidiform mole has a high incidence in women over 35.

Prenatal Teaching

Prenatal teaching with these women needs to be adjusted to fit their life style. If a woman has not planned on ever being pregnant, she may have isolated herself through the years from "mothering" activities so despite her years, know little about pregnancy and newborn care. She is knowledge-wise at the same level as a younger woman.

Chromosomal Assessment

Most obstetricians recommend that a woman over 35 years of age have a chorionic villi aspiration performed at 5 or 6 weeks or an amniocentesis performed at the fourteenth to sixteenth week of pregnancy for chromosomal analysis and a serum alpha-fetoprotein level drawn at the fifteenth week of pregnancy for detection of an open spinal cord defect (see Chapter 15). Be certain a woman is well prepared for these studies and receives support during them as they are very real "test" situations. Many women of this age group do not begin nest-building until these analysis points and confirmation that the child will probably be healthy are past. She may have a non-stress test scheduled for about the thirtieth or thirty-fourth week of pregnancy for evaluation of placental function.

Nutrition

Assess the number of meals a woman eats outside her home each week, including those she packs as a lunch or eats in restaurants. She may need some tips on how to adjust pregnancy nutrition so she can obtain the same nutrition whether she prepares meals at home or eats them at an office or school lunchroom. Be aware that many business luncheons or dinners are introduced with cocktails. Urge her to substitute a caffeine-free soft drink. In some offices a lot of time is spent drinking coffee. Urge her to substitute milk or juice. Many women this age drink little milk. Rather than changing her liquid intake habits, she may appreciate suggestions on other ways to ingest milk such as in puddings or yogurt.

Prenatal Classes

Because a pregnant woman over 35 is often "one of a kind" in her circle of friends, she may feel shut out of her usual group because of the pregnancy. She may be ripe, therefore, to join a preparation-for-childbirth class where she can be one of a group. Discussion at this type of class may center on how different she is from her friends and the stories they have told her about labor or delivery. Urge her to listen to her friends' memories of childbirth, but to also remember that if they are describing 15- to 20-year-old experiences, their impressions may have blurred over the years and at best they are not describing current obstetrical practices. Help her recognize that many of her friends delivered their children under a general anesthesia because that was once accepted practice, not because labor is so terrible that they needed anesthesia to endure it. Urge her sexual partner to attend prenatal classes; he may at first feel uncomfortable until he realizes that most men today feel that participating in labor is not only expected but a potential highlight of their life.

Be certain a woman plans (or they plan together as a couple) on set times during the day when she will do breathing exercises; otherwise, in a busy day she will never find time to include these preparations for labor.

Complications of Pregnancy

The complications of pregnancy that a woman over age 35 is most prone to are those related to a less competent circulatory system and less elastic body tissues.

Hemorrhoids

A woman over age 35 is very prone to hemorrhoids as she probably has some degree of rectal varicosities present at the beginning of pregnancy. Pain from rectal distention may, in fact, be one of her primary symptoms that she reports at a first visit. Urge her to *prevent* hemorrhoids or further hemorrhoidal distention by being certain to rest for at least an hour daily with her feet elevated and to sleep in a Sims' position at night for good rectal vein drainage. Assuming a knee-chest position for 15 minutes at noon and at bedtime is a good prophylactic measure for her as well. Help her plan how to arrange a "feet up, shoes off" time at work (she may have to pass up going to lunch with the office staff and eat a packed lunch at her desk or use a free classroom period, not standing duplicating material but resting with her feet elevated). Urge her to eat a diet high in fiber to avoid constipation and to manually replace protruding hemorrhoidal tissue following a bowel movement. You may need to suggest that her nurse-midwife or obstetrician prescribe a stool softener for her in order to keep constipation from adding to the problem of hemorrhoidal formation.

Varicosities

Varicosities, like hemorrhoids, develop readily in a woman over 35 because she may have some tendency toward them even before the pregnancy. As with hemorrhoids, her best measure during pregnancy is to *prevent* varicosities rather than to allow them to develop and then attempt to diminish them by resting daily with her feet elevated and sleeping in a Sims' position at night. Many business women who attend meetings each day spend their time sitting with their legs crossed. Urge a woman to refrain from this habit.

A woman's nurse-midwife or physician may prescribe support stockings during the later half of pregnancy in order to prevent further varicosity formation. Be certain she knows to put these on before she gets out of bed in the morning because once she is out of bed and walking the veins have already filled and the stockings are not as effective. This means she may have to adjust her hygiene pattern to a shower before bedtime instead of a shower in the morning. Because support stockings invariably do not look as delicate as nylon stockings, a business woman may be tempted to not wear them on "important" days. Check with her at visits how may days a week she is talking about. You may discover that she is omitting wearing the stockings half the time (which is her choice, but be certain she knows the possible consequences of permanent varicosities). Many women with extensive varicosities develop vulvar varicosities as pregnancy progresses. Urge a woman to wear loose undergarments for comfort. Resting with her feet elevated is also a good preventive measure.

Flag the chart of a woman with any degree of varicosity formation during pregnancy so nurses caring for her during the postpartal period can take special precautions to prevent thrombophlebitis. With venous stasis present, she is very prone to develop this problem.

Striae

A woman over 35 may develop more abdominal striae than a younger woman because of the relative inelasticity of her abdominal wall. These marks are often not as upsetting to her as to a younger woman, however: A younger woman worries about marks accumulating from a number of pregnancies; an older woman can foresee that she will have few additional pregnancies and so is not overly threatened by accumulating striae. She also has less tendency to wear revealing bathing suits or types of clothing that show abdominal marks.

Chloasma

Facial pigment may be distressing to a woman who earns her living meeting people daily in a business setting. She may need some help ap-preciating that everyone accepts these facial changes as part of pregnancy and indeed many people probably view her as more attractive—literally full of life. She can use makeup to cover these changes if they are distressing to her.

Pregnancy-Induced Hypertension

Women over 35 may have a higher incidence of pregnancy-induced hypertension than younger women, possibly related to inelasticity of blood vessels. The best way to reduce the symptoms of PIH is for a woman to rest a large portion of each day. A woman with a career may find this very difficult, not only because she feels she may "miss out" on a promotion or advancement at work if she is away from work for so long a time span but because she is used to accomplishing tasks during a day, not merely lying in bed. In order to allow her to rest effectively, you may need to help her plan activities she can accomplish on bedrest (rework her school course outline, restructure a software application), or work on a hobby such as embroidery that she has wished for years she could find time for.

If resting at home is not effective in reducing symptoms, she will be admitted to the hospital where bedrest can be better enforced and antihypertensives begun. Remember that a woman may be a new marriage partner so separation may cause a major strain on the new marriage. You may need to advocate for increased visiting time for her husband and provision of privacy for them as a couple so he does not feel shut away from her.

Iron Deficiency Anemia

Iron deficiency anemia is a potential problem of all women; as mentioned, if a woman had an IUD in place for contraception, it is a particular problem. Be certain the woman hangs a reminder sheet on her refrigerator door or bathroom mirror or at her office to remind her to take her iron supplement daily. A usually well organized woman may think she will be able to remember without help, but pregnancy distorts memory. Without a reminder sheet she may forget easily.

Labor

Labor in the "elderly" primipara may be prolonged as cervical dilatation may not occur as spontaneously as in the younger woman. Plotting labor on a Friedman graph is a good method of evaluating labor progress. A number of women this age will need to have a cesarean birth when labor becomes overly prolonged and the fetus becomes at risk. Urge women to ask for a regional anesthetic if possible for cesarean birth so they can stay awake. Urge a support person to view the birth even if a woman is anesthetized (it is his baby too).

Men over 35 may not be comfortable with participating in labor or watching the birth of their child. They may need increased urging to participate in labor and support to be an effective coach in labor.

The Postpartal Period

Women in the over-35 age group during the postpartal period may begin to have second thoughts about planning a pregnancy so late in life. The reality of the happening truly registers with them during this period. Although they have read a great deal during pregnancy about babies, they may wish they had read more or were as confident with this phase of their life as they are about the courtroom or school room they are in charge of. Review with women their plans for childcare and postpartal rest so they can balance their life. They may plan on returning to work almost immediately if their work policies do not allow a long maternity leave.

Hemorrhage

Just as the uterus at this age may not dilate as readily during labor, so it may not contract as readily postpartally. The woman is high-risk for a postpartal hemorrhage. Observe her closely as she also tends to be an independent woman who is interested in doing self-care. She may ask for few measures of care from you that would allow you to readily assess the amount of lochial flow.

Marriage

A problem of the adolescent who becomes pregnant is whether to marry or not; a problem of the older woman may be whether to *remain* married or not. If the pregnancy was the result of a new marriage, a woman may be very distressed if her partner has told her that he does not feel the same level of commitment to the new child she does. If the marriage has been a long-term commitment she may be surprised that, in the end, she and her partner seem to have so little in common. They might benefit from marriage counseling as neither of them may have been aware of how much stress a pregnancy entails and the level of concern it is causing in their lives. A woman needs time to discuss how she feels about a pregnancy; if still early in pregnancy, she may change her mind and decide to end the pregnancy. She should be made aware that placing the child for adoption is a possibility for her as it is for a younger woman. Once she is certain that she will continue the pregnancy and keep the child, she needs to problem solve how her life will change as the single parent of a child at this stage in her life.

Utilizing Nursing Process

Because women who are at age extremes are high risk for complications of pregnancy, labor, and the puerperium, nursing care during these times must be designed by the use of the nursing process in order to be comprehensive.

Assessment

Many adolescents feel that their world is totally separate from the adult world and, in order to keep it separate, do not share information voluntarily. They also resent adults who imply that they feel comfortable in a young world. Be certain in interviewing that you press for information that you need in order to assess safely and do not accept statements such as "I eat okay" as a nutrition history or "I'm a very active person" as a history of rest and activity. Women over 35 need their life style analyzed to see what modifications are necesary for pregnancy.

During a physical examination, be certain to explain findings for adolescents. A statement such as "Oh, you're starting to have colostrum," meant to be a positive finding of pregnancy, may be very frightening to an adolescent who does not know she is expected to have a breast discharge during pregnancy. Explaining not only a finding's presence but its meaning helps to make a pregnancy a growth experience for a girl.

Remember that a woman who has removed herself from the world of babies and homemaking to follow a career may, like the adolescent, have less awareness of normal pregnancy findings or healthful pregnancy practices than the average woman. Be certain that you do not equate knowledge in one field such as chemistry or law with knowledge about pregnancy.

Analysis

The nursing diagnoses associated with pregnancies at the age extremes are different in degree only, not substance, from the nursing diagnoses of all pregnancies. When establishing goals with adolescents, be certain they are realistic in relation to the girl's age. She cannot achieve goals that rely on her independently making decisions if such decisions are not hers to make.

Planning

A major problem with both the adolescent girl and the older woman is that they may not be interested in planning early in the pregnancy (hard time accepting the pregnancy as real). Adolescents are also at a point in life when inexperience makes problem solving difficult.

Implementation

A major reason that adolescents do not come for prenatal care is that they do not feel comfortable in a health care facility. Allowing adolescents as many independent decisions as they are capable of helps them to "fit in." A woman who is having her first baby late in life may be equally annoyed at having to wait at a prenatal visit because she is used to feeling in charge and may be certain she could organize your work more efficiently. Both these reactions reflect the difficulty a person is having integrating pregnancy into her life.

The mark of implementations for both these age groups is to *prevent* pregnancy complications so a great deal of implementation is concerned with teaching and allowing a woman to choose her best course depending on her particular needs.

Evaluation

Because bonding may be more difficult if a child arrives at a less-than-optimum point in life, evaluation of a woman at an age extreme should include evaluation of both the woman and her relationship to her new child. Evaluation may reveal that additional follow-up or referral is necessary to be certain that a woman truly chooses the time of her next pregnancy and that a child will be raised in an environment of love and healthy growth.

Nursing Care Planning

Kathy Benson is a 37-year-old woman having her first pregnancy.

Chief Concern. "I think I'm pregnant."

Assessment

Patient states she is "constantly tired"; LMP July 8; slight spotting July 30; now clear vaginal discharge present. Breasts tender and areola are darkened. Patient is married; registered nurse; works 12-hour shifts in an ICU 4 days/week.

States: "I can't stop work." Husband is partially disabled due to work accident. Patient supports husband and three children from husband's previous marriage. Admits to not eating breakfast because of early hour she leaves house.

P.E.: Breasts full and firm; venous congestion present. Fundal height 2 cm above symphysis; FHS at 140/minute by Doppler. Prominent varicosities present on left thigh and left vulva.

Analysis

Concern over maintaining life style related to pregnancy.

Locus of Decision Making. Patient.

Goal. Patient to maintain acceptable life style during pregnancy.

Criteria. Patient to continue work throughout pregnancy.

Nursing Orders

1. Urge patient to alert nursing supervisor to pregnancy.
2. Urge patient to ask for a change of unit assignment during pregnancy (12-hr days, with varicosities present, and level of X-ray exposure in ICU need to be reduced).
3. Plan ways that two rest periods can be provided daily (lunch, work breaks, etc.)
4. Review and strengthen pregnancy nutrition.
5. Urge support hose to reduce varicosity formation.

Questions for Review

Multiple Choice

1. Ann is a 15-year-old adolescent who is 6 months pregnant the first time she comes for prenatal care. She says she had no idea she was pregnant. You would assess this failure as more likely a manifestation of

   a. ignorance of pregnancy signs.
   b. denial of the pregnancy.
   c. general low intelligence.
   d. lack of signs of pregnancy present.

2. Ann asks you if her boyfriend (father of the baby) can come into the examining room with her. Based on his needs, your best response would be
   a. "Adolescent fathers have no legal right in regard to a child."
   b. "If you want him to come in."
   c. "If your mother approves."
   d. "Childbearing is only women's business, even in adolescence."

3. Ann develops hypertension of pregnancy and is confined to bedrest at home. Considering the developmental tasks of adolescence, which problem below is most apt to worry Ann at this point?
   a. difficulty determining what kind of person she is
   b. inability to participate in community activities
   c. inability to interact with younger brother and sisters
   d. concern over inability to complete a school project she started

4. In planning care for Ann, which procedure below would be most age appropriate?
   a. Insist that Ann have no further sexual relations during pregnancy.
   b. Ask Ann to delay schooling until the pregnancy is over.
   c. Permit Ann to decide on the total weight gain for her pregnancy.
   d. Allow Ann to weigh herself at clinic visits.

5. Nutrition counseling is a priority topic during an adolescent pregnancy. Which topic below could you anticipate you will need to cover?
   a. ways that Ann can learn how to cook her own food
   b. ways to obtain good pregnancy nutrition in restaurants
   c. ways to remember to take an iron supplement daily
   d. nutritional advantages of fresh foods over frozen

6. Ann is angry that she was denied permission to deliver her baby at an alternative birthing center. You would recognize the reason for refusal as
   a. alternative birth centers admit only married women.
   b. she must have been rude to the center director.
   c. she is high-risk for pelvic disproportion.
   d. her parents must have disapproved of the center.

7. Ann asks you if she should take a prepared-childbirth course. Your best response would be

   a. "Adolescents are generally poor students so do not do well in such courses."
   b. "Adolescent labor is so different from normal that the course material will not apply."
   c. "The chances for cesarean birth are so high the material would probably not be used."
   d. "Women of any age are well advised to begin labor with prepared childbirth."

8. Ann delivers an 8-pound boy after a 12-hour labor. In the postpartal period, which of the following would be a priority concern to assess for?
   a. postpartal hemorrhage
   b. endometritis
   c. thrombophlebitis
   d. amniotic embolus

9. Beverly is a 37-year-old woman you meet in a prenatal clinic. Which implementation below can you anticipate you will most likely be including in your plan of care?
   a. Helping Beverly decide on what clothing to wear during pregnancy.
   b. Evaluating Beverly's tolerance for pain.
   c. Scheduling Beverly for fetal chromosomal analysis.
   d. Scheduling Beverly for special electrolyte analysis.

10. Beverly states she has little time for pregnancy exercises. Which one below would you stress as most important for her to do?
    a. Jogging to strengthen thigh muscles.
    b. Sims' resting position to reduce varicosities.
    c. Tailor sitting to keep her lumbar spine flexible.
    d. Slow chest breathing to allow for uterine expansion.

Discussion

1. Helping adolescents to be responsible for their own health care aids achievement of a sense of identity. What are areas that even a very young girl could be responsible for during pregnancy?

2. A very young woman and an older woman have many similarities both psychologically and physiologically. What are ways in which they have similar needs?

3. Adolescents and older women both attend preparation for parenthood courses. How would you modify a class if the couples attending were mostly adolescents? Most over-age-35?

Suggested Readings

Burke, A. (1983). Community health model for pregnant teens. *M.C.N., 8,* 340.

Catrone, C., et al. (1984). A developmental mode for teenage parent education. *Journal of School Health, 54,* 63.

Cohen, S. J. (1983). Intentional teenage pregnancies. *Journal of School Health, 53,* 210.

Daniels, M. B., et al. (1983). A clinic for pregnant teens. *American Journal of Nursing, 83,* 68.

Donlen, J., et al. (1981). Teenage mother . . . high risk baby. *Nursing (Horsham), 11,* 51.

Green, K. W. (1983). Pregnancy in adolescence: Facts, risks and special considerations. *Consultant, 23,* 187.

Haire, M. F. (1982). Beyond 35 and pregnant: Every reason for optimism. *Perinatology/Neonatology, 6,* 57.

Holley, C. (1981). The older primipara: Implications for nurses. *J.O.G.N. Nursing, 10,* 182.

Horn, B. (1983). Cultural beliefs and teenage pregnancy . . . among ethnic groups in the United States. *Nurse Practitioner, 8,* 35.

Jacobson, H. N. (1983). Prevention of prematurity. *Perinatology/Neonatology, 7,* 17.

Mercer, R. T. (1983). Assessing and counseling teenage mothers during the perinatal period. *Nursing Clinics of North America, 18,* 293.

Neeson, J. D., et al. (1983). Pregnancy outcome for adolescents receiving prenatal care by nurse practitioners in extended roles. *Journal of Adolescent Health Care, 4,* 94.

Robinson, B. E., et al. (1982). Issues and problems related to the research on teenage fathers: A critical analysis. *Journal of School Health, 52,* 596.

Sacks, D. (1981). Pregnancy among teenagers. *Canadian Medical Association Journal, 124,* 960.

Sadovnick, A. D., et al. (1982). Maternal age-specific costs of detecting Down's syndrome and neural tube defects. *Canadian Journal of Public Health, 73,* 248.

Santangeli, B. (1984). Adolescent pregnancy. *Nursing Mirror, 158,* 32.

Sapala, S., & Strokosch, G. (1981). Adolescent sexuality: Use of a questionnaire for health teaching and counseling. *Pediatric Nursing, 7,* 33.

Schneider, S. (1982). Helping adolescents deal with pregnancy: A psychiatric approach. *Adolescence, 17,* 285.

Sewall, K. S. (1983). Peer group reality therapy for the pregnant adolescent. *M.C.N., 8,* 67.

Stein, A. (1983). Pregnancy in gravidas over age 35 years. *Journal of Nurse Midwifery, 28,* 17.

Ulvedal, S. K., et al. (1983). Profile: Pregnant teens who choose childbirth. *Journal of School Health, 53,* 229.

Weil, S. G. (1981). The unspoken needs of families during high-risk pregnancies. *American Journal of Nursing, 81,* 2047.

38

The Handicapped Woman

OBJECTIVES

Following mastery of the contents of this chapter you should be able to

1. Describe types of handicapping conditions that can influence pregnancy outcome.
2. Assess a woman with a handicap for assets that are important to childbearing and childrearing.
3. State a nursing diagnosis related to a problem of a woman with a handicap during pregnancy.
4. Plan nursing care that is specific to the needs and wishes of a woman with a handicap.
5. Implement nursing care that meets the special needs of a woman with a handicap.
6. Evaluate if goal criteria related to the needs of a woman with a handicap are met.
7. Analyze ways that nursing care could better meet the needs of a woman with a handicap during a childbearing year.
8. Synthesize knowledge of handicapping with nursing process to achieve quality maternal-newborn nursing care.

In the past, women with handicapping conditions such as vision or hearing impairment, mental retardation, spinal cord or orthopedic injuries were kept sheltered by their families to such an extent that even with a moderate handicap they did not become (and, it was believed, should not become) pregnant. Although care of a woman with a handicap was important to nursing as a whole, there was little application to the maternal-newborn area of care. Today, women with considerable degrees of handicapping attend public schools, work in offices, join community organizations, and so marry or establish sexual relationships. They also plan pregnancies. Because they face special problems due to their handicap during pregnancy (some of them have a support person who is also handicapped), nursing care during pregnancy must be specially designed to meet the individual woman's problems and needs. Discussed below is specific care for the woman with a sensory, motor, or intellectual handicap. General areas of care to be focused on are summarized in the box on page 859.

The Rights of the Handicapped

By federal law, handicapped persons must have freedom of access to or use of ramps or handrails in public buildings so they can enter or leave safely. You need to evaluate whether any health care agency that you work in is complying with these laws not only in terms of physical facilities but in the true spirit of the law (people are psychologically welcome as well as physically able to reach the inside of the building). By the same law, a hospital cannot deny care to a person with a handicap even though the handicapping condition considerably complicates care and may require extra personnel.

The Woman Who Is Visually Impaired

Although a number of visually impaired women of childbearing age have an impairment from an accidental injury in childhood, the average woman who is visually impaired has been so since birth. Some women are born with congenital eye defects such as lack of eye formation or cornea or lens destruction from rubella invasion while they were in utero; some of them were born prematurely and have retinal damage from the use of oxygen at their birth. When women have always been blind, they do not grieve for their lost eyesight but tend to have a positive "I can do it" attitude about their ability to accomplish. This is a positive characteristic to reinforce during pregnancy, and prenatal care is aimed at helping them find ways to complete a pregnancy safely and make plans for childrearing.

Degrees of Impairment

A designation of visual impairment means that a woman has some loss of vision; this could range from just loss of peripheral vision to full lack of eyesight, however. A woman with loss of peripheral vision will have few special problems during pregnancy, as by turning her head she can bring objects into her area of central vision. She may be unable to drive and be dependent on a support person for transportation. A woman is legally blind if her visual field is no greater than 20 degrees or central distance vision in her better eye is 20/200 or worse with the use of corrective lenses.

Areas of Planning Care for
Pregnant Handicapped Women

Area	Assessment
Transportation	Ask if a woman has transportation for prenatal care and for emergencies.
Pregnancy counseling	Assess the special modifications of care that will need to be made depending on a woman's special handicap. Use additional visual or sound aids in order to make your teaching points clear.
Support person	Assess who is the woman's support person. In some instances the woman's condition requires so much assistance during pregnancy that one support person will not be enough. If necessary, contact community agencies to lend second-ring support.
Health	Do not lose track of the fact that a woman has a primary health problem. The woman with cerebral palsy will need to continue an active muscle exercise program during pregnancy for her primary illness.
Work	Assess whether a woman works outside her home and, if this is discontinued during pregnancy, what she could substitute for a social contact activity. Many women with a handicapping condition are lonely because they do not have a wide range of friends or social contacts.
Recreation	Many women with a handicapping condition lead a rather sedentary life (partly because they do not have social contacts). Assess whether her level of activity is adequate and make concrete suggestions within her limitations.
Self-esteem	Assess a woman's level of self-esteem as it may be low due to repeated failure situations in her life. Give praise at prenatal visits to increase her confidence and allow pregnancy to be a growth experience for her.

A person with loss of central vision has greater difficulty because she is limited in more ways.

Prenatal Care

Visually impaired women need to come early and consistently for prenatal care because they may not be able to self-assess for some of the danger signs of pregnancy such as diplopia, blurriness of vision, or vaginal spotting. Because the woman may depend on her support person to furnish transportation to the health care facility, you may need to schedule appointments for her only at those times that this person is free to drive her or she will miss many visits. If a woman brings a guide dog with her, mark the dog's name as well as hers on the chart so you can also greet the dog by name. Although a guide dog's chief function is to offer her direction, its natural instincts cause it to become her protector. Caution small children of any other woman present in a waiting room not to pet the dog as, meaning to protect, it may snap at the sudden, unexpected movement of small children.

Health Assessment

In interviewing or health teaching, do not use your hands to illustrate points ("I'll need a urine sample of at least this much [measured with your fingers] urine"). Be careful not to raise your voice as you interview to make a point (the woman is visually impaired, not hearing impaired, and will still not understand your point). Do not use colors as descriptions of items ("put on the blue gown").

It is important to obtain a reason for a woman's

impaired vision at a health history, because the cause might suggest not only a genetic inheritance pattern but also a problem the woman is apt to be concerned about during pregnancy. If a woman is blind, for example, because she was born prematurely, she may be fearful that her baby will also be born early; she may be fearful at hearing her baby received even a wisp or two of oxygen at birth. If her lack of eyesight was caused by an inherited disorder, she has reason to worry that her child will inherit the same disease. If the cause of her lack of eyesight was rubella, she may be concerned if she develops even a mild upper respiratory illness during pregnancy.

Family Profile

Ask about a woman's financial resources (all persons legally blind are eligible for financial assistance through Social Security benefits) and whether this amount will be adequate for pregnancy expenses. Ask who else lives with her and who she turns to if she has a problem. Some women have met their husband or sexual partner through an agency for visually impaired persons and so have a life partner who is also blind. Investigate how the woman would contact the health care agency if she had an emergency such as ruptured membranes. If she is visually impaired but has some eyesight, write an emergency telephone number in large letters for her to tape over her telephone. If she has no vision, but reads braille, ask if she has access to a braille typewriter (she may own one or work in a sheltered workshop that has one). The number can then be written in braille for her. Ask who she could rely on for transportation in an emergency (possibly a neighbor or a friend).

Ask about the woman's education level. It is possible for a visually impaired woman to have finished college and even a doctoral program and to be very knowledgeable about body physiology and function. Do not make the common mistake of assuming that a handicap is associated with mental deficiency or a handicapped person has received poor schooling.

Pregnancy Counseling

If both a woman and her support person are fully visually impaired, use of pamphlets about pregnancy care is limited. If the woman's support person has vision, offering them to him and suggesting he read them to her as a shared activity will not only be helpful but will make him a more informed support person.

Schedule prenatal visits as needed in order to cover orally all the information she needs to learn to be informed about her pregnancy. Using three-

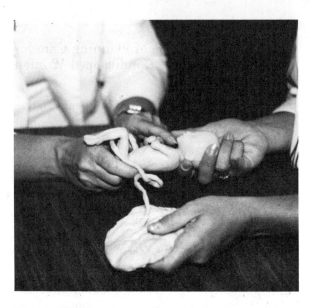

Figure 38-1 *Health teaching with handicapped women is modified to meet their particular needs. It often uses increased auditory or visual stimulation.*

dimensional models of anatomy or fetal growth is helpful in allowing a woman to appreciate how big her child is month by month (Figure 38-1). Many visually impaired women have a tape recorder that has been supplied free of charge to them from Recording for the Blind, a national, nonprofit, voluntary organization. Telephone the local association for the visually impaired and ask if they have any material already recorded on pregnancy or breast-feeding they could supply. If not, make a tape recording of any information you particularly want a woman to remember or she seems concerned about. You could supply the health care facility telephone number at the very beginning of the tape so in an emergency she could use this source for the emergency number; supply the date of her return visit this way also.

Discuss her level of activity during pregnancy. If she depends on the sound of a cane against sidewalks to direct her while she walks, she may not go out on days when there is snow or ice that obscures the sound. Stress that walking is important during pregnancy so if she cannot go outside then walking in her apartment or home achieves the same end in promoting venous return from lower extremities. Women with a visual impairment develop a keen sense of hearing and touch. At visits, use a Doppler instrument to listen to fetal heart sounds so she can hear them also; show her how to assess her ankles and fingers for edema as she will be able to assess for this danger sign of pregnancy very well.

When nutrition counseling, investigate her knowledge of good nutritional patterns. Investigate who does the cooking in her household. She may cook breakfast and lunch, preparing meals that do not require a stove; her support person may prepare a cooked evening meal. Nutritional counseling, for two meals daily, therefore, may need to center on foods that can be prepared without cooking. Do not be reluctant to use food names such as "green, leafy vegetables" or "oranges" when discussing food. Although these words are colors, they are also the only names these foods are known by.

Physical Assessment

When helping with or doing physical assessment, make a point that you are closing the room door or drawing a curtain to assure her that you are providing privacy. Always alert a woman that you are going to touch her before you do to avoid startling her. If the woman uses a guide dog who is lying at her feet during an interview or physical examination and you startle her by touching her unexpectedly, the dog may growl and rise to defend her.

Planning for Labor and Delivery

Encourage a woman to attend a preparation-for-childbirth class. Explain that a number of films may be used in the introductory session concerning childbirth and, although she will be unable to view these, the audio portion will still be helpful to her. She will be able to use breathing exercises as well as any other woman in labor; even if her support person is also visually impaired so he cannot time contractions by looking at a watch (most braille watches do not have second hands), he can count them out in seconds. Much of a support person's role in labor is not counting contraction lengths in any event, but simply being there as a supporting presence.

Planning for Childcare

Ask during pregnancy about the woman's plans for child care. Encourage a woman to breast-feed, which will be easier than preparing formula. If she chooses to formula feed, suggest she use ready-prepared formula that needs no dilution and can be poured into a clean bottle just before feeding in order to avoid sterilization of bottles and working with a hot stove. Caution her against propping bottles to avoid aspiration.

Explore with her how she will manage to supervise the child as he or she gets older and begins exploring the house. During pregnancy is the time for all women to remove harmful items from lower cupboards so if a child crawls or walks sooner than they anticipated they have already hidden dangerous substances.

Care During Labor and Delivery

Labor can be a confusing time for the visually impaired woman because she is able to function competently by arranging many measures in her life specific for herself or to stay "in charge" of situations. During labor she may feel she is losing this psychological edge as her body takes care of her. Be certain to explain any sound in a labor or birthing room such as the buzz of a central supply routing system, the fetal monitor, or the patient call light system: Hearing sounds and not being able to identify them is very frightening. Be certain that everyone who comes into her labor or birthing room introduces themselves (or you interrupt to introduce them) so she is not frightened by strangers' voices speaking to her. Remember that visually impaired women develop an acute sense of hearing. A woman can undoubtedly hear whispering in the hallway or laughing at the desk area that the average person would not hear.

At birth, be certain to give the baby to her as soon as possible so she can feel that the child is perfect. Describe the baby to her (long hair, pretty eyes, ten fingers, etc.). Even if she does not voice the fear she cannot help but have some concern that the baby is blind like herself. Assess whether the infant has a red reflex and whether he or she follows a moving light to assure her that the infant does see. (On the other hand, do not act too excited that the baby has sight. This reaction could be interpreted as a "putdown" of the mother herself.) Feeling the baby is much more satisfying for a new mother than your oral assurances. If chilling at birth is a problem because a delivery room is cold, be certain she understands that the reason you want to rewrap the infant is because of the cold, not because her touching is wrong or you are afraid she will discover something imperfect about the child you have not told her about yet.

The Postpartal Period

Be certain that a woman has her child with her for long stretches of time so she is used to such phenomena as the irregular pattern of breathing of a newborn (she may notice this because of her acute awareness of sound where others do not) and she is comfortable with changing diapers and feeding. As a rule, suggest a community health nurse visit her daily for the first few weeks she is home with the infant unless she has a seeing family member who will be home with her.

Many visually impaired people do not turn on lights because, of course, they do not appreciate the difference between light and dark. This is particularly true if two visually impaired persons live together. Urge the woman to turn on lights in rooms after dinnertime as the infant needs light to develop vision. Suggest she check with a neighbor monthly to see that light bulbs have not burnt out.

Teach her to look at the child to talk because making eye contact is important to the child in feeling secure. Be certain that she has an appointment for follow-up child health supervision and a return appointment for herself. Ask if she desires contraceptive information. She is probably aware that managing one infant will be a challenge for her; two small infants born close together might compromise her ability. She is not restricted to any special form of contraception because of a visual handicap.

The Woman Who Is Hearing Impaired

Hearing impairment ranges from having difficulty hearing whispered conversation to being totally deaf. A hearing loss of 30 dB means that a woman has some difficulty hearing normal instructions and questions. A loss of 50 dB or more is a severe hearing loss: This decibel level is used to conduct normal conversation. Many women with a hearing impairment also have a speech impairment. (The older term "deaf and dumb" is no longer used as it unfairly correlates a hearing impediment with mental retardation.)

Prenatal Care

The average woman of childbearing age with a hearing impairment has been hearing impaired since birth because of an infection such as rubella during intrauterine life, meningitis in early infancy, or a genetically inherited hearing disorder. These types of hearing losses are sensorineural; and they can be helped to some degree by a hearing aid, but hearing can never be fully restored. The loud music that many teenagers listen to is gradually causing a loss of hearing of this type in many of this age group.

A woman with a hearing impairment needs to come for a regular pattern of prenatal care. As she has missed the everyday discussions of pregnancy that other women have listened to or the spot announcements on television about avoiding alcohol or smoking during pregnancy, she may lack "savvy" about pregnancy and need more time at appointments so these areas can be discussed.

Health Assessment

Many hearing impaired women lip read readily so they can participate in an average conversation with little apparent difficulty. New words, however, such as amniotic, gestation, or edema cannot be deciphered this way. Make a habit of showing the woman the printed word so she can see what your lip motion represents. Speak slowly so she can follow your meaning. Remember that if she is lip reading she cannot understand your instruction or question if you turn away from her or hold a chart so she cannot see your lips. If she uses sign language she may bring an interpreter with her to translate. Be certain that you do not talk only to the interpreter and not to her (she is the patient).

Many women who have been hearing impaired since birth have difficulty enunciating words clearly because they have never heard the sounds they are trying to imitate. The more you listen to the woman the more adept you become at understanding her speech pattern. Do not be reluctant to explain that you do not understand a question she asked and ask her to repeat it so you can be certain she has all her concerns about pregnancy answered. After she repeats a question a second time, if you still have difficulty understanding it, ask her to write it out for you. Explore with the woman the reason for her hearing impairment; as with visual impairment, it may affect her concerns during pregnancy. If the cause of her loss of hearing is a genetic disorder, she may be concerned that her child will also develop this problem; if it occurred because of an intrauterine infection during her own pregnancy, she may be fearful all during pregnancy of developing an infection.

Family Profile

Ask who lives at home with her. Investigate whom she depends on for support in an emergency. How would she contact the health care facility if an emergency such as ruptured membranes occurred (most women have a neighbor they could call on to telephone for them). If she has partial hearing and can do this herself, review with her that the first person she contacts at the health care agency will be a switchboard operator; that she should begin her message with "Hello, I'm Mary Smith." Alert the switchboard operators and any department receptionist to the name and the degree of speech impairment present so they can forward the call quickly to you. Otherwise the woman may grow so frustrated by trying to explain who she wants to speak to or what her problem is that she stops trying. Plan with her how to contact help (perhaps a community 911 number) to use when the health care agency is not open. Ask about financial resources (most women with hearing impairment qualify for Social Security assistance).

Pregnancy Counseling

Use visual aids liberally (a picture is worth a thousand words) in order to explain the physiologic changes of pregnancy or what care is planned for her at a health visit.

Physical Assessment

Be certain you have a woman's attention before you touch her to avoid startling her. During a pelvic examination she may not be able to see the examiner's face so be aware that any questions or reassurances made during this time will not be heard.

Planning for Labor and Delivery

Encourage the woman to attend preparation-for-childbirth classes. She may not be able to hear the audio portion of any films used in class but the visual picture of a birth will be helpful to her. She can use breathing exercises during labor. As she will be unable to hear a coach say, "Contraction beginning," plan with her how her coach will alert her to relax (a hand on her forehead or her arm?).

Planning for Childcare

One of a woman's biggest worries is that she will not be able to hear her baby crying to tell her he or she is hungry and needs her, especially at night. Help her to plan to bring the infant's crib or bassinet close to her bed so she can feel the vibration of the baby's stirring and waking. Suggest she breast-feed (as you may suggest to all women) so if she misses the infant's first hungry demands, she can feed immediately without having to wait to warm or prepare formula.

Care During Labor and Delivery

Remember that the hearing impaired woman cannot hear how she is progressing in labor if a person is not directly facing her or she cannot see their face (as often happens with pelvic examinations). Remember that she cannot hear the infant cry at birth (which is how the average woman is reassured that her newborn is healthy); be sure she knows the baby is crying and breathing well.

Hearing impaired women have a strong need to see their infant as soon as possible to assure themselves that the infant is well. Even if they do not voice this fear, they are usually concerned that the infant is hearing impaired. You can assess for this disability by showing her how the infant startles at a loud noise such as clapping your hands. A better way is to show her how the baby quiets at the sound of your voice because you want to encourage her to talk to the baby. If she continues to test for hearing in the weeks to come, the latter is more preferable than encouraging her to test by making a loud startling noise (and, not accustomed to sound, she may not appreciate that one of these actions is frightening and one soothing).

The Postpartal Period

Be certain that a woman's nursing care plan is marked clearly that she is hearing impaired so people do not attempt to use an oral communication system to relay messages to her. Most women who are severely hearing impaired do not appreciate the comforting quality that speech has for children. Some women whose speech is severely affected are reluctant to speak to strangers. Assure her that her infant is not a stranger in this sense and will quiet readily to the sound of her voice. Unfortunately, the child may develop her speech pattern and need speech therapy during preschool years to learn to enunciate words clearly. Having been spoken to and sung to during the first year is important for overall development, however, so this is an unfortunate, but still preferable development to living in a world of silence.

Many women with a hearing impairment can sense what their infant needs (whether hungry or cold or lonely) more quickly than the average woman. The latter depends on an infant's verbal expression, while a woman with a hearing impairment has learned to assess other body mannerisms such as tense body posture or facial expression to understand people's needs.

Be certain that she has the child with her for a long enough time that she can tell from vibration that the infant is crying. Be certain that she has a follow-up health care appointment for both herself and her child. Ask the woman if she desires contraception information to space her children.

The Woman with a Spinal Cord Injury

Many women who have paraplegia (loss of sensory and motor control of their lower extremities) either have always had this difficulty because of a congenital spinal cord defect such as myomeningocele at their birth or suffered a violent accident such as being thrown from a horse or motorcycle during childhood or adolescence.

Prenatal Care

If a woman was born with a spinal cord defect she should be advised to have genetic counseling so she is aware that an infant of hers may also have a defect (about a 20 percent chance). She is advised to have an amniocentesis at the fourteenth to sixteenth week of pregnancy to see if alpha-fetoprotein can be detected in the amniotic fluid (its presence indicates an open spinal defect). If a spinal cord defect is suspected in the fetus, it may be very difficult for the woman to decide to abort (she is aborting a person like herself or admitting that she is somehow not as good as others). On the other hand, she may have very strong feelings about submitting a child to the limited life she has led.

Table 38-1 lists the expected level of ambulatory function expected with different levels of spinal cord injury.

Health Assessment

Explore in a health history the cause of a woman's physical problem and her general image of herself. Some women who are confined to wheelchairs maintain high self-esteem; they will be as able to deal with a complication of pregnancy as any woman. Others have a poor sense of self-esteem that would make an additional problem particularly difficult for them.

Table 38-1 Level of Function Anticipated Following Spinal Injury

Level of Spinal Cord Injury	Functional Abilities
C3–4	Manipulate electric wheelchair using mouthstick.
C5–7	Propel wheelchair with handrim on wheels.
T1–4	Propel wheelchair without special projections.
T5–L2	Use bilateral long leg braces and crutches.
L3–4	Use short leg braces with or without crutches.
L5–S3	Be ambulatory without aids.

Family Profile

Explore with a woman who lives at home and who she would count on for emergency transportation if an emergency of pregnancy should occur. Ask about her ability to reach a telephone if she is home alone (if she is upstairs and the only telephone is downstairs, what would she do?). Late in pregnancy, she might want to always rest near a telephone by sleeping on the couch or a sleeping bag on the kitchen floor so reaching a telephone would be less of a problem.

Physical Examination

Many examining tables are built fairly high with the comfort of the examiner in mind. The height makes it impossible to transfer from a wheelchair by simply sliding onto the table. In order for a woman to accomplish the switch, you may have to borrow a ramp from the physical therapy department and elevate the wheelchair to the level of the table. The woman may be unable to maintain her legs in a lithotomy position either due to hip flexion contracture or laxness of leg support; she may need to be examined in a dorsal recumbent rather than a lithotomy position.

Pregnancy Counseling

All women who use wheelchairs should be taught to press with their arms and lift their buttocks up off the seat of the wheelchair for 5 seconds every hour. This prevents decubiti of the buttocks and posterior thighs from forming because of continual pressure. It is important that a woman continues to take this precaution during pregnancy as the increased weight of her abdomen makes her even more prone to decubiti from compression.

The sharp bend of her hips as she sits in a wheelchair limits venous return from the lower extremities to some extent. Raising her buttocks this way every hour decreases this angle and allows better venous return. For this reason also it is important that she continues this task during pregnancy. For at least an hour morning and afternoon, she should elevate her feet to decrease the sharp bend at her knee, which provides venous return to prevent varicosities.

Women who have no sensation of voiding due to lack of bladder innervation have been taught to empty their bladder every 2 hours by using a Credé method (pressing on the upper anterior surface of the bladder to constrict it and empty it), self-catheterization every 2 hours, or a continuous indwelling catheter.

All women with an indwelling catheter in place have a high risk of urinary tract infection.

Urge a woman to continue good perineal care (washing her perineum well with soap and water two times a day and applying an antiseptic ointment such as Betadine to the insertion site). Be certain that when changing the catheter (a woman can do this herself by lying on her back and holding a hand mirror to view her perineum) she uses optimal sterile technique. Urge her to place a folded towel under one buttock to displace the uterus off the vena cava, which helps prevent supine hypotension. She may be unable to change her own catheter late in pregnancy, as her abdomen is so large she can no longer visualize her perineum and vulvar edema enlarges the labia so much that she needs a "third hand" to displace these to view the urethra opening. Discuss with her what arrangements she wants to make—for example, a support person can change the catheter, a community health nurse could visit, or she could make frequent prenatal visits).

The woman who does self-catheterization uses a clean, not a sterile catheter technique (washes her perineum with soap and water, inserts a clean catheter into the urethra, and allows urine to drain into a toilet). She then washes the catheter with soap and water and covers it with a plastic sandwich bag for use again in another 2 hours). Bladder infection does not occur with self-catheterization because, although only clean technique is used, it is done so frequently that bacteria do not remain in the bladder for a long enough time to grow in quantity. The size of a woman's abdomen may also interfere with self-catheterization; discuss her plans to solve the problem (change to a Credé method, have a support person catheterize for her?).

Planning for Childcare

During pregnancy, a woman needs to think through what problems she can anticipate while caring for an infant at home. Encourage her to breast-feed so she does not need to get up at night to go to the refrigerator for formula (some women may worry their bodies will fail them in this new function as it has in old ones). Discuss with her how breast innervation is not affected by her handicap so she should be successful (and being successful at breast-feeding may be a very satisfying accomplishment for her: It is one way that her body is equal to everyone else's).

Some infant crib rails are lowered by pressure on a foot pedal, some by a lever at a waist-high point. Urge a woman to test different makes of cribs to find one that she can manage from her wheelchair (otherwise, she will leave the crib rail down and her infant could suffer a serious fall).

Investigate how she anticipates carrying the infant (using an anterior baby backpack is usually effective with a wheelchair).

Care During Labor and Delivery

A woman who has no sensory involvement to her abdomen will not be able to feel uterine contractions. Remember that sensory innervation of the uterus is at the T10 spinal level; the motor innervation is at the T7 level. This means that a woman's uterus may begin to initiate contractions but the woman will not be able to feel them. Late in pregnancy she will need to periodically palpate her abdomen for tightening or the presence of contractions that she cannot otherwise feel. She may be admitted to a hospital at 38 weeks of gestation to have a uterine monitor put in place so uterine contractions can be detected. She may be scheduled for an amniocentesis to determine fetal maturity, followed by a cesarean birth if the fetus is mature. If she is unable to control abdominal muscles, she will be unable to push with the pelvic stage of labor: Cesarean birth may be necessary. If she has some abdominal muscle control, it may be possible for the infant to be delivered vaginally with forceps used to help descent and birth.

Following birth, a woman has a strong need to see the baby and assure herself that he or she is healthy. She undoubtedly wants to observe the child's back. Even in a chilly delivery room the woman can take the warm cover off the newborn as the inspection is so important to her. Point out to her how the infant spontaneously brings the knees up under the abdomen when you lie the baby prone, which proves to her that her child has full use of the legs.

The Postpartal Period

In the immediate postpartal period a woman with a high spinal cord injury (cervical or high thoracic) must be observed for *autonomic dysreflexia*. This is an exaggerated autonomic response to stimuli. Any irritating condition such as a distended bladder initiates the response; without upper motor neuron control to reverse the symptoms, extreme changes can occur. Severe hypertension (300/160) can result; the woman will have a throbbing headache, flushing of the skin and perfuse diaphoresis above the level of the spinal lesion, nausea, and bradycardia. Immediate action is necessary to protect against a cerebral vascular accident or intraocular damage. Elevate the woman's head to reduce cerebral pressure and locate the irritating stimulus (usually a distended bladder or bowel). Remove the bladder pressure by catheterizing if an indwelling catheter is not in place; check a catheter if it has failed to drain and unkink or flush it, thereby allowing urine to drain freely again.

As soon as the source of irritation is removed, symptoms fade quickly. It is a very frightening event for a woman, however, with the potential of causing severe, additional damage to her neurologic ability.

Be certain a woman carries out conscientious perineal care during the postpartal period (she does not sense pain in the area so a hematoma or an infection of a perineal suture line could occur without her being aware of it). Assess carefully for bladder filling in the postpartal period; again, the woman is not aware of bladder filling. She can return to her usual method of bladder emptying following delivery (Credé method, indwelling catheter, or self-catheterization).

Be certain the woman spends enough time with her infant so she begins to develop confidence in her ability to lift the newborn from a bassinet into the wheelchair and in diapering and feeding. Be certain she has a return appointment for health care for both herself and the infant. Ask if she desires contraceptive information as she is probably aware that two small children close together could be more of a challenge than she would be able to manage.

The Woman with Cerebral Palsy

In the most frequently occurring type of cerebral palsy, a woman has spasticity of all body muscles. This problem causes her to reach past objects and to walk unsteadily (her muscles overcontract on voluntary motion). Her speech is unclear as her facial and throat muscles are also affected. Cerebral palsy is caused by anoxia to brain cells either during intrauterine life or during labor and delivery. It may or may not be associated with mental retardation, depending on the extent of the anoxia. Cerebral palsy is a condition that ranges from only slight spasticity (difficulty with only fine motor control) to an extreme level where a woman would be limited to a wheelchair for ambulation and have difficulty performing simple tasks such as self-feeding. Evaluate each woman individually in order not to over- or underestimate her special needs during pregnancy.

Prenatal Care

Due to the muscle spasticity present, a woman with cerebral palsy may be limited to a wheel-chair, may walk with the aid of forearm-supported crutches, or may be ambulatory without aids (but with an unsteady gait). As pregnancy progresses, she may need a referral to a physical therapist for evaluation of her ability to maintain self-ambulation: The weight of her abdomen may necessitate the use of crutches if she did not use them before, the use of a wheelchair if she was ambulatory with crutches before pregnancy. Appreciate that a woman achieved the degree of ambulation that she first presents with only after years of physical therapy and strengthening of leg and arm muscles. Help her to see that reducing her degree of independence during pregnancy is not a step backward but a step forward in that it will allow her to have a safe pregnancy without repeated falls.

In order that a woman does not lose the strength of muscle groups or develop contractures due to reduced mobility, she needs to do active range of motion exercises twice daily and to spend about an hour daily walking in a physical therapy department with the support of parallel bars. Bringing her to a hospital daily may not be realistic in terms of the time her support person can commit. If necessary, help her to contact a community support group such as her church organization or a community organization for the handicapped to supply this transportation for her. Otherwise, she may continue to try to be independently ambulatory beyond her capacity or at the end of pregnancy discover that she can no longer be ambulatory beyond the limits of a wheelchair.

Health Assessment

Investigate who lives at home with the woman, how much school she attended, and whether she works outside her home for an estimation of her capabilities and her exposure to life activities such as pregnancy and childrearing. Do not mistake her inability to form words clearly for a lack of knowledge of what the words are or for a hearing impairment.

Ask if she knows the reason for her illness to determine if she is concerned that her illness will appear in her child (there is no reason to think it will except that she is a high-risk mother because of her instability and cerebral palsy occurs at a higher incidence in the infants of high-risk mothers).

Family Profile

Evaluate, if a woman's speech cannot be readily understood, how she can use a telephone to call for help if an emergency should occur. For many people with cerebral palsy, a push button telephone is easier to use than a dial type because pushing buttons requires less of a sustained motion than spinning a dial. Review with her that if she calls the health care facility to state her name first, "Hello, I'm Mary Smith," and then ask for help. Alert the main switchboard of the facility and any department receptionist of her status and the degree of speech impairment present so in an emergency she does not grow so frustrated trying to relay a message that she gives up the effort. Be certain that the woman knows how to summon help (perhaps a community 911 number) during any time the health care facility is closed.

Pregnancy Counseling

An important facet of pregnancy counseling for a woman with cerebral palsy is increasing her self-esteem. Her condition is one that comedians imitate and many people refer to callously with comments such as, "Don't get spastic." Children can be very cruel to a person who cannot control muscle motion smoothly so her years of schooling have probably been accumulated hurt. This pregnancy is a chance to accomplish; by having a healthy child, she will be equal to everyone who has made fun of her. She is an eager and excellent student, therefore, ready to learn all that you can teach her about how to make this pregnancy successful.

Allow time at prenatal visits for her to ask questions (she may be unable to write them out for you because of hand incoordination).

Physical Assessment

Women with cerebral palsy may find that lying on examining tables is uncomfortable because their muscle spasticity limits their ability to conform to a hard surface. They may have enough hip flexion contraction that they are unable to raise their feet comfortably into stirrups.

Preparation for Childbirth

Encourage a woman to attend a preparation-for-childbirth class although she may not be able to use breathing exercises effectively during labor because the spasticity of her muscles may not allow for a controlled breathing pattern. The general knowledge about labor and delivery, and a chance to participate in a shared experience with her life partner, will still be valuable.

Planning for Childcare

Help a woman to think through how she will carry a crying, struggling infant if she is unsteady on her feet or uses crutches to ambulate. She might be encouraged to use an infant backpack or to use a wheelchair with an anterior baby sling (so her hands are free to move the wheels or controls of the chair). If her home is not crowded for space she might consider using a toy wagon for pulling the infant. Some women lie on their back, place the infant on their chest, and slide across the floor by pushing with their feet. Impress on her that the way she chooses is not as important as the fact that it is done safely without danger of her falling on a small infant.

Encourage her to breast-feed, which will eliminate her having to walk an extra distance to warm or prepare formula. She may be reluctant because of lack of confidence in her body's functioning; and actually, if her spasticity is severe, she may not be successful at breast-feeding (the let-down reflex, which depends on muscle relaxation, may not occur).

Care During Labor and Delivery

Labor may be acutely painful for a woman with cerebral palsy because her abdominal muscles remain tight and the uterus grows tender raising and pressing against a tense abdomen with each contraction. She may not be able to use breathing exercises effectively to provide any pain relief for herself. Because she has ineffective use of abdominal muscles, she may not be able to push effectively during the pelvic division of labor, so fetal descent may not occur and cesarean birth or a forceps delivery may be necessary. She may be unable to assume a lithotomy position because of hip contractures and so must be vaginally delivered from a Sims' or a dorsal recumbent position.

She needs to see her baby immediately after birth to assure herself that he or she is healthy. If she received a high level of analgesia or anesthesia for labor or delivery, she needs to see the infant as soon as she is awake and aware. Cerebral palsy, as a rule, is not evident at birth but only at 3 or 4 months of age when the infant cannot accomplish expected tasks, such as reaching and grasping an object or pressing feet down against a flat surface when held in a standing position: Stress the things the child can do (follow a finger, suck well) to assure her of health.

The Postpartal Period

Help a woman to begin self-care at the level she is able. Mark her nursing care plan and her chart with a note that states clearly she has a speech impediment so people do not underestimate her intelligence and wait patiently for her to make her needs clear.

Urge her to use disposable diapers with the infant; a quick uncontrolled hand motion with a safety pin could injure the infant. Allow her adequate time to feed and hold the infant to become competent in the newborn's care.

Be certain that she has a return appointment for health care supervision for herself and the infant. Ask if she desires contraceptive information as she is probably aware that the year has been difficult for her and caring for one small infant will be a challenge; caring for two born close together might be beyond her capabilities.

The Woman with Mental Retardation

Young adults who are mentally retarded are generally affected in this way because of anoxia they suffered during their intrauterine life or shortly after birth. Most women with a chromosomal retardation syndrome such as Down's syndrome cannot reproduce and are not included in this group.

Like all handicapping conditions, mental retardation is always one of degree. Table 38-2 shows commonly used designations of mental retardation and the corresponding expected functional levels.

Some women with mental retardation who are pregnant were raised in an institution and only recently discharged to a halfway home or their own apartment. These women have difficulty making plans for childcare because they have never experienced normal family life and observed younger children being cared for. Some women have an additional problem because their pregnancy resulted from their being taken advantage of rather than from their own planning; some may have so little concept of how their bodies function that they do not know how they became pregnant. Some women come late for prenatal care because they do not realize that the changes they have noticed in their bodies indicate pregnancy.

Women with mental retardation need frequent and consistent prenatal care; they do not have the same judgment to determine if they are developing a complication of pregnancy as the average woman. They do not have the same level of "common pregnancy knowledge" as other women and need more teaching in order to complete their pregnancy safely.

Health Assessment

When interviewing a woman with mental retardation, ask her level of education as an indication of her degree of retardation. Many women, however, report that they finished high school, and indeed, they did attend school for 12 years, but their curriculum was limited. Be certain while interviewing that you limit your words to those a woman can easily understand. Keep the length of the interview time short (10 to 15 minutes) and the environment free of distractions because most persons with mental retardation have a short attention span and are easily distracted.

Family Profile

Investigate who lives at home with the woman, who would she turn to if she had a problem, and what is her source of financial support. The woman may be eligible for a Social Security assistance program but not be collecting it because of some such thing as a form she was not aware she needed to fill in. Ask if a woman has a telephone at her home and if she understands how to telephone the health care facility if she needs help.

Ask what she would do for transportation in an emergency (is there a neighbor, a family member, a friend who would drive her to the hospital?). If a family member accompanies the woman, ask the cause of the retardation (she may or may not know this herself).

Physical Assessment

Explain carefully any procedure such as blood drawing so a woman understands that this is a helping not a punishing procedure. She may not have had a pelvic examination done before and be very reluctant to reveal this portion of her body to a stranger. Give good support during the procedure.

Table 38-2 Levels of Mental Retardation

Level of Retardation	I.Q. Average	Abilities Expected
Mild	50–70	Educable; able to read and write well enough to carry out simple tasks and hold unskilled jobs.
Moderate	20–50	Trainable; able to learn the tasks of daily self-care.
Severe	Below 20	Requiring total care.

Pregnancy Counseling

Limit instructions to those few items about pregnancy that are crucial for safety (do not drink alcohol; do not take any medicine); use photos or drawings to illustrate your teaching points to increase understanding.

Help her to visualize from month to month (using drawings) how her baby is growing. Teach her as well what a newborn is like and a baby's capabilities. Without this information she may expect much more of the baby than he or she can do (to talk to her or play with her) and so not be prepared to give safe care.

Preparation for Childbirth

A woman with mental retardation may not be able to benefit from a preparation-for-childbirth class because her attention span is not long enough to enjoy the sessions or to profit from breathing exercises. If the retardation is not severe, she may benefit greatly from them. If she does not work or attend school, she has such ample time to practice breathing exercises that she may become very adept at using such a method to control pain in labor.

Planning for Childcare

Help a woman and her family plan realistically for child care. Encourage the woman to breast-feed, which will limit the chances of her misinterpreting instructions about formula preparation. If her attention span is short, however, she may not be a candidate for breast-feeding. If she is unable to grasp the importance of food for the child, she may put the child down when she is tired of feeding, not when the child has obtained enough milk. If she will actually not be the primary caregiver to the child because of severe retardation, she is probably advised to formula feed the infant.

If a woman has more than mild retardation, you have a legal obligation to help devise a safe plan of care for the child (she will move in with a friend, her mother will actually raise the child, etc.). Even though she is mentally retarded she has full rights to the child; the baby cannot be taken from her at birth without her consent. Likewise, she cannot be made to have an abortion to end the pregnancy unless that is her informed decision.

Care During Labor and Delivery

Labor may be a confusing time for a mentally handicapped woman because, although she had been told that she would have contractions, she was not fully prepared for the extent or length of labor contractions (overwhelming for even very intelligent women). She may need an anesthetic or sedation during labor in order to withstand this very strange experience.

Following birth of the infant, she needs to examine the infant immediately as the shift from "being pregnant" to "having a baby" may be difficult for her. If she is disappointed in the sex or appearance of the child, she might ask you to "give her another baby" because she does not fully understand the uniqueness of each child.

The Postpartal Period

During the postpartal period, allow a woman time to spend with the infant so she learns safe care. Using judgment for decisions as to how much to feed the baby or whether it is safe to lay the newborn on a bed alone may be difficult. Role model safe child care as a visual teaching strategy.

Ask if she desires contraceptive information. She may not be interested in preventing having another child at this time because a new baby is very cute and "doll-like." As a rule, suggest a community health nurse visit within a week to be certain that the child's environment is safe; mark on the referral if no contraceptive information was accepted as this might be advanced again when the community health nurse has established a relationship with her.

Be certain that she has a return appointment for both herself and the infant for follow-up care. Do not discharge the infant to her care until you are certain that she will be safe with the baby or another adult is assuming care. Otherwise, your action could be interpreted as child abuse.

Utilizing Nursing Process

In order that a woman with a handicap can successfully complete a pregnancy, nursing care during the pregnancy must include careful consideration of nursing process.

Assessment

As all handicapping conditions occur in degrees, each woman must be evaluated individually to determine both her assets and limitations. Be certain to assess not only her physical limitations and strengths but her psychosocial or emotional strengths as well. Her ability to adapt to pregnancy will depend partially on her physical capabilities and partially on her ability to persevere against odds and overcome what the average woman would think of as unsurmountable obstacles.

Analysis

Many diagnoses accepted by the North American Nursing Diagnosis Association apply to women with handicapping conditions. A number of these are: "Mobility, impairment of," "Injury, potential for," "Communication, impaired verbal," "Home maintenance management, impaired," and "Self-concept, disturbance in." When setting goals, be certain they are realistic in light of the circumstances. In some instances it may not be possible for a woman to carry a pregnancy through to completion as much as she may desire it. Some women may have to deliver their child by cesarean birth although this is not their preference.

Planning

The box on page 859 lists general areas of care that are important for planning for a woman with a handicap who is pregnant. Being certain that plans are established in all these areas helps to ensure that planning is comprehensive. If a woman is not totally independent in her care, you will have to do some planning with her support person, who may be the one to actually carry out the planned action. At the same time you are planning, be sure not to ignore the woman and "plan around her." Only if she approves of the plan can pregnancy be the enjoyable experience it should be for her.

As many women with handicaps have low self-esteem and little confidence in their body, plans should include ways to strengthen these areas. A mother needs both high self-esteem and confidence in order to mother well.

Include safe care of the newborn in plans during pregnancy. Once the infant is born it is too late to make these plans in a comprehensive manner.

Implementation

Many implementations with a woman who is handicapped are modifications of usual implementations during pregnancy, such as modifying a pelvic examination arrangement to not use table stirrups. Modifying procedures in this way for the handicapped woman enlarges your ability to adapt procedures and individualize them for all women, thereby improving your nursing care as a whole.

Evaluation

Successful evaluation must concern not only safe completion of the pregnancy but whether a woman grew from the experience in self-esteem and whether the environment for the infant will be safe and promote normal growth and development.

Nursing Care Planning

Ellen White is a 24-year-old woman who is mildly mentally retarded. She is 40 pounds above her ideal weight according to her height; she is brought to a prenatal clinic by her mother because a rehabilitation counselor suggested she might be pregnant. The following is a nursing care plan in relation to exercise during pregnancy you might devise for her.

Assessment

Patient completed 12 years of school in a mainstreamed setting. Now works 3 days a week in a sheltered workshop (independently takes bus to and from); her work is sitting cutting donated clothing into cleaning rags for industrial cleaning.

Attends a Sunday evening social club at the Cerebral Palsy Center (sessions include one action period of tumbling or games such as volleyball and one period of dancing).

Does not go out independently except for bus ride to workshop because she "wanders off" and cannot find her way home again.

Analysis

Potential for inadequate exercise during pregnancy related to sedentary life style.

Locus of Decision Making. Shared. Nurse, patient, and patient's mother.

Goal. Patient to maintain an exercise program during pregnancy to promote lower extremity venous return.

Criteria. Patient to accomplish some measure of promoting venous return daily.

Nursing Orders

1. Give patient a written list of instructions so mother can help evaluate suitable exercise.

2. Teach her to elevate her feet for 1 hour morning and afternoon.
3. Urge mother to walk with her a city block daily (weather permitting).

4. Urge to continue Sunday night social activities but advise to check with counselor if activity is suitable for her.

Questions for Review

Multiple Choice

1. Mrs. Martinez is a woman with a thoracic level spinal cord injury from a skiing accident. She is confined to a wheelchair for ambulation. An exercise you would remind her to do during pregnancy is to
   a. hold her breath to cause descent of her diaphragm hourly.
   b. tense her abdominal muscles hourly to maintain abdominal tone.
   c. raise her buttocks off the wheelchair seat hourly.
   d. do pelvic rocking hourly to maintain vertebral mobility.

2. Mrs. Martinez has a cesarean birth, after which an indwelling catheter was put in place. As you walk into her room you notice her face is reddened; she says she has a sharp headache. You take her blood pressure and discover it is 160/120. Your first action should be to
   a. lower her head and ask her to breathe slowly in and out.
   b. raise her head and assess the catheter for blockage.
   c. immediately cut and remove the indwelling catheter.
   d. sit her up abruptly and massage her lower back.

3. Mrs. Martinez is questioning whether she should breast-feed or not. Your best response to her would be,
   a. "Setting goals beyond your ability will cause you frustration."
   b. "You will not be able to do this because of your handicap."
   c. "You should have already made this decision during pregnancy."
   d. "All women should try breast-feeding, including you."

4. Mrs. O'Connor is a woman who has total vision impairment because of retrolental fibroplasia of prematurity. She delivers a girl weighing 6 pounds, 12 ounces, 2 weeks early according to her due date. Which statement below would you want to clarify for her?
   a. Retrolental fibroplasia cannot be detected until later in life.
   b. She should reveal anything she did that caused the early delivery.
   c. She need not feel guilty that her infant has been born prematurely.
   d. An infant born within 2 weeks of a due date is a term infant.

5. Mrs. O'Connor will return home after 7 days hospitalization. In discussing her plans for care of her newborn, which area below would you be most concerned about?
   a. if her home is "child-proofed"
   b. that she will not be able to detect jaundice in her newborn
   c. if she understands what jaundice entails even if she cannot see it
   d. that she will not be able to read to the child

6. Mrs. Nataro is severely hearing impaired. She poorly enunciates all syllables of words. You would suggest to her
   a. to tell her child not to imitate her speech.
   b. to speak and sing to her child as she gives care.
   c. not to speak to her newborn in order to discourage poor speech patterns.
   d. that listening to a radio will be a better source of sound for the child than her voice.

7. Mrs. Nataro is concerned that she will not wake at night to hear her newborn boy crying. You would recommend to her that
   a. she sleep with the newborn in bed with her so she can hear him.
   b. she feed him cereal at bedtime so he will not wake at night.
   c. if he wakes and cries but is not fed, he will not continue to wake at night.
   d. she sleep with her hand on his crib so she feels the vibration of his crying.

8. Mrs. Young is mildly mentally retarded. She is concerned that if her baby is floating in water inside her it will drown. Which teaching strategy below would you use to explain how it is safe for the baby to be in fluid in utero?
   a. Show her an illustration of a fetus in utero.
   b. Provide a taped explanation for her to play at home.
   c. Explain it is safe for a small baby to be under water.
   d. Caution her not to worry about things she cannot understand.

9. In planning home care for Mrs. Young and her infant, which factor below would be most important to assess?
   a. if she will be able to read stories to the child
   b. whether she has a support person available
   c. how she can most economically feed the child
   d. if she views education as important for the child

Discussion

1. Preparing a good pregnancy diet can be tiring for a woman with a neuromuscular illness. What suggestions could you make to a woman who tires easily in order to help her improve her nutrition?
2. Because many women with a handicap do not drive, they must rely on provided transportation. What facilities are available in your community a woman could call on?
3. The ability to secure help in an emergency varies from community to community. What are the ways in your community a woman who could not speak clearly could contact emergency help?

Suggested Readings

Aranosian, R. D. (1983). Better care for the mentally impaired. *Emergency Medicine, 15,* 123.

Asrael, W. (1982). An approach to motherhood for disabled women. *Rehabilitation Literature, 43,* 214.

Axel, S. J. (1982). Spinal cord injured women's concerns: Menstruation and pregnancy. *Rehabilitation Nursing, 7,* 10.

Baranowski, E. (1983). Childbirth education classes for expectant deaf parents. *M.C.N., 8,* 143.

Bogle, J., et al. (1979). *Family planning services are for disabled people, too: a manual for service providers.* Rockville, Md.: National Clearing House of Family Planning Information.

Caparulo, F., et al. (1981). Sexual health needs of the mentally retarded adolescent female. *Issues in Health Care of Women, 3,* 35.

Clifford, S., et al. (1983). Sex education . . . of mentally handicapped people. *Nursing Mirror, 157,* 36.

Craig, D. I., et al. (1983). Nursing care plan for a pregnant spinal cord injured patient. *Rehabilitation Nursing, 8,* 26.

Dickin, K. L., et al. (1983). Sterilization and the mentally retarded. *Canadian Mental Health Journal, 31,* 4.

Francis, R. A. (1983). The development of federal accessibility law: Physical access to public buildings. *Journal of Rehabilitation, 49,* 29.

Johnston, B. (1982). Pregnancy and childbirth in women with spinal cord injuries: A review of the literature. *Maternal-Child Nursing Journal, 11,* 41.

Kroeber, M. J. (1982). Sexuality and the physically disabled. *Journal of Enterostomal Therapy, 9,* 24.

Kutzler, D. L., et al. (1983). Maternity care for a profoundly handicapped woman: A team approach. *M.C.N., 8,* 290.

LaBan, M. M., et al. (1983). Pregnancy and the herniated lumbar disc. *Archives of Physical and Medical Rehabilitation, 64,* 319.

Levitt, R. (1981). Sex and physical disability. *Journal of Neurosurgical Nursing, 13,* 127.

Livneh, H. (1982). On the origin of negative attitudes toward people with disabilities. *Rehabilitation Literature, 43,* 338.

Longo, R. E., et al. (1981). Sexual assault of handicapped individuals. *Journal of Rehabilitation, 4,* 24.

McGrath, G., et al. (1981). The disabled and the nurse. *Lamp, 38,* 47.

Moss, M. (1984). Determined to be accepted . . . giving birth in hospital despite being blind. *Nursing Mirror, 158,* vii.

Peters, L. (1982). Woman's health care: Approaches in delivery to physically disabled women. *Nurse Practitioner, 7,* 34.

Rousso, H. (1982). Special considerations in counseling clients with cerebral palsy . . . the sexual aspects of their lives. *Sexual Disability, 5,* 78.

Salend, S. J., et al. (1982). Teaching proper health habits to mainstreamed students through positive reinforcement. *Journal of School Health, 52,* 539.

Sharkey, P. L., et al. (1982). Nursing care of the mentally retarded: Communication issues. *Issues in Mental Health Nursing, 4,* 191.

Shaw, M., et al. (1982). Changes in patterns of care of the mentally handicapped: Implications for nurses' perceptions of their roles and hospital decision-making process. *Journal of Advances in Nursing, 7,* 555.

Tabeek, E. S., et al. (1981). Teaching sexual awareness to the significantly disabled school-age child. *Pediatric Nursing, 7,* 21.

Weinberg, N. (1984). Physically disabled people assess the quality of their lives. *Rehabilitation Literature, 45,* 12.

Young, B. K., et al. (1983). Pregnancy after spinal cord injury: Altered maternal and fetal response to labor. *Obstetrics and Gynecology, 62,* 59.

Zamerowski, S. T. (1982). Helping families to cope with handicapped children. *Topics in Clinical Nursing, 4,* 41.

Ziff, S. F. (1981). The sexual concerns of the adolescent woman with cerebral palsy. *Issues in Health Care of Women, 3,* 55.

39

The Woman Who Develops a Complication of Pregnancy

OBJECTIVES

Following mastery of the content of this chapter, you should be able to

1. Identify common, unexpected complications of pregnancy such as bleeding during pregnancy, premature and postmature labor, multiple gestation, premature rupture of membranes, and hypertension of pregnancy.
2. Assess a woman with an unexpected complication of pregnancy as to her specific needs and risk assessment for a healthy pregnancy outcome.
3. State a nursing diagnosis related to an unexpected complication of pregnancy.
4. Plan nursing implementations specific for the unexpected pregnancy complication.
5. Implement nursing actions specific for the unexpected complication of pregnancy.
6. Evaluate goal criteria as to the effect of nursing implementations on pregnancy outcome.
7. Analyze ways that nurses can help prevent complications of pregnancy through health teaching and risk assessment.
8. Synthesize knowledge of unexpected complications of pregnancy with nursing process to achieve quality maternal-newborn nursing care.

MOST WOMEN ENTER pregnancy in apparent good health and achieve a normal pregnancy and newborn outcome without any complications. In a few women, however, for reasons that are usually unexplainable, unexpected deviations from the course of normal pregnancy do develop. Such a complication may threaten the pregnancy outcome, the woman's health, or both.

The leading causes of maternal death during pregnancy in order of occurrence are hemorrhage, infection, hypertension of pregnancy, anesthesia complications, ectopic pregnancy, heart disease,

and thromboembolism. Unexpected complications of pregnancy, therefore, cause more maternal deaths than do preexisting illnesses.

The advent of a complication can place a very severe burden on the woman and her family on top of the crisis situation of pregnancy. Any woman benefits from the support and the skill of a professional nurse who helps her work through the tasks of pregnancy, accepting it and preparing to become a mother. The support and skill of a professional nurse are essential to a woman who, in addition to the usual tasks of pregnancy, must question whether she will survive and whether her baby will be born well when conditions such as bleeding, premature rupture of membranes, pregnancy-induced hypertension, multiple gestation, hydramnios, blood incompatibility, or postmature or premature delivery occur.

Bleeding During Pregnancy

Vaginal bleeding is a deviation from the normal that may occur at any time during pregnancy. It is never normal, and it is always frightening. It may or may not be serious, but it must always be carefully investigated: If it occurs in sufficient amount or for sufficient cause, it can impair both the outcome of the pregnancy and the woman's life or future health.

Bleeding and the Development of Shock

The process of shock due to blood loss is shown in Figure 39-1. Note that because the uterus is a nonessential body organ, danger to the fetal blood supply occurs not as a last physiologic step but at the point the woman's body begins to decrease blood flow to nonessential organs (although the increased blood volume of pregnancy allows more-than-normal blood loss before hypovolemic shock occurs). Signs of hypovolemic shock (Table 39-1) will occur when 10 percent of blood volume or approximately 2 units of blood have been lost. It is important to know a baseline blood pressure for a pregnant woman because "normal" varies. Women should be told their blood pressure ("Your blood pressure is 110 over 70—that's normal"; not just "Your pressure is normal"). Then if blood loss should occur, a woman can be helpful in offering her baseline pressure.

A woman suspected of bleeding should have an intravenous fluid line begun with a large-gauge needle (18 or 19) for rapid fluid expansion and administration of a blood transfusion. She should have a hemoglobin, typing, and cross-matching for blood done. She may have a central venous

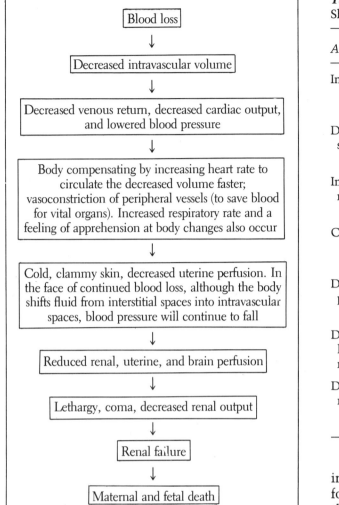

Figure 39-1 *The process of shock due to blood loss (hypovolemia).*

Table 39-1 Signs and Symptoms of Hemorrhagic Shock

Assessment	Significance
Increased pulse rate	Heart attempting to circulate decreased blood volume.
Decreased blood pressure	Less peripheral resistance because of decreased blood volume.
Increased respiratory rate	Increased gas exchange to better oxygenate decreased red blood cell volume.
Cold, clammy skin	Vasoconstriction occurs to maintain blood volume in central bloody core.
Decreased urine output	Inadequate blood is entering kidney due to decreased blood volume.
Dizziness or decreased level of consciousness	Inadequate blood is reaching cerebrum due to decreased blood volume.
Decreased central venous pressure	Decreased blood is returning to heart due to reduced blood volume.

pressure (CVP) catheter inserted. She should never lie flat on her back but in a lateral position so that there is minimal uterine pressure on the vena cava and as little blood as possible is trapped in the lower extremities. If respirations are rapid, oxygen by mask should be administered and blood gases drawn. Frequent assessments of vital signs and continuous fetal monitoring (by an external monitoring device) should be started. These steps are summarized in the box on page 876.

Central Venous Pressure

Central venous pressure is an estimation of the pressure or the amount of blood returning to the right atrium of the heart.

For a central venous pressure, a thin polyethylene catheter is inserted at the antecubital fossa into a vein or more directly into the subclavian or internal or external jugular vein. It is threaded forward until it rests in the vena cava just outside the right atrium. The distal end of the catheter is attached to a manometer. This is connected to a bottle and tubing of intravenous fluid (Figure 39-2). Tape the intravenous tubing and catheter connections securely. If the tubing should come unfastened, a woman could bleed profusely from the site or air could be introduced and form an air embolus. A chest X-ray may be ordered after the insertion to confirm proper catheter placement. Assure a woman that an X-ray is safe for her; be certain the X-ray technician provides a lead screen for her abdomen.

To obtain a CVP reading, ask the woman to lie on her back and lower the bed until it is flat. The 0 marking of the manometer must be at the midaxillary line of the woman's body (a level that is equal to the position of the right atrium). It is a good practice to mark this point on the woman's side with a marking pen so that everyone who will be taking readings uses the same level marker. Next, turn the stopcock on the manometer so intravenous fluid enters the manometer. Fill the manometer to a point over 15 cm H_2O. Next, turn the stopcock so the manometer fluid flows through the catheter into the woman. The fluid in

Emergency Interventions for Bleeding in Pregnancy

Interventions	*Rationale*
Alert health care team of emergency situation.	Provide for maximum coordination of care.
Place woman flat in bed on her side on bed rest.	Maintain optimal placental and renal function.
Begin IV fluid such as lactated Ringers with an 18- or 19-gauge needle.	Replace intravascular fluid volume; prepare IV line for blood replacement.
Withhold oral fluid.	Anticipation of emergency surgery.
Administer oxygen as necessary at 2–4 L/min.	Provide adequate fetal oxygenation despite lowered circulating blood volume.
Monitor uterine and fetal heart rate by external monitor.	Assess whether labor is present and fetal status; use external system to avoid cervical trauma.
Omit vaginal or rectal examinations.	If a rectal or vaginal exam is done with placenta previa, the placenta may be torn and hemorrhage occur.
Order type and cross-match of 2 units whole blood.	Prepare to restore circulating maternal blood volume.
Measure intake and output.	Assess renal function (will decrease with massive circulating volume loss).
Assess vital signs (pulse, respirations, and blood pressure) every 15 minutes.	Assess maternal response to blood loss.
Assist with placement of central venous pressure catheter.	Assess pressure of blood returning to heart.
Measure maternal blood loss by weighing perineal pads; save any clots passed.	Assess extent of continuing blood loss.
Set aside 5 ml of blood in a clean test tube and observe in 5 minutes for clot formation.	Assess for possible blood coagulation problem (disseminated intravascular coagulation). Suspect this if no clot forms within time limit.
Maintain a positive attitude toward fetal outcome.	Support mother-child bonding.
Support woman's self-esteem.	Problem solving is lessened by poor self-esteem.

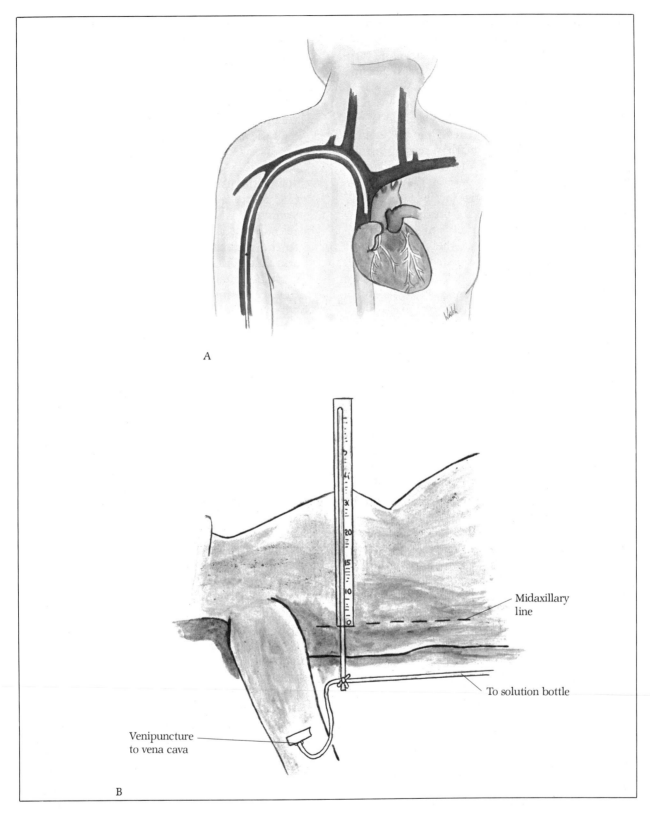

A

B

Midaxillary
line

To solution bottle

Venipuncture
to vena cava

Figure 39-2 *A. Placement of a central venous pressure catheter. B. The 0 marking on the manometer should be level with the midaxillary body line.*

the manometer will fall until it is equal with her central venous pressure. Read the manometer at this point. The column of fluid will never be completely stationary, as it fluctuates with respiratory movements.

Following a reading, change the stopcock position so the intravenous fluid infuses again to prevent the catheter from clotting. Urge the woman to turn onto her side rather than remain on her back so supine hypertension syndrome does not occur.

Normal CVP values range between 5 and 12 cm H_2O; 8 to 10 cm during pregnancy. A low reading indicates hypovolemia; a high reading indicates fluid overload or that the right atrium is unable to handle all the blood returning to it. Women admitted with shock from hemorrhage will have a low CVP reading; as they receive a great deal of intravenous fluid to replace blood loss, fluid overload is a possibility.

As important as the fact that the CVP values are within normal limits is the fact that they are not changing. A CVP reading that is gradually changing from 10 cm H_2O to 9 cm H_2O to 8 cm H_2O is still within normal limits. It suggests that bleeding and hypovolemia is occurring, however.

Check the insertion site of a CVP catheter daily to be certain that signs of infection (redness, tenderness) are not evident. Check connections to be certain that they are secure. If fluid tends to infuse slowly at any time it is generally due to one of two problems: There is a kink in the tubing or a clot is forming at the catheter tip. Check the tubing for kinking, and rearrange it to a free-flowing position as necessary. If clot forming appears to be the difficulty, attach a syringe to the catheter and aspirate to draw back the clot. Do not irrigate the catheter, as this might force a clot forward and cause an embolus. In most instances correcting the hypovolemia that occurs with bleeding in pregnancy can be accomplished quickly, so these long-term problems of CVP catheters do not usually occur.

First-Trimester Bleeding

The time during pregnancy at which bleeding occurs is usually important as an indication of its cause. The two most common causes of bleeding during the first trimester of pregnancy are abortion and ectopic pregnancy.

Abortion

An abortion is any interruption of a pregnancy before the fetus is viable. A fetus is said to be viable if the stage of development will enable the fetus to survive outside the uterus. A viable fetus is usually therefore defined as a fetus of at least 20 weeks' gestation age (some authorities use 24 weeks) or weighing 400 gm (600 gm at 24 weeks). A fetus born after this point would be considered a premature or immature birth.

An abortion is *early* if it occurs prior to the sixteenth week of pregnancy, *late* if it occurs between the sixteenth and twentieth weeks. For the first six weeks of pregnancy, the developing placenta is very tentatively attached to the decidua of the uterus; during the sixth and twelfth week a moderate degree of attachment to the myometrium is accomplished. After the twelfth week, the attachment is penetrating and deep into the uterine myometrium. Because of these varying degrees of attachment, it is important to try and establish the week of pregnancy at which bleeding became apparent. Bleeding before the sixth week is rarely severe; bleeding after the twelfth week can be very great in amount. Fortunately, at this time, with such deep placental implantation, the fetus is expelled as in natural childbirth before the placenta separates. Uterine contraction thus helps to control placental bleeding as it does postpartally. For some women, then, the stage of attachment between the sixth and twelfth weeks can lead to the most severe bleeding and threat to their life (the placenta delivers before the fetus; uterine contraction does not then occur readily and bleeding continues).

The most frequent cause of abortion in the first trimester of pregnancy is abnormal fetal formation, due either to a teratogenic factor or to a chromosomal aberration. About 60 percent of fetuses aborted early have structural abnormalities: 40 percent have grossly observable pathologic conditions (Pritchard, 1980). Early abortion may be thought of, therefore, as nature's way of preventing the birth of ill or deformed children.

Another common cause of early abortion is an implantation abnormality (about 50 percent of zygotes are never implanted). With inadequate implantation, the placental circulation will not be well established, and the fetus cannot grow normally. Poor implantation may result from inadequate endometrial formation or from an inappropriate site of implantation.

Abortion may occur if the corpus luteum fails to produce enough progesterone to maintain the decidua basalis. Progesterone may be used as therapy in a documented situation of this type.

Abortion may occur following trauma, such as a blow to the woman's abdomen in an automobile accident. The reason for the abortion in this instance is probably hemorrhage in the decidua basalis, resulting in placental detachment. It is always amazing, however, to discover how many women have accidents or falls during pregnancy without abortion. Such pregnancy histories provide good justification for the presence of the amniotic fluid; it truly serves as a buffer against fetal trauma.

There are many stories of women who have suffered abortion following a profound emotional shock. It is difficult to find documentation for these instances, and so they appear to be due to chance. Emotional causes of abortion cannot be totally discredited, however. Severe fright or stress could cause an elevation of maternal epinephrine sufficient to bring about extensive vasoconstriction, possibly leading to necrosis of the decidua basalis. Interference with circulation of the decidua basalis might lead to fetal death.

Infection in a woman may be another cause of abortion. Rubella and poliomyelitis viruses cross the placenta readily and may cause fetal death. *Mycoplasma* infections are implicated in both infertility and early abortion. Urinary tract infections may lead to early abortion. With failure of growth in the fetus due to illness, estrogen and progesterone production by the placenta falls; this leads to endometrial sloughing. With the sloughing, prostaglandins are released and uterine contraction and cervical dilatation and expulsion of the products of conception begin.

Most women want to know the exact reason for a spontaneous abortion. This gives them courage to attempt another pregnancy. Other women, strong believers in the theory that "what I don't know won't hurt me," would rather not know. In many instances, a reason for the abortion is not apparent.

Most couples find comfort in the theory that most early abortions occur because of aberrations in fetal development. However, some couples are so insecure about their ability to reproduce that they are demoralized to learn that they conceived a less-than-perfect child. Each couple and each woman need to be evaluated as individuals before deciding how much information should be given about the loss of a pregnancy.

Spontaneous Abortion. Spontaneous abortion is abortion that occurs from natural causes. It is popularly known as a *miscarriage*. Spontaneous abortions occur in about 10 percent of all pregnancies. The presenting symptom is almost always vaginal spotting, which is one of the danger signals of pregnancy. At the first indication of vaginal spotting, a woman should telephone her physician or nurse-midwife and describe what is happening. As a nurse is the person who often takes this initial call, you should be aware how to quickly assess vaginal bleeding during pregnancy.

The Nursing Care Highlight on page 880 outlines important questions for obtaining an accurate history of this condition.

The history of the episode is important in helping the physician or nurse-midwife form a diagnosis of the cause. The woman's actions are important to know about to make certain she has not made an attempt to self-abort. She may prefer not to mention such an attempt, but usually will if asked directly. Ask what she has done about the bleeding to be certain she has not inserted a tampon; a tampon can mask unknown amounts of blood loss, which a woman would report as only slight spotting.

Depending on the symptoms and the description of the bleeding or spotting the woman gives, the physician or nurse-midwife will make a decision as to whether or not the woman should be seen in the clinic, office, or hospital.

A nursing diagnosis related to spontaneous abortion is usually concerned with the woman's circulatory adjustment due to the blood loss or the woman's concern over the pregnancy loss. Because the entire family is affected by a pregnancy loss, it may speak to the family's rather the woman's individual concern.

Threatened Spontaneous Abortion. Threatened abortion is manifested by vaginal bleeding, usually bright red in color and moderate in amount. There are no associated symptoms such as cramping; there is no cervical dilatation present on vaginal examination. The only therapy advised for spontaneous abortion is to limit activities for 24 to 48 hours; complete bedrest is unnecessary. Complete bedrest may seem to stop the vaginal bleeding, but does not, because blood is pooling vaginally; when a woman does ambulate again, bleeding will recur. The woman is apt to be extremely upset (bleeding, perhaps watching a pregnancy end, and seeing hopes crushed are bound to be upsetting); she needs time to talk about how distressed she is with a sympathetic support or professional person.

It is important to convey concerned reassurance that the abortion happened spontaneously, not because of anything the woman did. A woman with a threatened abortion looks for reasons it happened and never fails to find them, such as running up a flight of stairs, forgetting to take an iron pill that morning, growing angry at an older child. Being told that none of these things causes abortions will help to free a woman of guilt.

Most women expect health personnel to have a cure for everything. They are disappointed to learn that there is nothing the physician can pre-

================= *Nursing Care Highlight* =================

Assessment of Vaginal Bleeding During Pregnancy

Assessment Factor	*Specific Questions to Ask*
Confirmation of pregnancy	Does she know for certain that she is pregnant (positive pregnancy test or physician/nurse-midwife confirmation)? A woman who has been pregnant before and states that she is sure she is pregnant is probably right even if she has not yet had this confirmed.
Pregnancy length	What is the length of the pregnancy in weeks?
Duration	How long did the bleeding episode last? Is it continuing?
Intensity	Was it just a few drops? A stream? Can she approximate the amount in teaspoons or cups?
Description	Was it mixed with amniotic fluid or mucus? Was it bright red (fresh blood) or dark (old blood)? Was it accompanied by tissue fragments or tissue resembling grape clusters? Was it odorous?
Frequency	Steady spotting? A single episode?
Associated symptoms	Cramping? Sharp pain? Dull pain? Has she ever had cervical surgery?
Action	Did anything happen that may have caused the bleeding? What has she done (if anything) to control the bleeding?

scribe for them to "hold the pregnancy" (they have heard this was done for their mother). No sure evidence supports giving estrogen or progesterone at the time of threatened abortion (as was done in the past), however, as a way to retain the pregnancy. The administration of diethylstilbestrol (DES), once prescribed to women at the time of threatened abortion, is an example of overtreatment. Its use did not improve the number of pregnancies that were retained, and daughters born of the DES-aided pregnancies are now in danger of developing vaginal cancer following adenosis, while male children have heightened susceptibility to cystic testicular development.

Keep your opinion about the outcome of a pregnancy to cautious optimism. If the spotting is going to stop, it usually does so within 24 to 48 hours of the time a woman begins to reduce her activity. After that, the woman can gradually resume normal activities. Coitus is usually restricted for 2 weeks following the bleeding episode to prevent the possibility of infection or induction of further bleeding.

About 50 percent of women with threatened abortion continue the pregnancy; in 50 percent, the threatened abortion changes to imminent or inevitable abortion.

Imminent Abortion. A threatened abortion becomes imminent if uterine contractions and cervical dilatation occur. With cervical dilatation, the loss of the products of conception is inevitable. A woman who reports cramping or uterine contractions is usually asked to come to a hospital, where she is examined. She should save and bring to the hospital with her any tissue fragments that she has passed. Any tissue fragments passed in the labor room should be saved, so that these as well as those the woman supplies can be examined for an abnormality, such as hydatidiform mole, or to assure the physician that all the products of conception have been removed from the uterus. Weighing perineal pads before and after use and subtracting the difference is a good way to accurately determine vaginal blood loss. In the hospital, if no fetal heart sounds are detected, a dilute solution of intravenous oxytocin may be begun to aid the cervix in dilatation and expulsion of the products of conception. A woman's physician may perform a dilatation and curettage (D&C) to ensure that all the products of conception are removed. Be certain a woman knows the pregnancy was lost at hospital admission and all procedures such as a D&C are to clean and ready the uterus for another pregnancy (forward-moving steps), not actually a cause of the pregnancy loss.

Complete Abortion. In a complete abortion, the entire contents of conception are expelled spontaneously without any assistance: fetus, membranes, and placenta. There is minimal, self-limiting bleeding.

Incomplete Abortion. In an incomplete abortion, part of the conceptus (usually the fetus) is expelled, but the membranes or placenta is retained in the uterus. *Incomplete* is a confusing term to many women. They may interpret it as indicating that because the abortion is only partial the pregnancy may continue. Be careful not to encourage false hopes by misinterpreting this term yourself.

In an incomplete abortion, there is a danger of maternal hemorrhage as long as part of the conceptus is retained in the uterus. A woman's physician will usually perform a D&C to evacuate the remainder of the conceptus. It is important that a woman be informed about what is happening, that she know the pregnancy is already lost, and that the procedure is being done only to protect her from hemorrhage and infection, not to end the pregnancy.

Missed Abortion. In a missed abortion, the fetus dies in utero but is not expelled. Women also find the term *missed* misleading. A missed abortion is usually discovered at a prenatal examination when the fundal height is measured and no increase in size can be demonstrated, or when previously heard fetal heart sounds are absent. A woman may have had symptoms of a threatened abortion (painless vaginal bleeding); she may have had no clinical symptoms.

A sonogram can establish that the fetus is dead; at that point the pregnancy will be ended by one of the same techniques used with induced abortion (see below). Within 2 weeks of death of a fetus, symptoms of abortion usually spontaneously occur and the fetus will deliver. There is a danger in allowing this normal course to happen, however, as disseminated intravascular coagulation, a coagulation defect, may develop if the dead (and possibly toxic) fetus remains too long in utero. Disseminated intravascular coagulation is a complication of other bleeding disorders in pregnancy as well (see page 905).

Most women hope until the moment the abortion is induced that the physician is mistaken, that their baby is alive. They need support in accepting the reality of the situation. They may need counseling in order to accept a future pregnancy, because of fears that whatever force struck silently and strangely in one pregnancy might strike again.

Induced Abortion. An induced abortion is a procedure performed by a physician in a controlled office or hospital setting to deliberately end a pregnancy. It is also referred to as a *therapeutic*, a *medical*, or a *planned* abortion. Nurses employed in a health care agency where induced abortions are performed, or by a physician who performs them, are asked to assist with the procedures as a part of their duties.

Induced abortions are done for a number of reasons: to end the pregnancy of a woman whose life is in danger because of the pregnancy (such as a woman with class IV heart disease), to prevent the growth of a fetus who has been found on amniocentesis to have a chromosomal defect, or to accede to the wishes of a woman who chooses not to have a child at this time in her life. The majority of induced abortions are performed for the last reason.

In 1973, the U.S. Supreme Court ruled that induced abortions must be offered in all states as long as the pregnancy is under 12 weeks in length. Whether induced abortions are performed after that point in pregnancy has been left to the individual states to determine. Whether an institution allows induced abortions in the facility depends on the policy and choice of the institution.

An abortion is a decision reached mutually by a woman and her physician. The consent of the father of the child for the procedure is not necessary. Most midtrimester abortions take place in hospitals; a hospital may require that the permission of a husband be obtained before the procedure is performed, but this is hospital policy only. Although the law is being debated, minors may consent to abortion without consent of their parents.

All women having induced abortions should have laboratory studies performed before the procedure. These usually include a pregnancy test, complete blood count, blood typing (including Rh factor), gonococcal smear, a serologic test for syphilis, urinalysis, and Pap smear.

Induced abortions involve a number of techniques, depending on the gestation age at the time the abortion is undertaken.

MENSTRUAL EXTRACTION. Menstrual extraction is the simplest type of abortion procedure. At 4 to 6 weeks following a menstrual period (before pregnancy tests are reliable enough to prove that a pregnancy exists), a woman voids and her perineum is washed with an antiseptic (shaving is not necessary), a speculum is introduced vaginally, the cervix is stabilized by a tenaculum, and then a narrow polyethylene catheter is introduced through the vagina into the cervix and uterus. By means of the vacuum pressure of a syringe, the lining of the uterus that would be shed with a normal menstrual flow is suctioned and removed. Because menstrual extractions are done before a pregnancy is confirmed, probably some women who have them done were not pregnant.

Menstrual extraction is an ambulatory procedure, completed quickly and with a minimum of discomfort (some abdominal cramping will occur when the tenaculum grasps the cervix and as the last of the endometrium is suctioned away). The woman should remain supine for about 15 minutes after the procedure to help uterine cramping quiet and to prevent hypotension on standing. She may be given an oral oxytocin to ensure full uterine contraction following the procedure. She can expect to have vaginal bleeding similar to her normal menstrual flow for a week following the procedure; she may have occasional spotting up to 2 weeks. She should not douche, use tampons, or resume coitus until after her 2-week checkup. She needs to return in 2 weeks' time for a pelvic examination and pregnancy test to be certain that the procedure was effective and her pregnancy effectively interrupted.

Menstrual extraction carries with it the same possibility of hemorrhage and infection as other abortion procedures. Because a pliable catheter is used, however, the possibility of uterine puncture is greatly reduced. A woman needs to know the danger signals to watch for following an abortion and who to telephone if any of these should be apparent (Table 39-2). She needs contraceptive counseling for more reliable reproductive life planning. Although some women's groups advocate menstrual extraction as a do-it-yourself procedure, too much risk is associated with it for this to be practical or encouraged.

DILATATION AND CURETTAGE. If the gestation age of the pregnancy is under 12 weeks, dilatation and curettage is often used as the procedure. A woman is admitted to a hospital or clinic for the procedure. If in the hospital, she may receive a general anesthetic, although a regional anesthetic such as a paracervical block works well for pain relief and is used in ambulatory settings. The use of a paracervical block does not completely obliterate pain but limits what a woman experiences to cramping and a feeling of pressure at her cervix.

Following voiding, cleaning of the perineum (shaving is unnecessary), and the anesthetic block, the cervix is dilated by graduated dilators until a uterine sound and a curet can be inserted through the cervical os. The uterus is then scraped clean with the curet, removing the zygote and trophoblast cells. Following the procedure, a woman should remain in the hospital or clinic for an hour, preferably 4 hours. She is given the same careful assessment of vital signs and perineal care as a woman in the postpartal period receives. An oxytocin medication ensures firm uterine contraction and minimizes bleeding. If there are no complications, she may return home after approximately 4 hours, following explanation of the danger signs of abortion (see Table 39-2) and pertinent contraceptive counseling.

Additional complications of D&C over menstrual extraction include uterine puncture from the instruments used and increased danger of uterine infection because of greater cervical dilatation.

DILATATION AND VACUUM EXTRACTION. In dilatation and vacuum extraction (D&E), as with dilatation and curettage, be certain a woman voids prior to the procedure; as with other uterine procedures, the perineum is washed but shaving is not necessary; and a paracervical block is carried out and the cervix is dilated. In some centers, dilatation of the cervix is accomplished by having a woman come into the center one day before and inserting a Laminaria "tent" into the cervix under sterile conditions. Laminaria is seaweed that has been dried and sterilized. In a moist body part, such as a cervix, it begins to absorb fluid and swell in size. Over a 24-hour period, gradually, painlessly, and untraumatically, it will dilate the cervix enough for a vacuum extractor tip to be inserted without further dilatation. There is some concern that frequent dilatation of the cervix leads to an incompetent cervix, or one that dilates so easily that it will not remain contracted during

Table 39-2 Danger Signals Following Induced Abortion

Signal	Possible Meaning
Heavy vaginal bleeding (more than two pads saturated in an hour)	Hemorrhage
Passing of clots	Hemorrhage
Abdominal pain	Infection (endometritis)
Abdominal tenderness	Infection (endometritis)
Fever over 100.4°F	Infection (endometritis)

pregnancy. This gentle dilatation procedure is often chosen for adolescent girls, therefore, who will perhaps have more than one abortion in their lifetime to try to safeguard their bodies for later childbearing. Antibiotic prophylaxis may be begun at the time of the Laminaria insertion to protect against infection. The woman is cautioned not to have sexual relations until the abortion is complete to reduce the possibility of infection being introduced.

Following either Laminaria dilatation or dilatation by traditional dilators, a narrow suction tip, specially designed for the incompletely dilated cervix, is introduced into the cervix. The negative pressure of a suction pump or vacuum container then gently evacuates the uterine contents in about 15 minutes time. A woman will feel pain if cervical dilatation is performed and some pressure and some cramps similar to menstrual cramps during the suction time, but D&E is not a markedly painful procedure.

Following the procedure, a woman should remain lying down for at least 15 minutes. While remaining in the hospital or clinic for about 4 hours, she is given the same careful assessment of vital signs and perineal care as a woman in the postpartal period receives. She usually receives an oxytocin medication to ensure firm uterine contraction and minimize bleeding. If there are no complications, she may return home after approximately 4 hours, following appropriate contraceptive counseling. She can expect to have bleeding comparable to a menstrual flow for the first week afterward, spotting up to 2 or 3 weeks afterward. Cramping may continue for 24 to 48 hours; she can be advised to take a mild analgesic such as acetaminophen (Tylenol) for this problem. She should not douche, use tampons, or resume sexual coitus until she returns for a 2-week examination; be certain she knows the danger signals shown in Table 39-2. If none of these is present, she can resume normal activities within 24 hours after the procedure.

Because of the rigid cannula used, a D&E has a potential for uterine puncture. In addition, because the cervix was dilated, there is a potential for infection following the procedure.

SALINE INDUCTION. If the gestation age of the pregnancy is between 14 and 16 weeks, a D&E may be used, but the technique generally chosen is saline or prostaglandin induction. Saline and prostaglandin methods are chosen for pregnancies between 16 and 24 weeks in length. Saline interferes with progesterone function, causing endometrium sloughing. A woman is admitted to the labor unit of a hospital. She should void im-

mediately before the procedure to reduce the size of her bladder so that it will not be accidentally punctured. Her abdominal wall is then prepared with an antiseptic solution and anesthetized by a local anesthetic.

A sterile spinal needle is inserted into the uterus through the abdominal wall, and 100 to 200 ml of amniotic fluid is removed by a sterile syringe with amniocentesis technique. A 20% hypertonic saline solution is then injected through the same needle through the abdominal wall into the amniotic fluid. The needle is withdrawn. Within 12 to 36 hours following the injection, labor contractions begin. Labor (which takes an additional 12–36 hours) may be assisted by administration of a dilute oxytocin intravenous solution. The woman is cared for like any woman in labor. She needs frequent explanations of what is happening; she needs her family or a support person with her; she needs medication for discomfort; she may find breathing exercises helpful to minimize discomfort; she needs to have health care personnel with her.

In most hospitals, women undergoing saline induction complete the abortion in a labor room and are not transferred to a delivery room. Because the products of conception are small, the actual delivery causes only a momentary stinging pain as the perineum is stretched. Women need to be reassured that it will not be dangerous for them to deliver in a labor room. They are not second-class patients because they are not being transferred to a delivery room; they simply do not need such a facility.

A possible serious complication of saline abortions is hypernatremia from accidental injection of the hypertonic saline solution into a blood vessel within the uterine cavity. The presence of such a concentrated salt solution in the bloodstream will cause body fluid to shift into the blood vessels in an attempt to equalize osmotic pressure. Serious dehydration of tissue will result. This is an intense reaction that occurs at the moment of injection and is manifested by increased pulse rate, flushed face, and severe headache. The injection must be stopped immediately in the event of such a reaction and an intravenous solution such as 5% dextrose begun to restore fluid balance.

If large amounts of oxytocin are necessary to induce labor with a saline abortion, the woman must be observed closely for signs of water intoxication or body fluid accumulating in body tissue due to oxytocin's antidiuretic effect. Signs of water intoxication are severe headache, confusion, drowsiness, edema, and decreased urinary output. These symptoms occur subtly at first, then grow in severity. Stopping the oxytocin drip is mandatory. Water intoxication will then decrease as body fluid shifts back to normal compartments. Always infuse oxytocin in a "piggy-back" method with abortion the same as in labor so you are able to stop the infusion of oxytocin quickly, yet maintain a fluid line for emergency drugs or fluid.

Such complications of saline abortions are unexpected for a woman. She envisioned a simple procedure and is overwhelmed with the amount of pain she is having and the seriousness of the complication. She needs reassurance that, although unexpected, these complications can be dealt with and she will be safe.

Following delivery of the products of conception, it is important that the tissue be examined to determine whether the entire conceptus has been delivered. The woman should be carefully observed for hemorrhage following delivery, just as if she had delivered at term. She is prone to the development of disseminated intravascular coagulation (see page 905); if this occurs she is very susceptible to hemorrhage. If she wishes to see the fetus, swaddle it as if it were a full-term infant and allow her to see it.

All women should have contraceptive counseling following the procedure and a follow-up examination in about 2 to 4 weeks after the abortion, so that it can be ascertained that the organs of reproduction have returned to their prepregnant state. Sexual relations and douching are generally contraindicated until the time of the post-abortion checkup or for 2 weeks. A woman can expect to have spotting for as long as 2 weeks and a menstrual flow 2 to 8 weeks following the procedure.

PROSTAGLANDIN INJECTION (PGF$_{2a}$). Second-trimester abortions can be done by the injection of PGF$_{2a}$ into the uterus through the abdominal wall in place of hypertonic saline. The woman's abdomen is prepared and anesthetized as with a saline injection. Because the amount of prostaglandin administered is small, no amniotic fluid needs to be removed prior to the injection. Uterine contractions begin much sooner after injection than with saline (½ to 1 hour). Generally, no oxytocin assistance is necessary for delivery to be accomplished.

Although prostaglandin injection is easier and contractions begin sooner, prostaglandins cause extreme nausea, vomiting, and diarrhea in some women and make them feel extremely ill. Their use is contraindicated if the woman has a respiratory disease or hypertension because they also cause vasoconstriction and bronchial constriction. They will induce a severe bronchospasm in women with asthma. A woman should be watched carefully for signs of respiratory distress as the medication is injected. Stopping the injection will fortunately reverse this effect quickly, as the half-life of PGF$_{2a}$ is very short.

A prostaglandin may be administered by vaginal suppository, repeated every 3 to 4 hours as necessary. To limit diarrhea and nausea, diphenoxylate hydrochloride (Lomotil) and prochlorperazine (Compazine) may be administered.

A prostaglandin may also be injected intramuscularly to effect uterine contractions and abortion. Newer methods also include transcervical insertion. Oral administration, once thought to be the answer to easy administration, appears to cause so much nausea, vomiting, shaking chills, and increased temperature that it is an unacceptable method of administration.

All women should have contraceptive counseling following the procedure and a follow-up examination in about 2 to 4 weeks after the abortion, so that it can be ascertained that the organs of reproduction have returned to their prepregnant state. Sexual relations and douching are generally contraindicated until the time of the post-abortion checkup or for 2 weeks. The woman can expect to have spotting for as long as 2 weeks and a menstrual flow 2 to 8 weeks following the procedure.

HYSTEROTOMY. If the gestation age is more than 16 to 18 weeks, a hysterotomy is the safest method of abortion. Since the uterus becomes resistant to the effect of oxytocin as it reaches this phase of pregnancy, it may not respond to saline induction or prostaglandin injection even with an oxytocin assist. Further, the chance is great at this gestation age that the uterus will not respond and contract afterward, leading to hemorrhage following a vaginal delivery. The technique for hysterotomy is the same as that for cesarean section (see Chapter 42).

PSYCHOLOGICAL ASPECTS OF INDUCED ABORTION. With the new abortion laws, women of all ages, married or unmarried, with and without previous children, request induced abortions. As mentioned, the majority of women choose to have an induced abortion to end an unwanted pregnancy. Some women who have been exposed to a disease such as rubella have not chosen the abortion willingly, but only as what seems to be the better of two bad alternatives. Others choose abortion because their pregnancy is the result of rape or incest and not of their choosing. These women may find the period of abortion extremely stressful because it may remind them of the original assault and violence.

Most women feel anxious when they appear at

a hospital or clinic for an abortion. Some of the anxiety comes from having made a difficult decision to reach this step. A great deal comes from having to face the unknown; they have never had an abortion before; they are worried that health care personnel may not be kind to them.

Women having induced abortions need the same kind of explanations that women in labor receive (often more, because women do not share abortion experiences with each other as they share labor experiences; and a woman attends no preparation-for-abortion class, so she may know very little about what will happen to her). During the hours when a woman is waiting for labor to begin after a saline injection, she is likely to behave in an introverted manner, perhaps because her progesterone level is beginning to fall, or perhaps because she feels that minimizing interaction with the health care facility staff prevents people from criticizing her for her decision.

Some nurses find caring for a woman who elects to have an induced abortion distasteful. They chose maternity nursing because they enjoy seeing children born; they do not prefer to care for women who will not allow their child to be born.

To have or not to have an abortion is a value judgment a woman has to make herself, however. She knows the situation in her home, her feelings, and her capabilities better than you or anyone else does. Furthermore, the goals of maternity care encompass more than helping to ensure the birth of healthy children. A child should not only be born healthy but be born into a loving environment. He or she will not have this kind of environment if born to a mother who is not ready for a child. Induced abortions, therefore, are one way of helping to guarantee parental love and concern to every child born.

A woman can choose whether she learns the sex of the child she aborts. Some women prefer not to know in order to prevent guilt or grief feelings in the future—if, for example, a woman aborts a girl, later to give birth only to boys (or vice versa). If she never learns the sex of the fetus she can hopefully prevent these negative feelings.

Freeman (Freeman, 1978) has demonstrated that the postabortion period is a time when the woman is ripe for contraceptive counseling. Table 39-3 contrasts the means of contraception used prior to abortion and after abortion by 106 women.

Women in this same study were asked the

Table 39-3 Percentage Distribution of Women Who Used Contraception Prior to Abortion and Four Months Postabortion, by Age and Method

Age	Total	No Method		Pill		IUD		Diaphragm	
		Pre	Post	Pre	Post	Pre	Post	Pre	Post
Total	100	41	7	5	60	5	7	5	7
15–17	10	36	9	9	73	0	9	0	0
18–19	17	61	11	0	83	0	0	0	0
20–21	22	52	17	4	52	4	4	4	13
22–29	31	27	3	6	61	9	12	3	6
30–39	9	10	0	0	30	10	10	30	20
Unknown	10	54	0	9	54	0	0	0	0

Age	Condom, Foam		Rhythm, Withdrawal		Sterilization		Other	
	Pre	Post	Pre	Post	Pre	Post	Pre	Post
Total	22	8	21	2	0	4	3	5
15–17	27	0	27	0	0	0	0	9
18–19	17	5	22	0	0	0	0	0
20–21	4	4	26	0	0	0	4	9
22–29	30	9	21	6	0	3	3	0
30–39	40	20	10	0	0	20	0	0
Unknown	18	18	9	0	0	9	9	18

Source: Freeman, E. W. (1978). Abortion: Subjective attitudes and feelings. *Family Planning Perspectives, 10*(3),151. Reprinted with permission.

Table 39-4 Percentage Distribution of 106 Reactions to Abortion 4 Months After the Experience

Reaction	Percent
It was a hard experience but I learned a lot.	42
The experience still troubles me: I think about it often.	29
It was an ordinary experience.	15
The experience was upsetting; I don't like to think about it.	9
It was a hard experience but I learned nothing.	3
No answer.	2

Source: Freeman, E. W. (1978). Abortion: Subjective attitudes and feelings. *Family Planning Perpectives, 10*(3), 151. Reprinted with permission.

open-ended question: What did you learn most about yourself as a result of your abortion experience? Typical answers were, "I learned that I could make up my own mind in a difficult situation," "I'm stronger than I thought," "I can get through difficult times."

The replies of women asked 4 months after the experience as to how they reacted to the abortion are shown in Table 39-4. Notice that only 15 percent of the women described the abortion as an "ordinary" experience.

Remembering that this is not a decision taken lightly and one that may be remembered by a woman for a long time to come, plan your nursing care to include interventions aimed at making the abortion as nontraumatic as possible.

Illegal Abortion. An illegal abortion is performed in an uncontrolled setting, usually by a person other than a physician, and without legal sanction. No follow-up care is provided, and unsafe and unsterile practices may be involved. Professional nurses are subject to loss of their nursing licenses if they participate in illegal abortions.

Complications of Abortion. Abortion or early termination of a pregnancy is a deviation from normal pregnancy in itself; in addition, it may lead to other deviations. In some instances, abortion may cause serious maternal complications. As with term childbirth, hemorrhage and infection are the chief complications following abortion. They may occur whether the abortion is induced, spontaneous, or illegal, but they occur most often with illegal abortions because of the lack of quality care and the use of less-than-sterile instrumentation. Some women are admitted to labor units with these complications after having undergone illegal abortions.

HEMORRHAGE. With a complete spontaneous abortion, serious or fatal hemorrhage is rare. With incomplete abortion or in a woman who has an accompanying coagulation defect (usually disseminated intravascular coagulation), major hemorrhage is a possibility. For an immediate measure, keep the woman flat and massage the uterine fundus to try and achieve contraction. The woman may need a dilatation and curettage to empty the uterus of the material that is preventing it from contracting and achieving hemostasis. She may need a transfusion to replace blood, and she may require direct replacement of fibrinogen to aid coagulation.

A woman who is being managed at home after a self-limiting complete abortion should telephone the physician's office or clinic daily for the first 3 or 4 days following the abortion to report her condition. Ask her about (a) the amount of bleeding she is having (in relation to that of a normal menstrual period), (b) the color (gradually changing to a dark color and then to the color of serous fluid, as it does with the postpartal woman), and (c) any unusual odor or passing of clots. If the physician has prescribed an oral medication such as ergonovine maleate to aid with contractions, check to see that she is taking it as prescribed. Some women want to forget the experience as quickly as possible; repression helps them to handle their anger or grief at the loss of the pregnancy most effectively. Be careful that in repressing the experience a woman does not also repress the memory of her medication. If a woman is hospitalized following an abortion, the same observations, plus careful recording of vital signs, are carried out.

If hemorrhage cannot be controlled by the measures that have been described, ligation of the hypogastric arteries or a hysterectomy may be necessary.

Hysterectomy is an extreme measure and always a difficult one for the woman to accept. Her feelings may range from anger (at the fetus, health care personnel, the child's father, herself, God, a contraceptive device that failed her), to grief (for loss of her body part, for loss of this unborn child and other unborn children), to pity for herself, to fright, bewilderment, and inadequacy. She needs strong support from her family and from the health care personnel around her if she is to weather a complication of this magnitude and put her life back together again.

INFECTION. Infection is a minimal possibility when the loss of conceptus occurs over a short period of time, bleeding is self-limiting, and instrumentation is limited.

Women should still be observed closely for signs of infection following abortion, including fever, local tenderness, and a foul vaginal discharge. Some women have a transient fever with abortion that is probably due to the period of lowered fluid intake preceding abortion in some instances. In other instances, the fever may be a systemic reaction to the abortion process. All fevers over 100.4°F should be evaluated carefully, however, so that a woman who is contracting an infection will not be overlooked.

Infection tends to occur in women who have lost appreciable amounts of blood due to the debilitating effect of blood loss. Such women need especially careful observation to rule out this second, possibly fatal, complication.

The organism responsible for infection following abortion is usually *Escherichia coli* (spread from the rectum forward into the vagina). A woman should be cautioned to wipe the perineal area from front to back after voiding and particularly after defecation, to prevent the spread of bacteria from the rectal area. Caution her not to use tampons to control vaginal discharge, since stasis of any body fluid increases the risk of infection. Be careful about statements such as "You'll have some vaginal flow now almost exactly like a menstrual flow." The woman may proceed to treat it as a menstrual flow and use tampons.

Endometritis is the infection that usually occurs following abortion. It may become more extensive, however, and parametritis, peritonitis, thrombophlebitis, and septicemia can occur (see Chapter 44). The management of these infections is the same as if they were occurring postpartum, after the safe delivery of a child.

Isoimmunization and Abortion. When the placenta is dislodged, either by spontaneous delivery or by dilatation and curettage at any point in pregnancy, blood from the placental villi (the fetal blood) may enter the maternal circulation. This occurrence has implications for the Rh-negative woman. Enough Rh-positive fetal blood may enter her circulation to cause isoimmunization—that is, the production by her immunologic system of antibodies against Rh-positive blood. If her next child should have Rh-positive blood, these antibodies would attempt to destroy the red blood cells of the fetus during the months of growth.

Following an abortion, because the blood type of the conceptus is unknown, all women with Rh-negative blood should receive RhO (D) immune globulin (RhoGAM) to prevent the buildup of antibodies in the event the conceptus was Rh-positive.

Recurrent Abortion. In the past, women who had three spontaneous abortions that occurred at the same time in pregnancy were called "habitual aborters." They were often advised that they were apparently too "nervous" or that something was so wrong with their hormones that childbearing was not for them. Today, a thorough investigation is done in women who lose one or more pregnancies to discover the cause and so to be able to predict more accurately whether or not the woman will be able to bear children. Habitual abortion usually occurs for the following reasons.

DEFECTIVE SPERMATOZOA OR OVA. A careful family history in such women may reveal a familial tendency to produce children with defects. If a woman has had more than one aborted fetus, a pathologic report and chromosomal karyotype on the fetus should be carried out to reveal a possible chromosomal abnormality. A chromosomal investigation of both parents will be done to see whether aberrant chromosomes can be detected in either the man's or the woman's karyotype. (Chromosomal abnormalities are discussed in Chapter 6). If such a chromosomal aberration is discovered, artificial insemination using donor sperm or donor embryo transfer can be suggested.

HORMONAL INFLUENCES. In women who have recurrent abortions, the progesterone produced by the corpus luteum or early placenta may be decreased, as revealed by a maternal serum analysis. If this problem is suspected as the cause of the abortions, the pregnandiol levels in maternal urine can be monitored during the woman's next pregnancy. Supplemental progesterone therapy might be indicated.

Ordinarily during pregnancy, the protein-bound iodine (PBI), butanol-extractable iodine (BEI), and globulin-bound iodine (GBI) are elevated. In women with recurrent abortions, these values may be lowered. Thyroid function is assessed by determining the woman's basal metabolic rate or other accompanying thyroid function tests. Poor thyroid function is a cause of infertility as well as of abortion. Thus, if the tests indicate poor thyroid function, the woman may be started on therapy to aid in conception as well as to help carry the next pregnancy to term.

NUTRITIONAL STATUS. Poor nutritional intake may add to the incidence of recurrent abortion.

Low levels of vitamins A, B complex, C, D, and E may contribute to fetal loss. A nutritional history, therefore, should be recorded for any woman with a history of recurrent abortions.

DEVIATIONS OF THE UTERUS. The uterus first forms in utero as an organ with a midseptum. As the organ matures, the septum atrophies and disappears. Occasionally, a woman reaches adulthood with a uterine septum still intact. The blood supply to the septum is not ordinarily as good as that of the endometrium covering the normal walls of the uterus. Placental implantation on the septum may result in an inadequate nutrient supply to the fetus and consequent abortion. The uterus may be only half the normal size because of the dividing septum, so the pregnancy may end prematurely.

A bicornuate uterus is one with sharp poles (horns). This abnormal shape may lead to abortion, although as high as 75 percent of women with bicornuate uteri carry pregnancies to term.

PSYCHOLOGICAL FACTORS. Although certainly not applicable to all women who have recurrent abortions, psychological factors may influence the outcome of pregnancy in some women. Personality factors of immaturity and extreme dependence have been found in women who have recurrent abortions. For these women psychiatric counseling and support may be effective in preventing further pregnancy loss. The exact influence of psychological factors is unproven, however, and it may be the guarded outcome of pregnancy that causes personality changes—not personality factors that influence pregnancy outcome.

BLOOD INCOMPATIBILITIES. Rh incompatibilities do not appear to cause abortions, but ABO incompatibilities may play a role in recurrent abortions. This factor should be considered in the overall assessment of a woman having recurrent abortions.

All women who have recurrent abortions should be thoroughly investigated to determine, if possible, the underlying cause. They no longer simply have to accept this loss as their fate, as they have been forced to do in the past. They need support during the assessment to maintain their self-esteem and confidence that the cause of their difficulty can be discovered and their next pregnancy can be brought to term.

Ectopic Pregnancy

In an ectopic pregnancy implantation occurs outside the uterine cavity. The implantation may

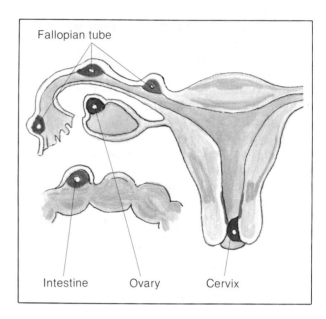

Figure 39-3 *Sites at which an ectopic pregnancy may occur.*

occur on the surface of the ovary, or in the cervix, but the most usual site (in about 95 percent of such pregnancies) is in the fallopian tube (Figure 39-3). Of these fallopian tube sites, about 60 percent occur in the ampullar portion, 25 percent in the isthmus, and 5 percent are interstitial. About 1 in every 200 pregnancies is ectopic; ectopic pregnancy is the second most frequent cause of bleeding early in pregnancy.

Normal fertilization takes place in the distal third of the fallopian tube, and immediately after the union of ovum and spermatozoon the zygote begins to divide and increase in size. If any obstruction is present, such as an adhesion of the fallopian tube from previous infection (chronic salpingitis), congenital malformations, scars from tubal surgery, or a uterine tumor pressing on the proximal end of the tube, the zygote is not able to traverse the course of the tube and will lodge at a strictured site along the tube and be implanted there instead of in the uterus. There is some evidence that intrauterine devices used for contraception may slow the transport of the zygote and lead to tubal or ovarian implantation. IUD devices tend to cause pelvic inflammatory disease so ultimately may cause fallopian tube scarring and increase the incidence of ectopic pregnancy.

Assessment. With ectopic pregnancy, there are no unusual symptoms at the time of implantation. The corpus luteum of the ovary continues to function as if the implantation were in the uterus. No menstrual flow occurs, and the woman may experience the nausea and vomiting of early pregnancy.

At the sixth and twelfth week of pregnancy (4 to 10 weeks following a missed menstrual period), the growing zygote ruptures the slender tube, or the growing trophoblast cells break through the narrow base of the fallopian tube, with resultant invasion and destruction of the blood vessels. The extent of the bleeding that occurs depends on the number and size of the ruptured vessels. If implantation is in the interstitial portion of the tube (where the tube joins the uterus), rupture will cause severe intraperitoneal bleeding. Fortunately, the incidence of tubal pregnancies is highest in the ampullar area (the distal third), where the blood vessels are smaller and profuse hemorrhage is less likely. However, the bleeding may in time result in a great loss of blood. Ruptured ectopic pregnancy is serious, no matter what the site of implantation.

The amount of bleeding *evident* with ectopic pregnancy is deceptive. The products of conception from the ruptured tube and the blood may be expelled into the pelvic cavity rather than into the uterus and then will not reach the vagina and become evident. The woman usually experiences a sharp, stabbing pain in one of the lower abdominal quadrants and notes a little vaginal spotting. (With placental dislodgement, progesterone secretion stops and the uterine decidua begins to slough, causing this bleeding.) She may experience light-headedness and rapid pulse, signs of shock.

The possibility of ectopic pregnancy is the reason it is important to ask all women when they call a health care agency in the first trimester of pregnancy reporting vaginal spotting whether or not there is any associated pain. Any woman with sharp pain and vaginal spotting must be seen, so that ectopic pregnancy can be ruled out.

Occasionally, a woman will move suddenly and pull the round ligament, the anterior uterine support. This will cause a sharp, momentary, innocent lower-quadrant pain. However, it would be very rare for this phenomenon to be reported in connection with vaginal spotting.

By the time a woman arrives at a hospital or physician's office, she may be in deep shock, with a rapid, thready pulse, rapid respirations, and falling blood pressure. Her abdomen gradually becomes rigid. If blood is slowly seeping into the peritoneal cavity, the umbilicus may develop a bluish tinge (Cullen's sign). She may have extensive vaginal and abdominal pain; movement of the cervix on pelvic examination causes excruciating pain. There may be pain in her shoulders from blood in the peritoneal cavity causing irritation to the phrenic nerve. A tender mass is usually palpable in the cul-de-sac of Douglas on vaginal examination. Leukocytosis may be present, not from infection but from the trauma. The temperature is usually normal.

Ectopic pregnancy must be considered an emergency situation. The woman's condition must be evaluated quickly, the amount of blood *evident* being a poor estimate of her actual blood loss. Blood must be drawn immediately for hemoglobin value, typing, and cross-matching. Blood is drawn for serum human chorionic gonadotropin (HCG) level for immediate pregnancy testing (or this is done by you by one of the short-term reporting techniques) if pregnancy has not been confirmed. Intravenous fluid to restore intravascular volume is begun (use a large-gauge needle so blood can be administered when available). If the diagnosis of ectopic pregnancy is in doubt, the physician may, under sterile conditions, insert a needle through the postvaginal fornix into the cul-de-sac to see whether blood that has collected there from internal bleeding can be aspirated. Either laparoscopy or culdoscopy can be used to visualize the fallopian tube if the symptoms alone do not reveal a clear-cut picture of what has happened. A sonogram may be helpful to show the ruptured tube and collecting pelvic blood.

Analysis. The nursing diagnosis established with a woman with ectopic pregnancy is usually related to the change in circulatory status due to hemorrhage (alteration in circulation related to blood loss from ectopic pregnancy). Because this is a stressful situation, the diagnosis may center on the anxiety level of the woman. As a major blood loss of this nature always poses an emergency condition, all goals established must reflect the urgency and short time frame in which the problem must be resolved. These are summarized in the Nursing Care Highlight on page 890. Outcome criteria should include a still fertile woman with high self-esteem.

Planning and Implementation. The medical therapy for ruptured ectopic pregnancy is laparotomy to ligate the bleeding vessels and to remove or repair the damaged fallopian tube. Previously, physicians attempted to "save" ruptured tubes to protect a woman's fertility. Now the ruptured tube is usually removed because a suture line on a fallopian tube may lead to another tubal pregnancy. This rationale should be explained to the woman. Otherwise, she may feel that she has not been given the correct treatment.

Following removal of one tube, a woman is theoretically only 50 percent fertile, since every

Nursing Care Highlight

The Woman with Ectopic Pregnancy

Goal	Nursing Concern
Aid assessment	Identify high-risk population: women with past tubal surgery, pelvic inflammatory disease, previous ectopic pregnancy.
	Ask at history taking if vaginal bleeding was associated with lower abdominal pain.
	Prepare woman for laparoscopy or colposcopy diagnostic procedures.
	Perform pregnancy test or send specimen to laboratory for test.
Maintain circulatory status	Begin intravenous fluid with large-gauge needle.
	Prepare to restore circulatory volume by general care measures shown in the box on page 876.
Support woman's self-esteem	Help woman to work through her grief at pregnancy loss.
	Help her to view childbearing in context—as only a part of one of her capabilities, not her only one.

other month, when she ovulates from the ovary adjoining the removed tube, the sperm cannot reach the ovum on that side. This cannot be counted on as a contraceptive measure, however. It has been shown in rabbits that translocation of ova can occur—that is, an ovum released from the right ovary can pass through the pelvic cavity to the opposite (left) fallopian tube, and vice versa.

Evaluation. A woman who has an ectopic pregnancy not only has grief stages to work through (she has lost a child) but may have problems of diminished self-image to resolve as well. She may believe that she is now half a woman if she equated childbearing with her femininity. She needs to verbalize concerns about future childbearing and concerns that her sexual partner may view her differently now that she is not fully fertile. The process of working through grief and role images takes weeks to months. It should begin in the hospital, where the woman has professional people to help her through the first days and estimate whether she will need counseling.

A woman who has had one ectopic pregnancy is more prone to have a second one because of the nature of ectopic pregnancies. Salpingitis that leaves scarring is usually bilateral. Congenital anomalies such as congenital webbing may also be bilateral. If chronic pelvic inflammatory disease (ordinarily a result of gonorrheal infection) was the reason for the ectopic pregnancy, a woman may feel that she is now being punished for previous sexual activity. She needs to verbalize her feelings, so that she does not leave the hospital feeling guilty and unworthy.

Very rarely—so rarely that the instances are difficult to document (although they have occurred)—after rupture, the product of conception will be expelled into the pelvic cavity with a minimum of bleeding. The placenta will continue to grow in the fallopian tube, spreading perhaps into the uterus for a better blood supply; or it may escape into the pelvic cavity and successfully implant on an organ such as an intestine. The fetus will grow in the pelvic cavity (an abdominal pregnancy). It is possible that such a pregnancy will reach term.

As with abortion, women with Rh-negative blood should receive RhO (D) immune globulin (RhoGAM) following an ectopic pregnancy for isoimmunization protection in future childbearing.

Abdominal Pregnancy

In abdominal pregnancy, the placenta is usually located posterior to the uterus on the intestines or in the cul-de-sac of Douglas. It may remain in the uterine fundus or the fallopian tube if the abdominal pregnancy resulted from a surviving fallopian pregnancy.

In an abdominal pregnancy, the fetal outline is not easily identified by palpation. The woman may not be as aware of movements as she would be normally or she may experience painful fetal movements and abdominal cramping with fetal movements.

Past history of the woman may include previous uterine surgery or the sudden pain of ectopic pregnancy earlier in the pregnancy. A sonogram may be used to reveal the fetus outside the uterus.

The danger of abdominal pregnancy is that the placenta will infiltrate and erode a major blood vessel in the abdomen, leading to hemorrhage. If implanted on the intestine, it may erode so deeply that it causes bowel perforation and a peritonitis. The risk to the fetus is also high. Fetal survival in an abdominal pregnancy is only 20 to 40 percent because of a poor nutrient supply due to abdominal placental implantation. In those infants who do survive there is an increased incidence of fetal deformity.

At term, the infant must be delivered by laparoscopy. The placenta is difficult to remove at delivery if it is implanted on an abdominal organ such as the intestine. If left in place, it will be absorbed spontaneously in 2 or 3 months (a follow-up sonogram can be used to detect whether this restoration has occurred).

Second-Trimester Bleeding

There are two main causes of bleeding during the second trimester: hydatidiform mole and incompetent cervix.

Hydatidiform Mole

Hydatidiform mole is proliferation and degeneration of trophoblast villi. As the cells degenerate, they become filled with fluid, appearing as fluid-filled, grape-sized vesicles; in this condition, the embryo fails to develop or dies before viability (Figure 39-4).

The incidence of hydatidiform mole is about 1 in every 2,000 pregnancies. This condition tends to occur most often in women from low socioeconomic groups who have a low protein intake, in young women (under 18 years of age), in women over 35 years of age, and in women of Oriental heritage. Women receiving clomiphene citrate (Clomid) to induce ovulation appear to have a higher number of hydatidiform mole formations than others.

Two types of molar growth can be identified by chromosome analysis. With a *complete* mole, all trophoblastic villi swell and become cystic. If an embryo forms it dies early at only 1 to 2 millimeters in size; no fetal blood is present in the villi. On chromosomal analysis, although the karyotype of the growth is a normal 46XY, this chromosome component was contributed only by the

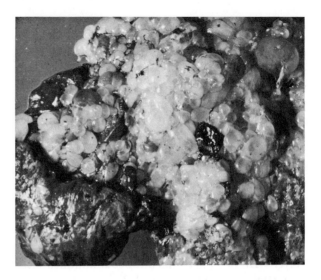

Figure 39-4 *Hydatidiform mole. From Crowley, L. (1974).* An introduction to clinical embryology. *Chicago: Year Book Medical Publishers. Reprinted by permission.*

paternal material or an "empty ovum" was fertilized and the chromosome material duplicated. This is shown in Figure 39-5A.

With a *partial* mole, some of the villi form normally; only the syncytiotrophoblast layer of affected villi is swollen and misshaped. Even though no embryo is present, fetal blood may be

Figure 39-5 *Formation of hydatidiform mole. A. Complete mole. B. Partial mole.*

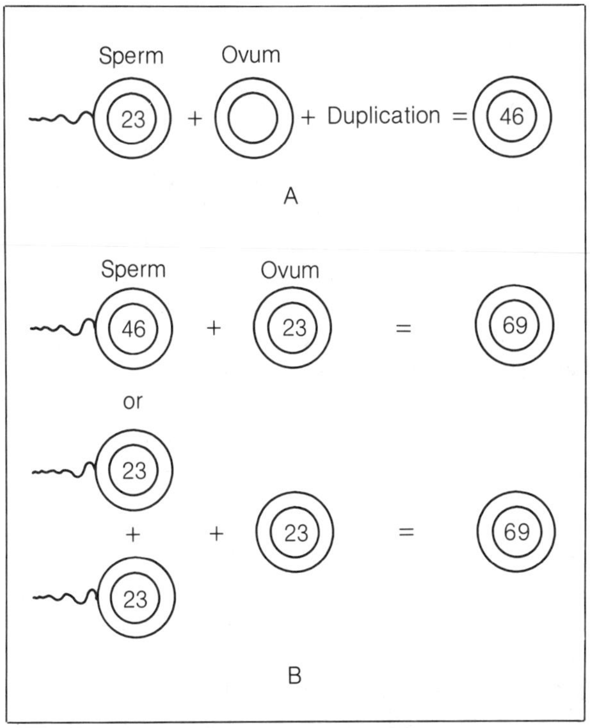

present in villi. A macerated embryo of about 9 weeks gestation may be present. A partial mole has 69 chromosomes (a triploid formation in which there are three chromosomes for every normal two, one set supplied by an ova which apparently was fertilized by two sperm or an ova fertilized by one sperm in which meiosis or reduction division did not occur). This could also occur if one set of 23 chromosomes was supplied by one sperm and an ova which did not undergo reduction division (Figure 39-5B).

HCG titers are lower in partial than complete moles; they return to normal faster after mole evacuation; partial moles rarely lead to choriocarcinoma. Preeclampsia symptoms are equal in severity with both patterns but occur a month later in partial mole (Szulman, 1984).

Assessment. Because the proliferation of the trophoblast cells occurs so rapidly with this condition, the uterus expands faster than it normally does. The uterus reaches its landmarks (just over the symphysis brim at 12 weeks, at the umbilicus at 20 to 24 weeks) before the usual time. This rapid development is also diagnostic of multiple pregnancy or miscalculated due date, however, so this finding must be evaluated carefully. No fetal heart sounds will be heard as there is no fetal or atrophied fetal formation. A blood or urine test for pregnancy will be strongly positive (1–2 million IU compared to a normal pregnancy level of 400,000 IU) because human chorionic gonadotropin hormone (the substance tested for in pregnancy tests) is produced by the trophoblast cells, which are overgrowing. Results continue to be strongly positive after the one-hundredth day of pregnancy, when the level normally would begin to decline. This fact must be evaluated carefully also, since highly positive test results are characteristic of multiple pregnancies with more than one placenta. Symptoms of hypertension of pregnancy (hypertension, edema, and proteinuria) are ordinarily not present before the twenty-fourth week of pregnancy; with a hydatidiform mole, they may appear before this time. A sonogram will show dense growth (typically a snowflake pattern), but no fetal growth in the uterus. The nausea and vomiting of early pregnancy is usually marked, probably due to the high HCG level present.

At about the sixteenth week of pregnancy, if the structure was not identified earlier by sonogram, it will identify itself with vaginal bleeding. This may begin as vaginal spotting of dark brown blood or as a profuse fresh flow. As the bleeding progresses, it is accompanied by discharge of the clear fluid-filled vesicles. This is one reason women who begin to abort at home should bring to the hospital any clots or tissue they have passed. The presence of clear, fluid-filled cysts changes the diagnosis immediately to hydatidiform mole.

Analysis. A nursing diagnosis related to hydatidiform mole often concerns the woman's distress at realizing she is not only not pregnant, as she thought, but a "tumor-like" structure has been growing inside her. If bleeding is heavy with the discharge of the mole, circulatory adjustment due to the blood loss may be a nursing diagnosis.

Planning and Implementations. Medical therapy for hydatidiform mole is induced abortion or dilatation and curettage to evacuate the mole. Although HCG levels are usually negative within a week following a normal pregnancy, the level remains high following hydatidiform mole. One half of women will still have a positive reading at 3 weeks; one fourth will still have a positive test result at 40 days.

The danger of hydatidiform mole is that retained trophoblastic tissue may convert to a malignant growth: choriocarcinoma. As a rule, women who still have a positive test result for HCG at 30 days are readmitted to the hospital for a repeat D&C and biopsy to check for the presence of choriocarcinoma.

Every woman who has had a hydatidiform mole should have a urine specimen or blood serum tested for HCG every month for a full year, so it can be ascertained whether new villi (suggesting the malignant transformation has occurred) are developing, and she should use a reliable contraceptive method during the year, so that a positive pregnancy test (the presence of HCG) resulting from a new pregnancy will not be confused with developing malignancy. Some physicians give women who have had a hydatidiform mole a prophylactic course of methotrexate, the drug of choice for choriocarcinoma. Since the drug has side effects that interfere with blood formation (leukopenia), however, the wisdom of prophylaxis must be weighed carefully.

After a year, if pregnancy test results are still negative, a woman is theoretically free of the risk of a malignancy developing; she could plan a second pregnancy at this time. Although the development of a hydatidiform mole means that a pregnancy never materialized, that a fetus never formed, a woman experiences the same reactions following its evacuation that she would following the loss of a true pregnancy. She did, after all, believe that she was pregnant. On top of losing the pregnancy, she has the added anxiety of being

Nursing Care Highlight
Hydatidiform Mole

Goal	Nursing Concerns
Aid assessment	Identify high-risk population groups: Oriental heritage, pregnancies at age extremes, low socioeconomic levels and clomiphene citrate users.
	Measure fundal height at all prenatal visits; compare to normal landmarks.
	Ask women if they have felt fetal movement at visits after 20 weeks' gestation.
Maintain circulatory status	Caution the woman to bring any tissue passed vaginally to the hospital with her so it can be analyzed for amount and abnormal villi.
	Prepare to restore circulatory volume by the general care measures shown in the box on page 876.
Detect malignant conversion	Counsel about reliable contraceptive method for 1-year use.
	Schedule monthly visits for serum HCG level for 1 year.
Assess future plans	Ask at visits how the woman is coping with delayed childbearing plans.
	Counsel regarding safety of future pregnancies.
Support self-esteem	Help the woman to work through her grief at the pregnancy loss.
	Help her to view childbearing as only one of her capabilities, not her only one.

aware that a malignancy may develop. She also must delay her childbearing plans for a full year. If, in addition, she has already put off having a child (so that she or her sexual partner could finish school or they could buy a house or she is over age 35), the year may seem to be the longest year of her life.

She needs to express her anger and sense of unfairness. She may also feel very inadequate because something went wrong with her pregnancy. She wonders whether it will happen again, whether she will ever be able to have children. Fortunately, the occurrence of a second hydatidiform mole is rare, and she can be assured of this low incidence. Goals of care for the woman with a hydaditiform mole are shown in the Nursing Care Highlight above.

Incompetent Cervix

An incompetent cervix is a cervix that dilates prematurely and therefore cannot hold a fetus until term. The dilation is usually painless. The first symptom is show (a pink-stained vaginal discharge), which is followed by rupture of the membranes and discharge of the amniotic fluid.

Uterine contractions begin, and after a short labor the fetus is born—but unfortunately at about the twentieth week of pregnancy, when the fetus is too immature to survive.

It is often difficult to explain in a particular instance what has caused incompetent cervix. Congenital developmental factors or endocrine factors may be responsible. Trauma to the cervix, such as might have occurred with a previous dilatation and curettage, is probably often the cause.

Following the loss of one child due to an incompetent cervix, a surgical operation termed *cervical cerclage* can be performed to prevent it from happening again. At about the fourteenth to eighteenth week of a new pregnancy, under anesthesia, a pursestring suture is placed in the cervix. This is called a McDonald or a Shirodkar-Barter procedure after the surgeons who perfected it. The sutures serve to strengthen the cervix and prevent it from dilating. Following a cerclage procedure, a woman can expect to notice mild uterine contractions from cervical manipulation and slight bright red vaginal spotting. The uterine contractions will end after several hours, the spotting after 1 or 2 days. She is cautioned to avoid coitus and douching for 2 weeks. If uterine contractions, vaginal bleeding, or rupture of membranes occurs, she must contact her health care provider immediately.

With either a McDonald or Shirodkar procedure, the sutures may be removed at the thirty-eighth to thirty-ninth week of pregnancy, so that the fetus may deliver vaginally or sutures may be left in place and the woman delivered by cesarean birth. The success rate with both of these procedures is between 65 and 80 percent.

Still newer techniques allow the pursestring sutures to be set before the woman is pregnant. This timing gives her the added assurance that she will not begin aborting before the fourteenth week of pregnancy (although the fourteenth week of pregnancy is chosen as this is beyond the point that spontaneous abortion from a defective embryo usually occurs).

It is important with these procedures that the suture be removed before vaginal delivery is attempted or the cervix will be torn. Be certain to ask women who are reporting painless bleeding (also the symptoms of spontaneous abortion) whether they have had past cervical operations.

Women with incompetent cervixes were formerly included in the category of habitual aborters and told to accept their fate. Their cervix was thought simply not strong enough to support a pregnancy. Today, the prognosis for a successful pregnancy in such women is favorable.

Third-Trimester Bleeding

Bleeding during late pregnancy occurs because of either placenta previa, premature separation of the placenta, or premature labor, all of which are serious conditions. Slight spotting late in pregnancy can be caused also by trauma from a pelvic examination, an innocent finding.

Placenta Previa

Placenta previa (Figure 39-6) is low implantation of the placenta. It occurs in three degrees: implantation in the lower rather than in the upper portion of the uterus (low implantation), implantation that occludes a portion of the cervical os (partial placenta previa), and implantation that totally obstructs the cervical os (total placenta previa). The degree to which the placenta covers the internal cervical os is generally estimated in percentages: 100 percent, 75 percent, 30 percent, and so forth.

Fibroid tumors of the uterus, uterine scars from surgery, or abnormal uterine position or shape might cause placenta previa, but generally the reason for the low implantation is not apparent. It occurs in women with increased parity or age, as if possibly the placenta must spread to seek adequate nutritional sources with a less elastic blood supply. The incidence in all pregnancies is about 1 in 200.

Assessment. Bleeding with placenta previa occurs when the lower uterine segment begins to differentiate from the upper segment late in pregnancy and the cervix begins to dilate. The bleeding is the result of the placenta's inability to stretch to accommodate the differing shape of the lower uterine segment or the cervix. Such bleeding generally occurs after the seventh month of pregnancy. The bleeding is usually abrupt and painless, and it is not associated with increased activity. It may stop as abruptly as it began, so that by the time a woman is seen at a hospital she is no longer bleeding; or it may slacken after the initial hemorrhage but remain as continuous spotting. The bleeding is usually acute and sudden enough to frighten a woman thoroughly. She telephones her physician or nurse-midwife, who instructs her to come to a hospital. She may ar-

Figure 39-6 *Degrees of placenta previa. (From Clinical Education Aid, No. 12, Ross Laboratories, Columbus, Ohio, 1963.)*

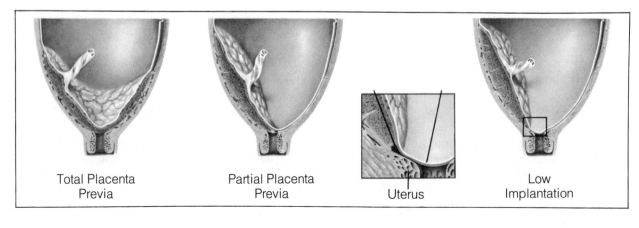

| Total Placenta Previa | Partial Placenta Previa | Uterus | Low Implantation |

rive by ambulance. In any event, she is frightened for herself and for her baby.

The bleeding of placenta previa, like that of ectopic pregnancy, is an emergency situation. The bleeding is from the uterine decidua (maternal blood), so the mother is in danger of hemorrhage. Because the placenta is loosened, the fetal oxygen supply may be compromised and the fetus be in threat also. Once more it is difficult to evaluate how much blood has been lost or whether bleeding is still occurring, since the blood may pool at the base of the uterus and not be apparent.

The woman requires immediate bedrest. You need to assess the following: the time the bleeding began; her estimation of the amount (ask her to estimate in terms of cupfuls or tablespoonfuls (a cup is 240 ml; a tablespoon is 15 ml); whether there was accompanying pain; the color of the blood (the redder the blood, the fresher it is); what she has done for the bleeding (it is important to know that she did not insert a tampon to halt the bleeding, or there may be hidden bleeding); whether there were prior episodes of bleeding during the pregnancy; and whether she had prior cervical surgery (do not mistake an incompetent cervix for placenta previa). To help determine management, you must know the duration of the pregnancy.

In the labor room, check the woman's perineum for bleeding. Estimate the present rate of blood loss. Weighing perineal pads before and after use and subtracting the difference is a good method to determine vaginal blood loss. *Never attempt a pelvic or rectal examination with painless bleeding late in pregnancy. Any agitation of the cervix when there is a placenta previa may initiate massive hemorrhage, fatal to both mother and child.* Take vital signs to determine whether symptoms of shock are present and to establish a baseline of information. Attach an external fetal monitor and begin recording fetal heart sounds. Obviously, any type of monitor that requires invasion of the cervix is completely contraindicated. Ascertain whether the uterus is contracting (whether the woman appears to be in labor).

Fetal heart sounds should be monitored continuously (by an external monitoring system; inserting an internal probe might sever the low-lying placenta); maternal pulse, respirations, and blood pressure should be taken every 15 minutes until it can be ascertained that they are stable. Oxygen equipment should be available in case the fetal heart sounds indicate fetal distress (bradycardia or tachycardia; late deceleration or variable deceleration dips, if the woman is in labor). The woman should have blood drawn for typing and cross-matching, and an intravenous fluid line for intravascular volume replacement should be begun. Vaginal delivery is always safest for an infant. Therefore, it is essential to locate the placenta as accurately as possible in the hope that its position will make vaginal delivery feasible.

On abdominal examination, the fetal head may be discovered to be nonengaged because of the interfering placenta. However, this finding gives little indication of how much of the placenta is obscuring the os and thus preventing the head from engaging.

The placenta may be located by sonogram scanning. A woman needs to be reassured that a sonogram does not use X-ray, and, although long term effects are not yet established, there is no evidence that the procedure will be harmful to her baby, and that the procedure will be painless for her. If a sonogram is not available, the placenta may be located by X-ray placentography. If the pregnancy is at term, this can be undertaken without risk to the fetus. Other, less-used techniques are amniography (instillation of radiopaque dye into the amniotic fluid), isotope injection, and thermography.

The woman's physician may attempt careful speculum examination of the vagina and cervix to rule out a source of bleeding such as ruptured varices or cervical trauma and to establish the percentage of placenta covering the os. If under 30 percent, it may be possible for the fetus to be delivered past it. If over 30 percent and the fetus is mature, the safest delivery method for both mother and baby will be a cesarean birth.

Vaginal examination (actual investigation of dilation) to determine whether placenta previa exists is done in an operating room only so that, if hemorrhage does occur with the manipulation, the woman may be immediately cesarean sectioned to remove the child and the bleeding placenta, contract the uterus, and save both the child and herself. Be careful when reporting the woman's symptoms to her physician on admission that you paint a clear picture of what has happened—Sudden gush of about 100 ml of red blood, no pain. Now a continuous trickle of vaginal blood in a woman 32 weeks' pregnant—so placenta previa will register quickly in his or her mind while skimming through the list of potential diagnoses. When you are working with inexperienced house staff, it is not unprofessional to suggest, "Do you want me to set up an operating room so you can do your vaginal exam there?" for the woman's safety.

Analysis. A nursing diagnosis established with a woman with placenta previa usually in-

Nursing Care Highlight

The Woman with Placenta Previa

Goal	Nursing Concern
Aid assessment	Ask at history taking if pain began episode; ask for an estimation of the amount of bleeding.
	Do not attempt a vaginal or rectal exam.
	Assess amount of vaginal bleeding; monitor maternal vital signs and fetal heart rate by external monitor.
Maintain circulatory status	Prepare to restore circulatory volume by the general care measures shown in the box on page 876.
Maintain self-esteem	Help the woman to grieve for the pregnancy loss if this occurs.
	Help the woman to view childbearing as only one of her capabilities, not her only one.

volves the insult to her circulatory status or her anxiety over the sudden pregnancy complication. In the postpartal period, she is susceptible to infection so a nursing diagnosis may address this problem. Placenta previa is an emergency situation. All goals should reflect its urgency and a short time frame for goal resolution. A summary of goals is shown in the Nursing Care Highlight above.

Planning and Implementations. Once a tentative diagnosis of placenta previa has been made, the age of the gestation will largely dictate the medical management. If labor has begun or bleeding is continuing or the fetus is being compromised (measured by the response of fetal heart rate to contractions), delivery must be accomplished irrespective of gestation age. If the bleeding has stopped, the fetal heart sounds are of good quality, maternal vital signs are good, and the fetus is not yet 36 weeks of age, the woman is usually managed by expectant watching. About a fourth of all women with bleeding from placenta previa are managed this way.

A woman remains in the hospital for close observation. Careful assessment of fetal heart sounds is carried out, and daily determination of hemoglobin or hematocrit is necessary for detection of hidden bleeding.

Placenta previa bleeding usually involves only one episode of painless bleeding as cervical preparation for labor begins. If the episode occurs early in the last trimester, the woman needs a clear explanation of what is happening and what is planned in the light of the fetal immaturity. It is difficult for a woman to wait for a pregnancy to come to term following placenta previa bleeding. She cannot stop wondering whether her infant is all right. She is very aware of fetal movement; asking her to count fetal movements may be helpful not only as a fetal assessment tool but as reassurance for her. Listening to fetal heart sounds and being told that they are in a healthy range is very helpful. She is afraid that the next bleeding she experiences may kill her, or her infant, or both.

She needs to be able to talk about her fears. She may become so worried about the safety of her child that she begins to think of her child as dead. She might neglect her diet or her supplementary vitamins because "it doesn't matter anymore." No matter what her outward appearance is during this time, she is under severe emotional stress.

Delivery. As soon as the fetus reaches 36 weeks of age (2,500 gm), an amniocentesis test for maturity shows a positive result, bleeding occurs again, labor begins, or the fetus shows symptoms of distress, the fetus will be delivered. A woman should be told during her weeks or days of waiting that delivery will probably be by cesarean birth because of the low implantation of the placenta. She must be told that her baby may have a low birth weight.

On her day of chosen delivery, she needs a great deal of support. It is one thing to talk about being ready for surgery; it is another to be truly ready. She is as frightened as she was the evening her bleeding first began.

If, at the time of the initial bleeding, the pregnancy is past 36 weeks, a delivery decision will generally be made immediately. If the placenta previa is found to be total, delivery through the placenta is impossible, and the baby must be delivered by cesarean birth. If the placenta previa is partial, the amount of the blood loss, the condition of the fetus, and the woman's parity will influence the delivery decision. When a cesarean birth is used in placenta previa, although the skin incision is still a transverse (bikini) one, because the uterine cut must be made high, it is made longitudinally above the low implantation site of the placenta.

Following delivery, whether by vaginal or cesarean birth, a mother will inspect her child very carefully, looking for defects. If the placenta was implanted wrongly, she thinks, there must surely be something wrong with her child as well. During the postpartal period, she needs long visiting periods with her child to make certain of normalcy.

Evaluation. Any woman who has had a placenta previa is prone to postpartal hemorrhage because the denuded placental site is in the lower uterine segment, a uterine segment which does not contract as efficiently as the upper segment. Also, because the uterine blood supply is less in the lower segment, the placenta tends to grow larger than it would normally. Thus a larger surface area is denuded when it is removed. A woman is liable to infection, too, because the placental site is close to the cervix, the portal of entry for pathogens.

Premature Separation of the Placenta (Abruptio Placentae)

Unlike placenta previa, in premature separation of the placenta (Figure 39-7), the placenta appears to have been implanted correctly. Suddenly,

however, it begins to separate and bleeding results. By definition, this occurs after the twentieth to twenty-fourth week of pregnancy; separation occurring earlier would be considered a spontaneous abortion. Although it generally takes place late in pregnancy, the condition may occur as late as during the first or second stage of labor.

The primary cause of premature separation is unknown, but certain predisposing factors contribute to it: chronic hypertensive disease, hypertension of pregnancy, or direct trauma, as in an automobile accident. Pressure on the vena cava from the enlarging uterus may contribute to the problem by putting tension on the uterus from back pressure. It tends to occur in women after their fifth pregnancy; it is associated with a low serum folic acid level.

Premature separation may follow a rapid decrease in uterine volume, as occurs with sudden release of amniotic fluid. Since the fetal head is usually so low in the pelvis that it prevents loss of the total volume of the amniotic fluid at one time, a rapid reduction in amniotic fluid does not normally occur.

Assessment. A woman may experience a sharp, stabbing pain high in the uterine fundus as the initial separation occurs. If labor begins with the separation, each contraction will be accompanied by pain over and above the pain of the contraction. In some women the pain is not evident with contractions but is felt on uterine palpation.

Heavy bleeding usually accompanies premature separation of the placenta, but it may not be readily apparent. There will be external bleeding if the placenta separates first at the edges and blood escapes freely from the cervix. If the center of the placenta separates first, however, blood

Figure 39-7 *Premature separation of the placenta. (From Clinical Education Aid, No. 12, Ross Laboratories, Columbus, Ohio, 1963.)*

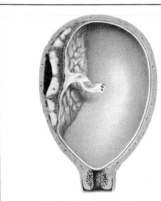 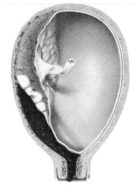 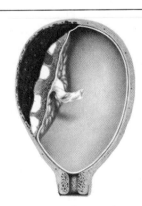

| Partial Separation (Concealed Hemorrhage) | Partial Separation (Apparent Hemorrhage) | Complete Separation (Concealed Hemorrhage) |

========================= *Nursing Care Highlight* =========================

The Woman with Premature Placental Separation

Goal	*Nursing Concerns*
Aid assessment	Identify high-risk population: women with high multiparity, trauma, rupture of membranes, hypertension.
	Assess amount of vaginal bleeding, monitor vital signs and fetal heart rate by external monitors.
Maintain circulatory status	Begin general measures to restore circulatory volume as shown in box on page 876.
Maintain self-esteem	Help the woman to work through her grief at pregnancy loss.
	Help her to view childbearing as only one of her capabilities, not her only one.

will pool under the placenta and be hidden from view. Blood may infiltrate the uterine musculature (*Couvelaire* uterus, or uteroplacental apoplexy), forming a hard, board-like uterus with no apparent, or minimally apparent, bleeding present. Signs of shock usually follow quickly because of the blood loss, and the uterus becomes tense and rigid to the touch.

If bleeding is extensive, a woman's reserve of blood fibrinogen may be used up in her body's attempt to accomplish effective clot formation or disseminated intravascular coagulation (DIC) syndrome occurs.

If a woman is being admitted after experiencing symptoms at home, you need to know the time the bleeding began, whether or not pain accompanied it, the amount and kind of bleeding, and the woman's actions. Initial blood work should include not only hemoglobin level, typing, and cross-matching but a fibrinogen level and fibrin breakdown products (FBP) test to detect the occurrence of DIC. For a quick assessment of blood clotting ability, draw 5 ml and place it in a clean, dry test tube. Stand it aside untouched for 5 minutes. At the end of this time period, if a clot has not formed, an interference with blood coagulation can be suspected. Because premature separation of the placenta may occur during an otherwise normal labor, you have to always be alert to the amount and kind of vaginal discharge a woman is having in labor. Listen to her description of the kind of pain she is having to detect this grave complication.

Analysis. A nursing diagnosis with premature separation of the placenta usually concerns the sudden interference with her circulatory status that has occurred; as the fetus depends on the placenta, the fetus is equally compromised, which suggests that a nursing diagnosis concerns fetal welfare also. As the fetal outcome of premature separation is guarded, a diagnosis may be related to the woman's need to grieve for a pregnancy brought so close to term. Premature separation of the placenta is an emergency situation. Goals established should reflect the crisis circumstances. A summary of goals for care is shown in the Nursing Care Highlight above.

Planning and Implementations. On her admission to the hospital, give oxygen by mask to the woman to limit fetal anoxia. Fetal heart sounds should be monitored by an external monitor, and maternal vital signs should be recorded to establish baselines and observe progress. The baseline fibrinogen determination is followed by additional determinations up to the time of delivery. Keep the woman in a lateral, not a supine, position to prevent pressure on the vena cava and additional compromising of fetal circulation. Do not do a vaginal or pelvic examination or give an enema in order not to disturb the injured placenta any further.

For better prediction of fetal and maternal outcome, the degrees of placental separation are graded, as shown in Table 39-5. Unless the separation is minimal (grades 0 and 1) the pregnancy must be terminated. If the premature separation occurs during active labor, rupturing the membranes or assisting labor with intravenous oxytocin may be the method of choice to speed delivery. Rupturing membranes keeps so much blood

Table 39-5 Premature Separation of the Placenta: Degrees of Separation

Grade	Criteria
0	No symptoms of separation were apparent from maternal or fetal signs. The diagnosis that a slight separation did occur is made after delivery when the placenta is examined and a segment of the placenta shows a recent adherent clot on the maternal surface.
1	This is minimal separation, but enough to cause vaginal bleeding and changes in the maternal vital signs. No fetal distress or hemorrhagic shock occurs, however.
2	This is moderate separation. There is evidence of fetal distress; the uterus is tense and painful on palpatation.
3	This is extreme separation. Without immediate interventions, maternal shock and fetal death will result.

from being trapped in the myometrium of the uterus wall that this prevents contractions of the uterus. Since membranes are ruptured with just a pinprick opening to allow a slow, steady escape of amniotic fluid, a sudden change in uterine pressure does not encourage more separation. If delivery does not seem imminent, cesarean birth is the method of choice.

If a woman has developed disseminated intravascular coagulation, surgery may be a grave risk for her because of the possibility that she will hemorrhage from the surgical incision. Her fibrinogen level must be elevated by the intravenous administration of fibrinogen or cryoprecipitate (which contains fibrinogen) or one of the other forms of therapy for DIC discussed on page 905.

Evaluation. Fetal prognosis depends on the extent of the placental separation and the degree of fetal hypoxia. Maternal prognosis depends on how promptly treatment is instituted. Maternal death is caused by massive hemorrhage leading to shock and circulatory collapse or renal failure from the circulatory collapse.

Any woman who has had bleeding prior to delivery is more prone to infection following delivery than the average woman. A woman with a history of premature separation of the placenta needs to be observed closely for the development of infection in the postpartal period.

Premature Labor

Preterm labor occurs in 6 to 7 percent of all pregnancies. Labor is premature if it occurs before the end of the thirty-seventh week of gestation or before the fetus weighs 2,500 gm. A woman is considered to be in premature labor if she is having uterine contractions of 30 seconds' duration as frequently as every 10 minutes for over 1 hour. Premature labor is always serious because it results in an immature infant and two thirds of all infant deaths in the neonatal period are related to low birth weight.

Why labor begins before the fetus is mature is not clear in most instances. Certain conditions are associated with premature labor. The chances of a woman delivering prematurely with these conditions are estimated in Table 39-6.

Halting Premature Labor. Until recent years, there were no measures available to halt premature labor. Today, if fetal membranes are intact, fetal heart sounds are good, there is no evidence that bleeding is occurring that will affect maternal or fetal welfare, the cervix is not dilated over 3 to 4 cm and effacement is not over 50 percent, medical attempts can be made to stop labor.

An agent that halts labor is a *tocolytic*. The first tocolytic agent used with considerable success was ethyl alcohol (ethanol) administered intravenously to the mother. Ethanol apparently blocks the release of oxytocin by the pituitary gland, thereby blocking, or at least delaying, labor contractions. It makes the mother mildly intoxicated, and she may experience light-headedness, vomiting, nausea, or restlessness. Unfortunately, the prescribed level of ethanol must be maintained over a long period of time to halt labor effectively. When administration is discontinued, labor may be initiated again.

New knowledge concerning the effect of alcohol on a growing fetus has now made halting labor by the administration of alcohol infusion questionable. An infant delivered while the maternal alcohol level is still elevated may be sleepy and have difficulty initiating respirations. He or she is more apt to develop respiratory distress syndrome than if the mother's blood alcohol level is allowed to return to normal before delivery.

Beta adrenergic drugs are the most frequently used tocolytic drugs today. Beta$_1$ receptor sites are found in adipose tissue, heart, liver, pancreatic islet cells and gastrointestinal smooth muscle. Beta$_2$ receptor sites are found in uterine smooth muscle, bronchial smooth muscle, and blood vessels. An ideal tocolytic drug acts entirely on only beta$_2$ receptor sites and does not cause any heart or GI symptoms. Beta adrenergic drugs act by cou-

Table 39-6 Risk for Preterm Delivery by Availability of Treatment

Risk Factor	Multiple by which Risk Is Increased	Estimated Chance that Patient Will Deliver Preterm
Average patient		1 in 15
Prevention possible		
Elective deliveries		
Acute pyelonephritis	3×	1 in 6
Rx may decrease risk		
Twins	5×	1 in 3
Severe preeclampsia	4×	1 in 4
Narcotic use	3×	1 in 5
Low-lying placenta	4×	1 in 4
Partial previa	7×	1 in 2
Total previa	12–13×	1 in 1
Premature rupture of membranes	2–3×	1 in 6
Incompetent cervix	10×	1 in 2
Intensive observation		
Previous stillborn	3×	1 in 5
Previous premature	3×	1 in 5
Previous neonatal death	2–3×	1 in 6
Habitual abortion	3–4×	1 in 4
Vaginal spotting	3–4×	1 in 4

Source: D'Angelo, L., & Sokol, R. J. (1978). Prematurity: Recognizing patients at risk. *Perinatal Care, 2,* 16.

pling with adrenergic receptors on the outer surface of the membrane of myometrial cells. This action releases adrenylcyclase, which triggers the conversion of adenosine triphosphate (ATP) into cyclic adenosine monophosphate (AMP). This substance is responsible for reducing the intracellular concentration of calcium by protein binding. With a lowered intracellular calcium concentration, muscle contraction is ineffective so uterine contractions halt.

Isoxsuprine hydrochloride (Vasodilan) is an adrenergic substance that acts on $beta_2$ receptor sites in the uterine myometrium to relax muscle and thereby halt uterine contractions. Unfortunately, isoxsuprine also acts on $beta_1$ receptor sites in heart muscle, causing the adverse cardiovascular side effects of extreme tachycardia and hypotension. Before it is administered intravenously, the woman must be well hydrated by an intravenous solution to reduce hypotension; and she must maintain a lateral position to aid blood return to the right side of the heart. Although isoxsuprine is an effective tocolytic, because it has such side effects it is little used today.

Ritodrine hydrochoride (Yutopar) is the tocolytic agent used most often today. Ritodrine acts almost totally on $beta_2$ receptor sites. Therefore, it has a milder hypotensive and tachycardiac effect. As the uterine muscle relaxes, however, so do blood vessels and bronchi: There is an increased heart rate in order to move blood more effectively. Hypokalemia may occur from a shift of potassium into cells; thus an increased blood glucose and accompanying plasma insulin level occurs. Pulmonary edema may occur. Headache, due to the dilatation of cerebral blood vessels, is a common side effect; nausea and emesis also may occur. Headache, nausea, and vomiting are side effects to be observed but are not reasons to discontinue therapy. Ritodrine is contraindicated with women with diabetes mellitus, thyroid dysfunction, cervical effacement over 50 percent, cervical dilatation over 4 cm, ruptured membranes, or vaginal bleeding.

ASSESSMENT. Before administration, baseline blood data (HCT, serum glucose, potassium, sodium, chloride, carbon dioxide) and an ECG (perhaps) are recorded. An external uterine and fetal monitor should be attached. Be certain a woman meets the criteria for labor (contractions 30 seconds in length, every 10 minutes for over an

Nursing Care Highlight

Premature Labor

Goal	*Implementations of Care*
Assess tocolytic criteria	Assess contraction rate is 30 seconds every 10 minutes for 1 hour.
	Membranes are intact (test vaginal pH).
	No temperature elevation is present.
	Fetal heart rate is 120–160/min.
	No vaginal bleeding is present.
	Cervical dilation is under 4 cm; effacement is under 50%.
Prevent uterine contraction	Assess pulse and blood pressure for baseline levels.
	Assess serum glucose, potassium, sodium, carbon dioxide, HCT.
	Begin IV infusion per M.D. order with microdrip and automatic pump as piggy-back to mainline IV.
	Increase infusion rate q10min until contractions halt.
	Assess pulse, blood pressure q15min during infusion.
	Assist woman to use controlled breathing exercises until contractions halt to make the experience a positive rehearsal for term labor.
Detect side effects	Discontinue IV infusion if chest pain, dyspnea, maternal heart rate over 120/min, arrhythmias, rales, or BP below 90/60 occur.
Maintain tocolytic effect	Teach woman to take her own radial pulse rate.
	Educate regarding the action of ritodrine hydrochloride.
	Educate to telephone health care facility if pulse rate is over 120/min, heart palpatations or extreme nervousness, rupture of membranes or temperature above 101°F occur.
Maintain self-esteem	Maintain an optimistic attitude.
	Support woman's measures for self-care.
	Encourage support person to remain with woman.

hour). Be certain she fulfills the safe criteria of no vaginal bleeding, no elevated temperature, and no cervical dilatation over 4 cm or effacement over 50 percent.

ANALYSIS. A nursing diagnosis with preterm labor is often focused on the physiologic process of halting contractions, or it may be centered on fetal well-being. As preterm labor is frightening, the diagnosis may speak to the loss of control a woman experiences. Be certain the goals established are realistic to the situation. Not all preterm labor can be halted; some infants will be born prematurely, with a consequent poor outcome. Goals of care are summarized in the Nursing Care Highlight above.

PLANNING AND IMPLEMENTATIONS. For administration, 150 mg of ritodrine is added to 500 ml of normal saline. Normal saline is used rather than a dextrose solution to prevent any unnecessary hyperglycemia. The drug should be administered as a piggy-back method connected to a mainline intravenous solution so it can be stopped immediately if effects such as tachycardia or arrhythmias occur. A microdrip and an automatic infusion pump should be used to ensure a constant infusion. Criteria for discontinuing an infusion are shown in the Nursing Care Highlight above.

An initial flow rate is calculated and begun. This initial flow rate will be increased every 10 minutes until uterine activity halts or a rate of 0.35 mg per minute (the maximum dose) is reached, side effects become extreme, or vaginal bleeding occurs. During administration, pulse and blood pressure should be assessed every 15 minutes during the time the flow rate is being increased, and every 30 minutes thereafter until contractions halt. Assess also for chest pain and dyspnea; auscultate the lungs for rales. Report promptly a pulse rate over 120 per minute, blood pressure below 90/60, chest pain, dyspnea, rales, or cardiac arrhythmias. Hematocrit determination and electrolytes may be drawn every 4 hours during administration. The fetal heart rate may decrease up to 9 beats per minute following the administration of ritodrine. Observe closely for late decelerations or variable decelerations that suggest possible uterine bleeding or the need for emergency delivery of the fetus rather than continuation of the pregnancy.

During administration, propranolol (Inderal) may be given to counteract the decreased blood pressure and allow the ritodrine infusion to continue. Hemodilution (revealed by a lowered HCT) precedes pulmonary edema. Weigh the woman daily as an increasing daily weight suggests heavy accumulation of edema.

Assess the total parenteral intake. With a measurement exceeding 100 ml per hour the woman may develop a fluid overload and pulmonary edema. Measure intake and output every hour during the infusion and then every 4 hours following the infusion.

For poorly understood reasons, the administration of a corticosteroid to the fetus appears to hurry the formation of lung surfactant. During the time labor is being chemically halted, therefore, a woman may be given a steroid (betamethasone) as well to attempt to hurry fetal lung maturity. Betamethasone used this way has a limited effect, so will need to be repeated weekly.

Following the halt of contractions, an infusion of ritodrine is continued for 12 to 24 hours, then oral administration is begun. The first oral dose to be administered is given 30 minutes before the intravenous infusion is discontinued to be certain no drop in serum concentration occurs. The oral dose is usually 10 mg followed by 10 mg every 2 hours for 24 hours, then 10 to 20 mg every 4 to 6 hours until 37 weeks' gestation or fetal lung maturity is established by amniocentesis. Teach a woman to take her pulse before each dose and to call for further advice if over 120 beats per minute or she experiences cardiac palpatation or extreme nervousness.

If membranes have ruptured or the cervix is over 50 percent effaced and 3 to 4 cm dilated, it is unlikely that labor can be halted. The rupturing of membranes, especially, can be thought of as a point of no return in stopping or delaying labor because of the risk of infection that begins with ruptured membranes.

It is important for a woman to call the health care facility immediately if she begins to experience labor contractions late in pregnancy. Some women wait, unwilling to face the fact that labor contractions have started (the ostrich phenomenon). Some diagnose their contractions as nothing more than extremely hard Braxton Hicks contractions and do not seek help until membranes rupture. Differentiating true contractions, however, is a judgment that the primigravida especially is unable to make. She should call her physician, who should make the evaluation. Today, when labor can be delayed until the fetus reaches a level of maturity that will allow survival in the outside environment, evaluation and the institution of therapy before membranes rupture is vitally important.

Labor that Cannot Be Halted. In some women, premature labor will be too far advanced when they are first seen in a health care facility to be halted. In these instances, labor may begin with rupture of the membranes or show from cervical dilatation. As show is often blood-tinged, initially a woman may report this condition as bleeding in pregnancy.

Most women assume that a premature labor will be shorter than normal labor. This is not necessarily so. The first stage of labor, the longest stage, proceeds exactly as it would with a term pregnancy. The second stage of labor *may* be shorter, because a small infant can be pushed through the dilated cervix and the birth canal much more easily than one of normal size. Since the second stage takes at most an hour, the difference will be not more than about a half hour to an hour. Unless they know these facts, women will worry during labor that not only is their labor premature but something is going wrong as well since it is taking so long.

Artificial rupture of the membranes is not performed as a rule in premature labor until the fetal head is firmly engaged because there is such a potential for prolapse of the cord around the small head. Delaying rupture of the membranes may prolong the first stage of labor.

Analgesic agents are administered with caution during premature labor. The immature infant will have enough difficulty breathing on his or her own at birth without the additional burden of being born sedated. If a woman wants anesthesia relief, an epidural, spinal, or infiltration anesthetic is preferable to a general anesthetic because they do not further compromise the infant's ability to initiate respirations at birth. Again, a woman needs to know why a particular method of anesthesia is chosen. She will bear a great deal of pain in the interest of her child's welfare. She will tolerate very little if she feels the choice of care is made for the convenience of the hospital staff.

Uterine contractions and fetal heart sounds should be monitored continually during labor. A woman is reassured by the evidence of monitor screen, graph, or projected sound; these monitors can tell her that, although her infant is likely to be small, the heart tones seem to be of good quality and the infant is reacting to labor well.

Most women also assume that because the infant's head will be small, an episiotomy will be unnecessary for delivery, and they can therefore escape the discomfort of postpartal stitches. Although the head of a premature infant is smaller than usual, it is also more fragile. Excessive pressure might result in a subarachnoid hemorrhage that could be fatal. A woman may therefore need an unusually large episiotomy incision. Forceps may be used for the same reason at delivery to reduce pressure on the fetal head.

The cord of the premature infant is usually clamped immediately, rather than after waiting for pulsations to cease. An immature infant has a difficult time excreting the large amount of bilirubin that will be formed if this extra blood is added to the circulation. The extra amount of blood may also overburden the circulatory system.

A woman in premature labor is undergoing an extreme crisis situation. She cannot help asking herself: What did I do to cause this? People who are looking for reasons find them. She may believe that the large meal she ate the night before is responsible because it "crowded out" the fetus. She may remember the old wives' tale that a woman should not raise her hands over her head during pregnancy and associates the premature labor with hanging curtains in the baby's room. She may worry that sexual relations the night before precipitated the premature labor. She needs to be assured that in no way is this happening her fault. Why labor begins at all is still a mystery. Why it sometimes begins prematurely is even more of a mystery.

In most instances, before giving advice or reassurance, it is wise to wait for a woman to bring up the topic at issue first: No one will listen to advice or counsel until ready. However, reassuring a woman in premature labor that the train of circumstances is not her fault is an exception to this rule. Whether or not a woman is voicing her concern, she is surely feeling it. While you are taking the initial history or timing contractions, you have an opportunity to bring the concern out in the open: "Did Dr. Smith explain to you that labor usually begins early this way without any

reason?" "Some women worry that they did something to bring on premature labor. Have you had any thoughts like that?"

Most women in premature labor are anxious to talk to someone who gives them any opening to express this concern. It is true that a child, if too immature, may die. He or she may have cerebral palsy or some other neurologic disorder common to low-birth-weight infants. Help a woman to be able to say to herself afterward: "I'm sorry this happened. I'd give anything to stop it from happening. I didn't mean for it to happen. *But it was not my fault.*"

Be careful, however, that you do not give false reassurances about the health or weight of the child in your effort to relieve a woman's guilt. On the other hand, do not be overly pessimistic. If she is going to establish a good mother-infant relationship, a woman needs to perceive her child as viable. Find a middle ground. "The baby's heartbeat is good. Labor is going well. Let's face one thing at a time."

A woman in premature labor needs a support person with her: her husband or the child's father. She is more concerned than the average person about being alone in labor. She imagines that the child will be delivered very easily and worries he or she may be born in the labor room; therefore, the woman should have health care personnel with her as well. She feels as if she has disappointed her unborn child, the child's father, and herself. She needs frequent assurance during labor that she is breathing well with contractions or just that she is "doing well." She may not yet have taken a preparation for labor class. She is not mentally prepared for labor, not keyed up to it because it has come unexpectedly. During the postpartal period she also needs reassurance that she is doing well. She must rid herself of guilt, in order to be ready to be a mother to her prematurely delivered child.

Other Causes of Bleeding During Pregnancy

Common causes of bleeding in pregnancy are summarized in Table 39-7. In addition to the causes of bleeding during pregnancy already discussed, a few others may occur.

Coexisting Disease

Cervical or vaginal polyps, vaginal varicosities, carcinoma of the cervix, or blood dyscrasias such as leukemia or decreased platelet levels may cause bleeding during any phase of pregnancy. These are not complications of pregnancy, how-

Table 39-7 Summary of Causes of Bleeding During Pregnancy

Time	Type	Cause	Assessment	Cautions
First trimester	Threatened abortion (early—under 16 weeks) (late—16 to 24 weeks)	Unknown; possibly chromosomal, uterine abnormalities	Vaginal spotting, perhaps slight cramping	
	Imminent (inevitable) abortion		Vaginal spotting, cramping, cervical dilatation	
	Missed abortion		Vaginal spotting, perhaps slight cramping; no apparent loss of pregnancy	Disseminated intravascular coagulation associated with missed abortion
	Incomplete abortion		Vaginal spotting, cramping, cervical dilatation, but incomplete expulsion of uterine contents	
	Complete abortion		Vaginal spotting, cramping, cervical dilatation, and complete expulsion of uterine contents	
	Ectopic (tubal) pregnancy	Implantation of zygote at site other than in uterus. Tubal constricture, adhesions associated	Sudden unilateral lower-abdominal-quadrant pain; minimal vaginal bleeding, possible signs of shock or hemorrhage	May have repeat ectopic pregnancy in future if tubal scarring is bilateral
Second trimester	Hydatidiform mole	Abnormal proliferation of trophoblast tissue; fertilization or division defect	Overgrowth of uterus; highly positive HCG test; no fetus present on sonogram; bleeding from vagina of old or fresh blood accompanied by cyst formation	Retained trophoblast tissue may become malignant (choriocarcinoma); follow for 1 year with HCG testing
	Incompetent cervix	Cervix begins to dilate, and pregnancy is lost at about 20 weeks; unknown cause, but cervical trauma from D&C may be associated	Painless bleeding leading to expulsion of fetus	Can have cervical sutures placed to ensure a second pregnancy
Third trimester	Placenta previa	Low implantation of placenta possibly due to uterine abnormality	Painless bleeding at beginning of cervical dilatation	No vaginal exams to minimize placental trauma
	Premature separation of the placenta (abruptio placentae)	Unknown cause; associated with hypertension	Sharp abdominal pain followed by uterine tenderness; vaginal bleeding; signs of maternal shock, fetal distress	Disseminated intravascular coagulation associated with condition
	Premature labor	Unknown cause; increased chance in multiple gestation, maternal illness	Show—pink-stained vaginal discharge accompanied by uterine contractions becoming regular and effective	Premature labor may possibly be halted up to the point that membranes rupture

ever, but the reverse: Pregnancy is a complication of the disease entity.

Cervical Ripening

Following a pelvic examination late in pregnancy, a woman may notice some slight vaginal spotting due to the manipulation of the cervix as cervical ripening is occurring. The bleeding should be slight and of short duration if this is the only cause.

Disseminated Intravascular Coagulation   DIC

Disseminated intravascular coagulation is an acquired disorder of blood clotting that results from excessive trauma or some similar underlying stimulus. Situations associated with childbirth that may cause this problem are premature separation of the placenta, hypertension of pregnancy, amniotic fluid embolism, placental retention, septic abortion, retention of a dead fetus, and saline abortion.

Blood clotting is a balance between the hemostatic (clotting) system and the fibrinolytic (dissolving) system of the bloodstream. Following a blood vessel injury, local vasoconstriction occurs rapidly to prevent additional blood loss at the site. With the tear in the vessel wall, the underlying collagen is exposed. Exposure to collagen causes changes in platelets (they swell, become adherent, and irregular in shape). They release adenosine diphosphate (ADP), which attracts additional platelets and binds them together (platelet aggregation). This phenomenon results in a platelet plug to seal the vessel. This plug is strengthened by fibrin threads forming as a result of an intrinsic and extrinsic coagulation process (Figure 39-8) into a firm, fixed structure. To prevent too much clotting from occurring, plasmin or fibrinolysin, a proteolytic enzyme, is formed from plasminogen; it digests fibrin threads and causes lysis of the clot along with consumption of blood clotting factors. As plasmin, fibrinogen, and fibrin are lysed, fibrin degradation products are formed. These products prevent the laying down of the fibrin network and platelet aggregation.

With DIC, an imbalance occurs between clotting activity and fibrinolysis. Extreme clotting due to endothelial damage begins at one point in the circulatory system, depleting the availability of clotting factors such as platelets and fibrin from the general circulation; a secondary initiation of fibrinolysis begins as well. A paradox exists: The person has both increased coagulation and a bleeding defect at the same time.

Assessment. A woman begins to have uncontrolled bleeding from puncture sites from injections or intravenous therapy; ecchymosis and petechiae form on her skin. The woman's toes and fingers may be cyanotic or mottled and cold as small blood vessels are so filled with coagulated blood that circulation to extremities is impaired. If coagulation is acute, neurologic or renal symptoms may occur from occlusion of vessels

Figure 39-8 *The mechanism of blood coagulation.*

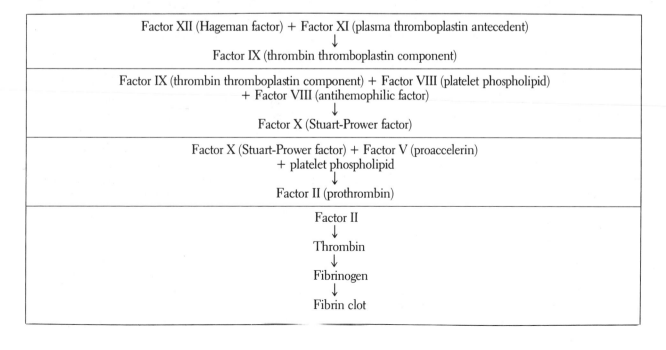

| Factor XII (Hageman factor) + Factor XI (plasma thromboplastin antecedent) ↓ Factor IX (thrombin thromboplastin component) |
| Factor IX (thrombin thromboplastin component) + Factor VIII (platelet phospholipid) + Factor VIII (antihemophilic factor) ↓ Factor X (Stuart-Prower factor) |
| Factor X (Stuart-Prower factor) + Factor V (proaccelerin) + platelet phospholipid ↓ Factor II (prothrombin) |
| Factor II ↓ Thrombin ↓ Fibrinogen ↓ Fibrin clot |

Nursing Care Highlight

Disseminated Intravascular Coagulation

Goal	Implementations of Care
Assess for DIC	Observe possible bleeding sites: gumline, injection sites.
	Mark chart of high-risk patients: premature separation of placenta, death of fetus, hypertension of pregnancy.
	Perform independent clotting test.
	Assess amount of vaginal bleeding during labor and the postpartal period.
Provide blood	Establish IV with lactated Ringers and large- (18 or 19) gauge needle or intracath for open fluid line.
Clotting factors	Draw blood sample for type and cross-match of blood.
	Administer fibrinogen, cryoprecipitate, or fresh frozen plasma per M.D. order.
	Compress injection sites to halt bleeding; handle gently to avoid petechiae and ecchymosis.

supplying the brain and kidneys. Observe all women with a complication of pregnancy carefully for signs of increased bleeding such as skin petechiae or oozing from blood-drawing sites.

Common blood coagulation values are shown in Appendix G. With DIC, laboratory tests usually show that the platelet count is depressed. The level depends on the rate at which bone marrow is able to replace the platelets. On a blood smear, many of the platelets appear large, evidence of their recent production, and they may appear fragmented from passing through meshes of collecting fibrin. As a rule, both the prothrombin time (PT) and the partial thromboplastin time (PTT) are prolonged. Fibrinogen, the final factor necessary to make the clot, will have a markedly low level in serum (under 100 mg/100 ml). Fibrin split (degradation) products (FSP or FDP) are elevated.

Analysis. A nursing diagnosis with disseminated intravascular coagulation is generally concerned with the physiologic phenomenon that is occurring; implementations are aimed at helping to halt the process and protect fetal welfare. As it is obviously frightening to have such a loss of blood coagulation, fear related to the phenomenon may be the center of the diagnosis. DIC is an emergency situation; goals must reflect its urgency. Goals of care are summarized in the Nursing Care Highlight above.

Planning and Implementation. To stop the process of disseminated intravascular coagulation, the underlying insult that began the phenomenon must be halted. When this happens with a complication of pregnancy, ending the pregnancy by delivering the fetus and placenta is therefore part of the answer. The marked coagulation can be stopped by the intravenous administration of heparin. Heparin must be given with caution close to delivery or postpartal hemorrhage may occur when the placenta is delivered. Although blood transfusion will be necessary to replace blood loss if bleeding during pregnancy is the beginning stimulus, it may be delayed until after heparin has been administered so that the new blood factors are not also consumed by the coagulation process. Fresh frozen plasma, fibrinogen, or cryoprecipitate (which contains fibrinogen) may be administered. If neither fibrinogen nor cryoprecipitate (cryoprecipitate is the blood product administered to a person with hemophilia and therefore may not be available in hospitals that do not routinely treat a large number of these patients) is at hand, fresh frozen plasma or platelets will aid in restoring clotting function.

It is bewildering to patients with a disorder such as premature separation of the placenta to have their physician tell them one minute that bleeding is the chief concern and the next minute that heparin has been ordered (or they may see you add heparin to their intravenous line). If they understand the action of heparin—to discourage blood coagulation—their need and the medication ordered seem directly contradictory. Be certain that a woman and her support person are given a full explanation: She has an increased risk of hemorrhaging because part of her system has begun coagulation—which you are stopping. This effort on your part will help maintain her confidence in her caregivers.

Evaluation. Evaluation is aimed at assessing whether a woman's blood coagulation studies are returning to normal and destruction has not occurred, particularly in renal or brain cells, from the occluded coagulated capillaries. Obviously, fetal assessment and, with delivery, newborn assessment is important to determine that placental circulation remained sufficient. As heparin does not cross the placenta, an infant does not need assessment for blood coagulation ability at birth related to this.

Premature Rupture of Membranes

Premature rupture of the membranes is a threat to the fetus: Uterine infection may follow. Premature labor may also result, posing the risk of immature birth to the fetus. Although the cause of premature rupture of the membranes is usually unknown, it is associated with advanced maternal age, nonwhite mother, multiparity, cigarette smoking, preterm labor, low pregnancy weight gain, instrumentation of the cervix before pregnancy, and recent coitus (Flood, 1983).

If a fetus is estimated to be mature enough to survive in an extrauterine environment at the time of rupture, and labor does not begin within 24 hours, it is usually induced by intravenous administration of oxytocin. Induction of labor is necessary in this situation because rupture of the membranes destroys the integrity of the uterus, allowing bacteria to enter the uterine cavity through the vagina and infect both mother and fetus (amnionitis). Rupture of the membranes also may permit prolapse of the umbilical cord (extension of the cord out of the uterine cavity into the vagina), particularly if it happens when the fetal head is still too small for a firm cervical fit.

Rupture of the membranes should be ascertained by the history. The woman will usually describe a sudden gush of clear fluid from the vagina, with continued minimal leakage. Occasionally, a woman will mistake urinary incontinence caused by exertion for rupture of the membranes. Amniotic fluid cannot be differentiated from urine by appearance. A Nitrazine paper test makes this differentiation, amniotic fluid giving an alkaline reaction and urine an acidic reaction. Smearing a sample of vaginal secretion on a slide, allowing it to dry, and observing it under a microscope for a ferning pattern is also helpful. Amniotic fluid has a high estrogen content and shows a ferning pattern; urine does not.

If, after premature rupture of the membranes, labor does not begin, the fetus is too young to survive outside the uterus, and the woman seems capable of following instructions conscientiously, she may be allowed to return home. She is instructed to take her temperature twice a day and to report a fever (temperature over 100.4°F) promptly. She should refrain from coitus and douching because of the danger of introducing infection. Her physician may prescribe a prophylactic antibiotic for her in order to prevent infection, although the actual effectiveness of antibiotic prophylaxis is not well documented.

Before a woman is discharged after an initial observation period, be certain that she knows how to read a thermometer (have her demonstrate her knowledge to you) and that she has specific instructions about what to report. Exactly what degree of temperature should she report? When should she report to her physician for her next checkup? Be certain she knows that as soon as the fetus is mature, she will be delivered by induction of labor.

There are old wives' tales about the agony of labor following premature rupture of the membranes (dry labor). A woman hopes every day that the fetus is at term and that labor will begin, ending the long wait, yet she is afraid to begin labor. She needs a great deal of support for the remainder of the pregnancy and reassurance that because amniotic fluid is always being formed, there is no such thing as "dry" labor.

Pregnancy-Induced Hypertension

Pregnancy-induced hypertension (PIH) (formerly termed *toxemia*) occurs in only 5 to 7 percent of all pregnancies in the United States, yet it is the third most frequent cause of maternal mortality, following only hemorrhage and infection. Despite years of research, the cause of hypertensive disease of pregnancy is still unknown. Originally it was called *toxemia* because researchers pictured a toxin of some kind being released by a woman in response to the foreign protein of the growing fetus. The toxin then supposedly led to the typical symptoms of hypertension, proteinuria, and edema. No toxin has been identified, however. Poor nutrition (particularly poor protein intake) is strongly correlated with the development of symptoms. A deficiency in pyridoxine (vitamin B₆) has also been suggested as a factor contributing to development of the condition. Parasitic invasion of a woman is also a possibility. According to a study by Lueck, et al. (1983), multiple forms of a parasitic organism were discovered in the blood samples and could be cultured from the surface of the placenta of women with hypertension of pregnancy. The organism, named *Hydatoci lualba,* was also located in the umbilical cord blood of infants born to such women. This study suggests that the cause of pregnancy-induced hypertension is basically infectious in nature. A genetic predisposition may be responsible (Chesley, 1980).

A basic cause of PIH's three symptoms is vascular spasm, but why the spasm occurs is difficult to prove. As the disorder tends to arise most often in primigravidas and has a high incidence in multiple pregnancy and the pregnancies of women with diabetes mellitus, uterine ischemia due to uterine stretching is a possibility. Normally, blood vessels during pregnancy are very resistant to the effects of pressor substances such as angiotensin and norepinephrine. With hypertension of pregnancy, this reduced responsiveness to blood pressure changes appears to be lost and so

blood pressure increases. Whether the change in responsiveness is a primary cause or a secondary result of the vasospasm is still unknown. Because hypertension of pregnancy occurs with one pregnancy is not an indication that it will occur with all a woman's pregnancies.

The vasospasm reduces the blood supply to organs as well as adding to or causing hypertension. This effect is most marked in the kidney, pancreas, liver, brain, and placenta. Ischemia in the pancreas may result in epigastric pain and an elevated amylase/creatinine ratio. Arteriolar spasm in the retina leads to vision changes; if hemorrhages occur, blindness can result. Tissue hypoxia may follow in the maternal vital organs; poor placental perfusion may reduce the fetal nutrient and oxygen supply.

Vasospasm in the kidney increases afferent arteriolar resistance and decreases glomeruli perfusion pressure. This change results in an elevated serum BUN, creatinine, and uric acid and a decreased creatinine clearance. The degenerative changes that develop in kidney glomeruli because of the vasospasm and local congestion lead to increased permeability of the glomerular membrane. This in turn allows the serum proteins albumin and globulin to cross into the urine (proteinuria). The degenerative changes also result in a decreased glomerular filtration rate and lowered urine output. Increased tubular reabsorption of

Figure 39-9 *Physiologic changes with pregnancy-induced hypertension.*

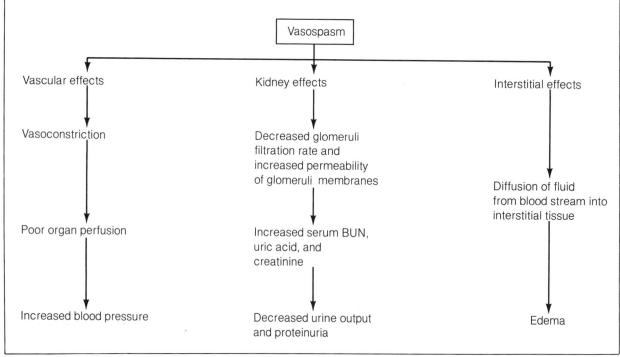

sodium occurs, causing edema. Edema is further increased as more protein is lost, the hydrostatic pressure of the circulating blood falls, and fluid diffuses from the circulatory system into the intracellular spaces to equalize the pressure (edema). Extreme edema will lead to brain edema and convulsions (eclampsia).

The arterial spasm causes the bulk of the blood volume in the maternal circulation to be pooled in the venous circulation so the woman has a deceptively low arterial intravascular volume. Measuring hematocrit levels helps to assess the extent of plasma lost to venous volume or the extent of the vasospasm. These physiologic changes are summarized in Figure 39-9.

Assessment

Pregnancy-induced hypertension tends to occur more frequently in certain women than in others: in primiparas under 20 years or over 30 years of age; in women from a low socioeconomic background (perhaps because of poor nutrition); in women who have had five or more pregnancies; in nonwhites; in multiple pregnancy; with hydramnios; with underlying disease such as heart disease, diabetes with vessel or renal involvement, and essential hypertension. If symptoms of hypertension of pregnancy are going to develop, they are rarely apparent before the twenty-fourth week of pregnancy. Symptoms occurring before this time suggests hydatidiform mole rather than PIH. Classification criteria for degrees of pregnancy induced hypertension are shown in Table 39-8.

Any woman who falls into one of the high-risk categories for pregnancy-induced hypertension should be observed especially carefully for symptoms at prenatal visits. She should be told the symptoms to watch for so that she can call and alert medical personnel.

A means of assessing blood pressure that is useful during pregnancy is mean arterial pressure (MAP). Mean arterial pressure is defined as one third of the pulse pressure (the difference between the systolic and diastolic pressure) plus 80. As an example, if a blood pressure is 120/70, the mean arterial pressure is $120 - 70 = 50$ divided by $3 = 16.6 + 80 = 96.6$ mm Hg. Mean arterial pressure demonstrates resistance to cardiac output; in other words, it is an index of cardiac work. The higher it is, the more vasospasm is present or the harder the heart has to work to push blood through narrowed arteries. Mean arterial pressure characteristically decreases slightly during the second trimester of pregnancy. For further differentiation, MAP[2] and MAP[3] determinations can be made. MAP[2] is an average of all blood pres-

sures taken during the fifth and sixth months of gestation. MAP[3] is the average of the highest two values separated by at least 6 hours during the third trimester of pregnancy (Chervenak, 1983). A MAP[2] over 90 mm Hg or a MAP[3] over 105 mm Hg is abnormal.

Table 39-8 Symptoms of Pregnancy-Induced Hypertension

Classification	Symptoms
Gestational hypertension	MAP[3] over 105 mm Hg or systolic pressure elevated 30 mm Hg or diastolic pressure elevated 15 mm Hg above pre-pregnancy level. No proteinuria.
Mild preeclampsia	MAP[3] over 105 mm Hg or systolic pressure elevated 30 mm Hg or diastolic pressure elevated 15 mm Hg above pre-pregnancy level or BP 140/90. Proteinuria of 1–2+ on a random sample. Weight gain over 2 lbs/wk in second trimester; 1 lb/wk, third trimester. Mild edema in upper extremities or face.
Severe preeclampsia	BP of 160/110 mm Hg. Proteinuria of 3–4+ on a random sample; 5 grams on a 24-hour sample. Oliguria (500 ml or under in 24 hr). Cerebral or visual disturbances (headache, blurred vision). Pulmonary edema. Extensive peripheral edema. Hepatic dysfunction. Thrombocytopenia.
Eclampsia	A convulsion occurs.

Gestational Hypertension

A woman is said to have gestational hypertension when she develops an elevated MAP[3] level, but had a normal MAP[2] and has no proteinuria. Perinatal mortality is not increased with simple gestational hypertension. Chronic hypertension may develop in these women later in life, however (Chervenak, 1983).

Preeclampsia

Mild Preeclampsia

A woman is said to be *mildly* preeclamptic when her blood pressure rises 30 mm Hg or more systolic or 15 mm Hg or more diastolic above her prepregnancy level, taken on two occasions at least 6 hours apart. The diastolic value of blood pressure is extremely important to note, as its rise indicates peripheral vascular spasm.

Formerly, a blood pressure of 140/90 was considered the criterion for preeclampsia and it is still a useful cutoff point. This general rule is obviously less meaningful than measuring each woman's blood pressure against her early pregnancy baseline. It is still a rule of thumb to keep in mind, however, if a woman comes for prenatal care for the first time late in pregnancy and there is thus no baseline pressure available for her.

Average blood pressures in American females are shown in Appendix G. Looking at the average pressure for young Caucasian women, you can see that a woman in the under-20 category could have a blood pressure of 98/61 and still be within normal limits. If her blood pressure were elevated 30 mm Hg systolic and 15 mm Hg diastolic, it would be only 128/76. This measure is well beneath the traditional warning point of 140/90, yet would be hypertension for her.

Using MAP criteria, a woman has developed preeclampsia when her MAP[2] is above 90 mm Hg or her MAP[3] is above 105 mm Hg and proteinuria is present.

Many women show a trace of protein in urine all during pregnancy. Actual proteinuria is said to exist when at least 1+ or more protein is evident on a reagent strip (representing a loss of 1 gm/liter).

Occasionally, women have orthostatic proteinuria (on long periods of standing, they excrete protein; at bedrest they do not). If a woman has no other signs of hypertension of pregnancy (no hypertension, no edema) and the urine she offers for testing is not her first morning one, but one she has voided in the health care facility, asking her to bring in a first morning urine may reveal that the actual problem is not pregnancy-induced hypertension.

Edema develops, as mentioned, because of the protein loss and a lowered glomerular filtration level. This swelling occurs in the upper part of the body rather than just in the ankles; and a woman has a gain in weight of more than 2 pounds a week in the second trimester and 1 pound in the last trimester, which usually indicates tissue fluid retention or beginning edema. This is likely to be the first symptom to appear and is discovered when a woman is weighed at a prenatal visit. Noticeable edema may or may not be present when this sudden increase in weight first occurs. The Perinatal Task Force for the Study of Pregnancy-Induced Hypertension demonstrated, however, that 85 percent of all gravidas have some edema during pregnancy and that the presence of edema alone does not change perinatal mortality. Edema with hypertension does not increase perinatal risk over the risk present by the hypertension alone; when both edema and proteinuria are present, perinatal mortality is increased (Chervenak, 1983).

Severe Preeclampsia

A woman has passed from mild to severe preeclampsia when her blood pressure has risen to 160 mm Hg systolic and 110 mm Hg diastolic or above on at least two occasions 6 hours apart at bedrest, marked proteinuria is found, and extensive edema is present. Marked proteinuria is a reading of 3 or 4+ on a random urine sample or over 5 gm in a 24-hour sample.

With a severe preeclampsia, the extreme edema will be noticeable in the woman's face and hands as "puffiness." It is most readily palpated over bony surfaces, where the sponginess of fluid-filled tissue can best be revealed. Palpating or pressing over the tibia on the anterior leg, the ulnar surface of the forearm, and the cheekbones is a good way to detect edema. Edema is nonpitting if you suspect swelling or puffiness at these points but you are unable to indent them with your finger. If you are able to indent tissue slightly, 1+ edema is present; moderate indentation, 2+; deep indentation, 3+; indentation so deep it remains as a pit after you remove your finger, 4+ pitting edema.

Further assess edema by asking a woman if she has been aware of any. Most women at the end of pregnancy have edema of the feet at the end of the day. They report this symptom as difficulty fitting into their bedroom slippers, or kicking off their shoes at dinnertime and then not being able to put them back on again. This is normal edema. Edema that has progressed to upper extremities or the face is abnormal and what you are listening for. Women report upper-extremity edema as "rings are so tight that I can't get them off," facial edema as "when I wake in the morning, my eyes are swollen shut" or "I'm unable to talk until I walk around awhile."

Some women have severe epigastric pain, nausea, and vomiting possibly due to abdominal

A roll-over test determines if pregnancy-induced hypertension is likely to occur. It should be done routinely on all women at the twenty-eighth to thirty-second week of pregnancy. Have a woman lie on her left side for 15 minutes and establish a baseline diastolic pressure for her (take two readings that have the same diastolic pressure), then have her turn to her back (supine) and measure her blood pressure in that position at 1 and 5 minutes after she turns. Use the last heard heart sound for the diastolic reading in both positions. A woman who has an increase of diastolic pressure of 20 mm Hg or more in the supine position will probably develop hypertension of pregnancy. She will need additional follow-up during pregnancy.

---

edema or ischemia to the pancreas and gastrointestinal tract. Pulmonary edema may cause them to feel short of breath. Cerebral edema will cause visual disturbances such as blurred vision or seeing spots before their eyes. Cerebral edema also gives symptoms of severe headache and marked hyperreflexia. This accumulating edema will reduce their urine output to about 400 to 600 ml per 24 hours.

At all prenatal visits, women should be screened for proteinuria, edema, increased blood pressure, and weight gain. They should be asked too about the symptoms of cerebral and visual disturbance: dizziness, spots before the eyes, or blurring of vision. The roll-over test (Gant, 1974) described in the Nursing Care Highlight above may be helpful in predicting which women will develop pregnancy-induced hypertension.

Analysis

A nursing diagnosis concerning pregnancy-induced hypertension is usually related to the physiologic elevation of blood pressure. Because bedrest is the most frequent therapy for an elevated blood pressure, the diagnosis may involve the problems concerned with requiring bedrest in an active woman with home and family responsibilities. Goals established should reflect the short time frame of the pregnancy and be realistic in terms of a woman's life style. Goals of care are summarized in the Nursing Care Highlight on page 912.

Planning and Implementations

Implementations for pregnancy-induced hypertension differ depending on whether the extent of the problem is mild or severe.

Mild Preeclampsia. Measures initiated with mild preeclampsia include bedrest, improved nutrition, and emotional support.

BEDREST. In a recumbent position, sodium tends to be excreted at a more rapid rate than during activity. Bedrest, therefore, is the best method of aiding increased evacuation of sodium and lowering levels of plasma sodium. With bedrest, diuresis occurs.

Rest should always be in a lateral recumbent position to avoid uterine pressure on the vena cava and supine hypotension syndrome. If a woman is able to rest at home, she can remain at home. If there is a question as to her compliance, she may be hospitalized even at this early date. In one study, when nulliparas with beginning signs of preeclampsia were hospitalized to ensure bedrest, the perinatal mortality rate was 9 per 1,000. Among women who left the hospital against advice, the perinatal mortality was 129 per 1,000 (Gant, 1978). The increased mortality may be due to more than the difference in bedrest because the reason the women left the hospital may reflect overall poor compliance to medical regimens.

NUTRITION. Because a woman is losing protein in the urine, she needs a high-protein diet. At one time stringent restriction of salt was advised in order to reduce edema. This suggestion is no longer made because stringent sodium restriction may activate the angiotensin system and result in increased blood pressure, compounding the problem.

EMOTIONAL SUPPORT. It is difficult for a woman to appreciate the potential seriousness of her symptoms because they seem so vague. Neither high blood pressure nor protein in urine is something that she can see or feel. She is aware that edema is present, but it seems unrelated to the pregnancy. It is her hands that are swollen, not a body area near her growing child. Many women therefore take instructions such as getting rest at this time rather lightly.

Nursing Care Highlight

Pregnancy-Induced Hypertension

Goal	*Implementation of Care*
Prevent eclampsia	Maintain bedrest; side rails elevated.
	Assign to darkened, quiet room.
	Administer sedative (such as phenobarbital) orally or IM as ordered.
	Maintain IV fluid line for emergency medication route.
	Administer loading dose of magnesium sulfate IV or IM as ordered.
	Continue magnesium sulfate IV or IM as ordered.
	Assess patellar reflex, urine volume, and respiratory rate before magnesium sulfate administration.
	Hematocrit daily to detect vasospasm.
	Assess urine output q1h.
Prevent hypertension	Administer antihypertensive as prescribed.
	Encourage high protein, moderate sodium diet.
Assess edema	Auscultate lungs for rales q4h.
	Weigh daily.
	Assess peripheral edema q4h.
	Maintain intake and output.
Promote fetal well-being	Monitor with external uterine and fetal monitor.
	Assess with nonstress test weekly.
	Keep side lying for improved placental perfusion.
	Collect 24-hr urine or serum level for estriol.
Provide emergency measures for convulsions	Keep turned to side.
	Administer oxygen by mask at 2–4 L (do not use nasal prongs or catheter as they are intrusive).
	Administer magnesium sulfate as prescribed.
	Assess for uterine contraction in postictal period.
Help determine delivery plans	Vaginal delivery is preferable to cesarean birth as the woman is high-risk for surgery.
Maintain self-esteem	Praise efforts to cooperate, maintain therapy.
	Maintain an optimistic pregnancy outcome.

Women are also used to having severe disorders treated with some form of medication, which does not happen with this problem. Then how can it be really serious? Furthermore, it is not always easy to comply with the instruction to get additional rest during the day. Almost fifty percent of women of childbearing age work outside their home. About half the women you talk to, therefore, are being asked to stop work in order to rest more. Physicians may give that instruction lightly, because they may not view a woman's earnings as adding greatly to a couple's basic income (only "frosting" or "egg money"). In reality, the contribution of most working women goes not for luxuries but for a good part of the mortgage or rent or car payments. If a woman is not married, her income is probably her sole support. Asking her to stop work, then, when she may be evicted, or have a loan or a house or a car foreclosed on because of missed payments, on the basis of a few vague symptoms—a little swelling, a little headache—is asking a great deal.

You cannot solve people's financial problems for them, but ask enough questions of a woman so that you can be aware of her problem. A question such as, "What will it mean to your family if you have to quit work?" brings it out in the open.

People can make arrangements with loan companies or banks to make partial payments or delayed payments during periods of hardship. A couple may have savings they were planning to use for the baby that can carry them over during this time (and still literally allows them to be used for the baby). Perhaps they can borrow money or change their living arrangements. In any event, they need to consider what extra rest during pregnancy will mean to them. People cannot begin to solve problems until they are aware of them.

A woman with other children must think through her day and make changes in order to get additional rest. The mother who spends considerable time chauffering school-age children to scouts, dancing lessons, and so forth may have to investigate car pooling. A mother may have to drop being a Brownie leader, or ask her husband to help her coach her neighborhood softball team. Again, a woman needs to understand that, although the symptoms she is experiencing are mild, they may be forecasting an extremely serious disorder. Ask, "What will it mean to your other children or your husband if you have to rest?" to allow her to face this problem.

Women with beginning signs of hypertension will be seen about every 2 weeks for the remainder of pregnancy. Be certain a woman understands that if symptoms worsen before 2 weeks she should not wait but call for an earlier appointment. There is little cure for eclampsia of pregnancy. Prevention at the early stage is what is important.

DIURETICS. For years, diuretics to evacuate fluid and decrease edema were routinely prescribed in preeclampsia, but their use in this condition is now contraindicated. Diuretics, particularly the thiazides, are effective in decreasing the reabsorption of sodium, thus lowering levels of sodium in the plasma. Fluid then shifts back from the extracellular spaces into the circulatory system and is excreted. Edema is thereby reduced, but plasma volume, which is already low, will be depleted even further and poor placental perfusion may result.

Diuretics also stimulate the release of renin. This action increases the permeability of glomerular vessels, leading to increased proteinuria and activating angiotensin, raising the blood pressure. Diuretics may therefore actually worsen preeclampsia, not improve it.

Severe Preeclampsia. If the preeclampsia is severe, hospitalization is strongly recommended. If the pregnancy is 36 weeks or more in length, or fetal maturity is confirmed by amniocentesis, induction of labor may be undertaken. If the pregnancy is less than 36 weeks in length, or the amniocentesis reveals immature lung function, interventions will be instituted to attempt to alleviate the symptoms and allow the fetus to come to term.

BEDREST. With hospitalization, bedrest can be enforced, and the woman can be observed closely. A woman with severe preeclampsia should be admitted to a private room so she may rest undisturbed by a roommate. She should lie in a left lateral recumbent position as much as possible. She should be away from the sound of women in labor or the crying of infants on a postpartal unit. A loud noise such as a crying baby or a dropped tray of equipment may be sufficient to trigger a convulsion, initiating eclampsia.

The room should be darkened; a bright light can also trigger convulsions. However, the room should not be so dark that you need to use a flashlight to make assessments. Having to shine a flashlight beam into a woman's eyes is the kind of stimulus you are trying to avoid.

Some physicians order *no visitors* for the woman, but this type of order needs to be evaluated individually. Social visitors should be restricted, but support people (husband, father of the child, mother, or older children) may enable her to rest more readily by assuring her that they are managing well at home and want the pregnancy as much as she does.

A woman hospitalized with severe hypertension needs almost constant nursing observation. Stress is a stimulus capable of increasing blood pressure and possibly evoking convulsions in a woman with severe preeclampsia. She should receive clear explanations of what is happening and what is planned for her. If she understands the importance of complete bedrest, she will tend not to cheat and get out of bed. She will accept the fact that, in the interest of maximal rest and minimal stimulation, visitors must be restricted to just her husband or to one person of her choice.

She must have opportunities to express how she feels about what is happening, how bewildered she is because the few simple symptoms she noticed 2 weeks ago (increase in weight, increasing edema) have now developed into a syndrome that may be lethal to her baby and possibly to her. She needs to talk about the things she did during pregnancy that she believes may have brought on her condition. Perhaps the night before her symptoms first became apparent she ate a half bag of potato chips. Could that have set off this event? The first 3 months of the pregnancy she wished she were not pregnant. Could that have been responsible?

A woman may want to discuss the financial impact of the hospitalization. She planned to work until the end of pregnancy. She planned on delivering her child at an alternative birthing center, and now she may be hospitalized for a month. She cannot afford a private room. Where is the money coming from?

Perhaps there are other children at home. Who will look after them? Who will remind them to brush their teeth? Who will remember that the youngest is afraid of the dark and the oldest needs help with his math homework? These are all real problems that prevent a woman from resting.

A woman with severe pregnancy-induced hypertension should not have a telephone in her room, because a ringing phone is a sudden, sharp stimulus and all such stimuli are to be avoided. She should be encouraged to write short notes to her children unless she is too heavily sedated. Her older children should be encouraged to send her notes or school drawings.

If the woman cannot be freed of these worries even with help, it is a fallacy to think that she is calmly waiting for her pregnancy to come to term.

MATERNAL MONITORING. The woman's blood pressure should be taken at least every 4 hours to detect any increase, which is a warning that her condition is worsening. If it is fluctuating, it may need to be assessed hourly. Blood studies (CBC, platelet count, liver function, uric acid, BUN, creatine and fibrin degradation products) may be taken daily to assess for renal and liver function and the development of disseminated intravascular coagulation. A woman may have a type and cross-match for blood done, as she is high-risk for premature separation of the placenta and hemorrhage.

A urinary catheter is usually inserted to allow accurate recording of output and comparison with intake. Urinary output should be over 600 ml per 24 hours (over 30 ml per hour); a lower output means that oliguria is present. Urinary proteins and specific gravity should be measured and recorded with voidings or hourly by catheter. Urine should be saved for 24-hour protein determinations and possibly for estriol determination to evaluate fetal well-being (see Chapter 15). A woman with mild preeclampsia spills between 0.5 gm to 1 gm of protein every 24 hours (1 + on a random sample); a woman with severe preeclampsia spills about 5 gm per 24 hours (3 to 4 + on an individual specimen).

Weight should be measured daily at the same time each day for evaluation of tissue fluid retention. A woman should bring a light duster or bathrobe with her to wear at every weighing, so that change in weight does not just reflect a change in the weight of her clothing. A daily hematocrit level should be determined to monitor blood concentration, an index of how well fluid is being retained in the intravascular system. Plasma estriol and electrolyte levels will also be measured frequently. The woman's optic fundus should be assessed daily for signs of arterial spasm, edema, or hemorrhage.

FETAL MONITORING. The fetal heart rate may be assessed by continuous fetal external monitor, but generally simple stethoscope auscultation at about 4-hour intervals is sufficient at this stage of management. A woman may have a nonstress test done once weekly to assess placental uterine sufficiency (see Chapter 15). Urinary estriol levels may be deceptively low in a woman with hypertension of pregnancy because her overall output is decreased and must be assessed in light of this reduced output.

SAFETY. The siderails on a woman's bed should be raised to keep her from falling should she have a convulsion. She needs to be told that the side rails have been raised not to imprison her but for her safety and the safety of her unborn child. With this explanation, a siderail rule is not difficult to enforce, and protection is provided when no nurse is present.

NUTRITION. A woman needs a high-protein, moderate-sodium diet to compensate for the protein she is losing in the urine.

MEDICATION. To encourage complete bedrest, a barbiturate such as phenobarbital orally or IM may be prescribed. A fluid line to serve as an emergency route for drug administration should be initiated and maintained. It is important that the insertion site be observed carefully for infiltration because if a woman is heavily sedated she may not be aware that the site is swelling and irritation from an infiltrated intravenous site is the sort of irritation that can trigger a convulsion in a severely preeclamptic woman.

A hypotensive drug such as hydralazine (Apresoline) may be prescribed to reduce the hypertension. Apresoline acts to lower blood pressure by peripheral dilatation and causes no interference with placental circulation. Apresoline may cause tachycardia; thus not only blood pressure but pulse as well should be assessed following its administration. Diazoxide (Hyperstat) or cryptenamine (Diatensen) may be used for their ability to produce rapid decreases in blood pressure. Diazoxide is not used for long-term administration as it tends to cause hyperglycemia. If vasopressors of this nature are used, diastolic pressure should not be lowered below 80–90 mm Hg or inadequate placental perfusion may occur.

Despite many new drugs suggested for the treatment of preeclampsia or eclampsia, magnesium sulfate is still the drug of choice. Magnesium sulfate is actually a cathartic. It reduces edema by causing a shift in fluid from the extracellular spaces into the intestine. It also has a central nervous system depressant action (it blocks peripheral neuromuscular transmissions) that lessens the possibility of convulsions. Although it has a minimal peripheral dilating effect, it does not greatly lower blood pressure, and it has no noticeable effect on labor contractions. Magnesium sulfate may be given intramuscularly or by a slow intravenous infusion.

To achieve immediate reduction of the blood pressure, magnesium sulfate is usually given intravenously in a loading or bolus dose (4 gm in 100 ml of 5% dextrose in water). Given intravenously over 5 to 20 minutes, the drug begins to act almost immediately but the effect lasts only 30 to 60 minutes.

Following the initial reduction of blood pressure, magnesium sulfate is then continued by slow intravenous infusion (1–2 gm/hr) or intramuscularly (5 gm of a 50% solution every 4 hours). Intravenously, the dose should be given piggy-backed to a main infusion line so it can be discontinued immediately without interfering with the main intravenous line; it should be administered with a microdrip and automatic pump to ensure safe and controlled administration. The intramuscular dose must be given deeply into a large muscle group so that absorption can take place. To reduce the pain of the injection, 0.5 ml of 1% procaine can be added to each injection.

In order for magnesium sulfate to act as an anticonvulsant, blood serum levels are maintained at 4.0 to 7 mg per 100 ml. If a blood serum level above this amount occurs, respiratory depression and cardiac arrhythmias and cardiac arrest follow. These serum levels are shown in Table 39-9.

Urine output must be observed carefully when a woman is receiving magnesium sulfate since magnesium is excreted from the body almost entirely through the urine. If severe oliguria occurs

Table 39-9 Effects of Increasing Magnesium Sulfate Serum Levels

Effect of Drug	Level of Occurence
Therapeutic range	4–7 mg/100 ml
Patellar reflex disappears	8–10 mg/100 ml
Respiratory depression occurs	10–12 mg/100 ml
Cardiac conduction defects occur	Over 15 mg/100 ml

(less than 100 ml in 4 hours), excessively high blood levels of magnesium will be seen. The most evident symptom of overdosage with magnesium sulfate is depression of respirations and deep tendon reflexes. Respirations should be above 16 per minute, and deep tendon reflexes should be checked before the next dose of drug is administered, or every hour if a continuous intravenous infusion is being used.

The easiest deep tendon reflex to check is the patellar reflex (knee jerk). Instructions for initiating this reflex are shown in the Nursing Care Highlight on page 916. If an epidural block has been given for labor anesthesia, you must assess a biceps or triceps reflex (Chapter 18).

A third assessment that should be done before further magnesium sulfate is administered is measurement of the urinary output. If not over 25 to 30 ml per hour (specific gravity 1.018 or better), the dose should be questioned.

Prevention of overdosing from magnesium sulfate therapy by conscientious checking of tendon reflexes, respiratory rate, and urine output is an important nursing responsibility. In addition to these measures, when magnesium sulfate is being given, a solution of 10 ml of a 10% calcium gluconate solution (1 gm) should be kept ready nearby for immediate intravenous administration. Calcium is the specific antidote for magnesium toxicity. Severe oliguria may be treated by IV infusion of salt-poor albumin. This high-colloid solution will "call" fluid into the intravascular space by osmotic pressure; the kidneys will then excrete the extra fluid along with magnesium sulfate levels.

At the time of delivery, the anesthesiologist must be alerted to the fact that a woman has been receiving magnesium sulfate. If magnesium sulfate is given intravenously within 2 hours of delivery, the baby may be born depressed because the drug crosses the placenta. Since this problem is rarely seen with intramuscular injection, however, that is the method of administration gener-

Nursing Care Highlight

Patellar Reflex

With a woman in a supine position, ask her to bend her knee slightly and to then relax her leg. Place your left hand under her knee to support the knee. Locate the patellar tendon in the mid- line just below the knee cap. Strike it firmly and quickly with a reflex hammer. The method by which deep tendon reflexes are scored is shown in Table 39-10.

---

ally used close to delivery. A fetus may show loss of beat-to-beat variability of fetal heart beat immediately following an intravenous loading dose. If this response persists for over 20 minutes, observe very carefully for other signs of fetal effects such as late deceleration.

Because magnesium sulfate is a neuromuscular blocking agent, the anesthesiologist must be cautious in administering other neuromuscular blocking agents such as succinylchloride (used to give relaxation for intubation with general anesthesia). Magnesium sulfate is continued for 12 to 24 hours following delivery to prevent eclampsia from occurring during this period. The dose is then tapered and discontinued; a woman should delay breast-feeding until the medication is discontinued.

Women who have had pregnancy-induced hypertension are generally not prescribed ergot compounds for milk suppression in the postpartal period: These compounds elevate blood pressure. A woman needs to be certain to return for a postpartal checkup to have her blood pressure evaluated for a return to normal and lack of chronic hypertension.

Eclampsia

This is the severest classification of hypertension of pregnancy. With it a woman has passed into the third stage in which cerebral edema is so acute that a convulsion occurs. With eclampsia, maternal mortality is as high as 15 percent.

Degeneration of the woman's condition from severe preeclampsia to eclampsia is usually marked by discernible signals. The woman's blood pressure may rise suddenly. Her temperature may rise sharply, to 39.4° or 40°C (103° to 104°F) from increased cerebral pressure. She may notice blurring of vision or severe headache (from the increased cerebral edema). She may have hyperactive reflexes. She may have a premonition that "something is happening." There may be epigastric pain and nausea as a result of vascular congestion of the liver or pancreas. Urinary output may slacken abruptly, to less than 30 ml per hour. Eclampsia has actually occurred, however, only when the woman convulses.

Grand Mal Convulsions. An eclamptic convulsion is a grand mal convulsion. With this type of convulsion, following the preliminary signals, all the muscles of a woman's body contract. Her back arches, her arms and legs stiffen, and her jaw closes abruptly. She may bite her tongue from the rapid closing of her jaw. Respirations will be halted, since her thoracic muscles are held in contraction. This phase of the convulsion, called the *tonic* phase, lasts about 20 seconds. It may seem longer because a woman may grow cyanotic from the cessation of respirations.

Oxygen administered by face mask may be needed to protect the fetus during this time interval. A woman should be turned on her side; or, even though she is almost at term, she can be placed on her abdomen to allow secretions to drain from her mouth to prevent aspiration. An external fetal heart monitor should be attached if it is not already in place to follow the condition of the fetus. Inserting a tongue blade between a woman's teeth to prevent her from biting her tongue is not recommended. The convulsion occurs suddenly, and thus the action that causes the jaw to clench shut has taken place before you can put a tongue blade between her teeth. Attempting to do so *after* the contraction has occurred rarely

Table 39-10 Scoring of Deep Tendon Reflexes

Score	Description
4+	Hyperactive; very brisk; abnormal
3+	Brisker than average but not abnormal
2+	Average response
1+	Somewhat diminished response but not abnormal
0	No response; hypoactive; abnormal

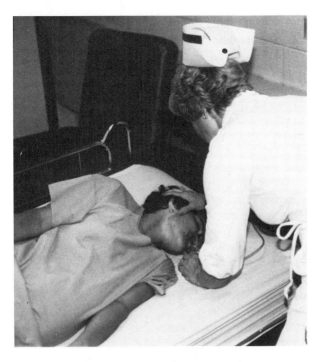

Figure 39-10 *During a convulsion, turn the woman's head to the side and administer oxygen as necessary.*

Table 39-11 Stages of a Grand Mal Convulsion

Stage	Appearance
Aura (momentary sensation)	Woman senses convulsion is beginning by seeing a bright light or smelling a sharp odor; epigastric pain from pancreatic ischemia may be present.
Tonic phase (20 seconds)	All muscles contract. Jaws will close; respirations stop. Woman appears stiff and cyanotic.
Clonic phase (20 seconds)	All muscles rhythmically contract and relax; respirations are noisy and uneven; breathing through collected saliva in mouth causes foaming of the mouth.
Postictal phase (1 hour)	Woman is semicomatose; rouses only to painful stimuli.

has any therapeutic effect and leads to broken teeth, scraped gums, bitten fingers, or broken tongue blades (Figure 39-10).

Following the tonic phase, all the muscles of the woman's body begin to contract and relax, contract and relax, causing a woman's extremities to flail wildly. She inhales and exhales irregularly as her thoracic muscles contract and relax. She may aspirate the saliva that collected in her mouth during the tonic phase if she was not placed on her side or abdomen. She blows through the collected saliva and any blood that is present in her mouth, causing the "foaming at the mouth" sometimes associated with convulsions. Her bladder and bowel muscles contract and relax; incontinence of urine and feces may occur.

Although she begins to breathe during this stage, the breathing is not entirely effective. Her color may remain cyanotic and she may need continued oxygen therapy, not for herself but for the fetus. This *clonic* stage of a convulsion lasts approximately 1 minute. Magnesium sulfate or diazepam (Valium) may be administered intravenously as an emergency measure at this time.

The third stage is a *postictal* state. The woman is semicomatose and cannot be roused except by painful stimuli for at least an hour and sometimes up to 4 hours. Extremely close observation is as necessary during the postictal stage as it is during the first two stages. Labor may begin during this period, but because the woman is unconscious,

she is unable to report the sensation of contractions. Also, the painful stimuli of contractions may initiate another convulsion. Fetal heart sounds should be continuously monitored. Check for uterine contractions by resting your hand on her abdomen and feeling for tenseness. A monitor to record uterine contractions may be attached to obtain this information, provided the device does not appear to irritate the woman. Check for vaginal bleeding every 15 minutes; the convulsion may have caused premature separation of the placenta. Evidence that separation may have occurred will appear first on the fetal heart sound record; vaginal bleeding will strengthen the presumption.

The woman should be regarded as and treated like any comatose patient. She should remain on her side, so that secretions can drain from her mouth. She should be given nothing to eat or drink. Remember that in coma hearing is the last sense lost and the first one regained. Be aware that when you are discussing a woman's condition she may be able to hear you even though she does not respond to you. A summary of the stages of grand mal convulsions is shown in Table 39-11.

Delivery

If the gestation age of the pregnancy is over 36 weeks, a delivery decision will be made as soon as the woman's condition stabilizes, which is usually 12 to 24 hours after a convulsion. There is some evidence that the fetus does not continue to grow after eclampsia occurs. Thus, terminating the pregnancy at this point is appropriate for both mother and child. For an unexplained reason, fetal lung maturity appears to advance rapidly with hypertension of pregnancy (possibly from the intrauterine stress), so even though the fetus is younger than 36 weeks, the lecithin/sphingomyelin (L/S) ration of amniotic fluid may be mature.

The preferred method for delivery is vaginal using a pudendal block. Because the vascular system is low in volume, a woman may become very hypotensive with conduction anesthesia such as an epidural block.

Cesarean birth is always more hazardous for the fetus, who may already be under sufficient strain. Further, a woman with eclampsia is not a good candidate for general anesthesia and surgery. Rupture of the membranes or induction of labor by intravenous oxytocin may be instituted. If this therapy is not effective and the fetus appears to be in imminent danger, cesarean birth will have to be done.

Evaluation. Eclampsia can result in death of the mother from cerebral hemorrhage, circulatory collapse, or renal failure. Fetal prognosis in eclampsia is poor because of hypoxia and consequent acidosis. If premature separation of the placenta occurs, the prognosis is even graver. If the fetus must be delivered before term, all the risks of the immature infant will be faced. In preeclampsia, perinatal mortality is approximately 10 percent. If eclampsia develops, the fetal mortality increases to about 25 percent.

Pregnancy-induced hypertension may occur up to 10 to 14 days after delivery, although most postpartal hypertension occurs in the first 48 hours following delivery. Women need follow-up care in the postpartal period to detect residual hypertensive or renal disease.

Chronic Hypertensive Vascular Disease

Women with chronic hypertensive disease come into pregnancy with an elevated blood pressure. Hypertension of this kind is usually associated with arteriosclerosis or renal disease. It tends to be a problem of the older pregnant woman. Retinal changes may be apparent on physical examination, caused by the chronic hypertension in retinal vessels. Deterioration of the renal glomeruli may have occurred, resulting in chronic proteinuria. There is a risk that fetal well-being may

be compromised by poor placental perfusion during the pregnancy.

Usually, a woman who enters pregnancy with slight hypertension will have an additional elevation of blood pressure with pregnancy and is prone to the development of edema and proteinuria. It is difficult to differentiate this increased blood pressure from developing preeclampsia if a woman comes to the health care facility late in pregnancy for her first prenatal visit.

Women with chronic hypertensive vascular disease must be followed by an internist during pregnancy as well as by an obstetrician. If the blood pressure becomes extremely elevated, complete bedrest for the entire pregnancy may be necessary, and the pregnancy may have to be terminated in order to prevent a cerebral vascular accident. The infants of women with chronic hypertension tend to have retarded fetal growth from poor placental perfusion. Since women with hypertension are advised not to take birth control pills, contraception may be a problem in the postpartal period.

Multiple Gestation

Multiple gestation is a complication of pregnancy: In addition to the effects of one fetus on a woman's body, her body must adjust to the effects of another fetus, or two others, or more.

Identical (monozygotic) twins begin with a single ovum and spermatozoon. In the process of fusion, or in one of the first cell divisions, the zygote divides into two identical individuals. Single-ovum twins usually have one placenta, one chorion, two amnions, and two umbilical cords. The twins are always of the same sex. Fraternal (dizygotic) (nonidentical) twins are the result of the fertilization of two separate ova by two separate spermatozoa. These twins are actually siblings growing at the same time in utero. Double-ova twins have two placentas, two chorions, two amnions, and two umbilical cords. The twins may be of the same or different sex.

It is sometimes difficult at delivery to discern whether twins are identical or fraternal because the two fraternal placentas may fuse and appear as one large placenta.

Multiple pregnancies of three, four, five, or six children may be single-ovum conceptions, multiple-ova conceptions, or a combination of two types. Multiple pregnancies are more frequent in nonwhites than in whites. The higher a woman's parity and age, the more likely she is to have a multiple gestation. Dizygotic twinning has a familial maternal pattern of occurrence.

Assessment

Multiple gestation is suspected early in pregnancy when the uterus begins to increase in size at a rate faster than usual. A sonogram will reveal multiple gestation sacs. At the time of quickening a woman may report flurries of action at different portions of her abdomen rather than at one consistent spot (where the feet are located). On auscultation of the abdomen, two sets of fetal heart sounds may be heard, unless one twin has his or her back positioned toward the woman's back. Diagnosis may be confirmed at term or after the twenty-eighth week by an X-ray if sonogram equipment is not available. On occasion, twinning is not discovered until after the birth of the first child when it is found that the uterus is not empty.

Because a woman is carrying a double weight during pregnancy, she notices extreme fatigue and backache. She may have increased difficulty resting or sleeping because of greater discomfort and increased fetal activity. As the growing uterus compresses her stomach, she may find her appetite decreasing and her intake falling. She may need to eat six small meals a day rather than three large ones to maintain adequate nutrition. She must take her iron, folic acid, and vitamin supplement.

Toward the end of pregnancy a woman may have extreme difficulty ambulating because of fatigue and backache. Her abdomen may become so stretched that she feels as if she were going to burst.

Analysis

A nursing diagnosis concerning a multiple gestation usually involves the extreme minor discomforts of pregnancy the woman notices, her need for increased rest and careful nutrition supervision, or her anxiety about carrying a multiple gestation. Goals established must be realistic in light of a woman's life style and her ability to compensate for this major life change.

Planning and Implementations

Women with a multiple gestation are more susceptible to such complications of pregnancy as pregnancy-induced hypertension, hydramnios, placenta previa, and anemia than women carrying one fetus; they are more prone to postpartal bleeding because of the additional uterine stretching. Since a multiple pregnancy usually ends before the normal term, immaturity of the newborns is a crisis superimposed at birth. The woman will need closer prenatal supervision than the woman with a single gestation in order to detect complications of pregnancy as early as possible. Spend time at health care visits reviewing with a woman her need for extra rest and "shoes off" times during the day. Most people are aware that a twin pregnancy will require special precautions and are willing to offer them to a woman as soon as she makes it known that two heart beats have been heard.

Many women with a multiple pregnancy are prescribed bedrest during the last 2 or 3 months of pregnancy. This precaution minimizes the number of falls and accidents that occur from body imbalance and increases the possibility that the pregnancy will come to term, or at least pass the thirty-sixth week, when the chances for survival of the fetuses rise markedly. A woman is usually urged to refrain from coitus during the last 2 or 3 months of pregnancy because the cervix may be dilating prematurely due to early onset of labor.

The woman with a multiple pregnancy has to work through two role changes during pregnancy rather than one. First, she is surprised to find that she is pregnant (pregnancy is almost always a surprise) and must work through to acceptance of being pregnant. By the twentieth week of pregnancy she is beginning to nest-build and show signs that she accepts the pregnancy, that she is preparing to become a mother, or the mother of four rather than of three. Suddenly, at a routine office visit, two sets of heart sounds are heard and many small body parts can be palpated. She is told that she has a twin pregnancy. Now, starting late in pregnancy, she has to work through a second role change: becoming a mother of two, not of one; a mother of five, not of four. This is difficult to complete in the 4 months of pregnancy remaining (possibly 3 months because multiple pregnancies usually end at 37 to 39 weeks). She may need postpartal follow-up counseling if she is to form a close mother-child relationship with her newborns (Figure 39-11).

In addition to having to rework a role change, a woman with a multiple pregnancy has more reason to fear for her life and the life of her babies than does the average woman. Most women worry at some time during a twin or multiple pregnancy that the infants will be born joined (like the Siamese twins she remembers seeing on an old circus poster). The chances of this event with twin pregnancy are so small that they can be discounted.

Every woman has also heard stories about twins being born so prematurely that they did not survive, and about the special danger for the second twin at delivery. If she has not already heard

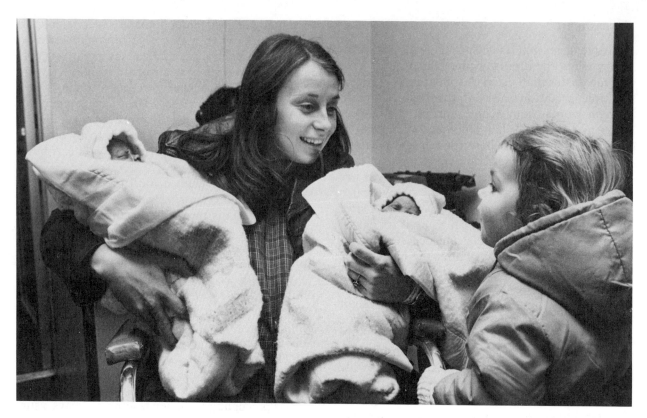

Figure 39-11 *Women need a great deal of support throughout a pregnancy when there are deviations from the normal. Here, a mother shows off twins to an older sibling. (Courtesy of the Department of Medical Photography, Children's Hospital, Buffalo, N.Y.)*

these stories, she will surely hear them before her due date. Unfortunately, they cannot simply be filed away under the heading of "old wives' tales." Both prematurity and high risk to the aftercoming twin are real hazards in multiple gestation. Although you cannot ignore them, you can help a woman to deal with these fears as positively as possible. You can tell her that there is no indication so far that her babies are in any danger; that right now it is best to continue doing the things that have to be done. If any problems should arise, you and the rest of the health care team and her family will be there to support her.

Sometimes a woman is so fearful that one or both of her twins will not survive that she makes no preparations for the infants or buys clothes and a crib for only one. This is an indication not so much that she does not accept the second child as that she lacks confidence in herself. She cannot imagine that she will be lucky enough or "good" enough to be able to carry a twin pregnancy to completion. She needs assurance during pregnancy that she is managing well, that she is following instructions well, so that her self-esteem is maintained at as high a level as possible. When her babies are born and both are healthy, the proof

she needs that she "deserved" this good fortune or was "capable" of it will be present in her arms. Then she will be free to begin interaction with the second child.

The problems that arise at delivery with multiple birth are discussed in Chapter 43.

Hydramnios

Hydramnios is excessive amniotic fluid formation. Amniotic fluid is usually 500 to 1,000 ml in amount at term. An amount over 2,000 ml is hydramnios.

That hydramnios is occurring will be evidenced by a more rapid enlargement of the uterus than is normal during pregnancy. The small parts of the fetus are difficult to palpate because the uterus is unusually tense. Auscultating fetal heart rate is difficult because of the increased amount of fluid surrounding the fetus.

A woman will begin to notice extreme shortness of breath as the overly distended uterus pushes up against her diaphragm. She may develop lower-extremity varicosities and hemorrhoids because of poor venous return from the extensive uterine pressure. She will have an increased weight gain.

Sonography will generally be ordered in an attempt to discover the reason for the excessive amount of fluid. Amniotic fluid is formed by the cells of the amniotic membrane. It is swallowed by the fetus, absorbed across the intestinal membrane into the fetal bloodstream, and transferred across the placenta. Accumulation of amniotic fluid suggests difficulty with the fetus's ability to swallow or absorb. This occurs in infants who are anencephalic or who have tracheoesophageal fistula with stenosis or intestinal obstruction. It tends to occur in diabetic women (hyperglycemia in the fetus draws fluid to the uterus by osmotic pressure).

It is possible to perform an amniocentesis to remove some of the extra fluid, which gives a woman some relief from the increasing pressure. Since amniotic fluid is replaced rapidly, however, this measure is only temporary.

In most instances of hydramnios there is premature rupture of the membranes due to excessive pressure, followed by premature labor. The infant must be assessed carefully in the newborn period for the factors that made him or her unable to swallow in utero.

Rh Incompatibility

About 15 percent of Caucasians and 10 percent of blacks in the United States are missing the Rh (D) factor in their blood, or have an Rh negative blood type. Although a blood incompatibility problem of this nature is basically a problem that affects the fetus, it causes such concern and apprehension in a woman during pregnancy that it becomes a maternal problem as well.

Blood incompatibility during pregnancy can be predicted when an Rh-negative mother (one negative for a D antigen or one with a dd genotype) is carrying a fetus with an Rh-positive blood type (DD or Dd genotype). For such a situation to occur, the father of the child must either be homozygous (DD) or heterozygous (Dd) Rh-positive (Figure 6-2). If the sexual partner is homozygous (DD) for the factor, 100 percent of the couple's children will be Rh positive (Dd). If the sexual partner is heterozygous for the trait, 50 percent of their children can be expected to be Rh positive (Dd).

It is easiest to understand how the Rh factor can endanger the fetus if you think of it as an antigen (which it is). People who have Rh-positive blood have a protein factor (the D antigen) that Rh-negative people do not. When an Rh-positive fetus begins to grow inside an Rh-negative mother, it is as though her body is being invaded by a foreign agent, or antigen. Her body reacts in the same manner it would if the invading factor were a foreign substance such as measles or mumps virus: It forms antibodies against the invading substance. The Rh factor exists as a portion of the red blood cell. In the case of Rh invasion, therefore, in order to destroy the antigen, the entire red cell must be destroyed. The maternal antibodies formed cause fetal red blood cell destruction (hemolysis). The fetus becomes so deficient in red blood cells that sufficient oxygen transport to body cells cannot be maintained. This condition is termed *hemolytic disease of the newborn* or *erythroblastosis fetalis*. Management of the infant born with this condition is discussed in Chapter 47.

Theoretically, there is no connection between fetal blood and maternal blood during pregnancy. In reality, an occasional villus ruptures, allowing a drop or two of fetal blood to enter the maternal circulation, which initiates the production of antibodies. As the placenta separates following delivery of the child, there is an active exchange of fetal and maternal blood from damaged villi. Therefore, most of the maternal antibodies formed against the Rh-positive blood are formed by the Rh-negative woman in the first 72 hours after delivery.

A woman with Rh-negative blood whose sexual partner is Rh-positive used to be advised that she could have no more than three children. This advice was based on the fact that during a first pregnancy, very little sensitivity to the foreign Rh antigen develops. However, as described, following termination of the first pregnancy, a large number of antibodies form and are in the maternal circulation when a second pregnancy begins. Many antibodies are formed at the end of the second pregnancy when the fetal-maternal exchange takes place. Thus, an even greater number—in many women, a lethal number—of antibodies are present when the third pregnancy begins.

Assessment

All women with Rh-negative blood should have an anti-D antibody titer done at their first pregnancy visit. If the results are normal or the titer is minimal (normal is 0), the test will be repeated at the twenty-eighth to thirty-eighth week of pregnancy. If there is no change in a woman's anti-D antibody titer at the twenty-eighth to thirty-eighth week of pregnancy, no special therapy need be undertaken.

If the woman's anti-D antibody titer is elevated

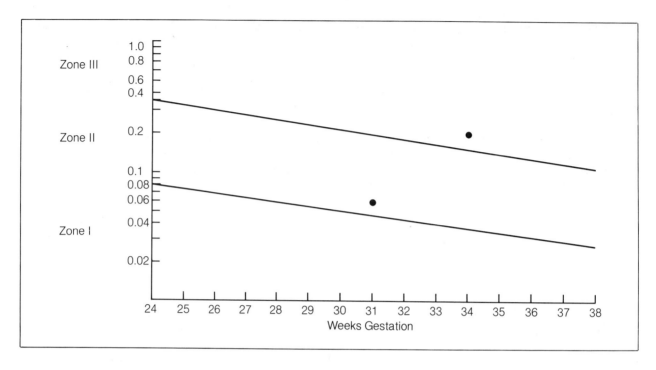

Figure 39-12 *A Liley graph to detect bilirubin content of amniotic fluid. At 30 weeks, level was in zone II; at 34 weeks, level has risen to zone III, a point of serious fetal involvement.*

at the sixteenth to twentieth week (over 1:8), showing Rh sensitization, the titer will be monitored about every 2 weeks during the remainder of the pregnancy. The well-being of the fetus in this potentially toxic environment will be monitored every 2 weeks (or oftener) by amniocentesis (see Chapter 15). Spectrophotometer readings are made of the amniotic fluid obtained by this technique to reveal the fluid density. If the readings (at 450 μ optical density) are plotted on a graph such as the one proposed by Liley (1964) and correlated with gestation age, the extent of involvement and the seriousness of the situation can be judged. A numerical value is obtained by the spectrophotometer analysis. This number is placed on a graph at the appropriate week of gestation.

If the fluid density remains low so that the plotted number falls into zone 1 of the graph during pregnancy (Figure 39-12), the fetus either is in no distress or, more likely, is an Rh-negative fetus. If the spectrophotometer reading is higher, so that the plotted number falls into zone 2 of the graph, preterm delivery by induction of labor at fetal maturity is indicated. If the reading is so high that the plotted number falls into zone 3 of the graph, the fetus is in imminent danger, and immediate delivery should be carried out or intrauterine transfusion begun. An antibody-D titer

of over 1:64 is also a critical point at which intrauterine transfusion may be initiated.

Analysis

A nursing diagnosis concerned with Rh incompatibility is usually related to the well-being of the fetus; or, because the concern the problem causes the mother (and family) is extreme, it may be related to her fear or concern. Be certain that goals established are realistic to the problem. The fetal outcome is seriously guarded in a woman who is sensitized to the Rh factor as she enters a pregnancy.

Planning and Implementations

Today, with the discovery of Rho (D) immune globulin (RhoGAM), the problem of maternal isoimmunization to an Rh-positive fetus should be eliminated. RhoGAM is a commercial preparation of passive antibodies against the Rh factor. If given by injection to the mother in the first 72 hours following delivery of an Rh-positive child, the Rh antigens present are immediately lysed and, therefore, the mother forms no natural antibodies. Since RhoGAM is passive antibody protection, it is transient, and in 2 weeks to 2 months the passive antibodies are destroyed.

Only those few antibodies that were formed during pregnancy are left.

Thus every pregnancy is like a first pregnancy in terms of the number of antibodies present, assuring a safe intrauterine environment for as many as the woman wishes to have. A newer technique of administering RhoGAM late in pregnancy (the seventh to ninth month) offers even more protection. RhoGAM does not cross the placenta late in pregnancy and destroy fetal red blood cells: The antibodies are not the IgG class, the only type that crosses the placenta. With prenatal administration, an additional injection must also be given within 72 hours after birth. RhoGAM is ineffective if a woman is already sensitized to the Rh factor.

Although in future years the problem of Rh sensitization will be greatly reduced, it remains a complication of pregnancy today. Some women of childbearing age began childbearing before RhoGAM was available and so have high Rh antibody titers in their blood. Some women do not receive RhoGAM injections following amniocentesis, abortions, or ectopic pregnancy as they should, and so antibody formation begins. Following an amniocentesis in which only a small amount of blood could have entered the maternal system, a micrhoGAM injection of a limited antibody amount can be administered.

Following delivery, an infant's blood type will be determined from a sample of the cord blood. If it is Rh-positive—Coombs-negative, indicating that a large number of antibodies are not present in the mother—the mother will receive a RhoGAM injection. If the newborn's blood type is Rh-negative, no antibodies have been formed in the mother's circulation during pregnancy and none will form. Thus, passive antibody injection is unnecessary.

The Rh-negative woman whose infant is Rh-positive needs a clear explanation of why she is receiving RhoGAM. If both infant and mother are Rh-negative, the woman should be told why RhoGAM is unnecessary. She needs to be assured that it is safe to have another baby if that is her wish.

Intrauterine Tranfusion

Formerly, although it was evident that the antibody titer was rising in pregnancy and fetal well-being was being threatened, nothing could be done until the fetus became mature enough to be delivered. Some infants were so affected by red cell destruction that they were stillborn; some died in the neonatal period of heart failure (erythroblastosis fetalis). Others suffered permanent brain damage with resulting motor and mental retardation from high bilirubin levels (kernicterus). The one measure that helps to combat the red cell destruction—exchange blood transfusion to remove the hemolyzed cells and replace them with healthy cells—could be done only after an infant was delivered. Today, blood transfusion, although not exchange transfusion, can be performed in utero through an amniocentesis technique. Intrauterine transfusion can also be done by fetoscopy. Although this technique may carry a greater risk for premature labor, it reduces the amount of X-ray exposure to the fetus.

For an amniocentesis technique, 2 or 3 hours before the transfusion is to begin, 50 ml of radiopaque dye is injected into the amniotic fluid by amniocentesis technique. A woman may be given a mild sedative to help her relax during this time of waiting. At the end of the waiting period, she is taken to the X-ray department of the hospital. Since the fetus swallowed amniotic fluid during the waiting time, the radiopaque dye was also swallowed and will be present in the intestines. On fluoroscopy, the fetal intestine or the location of the fetal abdomen will be clearly evident.

Fetal and placental location can also be located by sonogram. This method's advantage lies in not exposing the fetus to repeated X-rays.

Following location of the placenta by sonogram, the skin of the woman's abdomen is anesthetized with a local anesthetic. A large-bore needle and cannula are inserted into the amniotic fluid and guided gently under the observing eye of fluoroscope or sonogram into the fetal abdominal cavity. If fluoroscopy is being used, a small amount (about 2 ml) of radiopaque solution can be injected to confirm proper location of the cannula.

Blood used for transfusion in utero is group O negative because the fetal blood type is not known. It passes through the cannula into the fetal abdomen. From 75 to 150 ml of washed red cells will be used, depending on the age of the fetus. Following deposition of the blood in the fetal abdomen, the cannula is withdrawn, and the woman is urged to rest for about a half hour. Fetal heart sounds are recorded. The woman is discharged to her home to assume her usual routine.

The red blood cells are absorbed across the fetal peritoneum into the circulation and raise the level of functioning red blood cells in the fetus. Obviously, intrauterine transfusion is not without risk. The fetal liver or a major blood vessel may be lacerated by the needle or the uterus may be so irritated by the invasive procedure that labor contractions begin. For the fetus who is becoming severely affected by isoimmunization, however, such a risk is no greater than that of leaving the fetus untreated in the intrauterine environment.

Transfusion is sometimes done only once during pregnancy or it may be repeated every 2 weeks for five or six times. As soon as fetal maturity is reached, as shown by a mature lecithin/sphingomyelin ratio, delivery will be induced.

A woman in whom a high antibody titer is developing needs a great deal of support to help her reach the end of her pregnancy. She may feel she is somehow at fault, that she is responsible for literally destroying her child's blood. Often, a day-by-day approach is most helpful in managing such anxiety: "Today, everything seems to be going all right; Let's worry about tomorrow when it comes."

Following delivery, the infant may require an exchange transfusion to remove hemolyzed red blood cells and replace them with healthy blood cells (see Chapter 47). A woman needs to discuss her plans for further childbearing and to be provided with contraceptive information if she feels that the strain of this pregnancy, the constant feeling of wishing that everything was all right but never being certain that it was, is more than she can endure again.

Fetal Death

Obviously the severest complication of pregnancy that can occur is fetal death. If this event happens before the time of quickening, a woman will not be aware that the fetus has died because she was not able to feel fetal movements. This type of fetal death may be discovered at a routine prenatal visit when no fetal heartbeat can be heard; a real-time sonogram will reveal that no fetal heartbeat is present. Following fetal death, delivery will occur naturally but perhaps not until 4 to 5 weeks after the death. A dead fetus left in utero this long can initiate disseminated intravascular coagulation. To prevent this complication, once it is established by sonogram that the fetus is definitely dead, the pregnancy is terminated by oxytocin infusion.

A fetus's early death in intrauterine life may first be revealed by natural abortion. A woman begins painless spotting; this symptom gradually is accompanied by uterine contractions with cervical effacement and dilatation. No fetal heartbeat can be heard on assessment. The fetus is born lifeless and emaciated. Observe all women who deliver a dead fetus: If the fetus has been dead in utero for any length of time, her risk of developing DIC rises dramatically.

If a fetus dies in utero past the point of quickening, a woman is very aware that fetal movements are suddenly absent. She may lie down or sit in a position that she knows usually causes fetal movement; unable to believe that something could have happened, she may attribute the lack of movement to "sleeping" or "saving enough strength to be born." Because she is denying what is happening, it may be a full 24 hours before she telephones the health care facility to report the apparent lack of fetal movement. On assessment, no fetal heartbeat can be heard, and none will be revealed by a sonogram.

Labor for a fetus known to be dead is very difficult. The woman grieves for her dead child and her own ability to carry a pregnancy to completion. She cannot help but think she did something to cause this tragedy (forgot an iron supplement, painted a crib, wished too hard) and that she is basically not as good a woman as others (not as deserving of happiness as others). Give her opportunities to express how she feels about this loss. A statement such as "This must be a very difficult day for you" will open up the topic for discussion. If the death has occurred early in pregnancy before much bonding has taken place, the experience may be viewed as something that can be quickly handled so the woman can get on with childbearing. If it occurs after quickening, her grief is as real as if a newborn or another family member had died. Encourage her support person to remain with her during labor.

Labor will simulate term live labor as a live fetus is basically a passive participant during labor. It is difficult for a woman to use controlled breathing exercises although encouraging her is helpful in making the experience one of controllable pain. Maintain an attitude such as, "This is good practice for a future labor when your child will be well." If a woman wishes a high level of analgesia, she may have it because there is no fetus to protect from narcotic effects, although too much may lead to poor uterine involution in the postpartal period. Support the woman's choice of anesthesia. Some women want to remain awake for the delivery; some prefer a general anesthesia. Being awake is probably preferable because it makes the birth real, ends the pregnancy for the woman, and allows her to begin active grieving at an earlier time.

Ask if the parents wish to see the child. If they do, wash away obvious blood and swaddle the baby as if he or she were a well newborn. Point out that although dead for unknown reasons, the child is well formed (assuming this is so). Knowing that the child was perfect—that this death occurred for an unknown reason—gives the parents courage to attempt another pregnancy. If a child has a congenital anomaly that led to the death, prepare them for this anomaly before you bring the child to them and explain how the anomaly affected the child.

A woman need only remain for a short stay in the hospital, assuming uterine involution occurs within normal limits, for physiologic reasons. Be certain before she is discharged that she has a support person she can rely on during the following week or month when the full impact of the fetal loss registers with her. Be certain she has a return appointment for a gynecologic checkup so both her physiologic and psychological health can be evaluated.

Prepare her that the day the infant would have been born if the pregnancy had been carried to term may be very sad for her because the experience, perhaps for the first time, really becomes real. Communities have varying laws concerning whether burial for an immature fetus is necessary. Consult your local health department for the exact regulations in your community so you can serve as a resource person for parents.

The Postmature Pregnancy

A term pregnancy is 38 to 42 weeks long. A pregnancy that exceeds these limits is prolonged, or postmature. The infant of such a pregnancy is postgestational or postmature.

Some pregnancies appear to extend beyond the due date set for them because of a faulty due date. Women who have long menstrual cycles (40 to 45 days) do not ovulate on the fourteenth day as in a typical menstrual cycle; they ovulate 14 days from the end of their cycle, or on the twenty-sixth or thirty-first day. Thus their child will be "late" by 12 to 17 days.

In other instances the pregnancy is truly overdue. For some reason, the trigger that initiates labor did not work. Prolonged pregnancy can occur in a woman on a high dose of salicylates (for severe sinus headaches, rheumatoid arthritis) because salicylate interferes with the synthesis of prostaglandins. Prostaglandins may be responsible for the initiation of labor.

It is dangerous for a fetus to remain in utero more than 2 weeks beyond time to be born. A placenta seems to have a growth potential for only 40 to 42 weeks. After that time it is apparently too old to function adequately. A fetus still in utero will be forced to live with decreased blood perfusion. He or she may suffer from a lack of oxygen, fluid, and nutrients. Perinatal mortality is doubled for infants born at 43 weeks; it is three times greater at 44 weeks and four times greater at 46 weeks than for infants born at 42 weeks.

At each prenatal visit, the fundal height of a pregnancy should be compared to the standards in an attempt to predict the true gestation age. The gross size of the fetus is palpated to assess whether the infant seems to correlate in size to the month of gestation. If labor has not begun within 42 weeks, a woman may be asked to collect a 24-hour urine for estriol levels. She may be given a nonstress test. If the findings are normal and the physical estimation of size, perhaps checked by sonogram, suggests an infant smaller than normal term, the due date is recalculated. If the tests are abnormal or the physical examination or biparietal or abdominal diameter measured on sonogram suggests that the fetus is term size, the infant will be delivered by inducing labor. The fetal heart rate must be monitored closely during labor to be certain that placental insufficiency is not occurring from aging of the placenta. Problems at birth of the postmature infant are discussed in Chapter 48.

It is difficult for a woman to be pregnant past her due date. The same disappointed reaction occurs when a vacation trip is canceled or it rains on a Fourth of July picnic. She was promised something and now it is being withheld. She knows objectively that her distress is irrational; subjectively she is hurt and angry about what is happening to her.

At birth of the baby, she needs time to examine the child and assure herself that although he or she did not arrive on the day expected, everything is well and up to her expectations after all.

Hyperemesis Gravidarum

Hyperemesis gravidarum (sometimes called *pernicious vomiting*) is nausea and vomiting of pregnancy that is prolonged past the twelfth week or is so severe that dehydration, ketonuria, and significant weight loss occur within the first 12 weeks.

Assessment

The nausea and vomiting of normal pregnancy follows the rise in HCG beginning at about the sixth week of pregnancy and declining at about the twelfth week. Women with hyperemesis gravidarum have unexplained low HCG levels. Their difficulty may arise from sensitivity to estrogen.

A woman with the normal nausea and vomiting of pregnancy notices the nausea on arising in the morning; she shuns breakfast because she feels that she may vomit; she may vomit once during the morning. By noon the nausea has completely disappeared, and she is suddenly ravenously hungry. In other women (and still within a normal pattern), the nausea and vomiting occurs around dinnertime when they begin to prepare food and smell its odors, and also at the times of the day when they are most tired. Because normal nausea and vomiting last for only part of the day, a woman's nutrition, even without therapy such as an antiemetic, can be adequately maintained.

With hyperemesis gravidarum, a woman's electrolyte balance may be affected if vomiting is severe during the day or persists for an extended period. A woman may show an elevated hematocrit or hemoglobin concentration at her monthly prenatal visit—not because her hemoglobin level is so high, but because her inability to retain fluid has resulted in hemoconcentration. Concentrations of sodium, potassium, and chloride may be reduced, and hypokalemic alkalosis may result. In some women, polyneuritis, due to a deficiency of vitamin B, develops. A woman may lose weight. Her urine will test positive for ketones, evidence that her body is breaking down stored fat and protein for cell growth.

There may be a number of psychosocial factors involved in the development of pernicious vomiting. A woman with this condition may be ambivalent toward her pregnancy (but then, so are many women who do not have it). She may be psychosexually immature; she may be one of those persons who respond to stress through gastrointestinal symptoms (Figure 39-13).

Hyperemesis gravidarum must be stopped before starvation occurs and fetal damage results. Ask women at prenatal visits whether they are having nausea and vomiting. Determine exactly how much. Ask a woman to describe the events of the day before if she says it was a typical day. How late into the day did the nausea last? How many times did she vomit? What was the total amount of food she ate? Did she take adequate fluid?

Analysis

A nursing diagnosis concerned with hyperemesis gravidarum is usually related to the fluid and electrolyte imbalance that is apt to occur. It may be concerned with the family integrity problem

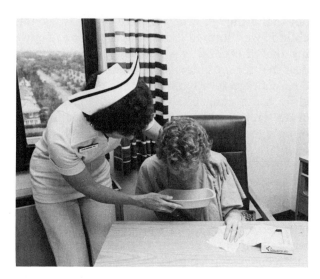

Figure 39-13 *Hyperemesis gravidarum is a serious disorder in pregnancy because it can rob the fetus of needed nutrients.*

that arises if the mother requires a long period of hospitalization for therapy. Be certain that goals established are realistic in relation to the basic problem. You may not be able to completely stop vomiting. Enough fluid can be supplemented, however, to counteract the loss of fluid with vomiting.

Planning and Implementations

For therapy of this condition, a woman needs to be hospitalized so that her intake, output, and blood chemistries can be monitored and dehydration prevented.

During the first 24 hours of the hospital admission, no food and fluid are allowed by mouth. A woman should receive approximately 3,000 ml of an intravenous solution such as lactated Ringers with added vitamin B. A sedative such as phenobarbital may be ordered to encourage rest, and an antiemetic may be prescribed. Almost all antiemetics carry risk early in pregnancy. Bendectin, the antiemetic most commonly prescribed in the past, has been withdrawn from the market by its manufacturer because of a possible danger of congenital anomaly.

Many physicians exclude all visitors for the first 24 hours or until the vomiting has ceased. If there is no vomiting after 24 hours, every 2 or 3 hours small quantities of dry toast, crackers, or cereal are given, and clear fluid (not over 100 ml at a time) is given at hours other than the dry foods. If no vomiting occurs, a woman is gradually advanced to a soft diet, then to a normal diet. If these measures are not effective, tube feeding may be tried. Total parenteral nutrition (hyperalimentation) may be attempted.

The normal nausea and vomiting of pregnancy are precipitated by fatigue and the smell of cooking, and so is pernicious vomiting. The portions of food served should be small, so that the amount does not appear overwhelming. Food should be attractively prepared. Hot foods should be hot and cold foods cold.

Although an emesis basin is an important piece of equipment for the person who is vomiting, put it out of sight so that the woman is not constantly reminded of vomiting. Be sure that food carts smelling of fish, bacon, coffee or other food odors are not parked outside her door at mealtimes.

A woman with hyperemesis gravidarum needs the opportunity to express how she feels about the strange thing that is happening to her. She needs to talk about how it feels to be pregnant; how it feels to live with the ever-present nausea. In some women, so many psychosocial factors are involved that psychological counseling is required to help them decide either to terminate the pregnancy or to accept it and allow it to go to completion.

Pseudocyesis

In pseudocyesis, nausea and vomiting, amenorrhea, and enlargement of the abdomen occur in a nonpregnant woman. In some women, the abdomen is so enlarged that they appear 7 or 8 months pregnant. This phenomenon is sometimes called *psychogenic* or *false pregnancy*. It tends to occur in women who are lonely, very desirous of having children, and perhaps infertile. A woman's body responds to her needs with physiologic symptoms. On physical examination, it is obvious the woman is not pregnant. Her abdominal wall is enlarged, but her uterus is not. No other signs of pregnancy but the amenorrhea, nausea, and vomiting are present. Such a woman needs psychotherapy to learn how to handle her needs on a sound mental health basis.

Utilizing Nursing Process

A complication of pregnancy is always a serious event because it not only threatens the health of the mother and the fetus but often interferes with the total family well-being. In order that nursing care related to pregnancy complications can be comprehensive, it should be organized using nursing process.

Assessment

Because nurses do health history interviewing at prenatal health care visits, they are often the first to be aware of a complication of pregnancy. Be certain at prenatal visits that enough time is provided so a woman can be interviewed for information such as headache, blurred vision, or vaginal spotting.

As important as asking a woman at prenatal visits for symptoms you can identify as a potential complication is her education; you want to be certain that she knows the symptoms of pregnancy complications so she can telephone the health care center if these occur. Assure women when giving this information that they are free to call; otherwise, they will wait until their symptoms are acute rather than call when they first notice them (not wanting to be a bother). Help women to report symptoms rather than handling the problem by ignoring it. Denial is a frequently used protective mechanism. Help a woman to see that no problem can be solved until it is faced.

Analysis

The North American Nursing Diagnosis Association has accepted no diagnosis specific to complications of pregnancy. Many diagnoses are applicable, however, such as fear related to guarded pregnancy outcome. Be certain that goals established reflect the short time frame of an emergency situation if one is present; be certain they speak to fetal as well as maternal welfare. Many times they may reflect family welfare.

Planning

Every health care facility should be equipped to deal with the complications of pregnancy. Be certain that protocols for bleeding, premature labor, and eclampsia are established, updated, and maintained. They should reflect a current nursing management level so your hands are not tied to waiting for a physician to begin intravenous fluid, monitoring, typing, and cross-matching of blood.

Implementations

Implementations with a complication of pregnancy include not only measures to maintain the physiologic functioning of the pregnancy but a woman's and family's psychological acceptance and maintenance of the pregnancy as well. In order that a woman does not begin anticipatory grieving for the fetus and halt the growth of bonding, maintain an optimistic attitude toward the fetal progress. If the complication can be sufficiently contained and the pregnancy continue uninterrupted, this approach will help protect the mental health of the child. If the pregnancy cannot be continued, be available to offer support to the family who grieves for the loss of the unborn child and, in rare instances, for the loss of future childbearing potential or of the woman's life.

Evaluation

Full evaluation of the outcome of a complication of pregnancy cannot be carried out until the child is born. Hopefully, evaluation at this time will reveal a healthy mother and healthy child. Be aware that following a complication of pregnancy, a woman cannot help but continue to worry during the remainder of the pregnancy that the complication will happen again or the original insult to the fetus was so severe that the infant will be born dead or malformed. Evaluate a woman's psychological attitude at each continuing health care visit as well as her physical status to be certain that she is coping with the fear and strain she lives under until the child is born.

Nursing Care Planning

Angie Bacco is a 42-year-old woman (para 7; gravida 8) admitted to the obstetrics unit for preeclampsia.

Assessment

Patient states: "I can't stay in the hospital long; I have children at home who need me." Reports a "continuous, nagging" headache she thinks is "sinusitis" (the only reason she agreed to hospitalization).

Blood pressure: 162/96. 4+ edema present in ankles and over tibia. 2+ edema in hands (no longer able to wear wedding ring). Urine tests 3+ on a random sample. Weight: 165 lbs (gained 3 lbs in last week).

Analysis

Fear regarding hospitalization related to family responsibilities.

Goal. Patient to accept therapy by 4 hours' time.

Criteria. Patient to accept bedrest and magnesium sulfate therapy.

Nursing Orders

1. Admit to room 204 (quiet, isolated room).
2. Maintain total bedrest.
3. Restrict visitors to husband and oldest daughter.
4. No radio, alarm clock, or telephone in room. Do not use intercom in room.
5. Insert indwelling urinary catheter to gravity drainage.
6. Intravenous therapy of lactated Ringers by M.D. order to be begun at 120 ml/hr.
7. Loading dose of magnesium sulfate (4 gm) to be administered intravenously followed by intramuscular administration (5 gm q4h).
8. Add 0.5 ml 1% Lidocaine to each magnesium sulfate IM injection.
9. Assess that patellar reflex is 2+ or better, urine output is over 30 ml/hr and respiration rate is over 16/min before additional magnesium sulfate injection.
10. Record intake and output; assess urine sample q4h for protein. Save total for daily 24-hour urine for protein and creatinine clearance.

Questions for Review

Multiple Choice

1. Mrs. Lloyd is diagnosed as having pregnancy-induced hypertension. The most typical symptom of pregnancy-induced hypertension you would anticipate discovering on assessment is
   a. ankle edema.
   b. weight loss.
   c. susceptibility to infection.
   d. protein in urine.

2. The underlying pathology of hypertension of pregnancy is
   a. vasospasm.
   b. interference with coagulation.
   c. heart failure.
   d. decreased glomerular filtration.

3. Mrs. Lloyd is treated with magnesium sulfate IM. An injection of magnesium sulfate should *not* be given if
   a. respirations are 20 per minute.
   b. blood pressure is 140/90.
   c. reflexes are hypoactive.
   d. she is tense and anxious.

4. Mrs. Whalen is admitted to the hospital with a diagnosis of placenta previa. On admission, your *best* action would be to
   a. perform a vaginal examination to assess the extent of bleeding.
   b. help Mrs. Whalen to remain ambulatory to reduce bleeding.
   c. assess fetal heart tones by use of an external monitor.
   d. assess uterine contractions by an internal pressure gauge.

5. The physiologic basis for a placenta previa is
   a. loose placental implantation.
   b. low placental implantation.
   c. a placenta with multiple lobes.
   d. a uterus with a midseptum.

6. Mrs. Sands is a woman admitted to the labor service in preterm labor. Her gestation length is 32 weeks. On your admission assessment, which finding below would cause you to question the administration of a tocolytic agent to Mrs. Sands?
   a. cervical dilation of 5 cm
   b. strong, regular contractions
   c. fetus in a breech presentation
   d. a spontaneous abortion in an earlier pregnancy

7. Mrs. Sands is begun on ritodrine hydrochloride. Which assessment would be most important to make prior to beginning the infusion?
   a. her respiratory rate
   b. her carotid pulse rate
   c. her digital filling time
   d. her apical pulse rate

8. Mrs. Sands develops the following effects from a ritodrine hydrochloride infusion. For which of the following would you slow or halt the infusion?
   a. headache
   b. chest pain
   c. nausea
   d. a leg cramp

9. Mrs. Rodrigues is a woman in labor who suddenly notices sharp fundal pain. She begins slight vaginal bleeding. Of the following, the most likely cause of these symptoms is
   a. premature separation of the placenta.
   b. preterm labor.
   c. placenta previa.
   d. possible fetal death.

10. Hyperemesis gravidarum is a complication of pregnancy because it most often leads to
    a. fluid intoxication.
    b. metabolic acidosis.
    c. metabolic alkalosis.
    d. proteinuria.

11. Mrs. Jones is a woman at 16 weeks' gestation who telephones you because she has passed some "berry-like" blood clots and now has continued dark brown vaginal bleeding. Which instruction below would be *best* to give her?
    a. "Maintain bedrest and count the number of perineal pads used."
    b. "Come to the health care facility if uterine contractions begin."
    c. "Continue normal activity but take your pulse every hour."
    d. "Come to the health care facility with any vaginal material passed."

12. Mrs. Collins is a 12-week pregnant woman who calls you because she has begun minimal fresh vaginal spotting. She is distressed because her physician says he is not going to do anything for her but "wait and see." Your best response to Mrs. Collins would be
    a. She would be well advised to ask for a second physician opinion.
    b. Administering medication to prolong a 12-week pregnancy is usually not advised.
    c. You're certain he meant for her to maintain strict bedrest by "wait and see."
    d. You would suggest she take an over-the-counter tocolytic just to feel secure.

13. Mrs. Wing is a woman with an Rh-negative blood type. She delivers an infant with Rh-positive blood. Following this, you administer her RhoGAM (D immune globulin). Its purpose is to
    a. promote maternal D antibody formation.
    b. prevent maternal D antibody formation.
    c. stimulate maternal D immune antigens.
    d. prevent fetal Rh blood formation.

14. Mrs. Wing asks you how many children she will be able to have before Rh incompatibility causes them to die in utero. Your best response would be
    a. No more than 3 children.
    b. As long as she receives RhoGAM there is no limit.
    c. Her next child will be affected.
    d. She will have to ask her physician.

Discussion

1. Both placenta previa and premature separation of the placenta occur as third trimester bleeding. How would you differentiate these two happenings in terms of pain, vaginal bleeding, and timing in pregnancy?
2. A quiet, darkened setting should be provided for the woman with severe preeclampsia. What factors would you need to consider in order to arrange for this at your work setting?
3. Discovery of a hydatidiform mole is always perplexing for a woman. How would you explain the development of this and the care the woman must take during the following year?

Suggested Readings

Boehm, F. H., et al. (1982). Genital herpes simplex during pregnancy. *Perinatology/Neonatology, 6,* 21.

Celebrezze, E. M. (1981). Third-trimester pre-delivery: Hemorrhage. *Emergency, 13,* 48.

Chervenak, F. A., et al. (1983). Pregnancy-induced hypertension. *Hospital Medicine, 19,* 169.

Chesley, L. C. (1980). Hypertension in pregnancy: definitions, familial factor, and remote prognosis. *Kidney International, 18,* 234.

Cousins, M. E. B. (1981). The reproductive risk potential of prolonged gestation. *Issues in Health Care of Women, 3,* 139.

Danis, D. M. (1981). Vaginal bleeding during pregnancy . . . aftercare instructions. *Journal of Emergency Nursing, 7,* 222.

Dickinson, C. L. (1984). Choriocarcinoma. *Oncology Nursing Forum, 11,* 32.

Ferris, T. F. (1983). Hypertensive and pregnant. *Emergency Medicine, 15,* 28.

Flood, B., & Naeye, R. L. (1983). Factors that predispose to premature rupture of the fetal membranes. *J.O.G.N. Nursing, 13,* 119.

Freeman, E. W. (1978). Abortion: subjective attitudes and feelings. *Family Planning Perspectives, 10,* 151.

Gant, N. F., et al. (1974). A clinical test useful for predicting the development of acute hypertension in pregnancy. *American Journal of Obstetrics and Gynecology, 120,* 1.

Gant, N. F., et al. (1978). Clinical management of pregnancy-induced hypertension. *Clinical Obstetrics and Gynecology, 21,* 397.

Hammer, R. M., et al. (1984). The prenatal use of Rho(D)Immune Globulin. *M.C.N., 9,* 29.

Harger, J. H. (1983). Cervical cerclage: patient selection, morbidity and success rate. *Clinics in Perinatology, 10,* 321.

Harris, J. L. (1984). Preterm labor: Who is at risk, who can be helped, and how. *Consultant, 24,* 256.

Hicks, E. C. (1982). Obstetrical emergencies: A systematic approach for nursing interventions. *Nursing Clinics of North America, 17,* 79.

Jacobs, M. K., et al. (1982). External pneumatic intermittent compression for treatment of dependent pregnancy edema. *Nursing Research, 31,* 159.

Jacobs, S. C. (1982). Urinary tract infection in pregnancy. *Infection Control, 6,* 25.

Jacobson, H. N. (1983). Prevention of prematurity. *Perinatology/Neonatology, 7,* 17.

Kelley, M., et al. (1982). Hypertension in pregnancy: Maternal position and blood pressure during pregnancy and delivery. *American Journal of Nursing, 82,* 809.

King, J. (1984). Vaginitis. *J.O.G.N. Nursing, 13,* 41.

Kuhn, P. L. (1983). Shirodkar and McDonald differentiation . . . surgical intervention in a pregnancy threatened by cervical incompetence. *Surgical Technology, 15,* 21.

Levin, A. A., et al. (1982). Ectopic pregnancy and prior induced abortion. *American Journal of Public Health, 72,* 253.

Liley, A. W. (1964). Amniocentesis and amniography in hemolytic disease. In J. P. Greenhill (Ed.). *Yearbook of obstetrics and gynecology,* Chicago: Yearbook.

Lipsit, E. R. (1982). Role of ultrasound in diagnosis of ectopic pregnancy. *Applied Radiology, 11,* 65.

Lueck, J., et al. (1983). Observation of an organism found in patients with gestational trophoblastic disease and in patients with toxemia of pregnancy. *American Journal of Obstetrics and Gynecology, 145,* 15.

Lynch, J. M. (1982). Helping patients through the recurring nightmare of herpes. *Nursing (Horsham), 12,* 52.

Mathewson, M. (1983). Women diagnosed with pregnancy-induced hypertension should be placed on a sodium restricted diet . . . fact or myth? *Critical Care Nurse, 3,* 114.

Morrison J. C. (1981). Heparin therapy for disseminated intravascular coagulopathies. *Perinatal Press, 5,* 10.

Patrick, J. D. (1982). Ectopic pregnancy: A brief review. *Annals of Emergency Medicine, 11,* 576.

Perley, N. Z., et al. (1983). Herpes genitalis and the childbearing cycle. *M.C.N., 8,* 213.

Peterson, G. (1983). Addressing complications of childbirth in the prenatal setting . . . discussion of birth complications should decrease fear. *Journal of Nurse Midwifery, 28,* 25.

Pritchard, J., & MacDonald, P. C. (1980). *Williams obstetrics* (16th ed). New York: Appleton-Century-Crofts.

Royko, M. A. (1982). An obstetric emergency: Abruptio placentae vs ruptured uterus . . . case review. *Journal of Emergency Nursing, 8,* 4.

Schneider, T. (1984). Voluntary termination of pregnancy. *J.O.G.N. Nursing, 13,* 77.

Shortridge, L. A. (1983). Using Ritodrine Hydrochloride to inhibit preterm labor. *M.C.N., 8,* 58.

Sonstegard, L. (1979). Pregnancy-induced hypertension: Prenatal nursing concerns. *M.C.N., 4,* 90.

Stenchever, M. A. (1981). Hypertension and pregnancy: Guiding your patient toward a safe delivery. *Consultant, 21,* 82.

Stewart, A. (1984). Intrauterine death. *Nursing Mirror, 158,* viii.

Sweeney, P. J. (1983). Genital herpes and pregnancy. *Perinatal Press, 7,* 19.

Szulman, A. E., & Surti, U. (1984). The syndromes of partial and complete molar gestation. *Clinical Obstetrics and Gynecology, 27,* 172.

Varner, M., et al. (1981). Perinatal infections. *Perinatology/Neonatology, 5,* 37.

Weil, S. G. (1981). The unspoken needs of families during high-risk pregnancies. *American Journal of Nursing, 81,* 2047.

White, M., et al. (1984). Psychological stressors in antepartum hospitalizaiton. *Maternal-Child Nursing Journal, 13,* 47.

Willis, S. E., et al. (1982). Hypertension in pregnancy: Prenatal detection and management. *American Journal of Nursing, 82,* 798.

40

Teratogens and Fetal Health

Infection

Infection During Pregnancy
Infections That Cause Illness at Birth

Drugs

Chemotherapeutic Agents
Thyroid Agents
Analgesics
Hormones
Diuretics
Sedatives
Antacids
Psychotropic Drugs
Hypotensive Agents
Antibiotics
Anticoagulants
Vitamins
Anticonvulsant Agents
Hypoglycemic Agents
Hallucinogenic Agents
Alcohol
Immunologic Agents
Labor and Delivery Medications

Environmental Teratogens

Radiation
Trauma
Smoking
Emotional Stress
Poor Nutrition
Hyperthermia and Hypothermia

Maternal Illness

Utilizing Nursing Process

Nursing Care Planning

Questions for Review

Suggested Readings

OBJECTIVES

Following mastery of the contents of this chapter, you should be able to

1. Define the term *teratogen.*
2. List common categories of teratogens.
3. Describe the ways that common teratogens cause fetal malformation.
4. Assess a woman and fetus for possible teratogen invasion and effect.
5. State a nursing diagnosis regarding teratogen effect and pregnancy.
6. Plan nursing care to prevent or counteract the effects of teratogen invasion.
7. Implement nursing care specific to effects of teratogen invasion.
8. Evaluate goal criteria to determine the expected outcome.
9. Analyze the potential for fetal harm from teratogens at various points in pregnancy.
10. Synthesize knowledge of teratogens with nursing process to achieve quality maternal-newborn nursing care.

A TERATOGEN is any factor, chemical or physical, that affects the fertilized ovum, the embryo, or the fetus adversely. The word is derived from the Greek *teratos,* which means "monster," and *genesis,* which means "production." Fetuses can reach maturity in optimal health only if they receive sound genes (see Chapter 6) from their parents and they develop in an optimal intrauterine environment, protected from the influence of teratogens.

At one time is was assumed that a fetus in utero was protected from injury due to the presence of amniotic fluid and the lack of direct exchange between mother and fetus at the placenta. Congenital disorders were attributed to the influence of "fate" or "bad luck" or, in primitive times, to evil spirits. Today it is acknowledged that a fetus is very vulnerable to injury and, although the causes of many anomalies occurring in utero are still unknown, many teratogenic factors can be isolated. Principles of teratogenic ac-

tion are shown in the Nursing Care Highlight on page 933.

Several factors influence the amount of damage a teratogen can cause. Strength is obviously one. Radiation is a known teratogen, but in small amounts (everyone is exposed to some radiation every day) it causes no damage. In large doses, however, such as a pregnant woman receives when being treated for cancer of the cervix, it can cause serious fetal defects or death. The amount of radiation received by a woman who works at a computer or word processor all day is now being seriously questioned in terms of teratogenicity (a number of word processor operators have delivered infants with congenital anomalies, particularly eye damage).

The timing of the teratogenic insult makes a significant difference. If a teratogen is introduced at the time when the main body systems are being formed (in the second to eighth week of embryonic life), more harm can be expected than if the teratogen is introduced at the eighth or ninth month of pregnancy when all the organs of the fetus are formed and are merely maturing. The times when different anatomic areas of the fetus are most likely to be affected by teratogens are given in Table 40-1.

Two known exceptions to the rule that deformities usually occur in early embryonic life are the effects caused by the organisms of syphilis and toxoplasmosis. These two infections can cause abnormalities in organs that were originally formed normally. This possibility has implications for a nurse working with pregnant women. A woman who contracts syphilis late in pregnancy needs treatment just as surely as the one who enters pregnancy with the infection. She should feel free to tell the health care personnel who care for her that she has been exposed to syphilis. If a nurse has made moral judgments

Table 40-1 Embryological Abnormalities by Time in Ovulation Weeks

Anatomic Tissue	Time (Approximate Range in Weeks)
Brain	2–11
Eyes	3–7
Cardiovascular	3–7
Renal	4–11
Genital	4–14
Lips and palate	7–10

Source: Adapted from Cavanagh, D., & Talisman, M. R. (1969). *Prematurity and the obstetrician.* New York: Appleton-Century-Crofts (Division of Prentice-Hall, Inc.).

Nursing Care Highlight

Principles of Teratogenic Action

1. The most vulnerable time period is that of organogenesis.
2. The more virile or potent the agent, the greater the damage.
3. Teratogens have specific affinity for specific tissue.
4. Teratogens may increase in effectiveness if a genetic predisposition for a defect is present.
5. A teratogen does not have to cause ill maternal effects to cause destructive fetal effects.

about a woman early in pregnancy, the woman will be unlikely to mention this new contact. Thus, the nurse, by lack of understanding and compassion, will have indirectly prevented the mother from receiving treatment and, in a way, acted as a human teratogen.

A third factor determining the effects of a teratogen is that each teratogen generally has an affinity for specific tissue, so that its effect can sometimes be predicted. Lead, for instance, attacks and disables nervous tissue. Thalidomide causes limb defects. Tetracycline causes tooth enamel deformities and possibly long bone deformities. The rubella virus, on the other hand, can affect many organs—the eyes, ears, heart, and brain being the four most commonly attacked.

Nurses who are involved in prenatal care should be familiar with the various categories of teratogens described in the sections that follow. Much screening done at prenatal visits is directly related to determining whether any teratogen interference could have occurred since the last visit (Figure 40-1). A great deal of prenatal health teaching is based on helping the mother-to-be

Figure 40-1 *A sonogram being recorded to detect fetal well-being. Notice how the woman's attention is focused on the screen.*

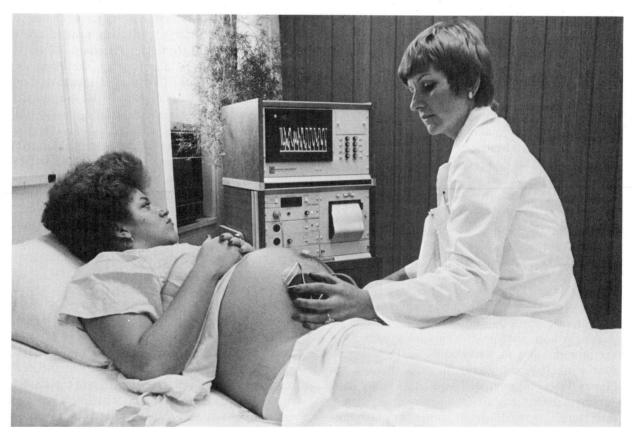

Table 40-2 Five Terms Used to Describe Teratogenic Effects

Term	Description
Disruption	Interference with growth in an originally normal developmental process. Example: cataract caused by rubella infection.
Malformation	An abnormality caused by an intrinsically abnormal developmental process. Example: polydactyly.
Deformation	Interference with growth caused by a mechanical force. Example: abnormal hand development caused by a cord wound tightly around the wrist.
Dysplasia	Abnormal organization of cells resulting in abnormal growth. Example: chondrodystrophy dwarfism in which all cartilage in the body is abnormal.
Polytropic field defect	An abnormality caused by interference of only one developmental tissue.

Source: Spranger, J., et al. (1982). Errors of morphogenesis: Concepts and terms. *Journal of Pediatrics, 100,* 160.

understand how to avoid teratogens. Terms used to describe teratogenic effects are shown in Table 40-2.

Infection

Bacterial, protozoan, and viral infections can all cause damage to a fetus; the infectious agent may cause an effect during pregnancy or at birth. Preventing and predicting fetal injury from infection is complicated, because a disease may be subclinical (without symptoms in the mother) and yet injure the fetus.

Infection During Pregnancy

The major infections which cause fetal damage during pregnancy are rubella, cytomegalic inclusion disease, syphilis, and toxoplasmosis.

A baby born with central nervous system damage or anomalies may have a TORCH (*t*oxoplasmosis, *r*ubella, *c*ytomegalic inclusion disease, and *h*erpes II) screen ordered. This is an immunologic survey to detect if antibodies against the common infectious teratogens are present in the newborn's

serum. A TORCH screen may also include assessment of serum for syphilis; it is ordered as TORSCH, or, alternatively, the O in TORCH can be assumed to include "other" infections or syphilis.

Rubella

The best (and worst) example of a viral infection that causes extensive fetal damage is the rubella (German measles) virus. Its teratogenic effects were first discovered following a rubella epidemic in Australia in 1939–1940. Because there had been no major rubella outbreak in the preceding 17 years, the majority of women of childbearing age had no immunity to the disease, and many contracted it during pregnancy. Of the infants born to these women, a large fraction had the classic sequelae: deafness, mental and motor retardation, cataracts, cardiac defects (patent ductus arteriosus and pulmonary stenosis being the most common), retarded intrauterine growth (small for gestation age), thrombocytopenic purpura, and dental and facial clefts, such as cleft lip and palate.

The greatest risk to the embryo from rubella virus is during the organogenesis period in early pregnancy. The frequency of defects is about 50 percent if infection occurs in the first 8 weeks of pregnancy, 20 percent in the ninth through the sixteenth weeks. The risk is minimal later in the second trimester and apparently nil thereafter. In addition, there is about a 30 percent chance of spontaneous abortion or stillbirth if the infection occurs in the first trimester (Pritchard, 1980).

All women of childbearing age should be immunized against rubella so that this teratogen can be eradicated. A woman who is not immunized before pregnancy cannot be immunized during pregnancy because the vaccine uses a live virus that would have effects similar to those occurring with a subclinical case of rubella. Following a rubella immunization, a woman is well advised to avoid becoming pregnant for 3 months' time. Immediately following a pregnancy, all women who have low rubella titers should be immunized so that they will have the needed protection against rubella during their next pregnancy. Screening postpartum mothers to discover those with low or unknown titers should be a responsibility of a nurse on a postpartum unit.

Infants who are born of mothers who had rubella during pregnancy may be capable of transmitting the disease for up to 12 months after birth. The infant should be isolated in the newborn period from other newborns, and the mother should be made aware of the possiblity that her infant might infect pregnant women. (Think of all the pregnant women who enjoy visiting a new baby, for a glimpse of what is to come.) Nurses with low rubella titers should avoid caring for these infants (and should act to have their serum titer elevated by immunization). Titer analysis is done by a hemagglutination inhibition assay (HAI). A titer of over 1:10 suggests immunity to rubella. A titer of less than this amount suggests that a woman is susceptible to invasion of the virus. If a titer increases greatly over a previous reading or the initial titer reading is extremely high, a recent infection has probably occurred.

Cytomegalic Inclusion Disease

Cytomegalic inclusion disease (CID) (salivary gland disease) is another viral disease (caused by the cytomegalovirus [CMV]) that can cause extensive damage to a fetus. It is transmitted by droplet infection from person to person. A mother has almost no symptoms and so is not aware that she has contracted an infection, yet the infant may be born with severe brain damage (hydrocephalus, microcephaly, spasticity), eye damage (optic atrophy, chorioretinitis), or chronic liver disease. The child's skin may be covered with large petechiae (blueberry muffin lesions). Diagnosis in the mother or infant can be established by the isolation of CMV antibodies in serum. There is unfortunately no treatment for the infection even if it presents with enough symptoms to be detected in the mother.

Other Viral Diseases

It is difficult to demonstrate other viral teratogens because of the phenomenon of subclinical infection, but the rubeola virus and the coxsackievirus are probably associated with defects; mumps, smallpox virus, and viral hepatitis (both A or B) may be related. Influenza virus is suspected of being a cause of heart defects, and poliomyelitis will cause poliomyelitis in the fetus. The rhinoviruses, which cause upper respiratory infections (the common cold), do not appear to be teratogenic although pregnant women may have more severe colds than nonpregnant women owing to reduced immunocompetence (which also keeps them from rejecting the foreign protein of the fetus).

Syphilis

Syphilis, a spirochete infection, is discussed in Chapter 36 because it has the potential for maternal as well as fetal illness. If contracted during pregnancy, syphilis can cause extensive damage to a fetus. This effect occurs after the eighteenth

week of intrauterine life, when the cytotrophoblastic layer of the placental villi has atrophied and no longer offers protection. Deafness, mental retardation, osteochondritis, and fetal death are possible effects. The placenta of infants with congenital syphilis is generally large in size, constituting about 25 to 30 percent of fetal body weight, as compared with the normal 16 to 20 percent. Women should have a serology determination for syphilis (a VDRL or RPR) at a first prenatal visit; it should be repeated close to term (the eighth month). Even when a woman has been treated with appropriate antibiotics, the serum titer remains high for over 200 days; an increasing titer, however, suggests an additional infection has occurred.

If treated at an early point in pregnancy (before 18 weeks), syphilis can be eradicated before it affects the fetus. If the infection is not detected or treated during pregnancy (with benzathine penicillin, a drug that may be given safely during pregnancy), the baby will be born with signs such as extreme rhinitis (snuffles) and a characteristic syphilitic rash, signs that help to identify the baby as high-risk at birth. The infant with the disease at birth should be isolated until treatment is effective and the infant is no longer infectious. The serologic test for syphilis (FTA-ABS) may remain positive in the infant for up to 3 months, even though the disease was treated therapeutically during pregnancy. Nursing care at birth is discussed in Chapter 47.

Toxoplasmosis

Toxoplasmosis, a protozoan infection, may be contracted by the mother by eating undercooked meat, although the organism is spread most commonly by contact with cat stool or with soil or cat litter. The mother has almost no symptoms of disease except for a few days of malaise and posterior cervical lymphadenopathy. Following placental transfer of the infection, however, the infant may be born with central nervous system damage, hydrocephalus, microcephaly, intracerebral calcification, or retinal deformities. Presence of the disease in the mother may be established by serum analysis. A course of sulfadiazine for a month may be begun during pregnancy if toxoplasmosis is identified, although its effectiveness in preventing fetal deformities is uncertain.

It is not necessary to remove a cat from a home during pregnancy as long as the cat is healthy; on the other hand, taking in a new cat is probably not wise. Pregnant women should be careful not to change a cat litter box or work in soil in an area where they notice cats defecate. They should be cautioned to avoid undercooked meat.

Infections That Cause Illness at Birth

A number of infections are not injurious to the fetus during pregnancy but are injurious if they are present at the time of birth.

Herpesvirus

Herpes I virus is the causative agent of the common cold sore. Herpes type II virus is generally the cause of genital lesions. The fetus is exposed to the herpes II virus not through placental transmission but at birth while passing through the birth canal and contacting infected genital secretions. Herpes type I virus can be contacted from an open lesion on the mother's mouth.

The infant appears well at birth but begins to develop fever, lethargy, and meningitis-encephalitis symptoms in a matter of hours. Although the prognosis for newborns who contract the infection is better than ever before, as many as 75 to 80 percent of infants will die or be left with extensive central nervous system damage. Women in labor should be observed closely to see whether herpes lesions (grouped, painful, pinpoint vesicles on an erythematous base) are present on the vulva or vagina. If they are, the baby should be delivered by cesarean birth to avoid virus contact. Because there is a close association between herpes simplex I and II virus, personnel with herpes infection should not work with newborn infants.

Varicella

Varicella, or chickenpox, is caused by a form of the herpes virus. Because there is no immunization for chickenpox and some women are not exposed to it as children, about 15 percent of women of childbearing age are susceptible to the disease. If a woman contracts this infection while pregnant, the fetus can be affected with accompanying cataracts, optic atrophy, and microcephaly. A fetus born without apparent ill effects may sequester the herpes virus and develop infantile herpes zoster (normally a very rare illness).

Gonorrhea

Gonorrhea is caused by the bacteria *Neisseria gonorrhoeae*. Because of the long-term health implications, the disease is discussed in Chapter 36.

If gonorrhea is present at the time of delivery, infected vaginal secretions can contaminate the fetal eyes as the child is born vaginally, causing a destructive conjunctivitis called *ophthalmia neonatorum*.

If a woman has a positive vaginal culture at the time of birth (or a yellow vaginal discharge suggestive of gonorrhea), the infant may be delivered by cesarean birth to rule out the possibility of fetal infection.

Candidiasis

If a monilial infection (*Candida albicans*) is present at the time of delivery, an infant can contract it while descending the birth canal, resulting in an oral monilial infection (thrush); it can also occur as a skin infection. A maternal monilial infection causes a cream cheese-like vaginal discharge; it can be identified by a quick microscopic test for fungal hyphae (see Chapter 36). Vaginal insertion of Nystatin or miconazole (Monistat) is curative.

Drugs

It is difficult to establish a drug as a teratogen because proof that a drug causes malformations or death in a fetus requires administration of the drug to a woman during pregnancy and observation of the effects on the fetus. Such experimentation is neither ethical nor legal.

Many women do not realize the danger of exposing their unborn child to drugs because they picture a placental barrier that acts as a shield against drugs. Others assume the rule of being cautious with drugs during pregnancy only applies to prescription drugs, and take over-the-counter drugs freely (Figure 40-2). Not all drugs

Figure 40-2 *In order to avoid the teratogenic effect of drugs, women should take no medication during pregnancy without the approval of their physician or nurse-midwife.*

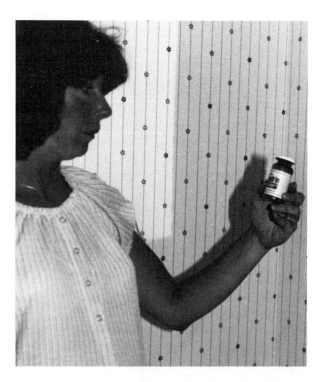

cross the placenta (heparin, for example, because of its large molecular size, does not), but most do.

The average number of drugs (over and above nutritional supplements and simple home remedies) that a woman takes during a pregnancy is about four. The most frequently consumed drugs are acetylsalicylic acid (aspirin), antihistamines, tranquilizers, antiemetics, laxatives, and nasal decongestants. In addition, a half ounce of pesticide per citizen per day is manufactured in the United States, and every day millions of cars and buses spew forth huge amounts of carbon monoxide. It seems highly likely that some of these substances affect women during pregnancy.

Over a dozen drugs and other substances are documented as being harmful to the fetus. More and more are identified every year. In order to identify drugs that are unsafe for ingestion during pregnancy, the Food and Drug Administration (FDA) has established five categories of safety, shown in Table 40-3. It is important to understand two principles relating to drug intake during pregnancy. First, any drug under certain circumstances may be detrimental to fetal welfare; therefore, during pregnancy, no woman should take any drug not prescribed by her physician or without consulting her physician or nurse-midwife. Second, no woman of childbearing age (14 through 40) should take any drug other than

Table 40-3 Categories of Potential Teratogenic Drugs

Category	Description
A	Well-controlled studies in women fail to demonstrate a risk to the fetus.
B	(a) Animal studies do not demonstrate a risk, but there are no studies in women; or (b) animal studies uncovered some risk but there are no adequate studies in women.
C	(a) Animal studies indicate adverse risk to the fetus, and there are no controlled studies in women; or (b) studies in women and animals are not available.
D	Human experience shows association of drug with a birth defect, but the potential benefits of a drug may be acceptable despite these risks.
X	These drugs are clearly contraindicated for use during pregnancy.

Source: Food and Drug Administration (1980). *Federal Register, 44,* 37434–67.

Table 40-4 Classifications of Drugs with Potential Teratogenic Effects

Classification	Example
Analgesics	Acetylsalicylic acid (aspirin)
Antacids	Products with bromide
Antibiotics	Tetracycline
Anticonvulsants	Phenytoin (Dilantin)
Anticoagulants	Coumarin
Chemotherapeutic agents	Amethopterine (Methotrexate)
Hallucinogenic agents	LSD (lysergic acid)
Diuretics	Thiazides
Hormones	Androgenic steroids
Hypotensive agents	Reserpine
Hypoglycemic agents	Tolbutamide
Immunologic agents	Live virus vaccines
Psychotropic agents	Diazepam (Valium)
Sedatives	Phenobarbital
Thyroid agents	Propylthiouracil
Vitamins	Vitamin A

those prescribed by a physician or nurse-midwife who is aware of her age, since a fetus is as endangered when a woman taking drugs becomes pregnant as when a pregnant woman takes drugs.

The most dramatic example of a drug that is known to affect fetal development is thalidomide, which causes amelia or phocomelia (total or partial absence of extremities) in 100 percent of instances if taken between the thirty-fourth and forty-fifth day of pregnancy. Interestingly, thalidomide caused no deformities in the rats on which it was tested, only in humans.

Other examples of drugs capable of being teratogenic are shown in Table 40-4 and are discussed below.

Chemotherapeutic Agents

The antimetabolites aminopterin, amethopterin (Methotrexate), chlorambucil, and 6-mercaptopurine are known to cause malformation and abortion. All the antimetabolite and cytotoxic drugs are suspected of causing fetal injury.

Thyroid Agents

Propylthiouracil and methimazole (Tapazole), thyroid inhibitors, can cause congenital goiter. Ingesting iodides, such as potassium iodide, may also enlarge the fetal thyroid gland. Excessive enlargement causes tracheal compression and difficulty with respiration at birth. Iodides are contained in many over-the-counter cough suppressants, often taken by women who are unaware that they are harmful. Radioactive iodine (^{131}I) is contraindicated in pregnancy because there will be uptake by the fetal thyroid as well as by the maternal thyroid, with destruction of the fetal thyroid.

Analgesics

Narcotics all cross the placenta readily. When given during labor, meperidine (Demerol) has been associated with decreased responsiveness in newborns, which may interfere with parent-child interaction. When women take narcotics continually during pregnancy, small-for-date infants and congenital anomalies may result. Infants from such pregnancies may be born as addicted as their mothers and may suffer extreme withdrawal reactions. This group includes infants born to mothers who have been placed on methadone for narcotic withdrawal (see Chapter 36 for a discussion on drug addiction during pregnancy).

Acetylsalicylic acid (aspirin), taken by many mothers for simple headaches (and not thought of by many as a drug, because it is so common), has been implicated in failure of labor to begin (resulting in postmature infants), prolonged bleeding time in the newborn (which could lead to intracranial hemorrhage from birth pressure), a decreased albumin-binding capacity (which may lead to hyperbilirubinemia in the newborn), and perhaps prolonged gestation (which can lead to impaired central nervous system function due to lack of fetal nutrition).

Hormones

Synthetic progestins (ethisterone, norethisterone) or androgenic steroids given to women during pregnancy tend to masculinize the female fetus. Diethylstilbestrol given during pregnancy has been associated with the development of vaginal cancer in females when they reach the age of puberty and cystic testicular formation in male children. Corticosteroids cause cleft palate deformities in animal models, although apparently not in humans. There is increasing evidence that exposure to sexual hormones in pregnancy may affect behavior in the child, influencing aggressiveness and athletic coordination.

Diuretics

The excessive use of diuretics such as the thiazides may lead to electrolyte imbalance in the infant. It would be unusual for a woman of child-bearing age to be on a diuretic except if she had accompanying kidney disease.

Sedatives

Infants of mothers who receive a barbiturate during labor may be born depressed. The infant of a mother who has taken barbiturates continually during pregnancy may be born addicted and have withdrawal symptoms. These withdrawal symptoms may occur 2 to 4 weeks after birth, when the infant is at home, away from medical care, and so tend to be extremely serious. Promethazine hydrochloride (Phenergan) is known to decrease the platelet count in the newborn, possibly leading to a clotting defect at birth.

Antacids

Antacids are not considered by many women to be drugs because they are largely over-the-counter medications. The sodium in them may lead to electrolyte disturbances in the mother and fetus, however. Products that contain bromides such as Bromo-Seltzer may cause bromide intoxication (lethargy, a bromide rash, mental retardation). Cimetidine hydrochloride (Tagamet) is proven teratogenic.

Psychotropic Drugs

Diazepam (Valium), one of the drugs prescribed to the general population to relieve anxiety, may cause infants to have poor sucking reflexes and hypotonia. Lithium, used by women with severe anxiety, has been implicated in congenital anomalies and in lethargy and cyanosis in the newborn.

Hypotensive Agents

Reserpine, given to women for treatment of high blood pressure during pregnancy, tends to cause nasal congestion, respiratory distress, cyanosis, and muscle flaccidity in the infant.

Antibiotics

Streptomycin may be associated with eighth cranial nerve deafness. The sulfonamides, given near term, interfere with bilirubin and may lead to kernicterus (high, destructive levels of bilirubin in brain tissue). Amphotericin B is associated with multiple congenital anomalies. Tetracycline may lead to brown-stained teeth and long bone deformities. Chloramphenicol, given near term, may cause shock and collapse in the newborn (the "gray baby" syndrome). Fortunately, ampicillin is a broad-spectrum antibiotic that can be given during pregnancy. It should be noted if mothers who are having urine collected for estriol levels are taking ampicillin, as it may reduce estriol excretion.

Anticoagulants

Coumarin may cause hemorrhage in the fetus or newborn. This effect can be severe enough to lead to fetal or newborn death.

Vitamins

Vitamins are another category of drugs that women may not consider medicine, yet vitamins A and D have been implicated in congenital deformities; excessive vitamin K can lead to hyperbilirubinemia in the newborn. Pyridoxine (vitamin B_6) may cause withdrawal seizures. Women with tuberculosis may take pyridoxine to complement the action of isoniazid. It is good to ask a pregnant woman not only whether she is taking the vitamin prescribed, but how many she is taking. A woman who is taking three or four tablets a day instead of the one prescribed for her (hoping that her infant will be the brightest, strongest baby ever) may actually be harming her infant.

Anticonvulsant Agents

Phenytoin (Dilantin) has been associated with congenital anomalies (cleft lip and palate, congenital heart disease). Trimethadione (Tridione) and paramethadione (Paradione) may lead to similar defects. It is difficult to evaluate the effects of anticonvulsants on fetuses because, if a woman has a seizure during pregnancy, the accompanying anoxia and acidosis may be the factors that lead to the fetal insult. Even though Dilantin, especially, may be responsible for a syndrome in infants very similar to the fetal alcohol syndrome (see below), women who have seizures uncontrolled except by such an agent may have no choice but to continue to take the drug during pregnancy.

Hypoglycemic Agents

Most diabetic women of childbearing age have juvenile diabetes (Type I) and therefore take injectable insulin rather than hypoglycemic agents. Insulin is one of the rare substances that does not cross the placenta because of its large molecular size. Oral hypoglycemic agents do cross the placenta. Tolbutamide (Orinase), a hypoglycemic agent, is associated with congenital anomalies.

All women with diabetes should use insulin for glucose regulation during pregnancy, not hypoglycemic agents.

Hallucinogenic Agents

Lysergic acid diethylamide (LSD) may cause breakage of chromosomes in the mother or father that will result in congenital deformities in children. Marijuana, on the other hand, a drug frequently attacked as being dangerous, has not been implicated in fetal deformities. It may, however, cause male impotence and thus be related to fertility problems.

Alcohol

It has been known for years ·that babies of mothers who consume a large quantity of alcohol during pregnancy have a high incidence of congenital deformities and mental retardation. It was assumed that the defects were the result of the mother's poor nutritional state (drinking alcohol rather than eating food), not the direct result of the alcohol.

Alcohol by itself has now been isolated as a teratogen: Due to immaturity, the fetus cannot remove the breakdown products of alcohol, particularly acetaldehyde, from his or her body. The large buildup of acetaldehyde leads to vitamin B_6 deficiency and accompanying neurologic damage.

Mothers who consume over 3 ounces of alcohol a day may have infants born with a *fetal alcohol syndrome*, which includes being small for gestation age, mental retardation, and a particular craniofacial deformity (short palpebral fissures, thin upper lip, and upturned nose). As there is no known "safe" level of alcohol ingestion during pregnancy, women should omit all alcohol. If this radical a change is not possible, women should be advised to limit consumption during pregnancy to under an ounce a day (remembering that they cannot save a week's limit for Saturday night and ingest it all then, because on that one day they could cause damage). This limitation of alcohol will be difficult for a woman whose life style includes the ingestion of alcohol daily or who is addicted to alcohol and feels the need for a large quantity daily.

Immunologic Agents

Live virus vaccines, such as measles, mumps, rubella, and poliomyelitis vaccines (Sabin type), are contraindicated during pregnancy because the actual virus infection can occur in the fetus. Care must be given to assess that adolescents are not pregnant before they are included in routine immunization programs. Women who work in biologic laboratories where vaccines are manufactured are well advised to not work with live virus products during pregnancy.

Labor and Delivery Medications

The use of oxytocin as a medicine to induce labor is now seriously limited because infants born after its use tend to develop electrolyte disturbances and hyperbilirubinemia due to competitive albumin binding. Depressive responses at birth have been associated with the use of analgesics in labor, particularly meperidine (Demerol) and morphine. The use of general anesthetics leads to anesthetized infants, as anesthetic agents cross the placenta readily and reach levels in the fetus equal to those in the mother. Local anesthesia injected as a paracervical block may lead to fetal bradycardia; injected as a spinal or caudal anesthetic, it may produce hypotension in the mother, resulting in reduced placental blood flow. The precautions necessary for using analgesics or anesthetics in labor are discussed in detail in Chapter 25.

Nurses working in operating room suites have a higher incidence of abortion and possibly congenital anomaly in children than nurses in other hospital areas, suggesting that breathing a low dose of anesthesia gases is teratogenic and an occupational hazard of nursing.

Environmental Teratogens

Teratogens that come from environmental sources can be as lethal to the fetus as those that are directly or deliberately ingested. Lead poisoning is generally considered a problem of early childhood. It is also a fetal hazard since lead is teratogenic if consumed by a woman during pregnancy. Preschool children ingest lead by eating paint chips or wall plaster; women ingest it by drinking moonshine liquor distilled in an apparatus using lead pipes or by sniffing gasoline (a form of drug abuse). Making moonshine is still a common practice in some rural areas of the southeastern United States. If you are caring for pregnant women in such an area, you should be aware that they may be ingesting lead from this source. Lead ingestion during pregnancy leads to mental retardation and central nervous system damage to the fetus. If a women is ingesting the lead through liquor, she needs counseling to decrease her alcohol intake.

Mercury can cause mental retardation and central nervous system motor damage in a fetus. Mercury is an ingredient of pesticides. Naphthalene, the ingredient of mothballs, if ingested, can cause hemolysis. Mothballs are sometimes ingested by girls attempting suicide or trying to cause an abortion. Carbon monoxide, if inhaled in sufficient quantites, can bring about severe fetal central nervous system damage because it replaces oxygen at the placental exchange site. Pregnant women should be cautious about driving cars that have defective mufflers or waiting for cars to be repaired in unventilated repair shops. Carbon monoxide fumes are given off from fire, so a pregnant woman who is burned often has effects of carbon monoxide inhalation.

The amount of the insecticide DDT that can be used as a pesticide today is severely limited because it can cause fetal deformities. Fluoride, in appropriate amounts, helps to strengthen teeth against cavities. In large amounts, fluoride stains teeth. Many city water supplies are fluoridated. A pregnant woman needs to use common sense and not take a fluoride supplement if fluoride is present in her drinking water.

Toxic wastes such as dioxin have been implicated in fetal malformation or the development of leukemia later in life. Obviously a woman should not deliberately expose herself to an environment where toxic wastes are processed or buried during pregnancy (and probably not at any time in life).

High altitude can be a teratogen if the oxygen content in the air is reduced. This effect is primarily a problem for women flying in unpressurized airplanes.

Radiation

Rapidly growing cells are extremely vulnerable to destruction by radiation (which is why radiation is used as a cancer therapy). Radiation's potency as a teratogen to unborn children results from the high proportion of rapidly growing cells present. It produces a range of malformations, depending on the stage of development of the embryo or fetus and on the strength and length of exposure. If the exposure occurs before implantation, it apparently kills the growing zygote; if the zygote is not killed, it survives apparently unharmed. The most damaging time is from implantation to 6 weeks after conception (during a time when many women are not yet aware that they are pregnant). The systemic nervous system, brain, and optic nerve are the organs most affected.

As a rule, therefore, all women of childbearing age should be exposed to X-rays only in the first 10 days of a menstrual cycle (a time when pregnancy is unlikely because ovulation has not yet occurred), except, of course, in emergency situations. A rapid serum assay pregnancy test should be done on all women who have reason to believe they might be pregnant before diagnostic tests involving X-ray are performed.

Radiation of the pelvis should be avoided if at all possible during pregnancy; it should be undertaken at term in pregnancy only if the data the X-ray will reveal cannot be obtained by any other means and will be important for delivery. Thus, X-ray examination is used to determine whether the fetal head can be delivered through the vaginal route or whether it is too large (X-ray pelvimetry); as a safeguard before using oxytocin for assistance in or induction of labor; and to verify suspected fetal malposition. Sonography is replacing X-ray examination for confirmation of situations such as multiple pregnancy, because although the long-term effects are not yet known, sonography does not appear to be teratogenic.

If a woman needs nonpelvic radiation during pregnancy (dental X-rays, a limb X-ray after a fall), her pelvis should be shielded by a lead apron during the procedure. Even fluoroscopy, which uses lower radiation doses than does regular X-ray photography, can cause deformation of the fetus and should be avoided during pregnancy—again, except in an emergency. Although the dosage of radiation that is apparently safe during pregnancy is 5 rads or less, the effect of long-term use of even slight radiation sources such as a word processor or computer is now being questioned; a number of infants with birth anomalies have been born to women working with word processors.

There is evidence that, in addition to immediate fetal damage, X-rays have long-lasting effects on the health of a child. Children exposed to X-rays while in utero seem to have an increased risk of cancer occurring before age 10 (Stewart, 1970). There is a possibility that the exposure of the fetal gonads could lead to a genetic mutation that would not be evident until the next generation.

These restrictions in the use of X-ray have special meaning for female nurses. If you are asked to assist with a patient in an X-ray room and you are in the postovulatory phase of a menstrual cycle, you have a right to demand lead shielding as pelvic protection. Do not be swayed when X-ray technicians say, "It's just one time," or "It's the buildup of radiation that counts." Protection that is suggested for women in general should be demanded by female nurses.

The use of nuclear magnetic resonance (NMR) scanning, which uses computer-controlled radio waves and magnetic fields to project a visual image on a screen with the same clarity as X-ray, is a new diagnostic tool found in major centers. It may be used safely during pregnancy for diagnostic studies.

Trauma

Trauma to a fetus may occur if a woman falls and strikes her abdomen; or it may happen from a blunt blow from an automobile accident or when a woman is battered. It can involve an actual puncture of the uterus from a knife or bullet. These situations may lead to spontaneous abortion, death, or handicapping of the fetus. As these situations also cause trauma to the woman, they are discussed in Chapter 41. Willful trauma to a fetus has legal implications because it can be viewed as a prenatal form of child abuse.

Smoking

Cigarette smoking by a pregnant woman has been shown to have teratogenic effects on the fetus. Although the teratogenic factor in cigarettes may be the nicotine (which causes vasoconstriction), cigarettes are discussed separately from other drugs because it is difficult for a woman who smokes to equate smoking with drug ingestion.

Although not proved, it is believed that the decrease in weight in infants of smoking mothers results from vasoconstriction of the uterine vessels, limiting the blood supply to the fetus. Part of the influence of cigarettes may come from carbon monoxide, which is inhaled. If this relationship is true, then inhaling the smoke of another person's cigarettes may be as harmful as actually smoking the cigarette. All prenatal health care settings should be posted with no-smoking signs for both personnel and patients.

Smoking may lead to premature rupture of the membranes. There is firm evidence that children born of cigarette-smoking mothers are smaller for gestation age than children born to nonsmoking mothers. There is further evidence that these children continue to be underweight for some time in early life. The effect is apparent when the mother smokes more than 10 cigarettes a day and thus is related to the quantity of cigarettes smoked. If a woman cannot stop smoking during pregnancy (and it is realistic to assume many cannot), reducing the number of cigarettes smoked per day will help diminish the adverse effects on the fetus.

A second sound reason women should at least limit the number of cigarettes smoked per day is to protect their own health. A child needs a well mother during the years of growing up. Losing a mother to lung cancer is as deleterious to the child's psychological health as the original smoking may be to his or her physical health.

Emotional Stress

There are many old wives' tales about the "marking" of infants in utero; if a woman sees a mouse during pregnancy, her child will be born with a furry or mole-like birthmark; eating strawberries causes strawberry birthmarks; looking at a handicapped child while pregnant will cause a child in utero to be handicapped the same way. Common sense and awareness of fetal-maternal physiology have dispelled these superstitions. There is growing evidence, however, that an emotionally disturbed pregnancy, one filled with anxiety and worry beyond the usual amount associated with pregnancy, may have some effect on an unborn child.

Anxiety produces physiologic changes through its effect on the sympathetic division of the autonomic nervous system. The main changes are an increase in heart rate, constriction of the blood vessels, a decrease in gastrointestinal motility, and dilation of coronary vessels. This effect is sometimes called the *fight or flight syndrome*. If the anxiety is prolonged, constriction of uterine vessels may interfere with the blood supply to the fetus.

These phenomena are characteristic only of long-term, extreme stress, not of the normal anxiety of pregnancy. Illness or death of a husband, difficulty with relatives, marital discord, and illness or death of another child are examples of stress situations that might provoke excessive anxiety.

Helping a woman resolve these problems during pregnancy is not easy, because they are usually complex. If maternal stress is a teratogen, however, securing counseling for the woman under emotional stress during pregnancy is as important as ensuring her good physical care.

Poor Nutrition

Although *excessive* intake of some nutrients, namely, vitamin A, riboflavin, zinc, caffeine, and manganese, has been shown to cause malformation in animals, the usual problem in human mothers is *under*nutrition.

Hypothyroidism (cretinism), for example, can occur in a fetus if the mother's iodine intake is inadequate during pregnancy. Lack of folic acid (necessary for cell formation and tissue growth) may result in malformations such as cleft lip or anencephaly. Lack of vitamin D may cause bone deformity (prenatal rickets).

General malnutrition results in babies that are small for their gestation ages and in an increase in low birth weight and fetal deaths. These effects may be related to deficiency of a number of nutrients in the fetus. There appears to be a strong correlation between the occurrence of iron deficiency anemia in the mother and low birth weight of the baby.

Protein intake in a mother is a major factor in maintaining the health of the unborn. The low-birth-weight rate of newborns increases when the maternal diet contains less than 50 gm of protein per day. The greatest damage from poor protein intake tends to occur in early pregnancy. This fact puts women of childbearing age on notice that it is essential to maintain themselves on an adequate protein diet. By the time they realize they are pregnant and begin to eat a proper diet, teratogenic effects may already be present.

Interestingly, more mentally retarded children are born in the late winter and early spring months (that is, were conceived the previous spring and summer) than at other times of the year. Perhaps in early pregnancy during hot weather a mother lowers her total intake, including her intake of protein.

Pica is not uncommon in the southern United States and is sometimes found in women who have migrated to the north. Clay, starch, and raw flour are the three substances most often eaten by pregnant women with pica. Few women can explain why they enjoy eating these substances. Some may use them to try to obtain relief from morning sickness; others simply feel a craving.

Clay eating may lead to iron deficiency anemia, since the presence of clay in the stomach interferes with the absorption of iron. Starch eating adds empty calories to a woman's diet and may prevent her from eating a nutritious diet during pregnancy. Pica in children is associated with iron deficiency, and children who are iron deficient tend to crave nonfood substances. Cause and effect is hard to determine: Is a woman iron deficient and so craves starch, or does she crave starch and then become iron deficient?

Pregnant women need guidance in selecting a healthy diet, in taking the vitamins, iron, and folic acid preparations prescribed for them by their physician or nurse-midwife, and in taking *only* those prescribed. Suggestions for nutrition counseling during pregnancy are given in Chapter 20.

Hyperthermia and Hypothermia

Hyperthermia to the fetus may be detrimental to growth. Hyperthermia can occur from the use of saunas or hot tubs or from a work environment next to a furnace, such as in welding or steel making. Maternal fever early in pregnancy (4 to 6 weeks) may cause abnormal brain development and possibly seizure disorders, hypotonia, and skeletal deformities.

The effect of hypothermia on pregnancy is not well known. Because the uterus is an internal organ, a woman's body temperature would have to be lowered significantly before a great deal of fetal change would result.

Maternal Illness

Certain disease states and other conditions in the mother can have teratogenic effects. Among them are maternal diabetes, maternal heart disease, and maternal blood incompatibility. Because these situations involve nursing care applicable to the mother as well as to the fetus, they are discussed in Chapter 36. Maternal age, either immaturity or postmaturity in relation to childbearing, may also affect fetal well-being.

Utilizing Nursing Process

Because fetuses are prone to injury from teratogens during pregnancy, they need well-designed nursing care in order to be kept safe from harm during pregnancy.

Assessment

Assessment of fetal growth and development is discussed in Chapter 15. Screening for the presence of teratogens is a nursing responsibility at all prenatal health visits.

Analysis

The North American Association of Nursing Diagnosis has accepted no diagnosis specific to the effect of teratogens. Commonly used diagnoses in the area are "Potential impairment of fetal growth related to cigarette smoking," "Fear related to early radiation exposure during pregnancy," and "Knowledge deficit related to the danger of alcohol ingestion during pregnancy."

When establishing goals for care with women, be certain that the goals established are realistic for the situation. The goal is almost automatically a long-term one in that it must last for the remainder of a pregnancy. A goal to *reduce* smoking in pregnancy, for example, may be more realistic than *stopping* smoking in pregnancy.

Planning

Helping a woman plan to avoid teratogens is often difficult because of the often drastic changes in life style required (not smoking, not drinking alcohol, changing a work environment, etc.). It is always amazing, however, how many things a woman will sacrifice in order to complete a pregnancy satisfactorily. With this level of motivation, planning becomes the task of determining what will be the best route to achieve a goal, not education for the need for goal attainment.

Implementation

Part of implementation in this area of nursing care involves good role modeling, such as not smoking in prenatal settings and evidencing a healthy life style in terms of nutrition or exercise. You should be certain that any medicine administered to a pregnant woman has been double checked for safe intake during pregnancy.

Evaluation

The ultimate evaluation point of teratogenicity is examination of an infant at birth. Adequate assessment and health promotion measures during pregnancy should encourage the birth of healthy newborns.

Nursing Care Planning

Mary Kraft is a 23-year-old woman you meet in an obstetrician's office.

Assessment

Heavy smoker—2 packs/day. Alcohol: 1–2 martinis/day. Takes Sudafed 60 mg daily for "sinus headache." Had one previous pregnancy, ending in spont. abortion (no known cause) 2 years ago.

Uterine height, not palpable above symphysis. No fetal heart sounds by Doppler.

Analysis

Potential impairment of fetal growth related to cigarette and alcohol use.

Locus of Decision Making. Patient.

Goal. Patient will safeguard fetal health for pregnancy duration.

Criteria:

1. Patient will decrease smoking to below 10 cigarettes daily.
2. Patient will omit all alcohol consumption during pregnancy.
3. Patient will carry pregnancy to term.

Nursing Orders

1. Refer to M.D. for evaluation of safety of sinus medication during pregnancy.
2. Urge to quit smoking or decrease number of cigarettes smoked per day to under 10.
3. Urge to eliminate alcohol consumption completely (substitute caffeine-free beverages).
4. Refer to M.D. if sonogram should be scheduled for fetal growth evaluation because of heavy smoking.

Questions for Review

Multiple Choice

1. Mrs. Gray is 2 months pregnant. She asks you when she can return to her usual habit of drinking a highball before dinner. Your best response would be
   a. any time after 6 weeks of pregnancy.
   b. any time after 3 months of pregnancy.
   c. she might consider permanently reducing her alcohol intake.
   d. not during the entire pregnancy.

2. Mrs. Gray takes aspirin daily for rheumatoid arthritis. She asks you why her physician suggested she discontinue this therapeutic measure 2 weeks prior to her estimated date of delivery. Your best response would be,
   a. "Aspirin can cause increased clotting late in pregnancy."
   b. "Aspirin can act to prolong a pregnancy."
   c. "Aspirin can increase the osmolarity of amniotic fluid."
   d. "Aspirin can cause eighth cranial nerve injury close to term."

3. At a seventh month health checkup, you interview Mrs. Gray for a health history. Which of the following diseases would give you the most concern if you learned she had been recently exposed to it?
   a. rubella
   b. syphilis
   c. pertussis (whooping cough)
   d. rhinovirus infection

4. Mrs. Gray is in an automobile accident and a physician in an emergency room wants to x-ray her wrist. She telephones you to ask what she should do. Your best response would be,
   a. "The X-ray will have to be delayed until the pregnancy's end."
   b. "You should insist on no X-rays until the ninth month of pregnancy."
   c. "The X-ray will be safe if the machine has been tested for environmental leakage."
   d. "You can safely have the X-ray if lead protection for your abdomen is provided."

5. Mrs. Gray's car was damaged in the accident. What damage, if she does not get it fixed immediately, would give you the most concern?
   a. The front seat is ripped so the seat stuffing is exposed.
   b. The windshield is cracked in two places.
   c. The gas tank cover is missing.
   d. The muffler is defective.

6. Mrs. Gray exercises at a local spa and then spends an hour in the sauna twice a week. She asks you if sauna heat could harm her fetus. Your best response would be,
   a. "Heat is dissipated by amniotic fluid so it is not teratogenic."
   b. "Excessive heat can be harmful."
   c. "Sauna heat is moist heat so it does not cross the adominal fat."
   d. "Heat increases the maturity of lung alveoli at term."

7. Mrs. Gray's oldest child brought home a kitten just before she became pregnant. She asks you what she should do concerning the kitten. Your best response would be,
   a. "Do not change the litter pan."
   b. "Your daughter will have to give the cat away."
   c. "Do not play with the cat so you will not be scratched."
   d. "Your daughter must feed the cat."

Discussion

1. Despite the proven effects of cigarette smoking on fetal welfare, many women still continue to smoke during pregnancy. What are ways that nurses can be helpful in educating women about this danger?
2. In order that women do not ingest alcohol during pregnancy, they must stop alcohol ingestion prior to conception. How can nurses be effective in educating this "prior to pregnancy" group of women?
3. Some women do not fill their prenatal vitamin prescription during pregnancy but take an over-the-counter vitamin source instead because this is more economical. What are disadvantages and possible teratogen effects of this practice?

Suggested Readings

Barr, K. (1984). Early fetal damage . . . can it be prevented? How much women know about early fetal development and fetal hazards. *Health Visitor, 57,* 78.

Baskett, T. F., et al. (1984). Antepartum fetal assessment using a fetal biophysical profile score. *American Journal of Obstetrics and Gynecology, 148,* 630.

Bennett, M. (1981). What do we know in advance? Antenatal diagnosis. *Nursing (Oxford), 1,* 907.

Burkart-Jayez, S. F. (1982). The effects of congenital rubella on the neonate. *Journal of Neurosurgical Nursing, 14,* 173.

Crelin, E. S. (1981). Development of the musculoskeletal system. *Clinical Symposia, 33,* 2.

Deibel, P. (1980). Effects of cigarette smoking on maternal nutrition and the fetus. *J.O.G.N. Nursing, 9,* 333.

Didolkar, S. M., et al. (1981). Tracing the heart action before birth. *Journal of Cardiovascular and Pulmonary Technology, 9,* 55.

Done, A. K. (1981). Babies' secondhand problems: Drugs or poisons that reach the infant indirectly transplacentally or through nursing. *Emergency Medicine, 13,* 75.

D'Souza, S. W., et al. (1981). Hearing speech and language in survivors of severe perinatal asphyxia. *Archives of Disease in Childhood, 56,* 245.

Erb, L., et al. (1981). Hyperactivity: A possible consequence of maternal alcohol consumption. *Pediatric Nursing, 7,* 30.

Finch, J. (1983). Law: Protection of the unborn child. *Nursing Mirror, 156,* 33.

Hays, D. P. (1981). Teratogenesis. A review of the basic principles with a discussion of selected agents. *Drug Intelligence and Clinical Pharmacy, 2,* 542.

Hazinski, M. F. (1983). Congenital heart disease in the neonate: Epidemiology, cardiac development and fetal circulation. *Neonatal Network, 1,* 29.

Ho, E. (1983). Fetal well being . . . the role of preconceptual care and the early and accurate detection of the fetus at risk. *Nursing Mirror, 12,* 156.

Levine, A. H., et al. (1982). Intrauterine treatment of fetal hydronephrosis. *Association of Operating Room Nurses Journal, 35,* 655.

Loper-Hunter, D. (1982). The beginning of the respiratory system . . . embryologic development. *Neonatal Network, 1,* 19.

Mattia, M. A. (1983). Hazards in the hospital environment: Anesthesia gases and methylmethacrylate. *American Journal of Nursing, 83,* 72.

Phillips, L. (1981). The effects of perinatal death. *Midwife Health Visitor and Community Nurse, 17,* 18.

Pritchard, J., & MacDonald, P. C. (1980). *Williams Obstetrics* (16th ed.). New York: Appleton-Century-Crofts.

Rayburn, W. F., et al. (1980). Drug use during pregnancy. Principles of perinatal pharmacology. *Perinatal Press, 4,* 115.

Roberts, A. (1981). Detection of fetal abnormality. *Nursing Mirror, 153,* vi.

Shepard, T. H. (1984). Teratogens: An update. *Hospital Practice, 19,* 191.

Stephens, C. J. (1981). The fetal-alcohol-syndrome: Cause for concern. *M.C.N., 6,* 251.

Stewart, A. (1984). Intrauterine death. *Nursing Mirror, 158,* viii.

Stewart, A., & Kneale, G. N. (1970). Radiation dose effects in relation to obstetric X-rays and childhood cancer. *Lancet, 1,* 1185.

Wharton, B., et al. (1982). Organogenesis, fetal growth and food. *Birth, 9,* 111.

Woodward, S. L. (1981). How does strenuous maternal exercise affect the fetus? *Birth and Family Journal, 8,* 17.

Wynn, M., et al. (1982). The importance of maternal nutrition in the weeks before and after conception. *Birth, 9,* 39.

41

Trauma and Pregnancy

OBJECTIVES

Following mastery of the contents of this chapter, you should be able to

1. Describe the most frequent types of trauma that occur in the young adult or childbearing age group.
2. Assess a pregnant woman following a traumatic accident.
3. State a nursing diagnosis in relation to trauma and pregnancy.
4. Plan care for a pregnant woman with a traumatic injury.
5. Implement care for a pregnant woman in regard to the special physiologic adjustments of pregnancy.
6. Evaluate the outcome criteria established following a traumatic injury.
7. Analyze ways that traumatic injuries could be prevented during pregnancy.
8. Synthesize knowledge of traumatic injury and nursing process to achieve quality maternal-newborn nursing care.

TRAUMA IS A PHENOMENON that seems remote from pregnancy because pregnancy is a time when a woman tries to protect her body and keep it from harm. Trauma occurs during pregnancy, however, because of its high incidence in the young adult or childbearing age group (automobile accidents, homicide, and suicide are the three leading causes of death in the young adult age group). Orthopedic injuries such as broken wrists or sprained ankles occur because a woman's sense of balance is not optimum. As many as 7 percent of all expectant women—or 250,000 women a year—suffer some form of trauma (Patterson, 1983).

In an automobile accident, a pregnant woman is often the front seat passenger. Statistics show a person in this position often receives the most severe injury in an accident. A pregnant woman may be the intended victim or an innocent bystander in a homicide incident. Unfortunately, pregnancy may be a reason for a young woman to attempt suicide. Finally, some women are seen in emergency rooms following a beating by their sexual partner or husband.

In an emergency situation, when care for trauma is given, the physiologic changes of pregnancy must be considered in order that both the woman and the fetus are adequately protected. A primary rule to remember is that following a traumatic injury, a woman's body will maintain her own homeostasis at the expense of the fetus. To maintain blood pressure in the face of hemorrhage, for example, a woman's body will use peripheral vasoconstriction. Because the uterus is a peripheral organ in a shock response, its blood supply will be greatly diminished and nutrient supply greatly compromised.

Physiologic Changes That Affect Assessment

A woman's total plasma volume increases during pregnancy from about 2,600 ml to 4,000 ml at term. This increase serves as a safeguard to the woman if trauma with bleeding should occur: She can lose up to 30 percent of her blood volume before hypovolemia is clinically evident. It also means, however, that fluid replacement volume will undoubtedly have to be high, as she needs more fluid than usual to fully restore her circulatory volume.

In order to accommodate this increased vascular load, cardiac output increases in pregnancy from 1 liter a minute early in pregnancy to 6 to 7 liters a minute in the second trimester. This volume circulates through the placenta at a rapid rate. About one sixth of total blood volume is present in the placenta at all times. If a uterine lesion occurs, therefore, a woman is prone to exsanguination.

In order to move this blood adequately through the circulation, the heart rate increases 15 to 20 beats above normal (a pulse rate of 80–95). It is important to remember that this elevated rate is normal so that a rapid pulse rate is not interpreted as a sign of hemorrhage when none is present. The heart is displaced by the elevated diaphragm, making interpretation of an ECG difficult.

Peripheral venous pressure in a pregnant woman is unchanged although it tends to be higher in lower extremities because of compression of the vena cava. This means that lacerations of the legs or perineum will bleed much more profusely than normally. Peripheral blood flow in general is increased due to decreased peripheral vascular resistance (the effect of estrogen and decreased sympathetic activity all through pregnancy). Pregnant women can be in severe shock and their extremities will still not feel cold and clammy.

The central venous pressure (normal 5–12 cm H_2O in a nonpregnant state) is increased to 8 to 10 cm H_2O. Although a woman needs a large amount of replacement fluid, her circulation is in increased danger of being overwhelmed by intravenous fluid infusion.

During pregnancy the leukocyte count rises (to 18,000 mm^3 at term), making it difficult to use this determination as a sign of infection following an open wound. Serum albumin level decreases during pregnancy, making the large loss that normally occurs with burns a more-serious-than-usual response. Serum liver levels remain the same during pregnancy (SGOT, SGPT, LDH); if these levels are elevated following trauma, liver trauma can be detected. Alkaline phosphatase, a substance also usually helpful in detecting liver trauma, is three to four times more abundant in pregnant women at term (from placenta origin), making this marker unreliable. Pancreatic amylase remains the same during pregnancy; lipase is decreased, so that the pancreas can be evaluated normally.

Because the stomach of a pregnant woman empties slowly, she should always be considered to have a full stomach. Automatically general anesthesia is a hazard for her. If she is anesthetized, a cuffed endotracheal tube must be used with cricoid pressure during insertion to prevent aspiration.

Abdominal pain is difficult to localize in a pregnant woman because, as the abdomen always feels tense during pregnancy, guarding and rigidity of the abdominal wall are lost as important findings. The position of organs is different because of the growing uterus. Bleeding into the abdominal cavity with an abdominal injury is apt to be forceful and extreme because of the increased pressure in the pelvic vessels. A procedure such as a needle paracentesis to assess for bleeding into the abdominal cavity is dangerous, because the bowel, dislocated from its usual position, can be easily punctured. *Culdocentesis*, or needle aspiration through the posterior vaginal fornix into the peritoneal cavity, may be done. Peritoneal lavage, or inserting a peritoneal dialysis catheter into the abdominal cavity, adding an amount of an isotonic solution, aspirating it again, and analyzing it for blood or urine may reveal bleeding best.

The bladder of pregnant women is very susceptible to rupture: It is the most anterior organ and is elevated abnormally. Following abdominal trauma, an indwelling bladder catheter is often inserted to assess for blood in urine.

Assessment Following Trauma

When a pregnant woman is seen at a health care facility because of an accident, she is both apprehensive and frightened, not only about herself but for the health of the fetus (Figure 41-1). She is worried not only about what *has* happened, but also about what *could* have happened (if the knife had slipped an inch further, if the auto accident had been even worse, if she had fallen even further from the stepladder) and concerned about what medical care will be required (does she need an X-ray; if she does will this be safe for the fetus?). She may feel very guilty about her carelessness (if she were really a good mother, she would have had her seatbelt fastened or not tried to stand on a stepladder to hang drapes alone).

A feeling of guilt lowers self-esteem and increases her level of stress. Remember that people under stress do not hear well and may not perceive correctly the information given to them; information given in an emergency room may be grossly misinterpreted. Always try to review information with them at a later date to be certain that they do have the facts of their injury in pro-

Figure 41-1 *Trauma in a pregnant woman is always serious; emergency care must address the needs of the fetus as well as the woman herself.*

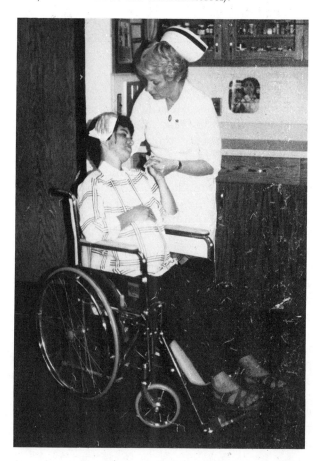

portion and they are accurate in their knowledge of follow-up care needed.

Health History

In an emergency situation, a few minutes spent attempting to calm a woman and move her past her initial fright is time well spent unless symptoms of major body system disturbances require that you direct your immediate efforts elsewhere. Being calm helps a woman cooperate with history giving and physical assessment procedures.

Take a brief pregnancy history (length of pregnancy, any complications). Ask if fetal heart tones have been heard by an examiner during the pregnancy. Ask if she has felt the fetus move since the accident. Ask if she has any sensation of tightening or pain in her abdomen that could be uterine contractions. Ask if she knows what her prepregnancy and pregnancy blood pressure have been to help evaluate the extent of blood loss she has had.

Take a brief history of the accident, documenting what happened, the time that has passed since the injury, signs and symptoms of injury the woman is experiencing, and actions she has taken to counteract these.

If a woman fell, how far did she fall (a fall from the top of a stepladder is more likely to be serious than a fall from a low rung). What body part did she land on (landing on her abdomen may be very serious, although she may be in less pain than if she injured an ankle in the fall). In an auto accident, ask how fast the car was traveling, if she was thrown from the car or not, or if the windshield broke or not (windshields are broken by heads striking them, so the woman needs to be assessed for a head injury).

Assess whether a woman's degree of injury is in proportion to that suggested by the trauma (a woman states her accident was tripping on a child's toy, yet all extremities are ecchymotic and her jaw is broken). Injuries out of proportion to the history suggest abuse (battering). Assess whether a woman was using a sensible degree of caution. If not, assess whether she might have wanted the pregnancy to end. A naive adolescent, for example, may attempt to end a pregnancy by a deliberate fall or poisoning she then reports as an accident.

Physical Examination

Accidents become fatal happenings when lung, heart, kidney, or brain function becomes inadequate; fetal health is injured when uterine function is impaired. These body systems must be evaluated first. The box on page 950 lists signs and symptoms to assess in order to evaluate function of these major body organs.

Be certain that a woman does not lie supine for an examination, which could cause supine hypotension syndrome. If it is necessary for her to lie on her back, manually displace the uterus from the vena cava with your hand or place rolled towels or blankets under her right side to tip her body about 15 degrees to the side. If surgery is necessary, an operating room table can be tipped to achieve this effect or a uterine displacement bar, a metal bar attached to the table that presses the uterus away from the vena cava, can be used.

If multiple trauma is present, a nasogastric tube is usually passed to empty the stomach. A Foley catheter is passed to assess for urine output and to rule out a ruptured bladder (blood would return or urine would be blood tinged if this were present).

Emergency Therapy

Failure to Breathe

If respirations are not present or are not effective, cardiopulmonary resuscitation should be begun with a pregnant woman as it would be with any person following trauma (Table 41-1). To be certain she has not just fainted, try to arouse her by calling her name or shaking her shoulders. If unsuccessful, assess whether her airway is obstructed by holding your cheek next to her nostrils and assessing for air exchange; look in her mouth for a foreign object. If she is not breathing, slightly extend her head and begin breathing for her, using either a mouth-to-mouth or a resuscitation bag technique.

Although an enlarged uterus puts considerable pressure on the diaphragm and consequently the lungs, unusual pressure in not necessary to fully inflate lungs in a resuscitation attempt. Assess cardiovascular function by palpating the carotid pulse. If this is not palpable or the pupils are fixed, heart function must also be supplemented. Begin external heart massage at a rate of two breaths to every 15 heart compressions (one rescuer) or one breath to five cardiac beats for two rescuers (the same as for all adults). Cardiac massage may be awkard late in pregnancy because of the size of the uterus, but undue pressure should not be necessary to create heart action.

Following assessment of the level of consciousness, cardiovascular and respiratory status, if there has been blood loss, a central venous pressure line is often inserted and lactated Ringers or

Important Assessments on Initial Examination

Body System	Assessment
Respiratory system	Quality of respirations (labored or even?)
	Rate of respirations?
	Sounds of obstruction (wheezing, retractions, coughing?)
	Color (cyanotic?)
	Oxygen hunger (inability to lie flat, nasal flaring?)
Cardiovascular system	Color (pallor from hemorrhage?)
	Gross bleeding?
	Pulse rate (increases with hemorrhage)
	Blood pressure (decreases with hemorrhage)
	Feeling of apprehension from altered vascular pressure?
Nervous system	Level of consciousness (woman answers questions coherently?)
	Pupils (equal and reacting to light?)
	Bruises or raised bump on head or spinal column?
	Loss of motion or sensory function in a body part?
Renal system	Bruising on anterior abdominal wall over bladder or on back over kidneys?
	Blood in urine?
Uterine-fetal system	Bradycardia, tachycardia or absence of fetal heart tones?
	Vaginal bleeding?
	Clear (amniotic) fluid leaking from vagina?
	Bruising on abdomen over uterus?

another isotonic solution infused to restore fluid volume or provide an open line for emergency medication.

If hypotension is present, it must be corrected quickly in order to maintain a pressure gradient across the placenta. Any antihypotensive agent, however, that achieves an increased blood pressure by causing peripheral vasoconstriction, is contraindicated. Ephedrine is the drug of choice with a pregnant woman to restore blood pressure as it has a minimal peripheral vasoconstriction effect. Dopamine in low doses is a second drug that can be used.

Following emergency implementations, care will be dependent on the specific injury or trauma present. Careful assessment that the pregnancy has not been harmed must be made, for a traumatic blow to the abdomen may cause dislodgement of the placenta (abruptio placentae); if uterine bleeding is occurring, it may begin premature labor. The uterus is palpated for any abnormal contours that would suggest edema or internal

bleeding. Fetal heart tones are counted. Using a Doppler technique is helpful to assure the woman that her fetus is all right. Real-time sonogram may also be helpful for this purpose and in assessing that the uterus or placenta are not torn.

A pelvic examination is performed to assess for vaginal bleeding or seepage of clear fluid that would suggest the amniotic membranes were ruptured from the force of an abdominal blow and amniotic fluid is beginning to leak vaginally. If a woman reports uterine contractions, a uterine and fetal monitor will be placed to estimate their strength and effect on the fetal heart rate and the possibility that premature labor has begun.

Choking

If a pregnant woman chokes on a piece of meat, or any foreign object blocks the airway, it can be dislodged by a sudden upward thrust to the upper abdomen (a Heimlich maneuver), as with any adult. This maneuver puts pressure on the dia-

Table 41-1 Cardiopulmonary Resuscitation During Pregnancy

Action	Technique
1. Shake and shout	Shake shoulders and attempt to rouse her to be certain woman has not fainted.
2. Position the airway	Put pressure on forehead with one hand while lifting with the other hand under the neck (slightly extend neck).
3. Establish lack of respirations	Assess if exhalations are occurring by placing your face next to woman's mouth.
4. Begin rescue breathing	Pinch nostrils and deliver four quick breaths to woman's mouth and lungs.
5. Assess cardiovascular status	Assess for presence of carotid pulse.
6. Begin heart massage	With one rescuer, place both hands on the lower sternum just above xyphoid process and deliver 15 chest compressions followed by two rescue breaths until cardiopulmonary function returns. With two rescuers, deliver five chest compressions followed by one breath.

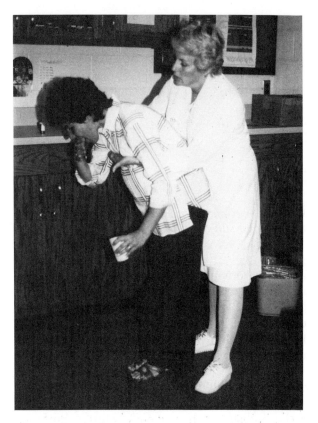

Figure 41-2 *A Heimlich maneuver during pregnancy is done with the side of the hand.*

phragm. As the diaphragm moves forcefully upward, air moves upward in the trachea, dislodging the object. A Heimlich maneuver is difficult to do late in pregnancy because of lack of space between the uterus and the end of the sternum, and it is difficult to do from the rear because you cannot reach around the woman's enlarged abdomen. To do this maneuver successfully during pregnancy, therefore, first strike the woman's back between her scapula four times: This action alone may be effective. Approach from the front, move the uterus slightly to one side manually; and use the side of your hand rather than a fist, which fits the limited upper abdomen space available, for a quick abdominal thrust (Figure 41-2).

Wounds

In order to prevent infection, open wounds should be thoroughly cleaned with soap and water or an antiseptic solution and sutured so the edges are approximated and healing is allowed to take place most rapidly. As mentioned, the white blood count is normally elevated during pregnancy and is a poor indicator of the presence or extent of infection in wounds.

Abrasions

Abrasions are superficial removal of a thickness of the skin (brush burns). The area should be washed and patted dry to remove obvious soil. Although painful and bright red in appearance, if abrasions are kept clean, they heal in a few days' time with no further therapy.

Lacerations

A laceration is a jagged cut. It may involve only the skin layer or penetrate to deeper subcutaneous tissue or tendons. Lacerations generally bleed profusely. Bleeding should be halted by pressure on the edge of the laceration (difficult to achieve in lower extremities because venous pressure is so great during pregnancy). Following cleaning, the area is sutured through each layer of tissue involved to approximate edges. In order for sutures to be used, a local anesthetic such as Xylocaine is necessary. Its local effect makes it safe during pregnancy. If the laceration is superficial

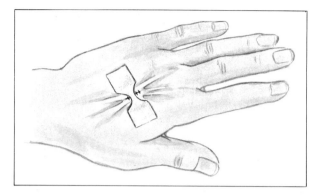

Figure 41-3 *A butterfly dressing may prevent the necessity for sutures during pregnancy.*

and the woman is nervous about the use of an anesthetic, the edges can be approximated by use of a butterfly strip made from a Band-Aid or a commercial adhesive strip (Figure 41-3). This method may allow it to heal with a slightly more noticeable scar, however.

Puncture Wounds

A puncture wound results from penetration of a sharp object such as a nail, splinter, knife, or nail file. Puncture marks bleed very little—an advantage in terms of minimizing blood loss but not advantageous in terms of wound cleaning. A puncture wound is usually not sutured to prevent a sealed, unoxygenated cavity from being created below the sutures; such a cavity can result in tetanus bacillus growth. If a woman has had a tetanus immunization within the last 10 years, tetanus toxoid is administered. Otherwise (and usually), tetanus toxoid plus immune tetanus globulin is administered; both these injections are safe during pregnancy.

Puncture wounds are frightening because most people know about tetanus and these wounds usually occur in association with a degree of violence. The uterus appears to have a natural resistance to infection: Even if punctured, infection in the uterus rarely occurs. Uterine puncture, however, could directly harm the fetus.

Stab Wounds

Stab wounds are deep penetrations made by an object such as a knife or a barbecue fork. A stab wound may easily reach the depth of the uterus and directly injure the fetus. Most stab wounds of the abdomen, however, occur in the upper quadrants above the height of the uterus. In order to determine the depth and extent of the wound, a *fistulogram* may be done. This technique involves insertion of a thin catheter into the wound; the wound is then filled with radiopaque solution; and an X-ray of the area the solution fills

reveals the extent of the puncture. If the peritoneal cavity was perforated, dye will outline the intestines. If there is suspicion of bleeding in the abdominal cavity, a *celiotomy*, or exploratory surgery into the abdominal cavity, may be performed. If the diaphragm was cut, intestine may herniate into the chest cavity (diaphragmatic hernia) due to the increased abdominal pressure from the enlarged uterus. Following surgical repair of an injured diaphragm, cesarean birth may be planned to avoid strain on the newly repaired diaphragm from pushing during labor.

Contusions

A contusion results from blunt trauma to underlying tissue; no visible break is present in the skin. Following the injury, the underlying tissue becomes edematous; broken underlying vessels ooze and form ecchymosis or a hematoma at the site.

The amount of blood seeping or formation of edema can be reduced by the application of ice for the first 24 hours. Following this, application of heat for 24 hours will clear the edema most quickly. Contusions can be very painful (out of proportion to their appearance) because of the tissue swelling and the pressure on nerves that results. If a woman strikes her abdomen in a fall, she may have contusions of the abdominal skin. She may be asked to remain overnight in the health care agency because compression of the uterus may have caused the placenta to separate (abruptio placentae). This condition also occurs for other reasons and is discussed in Chapter 39 along with other placental bleeding problems of pregnancy.

Gunshot Wounds

A woman may receive a gunshot wound either because she was an intended victim or because she was an innocent bystander; occasionally a woman attempts suicide with a gun. Assessment of a gunshot wound includes inspection not only for the point the bullet entered the woman's body but also the point that the bullet exited (the entry wound is small, the exit one is large because, as the bullet slows, it begins to tumble, enlarging the space it occupies). If the bullet entered high in the woman's abdomen, intestine will surely be injured; because so much is compressed above the uterus, intestine may sustain many tears from one bullet. The uterine wall is so thick during pregnancy that it may trap a bullet so there is no exit point from a woman's body.

Gunshot wounds are surgically cleaned and debrided and treated with a high concentration of antibiotics usually administered intravenously. Ampicillin is frequently ordered; fortunately, ampicillin administration is safe during pregnancy. Following the emergency therapy for the injury, investigate carefully the circumstances of the injury in order to help a woman learn safer use of firearms or to be certain that the injury was not deliberately induced. Gunshot wounds must be reported to the police. Stay with a woman as necessary while she recounts her history of the accident again for law enforcement officers.

Animal Bites

Pregnant women are rarely bitten by any animal but a dog. Animal bites are a form of puncture wounds, so if the rabies immunization status of the dog is known and is current, the wound can be washed and treated as a puncture wound. If the animal cannot be located or is proven to be rabid after 48 hours of observation, the woman must be administered a series of rabies immunizations. Although this vaccine has not been proven safe for the fetus, the woman's life depends on this protection.

Pregnant women should be advised to use caution with unfamiliar dogs or, if camping in a remote location, with taming or feeding wild animals such as squirrels and raccoons.

Poisoning

Pregnant women are not apt to swallow a poison, though it is possible if a woman wakes at night and attempts to take medicine in the dark. Poisoning in a pregnant woman should be managed as it would be for any individual. The woman should telephone the local poison control center, state what she accidentally swallowed, and follow the specific recommendations of personnel at the poison control center. Syrup of ipecac (30 ml) followed by a glass of water is the best emetic to cause vomiting and discharge of poison from her body and is safe for use during pregnancy.

After a woman has been treated and the emergency of the poisoning is over, investigate carefully the circumstances of the poisoning in order to help a woman learn safer habits of medicine taking or to discover if she could have intentionally meant to take a poison (to end the pregnancy or her life).

Orthopedic Injuries

Because a woman has poor balance late in pregnancy, she may trip more readily than usual; when she falls she automatically reaches out a hand to cushion the fall and prevent striking her abdomen. Ordinarily if a young adult falls this way, her wrist is not injured; but the extra weight that the pregnant woman carries puts a greater stress on the wrist so that more serious injuries can occur. Applying ice to the area decreases swelling as an immediate first-aid measure. An X-ray may be necessary to determine whether a fracture is present or not. You can assure women that an X-ray of an extremity is safe for them during pregnancy as long as their abdomen is shielded during the radiation exposure. Accompany a woman to the X-ray department and remain with her (outside the actual X-ray room) to both assure her that lead protection will be offered and to be available if signs of premature delivery should suddenly develop as a result of as-yet-undetected injury.

Because many adolescent girls are actively involved in sports or dancing activities, many develop trauma to their knee cartilage (torn or stretched cartilage). Once a knee injury has happened, the cartilage is more apt to be injured again. If a woman has a susceptible knee, therefore, she should be cautious during pregnancy (when she carries additional weight) about turning quickly: This twisting motion (foot planted and not turned) causes the most serious knee damage. This caution is particularly necessary late in pregnancy when all cartilage of her body is softened by the ovarian hormone relaxin. Following a torn ligament or dislocated kneecap, either a cast or a leg immobilizer will be applied, to be worn for 4 to 6 weeks (Figure 41-4).

A woman with a cast or immobilizer in place during pregnancy will be concerned as her delivery date approaches that the cast will interfere with a safe delivery (even with a full leg cast in

Figure 41-4 *Women who suffer knee dislocations during pregnancy may need to wear a leg immobilizer for the remainder of the pregnancy.*

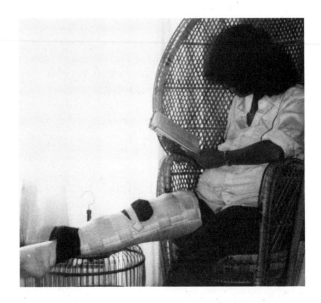

place she can be delivered safely) or interfere with care of the newborn. Plan with her ways that she will still be able to be active during pregnancy (on bedrest with a cast will increase the chance she will develop a thrombophlebitis) and ways that she will be able to manage in the postpartal period (ask a family member to live in with her for a few days and sleep downstairs so she does not have to attempt stairs, etc.). Because women of childbearing age are basically healthy, healing of fractures or torn ligaments occurs quickly and generally without complications. Be certain a woman has a good calcium intake if she has a fracture so both the fetus and herself have adequate calcium for new bone growth.

The laxness of body cartilage may also cause separation of the symphysis pubis if she falls with her legs outspread. This injury is very painful on walking or turning. To avoid pain and allow the cartilage to heal, a woman needs to remain on bedrest for 4 to 6 weeks—obviously very difficult for her, especially if close to delivery. A separation present at the time of delivery may cause labor to be very painful, especially the pelvic division when the fetus is pushed through the pelvic ring.

Burns

Burns are dangerous to a pregnant woman not only from the actual thermal injury that occurs but also if carbon monoxide gases from the fire are inhaled. Extreme fetal anoxia could result from carbon monoxide crossing the placenta in place of oxygen. Smoke is irritating to lung tissue and can cause extensive lung edema and anoxia from the lack of oxygen/carbon dioxide exchange space. The fluid and electrolyte loss is great with burns, and may lead to hypotension from hypovolemia or an electrolyte imbalance. A body response to a harsh trauma such as a burn is the production of prostaglandins, which could start premature labor.

Interestingly, pregnancy makes burn tissue heal more quickly, a phenomenon probably related to the generally increased metabolism and possibly to the increased cortisol serum level, which keeps inflammation and damage to tissue from the pressure of edema from occurring.

Postmortem Cesarean Birth

If a mother does not survive serious trauma, it may still be possible for her child to be delivered safely by a postmortem cesarean birth. This is usually attempted if the fetus is past 28 weeks,

and less than 20 minutes have passed since the mother expired. Infant survival is best in these circumstances if no longer than 10 minutes has passed. By general practice, no consent is necessary for this procedure, as the fetus is assumed to want to live but cannot give consent or make these wants known. A classic cesarean incision is used. Skilled health care personnel should be available to immediately resuscitate the newborn.

Safety and Pregnancy

Sensible precautions to take during pregnancy in order to avoid accidents and trauma should be included as part of pregnancy counseling. Although these recommendations (shown in Table 41-2) are largely commonsense actions, they are important to review during pregnancy. Accidents, as a category of events, occur more frequently in

Table 41-2 Safety Precautions to Take During Pregnancy

Area	Precaution
Home	Do not stand on stepstools or step ladders (difficult to maintain balance on a narrow base).
	Avoid throw rugs without a nonskid backing.
	Keep small items such as toys out of pathways (difficult for a pregnant woman to see her feet).
	Use caution stepping in and out of a bathtub (slippery).
	Do not overload electrical circuits (difficult for a pregnant woman to escape a fire because of poor mobility).
	Do not smoke to avoid falling asleep with a cigarette.
	Do not take medicine in the dark to avoid an error.
Work	Avoid handling toxic substances.
	Avoid working to a point of fatigue, which lowers judgment.
	Avoid long periods of standing, which can lead to orthostatic hypotension and fainting.
Automobile	Use a seat belt at all times.
	Refuse to ride with anyone who has been drinking alcohol or whose judgment might be impaired.

people under stress than in those who are stress-free. A pregnant woman is prone to accidents and injury unless she follows some sensible precautions for safety.

The Battered Woman

More than a million women in the United States are battered or beaten yearly. It is a problem at all socioeconomic levels. Battered women may be seen in prenatal settings because they are unable to resist sexual advances from their abusive partner, thereby becoming pregnant. The pregnancy may not be wanted; on the other hand, a woman may think that having a child will change her partner and make him a better person. She may be grateful, thinking that she will have an infant to love her. Beatings may increase during pregnancy because stress is often a trigger to beatings. A woman so nauseated that she cannot cook, so tired that she did not make a bed, is a convenient target for an unstable partner. A husband concerned about the hospital bill might resort to a beating to handle his frustration.

Wife abuse generally begins with a light level of abuse (stage I); if a woman does not leave at this point to end the relationship, it continues to become more frequent and more violent (by not stopping it, the woman is indirectly giving it permission to continue) until she may be killed. A fetus is in threat if the abusing is at stage II or III (see Table 41-3).

Women remain with abusive partners because at first the abuse is not great; the longer they stay, the more unable they are to leave as their self-esteem diminishes. They often feel that this state of affairs is their fault and if they were a better

person their partner would not resort to beating them. This guilt immobilizes them. They generally have no access to money because the abusing partner controls this; they feel that leaving the man would be worse than staying. Even if they have a skill—they were capable secretaries or lawyers once—their self-esteem has become so low that they no longer believe they can successfully put the skill to use. As the abuse becomes more violent, they may be afraid that the man will follow them if they leave and kill them. Other family members may be unwilling to shelter a woman for fear of being included in the man's violence. Police and social agencies may take the neutral stand that "domestic fighting" is strictly between the consenting adults involved.

Assessment

A battered woman may come late for pregnancy care because of lack of transportation (her husband controls the use of the car) or because she has tried to pretend that the pregnancy did not exist. "Not rocking the boat," keeping the stress level down, is her best defense against violence.

She may be noticeable in a prenatal setting by a failure to purchase clothing especially for the pregnancy (she has no funds for herself, and asking for money may incite violence). She may not go for laboratory tests if going involves transportation or money. She is different from women whose main problem is poverty. Even the poorest family will squeeze out money for one dress that will show off the pregnancy, or squeeze out money for laboratory tests to ensure a successful outcome to the pregnancy.

A woman may have difficulty following a pregnancy diet (she must cook what her partner wants or she will be beaten). She may leave at a prenatal visit before the nurse-midwife or physician sees her, or she may grow very anxious if her prenatal appointment is running late (she must be home to cook dinner or she will be beaten).

She may dress inappropriately for warm weather, wearing long-sleeved, tight-necked blouses to cover up bruises on her neck or arms. She may call and cancel appointments frequently (or simply not keep appointments) because she has an obvious black eye or a bleeding facial laceration she does not want to reveal.

A woman may be very anxious to listen to the baby's heartbeat at prenatal visits because her partner recently punched or kicked her abdomen and she is worried that the fetus has been hurt. If undressed for a physical examination, she may have bruises or lacerations on her breasts, her abdomen, or her back that she cannot explain. Her

Table 41-3 Levels of Wife Abuse

Level	Description
I	Abuse is occasional; consists of slapping, punching, kicking, verbal abuse. Contusions occur.
II	Abuse is becoming more frequent; beatings are sustained and cause fractures such as a broken jaw or ribs.
III	Abuse is even more frequent, perhaps daily. A weapon such as a gun, baseball bat, or broom handle may be used. Permanent disability or death from injuries such as intracranial hemorrhage or concussion may occur.

neck may reveal linear bruises from strangulation. Ask any woman with bruises to account for them. Listen to see whether the explanation seems to correlate with the extent and placement of the bruise.

Analysis

The North American Association on Nursing Diagnosis has accepted one diagnosis associated with trauma: Injury, potential for. With pregnancy, fear related to possible fetal harm or knowledge deficit related to pregnancy safety measures are often used. Be certain that goals established reflect the emergency situation present and are achievable within the woman's condition and life style.

Planning and Implementation

Working with battered women can be perplexing because it is hard to understand why they stay in their situation. Remember that fear of the abusive person (if they leave, he may find them and kill them) and the guilt and low self-esteem they feel (he has told them so many times that this is their fault and they deserve to be treated this way that they believe it) immobilize them. They are as paralyzed to do anything about their situation without outside help as if they were physically paralyzed. To compound the problem, their low self-esteem and depression lead them to think that no one would *want* to help them.

A woman needs help to make decisions. Support any ability to make constructive decisions that she has left. Be familiar with safe shelters for battered women in your community; help a woman to make arrangements to move to one or discuss with her how she could call the police at any time and they would take her there. Help her obtain a restraining order to keep the abusive person from coming near her again if this is necessary.

After the birth of the child, a woman may be depressed to realize how alone she is. She may have unreal expectations of the child, trying to make the newborn smile at her and interact with her more than is possible. She has a great need to be loved. Try to caution her that her newborn does love her but she has to give him or her time to grow. Show the mother all the things her child can do, such as attend to the sound of her voice or cuddle against her. Otherwise her unreal expectations may lead to disappointment and an interference with her mothering.

Do not leave a battered woman without a support system after birth of a child. If she was depending on you during pregnancy, you cannot abandon her afterwards without filling in the gap with another support system. A possible avenue is a social agency that deals specifically with battered women in your community; another is a community health nurse who will visit when the woman returns home. If she is left without a support person, her low self-esteem will not allow her to reach out and seek help. She may decide that suicide or returning to the person who abused her is her only resource.

Battered women need to be identified during pregnancy not only so they can be helped but to protect the mental health of the child. A child raised in a home where the mother is battered will learn that this interaction is acceptable conduct, and the battering may extend to yet another generation.

Rape

Rape is usually defined as the intrusion of the penis into the vagina by force. *Sexual assault* is used to refer to other forced sexual acts, such as oral-genital or anal-genital intrusion. Both rape and sexual assault are deviant behavior—acts of violence, not passion. They lack the components of privacy and consent that characterize "normal" sexual behavior. In contrast, rape and sexual assault are degrading and dehumanizing; they leave the victim feeling helpless.

The average rape victim is an adolescent girl, although the age range is from 1 to over 80. It can occur during pregnancy. In most instances the rapist is a stranger to the victim. The attacker is usually of young adult age with a background of amoral, aggressive behavior. Immediate self-gratification is a priority. A rapist's previous relationships with adult women have generally been poor, and he may rely on prostitutes for most of his sexual pleasure. An excessive amount of alcohol intake often precedes rape (Burgess, 1979).

Following rape, most women move through two stages of a *rape trauma syndrome:* disorganization and reorganization. In the initial phase, a woman feels a combination of humiliation, shame and guilt, embarrassment, anger, and desire for revenge. She feels her life has been completely disrupted by the crisis and her inability to prevent herself from being used in this way. She trembles from fear and may be in great pain from perineal or other lacerations. If pregnant, she is apt to bleed profusely from vaginal or perineal lacerations. She is apt to visibly start at the sound of anyone approaching or touching her: She needs effective support persons with her in the days following the event to allow her to feel safe. She may have nightmares of the attack occurring again.

This immediate stage of disruption and disorganization lasts about 3 days.

In the second stage, or reorganization, as they try to outlive this personal offense to their bodies, many rape victims change their residence at great sacrifice to both finances and convenience. They continue to report recurring nightmares, perhaps sexual dysfunction, and continuing inability to relate to men or face new and surprising situations. If rape occurs during pregnancy it may be so traumatic a happening that it interferes with maternal-infant bonding at the child's birth. Women may continue to have difficulty discussing the rape; if not offered constructive counsel they may continue to feel guilt or shame for many years.

Many more women do not report rape than do (as few as one in five are reported). Because these women do not receive any counseling, symptoms of what is termed *silent rape syndrome* may become manifest. When the subject of rape is mentioned, some women may grow emotionally disturbed; their behavior toward men, as seen in a health history, is altered at a set point in their life. Perhaps they began to resist getting out or being alone in a house following that point. This syndrome can be devastating to a woman's ability to maintain a work position or remain independent. She needs counseling as much as the woman who reports a rape.

In many instances of rape, the woman's sexual partner has difficulty being supportive—the rape may cause turmoil in his own feelings and self-image. Frequently, a relationship will deteriorate as a result of a sexual partner perceiving the woman as "dirty" or "soiled" following rape; he may mistakenly believe that women ask to be raped or actually enjoy the experience. A sexual partner may also become so overprotective of the woman following the incident (not allowing her to go out alone, checking on her constantly) that she is no longer free to maintain her identity. The man may be so filled with desire for revenge and anger that he cannot effectively relate with his sexual partner without his anger surfacing toward her as well as the attacker.

Emergency Room Care

Women are often confused by their treatment by police officers who respond to their call for help following rape if the officers imply that the woman provoked the attack or could have done more to resist or prevent the attack. This attitude increases the woman's feeling of shame and degradation: It reveals that people she has been taught to respect have no concept of the degree of fright she has experienced or the strength of her attacker. Health care providers who are the second group of people a woman sees following an attack need to be extremely cautious that they do not evidence any of the same callous behavior. A woman who has been raped is in the same category as a trauma victim who has been rescued from near drowning or crushed by a rolling truck. She needs both immediate physical care administered by warm caring people to ensure herself that she is now safe and away from danger and psychological counseling in order to survive the overwhelming insult she has suffered to her self-concept.

Most large cities are educating police officers to respect rape as a crime of intense violence, not one provoked by the woman; the understanding that women receive from the police department is now improving greatly. Most health care agencies where many rape victims are seen have a rape trauma team with specially educated counselors to talk to the victim immediately following the rape and to offer long-term counseling as needed. Any nurse, however, should be able to offer emergency support to the woman during the time before a specifically designated staff member arrives or if such a service is not available in the community.

One of the major needs of any accident victim following a violent act is to talk about what happened to them. A person who can describe an incident begins to "put a fence around the happening," which helps make the happening less frightening or overwhelming. This description brings the act down from "something terrible has happened to me," which leaves a person with a continuing high anxiety level, to "this specific thing has happened to me," which allows the traumatic event to be examined and dealt with. Something that is concrete and describable is rarely as frightening as "something out there."

Ask the woman to describe the incident to you, introducing the request with a statement such as "Most people find it helps to talk about what happened to them." The box on page 958 lists areas of information the woman needs to describe in order to reduce the incident to a psychologically workable size.

Because rape is a crime, the hospital chart of a rape victim is often displayed as part of a court procedure. In order that the woman can bring charges against her attacker, she needs to have information concerning her appearance and her history of the account detailed in the hospital chart. Be extremely careful that statements in a chart are accurate and unbiased. In recording a history, quote the woman's exact words whenever possible. Describe her physical appearance carefully, including the presence and location of injuries such as bruises, lacerations, teeth marks,

Areas to Explore in Rape Counseling

Area	*Concerns*
Circumstances	Where did the attack occur? What was happening at the time? This information is important for the victim to discuss and work through because any time she is in a similar circumstance she may experience an uncontrollable fear related to the identical circumstances of the attack. If she was walking home from work or waiting for an elevator in a public building, these are circumstances that will happen again. She can be assured that she was acting sensibly under the circumstances (a person should be able to walk home from work or wait for an elevator unharmed), that the rape was not her fault.
Assailant	Allowing the woman to review the description of the rapist may help her to realize that she may react to a man with the same build or description in negative ways in the future. If the man first approached her with a simple gesture, such as a hand on her shoulder, this circumstance will happen to her again; she needs to work through her revulsion for the act in order to handle what is usually a simple, friendly gesture.
Any conversation	Describing the conversation with the rapist is helpful for the woman to convince herself that she did not provoke the attack. She can realize that with hindsight everyone could improve on a conversation; but at the time, what she said or did not say was not really important. The rapist could not have been stopped.
Details of the assault	Describing the actual assault is extremely difficult for most women but doing so, again, allows the woman to work through the situation. Until the woman can describe the attack or the sexual act she was forced into, she may have difficulty performing these same acts with a person of her choice.
Resistance to the assault	Many women do not struggle during an assault because of fear of further harm. Later someone may say to a woman, "Didn't you do anything to try and fight him off?" and she will feel accused of provoking or accepting the attack. She needs reinforcement that no action was probably her best action and why she is still alive. Counseling that rape is a violent crime and that the strength of her attacker was probably far too great to resist helps to improve a woman's self-esteem.

or abrasions and the condition of her clothing. Ask the woman if she bathed or washed before coming for care; these can obscure evidence and obliterate the presence of sperm. Photographs should be taken as necessary to document the extent of injuries. Any clothing that is ripped or stained is evidence of violent assault and should be kept.

Following this preliminary observation, a gynecologic examination is used to evaluate the woman's physical condition, to document that rape occurred, and to confirm that the pregnancy has not been disrupted. A record should be kept of the existence of any vaginal or perineal lacerations and aspiration of sperm or acid phosphatase from the vagina. Acid phosphatase is a substance that is not normally present in vaginal secretions but is present in semen. Its presence is extremely important if the male is infertile or sterile (sperm may not be present); for the first 14 hours following the incident it forms the best proof that rape occurred. A vaginal culture for gonorrhea and a

Common Specimen Procedures Following Rape*

Procedure	*Purpose*
Oral washing	Patient rinses mouth with 5 ml sterile water; collected in test tube. Analyzed for blood group antigens or sperm of attacker.
Fingernail scraping	Scrape under all of patient's fingernails and place scrapings in envelope. Analyzed for blood, skin, and clothing fibers of attacker.
Blood VDRL	Draw blood for antibody titer for syphilis.
Blood typing	Patient's blood is typed to differentiate it from attacker's.
Pregnancy test	Either blood or a urine specimen may be obtained. Vaginal exam should be completed before woman voids.
Hair samples	Both scalp and pubic hairs of patient (about 10) are removed for comparison with attacker's and placed in envelope.
Vaginal smear	Vagina is swabbed with dry applicator and smeared onto slide. Allow to dry for analysis of sperm.
Gonococcus (GC) culture	Cervix, vagina, rectum are cultured (also throat if oral coitus was attempted).
Vaginal washing	5 ml of sterile saline is placed in vagina and aspirated. Analyzed to detect sperm and acid phosphatase.
Skin washings	Touch any dried stain of blood or semen on skin or clothing with a moistened cotton swab; drop into test tube. Analyzed for attacker's blood and semen.
Clothing care	Place any clothing stained or torn into a paper bag. Evidence of violent attack.

*Label all specimens carefully as to where they were obtained for both medical therapy and legal evidence.

Pap test are also taken. A VDRL is done for syphilis; blood should be drawn for a pregnancy test if pregnancy has not yet been established. Prophylactic administration of penicillin against gonorrhea and syphilis are also advisable and not contraindicated during pregnancy. If a woman is not pregnant at the time of rape, she is offered diethylstilbestrol as a contraceptive. If this medication is not effective in preventing a pregnancy, the child has a high probability of being born with DES defects (tendency toward vaginal carcinoma for girls and cystic testes for boys). It obviously should not be administered to a pregnant woman.

Although rape may include perineal and vaginal lacerations, it rarely involves cervical laceration or disrupts the pregnancy. Allow the woman to listen to fetal heart sounds so she can be assured the fetus is well. Assess for beginning signs of labor, especially premature rupture of membranes from trauma.

Be certain that during emergency care, a woman is offered privacy. A large number of people may want to ask her questions, such as police officers or detectives, her family, a rape trauma team, and an examining physician or nurse practitioner. Detailing the experience is good, but lack of privacy during a perineal examination or during a time with her important support person demonstrates little more concern for her self-esteem than her attacker provided her. Many women are uncomfortable with a male physician examining them following rape. It is helpful if a female nurse remains with the woman during this time, although a male nurse can be equally supportive. It is not the male-female contrast that a woman is seeking as much as an aggression-caring contrast, which both male physicians and male nurses can provide. The box above summarizes common tests and procedures for emergency care of rape victims.

Follow-Up Phase

A woman should be given the number of a counseling service before she leaves the emergency department. As genital bruising may not be apparent for 24 hours, she may be asked to return for a reexamination for purposes of documentation. Syphilis will not be apparent for up to 6 weeks in serum, so the woman should return for a repeat VDRL or this should be repeated at a routine prenatal visit at that time. Be certain that the woman has a support person to accompany her home and she is aware that if her distress becomes acute she can return as needed to the health care facility for additional care or counseling. Tell her about Women Against Rape (WAR), an organization active in many communities that has established follow-up counseling programs for rape victims.

Nurses working in emergency rooms may be asked to testify in court about a woman's appearance following an assault, although the documentation in the chart is generally all that is necessary. Many women do not press charges against their assailant because they were too frightened

Table 41-4 Measures to Prevent Rape

Your Home	Your Car	Your Work	Personal Actions
1. Do not advertise that you live alone by a single name on mailbox or telephone listing.	1. Avoid dark, isolated parking places; park near a building or parking attendant.	1. Do not enter an elevator with a stranger.	1. Do not wear chains around your neck that could be used to strangle you.
2. Ask for identification from metermen or repairmen before admitting them to a home.	2. Lock your car when sitting waiting in it or when you leave it parked.	2. Lock your office door and do not admit people you do not know when working alone at night.	2. Learn self-defense; scratch attacker's skin to get a skin and blood specimen under fingernails.
3. Insist on adequate lighting for hallways in an apartment building; install adequate light around your own home.	3. Look in the back seat before unlocking and entering your car.	3. Ask for security protection to walk out to your car.	3. Be aware that an attacker could take any weapon away and use it on you; use caution carrying a gun or Mace.
4. Have your house key in your hand when you approach your door; do not stand fumbling for it by the doorway.	4. Have your car key ready when you approach your car; do not stand fumbling for it.	4. Going to and from work, walk in the middle of the street rather than next to shrubs or dark buildings.	4. Use fighting or struggling cautiously to prevent further harm than the rape itself. Actions such as kicking or gouging eyes may not be effective and may cause more violence.
5. Keep your door and windows locked when you are alone at home.			5. If an attack occurs, observe the attacker's appearance, words he says, and any identifying mark such as a birthmark, scar, tattoo, or manner of speech. These will help you identify the man later.
			6. Fight back in court by pressing charges to make rape a crime of extreme magnitude.
			7. Work to provide rape prevention information and a united front against rape in your community.

at the time to observe his appearance (or he was masked). They may be unable to identify him later or be afraid that, by naming him in court, they are risking more violence. Whether the woman follows through with a legal action or not is her choice, but the incidence of rape might be reduced if rapists knew heavy penalties were attached to this crime. Taking a rapist to court may be the opportunity and appropriate time for a woman to "fight back"; in the end, she may not be as helpless as she was at the time of the actual attack. Be certain that the hospital chart is well documented for use in court if she decides to prosecute.

Rape Prevention

Health education of women needs to include precautions on how to help prevent rape. Common suggested precautions for women to take are shown in Table 41-4.

Utilizing Nursing Process

Trauma can be a major stressor to a pregnancy because of the potential threat to the cardiovascular system it always imposes. In order that nursing care can be adequate with such a major threat present, it must be planned using nursing process.

Assessment

Assessment of an injured woman must be done quickly yet thoroughly and include both the woman's psychological as well as her physical status. A pregnant woman may be so concerned with her fetus's health that she does not appreciate the fact that she is injured. In another woman, answering a question about fetal movement since the accident may be the first time she realizes her fetus could have been injured (she did not appreciate that a loss of blood from her leg would affect uterine blood flow). Assessment should be done concurrently with reassurance ("your blood pressure is low but the fetal heart beat sounds good"). Use a Doppler method of assessing fetal heart tones if possible to demonstrate to the woman as well as to yourself that the fetus appears to still be well.

In an emergency situation, a woman needs her support people around her; locate them as necessary; assess their reaction to the trauma also.

Analysis

In addition to the official diagnosis of trauma, potential for, accepted by NANDA, many diagnoses applicable to the specific situation can be used. Examples are "Fluid volume deficit, actual or potential," "Gas exchange, impaired," "Mobility, impaired, physical," "Comfort, alteration in," or "Respiratory dysfunction."

Planning

Planning in an emergency always has two phases: plans for immediate care, followed by plans for continuing care after the initial emergency phase is past. A woman may be unable to plan immediately following an accident or rape because of the shock of the accident. Be careful that you do not make all plans for her ("Your best plan would be to allow the doctor to put a cast in place as he suggested."); instead give a woman the alternatives available ("As the doctor suggested, there are two separate things to do for a dislocated knee; either have a cast put in place or you could use a knee immobilizer. Let me review with you the advantages and disadvantages of each therapy."). Allowing the woman to choose between alternatives helps her to select the kind of care she desires and will have to live with.

Most women who sustain a form of trauma during pregnancy need time after the emergency care is complete to talk about the event. They may feel very guilty that they were not more careful. In some instances, a woman's support person caused the injury (driving carelessly) so she feels a mixture of anger at his carelessness yet relief that he was not injured.

A couple can work through these emotions satisfactorily if the pregnancy progresses normally after this point and the fetus was not injured. If the fetus was injured or the pregnancy disrupted, it may be a happening too great for the relationship to survive. An important point for a couple to discuss is that many accidents are no one's fault, but the outcome of an action that at the time seemed sensible but now, with hindsight, seems foolish. It may help for a woman to try to put herself in her support person's place and ask if realistically she would have acted any differently under the same circumstances.

Implementation

Implementation in emergency situations must be done quickly yet always with the proviso that the woman's primary health condition is pregnancy. Be certain to guard against supine hypotension syndrome or abdominal pressure during procedures; remind personnel that a woman is pregnant before X-rays are taken.

Evaluation

Evaluation of a woman with trauma must include both the woman and the fetus; it is not complete until the pregnancy has ended and a well fetus is delivered. At birth the mother has reason to be especially worried about the baby's health. Be certain she spends enough time with the child to be able to see that he or she is well and healthy. She needs you to assess the infant with her in terms of ability to follow a finger and respond to the sound of your voice. Some fetal outcomes will not be optimal, however, so evaluation will then include the ability of the woman to adjust to care of an infant who is ill from the effect of trauma.

Nursing Care Planning

Mary Kraft is a 23-year-old woman in her thirty-sixth week of pregnancy you meet in an emergency room because she fell from a ladder at work (arranging books on shelves at the library).

Assessment

Patient reports she stepped down quickly from a 4-foot stepladder approx. 1 hour ago and her right knee "collapsed" underneath her. She fell to the floor, striking her right elbow and right "hip." Pain in her right knee was acute; kneecap of right knee was displaced to posterior surface of knee. A fellow worker realigned the kneecap for her manually.

Patient has not stepped on knee again following accident; knee is swollen; tender to palpation. Ecchymotic area forming on inferior portion. Patient unable to bend it voluntarily because of pain. Delayed coming to emergency room for fear an X-ray would be taken. Husband who accompanies her insisted on her coming because she is afraid to step on knee again.

Fetal heart rate: 120; no vaginal bleeding or discharge. No abdominal contractions by objective or subjective assessment. Ecchymotic area forming over right iliac crest.

Analysis

Mobility, impairment of, related to trauma.

Locus of Decision Making. Shared.

Goal. Patient's pregnancy to continue to term despite orthopedic trauma.

Criteria. No signs of premature labor occur related to accident.

Nursing Orders

1. Explain safety of X-ray for knee during pregnancy as long as lead shield to abdomen is provided.
2. Accompany to X-ray department to ensure pregnancy precautions are taken.
3. Discuss modifications that patient will have to make at work with leg immobilizer in place (no ladders, foot elevated for 1 hour 2× daily).
4. Plan ways that patient can maintain a level of exercise for remainder of pregnancy despite immobilization of leg.
5. Review signs of premature labor before discharge.
6. Review necessity of telephoning private M.D. if beginning signs of labor should occur.
7. Reassure that injury apparently caused no pregnancy interruption or harm to fetus.

Questions for Review

Multiple Choice

1. Mrs. Smith is a 26-year-old woman in her thirty-second week of pregnancy you see in an emergency room. She fell at the site of a new home she and her husband are having built and received a puncture wound of her leg from a nail. She states she has not had a tetanus immunization since infancy. Which question below in history taking would be most important to ask?

   a. What action has she taken since the accident?
   b. Is she certain she did not have a tetanus booster at age 12?
   c. How could she be so careless during pregnancy?
   d. Is she aware of the potential danger of puncture wounds?

2. Which action below would you expect to include in her plan of care?

   a. administration of tetanus immune globulin STAT
   b. analysis of her serum for tetanus antibodies
   c. inducing labor to avoid tetanus in the fetus
   d. administration of tetanus prophylaxis after delivery in 6 weeks

3. To evaluate the extent of blood loss from the wound, which physiologic change of pregnancy would be important to remember?

   a. Venous pressure in legs is increased during pregnancy.
   b. Increased vasoconstriction during pregnancy limits blood loss.

c. All antihypertensive drugs are unsafe during pregnancy.

d. Uterine pressure causes decreased venous pressure in lower extremities.

4. Mrs. Smith has contusions of her upper thighs from her fall. She is prescribed acetaminophen (Tylenol) and codeine for pain. She telephones after she returns home to tell you she is voiding "red-stained" urine. Your best response to her would be that

a. "codeine salts" are causing this reaction.

b. she is beginning labor and should telephone her obstetrician.

c. she will need to return to the emergency room for evaluation.

d. as long as she feels the fetus move, this is not important.

5. Mrs. Berman is a woman who is 36 weeks pregnant. She is brought to the emergency room because she was trapped in her upstairs apartment by a fire downstairs. Her breathing stops as she is moved to the examining table. Your best action at this point would be to

a. assess fetal heart tones to see they are above 100 per minute.

b. *not* exert pressure on her sternum to prevent uterine rupture.

c. administer four quick breaths of air to her by resuscitation bag.

d. press the uterine fundus to the side to allow diaphragm descent.

6. A physician arrives and works with you to perform cardiopulmonary resuscitation. The breathing/cardiac massage rate in a pregnant woman should be one breath for every

a. two heart compressions.

b. five heart compressions.

c. ten heart compressions.

d. fifteen heart compressions.

7. Following resuscitation, Mrs. Berman remains on oxygen administration. She says she is most grateful that she did not suffer burns in the fire. You would continue to assess fetal health carefully based on the knowledge that

a. fetal edema may occur from compression during resuscitation.

b. fetal heart tones may decrease with continued oxygen administration.

c. pulmonary edema may occur following smoke inhalation.

d. thermal burns may have occurred in the fetus within the mother.

8. Mrs. Henry is a 23-year-old woman, 20 weeks pregnant, who has a stab wound in her abdomen. She states she was slicing tomatoes with a butcher knife and the knife slipped; it entered her abdomen the full length of the blade. Ecchymotic areas on her arms she states are from the ambulance attendants handling her roughly. What could you conclude from this history?

a. She used poor judgment in using such a large knife.

b. She may be having hallucinations from hypertension of pregnancy.

c. The extent of her injury is out of proportion to the history.

d. She is angry at the ambulance attendants for bringing her there.

9. Mrs. Henry is diagnosed as being a "battered wife." Of the statements below, what is a frequent reason that a woman does not leave a man who is abusing her in this way?

a. She has too little self-esteem to believe she can live alone.

b. She is a "do-gooder" who believes she can change him.

c. She enjoys being abused and may even provoke attacks.

d. She hates men and feels this man is demeaning himself.

10. Eyonne Horner is a young pregnant woman who comes to the emergency room following rape. Which statement below by you is apt to be most therapeutic for her?

a. Try not to think about what happened.

b. Rape is a terrible crime.

c. Tell me about what happened.

d. Before the baby is born, you will need counseling.

11. Mrs. Horner's husband acts very coldly toward her in the emergency room. Which of the following is probably the basis for this behavior?

a. They do not have a close relationship.

b. He feels her injuries are minor so she does not need support.

c. Many support people need counseling as much as rape victims.

d. He is uncomfortable in an emergency room setting.

12. In the light of her pregnancy, which would be the most important assessment question to ask Mrs. Horner?

a. "Do you have any perineal bleeding?"

b. "Do you think rape is a sexual or violent crime?"

c. "Was any item of torn clothing expensive?"

d. "How could you have prevented this?"

Discussion

1. Because of the physiologic changes of pregnancy, pregnant women need special precautions following trauma. What are these precautions?

2. Following trauma, pregnant women are afraid for both their own safety and fetal safety. What are ways to assure a woman that the fetal health is not compromised?

3. Rape counseling is an important role in women's health care. What are important immediate steps to take for the woman who has been raped when she is first seen in the emergency department?

Suggested Readings

Aiken, M. M. (1983). When an employee tells you that she has been raped. *Occupational Health Nursing, 31,* 42.

Burgess, A. W., & Holmstrom, L. L. (1979). *Rape, Crisis and Recovery.* Bowie, MD: Robert J. Brady.

Cliff, K. (1982). Accidents—where the nurse fits in. *Nursing Mirror, 154,* 21.

Colver, A., et al. (1983). Home is where the danger lies . . . health education. *Health and Social Services Journal, 93,* 662.

Danis, S. M. (1981). An overview . . . aftercare instructions for patients discharged from the emergency department. *Journal of Emergency Nursing, 7,* 31.

Edlich, R. F., et al. (1981). Prehospital management of the trauma patient. *Emergency Medical Technician Journal, 5,* 186.

Ensinger, C. (1981). Don't panic . . . rapid emergency assessment guide. *R.N., 44,* 32.

Greany, G. D. (1984). Is she a battered woman? *American Journal of Nursing, 84,* 725.

Hass, J. (1980). Emergency management of soft tissue injuries. *Journal of Emergency Nursing, 6,* 20.

Haycock, C. E. (1982). Injury during pregnancy: Saving both mother and fetus. *Consultant, 22,* 269.

Heller, P. H. (1981). Bleeding disorders in the emergency room. *Emergency Medicine, 13,* 100.

Kess, R. C. (1980). Victims of rape—how can we help? *Journal of Emergency Nursing, 6,* 21.

Lauck, B. W., et al. (1983). Why patients follow through on referrals from the emergency room and why they don't. *Nursing Research, 32,* 186.

Lenehan, G. P., et al. (1983). Rape victim protocol and chart for use in the emergency department. *Journal of Emergency Nursing, 9,* 83.

McKennan, S., et al. (1983). First aid and home safety training in the community. *Occupational Health, 35,* 122.

Michaels, D., et al. (1982). Occupational safety: Why do accidents happen? *Occupational Health Nursing, 30,* 12.

Moynihan, B. A., et al. (1981). The role of the nurse in the care of the sexual assault victim. *Nursing Clinics of North America, 16,* 95.

Oliver, M., et al. (1983). Caring for the rape victim. *Emergency, 15,* 30.

Patterson, R. M., et al. (1983). Trauma during pregnancy. *Hospital Medicine, 19,* 33.

Penticuff, J. H. (1982). Psychologic implications in high-risk pregnancy. *Nursing Clinics of North America, 17,* 69.

Posey, V. M., et al. (1984). A timesaving flow sheet for life threatening emergencies. *Nursing 84, 14,* 76.

Ruch, L. O., et al. (1983). Sexual assault trauma and trauma change. *Women and Health, 8,* 5.

Smith, B. K., et al. (1983). Burns and pregnancy. *Clinics in Perinatology, 10,* 383.

Stafford, P. L. (1981). Protection of the pregnant woman in the emergency department. *Journal of Emergency Nursing, 7,* 97.

Van Oss, S. (1982). Emergency burn care: Those crucial first minutes. *R.N., 45,* 44.

Wein, S. G. (1981). The unspoken needs of families during high-risk pregnancies. *American Journal of Nursing, 81,* 2047.

Wetzel, S. K. (1982). Are we ignoring the needs of the woman with a spontaneous abortion? *M.C.N., 7,* 258.

Wright, B. (1981). The victims of violence. *Nursing Times, 77,* 2045.

42

Cesarean Birth

OBJECTIVES

Following mastery of the contents of this chapter, you should be able to

1. Describe the indications for cesarean birth.
2. Assess a woman in terms of surgical risk in order to plan nursing care preoperatively, intraoperatively, and postoperatively.
3. Describe preoperative teaching measures for cesarean birth.
4. Describe the experience a woman can expect to encounter in surgery.
5. Describe common preoperative and postoperative care measures.
6. Describe the importance of a support person being present for cesarean birth.
7. Analyze common complications of cesarean birth and measures used to prevent them.
8. Synthesize knowledge of cesarean birth with nursing process to achieve quality maternal-newborn nursing care.

CESAREAN BIRTH or birth through an abdominal incision into the uterus is one of the oldest types of surgical procedures known. Between 15 and 20 percent of deliveries in the United States today are accomplished by this method (Pritchard, 1980). Although cesarean birth has the potential to be more hazardous than vaginal birth for both mother and baby and has a maternal mortality twice that of vaginal birth (Amirikia, 1981), in comparison to other surgical procedures it is one of the safest types of surgery performed.

Originally (documented in early Roman literature), a cesarean procedure was done only postmortem in an attempt to deliver a viable fetus. When it was begun to be used on live women (during the nineteenth century), the operation always involved cesarean hysterectomy, or removal of the uterus with the child. In 1879, Max Sanger developed the classic cesarean birth, in which the uterus is saved. Today, cesarean birth is used most often as a prophylactic measure in order to alleviate problems from such conditions as those shown in Table 42-1. Contraindications to cesarean birth are fetal age under 28 weeks, immaturity by L/S ratio (the infant would not survive postuterine life), or a documented dead fetus (labor can be induced to avoid a surgical procedure).

The word *cesarean* is derived from the Latin *cedare* which means "to cut." At one time Julius Caesar was popularly believed to have been delivered by a cesarean birth (as a way to account for the name). Many people spell cesarean with an additional *a* as if it did come from Caesar (and the English spell it this way). There is little chance that Caesar could have actually been delivered by this method, however: With no antibiotics or sterile surgical technique, it seems unlikely that his mother, who is known to have been alive in his adult years, would have survived such a procedure.

Incidence of Cesarean Birth

A major concern in maternal-nursing nursing today is the increasing number of cesarean births being performed annually. As shown in Table 42-2, in 1965, only 4.5 percent of women had their infants delivered by cesarean birth; in 1981, 17.9 percent of women in all ages delivered by this method. In women over 35 years of age, 24.4 percent—almost one-fourth of all women this age—

Table 42-1 Conditions for Which Cesarean Birth Is Commonly Performed

Maternal Factors	Placental Factors	Fetal Factors
Cephalopelvic disproportion	Placenta previa	Transverse fetal lie
Severe hypertension of pregnancy	Premature separation of the placenta	Breech presentation
Genital herpes		Fetal distress
Previous cesarean birth		Large fetus
Handicapping conditions that prevent pushing to accomplish the pelvic division of labor		

Table 42-2 Cesarean Birth Rates for Nonfederal Short-Stay Hospitals by Age of Mother, United States, 1965–1981 (Rate per 100 Deliveries)

Year	All Ages	Under 20 Years	20–24 Years	25–29 Years	30–34 Years	Over 35 Years
1965	4.5	3.1	3.5	4.3	6.4	7.9
1970	5.5	3.9	4.9	5.9	7.5	8.3
1975	10.4	8.4	9.0	11.1	13.6	15.0
1979	16.4	13.7	15.6	16.4	19.5	21.1
1980	16.5	14.5	15.8	16.7	18.0	20.6
1981	17.9	13.2	16.0	19.4	21.3	24.4

Source: Placek, P. J., Taffel, S., & Moien, M. (1983). Cesarean section delivery rates: United States, 1981. *American Journal of Public Health, 73,* 861.

had a surgical delivery. This rate is rising partially due to justifiable reasons: the increasing safety of cesarean birth and the use of fetal monitors that discover when an infant in utero is not responding well to labor. It also may be unfortunately rising in response to fear of a malpractice suit: What if a fetus is allowed to deliver vaginally and is discovered to have suffered anoxia? Although the rising incidence of cesarean birth is a concern, the potential of the procedure for reducing the incidence of mental retardation or neurologic deformity in children must be weighed in the balance. Surely, no mother would feel that having a child by a vaginal birth is more important than having a healthy baby.

Types of Cesarean Birth

Two categories of women undergo cesarean birth—those who have known since the beginning of pregnancy that they would deliver by this method (elective or planned cesarean birth) and those who suddenly are told during labor they need a cesarean birth performed to make the birth safe for the fetus and/or themselves (emergency cesarean birth). In the first instance there is time for a thorough preparation for the experience. In the second instance preparation must be done much more rapidly, but with the same concern toward fully informing a woman and her support person about what circumstances have caused a problem and what will happen from that point on.

Cesarean birth should be mentioned in all preparation-for-childbirth classes so if it becomes

necessary at birth, a woman has at least heard that such a procedure may be used. Preparation-for-childbirth classes especially for women who know they will have a cesarean birth are available in many communities.

Elective Cesarean Birth

In the 1950s, cesarean birth became a status symbol of the very beautiful and very wealthy as Hollywood actresses asked to have cesarean birth to save themselves the strain of labor and in some instances to conveniently schedule the birth between movie contracts. The average woman came to think of cesarean birth as an easy method of painless childbirth. As the risk of cesarean birth is higher than of vaginal birth, this impression put both mothers and fetuses at greater risk than necessary. Scheduling cesarean births this freely, also, unfortunately, resulted in immature births. Today, the practice of truly elective cesarean birth is interesting only from an historical standpoint. In a reliable health care facility, a physical indication for a cesarean birth must be documented before one can be performed.

It is still common for women to ask if they can have an elective cesarean birth, as did their mother. If they have been raised thinking labor is so terrible their mother chose to avoid it by an elective surgical procedure, they may need a great deal of support during labor until they realize that contractions are bearable.

The need for cesarean birth can be anticipated in women who have a small pelvic inlet, who are apt to develop cephalopelvic disproportion, or who had previous cesarean birth with a classical uterine incision (with newer surgical techniques, "once a cesarean, always a cesarean" does not apply anymore).

Emergency Cesarean Birth

An emergency cesarean birth carries with it the risk of all emergency surgery: a woman who is not a prime candidate for anesthesia and a woman psychologically unprepared for the experience. In addition, the woman may have a fluid and electrolyte imbalance and be both physically and emotionally exhausted from a long labor.

Systemic Effects of Surgery

Any surgical procedure is a stress because even though it appears to involve only a small body area, surgery has systemic or holistic effects.

The Stress Response

Whenever a body is subjected to stress, either physical or psychosocial, it responds with measures to preserve the function of major body systems. Because a surgical experience involves both physical and psychosocial aspects, it readily activates this fight-or-flight mechanism.

A stress response results in release of epinephrine and norepinephrine from the adrenal gland medulla. Epinephrine causes an increased heart rate, bronchial dilatation, and elevation of blood glucose level. Norepinephrine leads to peripheral vasoconstriction, which forces a good blood supply to the central circulation and an increased blood pressure.

These normally positive responses (the person is tensed or ready for action with good heart and lung function and glucose for energy) may contradict anesthetic action (which is aimed at minimizing body activity). In the pregnant woman it may minimize blood supply to her lower extremities. Already prone to thrombophlebitis from stasis of blood flow, she faces a compounded or increased risk of this problem. Combined with interferences to major body systems, these effects can add to the risk of surgery.

Interference with Body Defenses

The skin serves as the primary line of defense against bacterial invasion. When skin is incised for a surgical procedure, this important line of defense is automatically lost. Strict adherence to aseptic technique during surgery and the days following the procedure must be maintained to compensate for the impaired defense. If cesarean birth is performed after membranes have been ruptured for hours, a woman is at double risk for infection.

Interference with Circulatory Function

The cutting of blood vessels is required in even the simplest of surgical procedures. Although incised vessels are immediately clamped and ligated during surgery, there will always be some blood loss. Extensive blood loss leads to hypovolemia and lowered blood pressure. This could lead to ineffective perfusion of all body tissues if the problem is not quickly recognized and corrected. The amount of blood lost in cesarean birth is comparatively high because pelvic vessels are congested with blood due to the amount needed to supply the placenta. Blood loss occurs freely due to this vessel pressure.

Interference with Body Organ Function

When any body organ is handled, cut, or repaired in surgery, it may respond with a temporary disruption in function. Pressure of edema or inflammation as fluid moves into the injured area will further impair function of the organ involved and that of surrounding organs. If blood vessels are compressed due to the edema, distant organs may be deprived of blood flow and thus function will be reduced in these organs. Following a surgical procedure, therefore, broad observation of not only the one organ involved but of total body function is necessary to assess the total degree of disruption present.

During cesarean birth, the uterus is obviously handled; it may not contract as well afterward. This can lead to postpartum hemorrhage. In order to reach the uterus, the bladder must be displaced anteriorly; enough pressure is exerted on intestine to cause a paralytic ileus or halting of intestine function. Following cesarean birth, therefore, not only uterine function, but bladder, intestine, and lower circulatory function must be carefully assessed.

Interference with Self-Image or Self-Esteem

Surgery always leaves an incisional scar that will be noticeable to some extent afterward. If the resulting scar from cesarean birth (a horizontal one across the lower abdomen or a vertical midline one) is very noticeable, its appearance may cause a woman to feel self-conscious. She may feel a loss of self-esteem if she feels she is marked as less competent than women who are able to give vaginal birth.

Admission of the Woman Anticipating a Cesarean Birth

The woman admitted to the hospital for an anticipated cesarean birth may be more worried about the procedure than a woman who is told during labor that an emergency procedure must be done: She has had a length of time to worry. She needs specific time put aside following routine admission procedures to talk about her fears; she needs encouragement to do as much as possible for herself preoperatively in order to feel in control of her body and reduce her fear.

A woman who is told during labor that an emergency procedure is necessary may be actually relieved that surgery has been suggested. She was having a great deal of pain with an abnormal labor and wants it alleviated. Although steps of preoperative care are done more quickly in such an emergency, the steps are still necessary in order to ensure safe care.

The woman needs to be oriented to her hospital room and her vital signs taken and recorded (an increased temperature may suggest an upper respiratory infection, which might make a general anesthetic inappropriate). An irregular heartbeat may suggest a heart evaluation before surgery, and carefully measuring weight and height will influence the amount and type of preoperative medication or anesthesia used.

A woman undergoing surgery cannot begin to relax as long as her support person is nervous and worried. Make a point of including this person in all explanations and admission routines.

The Preoperative Interview

Both a woman's physician and anesthesiologist will interview her preoperatively to obtain a medical history and make an assessment and decision for safe anesthetic use. In addition, a nursing interview should be held. Specific information you need to obtain is the woman's knowledge about (a) the procedure she will undergo (Does she view this as a major, serious but not major, or minor surgery? What will be done in surgery?), (b) the length of the hospitalization following surgery, (c) any postsurgical equipment that will be used, such as an indwelling catheter and intravenous fluid, and (d) her expectations for her infant. Cesarean birth is not without risk to the fetus. When a fetus is pushed through the birth canal, pressure on the chest appears to rid the lungs of lung fluid, making respirations more likely to be adequate at birth than if the fetus is not subjected to this pressure. About 5 percent of all infants delivered by cesarean birth have some degree of respiratory difficulty for a day or two after birth.

Determine as well whether a woman has had any past surgery, has any secondary illnesses, is currently taking any medication, or has any allergies to foods or drugs to help establish surgical risk.

Establishing Operative Risk

For any surgery to be performed safely, a person must be in the best possible physical and psychological state before surgery. People who are in less than optimal physical or psychological health are at risk for a complicated surgical outcome unless the risk factor is identified and special pre-cautions to lessen it are undertaken. Areas that create surgical risk include nutritional status, age, general health, fluid balance, psychological condition, extent of surgery, and facilities available.

Poor Nutritional Status

A woman who is obese or who has a protein or vitamin deficiency is at risk for surgery because such a condition interferes with wound healing. Tissue that contains an abundance of fatty cells is difficult to suture, so the incision may take longer to heal; an increased healing period invites infection and rupture of the incision (dehiscence). Such a person's heart may also have an increased workload; the physiologic shock of surgery may place too much stress on an already overworked organ. In addition, an obese person often has more difficulty moving and turning postoperatively than a person of normal weight and thus has an increased risk for developing respiratory or circulatory complications (pneumonia or thrombophlebitis).

Protein and vitamins C and D are necessary for new cell formation at the incision site. Vitamin K is necessary for blood clotting to effect hemostasis following surgery. Fortunately, pregnant women are a category of people who have, as a rule, been eating very sensibly for the last 9 months so they are nutritionally prepared for surgery. A woman who is iron deficient because she neglected to take an iron supplement or who has a multiple gestation that is requiring a great deal of iron may be high-risk in this category.

Age

Age affects surgical risk since it influences circulatory and renal function. Fortunately, again, most pregnant women fall within the young adult age group, and thus are excellent candidates for surgery. The young adolescent or the woman over 35 falls into age categories of slightly higher risk.

General Health

A person who has a secondary illness (cardiac disease, diabetes mellitus, anemia, kidney or liver disease) is at surgical risk depending on the extent of the primary disease. The pathology present from the secondary illness may not allow her to make the physiologic adjustments demanded by surgery. Women with secondary illness may also have accompanying nutritional or electrolyte imbalance related to their other illness.

Be certain to ask in your preoperative nursing history if a person has any secondary illnesses. Prior to surgery, people are under stress, which

Table 42-3 Drugs That May Result in Complications of Surgery

Type of Drug	Action
Antibiotics	Specific antibiotics may predispose to renal insufficiency or increase neuromuscular blockage.
Anticoagulants	May cause hemorrhage due to lack of hemostasis during surgery.
Anticonvulsants	May increase liver action and metabolism of anesthetic agent.
Antihypertensives	May result in hypotension following anesthesia.
Corticosteroids	May block body's response to shock and lead to lack of adrenal function.
Insulin	May lead to hypoglycemia during NPO period or hyperglycemia if a dextrose solution is administered.
Tranquilizers	May cause hypotension following anesthesia.

may limit their reasoning ability. It is not unusual for a person admitted for any type of surgery to state they are generally healthy and then minutes later ask if they will be receiving insulin on the day of surgery because they are diabetic.

Ask if the woman is currently taking any medication since some drugs will increase surgical risk by interfering with either the effect of the anesthetic or healing of tissue. A number of drugs that pregnant women might be taking and their potential complications are shown in Table 42-3.

Fluid and Electrolyte Balance

A woman who enters surgery with a lower-than-normal blood volume will feel the effect of normal blood loss more than a person with a normal blood volume. Hypovolemia may result from recent vomiting, diarrhea, or a poor fluid intake prior to surgery. The woman who began labor and now has been told she is to have a cesarean birth may easily fall into this category of a person with a poor fluid and electrolyte balance. She may have had nothing to eat or drink for almost 24 hours. To prevent fluid and electrolyte imbalances, many women are begun on intravenous fluid therapy preoperatively. Correction is continued postoperatively.

Psychological Condition

A woman who is frightened when anesthesia is administered is at greater risk for cardiac arrest than a person who is calm and relaxed. Elicit from women preoperatively their expectations of the procedure and their general attitudes toward it. Women who are extremely worried need a more detailed explanation of the procedure before they can enter surgery without intense fear.

In many instances, just helping a woman acknowledge that fear of surgery is normal is beneficial. The procedure does not become any less awesome but the woman can view herself as "normal" and competent because she feels this way.

Extent or Type of Surgery

Obviously a major surgical procedure carries more risk than a minor one; one performed under general anesthesia carries more risk than one performed under local anesthesia. Assuming there is no fetal distress, a cesarean birth carries more risk for a woman and fetus than vaginal birth. One reason is that a pregnant woman is very high-risk for aspiration during general anesthesia from the upward pressure on the stomach from the uterus.

Care Facilities and Staff Available

The risk of any surgery performed in a well-equipped operating suite with accompanying optimal preoperative and postoperative facilities and personnel available is less than that of surgery performed, for example, in battlefield conditions. Cesarean birth performed under emergency conditions must have special precautions taken to be certain that care is as safe as possible.

Preoperative Diagnostic Procedures

In order for surgery to be performed safely, adequate circulatory and renal function must be documented preoperatively. X-rays and an electrocardiogram (ECG) may also be ordered.

Urinalysis

All surgical patients have a urinalysis done prior to surgery to estimate metabolic and kidney function. It would be dangerous, for example, for a person with undetected diabetes to undergo surgery without extra precautions: Intravenous fluid containing glucose could be extremely dangerous to them during this time. This determination is especially important in pregnant women as gestational diabetes is a complication of pregnancy. It is equally dangerous for a person with poor kidney function to face the degree of physiologic shock of surgery unless special precautions are taken. Poor kidney function is revealed by the presence of protein, glucose, or abnormal specific gravity in urine.

Blood Studies

A number of blood studies are ordered prior to surgery in order to ensure adequate blood and kidney function. With poor kidney function, urea, the breakdown product of protein metabolism, accumulates in the bloodstream since it cannot be filtered and removed. Blood urea nitrogen (BUN) is a test to confirm or rule out poor kidney function.

A complete blood count (CBC) is routinely ordered before surgery to document that a woman has adequate blood components so that subsequent blood loss will not reduce her functioning blood components below a safe level. If a woman has a low hemoglobin level preoperatively, a blood loss that appears normal could be fatal. A woman with inadequate blood platelets will not have normal blood clotting ability and so blood loss will be appreciably more than usual. A person with an inadequate leukocyte count will have a difficult time resisting infection following surgery. A woman during pregnancy and particularly one who was in prolonged labor will have an elevated leukocyte count (up to 20,000 mm^3), so this finding is not necessarily as helpful with the pregnant woman as with others.

Cesarean birth involves a greater loss of blood than many other types of operation because of the blood loss that occurs with the placental removal. In order to safeguard the mother's circulatory competency, two units of blood are routinely typed and cross-matched.

Serum Electrolytes and pH

Women who have been NPO for labor may experience serious electrolyte imbalance. A woman who has been worried about surgery and has not been eating as well as usual may have a minimal electrolyte deficiency. In many hospitals serum electrolytes are ordered as a single battery of tests (an SMA-12 or SMA-18).

Chest X-ray

During surgery a person's respiratory level is decreased as respirations become slow and shallow due to anesthesia. A person with respiratory disease may suffer from anoxia at this time unless special precautions to institute good oxygen exchange are initiated. A health agency policy may require that chest X-rays be taken before surgery on all adults. Unless a woman has obvious lung pathology, this policy should not apply to pregnant women. A woman with accompanying lung disease can have a chest X-ray taken safely during pregnancy as long as she is provided a lead shield for her abdomen during the exposure. Be certain a nurse accompanies the woman to X-ray and that the shield is placed.

X-ray Pelvimetry

Because a frequent cause of cesarean birth is a cephalopelvic disproportion, many women will have an X-ray of their pelvis performed preparatory to surgery. You can assure them that this degree of X-ray exposure will not be harmful to their fetus and it is necessary to establish whether a cesarean birth will be necessary or not. Accompany the woman to the X-ray department and remain with her except for the time the X-ray is taken. One film is taken standing; a second is taken with her in a supine or lateral position. Help position her and make her comfortable on the hard X-ray table. If she is in active labor, take the fetal heart rate (FHR) every 15 minutes. Encourage the X-ray technician to speed the procedure as much as possible so she is away from the full emergency protection of the labor suite no longer than necessary.

Electrocardiogram

An electrocardiogram (ECG) may be ordered for all adults prior to surgery to detect any cardiac abnormalities; the effect of blood loss and physiologic shock could cause cardiac arrhythmia in a person with cardiac disease unless special precautions are undertaken. Because the heart is displaced by pregnancy, ECG recordings tend to be distorted during pregnancy, however, so this procedure is omitted in a woman admitted for a cesarean birth unless she has known heart disease.

Preoperative Teaching

Fear of the unknown is one of the hardest fears to conquer. Preoperative teaching is aimed at acquainting a woman with the procedure and any special equipment used so that she will be as informed about the surgery as possible. Activities to help maintain respiratory and skeletal function in order to prevent postsurgical complications from stasis of body secretions or circulation are also taught.

Be certain that you determine how much the woman already knows about surgery before you begin. The woman who had a cesarean birth for her first child and now is being admitted for a second procedure may have a better idea of what the surgery entails than you. Even so, she will undoubtedly appreciate having her memory refreshed and recall confirmed. Answer all specific questions and fill in gaps in knowledge.

Be certain that all information you offer is accurate as nothing is as confusing to women as being told something will not occur and then discovering it has (they worry a complication has occurred). Be certain not to use hospital jargon such as NPO. People under stress do not process information well. They cannot process at all what they do not understand. Have a woman demonstrate activities such as coughing and deep breathing to show you that she can do them well.

Use visual aids as necessary. Many women do not even know about body organs such as a ureter or diaphragm. Draw pictures or show illustrations of anatomy if necessary to help them understand exactly what the procedure involves. Do not leave textbooks that detail cesarean procedure techniques with a woman, however, because such books also detail cesarean procedure complications. A woman has to know possible complications of the procedure in order to sign an informed consent, but she may be frightened by reading about complications complete with colored illustrations.

Be certain to include the woman's support person in teaching. A support person's fears can reinfect the woman and render your preoperative teaching support ineffective.

Teaching Points

Explain preoperative measures that will be necessary such as use of an enema, surgical skin preparation, eating nothing to the time of surgery, premedication (if this will be used), and method of transport to surgery. Review the necessity for an indwelling catheter, intravenous fluid, and early ambulation afterward.

It is important that a woman understand the reason for the surgery. If she feels the operation is necessary because something is wrong with her child, she may later view the child as less than perfect. If the cesarean birth is being done because of a maternal problem (contracted pelvis, placenta previa, uterine dysfunction—the usual reasons), it is important in terms of a postpartal mother-child relationship that she understands the problem is hers, not the child's. "Your pelvis is too small to let the baby pass" may not seem very

different from "The baby's head is too big to pass through your pelvis," but the differing effects such statements have on a woman's postpartal attitude warrant such careful distinctions in wording.

Teaching to Prevent Complications

Women who cooperate to maintain good respiratory and circulatory function postoperatively will probably have a postoperative course freer of respiratory and circulatory complications than people who do not.

These preventive measures are best taught during the preoperative period, when a woman is free of incisional pain and can concentrate on your teaching. Such teaching also gives the woman a positive outlook about surgery (a sense of control as well as reassurance that, since you are taking time to teach her postoperative measures, you think she is going to recover safely from surgery). Her obstetrician and anesthesiologist both say to her, "I'll see you in the operating room in a few minutes." By teaching postoperative care, you are saying, "I'll see you and your new child safely back here in your room afterward," a message with comforting subliminal reassurance for a woman who has serious doubts that there will be an afterward—or at least one with a newborn.

Deep Breathing

Periodic deep breathing exercises fully aerate the lungs and help to prevent stasis of lung mucus (stasis tends to occur because the lungs are relatively quiet during surgery; mucus forms from irritation by anesthetic gases). Since stasis always has the potential for causing infection, it must be prevented as far as possible.

The woman will need to take five to ten deep breaths every hour for at least forty-eight hours following surgery. She does this simply by inhaling as deeply as possible, holding her breath for a second or two, and then exhaling as deeply as possible. She must be certain that she inhales and exhales fully or she will feel light-headed from hypoventilation.

Coughing

Coughing every hour helps move lung mucus and, again, prevent stasis. Teach a woman to inhale deeply, exhale deeply, inhale again, and attempt to cough. The irritation of air passing over bronchial mucus often spontaneously initiates the coughing reflex, which is why breathing in and out first is important. Coughing will hurt postoperatively because of her abdominal inci-

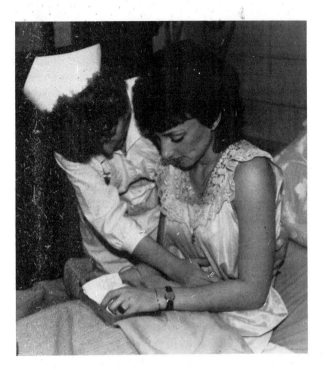

Figure 42-1 *Coughing and deep breathing exercises prevent lung stasis. Here a new mother allows a nurse to splint her operative incision for comfort.*

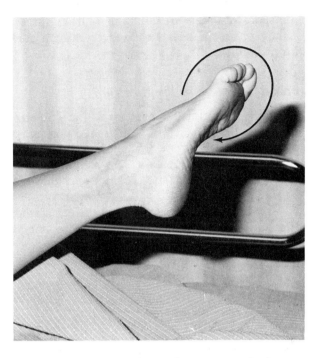

Figure 42-2 *Leg exercises, such as moving the leg in a circle, help to lessen the possibility of thrombophlebitis postoperatively.*

sion. Teach her to splint her incision area (or do this for her) with her interlaced hands or a pillow to reduce this "tugging" or "cutting" feeling (Figure 42-1).

Be certain that a woman not only clears her throat but uses her chest muscles when coughing. This action truly raises bronchial mucus. It is usually necessary to demonstrate a coughing technique to be certain a woman understands the depth of movement required.

Turning

Women do not need to practice turning side to side prior to surgery as this is very tiring for them while pregnant, but they should understand its importance (to prevent both respiratory and circulatory stasis).

Leg Exercises

Another means of preventing circulatory stasis postoperatively is ankle, knee, and hip flexion and extension about five times every hour. Lifting each foot off the mattress and moving it in a circle (circumduction) is also an effective motion to teach (Figure 42-2). Leg exercises are extremely important following cesarean birth as the edema of the low pelvic surgery compresses circulation to the lower extremities and makes the woman very prone to lower extremity circulatory stasis.

Obtaining Informed Consent

Obtaining operative consent is the surgeon's responsibility but seeing that it is obtained is everyone's responsibility. You are often asked to witness a woman's signature on such a form; be certain you agree that it was informed consent (the woman was explained the risks and benefits of the procedure in terms that she could understand) before signing as a witness.

Operative permit must be signed before the woman is given any preoperative medication since premedication makes her sleepy and her judgment questionable. Be familiar with the law regarding emancipated minors (girls under legal age who are pregnant or already the mother of a child) in your state; these individuals can sign their own surgical permission even though they are under age.

Immediate Preoperative Care Measures

If a woman is going to have a planned cesarean birth, the evening before surgery, measures toward preparing the woman' skin and gastrointestinal tract and promoting rest are performed. On the day of surgery, measures to safeguard the woman and her property, premedication, and transport to surgery are undertaken. If the surgery is done on an emergency basis, everything is done immediately prior to surgery.

Preoperative Skin Preparation

Reducing the number of bacteria on the skin prior to surgery automatically reduces the possibility of bacteria entering the incision at the time of surgery. Shaving away hair and washing the skin area over the incision site accomplishes this purpose.

The skin preparation area for a cesarean birth is shown in Figure 42-3. Traditionally skin preparations have been done the evening prior to surgery.

Figure 42-3 *Skin preparation for a cesarean birth extends from under the breasts and includes pelvic hair. (Courtesy of Johnson and Johnson, New Brunswick, N.J.)*

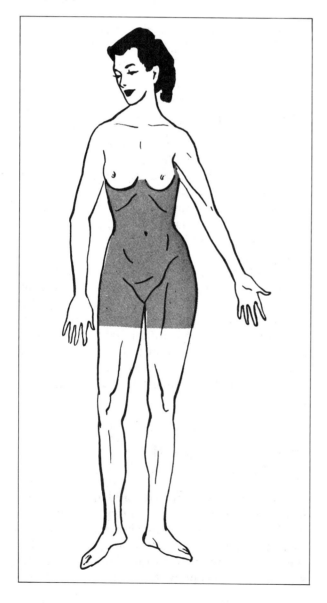

Many women scheduled for cesarean birth come to the hospital the morning of the procedure and, therefore, have this done at that time. A newer philosophy of preoperative care requires shaving to be done only minutes before a surgical procedure in order to make the best use of the antiseptic properties of the soap used and to achieve a surgical site most free of surface hair.

Review with a woman that a much wider skin area than the actual incision site is prepared to ensure a wide, safe area as free as possible from bacteria. Otherwise she may be alarmed that the procedure planned is more extensive than she had anticipated. Steps in preoperative skin preparation are shown in Procedure 42-1. To ensure that you do not cut or irritate skin, which would invite infection, use a generous supply of shaving lather or soap and a sharp razor. Use small, controlled, smooth strokes; shave with the grain of the hair shaft for comfort; provide a good light for yourself so you can accurately see that all hair has been removed from the area; use warm water to avoid causing uterine contractions.

Gastrointestinal Tract Preparation

A woman may have an enema ordered the evening before surgery in order to empty her lower bowel and allow the bowel a few day's rest during the first few days postsurgery when her abdominal muscles are nonfunctional due to the surgical incision. Be certain to administer an enema to a pregnant woman with gentle, gravity-only pressure. Provide a bedpan for her to expel the enema or remain with her and accompany her to the bathroom so she does not hurry to reach a bathroom and slip and fall.

Measures to Reduce Vomiting

An important measure to reduce vomiting in the woman following anesthetic administration is to restrict food and fluid intake for about 8 hours prior to surgery. In most instances this is achieved by preventing a woman who will have early morning surgery from eating or drinking after midnight. The woman who will have afternoon surgery may be allowed a light breakfast, then nothing more to eat until surgery.

Tell a woman the reason for this restriction; also make a point of actually removing all food and fluid from her room and cancel the diet order from the kitchen. Even though a woman knew the evening before surgery that she was not to drink anything the following morning, her level of anxiety may cause her to forget. If there is no water present on the bedside stand, she is reminded of the restriction. Mark the door and the

Procedure 42-1

Preoperative Skin Preparation

Purpose: To provide a skin area clear of body hair to reduce chance of infection at a surgical incision site.

Plan	*Principle*
1. Wash your hands; identify patient; explain procedure.	1. Prevent spread of microorganisms; ensure patient safety and cooperation
2. Assess patient status; analyze appropriateness of procedure; plan modifications as necessary.	2. Nursing care is always individualized according to patient needs.
3. Implement care by assembling supplies: safety razor with new blade, shaving soap or lather according to agency policy, waterproof pad, emesis basin, dry gauge sponges, good light source. Determine extent of skin area to be prepared.	3. A good light source is important to be certain that all hair is removed. Check with the surgeon or surgical suite if you are uncertain as to the extent of the preparation.
4. Provide privacy; fanfold covers as necessary to reveal body area to be prepared. Place waterproof pad under area to protect bed. Fill basin with warm water to use to rinse razor.	4. Protect against chilling; protect bed linen.
5. Lather area well with a moistened sponge, using predetermined soap or lather. Stretch skin taut; shave off all hair using short strokes in direction of hair shafts. Be careful not to nick skin.	5. Lather softens hair and reduces friction to skin. Any open area would be an invitation to infection.
6. Wipe away all removed hair; dry area well. Inspect it carefully for additional hair. Evaluate effectiveness, efficiency, cost, comfort, and safety of procedure. Plan health teaching as necessary; for example, inform the patient of the importance of remaining NPO prior to surgery.	6. Health teaching is an independent nursing action always included as part of care.
7. Leave patient comfortable. Chart area prepared and time of preparation.	7. Document patient status and nursing care.

bed area with an NPO sign and flag the nursing care plan so someone else does not offer fluid.

If a woman should accidentally eat or drink on the morning of surgery, the anesthesiologist and surgeon must be informed. A pregnant woman is at high risk for aspiration with a general anesthesia even with a supposedly empty stomach. If she did eat or drink, she is no longer a safe candidate for general anesthesia.

Some women who know they will deliver by cesarean birth are allowed to begin labor spontaneously (assuring their obstetrician that the pregnancy's natural time has ended or the chances that the fetus is mature are very high). Be certain such a woman has clear instructions that once she begins labor she should not eat or drink anything so her stomach is as empty as possible for surgery.

Promoting Sleep

A woman needs a good night's sleep the evening before surgery in order that her resources are at their optimum the morning of surgery. Most nonpregnant patients receive a sleeping medication the evening before surgery. Pregnant women do not ordinarily receive this aid because no unnecessary medication is given during pregnancy.

In order to help a woman sleep, allow some time for conversation before bedtime with the woman and her support person. Find out how she feels about her surgery in the morning and whether she has any special fears. Ask if she wants to talk with a clergyman before surgery. This type of surgery, like all surgery, has the potential of being detrimental to her hopes and expectations. Many women envision that, because their body is unable to deliver a child vaginally, they are somehow also inferior in terms of sheltering a fetus for 9 months. Pointing out that the two processes are not related helps her to feel confident about the outcome and be emotionally prepared for the morning's surgery.

Be certain the woman knows she can breast-feed if she wishes. There may be temporary difficulty with breast-feeding because her oral intake will be restricted for the first 2 days, and she will be uncomfortable because of incisional pain, but cesarean birth by itself is not a contraindication to breast-feeding.

Immediate Surgery Precautions

Immediate precautions before surgery include safeguarding the woman and her property.

Vital Signs

Assess vital signs (temperature, pulse, respiratory rate, blood pressure, and fetal heart rate) the morning of surgery; take particular care in temperature recording since an elevated temperature on the morning of surgery may be an indication of an upper respiratory tract infection. This will probably not cause the surgery to be postponed as cesarean birth is a timed event, but it might change the anesthetic used. Make certain that an increase in temperature or any variation in vital signs (including fetal heart rate) is reported promptly to the surgeon so that a new patient assessment can be made.

Morning Care

The woman needs to wash or shower on the morning of surgery to reduce the overall level of skin bacteria. Provide her with a clean hospital gown. Examine the skin preparation area to be certain that it is cleanly shaven. If the hair on a woman's head is long, encourage her to braid it or put it in a ponytail to more easily fit under the surgical cap she will wear in the operating room (hair contained by a cap is less likely to spread microorganisms than hair uncontained). Suggest she not use bobbypins in her hair since these can lacerate skin unnoticed while she is unconscious

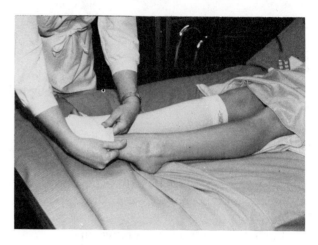

Figure 42-4 *When applying antiembolitic stockings, be certain they are applied with the woman in a supine position so veins are not full at the time of application.*

from anesthesia (even women who will be having surgery under a spinal anesthesia need to have these precautions followed; if a complication should occur during surgery, she may be instantly anesthetized while the emergency is managed).

Check the woman's nailbeds for nailpolish; if present, ask her to remove it from at least two fingers on each hand to allow nailbed color to be assessed during anesthesia administration. Caution the woman not to apply cosmetics on the morning of surgery since extreme paleness or cyanosis from lack of oxygen could be hidden by blush or lipstick. Have her remove all jewelry except a wedding ring (which could get lost during the time she is unconscious). Use adhesive tape to secure a loose wedding ring in place.

Some women may have elastic stockings ordered to be applied prior to surgery to ensure venous return during surgery. Apply these using gentle technique with the woman in a supine position (Figure 42-4).

Have her brush her teeth and rinse her mouth well so that her oral cavity is as clean as possible. If an endotracheal tube is passed through the mouth to the trachea, this precaution will lessen the number of organisms carried with it. Respiratory tract infection is a threat following surgery from stasis of secretions; do not introduce additional bacteria this way.

Check your hospital policy about dentures. When intubation tubes were fairly nonpliable, all dentures had to be removed prior to surgery (to many a person's embarrassment); now that newer anesthesia techniques are available, full dentures are sometimes left in place. Partial dentures and retainers (plastic appliances for additional correction following oral braces that many adolescents

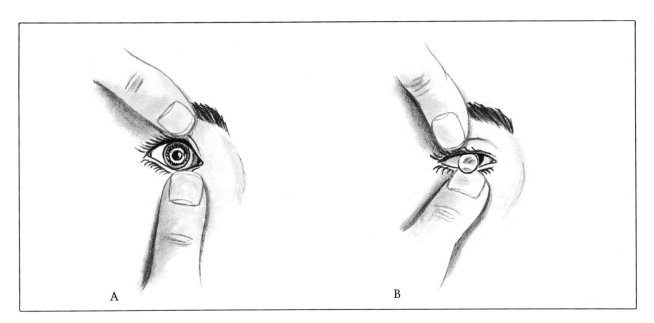

Figure 42-5 *Removal of contact lenses. A. Separate upper and lower eyelid. B. Exert pressure on lower eyelid and move upward to tip out lens.*

wear), which fit more loosely, generally need to be removed. Note on the chart if dentures are in place.

Ask a woman to remove contact lenses. In the eyes of an unconscious person, they might cause undetected corneal abrasions. If an intravenous fluid line has already been started in one of her hands before you think of this, you may have to remove the contacts for her. Procedure for removing contact lenses is shown in Figure 42-5. If a woman is to have a spinal anesthesia and needs eye glasses to be able to see her newborn clearly, be sure she wears these into the operating room.

Identification Insurance

Examine the woman's identification band to be certain that it is correct and secure. If the band is missing, secure a new one from the admissions department. Once unconscious, the woman has no way of identifying herself or guarding her well-being; that responsibility is yours.

Establishing Baseline Intake and Output Determinations

In order that the anterior bladder is reduced in size and away from the surgical field, a woman needs to have an indwelling catheter inserted prior to surgery. Bladder catheterization is reviewed in Procedure 29-2. Catheterizing a pregnant woman is difficult because of the pressure the fetal head puts on the urethra; the vulva may be swollen and distorted in shape from vulvar

varicosities or edema. Be certain to use a good light so the perineum is clearly revealed; take special care during the time of skin preparation to locate the urinary meatus. Use a gentle touch to avoid or minimize pain. Be certain following insertion of the catheter that urine is draining as fetal pressure may reduce the flow of urine considerably due to urethral pressure. Be certain during the transport time to surgery that the drainage bag is kept below the level of the woman's bladder so there is no backflow and introduction of microorganisms into the bladder.

If catheterization cannot be done easily prior to surgery, do not traumatize the urethra by repeated attempts. Catheterization can be done in the delivery room after the anesthetic for surgery is given. If there is a delay between the catheter insertion time and surgery, mark the drainage bag just prior to surgery with the amount in the bag or empty it so that presurgery urine can be differentiated from postsurgery urine. One of the gravest dangers of any surgery procedure is that kidneys may fail under the physiologic stress of surgery or lack of blood flow because of decreased blood pressure. All gynecologic surgery puts urethral flow at risk because of edema in the surgery area. Separating presurgical and postsurgical urine drainage allows you to accurately assess drainage following the procedure.

Maintaining Hydration

Most women have an intravenous fluid line begun prior to surgery in order that they are fully

Table 42-4 Preoperative Check List

Action	Completed
Patient concerns	
Skin preparation:	_____
Identification in place:	_____
Temperature, pulse, respiration _____	_____
Blood pressure _____	_____
Height _____ Weight _____	_____
Voided _____ Time _____ Amount _____	_____
NPO after _____	_____
Hospital gown	_____
Hairpins removed	_____
Nailpolish removed	_____
Jewelry removed	_____
Preoperative medication: _____	_____
Dentures removed _____ In place _____	_____
Contact lenses removed _____	_____
Prosthetic devices removed _____	_____
Chart concerns	
Addressograph plate attached	_____
Operative permit obtained	_____
Urinalysis	_____
Hematocrit	_____
Electrocardiogram	_____
Chest X-ray	_____
Blood order of _____	_____
Signature _____ R.N.	

hydrated and do not experience hypotension from the blood loss at delivery. Be certain this line is started in the woman's nondominant hand so that she will be able to hold her newborn immediately after surgery without interference.

Completing Patient Chart and Presurgery Checklist

You must finish your recording of nursing care up to the time the woman leaves the nursing care unit or labor room for the delivery room. Many hospitals use an additional preoperative checklist, such as that shown in Table 42-4, to remind you of all necessary measures to be taken. Checking and signing such a form indicates that you have completed the specific measures.

Preoperative Medication

A minimum of preoperative medication is used with a woman having a cesarean birth so that the fetal blood supply is not compromised due to hypotension and the newborn is wide awake at birth

and initiates respirations spontaneously. If a general anesthesia will be given, an atropine-like drug may be ordered to dry respiratory secretions and help prevent aspiration during anesthesia administration. Without sedative medication, a nurse has more responsibility to serve as a calming (sedative) influence.

If a general anesthesia will be given, antacid administration (30 ml Maalox) is usually ordered in order to neutralize the acid of the stomach secretions. In that way, if aspiration should occur (pregnant women are very high-risk because of the upward pressure on the stomach by the uterus and prolonged stomach emptying time if the woman is in labor) the secretions that enter the lungs will not be acid. Many women who are going to deliver by spinal anesthesia should also be given an antacid: They will be lying on their backs during the procedure and esophageal reflux is great during this time. Introduce this administration with a statement showing you realize the administration contradicts what you said previously. Otherwise it seems strange that you said for her to eat nothing and now you are telling her to drink something.

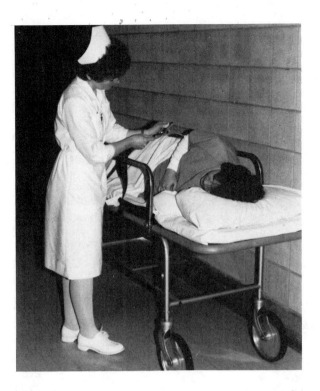

Figure 42-6 *To transport a pregnant woman, urge her to lie on her side to avoid supine hypotension syndrome.*

Transport to Surgery

To transfer a woman to surgery, she may either be taken in her bed or helped to move to a stretcher. Be certain that you hold the stretcher tightly against the side of the bed for safe transfer to the stretcher (she will be awkward in her movements due to pregnancy). Urge her to turn on her side to prevent supine hypotension syndrome. Use optimal safety features for transport (siderails up and cart straps secure) (Figure 42-6).

Cover her with a blanket as well as a sheet to prevent her from feeling chilled in the cool surgical suite. Her chart with the surgical checklist must accompany her. Check that her identification is secure one final time before she leaves the patient unit. Because you are standing in for her preoperative sedative, you should accompany her to the surgery suite.

Role of the Support Person

A support person should be as welcome to view a cesarean birth as a vaginal birth. This principle holds true even if the procedure is done under a general anesthesia (it is not just her baby; it is his also). You will need to help the support person scrub and gown and mask; he may be asked to remain outside until the anesthesia is given and the cover drapes and anesthesia screen are in place. Fortunately, this arrangement coincides well with the time it takes for a support person to wash and gown.

The Surgery Experience

Observing or participating in a cesarean birth offers you information about specific areas to explain to women before surgery and complications to watch for after surgery. In order to observe or participate, you must be free of infection, particularly cutaneous or respiratory infection. Before entering the operating room suite you must change to scrub clothing (cap, mask, gown, and shoe covers) and thoroughly wash your hands and arms. This procedure automatically reduces the level of bacteria in the operating room. Be certain that your surgical cap completely covers your hair; the mask should cover both your mouth and nose and should be pulled snugly against the edges of your face by ties at the back. In order that shoes do not conduct sparks, which could cause explosion of some anesthetic gases, they should be rubber-soled; covering them with a cloth or paper impregnated with a conduction strip further reduces their capacity to conduct electricity. If no flammable gases are being used, such a precaution may not be necessary.

In a typical operating room the operating table is located in the center under a large overhead light (Figure 42-7). The light is attached to a track so that it can be tilted or focused by means of an overhead handle. The table is built so that it can be tilted in many directions, allowing patients to be positioned with good support for different surgical approaches. Anesthesiology equipment (the portable machine for administering inhalation anesthesia with accompanying oxygen and suction equipment) is placed at the head of the table, and an instrument table at the foot. Additional equipment includes a small Mayo (over-the-table) stand for instruments that will be used first during surgery, a table for surgeon's gloves and gown, and kickbuckets (stainless steel buckets on wheels) for disposal of used sponges. The walls may be lined with cupboards with sterile supplies, additional intravenous equipment, and an X-ray viewer.

You need to assist a woman to move from the transport stretcher to the operating room table and remain with her while anesthesia is administered. If there will be a delay until the anesthesia is administered, encourage the woman to remain on her side. If she will have a spinal or epidural

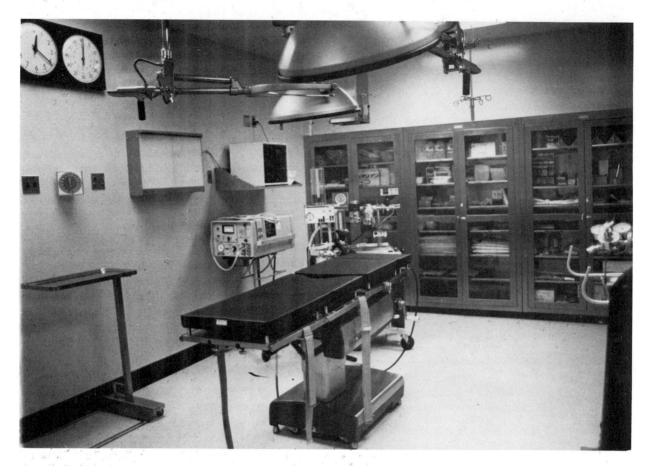

Figure 42-7 *Describe an operating room to a woman to reduce her apprehension; its sparse furnishings do not create a "friendly" place for her baby to be born. (Courtesy of the Department of Medical Photography, Children's Hospital, Buffalo, N.Y.)*

anesthetic, the anesthesiologist will administer it with the woman on her side. The anesthesiologist may ask you to help the woman curve her back so that vertebrae separate and the spinal needle will enter easily. If the woman is having uterine contractions, it is difficult for her to remain in this position. Talking to her while gently restraining her is most effective in helping her maintain this position.

If a general anesthetic will be given, the anesthesiologist will announce to the room at large that he or she is beginning anesthetic induction. The woman will then be asked to count backward from ten or some other such task while the anesthesiologist adds an intravenous medication to the woman's fluid line or administers anesthesia by a mask. As soon as the woman is unconscious, anesthesia is continued by placing an endotracheal tube through the woman's mouth into her proximal trachea. Because of the danger of aspiration from the pressure on the stomach by the full uterus, cricoid pressure must be exerted while the woman is intubated. The period during which a woman passes down through levels of anesthesia is one of the most dangerous times for her. Stand still and do not talk until the anesthesiologist announces that induction is complete: A loud noise at this point, such as dropping an instrument or talking suddenly, could be so shocking to the woman's nervous system that she might convulse or have a laryngospasm that compromises her airway. Stages of general anesthesia are summarized in Table 42-5.

Following anesthetic administration, the woman is tipped into a slight Trendelenburg's position to move other abdominal contents up away from the surgical field, and a metal screen is placed at the patient's shoulder level and covered with a sterile drape to block the flow of bacteria from the woman's respiratory tract to the incision site. The incision area on her abdomen is then scrubbed and appropriate drapes are placed around the area of incision so that only a small area of skin is left exposed. To shorten the time span of general anesthesia, this may be done before the anesthesia is administered.

Table 42-5 Stages of Anesthesia

Stage	Time Interval	Importance
I	From beginning of induction to loss of consciousness	Patient feels drowsy and then will remember nothing following this point.
II	From loss of consciousness to relaxation phase	Patient becomes excited; breathing is irregular; thrashing with extremities may occur. Stress at this point, e.g., from a loud noise or a change in position, might cause her to convulse.
III	From relaxation phase to loss of reflexes (surgery stage)	No auditory sensation present; breathing slow and regular; reflexes absent.
IV	Anesthesia stage is too deep and respiratory failure or cardiac arrest occur	No respiratory or cardiac action is present.

Role of the Support Person

For the average support person, watching a cesarean birth is the first surgery he has ever witnessed. He is often too overwhelmed by the procedure (and interested technically in it) to be of optimum support. He needs to remain behind the anesthesia screen with his partner and needs you near him to support him as well as the woman he may no longer be able to help. A support person may become worried that a great deal of manipulation and cutting appears to happen before the uterus itself is cut (assuming fetal distress is not extreme). You can review with him preoperatively that operating incisions are made with careful precautions against excess bleeding.

Just the skin layer is cut first and the capillaries there that begin to bleed are clamped with hemostats (small metal clamps); then sutures (strings of absorbable gut) are placed over each hemostat and tied to ligate (tie off) bleeding. The hemostats are then removed and returned to the Mayo stand. The layer of fat beneath the skin is cut and bleeders there are clamped and ligated in the same way. The incision is extended deeper and deeper through fascia and muscle using the same cut, clamp, ligate technique (in an emergency, hemostats are left in place and all ligating is done following the birth of the child).

Once the surgical incision is complete, retractors (long, metal curved instruments) are slipped into the incision. Gentle traction on the handles by an assistant keeps the incision spread apart and allows for good visualization of the uterus and the internal incision. Sterile towels may be placed in the incision to separate the uterus from other organs. The uterus itself is then cut and the child's head may be delivered manually or by the application of forceps (Figure 42-8). The mouth and nose of the baby are suctioned by a bulb syringe as in a vaginal delivery before the remainder of the child is delivered.

An oxytocin injection is given intramuscularly or intravenously to the mother as the child is delivered to increase uterine contraction and achieve hemostasis. Following full delivery, the uterus is pulled forward onto the abdomen and covered with moist gauze; the internal cavity of the uterus is inspected and the membranes and placenta are manually removed. Both uterine and skin incisions are then closed (remind parents that the process is long so they do not become concerned that something is wrong).

Observing the amount of abdominal manipulation that is accomplished during surgery allows you to appreciate how tender an abdomen will be afterward and how a postsurgery patient often has an overall "aching" feeling. It is not unusual for a fetus to be knicked by the scalpel blade because the uterine incision is made over the head area. You can assure parents this is a superficial scratch.

Types of Cesarean Incisions

The type of cesarean incision made depends on the presentation of the fetus and the speed with which the procedure will be performed.

Classical Cesarean Incision

In a classical cesarean incision, the incision is made vertically through both the abdominal skin and the uterus. The advantage of a classical incision is that it is high on the uterus so it can be used with a placental previa to avoid cutting the placenta; its disadvantage is that the incision leaves a wide skin scar and is through the active contractile portion of the uterus. The woman will be unable to have a subsequent vaginal delivery. A vertical uterine incision of this type may also be made through a horizontal skin incision described below.

Low Cervical Incision

A low cervical incision is made horizontally across the abdomen just over the symphysis pubis

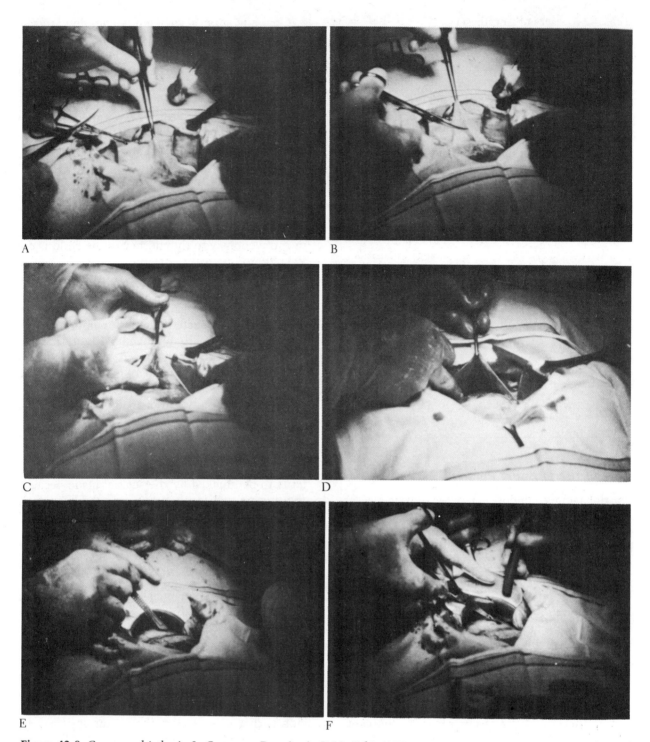

A

B

C

D

E

F

Figure 42-8 *Cesarean birth. A–L. Courtesy, Dansforth, D.N. (Ed.). (1971).* Text-book of obstetrics and gynecology *(2nd ed.). New York: Harper & Row.*

and also horizontally across the uterus just over the cervix (Figure 42-9). The most common type of cesarean incision made today, the incision is through the nonactive portion of the uterus. With this type of incision, the woman may labor and deliver vaginally with a subsequent pregnancy; this incision also has technical advantages of causing less blood loss, easier suturing, decreased postpartal uterine infections, and decreased incidence of postpartal gastrointestinal complications. For a woman it has the advantage of leaving only a small scar just over her pubic hair (often called a "bikini" incision because it will fit under a small bathing suit).

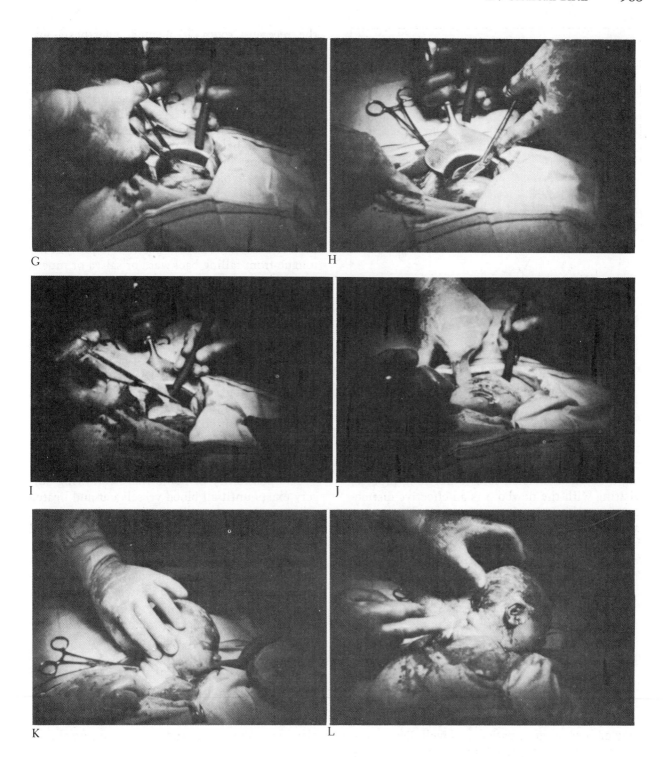

G

H

I

J

K

L

Anesthesia

Anesthesia for cesarean birth may be general, spinal, or epidural (in a true emergency, a classical incision can be performed under only local anesthesia). The use of a regional form such as epidural or spinal anesthetic is ideal because it allows a mother to be awake during surgery and simulates the excitement of a vaginal delivery for her. Having the mother awake puts added responsibility on you to be certain that she is well prepared and supported during the procedure. (All these types of anesthesia administration are discussed in Chapter 25.)

Introduction of the Newborn

Once he or she is breathing spontaneously, the newborn should be shown to the parents. The

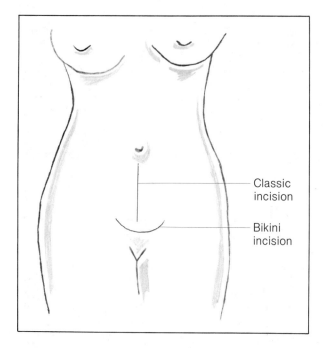

Figure 42-9 *Types of cesarean incisions.*

mother may not be able to hold the baby as she has intravenous fluid infusing into one hand and the surgical drapes are still in place. If the father chooses, he may hold his new child. Because closing a surgical incision is a rather long process, visiting with the newborn is an effective distraction in making the time of incision closure pass quickly; it also lays a firm foundation for bonding. Breast-feeding is usually delayed until a woman has been moved to a recovery room. Breast-feeding initiates uterine contraction and may interfere with suture placement, and it may be awkward with the anesthesia screen in place.

The Postpartal Phase

Women who deliver by cesarean birth have an additional care concern in the postpartal period because not only are they postpartal patients, they are postsurgical patients as well. Due to the strain of the unexpected procedure, they may have increased difficulty with bonding with their new infant. As with all postpartal women, this phase for a woman who delivers by cesarean birth can be divided into an immediate recovery period (the so-called *fourth stage of labor*) and an extended postpartal period.

The Immediate Postpartal Period

A woman is moved from the operating room table to a stretcher or recovery room bed for transfer to the recovery room. If a spinal anesthesia was used, be certain that she does not raise her head while assisting in the transfer in order to minimize the possibility of a postpartal spinal headache. You may need to use a roller for safe transfer. Remember that her legs are fully anesthetized so she cannot help you by moving them. The woman who had a general anesthesia will still be unconscious and must be rolled gently to the stretcher to avoid strain on the new suture line.

Positioning

If a general anesthesia was used, a woman will need to be kept in a Sims' position to prevent her tongue from falling backward or saliva or mucus from obstructing her airway until she is fully conscious again. Place a pillow securely behind her back to keep her in this position. Be certain the plastic airway placed by the anesthesiologist after removal of the endotracheal tube remains in place until the woman is conscious. A woman who delivered with a spinal anesthesia may lie in any position as long as she remains flat in bed. A woman who had epidural anesthesia is not limited to any position.

Hemorrhage

The possibility of hemorrhage following surgery exists until all blood vessels cut and ligated during surgery have thrombosed, sclerosed, and permanently sealed closed. The postpartal woman is at double threat: She may hemorrhage vaginally from an uncontracted uterus as well as internally from missed "bleeders," or blood vessels that were not securely ligated. The danger of hemorrhage is most acute in her first hour following surgery, and it remains an acute problem for the first 24 hours. Hemorrhage is revealed by a falling blood pressure, increased pulse, and rapid respirations. The woman may be restless and feel thirsty. Table 42-6 lists common vital sign "end points" to use as points of danger.

To detect the earliest signs of hemorrhage, blood pressure, pulse, and respiration rate should

Table 42-6 Postoperative Vital Sign Parameters

Fall in systolic blood pressure more than 20 mm Hg
Systolic blood pressure under 80 mm Hg
Blood pressure dropping 5 to 10 mm Hg over several readings
Pulse over 110 beats per minute or under 60 beats per minute

be taken every 15 minutes for the first hour after surgery, every 30 minutes for the next 2 hours, every hour for the next 4 hours, or as specifically ordered. The dressing over the surgical incision should be checked for blood staining, the perineal pad observed for lochia flow, and the fundal height palpated every time the vital signs are taken.

Lochial discharge may be decreased in amount in a woman following a cesarean birth, but it will always be present. A woman who had a spinal anesthesia will not experience pain on uterine palpation until the anesthesia has worn off (2 to 4 hours). A woman who delivered by a general anesthesia will feel pain with this procedure as soon as she is awake, however. Always palpate gently to avoid causing pain; be certain that you palpate thoroughly enough, however, to be certain that you know the uterine consistency. You are not doing a woman a favor by being gentle if postpartal hemorrhage is the result.

Be certain to turn the woman to look under her body for bleeding. Blood oozing from a surgical wound or vaginally can pool under a sedated patient unless you conscientiously check for it. At the same time you assess for uterine firmness, assess the remainder of the abdomen for softness; a hard, "guarded" abdomen is one of the first signs of peritonitis (peritoneal infection), a complication that may occur with any abdominal surgical procedure.

A woman's physician must be notified of changes in vital signs that might indicate hemorrhage in order that action can be taken to infuse additional fluid to replace loss or to return the patient to surgery. Remember that a minimal but continued change in vital signs (pulse steadily increasing, blood pressure steadily declining) is as ominous a sign of hemorrhage as a sudden alteration in these measurements.

Respiratory Obstruction

Women who had an intubation tube in place during surgery may have edema of the upper airway, which can compromise air exchange. An anesthetized woman does not have an operational gag reflex and so saliva from her mouth may pool in the back of her throat and flow into her trachea, causing obstruction or aspiration. The best way to prevent these complications is to be certain that the woman is positioned on her side in a Sims' position. Signs of obstruction are noisy respirations, restlessness, cyanosis, and increasing respiratory rate. Her throat often feels sore from intubation. As soon as she is able to take oral fluid, a few sips of cool liquid generally relieves these symptoms.

Extended Postpartal Period

The average woman who has delivered her child by cesarean birth will remain in the hospital for 5 to 7 days. During this period a number of interventions will promote healing and prevent postoperative complications as well as establish bonding with the new child.

Promotion of Adequate Respiratory Exchange

If a woman delivered under a general anesthesia, she breathed very shallowly during surgery. Following a return to consciousness, she may not breathe as deeply as normally in order to limit pain at the surgical site. This limited motion, along with increased respiratory secretions due to the irritation of the anesthetic and an endotracheal tube, may lead to an extreme pooling of fluid in the respiratory tract.

To prevent poor air exchange, begin encouraging deep breaths and coughing every hour. Be certain that the woman turns or is turned to a different position every 2 hours to further reduce fluid pooling.

Some women may have intermittent positive pressure breathing (IPPB) treatments ordered to encourage deep breathing. Give good instructions for the use of such equipment. Be certain the woman seals her lips around the mouthpiece; as she starts to breathe in, the machine "assists" her by pushing air into her lungs. This feeling may seem smothering at first. At the instant that a woman starts to breathe out, however, the machine clicks off. She controls the machine, rather than the other way around. A woman needs to be reassured of her control before beginning IPPB treatments (Figure 42-10).

Another device used postoperatively to encourage deep breathing is the incentive spirometer, a system of plastic tubes with colored Ping-Pong balls suspended in each tube, or a similar tube system that flashes lights. With most incentive spirometers, a woman places her lips around the mouthpiece and inhales. The harder she inhales, the further the Ping-Pong ball rises in the hollow tube (or the more the light flashes). Such an exerciser is fun to operate and gives a patient a sense of reward for the effort (Figure 42-11). Women need a good explanation before using an incentive spirometer since their initial impression is usually that the balls rise or lights flash as a result of blowing *into* the instrument. Its purpose is to cause a person to take deep breaths and fully aerate lung spaces, however, so most models are triggered by *inhalation*, not exhalation. Young adolescents may increase lung aeration best by being asked to blow up a balloon.

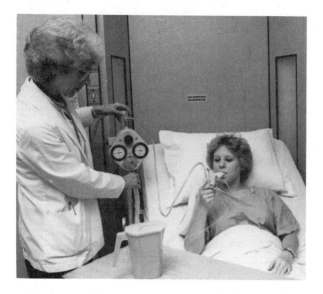

Figure 42-10 *IPPB treatments may be ordered post-operatively to prevent pulmonary stasis. (Courtesy of the Department of Medical Photography, Millard Fil-more Hospital, Buffalo, N.Y.)*

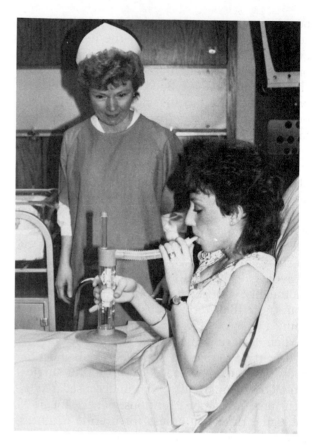

Figure 42-11 *Incentive spirometry is a helpful technique for encouraging deep breathing postoperatively.*

Promotion of Adequate Nutrition and Fluid Balance

To prevent aspiration, no woman should be given anything by mouth until she is wide awake from a general anesthesia used for surgery. Even if a spinal anesthesia was used, the handling of the intestine during surgery causes it to halt or slow in function; it takes about 24 to 48 hours before full function is restored.

A woman will be maintained on intravenous fluid until her gastrointestinal system has recovered from the handling of surgery to function competently again. Help a woman learn to "guard" the intravenous fluid line as she needs a high proportion of fluid during this time (she is a postpartal mother and all postpartal women are diuresing as a physiologic postpartal change). At the same time, do not urge such caution that a woman is afraid to turn or ambulate (she is high-risk for thrombophlebitis and must turn, do leg exercises, and ambulate early).

Assess a woman's abdomen once a nursing shift for bowel sounds (small "pinging" sounds heard on auscultation at a rate of 5 to 10 per minute that denote air and fluid are moving through intestines; ask if she is passing flatus as another indication that intestinal function is again active). As soon as these signs are present, the surgeon will order the intravenous fluid to be discontinued and sips of fluid to be begun (begin the fluid and wait an hour before removing the IV to be certain that the woman will not have nausea and need the intravenous fluid restarted).

Introduce fluid slowly (ice chips for the first hour, then sips of clear fluid such as ginger ale, Jell-O, tea, popsicles), and gradually return the woman to a soft and then regular diet as ordered. Some women assume that they will not be allowed to eat for a long time following surgery and are surprised (and suspicious) to learn that they can have something to drink only hours later. Other women try to drink and eat too soon and become nauseated. Help a woman to find the level that is right for her by introducing ice chips first. Because ice chips dissolve slowly, a person receives very little fluid from them; they feel cool, however, and quickly take away the cottony feeling caused by a preoperative agent or the soreness of the endotracheal tube.

Note carefully the time of a first bowel movement following surgery. If a woman has no bowel movement by the fourth or fifth day, her physician may order a stool softener, a suppository, or enema to assist with stool evacuation. Assure a woman who is not receiving much food yet that it is normal not to have bowel movements for 3 or 4 days postoperatively, especially if she had an enema administered prior to surgery.

Adequate fluid intake is important following surgery in order to replace blood loss and to maintain blood pressure and renal function. It must be monitored carefully to prevent too fast (which could lead to cardiac overload) or too slow (which could lead to inadequate circulatory compensation) a rate. Keep an accurate intake and output record for at least the first 48 hours to ascertain an adequate fluid balance.

Many physicians order an oxytocin such as Pitocin to be added to the first one or two 1,000 ml of fluid following cesarean birth in order to ensure firm uterine contraction. If the rate of fluid administration gets behind, be careful about "catch-up" administration. An oxytocin can elevate blood pressure due to vasoconstricton or cause water intoxication from antidiuresis. It may be safer to allow the fluid to remain a space of time behind rather than risk dangerously elevating blood pressure. At the point that the oxytocin is discontinued, be aware that the woman is very prone to hemorrhage: That point is the first time the uterus is really asked to maintain contraction on its own following the surgical procedure.

Promotion of Adequate Renal Function

Because the bladder was handled and displaced during surgery, its tone may be inadequate to initiate voiding later. The indwelling catheter placed before surgery will usually be left in place for about 24 hours in order to ensure good urine drainage. Make sure that the catheter is draining (a postpartal woman has a urine output of 3,000 to 5,000 ml per 24 hours; bladder distention will occur rapidly if the catheter becomes blocked). When helping the woman to ambulate, be certain the drainage bag remains below the level of her bladder to prevent reflux of urine into her bladder (Figure 42-12).

Before the catheter is removed, the physician may order a urine culture to be certain that a urinary infection did not occur. Such cultures are usually taken from the catheter port or tubing by a sterile syringe after the port has been cleaned with an antiseptic solution (Figure 42-13). This is reviewed in Procedure 42-2.

Following removal of the catheter the average woman voids in 4 to 8 hours. You can determine whether or not a bladder is filled by pressing lightly over the symphysis pubis to assess fullness and by percussion (an empty bladder sounds dull, a full bladder resonant, an extended bladder hyperresonant) (Figures 42-14 and 42-15). If a bladder has filled to capacity but cannot empty properly, the person may have "retention with overflow," or void 30 to 60 ml of urine every 15 to

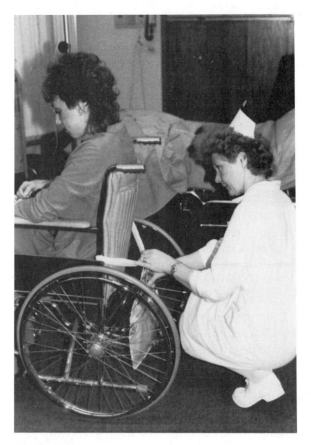

Figure 42-12 *To prevent urinary tract infection with an indwelling catheter, be certain to keep the drainage bag lower than the woman's bladder during transport.*

20 minutes. This voiding pattern is potentially dangerous because it means that the woman's bladder is held continuously under tension, which may result in permanent bladder damage if the condition is not detected. The constantly full bladder may prevent the uterus from contracting and increase postpartal hemorrhage.

Figure 42-13 *Removing a urine specimen for culture from an indwelling catheter.*

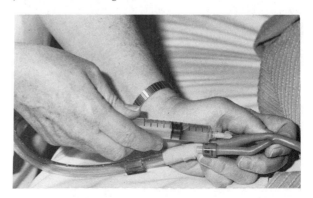

Procedure 42-2

Urine Culture from an Indwelling Urinary Catheter

Purpose: To obtain a urine specimen suitable for culture without contamination from tubing.

Plan	*Principle*
1. Wash your hands, identify patient; explain procedure.	1. Prevent spread of microorganisms; ensure patient safety and cooperation.
2. Assess patient condition; analyze appropriateness of procedure; plan modifications as necessary.	2. Nursing care is always individualized according to patient needs.
3. Implement procedure by assembling equipment: a sterile 5 ml syringe, a 25 gauge needle, alcohol swab, sterile urine container. Provide privacy.	3. Using a small needle prevents leakage of urine from puncture site following procedure.
4. Clamp urine tubing for 10–15 minutes.	4. Allow urine to collect in drainage tubing.
5. If no port is present, clean tubing just distal to bifurcation of balloon tubing; insert needle of syringe into tubing and withdraw urine with syringe. If a port is present, swab port and enter port.	5. Using an insertion site distal to bifurcation of balloon tubing prevents you from puncturing lumen of balloon tubing. Cleaning tubing prevents introduction of surface microorganisms.
6. Transfer urine obtained to sterile container.	6. Prepare specimen for laboratory processing.
7. Evaluate effectiveness, cost, comfort, and safety of procedure. Plan health teaching as needed, such as necessity to maintain a high fluid intake for urinary function.	7. Health teaching is an independent nursing action always included as a part of care.
8. Record on chart that specimen was obtained and when and where it was sent.	8. Document nursing care and patient status.

Measures to help women void include administration of an analgesic (helps to relax abdominal musculature), provision of privacy for voiding, helping the woman to walk to the bathroom, pouring warm water over her vulva (measure the amount of water used so that it can be differentiated from urine), and running water from a tap within hearing distance.

Voiding following surgery not only proves renal competency but also circulatory competency since the kidneys must have adequate blood flow through them to function.

Figure 42-14 *Assessing bladder filling by palpation.*

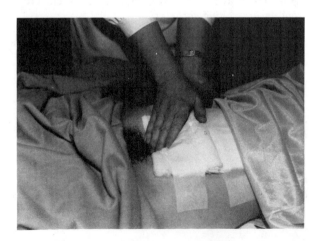

Figure 42-15 *Assessing bladder filling by percussion.*

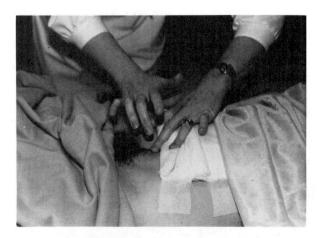

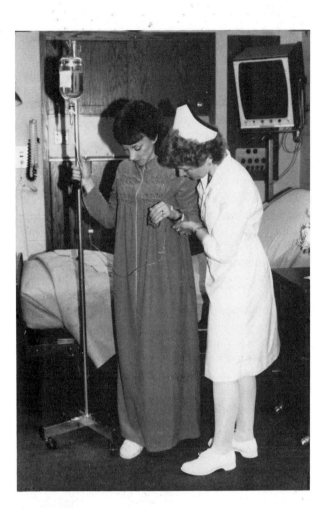

Figure 42-16 *Help a women to ambulate following a cesarean birth to prevent thrombophlebitis from venous stasis.*

Promotion of Adequate Circulation

Many women will have thromboembolic stockings, which promote venous return, ordered for them after surgery. Be certain these are placed with the woman supine in order to minimize venous distention at the time of application. Turning in bed, doing leg exercises such as flexing and extending her knee, and early ambulation are her best safeguards against circulatory problems (Figure 42-16). She may feel more comfortable turning and sitting up if she supports her abdomen with a hand. Because her abdominal muscles are so lax from having been stretched from pregnancy, abdominal contents tend to shift forward and put pressure on the suture line, causing pain and an uncomfortable feeling often described as "falling apart." If an abdominal binder is used to give abdominal support, be certain it is fastened from the top down to help the uterus contract, not from the bottom up. Always allow a woman time to sit on the edge of the bed for a few minutes before helping her to a standing position to prevent orthostatic hypotension.

Remember that when a postpartal woman moves from a supine to a standing position, lochia that has pooled in the vagina will be expelled and it will seem as if she is having a moment of excessive lochial discharge. Cautioning her in advance that this may happen reduces her surprise and worry.

Elicit a Homans' sign (pain in the calf of the leg on dorsiflexion of the foot) to detect if a blood clot is present in the calf before ambulation. It would be dangerous to ambulate anyone with this sign since a thrombus could shift and become an embolus, a potentially lethal situation.

It is difficult for women to appreciate how important it is for them to turn and ambulate as soon as possible following surgery. Still in pain and experiencing the taking-in postpartal phase (see Chapter 27), a woman would like to spend the first days following surgery just resting quietly in bed. Give analgesia as necessary in the first postoperative days so that movement and ambulation are possible.

Promotion of Psychological Well-Being

Many cesarean births are scheduled so quickly a woman does not have much time preoperatively to think how she will feel after surgery; most women are surprised to realize how overall well they do feel but also how quickly they become fatigued and how painful a simple surgical incision can be. Being assured that they are recovering well and that surgery is a physiologic shock to their system helps them to accept temporary discomforts.

Some women feel acute depression following cesarean birth because they were denied the experience of birth they had anticipated. If they received a general anesthesic they may feel a sense of loss that they did not hear the baby's first cry or see him immediately. Reviewing with the woman that her overall goal was for a safe pregnancy outcome and healthy newborn and she has achieved this helps modify this reaction.

If a woman's baby was born with a complication or has been transferred to a distant hospital, the postpartal course is very difficult. She experiences a great sense of loss, and depression slows all body functions as well as her ability to take hold in the postpartal period.

Be certain that a woman has ample time to hold and feed her child (Figure 42-17). She has some reason to think that her baby is not quite perfect—after all, delivery was not perfect—and thus she needs additional time to inspect and grow comfortable with her newborn. If she did not see the birth because a general anesthetic was used, review the identification system used with the baby with her; be certain that she sees the

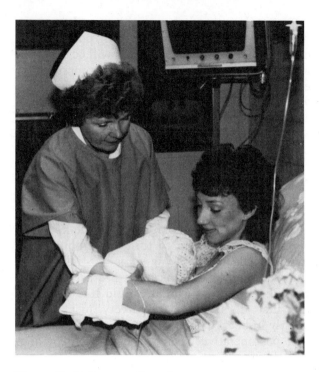

Figure 42-17 *Do not allow the equipment a postpartal woman has, such as intravenous therapy, to interfere with her interaction with her newborn, in order to promote bonding.*

baby as soon as she is awake from the anesthesia. (See the Nursing Research Highlight on page 991.)

Promotion of Activity and Rest

Early ambulation promotes both increased depth of respirations (helping to prevent respiratory complications) and circulatory function (helping to prevent venous stasis and promote wound healing). Encourage a woman to do as much for herself as she can as soon as possible following surgery in order to achieve these benefits of early movement. Many women are afraid to move following surgery, particularly from bed, because they are worried that their stitches will tear. This event is extremely unlikely, however, especially with a lower abdominal cesarean incision.

While a woman needs active movement after surgery, she also needs adequate rest. Many women proceed postsurgery to fully take care of both themselves and their infant because their excitement over their baby and their new role makes them oblivious to their symptoms of underlying fatigue. Extreme fatigue does not aid healing, however, and it makes the woman prone to postpartal infection. It will eventually interfere with bonding with the child, rather than promote it, if it does lead to postpartal complications. Help a woman plan a day that includes care of her new

child but periods of rest time for herself as well. Be certain at bedtime that she has adequate analgesic administered to allow her to be pain-free for the night. Provide a time in the middle of the morning and again in the afternoon for uninterrupted rest. Explore her plans for care at home to be certain that they seem realistic for a post-surgical-postpartal woman.

Promotion of Comfort

A major problem in a woman following cesarean birth is control of pain (although the average woman has an amazingly little amount in relationship to the extent of the incision). Pain is serious in the woman because it may lead to surgical complications such as pneumonia or thrombophlebitis because it prevents her from moving. It also may impair bonding if it hurts when she holds her child or the degree of pain is making the experience an intolerable circumstance for her.

The woman's physician generally orders a strong narcotic analgesic to be given IM for the first 24 to 48 hours after surgery, and then a less strong analgesic such as Tylenol or codeine orally. A woman who is concerned about her infant may experience more pain than the woman who is assured that her infant is doing well because a tense body posture causes pressure on sutures.

Be certain when administering analgesics following surgery that you supplement them with other comfort measures such as change of position or straightening of bed linen. Check for an uncomfortable distended abdomen, which suggests intestinal gas pain rather than incision pain. Always ask a woman what type of pain she is experiencing before administering an analgesic to be certain that she is describing incisional pain and not pain in a leg or some other body part that would suggest a complication.

Many women who are breast-feeding are reluctant to accept an analgesic especially just before breast-feeding for fear of it being passed in breast milk to the infant. It is true that most analgesics do pass in breast milk, but the infant takes such a small amount of breast milk (mainly colostrum) during this time that the amount received is negligible. Also, without the analgesic, the woman is so uncomfortable that she is unable to hold the infant and enjoy having the infant with her. Placing a pillow over her lap often deflects the weight of the infant off the suture line and lessens pain. Be certain to stay close by for the first 20 minutes after a narcotic is administered as she may notice some mild dizziness. She feels insecure holding her infant during this time and the safety of her holding the infant may be in doubt if the reaction is severe.

Nursing Research Highlight

Cesarean Birth

Maternal Attitudes in Prepared and Unprepared Cesarean Deliveries—Are They Different?

Hart (1980) found that women who were prepared for cesarean birth had a significantly greater desire for active participation in the delivery than women who were unprepared for the experience. The nurse who prepares women for the surgical procedure should be aware that many of these women desire active involvement in the procedure.

Reference

Hart, G. (1980). Maternal attitudes in prepared and unprepared cesarean deliveries. *J.O.G.N. Nursing, 9,* 243–245.

Do Women Who Have Cesarean Deliveries Have Lower Self-Esteem Than Do Women Who Deliver Vaginally?

One hundred women with cesarean deliveries and 100 women with vaginal deliveries were investigated at 1 month postpartum by Cox and Smith (1982). The group who had experienced cesarean births were found to have significantly lower levels of self-esteem. If it is assumed that increased self-esteem is desirable, then nursing interventions must focus on methods of increasing self-esteem for this group.

Reference

Cox, B., & Smith, E. (1982). The mother's self-esteem after a cesarean delivery. *M.C.N., 7,* 309–311.

Do Cesarean Birth Parents Have Special Needs?

In this study, 24 married middle-class couples, ranging in age from 22 to 42 years, were administered a questionnaire as to their needs during a cesarean birth experience. Both women and men identified extensive fatigue as a physical need especially if the woman had first been in labor. Women reported feelings of disappointment, anger, and resentment toward the experience and their delay in mothering ability; fathers noted a feeling of loss at being denied a coaching role during birth. All of these feelings were largely relieved, however, by a feeling of accomplishment over having a healthy baby.

Nursing implications would appear to be conservation of the couple's strength postpartally while focusing on the ultimate accomplishment: the healthy infant gained through this birth method.

Reference

Fawcett, J. (1981). Needs of cesarean birth parents. *J.O.G.N. Nursing, 10,* 372–376.

Transcutaneous Electrical Nerve Stimulation. Transcutaneous electrical nerve stimulation (TENS) is, as the name implies, the transmission of an electrical current across the skin. This is done by the application of electrodes to the surface of the skin. It is an effective method of controlling pain sensation because pain is carried by small affective (sensory) nerve fibers. Irritation or stimulation of the large afferent (sensory) nerve fibers blocks the ability of the cerebral cortex to interpret the incoming small afferent sensation (a gating theory). This is the same phenomenon that rubbing or scratching skin at the point of pain achieves.

For transcutaneous electrical stimulation, two electrodes are positioned, one on each side of the abdominal surgical incision, and taped in place under the surgical dressing in the operating room immediately following surgery. In the recovery room, the electrode leads are attached by cords to a monitor about the size of a transistor radio. This can be attached to the siderail of the bed or carried by the patient as she ambulates. When the unit is turned on, a mild electrical stimulation is transmitted to the skin. The woman controls the unit herself; stimulation for 30 minutes at a time as infrequently as 4 times a day is all that is necessary in most women to control pain for 24 hours.

In one research study with TENS (Vanderark & McGrath, 1975) for pain control in a group of 100 postsurgical patients, 77 percent of them were able to use no or very limited narcotic relief with the help of TENS. Postcesarean patients need to be able to reduce or eliminate narcotics because the side effects of these drugs are often transitory dizziness, hypotension, and sedation; and they are excreted to some degree in breast milk. The sedative and dizzying effects interfere with newborn care because a woman experiences such a loss of energy and stability; hypotension is potentially dangerous to any person who has had a surgical blood loss. Many postcesarean mothers breast-feed today, so potential contamination of breast milk is a concern.

TENS stimulation may allow a woman to ambulate earlier with less distress; because it allows her to cough and deep-breathe easier, postoperative complications such as thrombophlebitis may be lessened.

If a woman knows preoperatively that she will be having a cesarean birth and the use of TENS can be anticipated, the procedure should be explained to her preoperatively with other aspects of care, such as the need to cough and deep breath and turn. All women who plan to breast-feed should be given the option of using TENS therapy. Most people are concerned about the word *electric* and the possibility of a short in the system electrocuting them. At a point in time when they are psychologically guarding their body, their response to the method may be very uncomfortable. You might suggest that a woman allow the surgeon to place the electrodes, with their actual use left to her based on how much pain she has postoperatively. Stress that pain sensation differs greatly from one person to another and that she does not need to commit herself to only one form of pain relief. Narcotic administration will still be available if she needs it in addition to TENS stimulation.

Demonstrate the degree of stimulation the unit provides by applying an electrode to your hand (the feeling is a tingling, tickling one). Allow the support person to experience it if he likes. Both the woman and her support person might want to read the manufacturer's information booklet.

Because TENS therapy is not effective with all women, probably depending on the proportion of large and small afferent nerve fibers present, individual pain thresholds, and confidence in the therapy, you must continue to evaluate pain intensity during the postpartal period by observation. Watch the degree and ease with which a woman ambulates, her facial expression, and voiced concern. Be certain that the activation unit is removed when a woman showers or takes a sitz bath so that it is not submitted to water. Be certain to locate the cord before you help her turn in bed or get out of bed to avoid pulling the electrodes. If placed on the siderail, place the unit on the opposite side of the bed from the bedside stand and water glass so that an accidental spill of water will not wet it. Keep it on the opposite side from an IV infusion; in case the intravenous tubing loosens, and the bed becomes wet, the

unit is, again, not exposed to water. If electrodes should pull free, clean the electrode with an antiseptic solution or use a new sterile one and reattach it by lifting or changing the wound dressing. Do not replace the electrode without cleaning it; once it has been in the bed near lochia, it is potentially too contaminated to be replaced near an as-yet-unhealed surgical incision.

TENS therapy has some disadvantages. It increases the "unnaturalness" of cesarean birth by involvement of an electrical monitor and leads. The threat of electrical shock is too frightening for some people to tolerate. Lack of interest in self pain control may be apparent during the taking-in period and the accompanying euphoric effect that accompanies a drug such as Demerol may be helpful to some women with a minimal postpartal depression. Many postoperative patients are unable to use TENS because not only have they had surgery but they are ill. It appears to have its most appeal with postcesarean patients because although they are postsurgical, they are not ill and therefore are capable of a high level of self-care.

Promotion of Wound Healing

Surgical incisions heal by primary intention or by the gradual removal and replacement of dead or damaged cells at the wound site with new cells produced by the surrounding tissue. Assess the surgical incision once a nursing shift to be certain that the wound edges are approximated and no signs of infection such as erythema are present. As soon as a woman can walk steadily (the second postoperative day) she can take a shower, at the same time removing the dressing. Warm, clean water on the incision is healing to the incision area. Many obstetricians allow a woman to decide if she wants to continue to wear a dressing or not after this point (lack of a dressing prevents moisture at the incision site and decreases the possibility of infection). With a cesarean birth, healing will be complete enough that by the fifth to eighth day, skin sutures can be removed.

The Emergency Cesarean Birth

A woman who was scheduled for an emergency cesarean birth because a complication occurred during labor has even more reason to be concerned that her postpartal course will be difficult (labor was difficult) and that her infant is abnormal in some way. Be certain to review with her the reason for the surgery and to give assurance that she is doing well in the postpartal period. Be certain that both she and her support person have additional time with the infant to be able to assure themselves that the infant is well.

Continued Care

Be certain at discharge that a mother has a prescription for an analgesic to relieve pain while she is at home (propoxyphene [Darvon] is a common analgesic prescribed). Be certain she is aware of any restriction on exercise or activity (as a rule she should not lift any object over 10 pounds for the first 2 weeks). She should be aware of signs of possible complications directly related to the surgery—such as redness at the incision line, frequency or burning on urination—as well as normal postpartal concerns such as reddened, inflamed breast tissue and abnormal lochia flow. She can resume coitus as soon as the act is comfortable for her (as soon as 1 more week although many women feel discomfort through the 4th week) and she should have an appointment for a return visit for health assessment with her physician (arranged for 2 to 4 weeks).

Utilizing Nursing Process

Nursing care with a woman who has a cesarean birth must always be modified to some extent due to the addition of a surgical procedure. In order that two major life happenings—birth of a child and major abdominal surgery—can be integrated, careful planning of care must be done.

Assessment

The nurse is often the person on a health care team who is the first to suspect that a woman may need to be scheduled for a cesarean birth. He or she takes the initial pregnancy history and thus has the report of a past cephalopelvic disproportion; in labor the nurse is often the one who completes the first Leopold's maneuvers and detects a transverse lie or a breech lie or who realizes that fetal descent or cervical dilatation is not occurring due to plotting a Friedman graph.

Analysis

The Fourth Conference on Nursing Diagnosis accepted no nursing diagnosis specific to cesarean birth. Many diagnoses can be adapted to be specific for a cesarean experience, however: "Fear, related to impending surgery," "Pain related to a surgical incision," and "Fluid balance, inadequate, related to abdominal surgery" are examples. When setting an overall goal of care, the same major goal applies as with vaginal birth: a healthy mother and a healthy child.

Planning

Planning for any one cesarean birth is often limited to only a few minutes of time if it is initiated as an emergency procedure. In order to make cesarean birth safe, however, you must do anticipatory planning for *all* women in labor (What would you do that would be unique for this woman if a cesarean birth should be needed?).

Conditions for which cesarean birth were performed in one study are shown in Table 42-7. They can serve as a guideline to plan care.

Implementation

Every woman is aware that childbirth is a risk to her health. Superimposing major surgery on top of this risk makes it imperative that a woman and her support person feel confidence in the health care personnel caring for them, or they cannot emotionally survive the insult to their physiologic and psychological selves. When giving care to any woman in labor, be certain to establish a helping relationship with her so if a cesarean birth should become necessary she feels that she is among friends. Implementations often must be done with a degree of speed. Be certain that you do not associate speed with carelessness. Be very careful of sterile technique. A postpartal infection can be devastating to a woman who already has made many other physical adaptations.

Many implementations are teaching or supporting ones. The more a woman understands about what is happening to her, the more she can accept it. Be certain to provide adequate talk time following the procedure to allow a woman to review the procedure, work through the happening, and fit it in with other life occurrences. Other implementations involve coordination of health care team members (anesthesiologist, surgeon, pediatrician or neonatologist, recovery room or nursery personnel). This is particularly important if the surgery will be performed in a hospital surgery department rather than in the labor and delivery suite or if the infant will be transferred to a careful watch nursery or a distant site for intensive care following the birth.

Table 42-7 Cesarean Birth Rate and Rank for Complications of Pregnancy, Labor, and Delivery, United States, 1980

Complication	C-Birth Rate (per 100)	Rank	Complication	C-Birth Rate (per 100)	Rank
Disproportion, including contracted pelvis and fetopelvic disproportion.	93.8	1	Other complications, including edema and genitourinary infections.	47.0	8
Abnormality of organs, including uterine scar from previous surgery.	92.6	2	Infections and parasitic conditions.	46.5	9
Other indications for care, including failed induction.	65.2	3	Hypertension.	38.1	10
			Prolonged pregnancy.	34.0	11
Malposition of fetus, including breech presentation.	58.8	4	Multiple gestation.	34.0	12
Antepartum hemorrhage, abruptio placentae, and placenta previa.	54.1	5	Amniotic cavity problems and premature rupture of membranes.	31.9	13
			Other conditions including diabetes, anemia, etc.	31.6	14
Abnormal labor.	53.7	6	Obstructed labor.	26.1	15
Fetal and placental problems including fetal distress.	48.2	7	Early or threatened labor.	25.2	16

Source: Taffel, S., & Placek, P. (1983). Complications in cesarean and non-cesarean deliveries: United States, 1980. *American Journal of Public Health, 73,* 856.

Nursing Care Planning

Christine McFadden is a 15-year-old you care for. Because of a potential cephalopelvic disproportion she was allowed a trial labor. When labor did not progress, a cesarean birth was scheduled.

Problem Area. Emotional preparation for surgery.

Assessment
Patient states, "I don't want this. I'd rather die!" Mother is with her as support person, but a degree of mother-adolescent antagonism limits her effectiveness as a support person.

Analysis
Fear, related to impending cesarean birth.

Goal. Patient will accept surgery procedure by 15 minutes' time.

Criteria. Patient will sign informed consent for cesarean birth.

Nursing Orders
1. Review procedure with patient and support person (mother); allow time for ventilation of feelings.

2. Administer preoperative medication (atropine 1/150 grains, SC).
3. Insert indwelling catheter to gravity drainage.
4. Maintain NPO status.
5. Administer 30 ml Amphojel orally.
6. Remove oral retainer; remove nailpolish from 2 fingers, 2 toes.
7. Skin preparation: from beneath breasts to perineum.
8. Continue FHR monitoring until transfer to operating room.
9. Review coughing and deep breathing, leg exercises for postpartal period.

Following the cesarean birth of a 6-pound girl, you design the following postpartal care plan.

Problem Area. Comfort.

Assessment
Patient states, "I hurt all over. I can't breathe I have so much pain!" Holding hands over abdomen. Barely moving in bed.

Analysis
Discomfort related to cesarean incision.

Goal. Patient to reach an acceptable level of comfort by 20 minutes' time.

Criteria. Patient voices she has reduced pain; no discernible tension present by facial expression or posture.

Nursing Orders
1. Administer Demerol 50 mg IM q4h per M.D. order.
2. Straighten bed; urge patient to rest.
3. Review that pain is expected postsurgically but analgesia will be effective in reducing pain.

Problem Area. Fluid and electrolyte balance.

Assessment
Patient states, "Mouth is like sand." Urinary output 100 ml/last hour. Skin turgor good.

Anaysis
Potential for fluid and electrolyte imbalance related to combined surgical and postpartal influences.

Goal. Patient to maintain fluid and electrolyte balance.

Criteria. Specific gravity and urine will remain within normal level (1.003 to 1.030).

Nursing Orders
1. Infuse 3,000 ml of lactated Ringer's at 125 ml/hr per M.D. order.
2. Add 1 ml of Pitocin to first 1,000 ml of fluid per M.D. order.
3. Strict I&O.
4. Remove Foley at 12 hours pp following culture of urine. Measure next two voidings for amount and S.G.
5. Assess for bowel sounds q8h until return.
6. Begin ice chips when bowel sounds are present.
7. Blood pressure and pulse q15min, × 1h, then q1h × 4, then q8h × 24h.

Problem Area. Promote healing and involution.

Assessment
Blood pressure: 110/80; respirations: 22; temperature 98.6 orally. Dressing dry and intact. Scant lochia discharge. Uterus firm and 1F below umbilicus. Abdomen soft.

Analysis
Potential for interference with involution related to cesarean birth.

Goal. Patient's postpartal course to remain within normal parameters.

Criteria. Uterus involution to progress at "finger" rate daily; lochia to gradually become lessened. Incision to remain noninflamed and intact.

Nursing Orders
1. Assess dressing for drainage q1h.
2. Assess abdominal softness with uterus assessment.
3. Encourage turning side to side and not crossing legs.
4. Ambulate at 12 hours.
5. Schedule Hct and HGB at 4h and 24h postprocedure.
6. Cough and deep breathe q1h.
7. Support incision with movement or coughing.
8. Use no knee gatch on bed to prevent thrombophlebitis.

Problem Area. Bonding.

Assessment
Patient states, "I'm glad I had a girl." Held her for only a moment in the delivery room. Stated she feels too tired to feed her now; will "try it later."

Analysis
Potential for bonding interference related to cesarean birth.

Goal. Bonding will progress satisfactorily by 1 week's time.

Criteria. Patient will hold infant warmly and speak of her in a positive light.

Nursing Orders
1. Encourage patient to keep infant in room with her for extended periods of time.
2. Help her to handle and feed infant with support.
3. Review normal growth and development of newborns and point out positive points (long hair, alert expression).
4. Attempt to increase mother's self-esteem by praising for managing so well despite a very difficult time in her life.

Questions for Review

Multiple Choice

1. Mrs. Allen is a primigravida whose baby is presenting breech. She is scheduled to have a cesarean birth. Which postoperative procedure would you prepare her for?
   a. presence of an indwelling catheter
   b. bedrest for the first 4 days
   c. presence of a nasogastric tube
   d. separation from her infant for 72 hours

2. Mrs. Allen will have a general anesthesia for the procedure. What preoperative preparation will you anticipate including in your plan of care?
   a. administering intravenous phenobarbital
   b. administering an oral antacid
   c. administration of morphine sulfate IM
   d. administering sips of water orally

3. Mrs. Allen asks you if she will have any difficulty breast-feeding following the procedure. Your best response would be that
   a. you don't recommend she try to breast-feed following a cesarean birth.
   b. there is no comfortable position to hold a newborn with an abdominal incision.
   c. she will need too much analgesia postoperatively to make breast-feeding safe.
   d. You will help her find a comfortable position for breast-feeding her infant.

4. Mr. Allen asks if he can view the birth. A modern policy on this subject is
   a. surgery is too distressing for fathers to view.
   b. viewing the surgery ruins the surprise of the child's sex.
   c. he can view it if he chooses even though his wife is not awake.
   d. his wife will be in too much pain for him to be comfortable.

5. Following the cesarean birth, Mrs. Allen has 3,000 ml of intravenous fluid ordered. You would anticipate in your plan of care that she will be kept NPO except for minimal ice chips until which time?
   a. 24 hours postprocedure
   b. 48 hours postprocedure
   c. until bowel sounds have returned
   d. until her bladder tone has returned

6. In order to prevent thrombophlebitis following birth, which implementation would be most important?
   a. Urge her to cough and deep breathe.
   b. Urge her to ambulate.
   c. Urge her to not dislodge the IV fluid.
   d. Urge her to press inward on her abdomen periodically.

Discussion

1. Many cesarean births are done on an emergency basis. What are measures that you would use to assure a woman that although procedures are being done quickly both she and her infant are being protected?

2. In some instances the father of the fetus is not allowed to observe a cesarean birth. What are measures you could use to help the father still feel a part of the birth of his child?

3. Women are generally fatigued following cesarean birth. What are ways that you could both encourage rest and yet initiate mother-child bonding?

Suggested Readings

Adams, J. L. (1983). The use of obstetrical procedures in the care of low-risk women. *Women Health*, 8, 25.

Allen, A. (1981). Preoperative teaching for cesarean birth. *Association of Operating Room Nurses Journal*, 34, 846.

Amirikia, H., et al. (1981). Cesarean section: A 15-year review of changing incidence, indications, and risks. *American Journal of Obstetrics and Gynecology*, 140, 81.

Bacon, K. K., et al. (1981). Care of the neonate after cesarean section. *Association of Operating Room Nurses Journal*, 34, 860.

Baudy, P. (1980). Preparation for childbirth: A cesarean birth series. *Issues in Health Care of Women*, 2, 15.

Boyd, S. T., & Mahon, P. (1980). The family-centered cesarean delivery. *M.C.N.*, 5, 176.

Bradley, C. F., et al. (1983). A prospective study of mother's attitudes and feelings following cesarean and vaginal births. *Birth*, 10, 79.

Brumbaugh, P. (1982). Self-esteem—a concern . . . about cesarean-delivered mothers. *M.C.N.*, 7, 312.

Coady, D. J. (1980). Cesarean section: Trends in rates and indications. *Women and Health*, 5, 9.

Cox, B. E., & Smith, E. C. (1982). The mother's self-esteem after a cesarean delivery. *M.C.N.*, 7, 309.

Cranley, M. S., et al. (1983). Women's perceptions of vaginal and cesarean deliveries. *Nursing Research*, 32, 10.

Davies, K. (1982). A conflict of roles . . . the physical and psychological hazards of . . . caesarean section. *Nursing Mirror*, 7, 155.

Faulconer, D. R., et al. (1983). Decentralizing cesarean births to labor and delivery. *Today's OR Nurse*, 5, 10.

Fawcett, J. (1981). Needs of cesarean birth parents. *J.O.G.N. Nursing*, 10, 372.

Flynn, M. E., et al. (1982). Promoting wound healing. *American Journal of Nursing*, 82, 1543.

Foote, J. A. (1981). Special needs of teenage cesarean patients. *Association of Operating Room Nurses Journal*, 43, 855.

Gibbs, C. E. (1980). Planned vaginal delivery following

cesarean section. *Clinical Obstetrics and Gynecology, 23,* 507.

Hallmark, G., et al. (1982). Cesarean birth in the operating room . . . the goal should be that of a positive birth experience. *Associaiton of Operating Room Nurses Journal, 36,* 978.

Harris, J. K. (1980). Self-care is possible after cesarean section. *Nursing Clinics of North America, 15,* 191.

Hart, G. (1980). Maternal attitudes in prepared and unprepared cesarean deliveries. *J.O.G.N. Nursing, 9,* 243.

Jackson, S. H., et al. (1982). Effect of fathers at cesarean birth on postpartum infection rates. *Association of Operating Room Nurses Journal, 36,* 973.

Kehoe, C. F. (1981). *The cesarean experience.* New York: Appleton-Century-Crofts.

Kurzel, R. B., et al. (1981). When to do a cesarean section. *Perinatology/Neonatology, 5,* 19.

Leach, L., et al. (1984). Meeting the challenge of cesarean births. *J.O.G.N. Nursing, 13,* 191.

Leonard, L., et al. (1982). And father makes three— should fathers attend cesarean deliveries? *Canadian Nurse, 78,* 38.

Lipson, J. G. (1984). Repeat cesarean births: Social and psychological issues. *J.O.G.N. Nursing, 13,* 157.

Loughlin, N. (1982). Cesarean childbirth: Current perspectives. *Today's OR Nurse, 4,* 8.

Morrison, J. C., et al. (1982). Cesarean section: What's behind the dramatic rise? *Perinatology/Neonatology, 6,* 87.

Ott, W. J., et al. (1981). Paternal observation of a cesarean section. *Perinatology/Neonatology, 5,* 63.

Petrie, R. H., et al. (1981). Why so many cesarean deliveries—are they justified? *Consultant, 21,* 88.

Placek, P. J., et al. (1983). Cesarean section delivery rates: United States, 1981. *American Journal of Public Health, 73,* 861.

Pritchard, J., & MacDonald, P. C. (1980). *Williams Obstetrics* (16th ed.). New York: Appleton-Century-Crofts.

Quilligan, E. J., et al. (1981). Cesarean section: Some important considerations. *Perinatal Press, 5,* 111.

Richards, M. P. M. (1983). Casearean birth and the development of children. *Midwife Health Visitor and Community Nurse, 19,* 368.

Riley, J. E. (1982). The impact of transcutaneous electrical nerve stimulation on the postcesarean patient. *J.O.G.N. Nursing, 11,* 325.

Shearer, E. C. (1982). Education for vaginal birth after cesarean. *Birth, 9,* 31.

Shearer, E. C. (1983). How do parents really feel after cesarean birth? *Birth, 10,* 91.

Taffel, S. M., et al. (1983). Complications in cesarean and non-cesarean deliveries: United States, 1980. *American Journal of Public Health, 73,* 856.

Vanderark, G., & McGrath, K. (1975). Transcutaneous electrical stimulation in treatment of postoperative pain. *American Journal of Surgery, 130,* 335.

Weinstein, L. (1983). Antibiotic prophylaxis in cesarean section. *Perinatology/Neonatology, 7,* 29.

43

The Woman Who Develops a Complication During Labor or Delivery

OBJECTIVES

Following mastery of the contents of this chapter, you should be able to

1. Define the general term *dystocia.*
2. Describe deviations of the force of labor, the fetus, or pelvic configurations that cause dystocia.
3. Assess a woman in labor and during delivery for deviations from the normal labor process.
4. State a nursing diagnosis and goals related to a deviation from normal in labor and delivery.
5. Plan nursing implementations with a woman and her support person that will help her meet her established goals.
6. Describe implementations of care related to such deviations from the normal as breech presentation, multiple gestation, fetal distress, and prolapsed cord.
7. Evaluate the fulfillment of goals related to deviations from the normal in labor and delivery.
8. Analyze measures to prevent deviations from the normal in labor and delivery.
9. Synthesize the knowledge of deviations of normal in labor and delivery with nursing process to achieve quality maternal-newborn nursing care.

THE HOURS OF LABOR are hours of stress for a woman and the father of her child. It is such a stressful time that a woman needs to be assured from time to time that everything is going smoothly, that both she and the infant appear to be doing well.

If a complication occurs and such assurances cannot be given so freely, the stress for a woman increases a hundredfold. How unfair it is to carry a child for 9 months and have something go wrong now. How much she wants to protect the life inside her. How helpless she is to do anything about the heartbeat that she knows is fading. How real become the thoughts that flickered across her mind when she first realized she was in labor: "This may be the day my baby dies; this may be the night *I* die."

Every woman in labor should have with her a nurse who is highly skilled both in the physical aspects of her care and in interpersonal relationships. The woman who realizes she is having a complication in labor, who wills her body to complete successfully the job it started 9 months before, who knows she has no real control over these last few hours before birth, needs someone who understands her fears and her feelings of helplessness.

There is no better definition of a professional nurse than one who is able to support and care for a woman both physically and emotionally during a complication of labor and delivery such as when dystocia exists or induction of labor is necessary.

Dystocia

Dystocia is a broad term for difficult or abnormal labor. Labor is basically a simple concept: It is the process in which the fetus and its accompanying structures (placenta, cord, membranes, and amniotic fluid) are pushed through the birth canal by a force to the outside world. Any difficulty that occurs, therefore, must involve one or more of the terms of this proposition; that is, a complication with the force that propels the fetus (the uterine contractions), the fetus (the passenger), or the birth canal (the passageway). See Chapter 23 for a full discussion of the labor process.

Uterine Dysfunction: Difficulty with the Force

The contractions of the uterus are the basic force that dilates the cervix and moves the fetus through the birth canal.

Abnormal Uterine Contractions

Uterine contractions occur because of the interplay of contractile hormones (adenosine triphosphate, ATP); estrogen and progesterone; the influence of major electrolytes such as calcium, sodium, and potassium; specific contractile proteins (actin and myosin); epinephrine and norepinephrine; oxytocin; and prostaglandins. Three types of abnormal contractions can be described.

Hypotonic Contractions. With hypotonic contractions the number of contractions is usually low or infrequent (not increasing beyond 2 or 3 in a 10-minute time period). The resting tone of the uterus remains under 10 mm Hg (Figure 43-1A).

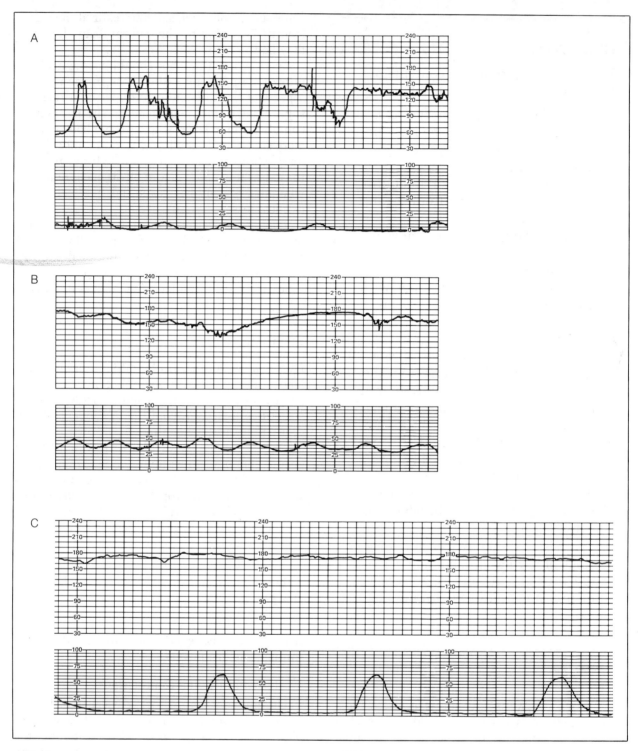

Figure 43-1 *A. Hypotonic contractions. Notice that the fetal heart rate on this strip shows late decelerations even with these ineffective contractions of no more than 10 mm Hg pressure. B. Hypertonic contractions. Notice the high resting pressure (40–50 mm Hg). FHR is rapid (170) with variable decelerations. C. Normal uterine contractions.*

Hypotonic contractions of this kind tend to occur when analgesia is administered too early in labor (before cervical dilatation of 3–4 cm) or when bowel or bladder distention is present, preventing descent or firm engagement of the fetus. It may occur in a uterus overstretched by a multiple gestation, a larger-than-usual single fetus, or hydramnios, or in a lax uterus from grand multiparity. Such contractions are not exceedingly painful because of the lack of intensity (pain is a subjective symptom, however, so an individual woman could interpret them as very painful).

An infusion of oxytocin to "assist" labor is usually helpful to strengthen hypotonic contractions and increase their effectiveness. If not assisted to become stronger, hypotonic contractions increase the length of labor because so many of them are necessary to achieve cervical dilatation. The mother becomes generally exhausted (which in turn causes increased uterine exhaustion). During the postpartal period, the uterus, exhausted from a long labor, may continue to contract ineffectively and so a woman's chance for postpartal hemorrhage increases. With the cervix dilated for a long period of time, both the uterus and the fetus are prone to infection.

Mark a woman's chart that hypotonic contractions occurred. In the first hour following labor, the uterus needs to be palpated every 15 minutes and lochia carefully assessed to be certain that postpartal contractions are adequate.

Hyptertonic Contractions. Hypertonic uterine contractions are marked by an increase in resting tone above 15 mm Hg (Figure 43-1B). The intensity of the contraction apex may be no stronger than with a hypotonic contraction however. This type of contraction occurs because repolarization of the muscle fibers of the myometrium does not occur following a contraction. Repolarization serves the purpose of "wiping the muscle cells clean" to accept a new pacemaker stimulus. Hypertonic contractions tend to become very painful as the myometrium becomes tender due to constant lack of relaxation and anoxia of uterine cells. A woman may become frustrated or disappointed with her breathing exercises for childbirth because they are not effective in keeping her pain-free. Telling her to relax and "breathe with" contractions is ineffective because the problem is reversed: The lack of relaxation makes it impossible for her to breathe effectively.

The lack of relaxation between contractions does not allow optimal uterine artery filling so the fetus may begin to suffer anoxia early in the latent phase of labor. Any woman whose pain seems out of proportion to the quality of her contractions should have both a uterine and fetal external monitor applied for at least a 15-minute interval to be certain the resting phase of the contractions is adequate and the fetal pattern is not showing late deceleration.

Oxytocin is not effective with hypertonic contractions; to strengthen them, the woman needs rest and possibly sedation. Change linen and her patient gown; darken room lights and decrease noise and stimulation. Both the woman and her support person need support to understand why the contractions, which feel as if they must be very effective because they feel strong, are in reality very ineffective and not achieving cervical dilatation.

Uncoordinated Contractions. Normally one point in the uterus acts as the initiating point of all contractions. The contraction sweeps down over the uterus, encircling it. Repolarization occurs, a low resting tone is achieved, and another contraction begins. With uncoordinated contractions more than one contraction may be initiated at the same time, or receptor points in the uterus myometrium are acting independently of each other. Uncoordinated contractions may occur so closely together that they do not allow good cotyledon filling. They make it difficult for a woman to rest between contractions and to use breathing exercises because they occur so erratically (one on top of another and then a long space of time without any and so forth).

Apply a fetal and uterine external monitor and assess the rate, pattern, resting tone, and fetal response to contractions for at least a 15-minute interval (a longer time may be necessary to show the disorganized pattern in early labor).

Oxytocin administration may be helpful in uncoordinated labor to stimulate a more effective and consistent pattern of contractions with a better lower resting tone.

Uterine Inertia (Dysfunctional Labor)

Inertia is a time-honored term to denote that sluggishness of contractions has occurred. This is more often today termed *dysfunctional labor.* Dysfunction can occur at any point but is generally classified as *primary* (occurring at the onset of labor) or *secondary* (occurring later in labor). The incidence of postpartal infection and hemorrhage in the mother and mortality in the infant is higher in women who have a prolonged labor than in those who do not: Recognizing and preventing dysfunctional labor is vitally important.

Uterine inertia appears to result from a number of factors, which are summarized in Table 43-1.

Table 43-1 Factors That Lead to Dysfunctional Labor

Inappropriate use of analgesia (excessive or too early administration).
Pelvic bone contraction, such as might have occurred from rickets, that has so narrowed the pelvic diameter that the fetus cannot pass.
Poor fetal position (a posterior rather than an anterior position).
Extension rather than flexion of the fetal head.
Overdistention of the uterus, as with multiple pregnancy, hydramnios, or an excessively oversized fetus.
Cervical rigidity, such as may occur in an elderly primipara.
Presence of a full rectum or urinary bladder that impedes fetal descent.
Mother becoming exhausted from labor.
Primigravida.

Hypotonic, hypertonic, and uncoordinated contractions all play roles in dysfunctional labor.

Dysfunction of the Preparatory Division of Labor.

The major dysfunction of the preparatory division is a prolonged latent phase. Figure 24-18 shows a normal graph of labor, depicting the latent phase, acceleration phase, phase of maximum slope, deceleration phase, and maximum slope of descent. If labor is plotted in this way, when dystocia occurs it can be recognized.

PROLONGED LATENT PHASE. A prolonged latent phase, defined as a latent phase that is longer than 20 hours in a primipara and 14 hours in a multipara, may happen if the cervix is not ripe at the beginning of labor and so time has to be spent truly getting ready for labor. It may reflect dysfunctional labor. With a prolonged latent phase, the uterus tends to be in a hypertonic state. Relaxation between contractions is inadequate, and the contractions themselves are only mild (under 15 mm Hg on a monitor printout) and therefore ineffective. One segment of the uterus may contract with more force than another segment.

This unequal, irregular pattern of contractions with poor relaxation in between is very painful and very frightening to the woman in labor. She has no pain-free periods; she cannot time contractions; she senses that something is not right and her worry and tension make the contractions seem more painful. The situation is potentially harmful to the fetus, because the lack of uterine relaxation does not allow the maternal cotyledons to refill with freshly oxygenated blood between contractions, and so fetal anoxia may occur.

It is important in early labor to assess the strength and intensity of contractions and establish that a relaxation phase is occurring. Contractions and fetal heart sounds should be monitored throughout labor to detect fetal distress.

Management of a prolonged latent phase in labor is aimed toward helping the uterus to rest and administering adequate fluid to a woman to prevent dehydration. It may be wisest to administer the fluid intravenously to keep the woman's gastrointestinal tract free of fluid in case anesthesia is necessary for delivery. Administration of morphine may relax hypertonicity. When the woman awakens from a short sleep, labor usually becomes effective and begins to progress. If it does not, the infant may have to be delivered by cesarean birth or labor assisted with amniotomy and oxytocin infusion. A diagram of a prolonged latent phase is shown in Figure 43-2.

Dysfunctions of the Dilatational Division of Labor.

The major dysfunctions of labor that occur during the dilatational division of labor are the prolonged active phase and protracted descent.

PROLONGED ACTIVE PHASE. A prolonged active phase is usually associated with cephalopelvic disproportion or fetal malposition, although it may reflect ineffective myometrial activity. The phase is prolonged if the phase of maximum slope is not 1.2 cm or more per hour in a nullipara or 1.5 cm or more per hour in a multipara. If the cause of the delay in dilatation is fetal malposition or cephalopelvic disproportion, cesarean birth may have to be initiated to effect delivery. Dysfunctional labor during the dilatational division tends to be hypotonic in contrast to the hypertonic action at the beginning of labor. This is shown in Figure 43-2.

Figure 43-2 *A prolonged latent phase pattern (A) and a protracted active phase pattern (B) compared to a normal labor pattern (C).*

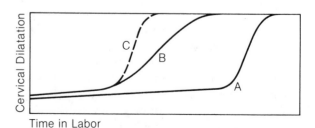

PROTRACTED DESCENT. A woman is having a protracted descent phase of labor if descent is occurring at a rate of less than 1 cm per hour in a nullipara or less than 2 cm per hour in a multipara.

With both a prolonged active phase of dilatation and protracted descent, contractions have been of good quality and proper duration, and effacement and beginning dilatation have occurred; but then the contractions gradually become infrequent and of poor quality, and dilatation stops. If everything except the suddenly faulty contractions is normal (cephalopelvic disproportion or poor fetal presentation has been ruled out by X-ray or sonogram), then rest and fluid intake, as advocated for hypertonic contractions, are applicable here also. If membranes have not ruptured, rupturing them at this point may be helpful. Intravenous oxytocin may be used to induce the uterus to contract effectively.

Whether the dysfunctional labor occurs in the preparatory or the dilatational division of labor, the effect on the woman and her support person will be the same: anxiety, fear, discouragement. A woman needs a running explanation of what is happening: "We're going to take an X-ray to check the baby's position." "This is a drug to urge your uterus into stronger contractions." "I know resting is the last thing you feel like doing, but that is what I want you to try to do."

Dysfunctions of the Pelvic Division of Labor.
Four disorders—prolonged deceleration phase, secondary arrest of dilatation, arrest of descent, and failure of descent—may occur with the pelvic division of labor.

PROLONGED DECELERATION PHASE. A deceleration phase has become prolonged when it extends beyond 3 hours in a nullipara, 1 hour in a multipara.

SECONDARY ARREST OF DILATATION. A secondary arrest of dilatation has occurred when there is no progress in cervical dilatation for more than 2 hours.

ARREST OF DESCENT. Arrest of descent is present when no descent has occurred in 1 hour.

FAILURE OF DESCENT. Failure of descent has occurred when expected descent of the fetus does not begin.

The most likely cause for arrest in labor during the pelvic division is cephalopelvic disproportion. Cesarean birth is generally chosen as the method of delivery of the infant. If there is no contraindi-

cation to vaginal delivery, oxytocin may be used to assist in labor.

Prevention of Dysfunctional Labor.
It is impossible to prevent all dysfunctional labor as it is impossible to determine fetal size exactly without a technique such as sonogram or X-ray, and it is impossible to predict anyone's hormone system or individual response to labor. There are a number of factors that are always helpful, however.

MAINTAINING A SERUM GLUCOSE LEVEL. Because labor is such hard work, a woman can quickly deplete her glucose stores during labor. Assess on admission to a birthing room how likely this is to happen by being certain to ask when was the last time the woman ate. If she ate breakfast at 8 A.M. and then began labor, by 2 P.M. she is only 6 hours away from a full meal. If she last ate at 5:00 the following evening, and because she woke with labor in the morning, ate no breakfast, she is 11 hours away from a full meal. The chance that she will deplete glucose stores is three times greater. Alert the physician or nurse-midwife and, if she is still in early labor, she may be allowed some high carbohydrate fluid such as orange juice. An intravenous solution to provide glucose may also be started.

Many women react poorly to the suggestion of intravenous fluid. They picture themselves being submitted to intense pain and totally immobilized; they perceive it as losing control over their bodies, of having the naturalness of labor and delivery taken away from them. Introduce the suggestion of intravenous fluid and explain its purpose before you arrive with a bag of fluid and tubing. Assure a woman that although the needle will sting momentarily (a pinprick) as the needle is inserted, there is no discomfort after that. Because women of childbearing age are young and healthy, placing the needle is usually a simple procedure, not one involving many painful efforts. Be certain it is placed in the nondominant hand and only a small "reminder" handboard is used rather than a long one.

Assure a woman that she can be out of bed and walking, can turn freely, squat, sit, or whatever position she prefers; that none of these acts will interfere with the infusion (Figure 43-3). Letting the woman choose the site for the infusion and agree to the procedure rather than suddenly looking up to see you with the equipment helps her to feel in charge. In some instances you may need to stress the purpose of the fluid—to provide sugar for energy for the uterus so that it can continue with labor and she can deliver "naturally."

Most physicians and nurse-midwives allow

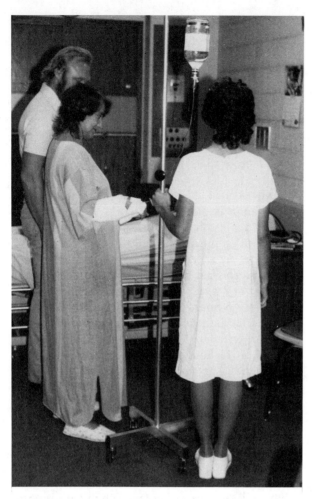

Figure 43-3 *Many women with dysfunctional labor have an intravenous fluid line inserted. Help them to ambulate with this in place if walking makes labor easier for them.*

women to have lollipops or sourballs to suck on during labor to supply glucose.

PREVENTING FLUID AND ELECTROLYTE LOSS. Low levels of serum electrolytes or body fluid can occur in labor for the same reason as a decreased glucose level: a long interval between eating and the present time. Such losses can be worsened by the vomiting and diarrhea that occasionally occur as an accompaniment to labor. Ask if these occurred and their extent (one episode of a small amount of diarrhea or diarrhea for a full half hour's time). Perfuse diaphoresis and hyperventilation that occur with labor increase these problems further through insensible water loss. Test all voidings during labor for glucose, protein, ketones, and specific gravity (place a urine collector container on the bathroom toilet if a mother is going to use the toilet). Ketones suggest starvation ketosis; a concentrated specific gravity sug-

gests a lack of fluid. Extreme dehydration leads to increased blood viscosity; this may increase the possibility of thrombophlebitis during the postpartal period. Fluid administration then may not only prevent dystocia but postpartal complications as well.

REDUCING PSYCHOLOGICAL STRESS. A cervix dilates more rapidly and therefore labor is shortened if the woman is not tense and frightened during labor. Manage stress by making the transfer from home to health care facility as nontraumatic as possible. Ask directly if there is anything the woman is concerned about. Offer explanations of all procedures. Make the support person just as welcome and comfortable as the woman herself. A question such as, "Is labor what you thought it would be?" to both the woman and her support person often helps them to express whatever is causing concern.

SUPPORTING MEASURES TO REDUCE PAIN. Pain is an exhausting phenomenon. Praise breathing attempts; breathe with the woman, give back rubs, change sheets, use cool washcloths, etc. If breathing exercises can be effective, the need for analgesia (which can lead to hypotonic contractions) can be reduced.

MAINTAINING A SIDE-LYING POSITION. To increase the blood supply to the uterus and prevent hypotension, urge a woman to lie on her side so the uterus is lifted off the vena cava. If a woman insists on lying supine, place a hip roll under one or the other buttock to cause her pelvis to "tip" and, at least to some extent, move the uterus to the side.

KEEPING THE BLADDER EMPTY. A full bladder prevents descent of the fetus and perhaps impedes uterine contractions. Urge a woman who is high-risk for dysfunctional labor to void every 2 hours during labor to keep the bladder empty.

Precipitate Delivery

A precipitate labor and delivery occurs when uterine contractions are so strong that a woman delivers with only a few rapidly occurring contractions. It is often defined as a labor that is completed in less than 3 hours. Such rapid labor is likely to occur with multiparity and may follow induction of labor by oxytocin or amniotomy. Rapid labor poses risk to the fetus because subdural hemorrhage may result from the sudden release of pressure on the head; the woman may sustain lacerations of the birth canal from tearing rather than stretching of tissue. Forceful contractions may lead to premature separation of the placenta and both maternal and fetal risk.

Assessment. A precipitate labor can be predicted from a labor graph if, during the active phase of dilatation, the rate is greater than 5 cm per hour (1 cm every 12 minutes) in a primipara and over 10 cm per hour (1 cm every 6 minutes) in a multipara.

Implementations. The woman with multiparity should be told by the twenty-eighth week of pregnancy that she can expect each labor to be shorter than the one before so she can make plans for rapid transportation to the hospital or alternate birthing center. Women who had a prior precipitate labor and delivery should be alerted that they may well deliver this way again. Both grand multiparas and women with histories of precipitate labor should be taken to the delivery room or have the birthing room converted to delivery readiness before full dilatation; even a rapid delivery can then be accomplished in controlled surroundings.

Pathologic Retraction Ring

The development of a pathologic retraction ring (Bandl's ring) at the juncture of the upper and lower uterine segments is a warning sign that severe dysfunctional labor is occurring.

Assessment. The ring appears as a horizontal indentation across the abdomen (Figure 43-4). It occurs in early labor when there are uncoordinated contractions. When it happens in the dilatational division of labor, it is usually caused by obstetrical manipulation or is the result of the administration of oxytocin. With fetal monitors in place, there is a tendency not to observe a woman's abdomen in labor as often as when fetal heart sounds are being auscultated by stethoscope. You must observe a woman's abdomen if you are to detect a pathologic retraction ring, which is a forewarning of uterine rupture.

A fetus is gripped by a retraction ring and cannot advance beyond that point. The undelivered placenta will also be held at that point after delivery of the infant.

Implementations. Report such a finding promptly. Administration of intravenous morphine sulfate or of amyl nitrite may relieve the retraction ring. If not, uterine rupture and death of the fetus may occur. In the placental stage, massive maternal hemorrhage may result, because the placenta is loosened but not delivered, and so the uterus cannot contract.

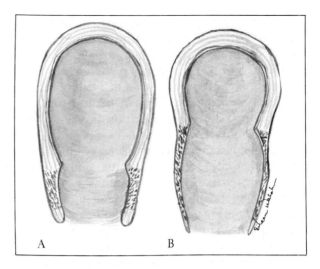

Figure 43-4 *Pathologic retraction ring. A. Uterus in the normal second stage of labor. Notice how the upper uterine segment is becoming thicker and the lower uterine segment is thinning. A physiologic retraction ring is normally formed at the division of the upper and lower uterine segments. B. Uterus with a pathologic retraction ring (Bandl's ring). The wall below the ring is thin and overdistended, and the ring rises against the abdominal wall. This constriction is caused by obstructed labor and is a warning sign that, if the obstruction is not relieved, the lower segment may rupture.*

Cesarean birth may be chosen to effect safe delivery of the fetus. Manual removal of the placenta under general anesthesia may be necessary for a placental-stage pathologic retraction ring.

Rupture of the Uterus

Rupture of the uterus during labor, although rare, is a possibility that should always be kept in mind. A uterus ruptures when it undergoes more strain than it is capable of sustaining. Rupture occurs most commonly when a scar from a previous cesarean birth, hysterotomy, or plastic repair of the uterus tears. However, prolonged labor, faulty presentation, multiple gestation, unwise use of oxytocin, obstructed labor, and traumatic maneuvers using forceps or traction are contributing factors.

Assessment. Impending rupture is suggested by a pathologic retraction ring. Strong uterine contractions without any cervical dilatation are present.

Implementations. To prevent rupture, a cesarean birth must be immediately scheduled. When a uterus ruptures, a woman experiences a sudden, severe pain during a strong labor contraction. With complete rupture, uterine contractions will stop. There is hemorrhage from the torn uterus into the abdominal cavity and possibly into the vagina. Signs of shock begin, including rapid, weak pulse, falling blood pressure, cold and clammy skin, and dilatation of the nostrils from air hunger. The woman's abdomen will change in contour, and two distinct swellings will be visible: the retracted uterus and the extrauterine fetus. Fetal heart sounds halt. If the rupture is incomplete (the placenta is not damaged), the signs are less evident than in complete rupture. The woman experiences a localized tenderness and a persistent aching pain over the area of the lower segment; contractions usually cease; and fetal heart sounds and the woman's vital signs will gradually reveal fetal and maternal distress.

Because the uterus at the end of pregnancy is such a vascular organ, uterine rupture is an intense emergency situation comparable to splenic or hepatic rupture. Emergency fluid replacement must be administered; a laparotomy must be scheduled as an emergency measure to control bleeding and effect a repair. The viability of the fetus will depend on the extent of the rupture and the time that elapses between the rupture and abdominal extraction. The woman's prognosis will depend on the extent of the rupture and blood loss.

Since it is not advisable for a woman who has a rupture of the uterus (unless it occurred in the inactive lower segment) to conceive again, she is usually sterilized, either by removal of the damaged uterus (hysterectomy) or by tubal ligation at the time of the laparotomy. This procedure may be very difficult for her to accept: At the moment she is given anesthesia, the health of the fetus is unknown. If blood loss was immediately acute, she may be unconscious from hypotension, and her support person may have to give this consent, relying on the integrity and skill of the operating surgeon.

Be prepared to offer understanding to the support person and to inform him as soon as possible about the fetal outcome, the extent of the surgery, and the woman's safety. The woman and her support person are immediately grateful, obviously, for having her life saved; she may become almost immediately angry, however, that the rupture occurred, especially if the fetus died and she cannot have any further children. Allow her time to express these justifiable emotions without feeling threatened. She grieves for the loss of both the child and her own fertility even if she was not planning on having other children. Being forced to become infertile is not the same as choosing to be infertile.

Amniotic Fluid Embolism

Amniotic fluid embolism occurs when amniotic fluid is forced into an open maternal uterine blood sinus through some defect in the membranes or after membrane rupture or partial premature separation of the placenta. Solid particles (such as skin cells) in the amniotic fluid enter the maternal circulation and reach the lungs as small emboli. They produce a pulmonary embolism whose severity is out of proportion to the size of the particles.

Assessment. The clinical picture is dramatic. The woman, in strong labor, sits up suddenly and grasps her chest because of inability to breathe and sharp pain. She pales and then turns the typical bluish gray associated with pulmonary embolism and lack of blood flow to the lungs.

Implementations. The immediate management is oxygen administration by face mask or cannula. Within minutes the woman needs cardiopulmonary resuscitation. This technique may not be effective, however, as these procedures (inflating the lungs and massaging the heart) do not move the emboli to allow blood to circulate to the lungs. Death may occur in minutes.

If death is not immediate, she will be moved to an intensive care unit for continued critical care. She is prone to develop disseminated intravascular coagulation (DIC) as a further complication.

A woman's prognosis depends on the size of the embolism and the skill and speed of the emergency aid available to her. Even if she survives the initial insult, the incidence of disseminated intravascular coagulation developing to further compound her condition is high.

Uterine Inversion

Inversion of the uterus is the turning of the uterus inside out. This rare happening occurs following the birth of an infant if traction is applied to the umbilical cord to remove the placenta or pressure is applied to the uterine fundus when the uterus is in a noncontracted state (see the Nursing Care Highlight on page 1007). It may occur with insertion of the placenta at the fundus so that, as the fetus is delivered, it pulls the fundus down; or atony of the uterus is so extreme that coughing or sneezing forces the fundus outward.

Assessment. Inversion occurs in various degrees. The inverted fundus may lie within the

Nursing Care Highlight

The Woman with Uterine Inversion

Uterine inversion is a grave complication. If the situation is not immediately corrected, emergency hysterectomy is necessary to save the woman's life. Almost all occurrence of uterine inversion can be avoided by two axioms of care: *Do not put pressure on an uncontracted fundus* *immediately postpartum* (massage first to cause it to contract), and *Do not exert pressure on an umbilical cord to achieve placental delivery.* Patience will achieve the same result in most instances and do it safely.

---

uterine cavity or the vagina or, in total inversion, protrude from the vagina. When an inversion occurs, there is a large, sudden gush of blood from the vagina; the fundus is no longer palpable in the abdomen. If the loss of blood continues unchecked for more than a few minutes, the woman will immediately show signs of blood loss: hypotension, dizziness, paleness, diaphoresis. The uterus is not contracted in this position and so the bleeding continues unchecked. A woman will exsanguinate within a time period as short as 10 minutes.

Implementations. Never attempt to replace the inversion; without good pelvic relaxation this may only increase bleeding. Never attempt to remove the placenta if it is still attached; this will only create a larger bleeding area. The administration of an oxytocic drug only compounds the inversion. The woman needs to be given a general anesthesia immediately for pelvic relaxation; the delivering physician then replaces the fundus manually.

An intravenous fluid line needs to be started if one is not already present (use a 19- or 18-gauge needle because blood will need to be replaced); a present fluid line should be opened to achieve optimal flow of fluid in order to restore fluid volume. Administer oxygen by mask and assess vital signs. Be prepared to perform cardiopulmonary resuscitation if the woman's heart should fail from the sudden blood loss.

The Fetus: Difficulty with the Passenger

Difficulty with the fetus will occur if it is malpositioned to the canal, is too large for the birth canal, or is malformed, or if more than one fetus is present.

Many high-risk fetuses will have their heart rate monitored internally by insertion of fetal scalp electrodes during labor. In addition, in order to establish that a long or difficult labor is not causing detrimental fetal effects, many high-risk fetuses undergo internal fetal blood sampling during labor.

The oxygen saturation, PO_2, PCO_2, pH, and hematocrit of fetal blood may all be determined during labor if a sample of capillary blood is taken from the fetal scalp as it presents at the dilated cervix. The fetal scalp is first prepared with iodine before a scalpel is introduced for the actual puncture. The amount of blood obtained (collected by a capillary tube) is usually so small that the pH level of the blood is the only determination that can be evaluated. This averages 7.25. A range of 7.20 to 7.30 is considered normal during labor. A fetus with a lower level (acidotic) is suffering anoxia.

Serial readings should be determined, as a *change* in pH may provide information on fetal welfare before an *abnormal* pH exists. Following the procedure, the infant's scalp should be observed following two contractions to be certain that bleeding at the puncture site has halted. Infants who have had internal scalp blood samples taken should not be delivered by vacuum extraction, which can lead to renewed bleeding at the puncture site.

A woman needs a clear explanation of what is being attempted before fetal blood samples are obtained. Otherwise she may worry that the scalpel used will press into the baby's brain or by accident invade an eye or ear or cut her vaginally. She cannot relax to allow for vaginal manipulations of this nature if she is concerned about her child's welfare to this extent.

Problems of Position or Presentation

Prolapse of the Umbilical Cord. In prolapse of the cord, a loop of the umbilical cord slips down in front of the presenting fetal part (Figure 43-5). Prolapse may occur at any time after the membranes rupture and if the presenting part is not fitted firmly into the cervix. It thus tends to

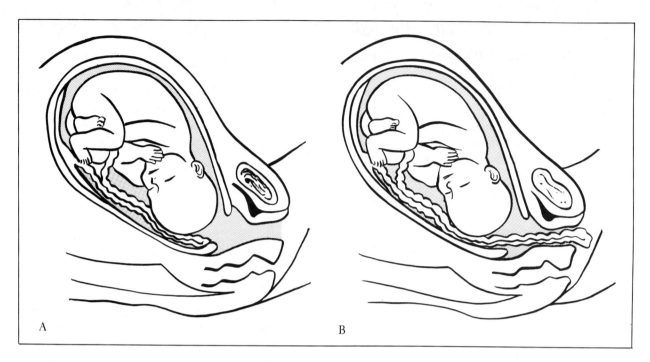

Figure 43-5 *Prolapse of the umbilical cord. A. The cord is prolapsed but still within the uterus. B. The cord is visible at the vulva. In both instances the fetal nutrient supply is being compromised. Although only a cord such as that in B would be visible, both prolapses could be detected by fetal monitoring equipment.*

occur most often with the conditions shown in Table 43-2.

ASSESSMENT. Very rarely, the cord may be felt as the presenting part on vaginal examination. You will feel the cord pulsating as you are examining for dilatation or trying to identify fontanelles. In the event of this presentation, cesarean birth will be necessary before rupture of the membranes occurs; otherwise, with rupture, the cord will surely be flushed down into the vagina. More often, however, cord prolapse is first discovered when the variable deceleration pattern of cord compression suddenly becomes apparent on a fetal monitor. The cord may then be visible at the vulva although, if it is held against the pelvic brim, it may not be apparent.

Table 43-2 High-Risk Conditions for Prolapsed Cord

Premature rupture of the membranes.
Fetal position other than cephalic presentations.
Placenta previa.
Intrauterine tumors that prevent the presenting part from engaging.
A small fetus.
Cephalopelvic disproportion that prevents firm engagement.

To rule out cord prolapse, fetal heart sounds should always be recorded immediately following rupture of the membranes, whether this occurs spontaneously or by amniotomy.

IMPLEMENTATIONS. Cord prolapse automatically leads to cord compression as the fetal presenting part presses against the cord at the pelvic brim. Management is aimed toward relieving pressure on the cord and thereby relieving the compression and the resulting fetal anoxia. This goal may be reached by having a woman assume a knee-chest position, which causes the presenting part to fall back from the cord. You may need to press pillows under the woman's abdomen to allow her to remain in this position in active labor. You may be able to relieve compression on the cord by turning the woman supine and pressing on the fetal head by a gloved hand in the vagina to press the head off the cord. It is easier to prepare the woman for cesarean birth in this position.

If the cord is exposed to room air, drying will begin, and with the drying, the umbilical vessels will start to atrophy. Do not attempt to push any exposed cord back into the vagina, however, or you may add to the compression by causing knotting or kinking. Instead, cover any exposed portion with a sterile saline compress to prevent drying (see the Nursing Care Highlight on page 1009).

Nursing Care Highlight

The Woman with a Prolapsed Cord

Prolapse of the cord is an emergency situation that requires prompt action. Often, you are the person with the woman when this occurs. Carry out measures such as a knee-chest position to relieve cord compression quickly. With cord prolapse, you are the first line of defense against permanent brain damage in the child. You have less than 5 minutes to institute relief measures to prevent irreparable central nervous system damage to the infant.

If the cervix is fully dilated at the time of the prolapse, the physician may choose to deliver the infant rapidly, possibly with forceps, to prevent a lengthy period of anoxia. If dilatation is not complete, cesarean birth will be the delivery method of choice.

Occipitoposterior Position. Normal fetal position is discussed in Chapter 23. In approximately a tenth of all labors, the fetal position is posterior rather than anterior; that is, the occiput (assuming the presentation is vertex) is directed diagonally and posteriorly: right occipitoposterior (ROP) or left occipitoposterior (LOP). In these positions, in the process of internal rotation, the fetal head must rotate not through a 90° arc but through an arc of approximately 135° (Figures 43-6 and 43-7).

ASSESSMENT. Posterior positions tend to occur in women with android, anthropoid, or contracted pelves. That a posterior position exists

Figure 43-6 *Left occipitoanterior (LOA) rotation. A. A fetus in a cephalic presentation, LOA position. View is from the outlet. The fetus rotates 90 degrees from this position. B. Descent and flexion. C. Internal rotation complete. D. Extension. The face and chin are born.*

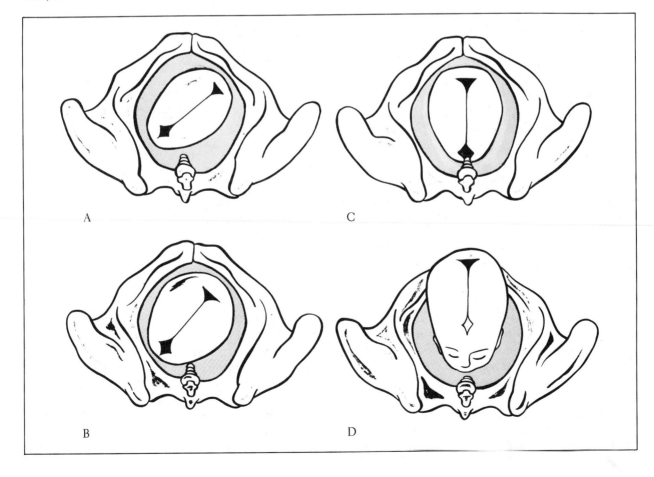

A

C

B

D

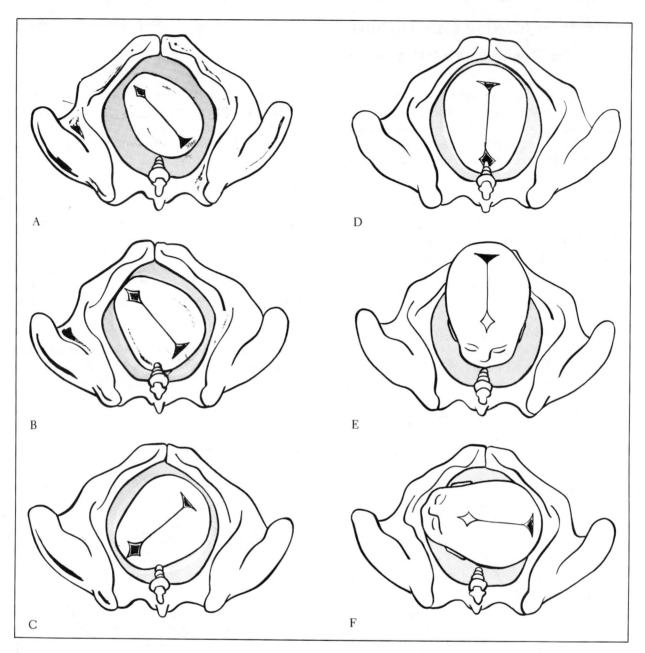

Figure 43-7 *Left occipitoposterior (LOP) rotation. A. Fetus in a cephalic presentation, LOP position. View is from the outlet. The fetus rotates 135° from this position. B. Descent and flexion. C. Internal rotation beginning. Because of the posterior position, the head will rotate in a longer arc than if it were in an anterior position. D. Internal rotation complete. E. Extension. The face and chin are born. F. External rotation. The fetus rotates to place the shoulders in an anteroposterior position.*

may be suggested by a dysfunctional labor pattern such as a prolonged active phase, arrested descent, or fetal heart sounds heard best at the lateral sides of the abdomen. The position of the fetus is confirmed on vaginal examination.

IMPLEMENTATIONS. A posteriorly presenting head does not fit the cervix as snugly as one in an anterior position, increasing the risk of prolapse of the umbilical cord, which must be assessed for all during labor. If uterine contractions are forceful and the fetus is of average size and in good flexion, the majority of infants presenting with these posterior positions will rotate through the large arc, will arrive at a good delivery position for the pelvic outlet, and will be delivered satisfactorily with only increased molding and caput formation. Because the arc of rotation is greater, it is

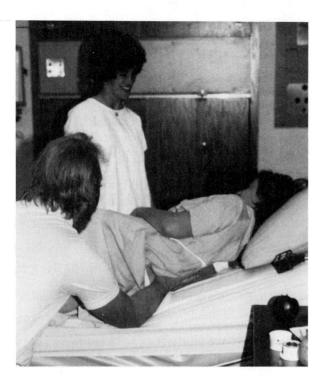

Figure 43-8 *With a posterior fetal position,.the woman may feel extensive back pressure. Pressure on her lower back by her support person may help relieve this problem.*

usual for the labor to be somewhat prolonged. Because the fetal head rotates against the sacrum, the woman may experience pressure and pain in her lower back from sacral nerve compression during labor, which may be so intense that she asks for medication for relief, not for her contractions, but for the intense back pressure and pain she is feeling. Sacral pressure such as that afforded by a back rub or a change of position may be helpful in relieving a portion of the pain (Figure 43-8). During a long labor, be certain that a woman voids about every 2 hours to keep her bladder empty; a full bladder impedes descent of the fetus. Be aware how long it has been since she last ate; she may need intravenous glucose to ward off uterine dysfunction.

If contractions are not effective, or the infant is above average size or not in good flexion, rotation through the 135° arc may not be accomplished. Uterine dysfunction may result from maternal exhaustion. The head may arrest in the transverse position (transverse arrest). Rotation may not take place (persistent occipitoposterior position). In both instances, if the fetus has reached the midportion of the pelvis, the fetus may be rotated to an anterior position with forceps and then delivered. With the woman on the delivery room table and appropriate anesthesia administered, the physician applies forceps to the fetal head and

rotates the head to the anterior position, removes the forceps, reapplies them, and delivers the infant in an occipitoanterior position (*Scanzoni's maneuver*). A small-sized infant might be delivered from the original posterior position (face-to-pubis delivery). Today, cesarean birth is often elected over rotation and extraction as the risk of a midforceps maneuver exceeds or is equal to the risk of a cesarean birth.

A woman who has had a long labor is more prone to postpartal hemorrhage and infection than others. If forceps were used for delivery, she is at risk for reproductive tract lacerations. During labor, she needs a great deal of support to prevent her from becoming panicky over the length of the labor, and she needs practical explanations of what is happening, step by step. Paradoxically, women who are best prepared for labor are often most frightened when deviations occur. Things are not going "by the book," not happening just as described by the instructor of the course they attended. Such women should have frequent reassurance that although their pattern of labor is not textbook, it is still within safe, controlled limits.

Breech Presentation. The majority of fetuses are in a breech presentation early in pregnancy. By the thirty-eighth week of gestation, however, the fetus normally turns to a cephalic presentation. Although the fetal head is the widest single diameter, the fetus's buttocks (breech), plus the lower extremities, actually take up more space. The fact that the fundus of the uterus is the largest part probably accounts for the fact that in about 97 percent of all pregnancies the fetus turns so that the buttocks and lower extremities are in the fundus.

There are several types of breech presentations. These are shown in Table 43-3. Breech presentation may occur for any of the reasons shown in Table 43-4. There are many old wives' tales about breech delivery (they are more painful, much longer, they crush the fetal head, the woman is horribly torn, and so forth). For this reason, some physicians do not tell a woman that her baby is in a breech presentation. If this choice has been made, be certain that you are not the person who reveals the information. A more current theory is to educate a woman about the actual circumstances of a breech presentation, which allows her to be a more active participant in labor.

Prolapse of the umbilical cord is more likely to occur with breech delivery than with cephalic delivery because the breech does not engage the cervix as snugly as the head does. Early rupture of the membranes tends to occur because of the poor fit of the presenting part. The inevitable contrac-

Table 43-3 Classification of Breech Presentations

Type	Description
Complete	Feet and legs are flexed on thighs; thighs are flexed on abdomen; buttocks and feet are the presenting parts.
Frank	Legs are extended and lie against abdomen and chest; feet are at the level of shoulders; buttocks are the presenting part.
Double footling	Legs are unflexed and extended; feet are the presenting part.
Single footling	One leg is unflexed and extended; one foot is the presenting part.

Table 43-4 Causes of Breech Presentation

1. Gestational age under 40 weeks.
2. Abnormality in the fetus, such as anencephaly, hydrocephalus, or meningocele. (In a fetus with hydrocephalus, the widest fetal diameter is the head, and so it retains the most "comfortable" position.)
3. Hydramnios that allows for free fetal movement, so that the fetus does not have to make a "most comfortable" choice.
4. Congenital abnormality of the uterus, such as a midseptum that traps the fetus in a breech position.
5. Any space-occupying mass in the pelvis, such as a fibroid tumor of the uterus or a placenta previa, that does not allow the head to present.
6. Pendulous abdomen. If the abdominal muscles are very lax, the uterus may fall so far forward that the fetal head comes to lie outside the pelvic brim, and so the breech presents.
7. Multiple gestation. The presenting twin cannot turn to a vertex position.
8. Unknown factors.

tion of the buttocks often causes meconium to be extruded before delivery. This is not indicative of fetal distress but is expected from the buttock's pressure. Such meconium excretion, however, can lead to meconium aspiration if the infant breaths in any amniotic fluid.

An additional complication of breech labor might occur because the breech is able to pass through the cervix before full dilatation is reached. The breech may be evident at the vulva (crowning) before the first stage of labor is complete. A woman must not push with contractions with a breech delivery until vaginal examination shows that full dilatation has been reached. If she pushes when the breech is at the vulva but cervical dilatation is not complete, the fetus may deliver up to its neck, then be unable to pass through the incompletely dilated cervix. Waiting for delivery of the aftercoming head may be lethal to the fetus from pressure of the head against the cord during the time it is awaiting dilatation. A woman may need inhalation analgesia with each contraction to keep from pushing; it is an almost uncontrollable reflex when the presenting part is at the perineum.

Breech presentation is more hazardous than a cephalic presentation as there is a higher risk for anoxia from prolapsed cord, traumatic injury to the aftercoming head (that can result in intracranial hemorrhage or anoxia), or fracture of the spine or arm. Dysfunctional labor may result because the presenting part does not fit the cervix snugly.

ASSESSMENT. With a breech presentation, the fetal heart sounds are heard high in the abdomen. Leopold's maneuvers and a vaginal examination will reveal a breech presentation. If the breech is complete and firmly engaged, the tightly stretched gluteal muscles may be mistaken on vaginal examination for a head; the natal cleft may be mistaken for the sagittal suture line. Confirmation of a breech presentation may be made either by X-ray or by sonography. Such studies also give information on pelvic diameters, fetal skull diameters, and whether a placenta previa exists or not. Also revealed is any bony fetal abnormality (such as hydrocephalus) that will make vaginal delivery impossible.

With every breech presentation, a fetal monitor and uterine contraction monitor should be in place during labor. They may make possible detection of fetal distress from a complication such as a prolapsed cord at the earliest possible moment.

DELIVERY. Cesarean birth is more and more becoming the preferred method of delivery for babies in breech presentation in order to provide the safest form of birth possible.

Even though few infants are allowed to deliver vaginally from a breech presentation, it is helpful to understand the mechanism of breech delivery. In a breech delivery, the same stages of flexion, descent, internal rotation, expulsion, and external rotation occur as in a vertex delivery (Figure 43-9).

When full dilatation is reached, a woman is allowed to push, and the breech, trunk, and shoulders are delivered. As the breech spontaneously

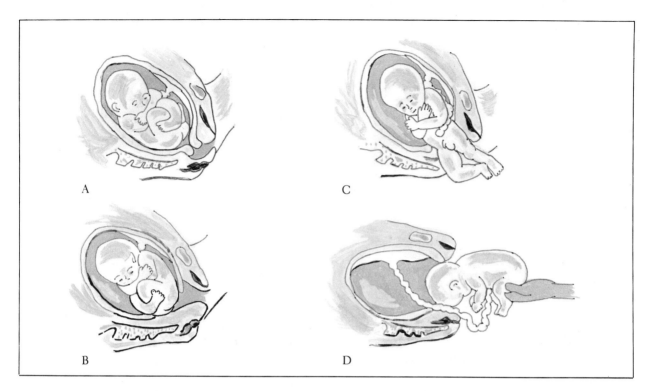

Figure 43-9 *Breech delivery. A. Position prior to labor: LSP. B. Descent and internal rotation. C. Legs being born. Note the anterior-posterior diameter best accommodates the shoulders. D. The head is born. External rotation has put the anterior-posterior diameter of the head in line with the anterior-posterior diameter of the mother's pelvis.*

emerges from the birth canal, it is steadied and supported by a sterile towel held against the infant's inferior surface. The shoulders present to the outlet with their widest diameter anteroposterior. If they do not deliver readily, the arm of the posterior shoulder may be drawn down by passing two fingers over the infant's shoulder and down the arm to the elbow, then sweeping the flexed arm across the infant's face and chest and out. The other arm is delivered in the same way. External rotation is allowed to occur to bring the head into the best outlet diameter.

Delivery of the head is the most hazardous part of the breech delivery. The umbilicus precedes the head, and a loop of cord passes down alongside the head. This loop of cord will automatically be compressed by the pressure of the head against the pelvic brim. A healthy, noncompromised fetus can survive as long as 10 minutes of cord compression. If compromising factors, such as maternal preeclampsia or hypertension or an exceptionally long first stage of labor, are present, the length of time in which the fetus may be safely delivered becomes considerably shorter.

A second danger of a breech delivery is intracranial hemorrhage. With a cephalic presentation, molding to the confines of the birth canal takes place over hours; with a breech delivery, pressure changes occur instantaneously. The result may be tentorial tears, which can cause gross motor and mental incapacity or lethal damage to the fetus. The infant who is delivered suddenly to reduce the amount of time during which there is cord compression may suffer an intracranial hemorrhage, the infant who is delivered gradually to reduce the possibility of intracranial injury may suffer hypoxia. Delivery of an aftercoming head involves a great deal of judgment and skill.

To aid delivery of the head, the trunk of the infant is usually straddled over the physician's right forearm. Two fingers of the physician's right hand are placed in the infant's mouth (Figure 43-10). The left hand is slid into the vagina, palm down, along the infant's back. Pressure is applied to the occiput to flex the head fully. Gentle traction applied to the shoulders (upward and outward) delivers the head. An aftercoming head may be delivered by the aid of Piper forceps to control the flexion and rate of descent (Figure 43-11).

EVALUATION. A mother usually inspects a breech baby following birth very closely. She is looking for the reason that made the presentation

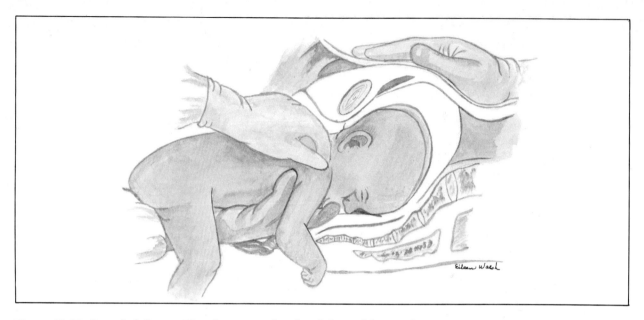

Figure 43-10. *Breech delivery. The aftercoming head is delivered by gentle pressure to flex the head fully and by gentle traction to the shoulders upward and outward. Additional pressure might be applied by an assistant to the abdominal wall to ensure head flexion.*

Figure 43-11 *Breech delivery by means of Piper forceps. With Piper forceps, traction is applied directly to the head, and damage to the infant's neck is avoided.*

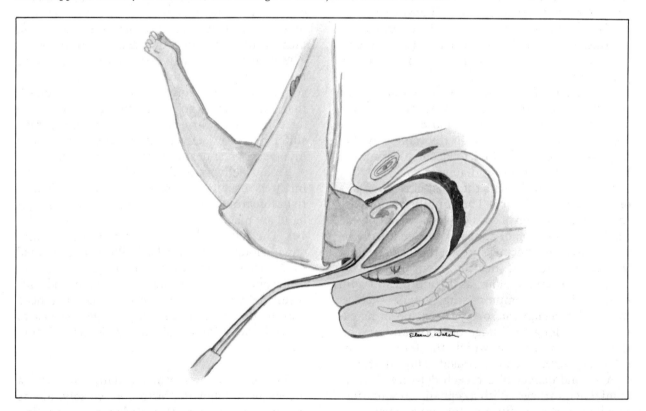

breech, as will the health care personnel who make the initial physical assessment of the infant. An infant who presented in a frank breech lie may tend to keep the legs extended and at the level of the face for the first 2 or 3 days of life; the infant who was a footling breech may tend to keep the legs extended in a footling position for the first few days. It is good to point this out to the mother, so that she does not misinterpret the strange posture of her infant.

BREECH VERSION. Because fetal risk in a breech delivery is two or three times higher than in a cephalic delivery, some physicians will attempt to change a breech position to a cephalic position at about the thirty-seventh to thirty-eighth week of gestation by external cephalic version. With the woman in a lithotomy position, the physician exerts pressure on the cervix to disengage the breech. Then, applying pressure to the woman's external abdomen, he or she attempts to turn the fetus to a cephalic presentation. This must be done with the pressure (that turns the fetus) toward the cord, to prevent tearing of the cord and placenta.

External version is not without risk. The cord may become wound around the neck of the fetus and impede fetal circulation. The maneuver may also result in premature rupture of the membranes, premature labor, or infection. In the rare instance of a short cord, the placenta may become separated, with resultant fetal anoxia and maternal blood loss. If extreme force is used, uterine rupture is a possibility. For this reason, external version is contraindicated in women with uterine scars from hysterotomy or cesarean birth.

A version will not be successful if (a) the uterine and abdominal tone is too high to effect relaxation, (b) the uterus has a septum, or (c) the fetus is so large that there is no room to turn. Even if a version is accomplished, there is no guarantee that the fetus will not revert to a breech presentation before delivery. Persistent breech presentation arouses suspicion of a bicornuate uterus, placenta previa, or a fetal abnormality such as hydrocephalus.

Face Presentation. Face (chin, or mentum) presentation is rare, but when it does occur, the diameter the fetus presents to the pelvis is often too large for delivery to proceed. A face presentation is suggested by a head that feels more prominent than normal and with no engagement apparent on Leopold's maneuvers. It is also suggested when the head and back are both felt on the same side of the uterus by the same maneuver. The

back is difficult to outline in this presentation because it is concave.

If the back is extremely concave, fetal heart tones may be transmitted to the forward thrusted chest so they may be heard on the side of the fetus where you located feet and arms. A face presentation is confirmed by vaginal examination, when the nose, mouth, or chin can be felt as the presenting part.

A fetus in a posterior position, instead of flexing the head as labor proceeds, may extend the head, resulting in a face (chin) presentation. The usual situation of occurrence is in a woman with a contracted pelvis or in the presence of a placenta previa. It may occur in the relaxed uterus of a multipara or with prematurity, hydramnios, and fetal malformation. It is a warning signal: Something abnormal is causing the chin presentation.

When a face presentation is suspected, an X-ray film or sonogram will be made to confirm it and indicate the measurements of the pelvic diameters. If the chin is anterior and the pelvic diameters are within normal limits, the infant may be delivered without difficulty (perhaps following a long first stage of labor, because the face does not mold well to make a snugly engaging part). If the chin is posterior, cesarean birth may be the choice of delivery; otherwise, it would be necessary to wait for a long posterior-to-anterior rotation to occur. Such rotation can result in uterine dysfunction or a transverse arrest.

Babies born following a chin presentation have a great deal of facial edema; their faces may be purple from ecchymotic bruising. Lip edema may be so severe that the infants are unable to nurse for a day or two. They may have to have gavage feedings to obtain enough fluid until they can suck effectively. They must be observed closely for a patent airway, and thus usually are transferred for the first 24 hours to a careful watch nursery. A mother needs to be assured that the edema is a result of the delivery and nothing else; it is transient and will disappear in a few days, with no aftermath.

Brow Presentation. A brow presentation is the rarest of the presentations. It occurs with a multipara or relaxed abdominal muscles. It almost invariably results in obstructed labor, since the head becomes jammed in the brim of the pelvis as the occipitomental diameter presents. Unless the presentation spontaneously corrects, cesarean birth will be necessary to deliver the infant safely. Brow presentations also leave the infant with extreme ecchymotic bruising on the face. Knowing that the anterior fontanelle or "soft spot" is underneath the injury, parents may need additional reassurance that the child is normal following delivery.

Transverse Lie. Transverse lie occurs in women with pendulous abdomens, with uterine masses such as fibroid tumors obstructing the lower uterine segment, with contraction of the pelvic brim, with congenital abnormalities of the uterus, or with hydramnios. It may occur in infants with hydrocephalus or other gross abnormalities that prevent the head from engaging. It may occur in prematurity, when the infant has room for free movement; in multiple gestation (particularly of the second twin); or when there is a short umbilical cord.

A transverse lie is usually obvious on inspection, when the ovoid of the uterus is found to be more horizontal than vertical. By means of Leopold's maneuvers the abnormal presentation will be detected. An X-ray film or sonogram may be taken to confirm the abnormal lie and to give information such as pelvic size.

A mature fetus cannot be delivered vaginally from this presentation. Often, the membranes rupture. Because there is no firm presenting part, the cord prolapses, or an arm may prolapse, or the shoulder obstructs the cervix. Cesarean birth is necessary.

In a grand multipara, if the X-ray film reveals no apparent abnormality, such as placenta previa or contracted pelvis, or an abnormality with the fetus, the physician may externally rotate the fetus to a cephalic presentation at the beginning of labor. If the fetus "holds" that presentation through descent, a normal delivery will result. It is important that a transverse lie be detected before the membranes rupture and the chance for a prolapsed cord occurs. Since the nurse is the first person to observe a woman on her admission to a health care facility, such an abnormal presentation could be identified almost immediately if you take the responsibility to look with Leopold's maneuvers.

Oversized Fetus (Macrosomia)

Size may become a problem in a fetus who weighs more than 4,500 gm (10 pounds); a lower weight is not likely to cause difficulty. Only 1 in 100 infants weighs this much at birth (weights up to 17 pounds have been reported). Babies of this size are most frequently born to women who are diabetic. Large babies may be associated with multiparity, as each infant born to a woman tends to be slightly larger than the one born just before.

An oversized infant may cause uterine dysfunction during labor or at delivery due to the overstretching of the fibers of the myometrium. The wide shoulders may pose a problem at delivery and cause cephalopelvic disproportion or even uterine rupture from obstruction. The large size of the fetus may be missed in an obese woman because the fetal contours are difficult to palpate. Because she is obese does not mean that she has a larger-than-usual pelvis. Pelvimetry or sonography can be used to compare the fetal size to the woman's pelvic capacity. If the infant is so oversized that vaginal delivery is not possible, cesarean birth becomes the method of choice.

There is a sizable increase in the perinatal mortality of larger infants (15 percent versus the normal 4 percent). The large-sized infant who is born vaginally has a higher risk of cervical nerve palsy, diaphragmatic nerve injury, or fractured clavicle. The mother in the postpartal period has a higher-than-usual chance of hemorrhage because the overdistended uterus may not contract as readily.

Fetal Anomalies

Fetal anomalies of the head or spine can interfere with presentation. Although these congenital anomalies are rare, the possibility they may be present should be considered with dysfunctional labor or malposition.

Hydrocephalus. Hydrocephalus, or fluid-filled, enlarged ventricles, is most frequently caused by congenital obstruction of the narrow aqueduct of Sylvius, causing cerebral spinal fluid to accumulate in the forward ventricles of the brain. As the fluid grows in amount, pressure is exerted on the brain and skull. The skull expands at the fontanelles and cartilage suture lines and the entire skull grows in size. Head growth with hydrocephalus is rare in utero, however. The head of the infant is most often normal size at birth but then begins to grow in the first few weeks of life. This phenomenon is probably related to the pressure exerted on the fetal head by the amniotic fluid and membranes. If hydrocephalus should occur in utero, vaginal delivery of the enlarged head is difficult; full obstruction and uterine rupture can occur.

Hydrocephalus can be detected in utero by palpation of the abnormally sized head. A sonogram during pregnancy or an X-ray film at term will reveal excess fluid–filled ventricles. In many instances the fetus with hydrocephalus presents breech because the largest bulk of the fetus (in this instance, the enlarged head) accommodates to the larger size of the uterine fundus. If the presentation is vertex, the head will be unengaged because it is too large to enter the pelvic inlet.

If hydrocephalus is detected by sonogram during pregnancy, the parents may elect to abort the pregnancy. If the hydrocephalus does not appear to be associated with other anomalies, however, and it is not yet at a point where brain tissue appears to be compressed, the fluid may be reduced by insertion of a catheter into the fetal ventricles by fetoscopy technique. If done just prior to delivery, vaginal delivery can be achieved with the usual close monitoring necessary for any high-risk birth. If the hydrocephalus is first detected during early labor, such a procedure is still technically possible.

If this technique is not effective in compressing the head, the infant must be delivered by cesarean birth. If the sonogram suggests that the fetus has extreme neurologic damage from brain compression or there are a multitude of congenital anomalies, the fetal head may be compressed by a needle and syringe inserted vaginally into the posterior fontanelle (in a cephalic presentation). In a breech presentation, head decompression can only be achieved when the aftercoming head has reached the perineum. These are destructive procedures. As the fluid is removed quickly, intracranial bleeding frequently results and the respiratory and circulatory centers may be destroyed.

Be certain that parents who sign permission for such a decompression are informed about what they are actually consenting to (death of the fetus). Be certain that parents who are having fetoscopy procedures done to gently and therapeutically remove cerebral spinal fluid are not told by well-meaning friends that the procedure will kill the infant (the risk of premature labor is present, but at no greater incidence than with other fetoscopy procedures).

Hydrocephalus is a bewildering congenital anomaly; why it occurs is rarely known. Fortunately it is rarely a problem associated with labor but more often with the first weeks of life, when a shunting procedure to direct the excessive fluid into the peritoneal cavity can be performed (see Chapter 46). The mother who delivers a child with hydrocephalus needs close observation in the postpartal period for hemorrhage as the enlarged head has stretched the uterus more than normally. She is usually referred for genetic counseling before she undergoes a second pregnancy although, because environmental influences can cause the defect, in most instances no genetic cause will be found.

Anencephaly. Anencephaly is absence of the cranium or top portion of the fetal head. Labor may be prolonged because without a normal sized head, there is a lack of firm cervical dilatation.

The infant's shoulders may present obstruction and perineal tearing as the cervix did not dilate wide enough for them to pass. Hydramnios may occur during the pregnancy as swallowing is governed by an intact neurologic system. The parents need to be referred for genetic counseling before they attempt another pregnancy, although in many instances, as with hydrocephalus, no genetic cause may be found.

Multiple Gestation

Twin gestations occur about 1 in every 99 conceptions. The thought of having a woman in labor with a multiple gestation causes a flurry of excitement in most people. Additional personnel have to be assembled for the delivery (two nurses to attend to possibly immature infants, a pediatrician for immature care). In the middle of all the preparatory activity it is easy to forget that a woman may be more frightened than excited. Be careful that the air of anticipation around her is not interpreted as everyone having fun but her, everyone invited to a party but her.

The first stage of labor during a multiple gestation does not differ from the first stage of a single gestation labor, except that the mother is usually instructed to come to the hospital early in labor and you should try to monitor both fetal heart rates by separate fetal monitors if possible. Coming to a hospital this early in labor will make labor seem long; urge a woman to spend the early hours of labor with an activity such as playing cards or backgammon to make the time pass quicker (Figure 43-12).

Because the babies are usually small, cord prolapse is an increased possibility after rupture of

Figure 43-12 *Labor with a multiple gestation may seem long because the couple is asked to come to the hospital early in labor. Encourage them to keep active early in labor by an activity such as cards or here, backgammon.*

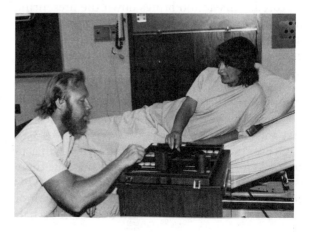

the membranes. Uterine dysfunction and premature separation of the placenta may be more common. Because of the multiple fetuses, abnormal fetal presentation may occur. Analgesia administration should be conservative, so that it will not add to any respiratory difficulties the infants may have at birth because of their immaturity. To avoid the need for analgesia or anesthesia, support breathing exercises. A woman may not have practiced well during pregnancy, anticipating that the usual methods would not apply to her because she is laboring with twins; she may need help to understand that labor contractions are the same no matter how many infants are in the uterus. The mother may have anemia and has a greater chance of developing hypertension during the pregnancy; she needs her hematocrit level and blood pressure assessed conscientiously during labor.

The first twin is usually delivered normally. Both ends of the cord of the first twin are tied or permanently clamped; if a common placenta is shared and a cord clamp should slip it should be replaced immediately or the second twin will hemorrhage through the open cord. The first twin is identified as Twin I or Twin A depending on the hospital's policy. Newborn care is begun for the first twin, but an oxytocin to begin uterine involution is not given to the mother in order to prevent compromising the circulation of the second twin.

If the presence of twins had been undetected and an oxytocic drug was given at the same time the shoulder of the first twin was delivered, the resulting tonic contractions may prevent delivery of the second twin. More often, the forceful contractions from the oxytocin cause the second twin to be delivered extremely rapidly.

The lie of the second twin is determined by external abdominal palpation. If the lie is not longitudinal, external version is attempted to make it so. The presentation is confirmed by vaginal examination, and the second set of membranes is ruptured. This action brings down the presenting part of the second twin and may initiate contractions if they are not already active. An oxytocin infusion may be begun to assist uterine contractions so that a long time span does not occur between the times of delivery. Most twin pregnancies present with both twins vertex, followed in frequency by vertex and breech, breech and vertex, and then breech and breech (Figure 43-13).

Occasionally, the placenta of the first twin separates before the second twin is born, and there is sudden, profuse bleeding at the vagina. This creates a risk for the woman; the uterus cannot contract as it normally would and thereby halt the bleeding because it is still filled with the second baby. If the separation of the first placenta caused loosening of the second placenta, or if a common placenta is involved, the fetal heart sounds of the second twin will immediately register distress, and he or she will have to be delivered at once for survival.

Mothers usually want to inspect twins thoroughly following the births. The time allowed for this inspection will depend on the infants' weights and conditions. Most mothers of twins worry that the hospital will confuse the two through improper identification. Review with her and her support person the careful measures that are being taken to ensure correct identification.

Most women who have a multiple birth have difficulty believing that it is real. They need to recount over and over their surprise and to view both their infants together to prove to themselves that it is true. If they were not able to inspect the infants thoroughly immediately following birth because of their low birth weight and the danger of chilling, they need the time to do so as soon as possible, to dispel all the fears they had throughout pregnancy that the babies would be born joined or deformed.

The mother needs to be observed very carefully in the immediate postpartal period because, overdistended, her uterus may have difficulty contracting; she is prone to postpartal hemorrhage from uterine atony. The infants need careful assessment to determine their true gestational age and whether a phenomenon such as twin-to-twin transfusion has occurred (see Chapter 47).

The Birth Canal: Difficulty with the Passageway

The third problem that can cause dystocia is a contraction or narrowing of the passageway, or the birth canal. The pelvis may be contracted (narrow) at the inlet, the midpelvis, or the outlet. This complication is termed *cephalopelvic disproportion* (CPD), or a disproportion between the size of the normal fetal head and the pelvic diameters.

Inlet Contraction

Inlet contraction is ordinarily due to rickets in early life or an inherited small pelvis. Rickets is more common in black women than in Caucasians and at the lower socioeconomic levels. However, it is a fallacy to believe that all people are eating adequate diets just because they have the money to afford them, or that rickets occurs only in low socioeconomic groups.

Inlet contraction is defined as narrowing of the

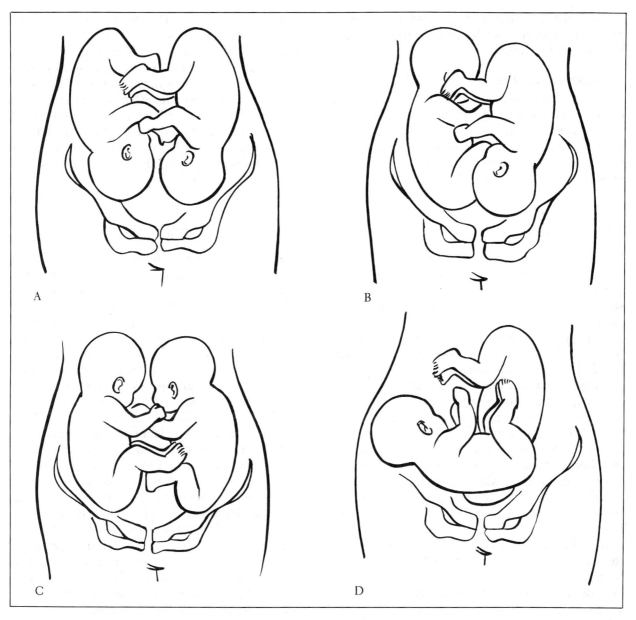

Figure 43-13 *Four different twin presentations. A. Both infants vertex. B. One infant vertex and one breech. C. Both infants breech. D. One infant vertex and one in a transverse lie.*

anteroposterior diameter to less than 11 cm, or of a maximum transverse diameter of 12 cm or less. In primigravidas, the fetal head normally engages at the thirty-sixth to thirty-eighth week of pregnancy. This event occurring before labor begins is proof that the pelvic inlet is adequate. Following the general rule that "what goes in, comes out," a head that engages, or proves it fits into the pelvic brim, will probably also be able to pass through the midpelvis and through the outlet.

A woman who has delivered a previous infant vaginally without problems has proved that her birth canal is adequate. When engagement does not occur in a primigravida, suspicion should be very high that either a fetal abnormality (larger-than-usual head) or a pelvic abnormality (smaller-than-usual pelvis) is causing the lack of engagement. As a rule, engagement does not take place in multigravidas until labor begins.

Every primigravida should have pelvic measurements taken and recorded before the twenty-fourth week of pregnancy, so that a delivery decision can be made, based on these measurements and on the assumption that the fetus will be of average size.

With cephalopelvic disproportion, because the fetus does not engage but remains "floating," malposition may occur that compounds an already difficult situation. The possibility of cord prolapse is very high with a floating head if membranes should rupture.

Outlet Contraction

Outlet contraction is defined as the narrowing of the transverse diameter of the lower portion of the pelvis to less than 11 cm. This is the distance between the ischial tuberosities, a measurement that is easy to make during a prenatal visit so can be anticipated before labor begins.

Trial Labor

If a woman has a borderline (just adequate) inlet measurement, and the fetal lie and position are good, her physician may allow her a trial labor to see whether labor can progress normally; this is allowed to continue as long as descent of the presenting part and dilation of the cervix are occurring. Fetal heart sounds and uterine contractions should be monitored during a trial labor. It is especially important that the urinary bladder be kept emptied to allow all the space available to be used by the fetal head (urge a woman to void every 2 hours). Assess fetal heart rate carefully following rupture of the membranes as, if the fetal head is high, there is increased danger of prolapsed cord and anoxia in the fetus. If after a definite period (6 to 12 hours) inadequate progress is made in labor, the woman will be scheduled for a cesarean birth.

It is difficult for women to undertake a labor they know they may not be able to complete. Some physicians let a woman know that the labor is a trial one; others feel that it goes better if she does not know because she prepares better and relaxes more.

It is important that a woman does not interpret a trial labor as a whim of her physician. Labor is painful, and a woman cannot have much confidence in her physician if she thinks that he or she is putting her through pain "just for the fun of it." Emphasize that it is best for the baby to be born vaginally. However, do not overstress this fact. If the trial labor fails and cesarean birth is scheduled, you will need to explain why a cesarean birth will be good for the baby.

Some women having a trial labor feel very much as if they themselves are on trial. When dilatation does not occur, they feel discouraged and inadequate, as if they have failed. A woman may not even have realized how much she wanted this trial labor to work, until she is told that it is not working. The father is as frightened and feels as helpless as his partner when a devia-

tion occurs in labor. He makes comments such as, "The doctor knows best" or "This is a good hospital, and nothing bad is going to happen to the baby," but his reassurances sound as false to him and the woman as they do to you. The couple needs assurance from health care personnel that a cesarean birth is not an inferior method of delivery but an alternative method; in this instance, it is the method of choice. A cesarean birth will secure for them the goal they and you both seek: a healthy mother and a healthy child.

Induction of Labor

Inducing labor is an attempt to initiate labor (a) before the time when it would have occurred spontaneously because the fetus is in danger, or (b) because it does not occur spontaneously, and the fetus appears to be at term. The primary reasons for inducing labor are the presence of preeclampsia, eclampsia, severe hypertension or diabetes, Rh sensitization, premature rupture of the membranes, intrauterine growth retardation, and postmaturity (situations in which it seems risky for the fetus to remain in utero).

Before induction of labor is begun, the following conditions should be present: The fetus is in a longitudinal lie and at a point of extrauterine viability; the cervix is ripe, or ready for delivery; a presenting part is engaged; and there is no cephalopelvic disproportion. The procedure should be used cautiously with multiple gestation, hydramnios, grand parity, maternal age over 35 years, and in the presence of previous uterine scars. It carries a risk of uterine rupture, a decrease in the fetal blood supply from poor cotyledon filling, and premature separation of the placenta.

To determine whether a cervix is ripe, Bishop (1964) has devised a method of scoring certain criteria for ripeness (Table 43-5). If a woman's total score is 9 or above on the items in the table, the cervix is considered ripe and should respond to induction. In addition, a fetal estimation of maturity should be made, such as an L/S ratio or sonogram biparietal diameter.

Induction of Labor by Oxytocin

Oxytocin initiates contractions in a uterus at a pregnancy's term. Aside from fetal risk, induction by oxytocin is always a procedure with some degree of associated risk for the mother because each woman responds to the drug to a different degree. An oxytocin is never administered intramuscularly during labor in order to control the length of its effect. The half-life, its functioning

Table 43-5 Scoring of Cervix for Readiness for Elective Induction

	Score			
Factor	0	1	2	3
Dilatation (in cm)	0	1–2	3–4	5–6
Effacement (%)	0–30	40–50	60–70	80
Station	−3	−2	−1 to 0	+1 to +2
Consistency	Firm	Medium	Soft	—
Position	Posterior	Mid	Anterior	—

Source: Bishop, E. (1964). Pelvic scoring for elective induction. *Obstetrics and Gynecology, 24,* 266.

length, of oxytocin is about 3 minutes with intravenous administration. With intramuscular administration, hours might pass before the serum level decreases.

Induction is begun by the administration of a dilute intravenous form of oxytocin such as Pitocin or Syntocinon. The drug is used in the proportion of approximately 10 IU in 1,000 ml of normal saline. Since 10 IU of oxytocin is the same as 10,000 *milliunits* (mU), each milliliter of this solution will contain 10 *milliunits* of oxytocin; and each 0.1 ml contains 1 mU. Physician's orders for administration of oxytocin for induction generally designate the number of milliunits to be administered per minute. The oxytocin solution must be piggy-backed with a maintenance intravenous solution such as 5% dextrose and water; then if the oxytocin needs to be turned off abruptly during the induction, the intravenous line will not be lost. A minidrip regulator and a constant infusion pump should both be used to control the small amount of fluid given and to ensure a uniform infusion rate even when the woman changes position (Figure 43-14). A physician should be immediately available during the entire procedure to ensure safety.

Infusions are usually begun at a rate of 1 or 2 mU per minute. If there is no response, the infusion is gradually increased in amount every 15 to 30 minutes by small increments of 2 to 4 mU until contractions do begin. The rate should not be increased over 16 mU per minute without checking for further instructions. Such a rapid rate is apt to cause tetanic contractions.

Both fetal heart sounds and uterine contractions should be continuously monitored during the procedure. A woman's pulse and blood pressure and the fetal heart rate should be taken every 15 minutes. When cervical dilation reaches 4 cm,

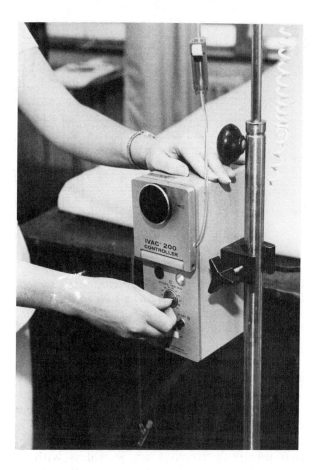

Figure 43-14 *Oxytocin infused to induce labor needs special precautions taken in order to be administered safely. Always use an infusion pump for accuracy. (Courtesy of the Department of Medical Photography, Children's Hospital, Buffalo, N.Y.)*

artificial rupture of the membranes will further induce labor; the infusion can usually be discontinued at that point.

Women who are having labor induced should never be left alone. Excessive stimulation of the uterus by oxytocin may lead to tonic uterine contractions, with fetal death or, in extreme instances, rupture of the uterus. Contractions should occur no more than every 2 minutes, should not be over 50 mm Hg pressure, and should last no more than 70 seconds. The resting pressure between contractions should not exceed 15 mm Hg by monitor (Figure 43-15). If contractions become more frequent or longer in duration than these safe limits or signs of fetal distress occur, stop the intravenous infusion and seek help. It is better for contractions to slow from a period of inadequate oxytocin administration because you stopped the infusion unnecessarily than for tonic contractions to continue because you are unsure of whether to proceed. As mentioned, because of the short half-life of oxytocin,

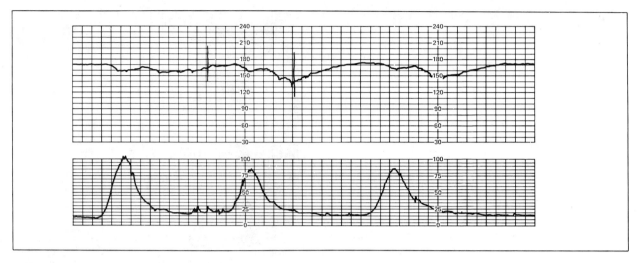

Figure 43-15 *Hypertonic uterine contractions caused by an oxytocin infusion. Contractions are as high as 100 mg Hg intensity. Late decelerations and a FHR of 170 are present. From Paul, R. H. (1971).* Fetal intensive care, *Los Angeles, Calif.: University of Southern California.*

stopping the flow rate almost immediately stops the oxytocin effect.

Women have heard many scare stories about induction of labor. They have been told that it is more painful, "so different" from normal labor that breathing exercises are worthless with it; that it goes very fast and so is harmful to the fetus, or goes very slowly and therefore is harmful to the fetus. In fact, induced labors tend to have a slightly shorter first stage than the average, unassisted labor. This is an advantage to the woman, however, not a disadvantage. Once contractions begin by this method, they are basically normal uterine contractions. A woman needs to be assured of this normality so that she does not fight them, become unnecessarily tense, and then be unable to use her breathing techniques effectively. She should be encouraged to begin breathing exercises with beginning contractions.

Because oxytocin has an antidiuretic effect, there will be a decreased urine flow during its administration. The result may be water intoxication in the woman, first manifested by headache and vomiting. If these danger signals are observed during induction of labor, they should be reported and the infusion discontinued. Water intoxication in its severest form can lead to convulsions, coma, and death because of the shift in interstitial tissue fluid it causes. Keep an accurate intake and output record and test and record specific gravity of urine to detect discrepancies in the pattern. Limit the amount of intravenous fluid to 150 ml per hour by being certain that the mainline intravenous fluid flows at a slow rate (not over 2.5 ml per minute).

Because induction of labor with oxytocin may predispose a newborn to hyperbilirubinemia and jaundice, and because water intoxication in a woman may occur especially if a balanced electrolyte solution is not used, induction is no longer an elective procedure. It should be used only when delivery of an infant in this way is less hazardous than the fetus's remaining in utero. Important considerations of induction are shown in the Nursing Care Highlight on page 1023.

Augmentation by Oxytocin

Augmentation of labor indicates that labor contractions began spontaneously but then were so weak, irregular, and ineffective that an oxytocin augmentation or assist was needed to strengthen them.

The same precautions regarding oxytocin assist are used as for primary induction of labor. A uterus may be very responsive to oxytocin when it is used as an assist. Be certain that it is increased in small increments only and fetal heart sounds are well monitored during the procedure.

Induction of Labor by Prostaglandins

Labor may be induced by the use of prostaglandins such as PGE_2 and PGF_{2a}. These are most often administered by vaginal suppository. Unfortunately, prostaglandins cause nausea and vomiting in most women. Induction of labor thus becomes an uncomfortable procedure, with the woman so ill that she cannot enjoy it. Prostaglandin administration will not be a preferable

Nursing Care Highlight
The Woman Having Induction of Labor

1. Be certain that a woman meets the criteria for labor induction before preparing the solution: No cephalopelvic disproportion is suspected; the fetal head is engaged and the cervix is ripe.
2. Always prepare oxytocin as a piggy-back solution, being extremely careful of the dose used.
3. Both a uterine and fetal heart rate monitor should be used continuously during labor induction.
4. Observe that contractions occur no less than 2 minutes apart and are no longer than 70 seconds in duration.
5. Increase oxytocin flow only in increments of 2 to 4 mU to avoid causing hypertonic contractions or uterine tetany.
6. Urge and support a woman to use breathing exercises and to remain on her left side during labor to offer a good blood supply to the uterine muscle.
7. If uterine contractions should become too strong or too frequent or fetal bradycardia, tachycardia, or abnormal decelerations should occur, discontinue oxytocin solution immediately.
8. Do not increase the rate over 16 mU per minute without specific directions; this high a flow rate invariably leads to tonic uterine contractions.

---

method for induction until it can be refined to eliminate these side effects.

Forceps Delivery

If a woman is unable to push with contractions in the pelvic division of labor (such as after regional anesthesia), cessation of progress in the second stage of labor occurs; if the fetus is in an abnormal position, forceps application will be necessary to deliver the baby. A fetus in distress from a complication such as prolapsed cord can be delivered more quickly by the use of forceps. Their use can reduce the work a woman has to accomplish during labor by cutting down the amount of pushing she must do. Forceps are designed to prevent pressure from being exerted on the fetal head. They may be used as the fetal head reaches the perineum to reduce pressure and avoid subdural hemorrhage in the fetus from too much force.

Forceps are steel instruments constructed of two blades that slide together at their shaft to form a handle. Forceps are applied first by one blade being slipped into a woman's vagina next to the fetal head, then the other side being slipped into place. Next, the shafts of the instrument are brought together in the midline to form the handle.

A forceps delivery is an *outlet* procedure when the forceps are applied once the fetal head reaches the perineum. When the fetal head is at the level of the ischial spines and the biparietal diameter is through the inlet (engaged), this is a *midforceps* delivery. Cesarean birth today carries less risk to the fetus than does the use of midforceps, so such a procedure is rarely seen. If forceps are applied to a nonengaged head, this is *high* forceps use. High forceps are not used in preference to cesarean birth today. Some anesthesia, at least a pudendal block, is necessary for forceps application to achieve pelvic relaxation and reduce pain.

If the obstetrician doing the procedure is teaching a house staff officer or a medical student and so is detailing and explaining the procedure while working, the mother and father may become frightened at hearing that blades are being slipped past their baby's head. Listen for this kind of exchange and alleviate worries by explaining terms (they are not really blades but blunt, pointed handles).

Four common types of forceps are described in Table 43-6. In order to apply forceps, membranes must be ruptured, no cephalopelvic disproportion must be present, the cervix must be fully dilated, and the woman's bladder must be empty. An episiotomy is usually used to prevent perineal tearing from pressure on the perineum.

Vacuum Extraction

A fetus may be delivered by means of a vacuum extractor in place of forceps. With the fetal head at the perineum, a disk-shaped cup is pressed against the fetal scalp over the posterior fon-

Table 43-6 Common Types of Delivery Forceps

Name	Description
Barton	Forceps with a hinge in the right blade used to rotate the fetal head to a more favorable position, such as ROP to OA.
Kielland	Forceps with short handles and a marked cephalic curve used to rotate the fetal head to a more favorable position, such as ROP to OA.
Piper	Used to deliver the head in a breech presentation.
Simpson	Forceps used most commonly as outlet forceps.
Tarnier	Axis traction forceps.

tanelle. When vacuum pressure is applied, air beneath the cup is sucked out and the cup then adheres so tightly to the fetal scalp that traction on the cord leading to the cup will deliver the fetus.

Vacuum extraction has the advantage over forceps delivery in that little anesthesia is necessary and it causes fewer lacerations of the birth canal. With less anesthesia, the infant is less depressed at birth. It has a disadvantage of causing a marked caput that may still be noticeable as long as 7 days after birth. A mother may need to be assured that this swelling will decrease rapidly and is harmless to her infant. Vacuum extraction should not be used as a method of delivery if scalp blood sampling was done; the suction pressure can cause severe bleeding. Nor is it advantageous for preterm infants because of the softness of the preterm skull.

Although vacuum extraction is not used extensively in the United States, it is popular in Europe and the developing countries. In these locales, it may be used not only as an outlet procedure but to aid descent after full dilatation has occurred.

Anomalies of the Placenta and Cord

The placenta and cord are always examined following birth to ascertain whether any abnormalities are present. The normal placenta weighs about 500 gm and is 15 to 20 cm in diameter and 1.5 to 3.0 cm thick. Its weight is about one sixth that of the fetus. A placenta may be unusually enlarged in a woman with diabetes. In certain diseases, such as syphilis or erythroblastosis, the placenta may be so large that it weighs half as much as the fetus. If the uterus has scars or a septum, the placenta may be wide in diameter, as it was forced to spread out to find implantation space.

Placenta Succenturiata

A succenturiate placenta (Figure 43-16A) has one or more accessory lobes connected to the main placenta by blood vessels. No fetal abnormality is associated with it. However, it is important that it be recognized, because the small lobes may be retained in the uterus at delivery, leading to severe maternal hemorrhage. On inspection, the

Figure 43-16 *Abnormal placental formation. A. Placenta succenturiata. B. Placenta circumvallata. C. Battledore placenta. (From Clinical Education Aid, No. 12, Ross Laboratories, Columbus, Ohio, 1963.)*

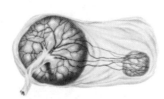
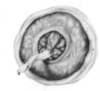
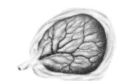

Placenta Succenturiata   Placenta Circumvallata   Battledore Placenta

A   B   C

placenta will appear torn at the edge, or torn blood vessels may extend beyond the edge of the placenta. The remaining lobes must be removed from the uterus manually to prevent hemorrhage in the mother from poor uterine contraction.

Placenta Circumvallata

Ordinarily, the chorion membrane begins at the edge of the placenta and spreads to envelop the fetus, and no chorion covers the fetal side of the placenta. In placenta circumvallata, the fetal side of the placenta is covered to some extent with chorion (Figure 43-16B). The umbilical cord enters the placenta at the usual midpoint, and large vessels spread out from there. They end abruptly at the point where the chorion folds back onto the surface, however. (In *placenta marginata*, the fold of chorion reaches just to the edge of the placenta.) Although, again, no abnormalities are associated with this type of placenta, its presence should be noted.

Battledore Placenta

In a battledore placenta, the cord is inserted marginally rather than centrally (Figure 43-16C). This anomaly is rare and has no known clinical significance.

Velamentous Insertion of the Cord

In this situation, the cord, instead of entering the placenta directly, separates into small vessels that reach the placenta by spreading across a fold of amnion. This form of cord insertion is most frequently found with multiple pregnancy. It can lead to exsanguination of the fetus if these cord vessels are torn when the membranes rupture. Its presence is yet another reason for the fetal heart rate to be monitored following rupture of the membranes.

Placenta Accreta

Placenta accreta is unusually deep attachment of the placenta to the uterine myometrium. The placenta will not loosen and deliver; attempts to remove it manually may lead to extreme hemor-

rhage because of the deep attachment. Hysterectomy may be necessary at that point.

Vasa Previa

The umbilical vessels of a velamentous cord insertion can cross the cervical os and be delivered prior to the fetus. In this arrangement, the vessels may tear with cervical dilatation just as with placenta previa. Sudden fetal blood loss would result. Before the use of any instrument, such as an internal fetal monitor, structures should be identified to prevent accidental tearing of a vasa previa. Such an infant needs to be delivered by cesarean birth.

A Two-Vessel Cord

The absence of one of the umbilical arteries is associated with congenital heart and kidney anomalies. The insult that caused the loss of the vessel probably affected other mesoderm germ layer structures as well. The absence of the vessel is noticed as the cord is inspected immediately following birth. Mark prominently on the infant's chart that only two vessels are present. Many people draw a circle with three smaller circles inside to indicate a three-vessel cord (Figure 34-7). Do not mistake this important mark on a chart for only a cute smiling face.

The child needs to be observed carefully for other anomalies in the newborn period. Inspection of a cord must be made immediately as it begins to dry quickly, and the cut surface will then be distorted in appearance.

Unusual Cord Length

An unusually short umbilical cord can result in premature separation of the placenta or an abnormal fetal lie. An unusually long cord can be compromised more easily due to a tendency to twist or knot. The length of the umbilical cord rarely varies to these extremes, however. An occasional cord will actually form a knot, but the natural pulsations of the blood through the vessels and their muscle walls keep the blood flow adequate. It is not unusual for a cord to wrap once around the fetal neck—again, with no interference to fetal circulation.

Utilizing Nursing Process

Nursing care organization and planning is essential when a complication of labor and delivery occurs. Many times a nurse first detects a devia-

tion from normal and thus is the first person capable of preventing fetal distress or injury to the mother.

Assessment

One of the chief assessment measures to detect deviations from normal during labor and delivery is fetal and uterine monitoring. Working with such apparatus involves explaining to parents its importance, winning their cooperation, and using judgment to read the various patterns. Monitoring with high-risk mothers entails problems not found in other high-risk areas, such as intensive care units. In the latter situation, the person being monitored is admitted to the unit because he or she is very ill; the person, knowing the seriousness of the illness, accepts almost any monitoring or other procedure without protest. He or she lies still to prevent artifacts on the tracing.

A woman in labor feels well; she has pain but it is controllable pain. She moves more and so may feel "trapped" by monitoring equipment. Her movement causes artifacts on tracings and necessitates frequent adjustment of equipment to achieve a clear tracing. Learn to accept this problem as the result of caring for basically well women; accept it as a favorable circumstance, not an unfavorable one.

Analysis

The North American Association of Nursing Diagnosis has accepted no diagnosis specific to the deviations of labor and delivery. Many nursing diagnoses can be modified, however, to become specific to these hours. "Fear related to a complication of labor," "Potential for ineffective labor related to fatigue," or "Fetal tachycardia related to cord compression" are examples of nursing diagnoses that reflect the problems caused by deviations from the normal in labor and delivery. Goal setting during this time is often difficult, and one of the ways that you may be most helpful to a couple is to help them define their goal. A woman typically says early in labor that having no monitoring equipment used or no episiotomy is her goal in labor. When the baby is detected to be in a breech lie, however, discussing with her that what she really wants is a healthy baby will allow her to agree to these implementations.

Planning

A complication of labor and delivery invariably becomes, if not an emergency situation, at least a priority action one. Planning must be done efficiently based on the individual circumstance so that when the moment of action is at hand, delivery can be accomplished without hesitation or failure.

Implementations

Implementations during a high-risk situation in labor and delivery involve dependent, independent, and interdependent actions. All actions must safeguard both the woman and the fetus while providing psychological reassurance for the woman and her support person.

Evaluation

Evaluation of patient care goals may be a sad period because not every couple who experiences a deviation from the normal in labor and delivery will be able to have a perfect child. Some deviations will be too extreme; some implementations will not be maximally effective due to individual circumstances. Some infants will die; some women will be left unable to bear future children. Evaluation will lead to new analysis that the couple's chief need at that point is to grieve for the child and life style that can no longer be theirs.

Nursing Care Planning

Angie Baco is a 42-year-old woman you care for in labor. The following is a nursing care plan you might design for her at admission.

Problem Area. Gestational diabetes.

Assessment

Patient awoke with labor contractions this morning. Called M.D. and told to take no insulin; report to hospital instead. Routinely takes 10 units NPH and 4 units regular insulin daily. Concerned now because it is about an hour past her usual time of injection. Had a negative nonstress test 2 days ago; asking if 38 weeks' gestation has been long enough that baby will not be immature. Husband with her. Asked if fetal monitor will reveal whether fetus has a heart defect or not (previous child had congenital heart disease and died at birth).

Urine 2+, neg. FHR: 130. Contractions: 30-second duration, 30 minute frequency; intensity, 30–45 mm Hg on monitor.

Analysis

Fear related to compound problem of gestational diabetes, 38-week gestation, and previous child with CHD.

Locus of Decision Making. Shared.

Goal. Patient to deliver well child vaginally.

Criteria.

1. Fetal heart tones to remain within normal limits by monitor.
2. Insulin-glucose levels to be maintained by continuous insulin infusion per M.D. order.
3. Blood sugars to be monitored q2h and to be within normal limits.

Nursing Orders

1. Explain purpose of monitors (external until membranes are ruptured, then internal).
2. Expain purpose of intravenous infusion and balance of glucose and insulin.
3. Maintain NPO.
4. Fasting blood sugar drawn. Repeat q2h.
5. Catheter inserted for urine testing q2h.
6. Schedule pelvimetry by X-ray for cephalopelvic disproportion per M.D. order.
7. Routine temperature, pulse and respiration recordings.

————————

At 4 hours into labor, you make the following additional assessments: Patient asking if blood sugar level is all right. A friend told her that if her baby was going to die, this is the time (in labor) that it would happen. Very apprehensive of any change in sound of fetal monitor. Asking for something to eat "to keep up energy."

Assessment
Internal monitor inserted. FHR baseline 120–130; beat-to-beat variability 5–10 bpm. Contractions still minimal; 30–45 mm Hg by monitor; duration, 30 seconds; frequency, 20 minutes.

Continuous IV infusion of regular insulin and normal saline infusing at 2 minidrops/min by IVAC. Second IV of 5% dextrose in Ringer's lactate infusing at 30 drops/min.

Blood sugars: fasting: 100 mg/100 ml; 2h: 92 mg/100 ml.

Pelvimetry report; No difficulty with vaginal delivery expected.

Analysis
Increased concern related to well-meant but unfortunate remark of friend.

Goal. Unchanged.

Criteria. Unchanged.

Nursing Orders
1. Continue to reassure that fetal heart tones are good.
2. Continue IV infusion; blood sugars and urine testing q2h per M.D. order.
3. Explain reason for NPO as glucose solution is infusing.

————————

Mrs. Baco's labor progresses slowly; after an additional 2 hours, her physician orders an oxytocin infusion begun to assist with contractions.

Assessment
Both parents growing discouraged with labor progress. Happy to hear that oxytocin assist will be started to strengthen contractions.

Both parents are watching monitor patterns carefully; noticeably apprehensive.

Analysis
Unchanged.

Goal. Unchanged.

Criteria. Unchanged.

Nursing Orders
1. Explain all new equipment used with both parents.
2. Syntocinon IV (10,000 mU in 1,000 ml 0.9 saline) begun at 12 minidrops per minute (2 mU per minute) added on to existing IV.
3. Internal fetal and uterine monitors in place.
4. FHR, BP, pulse, and respirations to be taken every 15 minutes.
5. Duration, frequency, and strength of contractions to be noted every 15 minutes.
6. Oxytocin infusion to be advanced in 2 mU per minute increments (up to 16 mU per minute) until contractions reach 60-second duration, 2-minute frequency per M.D. order.
7. Oxytocin to be discontinued and M.D. notified if FHR is above 160 or below 120; baseline variability is under 5 bpm; late decelerations occur; contractions are longer than 60 seconds; resting pressure of contractions is over 15 mm Hg; frequency is less than 2 minutes; general apprehension, confusion, or headache is present.

Questions for Review

Multiple Choice

1. Mrs. Martin is a woman you care for in labor. Her contractions are 2 minutes apart but rarely are over 50 mm Hg in strength; the resting tone is high: 20 to 25 mm Hg. She asks you what she can do to make contractions more effective. Based on the following, your response would be that
   a. she needs to rest because her contractions are hypertonic.
   b. her physician will order oxytocin to strengthen contractions.
   c. hypotonic contractions of this kind will strengthen by themselves.
   d. walking around will make hypertonic contractions more regular.

2. Mrs. Martin has an intravenous infusion of 5% dextrose/water begun. Following this, which advice below would you give her?
   a. lie perfectly still so as not to dislodge the needle
   b. not to get out of bed once the needle is in place
   c. lie on her back to allow for optimal flow
   d. try to forget the fluid line is in place

3. Mrs. Martin's contractions become effective and dilatation begins. At 8 cm dilatation, fetal heart rate suddenly slows. On perineal inspection you observe the fetal cord has prolapsed. Your first action should be to
   a. turn her to her left side.
   b. place her in a knee-chest position.
   c. replace the cord with gentle pressure.
   d. cover the exposed cord with a dry, sterile wrap.

4. Mrs. Wheeler is a woman in labor with diabetes mellitus. She is 37 weeks' pregnant and going to be induced with oxytocin. Which statement below reflects the induction technique you would anticipate her physician will order?
   a. administer Pitocin as a 20 cc bolus of saline
   b. administer the Pitocin in two divided intramuscular sites
   c. administer the oxytocin dilated in 1,000 ml intravenous fluid
   d. infuse at least 1,000 ml of fluid hourly to maintain blood pressure

5. After an hour of oxytocin therapy, Mrs. Wheeler states she is becoming dizzy and nauseated. Your best action would be to
   a. assess the rate of flow of the oxytocin infusion.
   b. discontinue the oxytocin infusion.
   c. assess her vaginally for full dilatation.
   d. instruct her to breathe in and out rapidly.

6. After an additional hour of Pitocin administration by intravenous route, you assess Mrs. Wheeler's contractions to be 80 seconds in length. Your first action should be to
   a. slow the infusion to under 10 gtts per minute.
   b. increase the flow rate of piggy-backed dextrose/water infusion.
   c. discontinue the Pitocin infusion.
   d. discontinue the entire intravenous infusion.

7. Mrs. Wheeler develops a pathologic retraction ring. On assessment, you would expect to find its appearance as
   a. mottling, surrounding the cervix.
   b. an ecchymotic area over the symphysis pubis.
   c. a line of indentation over the lower abdomen.
   d. a protruding circle over the uterine fundus.

8. The importance of the development of a pathologic retraction ring in terms of planning care is that
   a. it precedes uterine rupture.
   b. it suggests cesarean birth is no longer possible.
   c. it denotes a multiple pregnancy is present.
   d. it means the pelvic division of labor is beginning.

9. Mrs. Young is a para 6, gravida 7. She is only in the hospital 15 minutes when she begins to deliver precipitously. The fetal head begins to deliver as you walk into the labor room. Your best action would be to
   a. place a hand gently on the fetal head to guide delivery.
   b. ask her to push with the next contraction so delivery is rapid.
   c. assess blood pressure and pulse to detect placental bleeding.
   d. attach a fetal monitor to determine fetal status.

Discussion

1. Mrs. Taylor is a woman whose fetus is found to be in a breech presentation and thus will be delivered by a cesarean birth. What are the reasons that cesarean birth is most often the choice for a breech presentation today?
2. A lengthy labor is both a physical and psychological stress to a woman and her support person. What measures could you take to lessen the couple's stress?
3. While caring for Mrs. Herman in labor, you notice a prolapsed cord has occurred. What emergency care actions would you take?

Suggested Readings

Angelini, O. J. (1980). Intrapartum management of the large infant. *Issues in Health Care of Woman, 2,* 83.

Artinian, B. (1984). Collaborative planning—prenatal, labor, delivery, and neonatal settings. *J.O.G.N. Nursing, 13,* 105.

Bishop, E. (1964). Pelvic scoring for elective induction. *Obstetrics and Gynecology, 24,* 266.

Brengman, S. L., et al. (1983). Ritodrine hydrochloride and preterm labor. *American Journal of Nursing, 83,* 537.

Calvert, J. (1981). Breech presentation. *Nursing Mirror, 153,* V.

Cranley, M. S. (1983). Prenatal risk. *J.O.G.N. Nursing, 12,* 13.

Harris, J. L. (1984). Preterm labor: Who is at risk, who can be helped, and how. *Consultant, 24,* 256.

Heffron, C. H., et al. (1978). Abnormal labor: Diagnosis and management. *Perinatal Care, 2,* 14.

Hibbard, B. (1981). Shock in obstetrics. *Nursing Mirror, 153,* IX.

Hugh, A., et al. (1978). Monitoring fetal arterial oxygen continually during labor. *Contemporary Obstetrics and Gynecology, 12,* 73.

Ishida, Y. (1980). How to deal with grief in childbirth. *Female Patient, 5,* 74.

Kelley, M., et al. (1982). Hypertension in pregnancy, labor, delivery and postpartum. *American Journal of Nursing, 82,* 813.

Lamont, R. F. (1982). Management of preterm labour. *Midwife Health Visitor and Community Nurse, 18,* 282.

Mead, P. B. (1982). Maternal and fetal infection related to internal fetal monitoring. *Perinatal Press, 6,* 127.

Peterson, G. (1983). Addressing complications of childbirth in the prenatal setting . . . discussion of birth complications should decrease fear. *Journal of Nurse Midwifery, 28,* 25.

Phillips, L. (1981). The effects of perinatal death. *Midwife Health Visitor and Community Nurse, 17,* 18.

Quilligan, E. J. (1979). Identifying true fetal distress. *Contemporary Obstetrics and Gynecology, 13,* 89.

Shearer, E. C. (1982). Education for vaginal birth after cesarean. *Birth, 9,* 31.

44

The Woman Who Develops a Complication During the Puerperium

OBJECTIVES

Following mastery of the contents of this chapter, you should be able to

1. Describe common deviations from normal during the puerperium.
2. Assess a woman for deviations from the normal during the puerperium.
3. State a nursing diagnosis related to deviations from the normal during the puerperium.
4. Plan implementations that meet the special and individual needs of a postpartum mother with a complication.
5. Describe implementations for the care of a woman with a puerperium complication such as hemorrhage, infection, hypertension of pregnancy, or postpartal psychosis.
6. Evaluate the goal outcomes based on established criteria.
7. Analyze the meaning of postpartal complications to a woman, her family, and her bonding relationship.
8. Synthesize knowledge of puerperium complications with nursing process to achieve quality maternal-newborn nursing care.

THE MAJORITY OF COMPLICATIONS of the puerperium are preventable, a concept to keep in mind when caring for a postpartal woman. Complications must be prevented because they automatically submit a woman to an experience that can be frightening and painful—and may leave her afraid of or physically incapable of bearing more children. As a category, they *are avoidable*. Major complications which occur are hemorrhage, infection, and psychological depression.

Hemorrhage

Hemorrhage, the leading cause of maternal mortality associated with childbearing, is possible all through pregnancy, but it is a major danger in the immediate postpartal period. In a normal delivery, the average blood loss is 300 to 350 ml. Postpartal hemorrhage is defined as any blood loss from the uterus greater than 500 ml within a 24-hour period. Hemorrhage may be either immediate, that is, occurring in the first 24 hours, or late, occurring during the remaining days of the 6-week puerperium. The greatest danger of bleeding is in the first 24 hours because of the grossly denuded and unprotected area left after detachment of the placenta.

There are four main reasons for postpartal hemorrhage: uterine atony, lacerations, retained placental fragments, and disseminated intravascular coagulation. The primary nursing diagnosis concerned with any hemorrhage is loss of circulation related to the hypovolemia present. Loss of self-esteem and a potential for bonding interference may be problems. A woman in this situation senses her body's control systems are failing her and she may blame the newborn for this complication.

When planning care, remember that any woman is exhausted after delivery. If a woman hemorrhages in the immediate postpartal period, she feels even more exhausted. The last thing she wants is someone pushing a hand into her abdomen to check her uterus or tightening a blood pressure cuff on her arm every 15 minutes. As she looks around a recovery room and sees that she is the only one receiving this concentrated attention for such a long period of time, she will become more and more frightened. You need to explain that the measures you are taking, although disturbing, are to ensure her health. Make the recordings as quickly and gently as possible, so that a woman has a minimum of discomfort and time to nap between observations.

Due to this exhaustion, women who have a postpartal hemorrhage tend to have a postpartal recovery that is longer than average. A number of blood transfusions may be necessary in order to restore a functioning hemoglobin level. The woman's physician will usually place her on a course of iron therapy to ensure good hemoglobin formation. She will probably have special orders concerning the amount of exertion and postpartal exercise she can safely undertake.

You should discuss with her the possibility of having someone with her at home at least for the first week to help her with housework and the care of her new baby. An exhausted mother cannot enjoy childcare and exhaustion may turn childbearing into a less than satisfying event and interfere with infant bonding. Extensive blood loss is one of the precursors of postpartal infection. Any woman who has undergone more than the normal blood loss should be observed closely for changes in lochia discharge, and her temperature should be monitored closely in the postpartal

Conditions that Make Women High-Risk for Postpartal Hemorrhage

Condition	Cause
Distention of the uterus beyond average capacity	Multiple gestation Hydramnios (excessive amount of amniotic fluid) Large baby (over 9 pounds) Presence of uterine myomas (fibroid tumors)
Tears in uterus	Operative delivery Rapid delivery
Unusual placental attachment	Placenta previa Premature separation of the placenta
Exhaustion of uterus that prevents ready contraction	Deep anesthesia or analgesia Labor initiated or assisted with an oxytocin agent Maternal age over 30 years High parity Prolonged and difficult labor Secondary maternal illness such as anemia

period to detect the earliest signs of developing infection. Conditions that make a woman high-risk for postpartal hemorrhage are given in the box above. Goals of care for the woman who hemorrhages postpartally are shown in the Nursing Care Highlight on page 1033.

Uterine Atony

Uterine atony is the most frequent cause of postpartal hemorrhage. As mentioned in the discussion of involutional changes (Chapter 28), the uterus must remain in a contracted state after delivery if the open vessels at the placental site are to be sealed. Those factors that predispose to poor uterine tone and an inability to maintain a contracted state are summarized in the box above. When you are caring for a patient in whom any of these conditions are present, be especially cautious in your immediate observations and on guard for signs of uterine bleeding.

Assessment

If the uterus suddenly relaxes, blood abruptly gushes from the placental site, with vaginal bleeding and symptoms of shock and blood loss. With uterine atony, it is more common for the uterus to become uncontracted gradually, so that the bleeding that is seen from the vagina is seep-

age, not a gush. Over a period of hours, however, this seepage can result in a condition as lethal as a sudden release of blood.

Estimating the amount of blood loss in the postpartal period is difficult because it is likewise hard to estimate the amount of blood necessary to saturate a perineal pad; the figure is somewhere between 25 and 50 ml. By counting the perineal pads saturated in given lengths of time, say half-hour intervals, you can form a rough estimate of blood loss. Five pads saturated in half an hour is obviously a different situation from five pads saturated in 8 hours. However, in either situation, a woman will have lost upward of 250 ml of blood in that time interval; if either rate of flow is allowed to continue untended, she will be in grave danger.

Be sure you differentiate between *saturated* and *used* when counting pads; *used* in this context is meaningless. Weighing perineal pads before and after use and substracting the difference is an accurate way to measure vaginal discharge. In weighing, 1 gm of weight equals 1 ml of blood as a gram and a milliliter are comparable measures. Whether a woman is losing blood rapidly or slowly, always ask her to turn on her side when estimating blood loss so you can be certain that large amounts are not pooling undetected underneath her.

Nursing Care Highlight

The Woman Who Hemorrhages Postpartally

Goal	Implementations
Detect systemic vascular changes	1. Assess lochia meaningfully by counting the number of saturated pads or weighing pads (1 gm weight equals 1 ml fluid). 2. Assess lochia for clots, which suggest intense bleeding. 3. Remember that a slow, steady change in vital signs is as meaningful as a sudden change because the vascular system compensates well during beginning blood loss. 4. Always turn a woman to assess for postpartal bleeding so blood does not pool unnoticed underneath her. 5. Blood flow increases on ambulation (or vaginal blood drains). The true amount of lochial flow may only be appreciated with ambulation.
Maintain adequate circulation	1. Keep the woman with excess blood loss flat to supply blood to heart and brain. 2. Do not place a woman in a Trendelenburg's position unless specifically ordered. This may deprive the kidneys of blood and cause the uterus to become uncontracted. 3. Set up for an intravenous infusion of lactated Ringer's or saline. 4. Check that cross-matching has been completed for blood replacement. 5. Oxytocins may be prescribed to aid uterine contraction. Remember that Methergine increases blood pressure (at the point that blood pressure is again restored, it can cause hypertension or a secondary problem).
Maintain self-esteem	1. Provide explanations of all happenings. 2. Maintain every effort to promote mother-child bonding.

Palpating the uterine fundus at frequent intervals in the postpartal hours to ascertain that the uterus is remaining in a state of contraction is the best preventive measure against immediate hemorrhage. Frequent checks of lochia and vital signs, particularly of pulse and blood pressure, are equally important. If you reach to massage a fundus and are unsure you have located it, the uterus is probably in a state of relaxation. Under normal circumstances, a well-contracted uterus is firm and easily recognized and feels like no other abdominal structure.

If a woman is losing continuous blood, the circulatory system compensates for a long time, and as a result little change can be found in pulse and blood pressure at first. Suddenly the system can compensate no more, and the pulse rate rises rapidly. The pulse becomes weak and thready, and the blood pressure drops abruptly. The woman's skin becomes cold and clammy and shows obvious signs of shock. If you are taking frequent vital signs and are carefully monitoring lochia flow, you should be able to detect blood loss before this point is ever reached; detecting uterine relaxation should be your first assessment.

Implementations

The first step in controlling hemorrhage in the event of uterine atony is to attempt uterine massage to encourage contraction. Place one hand on the woman's symphysis pubis to give good support to the base of the uterus, then grasp the fundus of the uterus with your other hand and massage gently. Unless the uterus is extremely lacking in tone, massage is usually effective in causing contraction, and after a few seconds the uterus will assume its healthy grapefruit-like feel.

However, the fact that the uterus responds well to massage does not mean that the problem is solved. A few minutes after you remove your hand from the fundus, the uterus may relax, and the lethal seepage may begin again. You must therefore stay continuously with the patient for at least an hour following massage and then observe her closely for the next 4 hours.

A full bladder pushes an uncontracted uterus into an even more uncontracted state. Offer a bedpan at least every 4 hours to keep a woman's bladder empty. In order to reduce bladder pressure, the woman's physician may order insertion of a urinary catheter. Drawing blood for a clotting time may be ordered.

If the uterus does not remain contracted, a physician will invariably order an oxytocin to be begun by intravenous infusion to help the uterus maintain tone. Oxytocins must be kept readily available on a postpartal unit for instant use in the event of postpartal hemorrhage. Be prepared for this eventuality. If a woman is having respiratory distress, administer oxygen by face mask. Keep her flat to allow adequate blood flow to her brain.

The oxytocin most often given intravenously is Syntocinon because its action is immediate; be aware, however, that Syntocinon does not have a sustained action (only about an hour), so symptoms of uterine atony can recur quickly following administration of only a single dose. Methergine is an oxytocin that may be given orally (action begins in 5 to 10 minutes) or intramuscularly (action begins in 2 to 5 minutes). The duration of action with this drug is 3 to 4 hours, a considerable increase over that achieved with Syntocinon. Methergine has the side effect of causing hypertension and thus never should be administered if a woman's blood pressure is over 140/90; always assess for this high a rate before administration. The drug is rarely given intravenously because the hypertensive effect is so extreme with this method of administration.

Be certain with uterine atony that vital signs are not only taken frequently but interpreted intelligently during the immediate postpartal period. The pulse rate, for example, may increase only a point or so at each recording; if you do not look at the entire picture, the slow rise will mask the *continual* rise.

You can anticipate that any woman who has had a blood loss over 500 ml may have to have blood replaced. Check to be certain that blood has been drawn for a cross-matching, so that blood of her specific type can be made ready. Be sure that your hands are not tied by hospital policies on ordering blood for replacement. Hemorrhaging women need replacement, and you should have the authority to request that cross-matching and blood-readying procedures be started. If the necessary forms require a physician's signature, valuable time could be lost in waiting.

If uterine massage and intravenous oxytocin are not effective in stopping uterine bleeding, a physician may attempt bimanual compression (one hand inserted in the vagina, the other pushing against the fundus through the abdominal wall). It may be necessary to return a woman to the delivery room, so that the physician can explore her uterine cavity manually for retained placental fragments that may be preventing good contraction.

Bimanual compression is effective in halting bleeding in all but extremely atonic uteruses. In the latter, rare instance, a hysterectomy may have to be performed. Appreciate the fact that this measure is carried out as a last resort only. Despite the emergency conditions, try to comfort and give support to a woman at this time. Neither she nor her support person will be prepared for this totally unexpected outcome of childbearing.

Following hysterectomy, a woman will usually want to talk about what happened, why surgery was necessary, and how she feels now that she can no longer bear children. She needs to discuss her feelings with a person who will listen quietly and help her sort through her "why me?" feelings. She usually has ambiguous feelings because she wanted to have more children (or at least have the ability to have more) but she also wanted to live. She is grateful to her physician and the hospital personnel for saving her life, but she may feel resentful that you were not skilled enough to leave her capable of future childbearing. She may grieve (very genuinely) for her children who will not be born. If she delivered outside the hospital and was brought there under emergency circumstances, she has a need to talk about her choice of location for childbirth and perhaps some help with guilt that she did not choose the best place considering the circumstances.

Open lines of communication between a couple and the hospital staff, so that the family can vent its feelings, will be most helpful to the couple in this crisis. Grieving for future children who will not be born can interfere with bonding with the newborn.

Lacerations

Small lacerations or tears of the birth canal are so common they can be considered a normal consequence of childbearing. Large lacerations occur most often with difficult or precipitate deliveries, in primigravidas, with the birth of a large infant (over 9 pounds), and if a lithotomy position and instruments were used for delivery. They can occur in the cervix, vagina, or perineum. Any time the uterus is firm following delivery and yet bleeding persists, a laceration at one of these three sites should be suspected.

Cervical Tears

Assessment. Lacerations of the cervix are usually found on the sides near the branches of the uterine artery. The amount of blood loss is usually great, and this arterial blood will be brighter red than the venous blood lost from uterine atony. The force of the blood is such that it often gushes from the vaginal opening. Fortunately, this bleeding ordinarily occurs immediately following delivery of the placenta, when the mother is still on the delivery table and the physician or nurse-midwife is still in attendance.

Implementations. Repair of a cervical laceration is difficult because the bleeding is so intense it obstructs visualization of the area. Be certain the physician has adequate space to work and adequate sponges and suture supplies. A woman is not always aware of what is happening but she will respond to the tone of activity in the room. Try to maintain an air of calm and, if possible, stand beside her at the head of the table. She may be worried that the extra activity in the room has something to do with her baby. She needs to be assured that the baby is fine. The problem is with the opening from her uterus; use an explanation such as "you will need to stay in the delivery room a little longer than expected while the doctor places additional stitches." Remember that mothers transfer the protective attitude toward their bodies they felt all during pregnancy onto the baby at birth. Learning that the problem is theirs, not the infant's, is generally good news.

If a laceration appears to be extensive or difficult to repair, the physician may ask for a general anesthetic for relaxation of the uterine muscle and to prevent pain. Be certain to give good explanations to the father, assuming he is still present in the room, concerning the need for an anesthetic and the procedures being carried out.

Vaginal Tears

Assessment. Lacerations in the vagina are more rare but easier to diagnose because they are easier to view.

Implementations. Since vaginal tissue is friable, however, such lacerations are also hard to repair. Some oozing often follows a repair here, and the vagina may be packed to maintain pressure on the suture line. Be certain that the patient's chart and the nursing care plan are both marked to show that packing is in place. Packing is usually removed after 24 to 48 hours and it will be the physician's responsibility to remove it. However, by careful recording of the packing's existence and making sure that it is removed, you serve as the woman's first line of defense against infection. Packing left in place too long tends to cause stasis and infection similar to toxic shock syndrome.

Perineal Tears

Assessment. Lacerations of the perineum usually occur when a woman is delivered from a lithotomy position and an episiotomy was not performed. Occasionally they are an extension of an episiotomy incision. Perineal lacerations are classified into four categories, depending on the extent and depth of the tissue involved. These are shown in Table 44-1.

Implementations. Perineal lacerations are sutured and treated as an episiotomy repair. It is often difficult to distinguish a repaired perineal laceration from an episiotomy, except that lacerations tend to heal more slowly because the edges of the suture line are ragged. Any woman who has a third- or fourth-degree laceration should not be given an enema or a rectal suppository and her temperature should not be taken rectally; the sutures involve the rectal sphincter, and the hard tips of equipment could open them. To prevent constipation and hard stools that could break the sutures, a woman should have a diet high in fluid and is usually given a stool softener for the first week of the puerperium. Make certain that the

Table 44-1 Classification of Perineal Lacerations

Classification	Description
First degree	These involve the vaginal mucous membrane and the skin of the perineum to the fourchette.
Second degree	These involve the vagina, perineal skin, fascia, levator ani muscle, and perineal body.
Third degree	These involve the entire perineum and the external sphincter of the rectum, either partially or completely.
Fourth degree	These involve the entire perineum, rectal sphincter, and some of the mucous membrane of the rectum.

degree of the laceration is marked on her nursing care plan; ancillary caregivers such as aides have no appreciation of why rectal temperatures are contraindicated unless informed.

Retained Placental Fragments

Occasionally, the placenta does not deliver in its entirety, leaving fragments behind. Since the portion retained keeps the uterus from contracting fully, uterine bleeding ocurs. This is most likely to happen with a succenturiate placenta (see Chapter 43), but it can happen in any instance. A placenta accreta has fused with the myometrium due to an abnormal decidua basalis layer. Sections of this type of placenta will remain following delivery and may need to be surgically incised. To detect the complication of retained placenta, every placenta should be inspected carefully following birth to see if it is complete.

Assessment

If a retained fragment is large, the bleeding will be apparent in the immediate postpartal period. If the fragment is small, bleeding may not be detected until the sixth or tenth day postpartum, when the mother notices an abrupt discharge of a large amount of blood.

On examination, the uterus is usually found to be not fully contracted. If the bleeding does not appear to be major, the physician may order a pregnancy test, preferably an immunologic test, which gives the results in a matter of minutes or hours. If placental tissue is still present in the woman's body, human chorionic gonadotropin will also be present; even though the woman is no longer pregnant, the test will be positive. Retained placental fragments may also be detected by sonogram.

Implementations

A woman will be given a supportive blood transfusion if necessary, and then taken to a delivery room where a D&C will be performed to remove the offending placental fragment. Because hemorrhage from retained fragments is often delayed until after women go home, they must be instructed to observe the color of lochia discharge and report to their physician any tendency for the discharge to change from lochia alba to rubra.

Disseminated Intravascular Coagulation

Disseminated intravascular coagulation, a deficiency in clotting caused by a low level of fibrinogen (see Chapter 39), may occur in any woman in the postpartal period but is usually associated with women who had premature separation of the placenta, missed abortion, or fetal death in utero.

Assessment

DIC should be suspected when the usual measures to induce uterine contraction fail to stop the blood flow. Oozing from an intravenous site or difficulty in stopping blood from flowing from a blood-drawing site is highly suggestive that a level of low fibrinogen exists.

Implementations

A maternity service should maintain a supply of fibrinogen to be used for treatment of this condition. Increasing the woman's supply of fibrinogen usually decreases bleeding dramatically if hypofibrinogenemia is the underlying cause. Heparin may also be used as therapy since it prevents massive clotting and further lowering of the fibrinogen level. DIC is explained more fully in Chapter 39 as a complication of pregnancy.

Other Problems of Hemorrhage

Subinvolution

Subinvolution is incomplete return of the uterus to its prepregnant size and shape. At a 4- or 6-week postpartal checkup, the uterus is still enlarged and soft and the woman still has a lochial discharge. Subinvolution may result from a small retained placental fragment, a mild endometritis, or an accompanying problem such as a myoma that is interfering with complete contraction. Oral administration of Methergine (0.2 mg four times a day) is generally prescribed to improve uterine tone and complete involution. If the uterus is tender to palpation, suggesting endometritis, an oral antibiotic may be prescribed. Be certain that women know at discharge from a health care facility the normal process of involution and lochial discharge. Otherwise they could wait a long time before seeking health care advice and their chronic loss of blood could result in anemia and lack of energy and possibly interfere with bonding through exhaustion.

Hematomas

A hematoma is a collection of blood in the subcutaneous layer of tissue. Such blood collection may occur in the perineum as a result of injury to blood vessels in the perineum during delivery. Hematomas are most likely to occur in rapid, spontaneous deliveries and in women who have perineal varicosities. They may occur at an episiotomy repair site or a laceration repair site if a vein is pricked during repair. They can cause the mother acute discomfort and concern but, fortunately, they usually represent only minor bleeding.

Assessment. Perineal sutures almost always give a postpartal woman some discomfort. When she complains of severe pain in the perineal area or a feeling of pressure between her legs, inspect the perineal area for a hematoma. If one is present, it appears as an area of purplish discoloration and obvious swelling anywhere from 1 inch to as much as 4 inches in diameter. The area is tender to palpation, and it may at first feel fluctuant. As seepage into the area continues and tissue is drawn taut, it palpates as a firm globe. The overlying skin, as a rule, is intact without noticeable trauma.

Implementations. Report to the physician or nurse-midwife the presence of the hematoma, its size, the degree of discomfort it is causing the woman, as well as any increase in size you notice. Administer a mild analgesic as ordered for pain relief. Applying an ice pack (covered with a towel to prevent a thermal injury to the skin) may limit further bleeding, and the hematoma will then be absorbed over the next 3 or 4 days. If the hematoma is very large when discovered or continues to grow in size, the woman may have to be returned to the delivery room to have the site incised and the bleeding vessel ligated. Be certain you assess the size of the hematoma by measuring it in centimeters each time you inspect the perineum and record this measurement as well as the general appearance in a meaningful way. Describing a hematoma as "large" or "small" gives little information to the nurse relieving you or to the physician or nurse-midwife about the hematoma's actual size. Describing the lesion as 5 cm across—or the size of a quarter or a half dollar—is meaningful since it establishes a basis for comparison.

A mother can be reassured that unless the hematoma is extremely extensive, although the hematoma may give her considerable discomfort, her hospital stay will probably not be lengthened by its occurrence. She can also be told that the hematoma will absorb over the next 6 weeks, causing no further difficulty. If an episiotomy incision line is opened in order to drain a hematoma, it may be left open and packed with gauze. Be certain this packing is recorded on the woman's chart and nursing care plan so that you can check its removal (at about 24 to 48 hours). A suture line opened this way heals by tertiary intention, in other words, slower than a first-degree intention suture line.

Vulvar Edema

Some vulvar edema is always present following vaginal delivery from the pressure of the fetal head on the perineum and the stretching of the vagina to accommodate birth. Extensive edema of the vulva has been reported following local and regional anesthesia. This atypical edema occurs on the second postpartal day and rapidly spreads to include not only the vulva, but gluteal and inner pelvic areas as well. Fever is present. A woman may have an elevated white blood count. The edema may become so involved that vascular collapse and death occur. Although the etiology of this edematous process is not understood, massive administration of antibiotics appears to be helpful, suggesting that it has an infectious basis. In any event, close assessment of the vulvar area for edema as well as for hematomas will reveal this condition at its first appearance.

Postpartal Anterior Pituitary Necrosis

Postpartal anterior pituitary necrosis (also termed *Sheehan's syndrome*) is a rare disorder that may occur in a woman following severe hemorrhage. The pituitary gland appears to be so damaged by the abrupt hypovolemia that it does not function adequately. This condition is revealed by signs of decreased or absent lactation, genital and breast atrophy, and loss of pubic and axillary hair; myxedema or symptoms of thyroid dysfunction may result.

A woman with this syndrome needs hormone therapy to replace hormones that her body has difficulty producing, most noticeably estrogen, cortisone, and thyroid. Because of decreased stimulation to the ovaries, the woman may be infertile or sterile following this pituitary insult.

Puerperal Infection

Infection of the reproductive tract is the second most common cause of maternal mortality associated with childbearing. The factors that predispose to infection in the postpartal period are shown in the box on page 1038. When caring for a woman who has any of these circumstances, be extremely aware that postpartal infection is apt to occur.

The uterus is theoretically sterile during pregnancy and until the membranes rupture. It is capable of being invaded by pathogens after that point; there is greater risk if tissue edema and trauma are present. When infection occurs, the

Conditions That Make Women High-Risk for Postpartal Infection

1. Rupture of the membranes over 24 hours before delivery (bacteria may have started to invade the uterus while the fetus was still in utero).
2. Placental fragments that have been retained within the uterus (the tissue necroses and serves as an excellent bed for bacterial growth).
3. Postpartal hemorrhage (a woman's general condition is weakened).
4. Preexisting anemia (the body's defense against infection is lowered).
5. Prolonged and difficult labor, particularly instrument deliveries (trauma to the tissue may leave lacerations, fissures, or easy portals of entry for infection).
6. Internal fetal heart monitoring (contamination may have been introduced with the placement of the scalp electrode).
7. Local vaginal infection was present at the time of delivery (direct spread of infection occurred).
8. The uterus was explored following delivery for a retained placenta or abnormal bleeding site (infection was introduced with exploration).

prognosis for complete recovery depends on the virulence of the invading organism, the general health of the woman, the portal of entry and specifically the degree of involution, and presence of lacerations in the reproductive tract. A puerperal infection is always serious because, although it usually begins as only a local infection, it can spread to involve the peritoneum (peritonitis) or circulatory system (septicemia)—conditions that can be fatal in a woman already stressed from childbirth.

Because the uterus is a closed space, anaerobic organisms that invade the uterus rapidly grow within its denuded folds. Most postpartal infections are caused by invading anaerobic streptococci, although anaerobic staphylococci infections are becoming more and more common. Staphylococci infections are the cause of toxic shock syndrome, an infection not unlike puerperal infection in its ability to cause death and morbidity.

Some bacteria, such as anaerobic streptococci, are normal inhabitants of the birth canal. Ordinarily, they are nonpathogenic and give no evidence of their presence. In the face of traumatized, devitalized tissue, however, such as might be present following a difficult delivery, they become pathogenic, invade the tissue, and lead to infection.

Some bacteria are transferred to a woman as a result of nasopharyngeal infection in hospital personnel. At delivery, all persons in the delivery room or birthing room should be masked (nose and mouth). Any article (glove, instruments, and so on) introduced into the birth canal during labor, delivery, and the postpartal period must be sterile. A woman must be given good instruction in perineal care, so that she does not bring *Escherichia coli* organisms forward from the rectum. When you are giving perineal care, be certain that you wash your hands before the procedure and do not open the labia, permitting contaminated water to enter the vagina. Each maternity patient should have her own bedpan and perineal supplies to prevent transfer of pathogens. Equipment that is used by many women (e.g., bathtubs, heat lamps) must be cleaned between patients.

Assessment

The white blood count of a postpartal woman is normally increased to 20,000 to 30,000 per cubic millimeter. Thus, this conventional method of detecting infection is not of great value in the puerperium. An increase in oral temperature above 100.4°F (38.0°C) for two consecutive 24-hour periods, excluding the first 24-hour period following birth, is defined by the Joint Committee on Maternal Welfare as a febrile condition suggesting infection. All women with temperatures within this range should be suspected of having a postpartal infection until it is proved otherwise.

Analysis

The nursing diagnoses established with a woman with a postpartal hemorrhage are generally concerned with restoration of body defenses and interference with bonding. The mother may

Nursing Care Highlight

The Mother with a Postpartal Infection

1. As a rule, the baby of a mother with an increased temperature (100.4°F or 38.0°C) for two consecutive 24-hour periods exclusive of the first 24 hours should be excluded from her room until the cause of the infection is determined. The mother may have an upper respiratory or a gastrointestinal infection unrelated to childbearing—but one that is transmittable to the newborn.

2. If the cause of the fever is found to be related to childbirth but involves a closed infection such as thrombophlebitis, where there would be no danger of the baby's contracting the disease, the mother can care for her child as long as she maintains bedrest in the prescribed position while doing so.

3. If the infection involves drainage (e.g., endometritis, perineal abscess), newborn visiting may be contraindicated. If the mother is allowed to feed her child, she should wash her hands thoroughly before holding the infant. She should never place the baby on the bottom bed sheet, where there may be some infected drainage from her perineal pad (furnish a clean sheet to spread over the covers when you bring in the baby).

4. Most hospitals are reluctant to return to a central nursery a baby who has visited in a room where there is an infection. The hospital should provide small nurseries that may be used as isolation nurseries for these situations. Otherwise a baby can be placed in a closed Isolette in a central nursery or cared for in the mother's room.

5. If the mother has a high fever, breast milk may be deficient. With modern antimicrobial therapy, puerperal infections are limited, and the period of high fever will be transient. If the mother is too ill to nurse the baby during this time, or is receiving an anticoagulant or antibiotic such as tetracycline that is passed in breast milk, the infant should be fed by a supplementary milk formula. The woman's breast milk should be manually expressed to maintain the production of milk so that it will be available when she is again able to nurse. You may need to assist her because she fatigues easily and her energy level may not be enough to support her good intentions. If it appears that the course of the infection will be long, the mother may choose to, or may be advised to, discontinue breast-feeding. In these instances, the physician will usually prescribe a lactation-suppressing drug to discourage breast engorgement. Once lactation is well established, however, these drugs are not effective in suppressing lactation so engorgement may be painful.

6. If it is necessary for the woman to discontinue breast-feeding, she needs to be assured that she can meet the needs of the child through bottle-feeding and that she has not become a bad or inadequate mother because of the complication.

7. If the woman is going to be hospitalized for a period of time, she may have to make arrangements for the discharge and care of the baby. She may be interested in a homemaker service or temporary foster care if she has no close friends or family. If she has older children at home, she needs to keep in close contact with them, calling them on the telephone or writing them short notes if possible. She needs to see a photo of the newborn (a Polaroid camera should be a piece of equipment on every postpartal unit) and hear daily reports of the baby's progress and well-being.

---

need to be separated from her infant to protect the infant from contracting the infection.

Planning and Implementations

Whether or not a mother who has an infection should be allowed to feed and care for her baby is always a concern on postpartal units. Most hospitals have well-defined guidelines in this area for you to follow. The Nursing Care Highlight above summarizes these common guidelines.

When planning care, appreciate that a mother with an infection is always anxious. She quickly realizes that her care is different from that of the other women on the unit. She is confined to bed while the other women are ambulatory. She is still uncomfortable while they are not.

Good nursing care is important. Ice bags used to minimize perineal discomfort must not be allowed to saturate the bed, making the woman feel chilled or otherwise uncomfortable. If isolated, she must not feel separated from the hospital staff or her family. Although you must use scrupulous infection technique, be certain you do not give a woman the impression that she is contaminated or dirty in any way.

This is a point in life when a woman is adjusting to a new life role—difficult enough to accomplish when things are going well. When she is segregated, denied the pleasure of holding and feeding her baby, and frightened by her condition, the struggle may be more than she is prepared to tolerate. She needs friendly, understanding support from hospital personnel who give her care. Infection may involve the perineum, or uterus, or spread to the vascular system or peritoneum.

Infection of the Perineum

A suture line on the perineum from an episiotomy or a laceration repair is a ready portal of entry for bacterial invasion. Infections of the perineum generally remain localized and so manifest the symptoms of any suture line infection: pain, heat, and a feeling of pressure. The woman may or may not have an elevated temperature, depending on the systemic effect and spread.

Assessment

Inspection of the suture line reveals inflammation. One or two stitches may be sloughed away or an area of the suture line may be open, with pus present. Notify the woman's physician or nurse-midwife of the localized symptoms and culture the discharge by a sterile, cotton-tipped applicator touched to the secretion.

Implementations

The woman's physician or nurse-midwife may choose to remove the perineal sutures in order to open the area and allow for drainage. A packing such as iodiform gauze may be placed in the lesion to keep it open and guard its ability to drain. Be certain the woman is aware that the packing is in place and that each time she changes her perineal pad she must be careful not to dislodge it.

An antibiotic will be ordered even before the culture report is returned, along with an analgesic for discomfort. Sitz baths or warm compresses may be ordered to hasten drainage and cleanse the area. Remind a woman to change perineal pads frequently, since they are contaminated by seropurulent drainage. If left in place for long periods

of time, they might cause vaginal contamination or reinfection. A woman should be instructed to wash her hands (and you want to be certain to do this also) after handling perineal pads. Be certain she wipes front to back following a bowel movement so feces are not brought forward onto the healing area.

Evaluation

Local infection of this nature (if extensive) may lengthen a woman's hospital stay by 3 or 4 days because the incision site, once opened, must then heal by tertiary rather than primary intention. Infections of this nature are annoying and painful to the mother out of proportion to their size. Fortunately, with the use of improved techniques during parturition and the puerperium, perineal infections are not seen as commonly as they used to be. Because they are localized, they generally respond well to a regimen of oral antibiotics and warm, moist heat three or four times a day.

Because the infection is localized, there is no need to exclude the infant from the mother as long as she washes her hands well first. Be certain not to place an infant on the mother's bottom bed sheet in possible contact with pathogenic bacteria. Be certain that she continues to ambulate even though the pain from an infected suture line can be severe. Assess the mouth of an infant for thrush (oral candidiasis), and check the infant's skin if a mother is breastfeeding while taking an antibiotic. A portion of the antibiotic passes into breast milk and overgrowth of fungal organisms may occur with a decrease of bacteria. Assess an infant well for easy bruising; a decrease of microorganisms in the bowel may lead to insufficient vitamin K formation and decreased blood-clotting ability.

Endometritis

Endometritis is an infection of the endometrium, the lining of the uterus. Bacteria gain access to the uterus through the vagina either at the time of delivery or during the postpartal period.

Assessment

Endometritis usually manifests itself on the third or fourth day of the puerperium, suggesting that a great deal of the invasion occurs during labor or delivery.

As a rule, a mother demonstrates a rise in temperature. A temperature on the third or fourth day postpartum coincides with the days that breast milk comes in. Do not be led astray by the old wives' tale of "milk fever." Fever on the third or fourth day postpartum should be considered possible endometritis until proven otherwise.

Depending on the severity of the infection, a woman may have chills, loss of appetite, and general malaise. Most women experience some abdominal tenderness. The uterus is generally not well contracted and is painful to the touch. A woman may have strong afterpains. Lochia will usually be dark brown in color and have a foul odor. It may be increased in amount because of poor uterine contractions. However, if the infection is accompanied by high fever, lochia may be scant or absent.

Treatment of endometritis consists of the administration of an appropriate antibiotic determined by a culture of the lochia (take a culture from the vagina by a sterile swab rather than from a perineal pad so you are certain you are culturing the endometrial infectious organism, not an unrelated one from the pad), accompanied by an oxytocic agent to encourage uterine contraction. A woman requires additional fluid to combat the fever. If strong afterpains and abdominal discomfort are present, she needs an analgesic for pain relief.

Fowler's position or ambulating upright are best for the woman with endometritis because these positions encourage lochia drainage due to gravity and prevent pooling of infected fluid. Both you and the woman must use good hand washing techniques after handling perineal pads because the pads contain contaminated discharge. A woman may be isolated from other patients to reduce the chances of spreading infection.

Evaluation

As with any infection, endometritis can be contained best if it is discovered early in the disease process. If you can intelligently interpret the color, quantity, and odor of lochia discharge, and the size, consistency, and tenderness of a postpartal uterus in connection with an increased temperature, you may be the first person to recognize that disease is present.

If an infection is limited to the endometrium, the course of infection will be 7 to 10 days. The mother may have to make arrangements for her baby's discharge prior to her own, since her hospital stay will be extended about 2 weeks. Endometritis can lead to tubal scarring and interference with future fertility. At the point when she desires more children, the woman should ask for a fertility assessment (including a hysterosalpingogram) for tubal patency if after a 6-month period she has not conceived. With mild endometritis, this is usually not a problem, but a woman should be forewarned and told the steps to take in case it does occur.

Thrombophlebitis

Phlebitis is an inflammation of the lining of a blood vessel; thrombophlebitis is inflammation of the lining of a blood vessel with the formation of blood clots. Thrombophlebitis usually occurs in the postpartal period as an extension of an endometrial infection. It is prone to occur in the postpartal period because blood clotting ability is high due to increased fibrinogen, veins are dilated due to pressure of the fetal head during pregnancy and birth, and the relative inactivity of the period leads to pooling, stasis, and clotting of blood in the lower extremities. Women most prone to thrombophlebitis have varicose veins, are taking an estrogen supplement, are obese, have had a previous thrombophlebitis, are over 30 years old, have increased parity, were in a stirrups position for a long time during labor, or have a high incidence of thrombophlebotic disease in their family.

Thrombophlebitis is of two types: (a) femoral, in which the femoral, saphenous, or popliteal veins are involved, and (b) pelvic, in which the ovarian, uterine, and hypogastric veins are involved. An older term for the former type of involvement is *milk leg* or *phlegmasia alba dolens* (white inflammation).

Femoral Thrombophlebitis

The infection site in thrombophlebitis is a vein, but an accompanying arterial spasm diminishes arterial circulation to the legs as well. The decreased circulation, along with edema, gives the leg a white or drained appearance. As a woman's temperature rises because of the infection, her supply of breast milk tends to decrease (the body attempts to save fluid). It was formerly believed that breast milk was going into the leg, giving it its white appearance (milk leg).

As with the other complications of the postpartal period, thrombophlebitis is largely preventable. Goals of care are summarized in the Nursing Care Highlight on page 1042. Prevention of endometritis by use of good aseptic technique prevents thrombophlebitis as well. Early ambulation encourages circulation in the lower extremities and decreases clot formation. If a woman cannot be out of bed following childbirth for any reason, begin leg exercises with her (flexing and straightening her knee, raising the leg and drawing a circle in the air) by 8 hours postbirth.

Be certain the stirrups of examining and deliv-

=== *Nursing Care Highlight* ===

The Woman with a Thrombophlebitis

Goal	*Implementations*
Prevent the development of thrombophlebitis	1. Pad delivery table stirrups to prevent sharp calf pressure. 2. Do not allow a woman to remain in a lithotomy position over an hour. 3. Assist with early ambulation to promote lower extremity circulation. 4. If a woman cannot be ambulatory, begin leg exercises 8 hours postbirth. 5. Recommend support stockings for any woman with varicosities or a past history of thrombophlebitis.
Promotion of comfort	1. A thrombophlebitis is painful. Give analgesics as needed. 2. Be certain acetylsalicylic acid as an analgesic, which increases coagulation time, and an anticoagulant are not combined. 3. Use a bed cradle to keep covers off leg for comfort. 4. Warmth from a heated cradle or warm compresses is comforting and increases circulation to the leg. Be certain that the light bulb of the cradle is 15 to 18 inches away from leg. 5. Be certain that moist, warm compresses are not too hot (heat sensation is decreased in leg due to edema). 6. Do not rub calf of leg for comfort. This action can cause a pulmonary embolism.
Establishment of improved circulation	1. Assess that prothrombin or clotting level is determined before administration of an anticoagulant. 2. Assess q4h for amount of lochia (excessive if saturating over 1 pad in 45 minutes). 3. Weigh perineal pads as necessary to obtain accurate amount of lochia flow. 4. Assess for bleeding gums, ecchymotic spots, and oozing from episiotomy sutures as other indications of low clotting level. 5. Dicumarol is passed in breast milk. Help a mother understand reason for discontinuing breast-feeding and importance of manually expressing breast milk to maintain milk supply. 6. Encourage a good fluid intake to increase viscosity of blood (at least 3,000 to 4,000 ml daily).

ery tables are well padded so a woman does not have sharp pressure against the calves of her legs. Women should not remain any longer than an hour in a lithotomy and stirrups position. If a woman had varicose veins during pregnancy, wearing support stockings for the first 2 weeks postpartum will increase venous circulation and help prevent stasis (Figure 44-1). Assess all women for varicosities immediately postpartum and make recommendations to physicians or nurse-midwives for these stockings. Be certain a woman puts them on before she rises in the morning; if she waits until she is already up and walking, venous congestion has already occurred.

Remove support stockings twice daily and assess the skin underneath them for mottling or inflammation that would suggest inflammation of veins.

Assessment. Femoral thrombophlebitis is manifested on about the tenth day after delivery by an elevated temperature, chills, stiffness, pain, and redness in the affected part. The leg begins to swell below the lesion, since venous circulation is blocked. The skin becomes stretched to a point of shiny whiteness. Homans' sign (pain in the calf on dorsiflexion of the foot) will be positive (Figure 29-8). Measure the diameter of the leg above and

Nursing Care Highlight
Femoral Thrombophlebitis

Legs with a phlebitis or thrombophlebitis should never be rubbed or massaged or the clot may move and become a pulmonary embolus, a possibly fatal complication.

---

below the knee so you will be able to tell in following days if it is decreasing or increasing in size.

Implementations. Treatment consists of bedrest with the affected leg elevated, administration of anticoagulants, and application of heat. Never massage the leg (see the Nursing Care Highlight above). Women who have been discharged from the hospital will need to return so that strict bedrest can be enforced. A cradle should be used to keep the pressure of the bedclothes off the affected leg, both to decrease the sensitivity of the leg and to improve the circulation (Figure 44-2). A

light bulb used with the cradle can supply continual heat to the leg or heat may be supplied by means of moist, warm compresses.

Warm, wet dressings are one of the most technically difficult treatments to arrange because dressings invariably dry and therefore are not moist very long, or become cold and therefore are not warm after a short time. Dressings may be applied by simple gauze squares wet in a warmed solution. Compresses and water do not have to be sterile because with thrombophlebitis there is no break in the skin present. Be certain to test water temperature by dipping your inner wrist in the water prior to soaking the sponges to be certain that it is not too warm (sensation in a woman's leg is decreased due to edema so she can be burnt easily). Always cover wet, warm dressings with a plastic pad to hold in heat and moisture. Additional measures such as K-pads (with circulating heating coils) or hot water bottles may be positioned over the plastic to ensure the soaks stay warm. Be certain that the weight of a hot water bottle or pad does not rest on the leg, obstructing the flow of blood by its weight. A newer type of apparatus (a Gaymar pump) keeps a pad that is

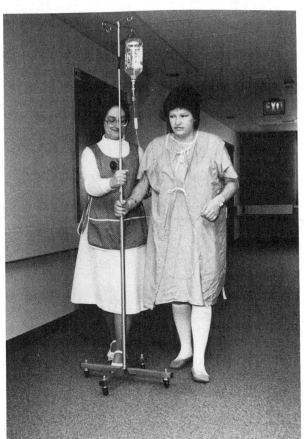

Figure 44-1 *Ambulation helps to prevent thromboembolism. Notice the thromboembolitic stockings in place.*

Figure 44-2 *A bed cradle used to lift the weight of bedclothes off the legs.*

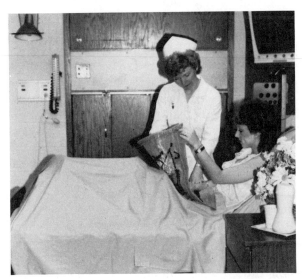

moistened about every 8 hours warm by a circulating flow of water through the attached pump.

Check a woman's bed frequently when wet compresses are being used to be certain that the bed is not wet from seeping water. In order for soaks to stay in place, a woman must keep her leg fairly immobile. Be certain she does not interpret this instruction as meaning she cannot turn, however. Providing activities for a woman so she does not become restless helps to keep dressings in place. Figure 44-3 shows a crossword puzzle concerning newborn care that is the sort of activity which not only helps a woman maintain bedrest but educates her about infant care as well. Provide good back and buttocks care for the woman; check for bed wrinkles so that she does not develop a secondary problem of a decubitus while remaining still in bed.

The pain of a thrombophlebitis is usually severe enough to require administration of analgesics. An appropriate antibiotic and often an anticoagulant (Dicumarol or heparin) will be ordered to prevent further formation of clots. A woman will have daily prothrombin or clotting level determinations before administration of the anticoagulant each day. Lochia will usually increase in amount in a woman who is receiving an anticoagulant. Be sure to keep a meaningful record of the amount of this discharge so it can be estimated. "Lochia serosa with scattered pinpoint clots; three perineal pads saturated in 8 hours" is far more meaningful than "large amount of lochia." Weighing perineal pads before and after use and subtracting the difference is an accurate way to determine the amount of vaginal bleeding (1 gm weight equals 1 ml fluid). Also assess other possible signs of bleeding such as bleeding gums, ecchymotic spots on the skin, or oozing from an episiotomy suture line.

The Dicumarol anticoagulants are passed in breast milk, so a mother will have to discontinue breast-feeding during a course of therapy. If the infection does not seem to be severe and the mother wants to reinstate breast-feeding after the course of anticoagulant (about 10 days), she should manually express breast milk at the time of normal feedings in order to maintain a good milk supply. Heparin is one of the few drugs that does not pass into breast milk. If this anticoagulant is chosen, breast-feeding does not need to be halted. Protomine sulfate is the antagonist for heparin and should be readily available—check the nursing unit's emergency cart any time heparin is being administered.

Acetylsalicylic acid tends to increase coagulation time. Some women may be given aspirin

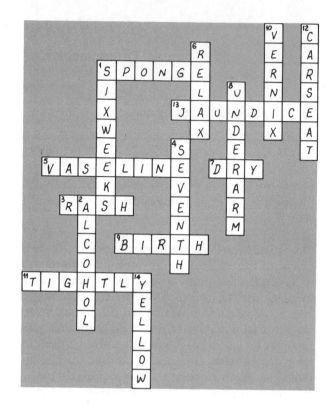

Across

1. Type of bath to give until cord falls off.
3. Consequence of not washing buttocks after bowel movement.
5. Ointment usually applied to circumcision at home.
7. Condition in which to keep umbilical cord.
9. Age at which a newborn sees.
11. Manner in which newborns like to be wrapped.
13. Name of yellow tinge to newborn skin.

Down

1. Age at which infant first smiles.
2. Antiseptic usually applied to cord at home.
4. First day cord can be expected to fall off.
6. Important rule for breastfeeding.
8. Best place to take an infant's temperature.
10. Name of white cream cheese-like substance on newborns.
12. Important piece of safety equipment with newborns.
14. Typical color of infant stool.

Figure 44-3 *A crossword puzzle designed to be both an activity and a learning aid to a postpartal woman on bedrest.*

every 4 hours to act in this capacity. Be certain that you do not interpret aspirin used this way as a PRN analgesia order and withhold it depending on the woman's level of pain. If an anticoagulant is ordered, as a rule, a woman should not be given both aspirin and anticoagulants in conjunction. Make it your responsibility to check the orders for aspirin or an aspirin compound as an analgesic if an anticoagulant is ordered.

With proper treatment, the acute symptoms of femoral thrombophlebitis last only a few days, but the full course of the disease takes 4 to 6 weeks before it is resolved. The affected leg may never return to its former size and may always cause discomfort after long periods of standing.

Pelvic Thrombophlebitis

Pelvic thrombophlebitis occurs later than femoral thrombophlebitis, often around the fourteenth or fifteenth day of the puerperium. The infection may necrose the vein and result in a pelvic abscess.

Assessment. A woman is suddenly extremely ill, with a high fever, chills, and general malaise.

Implementations. If a woman has been discharged from the hospital, she must be readmitted, as she would be with femoral thrombophlebitis, for total bedrest and antibiotics and anticoagulant treatment. Because major veins are involved in this disease, the infection can become systemic and result in a lung, kidney, or heart valve abscess.

Evaluation. The disease runs a long course of 6 to 8 weeks and, if an abscess forms, may have a fatal outcome (although this can be located and incised by laparotomy if necessary). An inflammation of this extent may leave tubal scarring and interfere with future fertility. A woman may need surgery to remove the affected vessel before attempting to become pregnant again. If she should be pregnant in the future, she needs to be careful not to wear constricting clothing, to rest with feet elevated, and to ambulate daily during pregnancy. She should be cautioned to tell the physician or nurse-midwife at her next delivery of the difficulty she experienced so extra precautions to prevent thrombophlebitis can be taken.

Pulmonary Embolus

The signs of pulmonary embolus are sudden, sharp chest pain, tachypnea, tachycardia, orthopnea (inability to breathe except in an upright position), and cyanosis (the blood clot is obstructing the pulmonary artery, preventing blood flow to the lungs and return to the heart). This is an emergency condition. The woman needs oxygen administered immediately; she may almost immediately need cardiopulmonary resuscitation. Her condition is extremely guarded until the clot is lysed or adheres to the pulmonary artery wall

and is reabsorbed. A woman with this degree of postpartal complication is transferred to an intensive care unit for continuing care.

Because this level of complication may occur, thrombophlebitis must be prevented; if it should occur, it should be respected as a potentially serious disorder.

Peritonitis

Peritonitis or infection of the peritoneal cavity is usually an extension of endometritis. It is one of the gravest complications of childbearing and accounts for a third of all deaths from puerperal infection. The infection spreads through the lymphatic system or directly through the fallopian tubes or uterine wall to the peritoneal cavity. An abscess may form in the cul-de-sac of Douglas, which is the lowest point of the peritoneal cavity.

Assessment

The symptoms are the same as those caused by any peritoneal infection: rigid abdomen, abdominal pain, high fever, rapid pulse, vomiting, and the appearance of being acutely ill. It is important when assessing the abdomen of postpartal women that you notice not only whether the uterus is well contracted but whether it is tender to touch and the remainder of the abdomen is soft. The occurrence of a rigid abdomen (guarding) is one of the first symptoms of peritonitis.

With peritonitis, paralytic ilius occurs, so a nasogastric tube will be inserted; and a woman will need intravenous fluid or total parenteral nutrition while she is unable to take food orally because of the intestinal paralysis. She will need analgesics for pain relief. She will be placed on large doses of antibiotics. Her hospital stay will be lengthy, and her prognosis is guarded. A peritonitis may interfere with future fertility by leaving scarring and adhesions in the peritoneum. Adhesions may separate the fallopian tubes from the ovaries so that ova can no longer easily enter the tubes.

Mastitis

Mastitis (infection of the breast) may occur as early as the seventh postpartal day or may not occur until the baby is weeks or months old. The organism causing the infection usually enters through cracked and fissured nipples. Thus, the measures that prevent cracked and fissured nipples also prevent mastitis. These include not leaving the baby too long at the breast, making certain that the baby grasps the nipple properly, both nipple and areola, releasing the baby's grasp on the nipple before removing the baby from a breast, washing hands between handling perineal pads and breasts, exposing nipples to air for at least part of every day, and using a vitamin E- or lanolin-based ointment or A&D ointment to soften nipples daily.

Occasionally, the organism that causes the infection comes from the nasal-oral cavity of the infant. In these instances the infant has usually acquired a staphylococcal or streptococcal infection while in the hospital nursery. Sucking on the nipple, the infant introduces the organisms into the milk ducts, where they proliferate (milk is an excellent medium for bacterial growth). This is an epidemic breast abscess; it is usually found that several mothers discharged from the health care facility at the same time have similar infections.

Assessment

Mastitis is usually unilateral, although epidemic mastitis (because it originates with the infant) may be bilateral. The affected breast shows localized pain, swelling, and redness. Fever accompanies the first symptoms within a matter of hours, and breast milk becomes scant.

Implementations

A mother will be placed on a broad-spectrum antibiotic. Breast-feeding is continued because keeping the breast emptied of milk helps to prevent growth of bacteria. Some mothers may find the breast too painful to allow the infant to suck and may prefer to manually express milk from the affected breast for two or three days until the antibiotic has taken effect and the mastitis has faded (about 3 days). Ice compresses and good bra support give a great deal of pain relief until the process improves. Warm, wet compresses may be ordered to reduce inflammation and decrease edema.

If therapy is started as soon as symptoms are apparent, the condition will run a short course, about 48 hours. If untreated, a breast infection may become a localized abscess. This may involve a large portion of the breast and rupture through the skin, with thick, purulent drainage. A mother will need to be readmitted to the hospital for incision and drainage of the abscess. If an abscess forms, breast-feeding is discontinued but mothers are encouraged to continue to pump breast milk until the abscess has revolved in order to preserve breast-feeding. Some women may feel that the breast is too tender to do this; these women can be assured that formula-feeding is an alternative acceptable feeding method.

Evaluation

Neither mastitis or breast abscess leave any permanent breast disease. A woman can be assured that such an incident has no association with development of breast cancer or interference with future breast-feeding potential.

Urinary Problems

Urinary Retention

Urinary retention implies inadequate bladder emptying. It occurs following childbirth because of decreased bladder sensation for voiding due to edema of the bladder from the pressure of birth. Unable to empty, the bladder fills to overdistention. When a woman does void, instead of emptying completely, the bladder only empties a small portion of its contents. It may quickly, therefore, become overdistended again (retention with overflow). Overdistention is potentially serious because, if it is allowed to continue for a long period of time, permanent damage can occur such as permanent incontinence.

In a postpartal woman urinary retention with overflow is less easy to detect than primary overdistention because, with overdistention, a woman does not void at all. It is easy to detect that a longer-than-usual time (over 8 hours) has passed following delivery or between voids. Assessment by percussion or palpation of the bladder reveals the distention.

With urinary overflow, however, a woman is not only voiding but is voiding very frequently (suggesting that her output must be adequate). Unfortunately, her bladder is never emptied by these overflow voidings so is never relieved of pressure. It is a good practice to measure the amount of the first voiding following delivery by asking a woman who is not yet ambulatory to use a bedpan or putting a measuring container on the toilet seat in the bathroom of a woman who is ambulatory so you can collect and measure voidings. As a rule, if a voiding is less than 50 ml, urinary retention should be suspected.

Urinary retention is proved by catheterizing a woman immediately following a voiding. If the amount of urine left in the bladder following a voiding is over 100 ml, the woman has retention above the normal amount. As a rule, a physician or nurse-midwife writes an order to read: Catheterize for residual urine; if this is over 100 ml, leave indwelling catheter in place. Always use a Foley (indwelling) catheter to catheterize for a residual urine, therefore, in order that you have the proper catheter in place if it needs to be left in. Be very careful to use absolutely aseptic technique so that you do not introduce pathogenic bacteria and cause a urinary tract infection with catheterization.

The procedure for catheterization is shown in Procedure 29-2. Catheterizing a woman during the early postpartal period is often difficult from a procedural standpoint because vulvar edema distorts the position and appearance of the urinary meatus. Use a gentle technique as a woman's perineum is apt to feel tender to touch.

How much urine to remove from an overdistended bladder at one time is controversial. Removing more than 750 to 1,000 ml of urine at any one time will seemingly create a great pressure change not only in the bladder but in the lower abdomen. This decreased pressure in the lower abdomen may cause blood to flow into the area, creating supine hypotension. There are few actual documented occurrences of this happening, however. Particularly in the postpartal period, when a bladder easily distends and the uterus is larger than normal, this shift in pressure may not be as important. Follow health care agency policy in regard to how much urine to remove from a full bladder at catheterization.

If a catheter will be left in place, be certain to explain its principle and draw a picture or explain how the balloon is inflated to hold it in place. The average woman is not aware of the balloon on the catheter and thinks that she has to lie very still or it will become dislodged. This misunderstanding limits her amount of activity and may lead to other complications such as thrombophlebitis. Catheterization is a procedure that has a bad reputation as being extremely painful. You can assure women that, as a rule, it involves only a momentary sting (like a pinprick) as the catheter is inserted. Once the catheter is in place, there is no more pain. The pain sensation of tissue that is edematous is decreased so in the woman with extreme vulvar edema, the pain experienced may be barely noticeable.

After 24 hours, an indwelling catheter is usually ordered to be removed. Encourage a woman to void at the end of 6 hours after removal by offering fluid, administering an analgesic so she can relax, assisting her to the bathroom as necessary, and trying time-honored solutions such as running water at the sink or letting her hold her hand under running water. In the majority of women, bladder and vulvar edema have decreased to such an extent by this time that a woman is able to void without further difficulty. If she has not voided by 8 hours after catheter removal, the physician or nurse-midwife may suggest another catheter be inserted for an additional 24 hours or the administration of a cholinergic drug such as bethanechol chloride (Urecholine) to cause bladder constriction and improved tone.

Difficulty with bladder function following childbirth is becoming less of a problem as less anesthesia and fewer forceps are used at delivery, lessening bladder and vulvar pressure. It is a difficult problem for the woman to accept because bladder elimination is a basic step of self-care. It is disappointing and discouraging to a woman who wants not only to be able to care for herself but to care for a new infant. Assure women that bladder complications are not that uncommon but invariably are no longer present by 48 hours postpartum. Once the difficulty has passed it will not recur, so she does not need to worry about it any longer and can proceed to focus her attention away from her body to that of her new child.

Urinary Tract Infection

Many women have difficulty voiding in the postpartal period because of vulvar edema and loss of bladder tone from the pressure of the fetal head during delivery. Other women seemingly void without difficulty, but their bladder does not fully empty each time (increased residual volume or urinary retention). In both instances, urine remains in the bladder for a longer-than-normal time. Stasis of any body fluid leads to infection.

A woman who was catheterized at the time of delivery or who is catheterized in the postpartal period is very prone to developing a urinary tract infection because bacteria may be introduced into the bladder at the time of catheterization.

Assessment

When a urinary tract infection develops, a woman notices symptoms of burning on urination, possibly blood in the urine (hematuria), and a feeling of frequency (always having to void). The pain is so sharp on voiding that she may resist doing so and thus compound the problem of urinary stasis. She may have a low-grade fever and discomfort from lower abdominal pain.

A woman with any symptoms of urinary tract infection should have a clean-catch urine obtained (do this as an independent nursing action). The procedure for obtaining a clean-catch urine specimen is shown in Procedure 18-1. In order to prevent lochia from contaminating the specimen, be certain to supply a sterile cotton ball for the woman to tuck in her vagina following perineal

========== *Nursing Care Highlight* ==========

Suggestions to Prevent Urinary Tract Infection

1. Maintain a good fluid intake daily (3,000 to 4,000 ml).
2. Void frequently (about every 4 hours).
3. Avoid the use of bath salts or feminine hygiene sprays.

4. Following voiding or defecation, wipe the perineum from front to back to avoid moving organisms from the rectum forward.
5. Void following sexual coitus to expel any organisms in the urethra.

---

cleansing. Be certain to ask if a woman removed the vaginal cotton ball following the procedure; otherwise it will cause stasis of vaginal secretions and possibly endometritis. Mark the specimen *possibly contaminated by lochia* so any blood in the specimen will not be overly interpreted by the laboratory technician.

Implementations

A woman will be started on a broad-spectrum antibiotic such as ampicillin to treat the infection. Encourage her to drink large amounts of fluid (a glass every hour) to help flush the infection from her bladder. She may need an analgesic to reduce the pain of urination for the next few times she voids until the antibiotic begins to work and the burning sensation disappears. Otherwise, she will not drink the fluid you suggest, knowing that will increase the number of times she will need to void, and the voiding is painful.

Although symptoms of urinary tract infection decrease quickly, a woman will need to continue to take the antibiotic for a full 10 days to completely eradicate the infection. Once symptoms have disappeared, particularly if a person is busy—and a new mother at home with a baby is *very* busy—people are usually poor medicine takers. Make a chart for the woman's refrigerator door for her to take home to remind her to continue to take her medication. Otherwise, bacteria in the urine will begin to multiply again, and in another week, symptoms and the active infection will recur. Be certain that she is aware of common methods all women should use to prevent urinary tract infections. (See the Nursing Care Highlight above.)

If a woman is breast-feeding she should temporarily discontinue this if her antibiotic is tetracycline or a sulfonamide. Or you should ask her physician if her antibiotic could be changed to one safe for breast-feeding, such as ampicillin. Otherwise, she may decide to breast-feed once

she is home and not take the prescribed antibiotic.

Postpartal Pregnancy-Induced Hypertension

Mild preexisting hypertension of pregnancy (see Chapter 39) may increase in severity during the first few hours or days after delivery. Rarely, hypertension of pregnancy develops for the first time in a woman who has had no prenatal or intranatal symptoms.

Assessment

The cardinal symptoms are those of prepartal hypertension of pregnancy, namely, proteinuria, edema, and hypertension.

Implementations

The treatment measures will also be the same: bedrest, a quiet atmosphere, and sedatives or antitensives. A woman will need frequent monitoring of her vital signs and urine output. She may be returned to surgery to have a D&C to ascertain that all placental fragments have been removed from the uterus or that none of the pregnancy is still existing. Following a D&C, her blood pressure often dramatically falls to normal.

If convulsions are going to occur with postpartal hypertension of pregnancy, they invariably develop 6 to 24 hours after delivery. Convulsions occurring more than 72 hours after delivery are probably not due to eclampsia but to some cause unrelated to childbearing.

Women in whom postpartal hypertension develops are bewildered by what is happening to them. If convulsions occur, they are frightened to discover how little control they have over their body. They worry that convulsions will occur after they are home while they are working at a hot stove or holding the baby.

A woman should be assured that hypertension

of pregnancy, although appearing late, is a condition of pregnancy; now that she is no longer pregnant, it need give her no further cause for concern. Because eclampsia or preeclampsia occurs with one pregnancy, there is no statistical reason to believe it will occur with a future pregnancy (unless chronic hypertension persists).

The Woman with Reproductive Tract Displacement

If the support systems of the uterus are weakened because of pregnancy, the ligaments will no longer be able to maintain the uterus in its usual position or level following pregnancy and problems of retroflexion, anteflexion, retroversion, and anteversion or prolapse of the uterus may occur. These uterine displacement disorders not only may interfere with future childbearing and fertility but they also cause continued pain or a feeling of lower abdominal heaviness or discomfort.

If the walls of the vagina are weakened, a cystocele (outpouching of the bladder into the vaginal wall) or a rectocele (outpouching of the rectum into the vaginal wall) may occur. Stress incontinence (involuntary voiding on exertion) may occur. These problems tend to occur most frequently in women with a high parity and following operative delivery such as forceps delivery. They are discussed in Chapter 18 with other gynecologic problems.

Separation of the Symphysis Pubis

During pregnancy, many women feel some discomfort at the symphysis pubis because of relaxation of the joint preparatory to delivery. If the fetus is unusually large or fetal position is not optimal, the ligaments of the symphysis pubis may be so stretched by delivery that they actually tear.

Following labor, a woman feels acute pain on turning or walking; her legs tend to externally rotate, giving her a "waddling" gait. A defect over the symphysis pubis can be palpated; the area is swollen and tender to touch.

Bedrest and the application of a tight pelvic binder to immobilize the joint are necessary to relieve pain and allow healing. As with all ligament injuries, a 4- to 6-week period is necessary for healing to take place. The woman will need to arrange for some type of childcare help at home and must avoid heavy lifting for an extended time until healing in the ligaments is complete. It may

be advised that in a future pregnancy she be considered a candidate for cesarean birth.

Psychological Considerations

Any woman who delivers an infant who in any way does not meet her expectations (wrong sex, not as pretty as she had hoped for, handicapped, ill) may have difficulty establishing bonding with the infant. Inability to bond is a postpartal complication with far-reaching implications as it affects the future health of the entire family.

The Woman Whose Child Is Born Handicapped

The nurse who works on a postpartal unit has usually chosen this type of nursing because she enjoys the feeling of happiness that pervades this area. She enjoys holding and feeding babies and teaching in an area of primary prevention care. She may therefore find herself ill at ease when the atmosphere in a patient's room turns to sadness, when a mother needs instructions different from the usual ones because her child has been born handicapped. The professional nurse should have enough skill and enough ability in relating to patients to meet this woman's needs, however, in the same way that she would for other patients.

Most women say during pregnancy that they do not care about the sex of the child as long as the child is normal. How cheated they feel when this one requirement is not met. They are angry, hurt, and disappointed. They may feel a loss of self-respect: they have given birth to an imperfect child, and so they see themselves as imperfect. A mother sometimes responds with a grief reaction, as if the child has died. This is normal, because the "perfect" child she thought she was carrying *has* died.

The average woman has difficulty during the period immediately after delivery believing that her child is real. How much greater is the difficulty for the mother of a handicapped child. She must not only grasp the fact that the baby has been born but understand that the baby she has delivered is less than what she wished for.

At one time, the mother of a child born with a handicap was put under deep anesthesia at delivery, and 24 hours later, when she was "stronger" and "better able to accept the situation," the extent of the handicap was explained to her and she was then shown the baby. This method of dealing with the problem seems to have little merit. The mother cannot begin to accept her situation and work through the problem associated with it un-

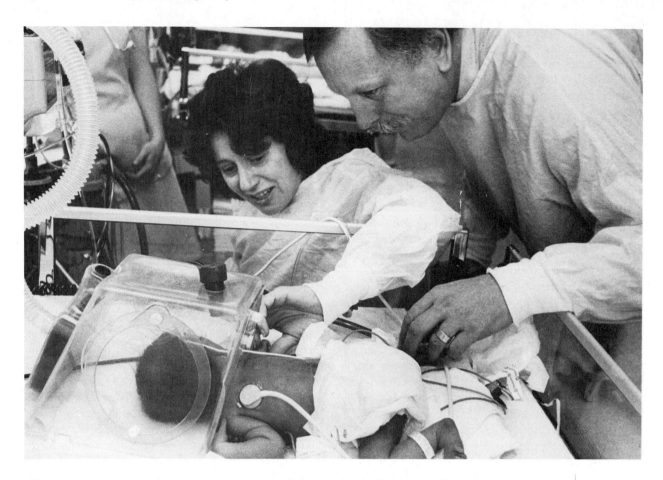

Figure 44-4 *Be certain that women with a complication of pregnancy or with an ill newborn have adequate care time with their newborn if at all possible. (Courtesy, Department of Medical Photography, Children's Hospital, Buffalo, N.Y.).*

til she knows what she is facing. She will worry about the baby she does not see. She will imagine a state of affairs much worse than it actually may be. The baby may only have a deformed finger, but in her mind he or she may be totally deformed or even dead.

Most women are now shown their child moments after birth, and the handicap is immediately explained to them. The same procedure is followed for the father as well. This timing shocks couples, but they are not left feeling they have been deceived by the health center staff. Families are not happy over their child's handicap, but they appreciate having honest friends who dare to face the problem with them when it first becomes apparent.

You should be familiar with the common birth defects and with the treatment that is available for them. Physicians or nurse-midwives will usually make it their responsibility to tell parents of defects, but you must be prepared to reinforce this information or review the problem. People who are under stress are not good listeners and need

explanations repeated several times before they are sure they understand.

A mother should be allowed to care for her child during the postpartal period if the child's condition makes it possible (Figure 44-4). If the infant has a heart defect or respiratory problem that requires being kept in an Isolette, separated from the mother, she should be taken to the nursery and allowed to see the infant and talk with the personnel who are caring for her baby. She should be permitted to handle her child in the Isolette if at all possible—to begin to touch, relate to, and "claim" her infant in as nearly normal a manner as possible. Many women wait until their support person visits to do this so visiting with their newborn is a family activity.

When you handle an infant, be certain that you do so with tender loving care. If you treat the baby as if you find him or her a desirable, attractive child despite the handicap, the mother will find holding and accepting the child an easier task.

Open lines of communication between the parents and the hospital staff that allow for free discussion of feelings and fears will do much to strengthen parent-child relationships when a child is born handicapped.

The Mother Whose Child Is Born Prematurely

The care of the low-birth-weight child is discussed in Chapter 48. The focus here is on the family of the low-birth-weight child in the postpartal period. This family reacts in much the same way as the family whose child has been born handicapped. There is likely to be a loss of self-esteem. The mother could not carry a baby to term; she has somehow "failed."

Despite a child's small size, a woman needs to touch and hold the baby daily, even if in an Isolette. In the past, it was traditional to separate low-birth-weight infants from their mothers on the grounds of preventing infection. Mothers felt unwelcome in high-risk nurseries because of the amount of seemingly complicated equipment and the caps and gowns of hospital personnel. After a simple explanation of the purposes of the equipment and how it works, however, a mother can care for an infant in an Isolette with the same relaxation and skill as a beginning health care provider.

A woman should be given honest appraisals of the child's progress. This policy will help to avoid situations in which a woman is told that her infant is doing well and then must be told later that the child has died. Mothers who are told their child has little chance of living have equally serious problems, however. They do not begin to form a relationship with the new child because they do not want to offer love, knowing that in a matter of hours or days they will be hurt by the newborn's death. This is grieving in anticipation of death, or anticipatory grief. If the child does well and lives, these mothers may have difficulty binding-in their child. They may act as if their child died (he did die in their minds) and the child offered to them is a stranger. They need to spend extra time with their child so they can grasp the concept that he or she is now doing well.

If a newborn is transported from a local hospital or birthing center to a regional center for care, the transport team should leave behind a Polaroid photograph of the infant so the woman and her support person have something tangible to relate to until they are able to see the infant again.

When a mother is discharged from the hospital she should be allowed to telephone the intensive-care nursery daily to ask about her child's progress. She should be able to visit as often and for as long as she wishes.

Low-birth-weight children sometimes remain in the hospital so long that nursing personnel begin to think of them as "their" babies. They may need to be reminded that a child is not theirs and is only under their temporary care. The mother needs to be offered every opportunity available to feel like the child's mother, to begin a relationship with the child that allows her to bind-in warmly despite the child's small size. It often helps her to know that low-birth-weight infants are usually strong and durable despite their small size.

The Woman Whose Child Has Died

The woman who loses a child always has questions about what happened. She is likely to feel bewildered, perhaps bitter, perhaps resentful that the hospital staff could not save the child. "Why me? Out of all the women here, why did my baby die?"

You should be familiar with the forms the mother or father will have to sign when a baby dies or is born dead, and you should know whether or not in your state stillborn infants have to be given a name and to have a funeral.

Other women on the unit tend to stay away from a woman whose child has died, as if what has happened to her were contagious. It is easy to rationalize that a woman's emotions are too raw at this point for anyone outside her family to be of any help. Mothers who have gone through the experience express an opposite view, however. They find that friends and relatives are equally unable to talk about the situation with them, and they want to face what has happened to them in the health care facility, where it happened. They want a nurse to approach them and say, "Do you want to talk about it?" or "Would it help to talk about it?"

No matter how crowded a maternity service is, a woman whose child has died should never be placed in a room with a mother who has had a healthy child. This contrast is too much to ask her to bear. A private room allows the woman an opportunity to express herself. She does not have to keep up a front for a roommate and the hospital staff can bend visiting rules for her. She needs her family with her to fill a portion of the void left by her loss.

Nurses accept the fact that women have physical complications of childbearing. They learn to care for a woman who hemorrhages or acquires an infection. They must become as skilled at caring for a woman whose complication is grief because she is not a mother.

Postpartal Neurosis

Almost every woman notices some immediate postpartal depression or a feeling of sadness (postpartal "blues") following delivery. This occurs as a response to the anticlimactic feeling following labor and probably is related to hormone shifts as estrogen and progesterone levels in her body decline.

In a few women this depression continues beyond the 1 or 2 days of the immediate postpartal period. In addition to an overall feeling of sadness, a woman may have extreme fatigue, an inability to stop crying, increased anxiety about her own or her infant's health, insecurity (unwilling to be left alone or unable to make decisions), and psychosomatic symptoms (nausea and vomiting, diarrhea). Depression that continues beyond a few days may reflect a neurotic process. The woman often has a multitude of related concerns such as lack of effective support people. She needs counseling in order to integrate the experience of childbirth into her life. Ask at postpartal return visits for symptoms that would suggest neurosis that needs appropriate referral.

Postpartal Psychosis

As many as 1 woman in 500 presents enough symptoms in the year after delivery of a child to be considered psychiatrically ill (the current rate of overall mental illness). In about two thirds of these women, the illness develops during the first 6 weeks after delivery. Because the illness coincides with the postpartal period, it has been called *postpartal psychosis* in the past. Rather than being a response to the physical aspects of childbearing, however, it is probably a response to the *crisis* of childbearing. Nearly a third of these women will have had symptoms of mental illness prior to the pregnancy. If the pregnancy had not precipitated the illness, a death in the family, the loss of a husband's job, a divorce, or some other major life crisis would probably have precipitated it.

Symptoms that usually occur are a dysphoric mood (depression, anxiety, or irritability); poor appetite or significant weight loss or increased appetite or significant weight gain; insomnia or hypersomnia; psychomotor agitation or retardation; loss of interest or pleasure in usual activities or decrease in sexual drive; feelings of worthlessness, self-reproach, or excessive or inappropriate guilt; complaints or evidence of diminished ability to think or concentrate; recurrent thoughts of death, suicide, wishes to be dead or suicide attempt (Spitzer, 1980).

By definition, psychosis exists when a person has lost contact with reality. A mother with a childbearing psychosis may deny that she has had a child and, when the child is brought to her, insist that she was never pregnant. A psychosis is a severe mental illness that requires professional psychiatric counseling in order to establish better coping mechanisms against stress. When observations tell you that a woman is not functioning in reality, you cannot improve her concept of reality by a simple measure such as explaining a correct perception. Her sensory input is too disturbed to enable her to comprehend this, and she may interpret your attempt as a threat. She may respond with anger or become equally threatening.

Women with postpartal psychosis need referral to a psychiatric counseling service or resource person. While waiting for such a skilled professional to arrive, do not leave her alone (distorted perception might lead to self-harm). Do not leave her alone with her infant.

Puerperal psychosis may occur after a woman is discharged from the health care facility. Always keep in mind that, although rare, the phenomenon does exist; that childbearing can lead to this degree of mental illness helps you to put childbearing into perspective. If it is a crisis important enough to trigger mental illness in some people, it cannot be considered an everyday incident in anyone's life.

Utilizing Nursing Process

A woman who has a postpartal complication is always at threat from two points of view—her own health and future childbearing potential and her ability to bond with her new infant. A complication at this point of time also invariably causes a family disruption because of increased separation of family members due to an unexpected hospitalization. Extended childcare may need to be arranged, making financial difficulties paramount. Pregnancy, labor, and delivery themselves create a crisis situation. If a crisis is not resolved but continues, it grows immeasurably in proportion and in the difficulty the woman has in coping.

Assessment

Postpartal complications invariably begin with subtle signs such as tenderness in the calf of the leg, slightly increased pain, a slightly elevated temperature, and a slightly increased amount of lochia. Because the average woman has no postpartal complications, it is easy to perform postpartal assessments with a degree of routine. It is important when doing these assessments, however, to bear in mind anything you will categorize as "more than usual" or "more reddened than normal." These are very subjective judgments and it is easy to be misled. Do not rely on a mother's reports of perineal healing or amount of lochia—be certain to observe the perineum yourself. The report of "feels fine" may be very deceptive (she expected to have pain and so reports extreme pain as nothing out of the norm; she has no knowledge of what is "normal" lochia or fundal height and so reports these erroneously).

An increased temperature exclusive of the first 24 hours following delivery is a very serious finding. Women may try to explain away an increased temperature because they know that if they have an elevated temperature they may not be allowed to feed their infant. Do not be misled by such rationalizations as "I was smoking a cigarette just before the temperature was recorded," "The room is warm," "I just had some coffee." Although these factors may make a slight difference (part of a degree) in temperature level, they do not affect it enough to account for a temperature over 100.4°F.

Analysis

The North American Association on Nursing Diagnosis has accepted no diagnoses specific to a complication of the postpartal period, but many diagnoses are applicable to the period. Some examples of diagnoses during this time might be "Alteration in fluid balance related to increased lochia flow," "Alteration in body defense related to infection of perineal incision," or "Alteration in circulation related to thrombophlebitis."

Setting goals of care with a woman may be particularly difficult during this time because, although she wants to do everything necessary to become well again, she also does not want to plan anything or allow anything that will interfere with her being able to relate to her child. During the stage of postpartal taking-in, she may not be interested in doing things for herself; during the second stage of taking-hold she may not be interested in your doing procedures for her. As a rule, however, never underestimate the degree of pain, inconvenience, or sacrifice that a woman will undergo in order to prepare herself to care for her child. That quality is the essence of motherhood.

Planning

Be certain in making plans for a postpartal woman that you provide for both areas of involvement: that which will restore her most quickly to health again, plus that which will continue contact between herself and her child and between her and her support person and family. "Contact" cannot always be physical, but it can always include frequent reports of the infant's health and preferences. This information can be passed on by planning for a nursery nurse to contact a mother at least once a nursing shift during the taking-in period and for telephone calls initiated by the mother during the taking-hold phase. Supplying Polaroid photos of the infant offers a woman something concrete to relate to. Many mothers respond well to notes written as if they were from the child: "Hi, Mom. Just a note to say hello. I'm drinking well but I miss you and can't wait for you to get better and be allowed to take care of me again. Love, Susan Marie." Such a note serves to relieve the mother's concern for the child (who is doing well) and also helps her to feel both more importance and more self-esteem, which helps bonding.

Implementation

Implementation of care for a mother with a complication of the postpartal period must be accompanied by teaching of child care and stressing that the complication is a transitory one (assuming that is true). Continuing to review well-child care with a mother helps her to accept the situation as temporary (If it were not, why would you be stressing her ability to return home shortly and care for the child?).

Evaluation

Evaluation of a woman with a postpartal complication should address both life aspects that are affected: Has the mother returned to optimal health? Is her bonding with her child adequate? Evaluation may suggest that follow-up care by a community health nurse may be necessary in order for a woman to cope with the responsibility of childcare and integrating the child into the family in the face of reduced energy.

Nursing Care Planning

Angie Baco is a 42-year-old woman you care for during the postpartal period. She had gestational diabetes during pregnancy. She is concerned now because her right leg has pain on movement.

Problem Area. Gestational diabetes.

Assessment

Asking whether urine tests are showing any glucose spillage, apprehensive that diabetes will not end with the pregnancy. Asking whether dieting will reduce possibility of diabetes. No subjective symptoms, no thirst, dizziness, lethargy. Voiding frequently (100 ml per hour) since Foley catheter removed. On regular diet.

Urine neg, neg for protein and ketones. Two-hour postprandial blood sugar = 120 (Normal).

Analysis

Fear related to concern that gestational diabetes will not be transient.

Locus of Decision Making. Shared.

Goal. Patient is familiar with normal postpartal course following gestational diabetes.

Criteria.

1. Patient does not confuse a postpartal symptom such as polyuria with a diabetic symptom.
2. Patient maintains health supervision.

Nursing Orders

1. Continue to assess urine before meals for glucose and acetone (double-voided specimens).
2. Instruct to return to prepregnancy diet during postpartal period rather than dieting now.

Problem Area. Pain in right calf.

Assessment

Patient states that her right calf is tender to touch; skin over area is white and shiny. She first noticed symptom this morning when she awoke (20 minutes ago). Homan's sign positive; right calf larger than left calf by 2 cm diameter. Toes blanch equally well in both feet. Temperature: 99.6°F orally.

Analysis

Circulatory interference related to femoral thrombophlebitis (M.D. confirmed).

Goal. Patient to complete postpartal course without further leg involvement.

Locus of Decision Making. Shared.

Criteria. Erythema and pain in leg to resolve.

Nursing Orders

1. Complete bedrest with cradle.
2. Position infant crib next to bed so she can reach infant easily.
3. Warm, wet dressings with Gaymar pump continually.
4. Assess leg for diameter and Homans' sign b.i.d.
5. Encourage good fluid intake (3,000 to 4,000 ml daily) to decrease blood viscosity.
6. Use acetaminophen (Tylenol) for pain relief in place of aspirin (both are ordered).
7. Heparin to be administered daily based on prothrombin level report. Schedule prothrombin level daily at 6 A.M.
8. Is allowed to formula-feed infant as infection is contained. Be certain she is comfortable holding infant without pressure on leg.
9. Remind patient not to rub right leg; no massage by nursing staff of right leg.
10. Ask husband to bring in an activity such as knitting for her as she will remain in hospital for an additional 3 or 4 days.

Questions for Review

Multiple Choice

1. Mrs. Smith is a woman you care for in the postpartal period. Which assessment below would lead you to believe she is developing a urinary complication?
   a. At 8 hours postdelivery she has voided 100 ml in four small voidings.
   b. She has voided 1,000 ml in two voidings each spaced 1 hour apart.
   c. She tells you she is extremely thirsty.
   d. Her perineum is obviously edematous to inspection.

2. You assess Mrs. Smith and discover she has saturated two perineal pads in 15 minutes; she looks extremely pale. Which of the following measures would be your best first action?
   a. assess her blood pressure and pulse
   b. assess and massage her uterus
   c. turn her onto her left side
   d. raise the head of her bed.

3. You administer Methergine 0.2 mg to Mrs. Smith to achieve increased uterine contraction. Which as-

sessment below should you make prior to administering this medication?

   a. Her urine output is over 50 ml per hour.

   b. Her blood pressure is below 140/90.

   c. She can walk without experiencing dizziness.

   d. Her hematocrit level is over 45 percent.

4. Which assessment on the third postpartal day would make you evaluate Mrs. Smith as having uterine subinvolution?

   a. Her uterus is 2 cm above the symphysis pubis.

   b. Her uterus is three fingerwidths under the umbilicus.

   c. Her uterus is at the level of the umbilicus.

   d. She experiences "pulling" pain while breast-feeding.

5. On the third day postpartum, which temperature level below is internationally defined as a postpartal infection?

   a. 99.6°F

   b. 100.4°F

   c. 102.4°F

   d. 104.2°F

6. Mrs. Smith is diagnosed as having endometritis. Which position would you place her in based on this diagnosis?

   a. flat in bed

   b. on her left side

   c. Trendelenburg's

   d. semi-Fowler's

7. Mrs. Smith's physician tells you he suspects she is also developing a thrombophlebitis in her right leg. Which assessment below would you make with her to detect this?

   a. Bend her knee and palpate her calf for pain.

   b. Ask her to raise her foot and draw a circle.

   c. Blanch a toe and count the seconds it takes to color again.

   d. Dorsiflex her right foot and ask if she has pain in her calf.

8. Mrs. Smith is placed on an anticoagulant to prevent further clot formation. She asks you if she will be able to continue breast-feeding. Your best response would be that

   a. all anticoagulants pass in breast milk so she will have to stop.

   b. anticoagulants pass in breast milk but not in amounts to cause harm.

   c. the effect of anticoagulants is counteracted by infant gastric juices.

   d. your answer depends on the type of anticoagulant she is taking.

9. Mrs. Smith states that her leg is very painful. Which action below would be most appropriate to relieive this pain?

   a. Massage the calf of her leg.

   b. Keep covers off the leg.

   c. Apply ice to her leg above the knee.

   d. Urge her to walk to relieve muscle spasm.

Discussion

1. Hemorrhage is a serious complication following childbirth. What steps would you take if you discovered a woman with vaginal hemorrhage at the first hour following childbirth?

2. Infection in the postpartal period generally occurs because of contamination during delivery. What precautions should you always observe during delivery to prevent postpartal infection?

3. Symptoms of postpartal depression may be subtle. What specific observations would you make to detect whether this has occurred?

Suggested Readings

Atkinson, S., et al. (1983). Puerperal psychosis—a personal experience. *Health Visitor, 56,* 17.

Davis, J. H., et al. (1984). Sorting out new mother's learning priorities on home visits. *Home Health Visitor and Community Nurse, 2,* 38.

Devancy, S. W., et al. (1980). Nursing care for the relinquishing mother. *J.O.G.N. Nursing, 9,* 375.

Ewing, T. L., et al. (1979). Maternal deaths associated with postpartum vulvar edema. *American Journal of Obstetrics and Gynecology, 134,* 173.

Henderson, K. J., & Newton, L. D. (1978). Helping nursing mothers maintain lactation while separated from their infants. *M.C.N., 3,* 352.

Huffman, M. H. (1983). Acute care of the patient with a pulmonary embolism due to venous thromboemboli. *Critical Care Nurse, 3,* 70.

Ishida, Y. (1980). How to deal with grief in childbirth. *Female Patient, 5,* 74.

Kelley, M., et al. (1982). Hypertension in pregnancy: Labor, delivery and postpartum. *American Journal of Nursing, 82,* 813.

Martell, L. K., et al. (1984). Rubin's "puerperal change" reconsidered. *J.O.G.N. Nursing, 13,* 145.

Nyman, J. E. (1980). Thrombophlebitis in pregnancy. *American Journal of Nursing, 80,* 90.

Oakley, A. (1981). Adjustment of women to motherhood. *Nursing (Oxford), 1,* 939.

Petrick, J. M. (1984). Postpartum depression, *J.O.G.N. Nursing, 13,* 37.

Rancillo, N. (1979). When a woman is diabetic: Postpartal care. *American Journal of Nursing, 79,* 453.

Scupholme, A. (1982). Puerperal inversion of the uterus: A case report. *Journal of Nurse Midwifery, 27,* 37.

Spitzer, R. L. (1980). *Diagnostic and statistical manual of mental disorders* (3rd ed.). Washington, D.C.: American Psychiatric Association.

Swanson, J. (1978). Nursing intervention to facilitate maternal-infant attachment. *J.O.G.N. Nursing, 7,* 35.

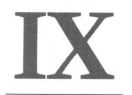

The High-Risk Newborn

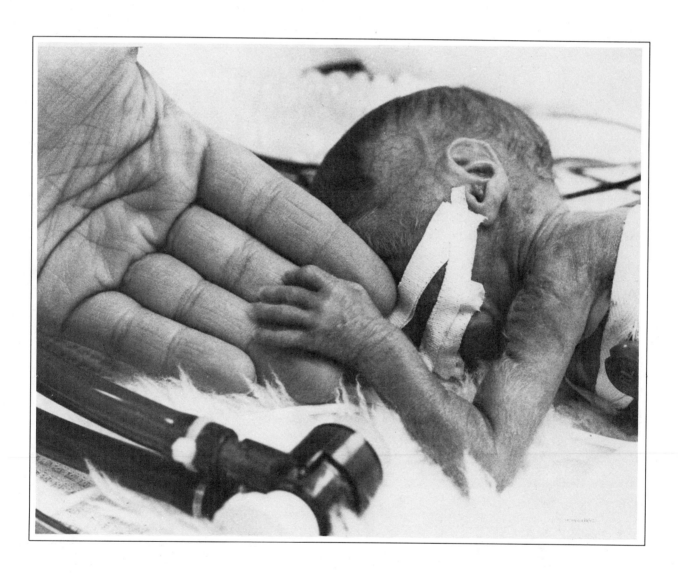

45

Identifying the High-Risk Infant

OBJECTIVES

Following mastery of the contents of this chapter, you should be able to

1. Define a high-risk infant and give examples of infants who would be categorized as such.
2. Describe the concept of regionalization and maternal and infant transport in care of the high-risk infant.
3. Analyze the basis for nursing care important to all high-risk infants.
4. Synthesize knowledge of the high-risk newborn with nursing process in order to achieve quality maternal-newborn nursing care.

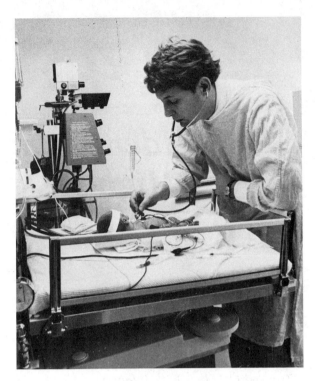

Figure 45-1 *Infants are classified as high-risk for many reasons. (Courtesy of the Department of Medical Photography, Children's Hospital, Buffalo, N.Y.)*

A HIGH-RISK INFANT is one born with less-than-average ability or fewer chances to survive or a greater chance of being left with a permanent handicap either psychosocially or physiologically. About 60 percent of the time the pregnancy history suggests a high-risk infant will be born (amniotic membranes have been ruptured for over 24 hours, maternal bleeding occurred or small intrauterine growth has been documented, as examples). Other infants are categorized as high-risk at birth because, on physical examination, it is apparent that they have a congenital anomaly or are low birth weight or small for gestation age (Figure 45-1).

Still other infants appear to be healthy at birth but then, as early as at 5 minutes of life, have difficulty establishing effective respirations. There are still more infants who are categorized as high-risk because economic or psychosocial factors of their family have the potential to interfere with optimum growth or development. Common causes of high risk in infants are categorized in Table 45-1. Important concerns of nurses are the identification, transport, and care of such infants.

The nursing care of high-risk infants has special demands including a total commitment to keep the family involved in care, unique considerations for the small size of the child, and participation as a member of a perinatal health care team (often consisting of a neonatalogist or pediatrician with special extended education, a respiratory care therapist, social worker, nutritionist, psychologist, chaplain, neonatal care practition-

ers and obstetricians, nurse-midwives, and maternal-newborn nurse practitioners). Because care of these smallest patients is so unique and specialized, this number of people is needed in order to make care complete and comprehensive.

Regionalization of Perinatal Care

Providing safe care for infants with perinatal problems is best accomplished by a regionalization care system. This system of care originated because caring for high-risk infants requires such high expenditures for personnel and equipment that not all hospitals can afford to provide for high-risk infant care. To initiate the system, levels of care that can be given safely at each hospital within a health systems area are evaluated, and hospital nurseries are then designated as level I, II, or III, depending on the amount and type of care available at that particular site. Descriptions of these three levels are listed in Table 45-2.

It is important that health care facilities not attempt to provide care beyond their capabilities or rating. High-risk nurseries that are high-risk in name only do not provide safe care and may actually be more unsafe than a regular nursery.

In order for regionalization to operate effectively, a number of important subsystems must

Table 45-1 Common Factors Causing Infants To Be Categorized as High-Risk

Factor	Possible Consequence in Infant
Antenatal Factors	
Pregnancy-induced hypertension	May be small for gestation age; hypoglycemia and polycythemia.
Cardiac disease	May have intrapartal anoxia; small for gestation age.
Poor nutrition	Small for gestation age; hypoglycemia.
Diabetes	Respiratory distress syndrome; large for gestation age; hypoglycemia. If diabetes is class D, infants may be small for gestation age.
Rh isoimmunization	Anemia, hyperbilirubinemia.
Maternal age more than 35	Genetic malformations; dysfunctional labor patterns leading to fetal anoxia.
Maternal age less than 16	Small for gestation age; effects of hypertension of pregnancy, premature labor, or inadequate pelvis.
Anemia	Anoxia; small for gestation age.
Maternal infections	Congenital anomalies; neurologic disorders.
Chronic renal, vascular, or collagen disease	Small for gestation age; specific problem related to maternal drug use.
Maternal drug use	Small for gestation age; neurologic and metabolic disorders.
Multiple gestation	Small for gestation age; birth trauma, anoxia.
Prolonged pregnancy	Anoxia, birth injury, neurologic disorders.
Hydramnios	Tracheoesophageal fistula; anencephaly.
Natal Factors	
Prolonged rupture of membranes	Infection.
Premature labor	Anoxia, respiratory distress syndrome, intrapartal injury.

Factor	Possible Consequence in Infant
Abnormal presentation	Birth trauma, anoxia.
Cesarean section	Respiratory distress syndrome.
Premature separation of placenta	Anoxia.
Placenta previa	Severe anemia, anoxia.
Oxytocin and/or epidural anesthesia	Anoxia.
Meconium-stained amniotic fluid	Anoxia.
Prolapsed cord	Anoxia.
Prolonged labor	Anoxia.

be well designed and functional: ability of level I and II nurses to identify infants too ill for these levels of care, a system to transport infants to level III settings, a system of support for parents while their child is cared for at a distant site, and follow-up care of the infant as he or she regains health at either a facility closer to home or at home.

Identification of Ill Infants

As nurses are the health care providers who are often in the best position to assess changes in the health of neonates because they provide the most consistent care, they often are the ones most likely to identify a child's condition as changing, justifying transport to another level of care. Identifying their needs is the responsibility of nurses in level I and level II nurseries; providing educational programs on high risk identification is generally regarded as the responsibility of the level III facility.

Maternal Transport

Women who are transported to special care centers are those who are severely preeclamptic, those who have had an episode of beginning premature labor (now halted), or women with an anticipated multiple birth. It is difficult for a woman to leave a local community hospital and be transported to a level III center for care as they have confidence in the care givers at the local facility but not in the people at the specialized center.

Table 45-2 Levels of Care

Level	Description
I	Hospital provides services for uncomplicated deliveries and normal newborn infants. The number of births at the facility is small. Initial newborn management such as resuscitation and short-term assisted ventilation is available while transport to a level II or III facility is awaited.
II	Hospital provides services for both the normal and high-risk pregnant patient and for the management of selected neonatal illnesses. The facility is capable of resuscitation, short-term assisted ventilation with bag and mask or endotracheal tube, intravenous therapy with infusion pumps, arterial blood gas monitoring, continuous cardiorespiratory monitoring with appropriate equipment, performance of exchange transfusion, and oxygen administration.
III	Hospital serves as a regional center and provides all aspects of perinatal care, including intensive care and a broad range of continuously available subspecialty consultation. The facility provides educational programs, consultation services, and back-up support for level I and II facilities. The facility provides transport service and transport personnel for the infant in need of such care.

Source: American Academy of Pediatrics. (1977). *Standards and recommendations for hospital care of newborn infants* (6th ed.). Evanston, Ill.: The Academy. Copyright American Academy of Pediatrics 1977.

If you are a member of the community hospital staff, make an effort to convey a feeling of welcome to the transport team; your obvious acceptance of them helps the woman to accept them also. If you are a member of a transport team, be certain to introduce yourself and take time to become acquainted with the woman and her support person before transport in order to help the woman feel that what you are providing is continuity of care, or at least that she is not among strangers.

Prior to a maternal transport, the woman must be evaluated to be certain that transport will be safe for both her and her fetus. Vital signs, including fetal heart rate, should be recorded. If the woman had premature labor halted, a uterine contraction monitor should be used to assure that no further labor contractions are present. Supplies needed to accompany her are an emergency delivery pack, a warmed Isolette, and emergency drugs including magnesium sulfate and a tocolytic. An external fetal monitor can be attached or frequent (every 10 minute) fetal heart rate determinations made by stethoscope or Doppler.

A fluid line should be inserted as a safety measure during transport. The type of intravenous pump used should be evaluated as to its capacity to remain accurate while an ambulance is in motion (e.g., a type using a drop sensing "eye" may not be the appropriate choice [Reedy, 1984]). Ideally, the transport ambulance should have room for the woman's support person to accompany her to the special care center. If this is not possible be certain the support person has detailed instructions as to where the woman is being transported and where in the new facility she can be located.

Transport of High-Risk Infants

Infants who are born at level I and II facilities but require level III care must be transported for such care. If it is known before birth that the infant will need level III care (premature rupture of the membranes at 30 weeks' gestation, for example), ideally the mother is transported to the level III health care facility before birth so that the infant can immediately have the benefit of that level care. If hospitalizing the woman is not feasible in advance (the woman is admitted to a level I hospital in active labor and delivers before transport is available or advisable), transporting the infant as soon as he or she is stabilized after birth is the next best approach to providing care.

The philosophy of transporting ill newborns has swung full cycle in recent years, from one of not transporting in the early hours of life (to stress the child the least amount possible in these first critical hours), to one of transporting immediately no matter what the baby's condition, to one of transporting as soon as possible but only after stabilizing the infant's condition. This is an important philosophy for the parents of a child to understand. They may envision a transport team hurrying into the community hospital and immediately swooping up their child and leaving for the regional center. Instead, the transport team delays to insert an intravenous line and an oral-gastric tube and perhaps intubate. They worry that their child is sicker than they were first told (or the transport team is not very efficient). They need to be told that stabilizing infants before transport safeguards them during transport. Inserting an intravenous line in a rocking ambu-

Helpful Information on Infants for Transport Team

Estimated gestation age (from date of confinement and physical examination)

Birth weight

Health disorders during the pregnancy

Unusual aspects of labor or delivery

Infant temperature and measures being employed to keep temperature in neutral zone

Infant color

Oxygen requirement (documented by arterial blood gas if possible) and measures employed to keep the infant's PO_2 at that level

Respiratory assessment (apnea, retractions, etc.)

Blood glucose or Dextrostix reading

Blood pressure (if there is equipment to take it accurately)

Chest X-ray findings and hematocrit on any infant with respiratory distress, cyanosis, or shock

---

lance at the point a child needs it is obviously more hazardous than inserting it prophylactically in a warmed, well-lighted, firmly grounded nursery.

The role of nurses in transporting infants has also come full circle—from their being the only ones involved, to giving up the role to physicians, to specially prepared nurses (neonatal clinicians) taking it on. In order to safely transport infants, a clinician must be able to offer emotional support to extremely stressed parents as well as to perform such skills as inserting intravenous lines, inserting umbilical catheters, and intubation. He or she must be extremely aware of drug use and dosages and temperature stabilization measures. In order to do this safely the nurse clinician should have access to a telephone line for physician consultation as necessary.

Transport service must be available 24 hours a day. In many institutions, calling for transport service is the physician's responsibility. In others, after the need for transport has been confirmed by a physician, the nurse actually sets the process in motion. If you are working at an alternative birthing center, although you anticipate that all infants will be well at birth because of careful screening to eliminate high-risk mothers, you need to be aware of how to contact a level III facility for those few instances when an infant is not well at birth. This preparation may be particularly important as, at a wellness-oriented setting, there may not be equipment available for sustaining an ill infant for any length of time.

In order that a transport team can anticipate what equipment will be needed to stabilize and transport a particular infant, accurate clinical data on the infant must be reported to its members. The type of information that transport personnel find helpful is shown in the box above. On the basis of this information, the transporting facility may suggest further measures that should be taken before they arrive.

Vitamin K and eye prophylaxis should be routinely administered unless contraindicated by unusual circumstances. Copies of both the mother's and infant's charts should be prepared to accompany the infant. About 10 ml of clotted maternal blood, an equal cord blood sample, and the placenta, if applicable, should accompany the infant also so that the level III facility can perform blood analysis without delay.

It is important that an infant be transported in an incubator with a source of oxygen, easy access to the infant, ability to provide heat, and good visibility (Figure 45-2). Parents need to see their infant and touch him or her if at all possible before transport. If parents are not allowed to see their child, the birth does not seem real or such parents may be left imagining that the child has even greater problems than actually exist (not only is the baby small, but there must be physical defects as well). Otherwise, why were they not allowed to see their baby? Such thoughts "turn off" parent-child bonding. If it is not possible for a mother to see her infant (she delivered under general anesthetic and is not yet awake), she should be shown a Polaroid photograph of the baby as soon as she is awake. If the infant must be transported so far that it will be difficult for the woman to visit, this picture will leave her some-

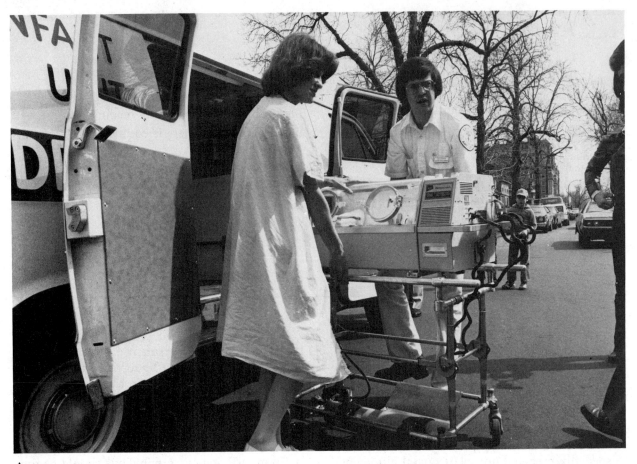

A

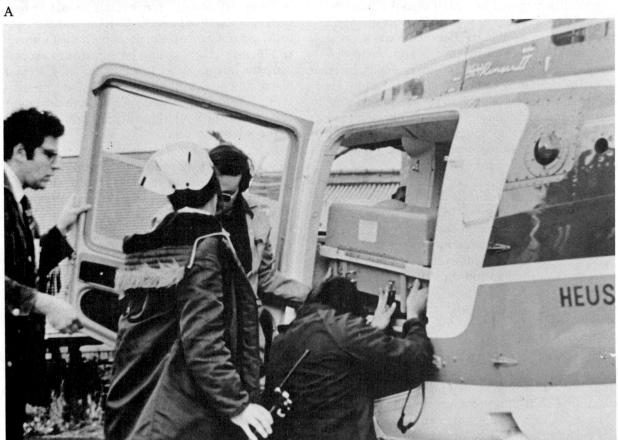

B

thing tangible to bind to until she can visit and care for her child.

Parent-Child Bonding

There appears to be a sensitive period in the first few days of life when women bond with their infants most easily (Klaus, 1982). It is therefore just as important that mothers of high-risk infants have the opportunity to hold and touch their infants as it is for mothers of well infants. It is frightening for parents to walk into intensive care units. The number of machines, the concentration of personnel, the fragile appearance of their newborn make it very hard for them to say, "I want to hold my baby." If not given active support, they will come no closer to their child than looking through a glass window in the hallway. In most level III facilities, parents are allowed to visit or call any time during the day or night.

Some intensive care facilities encourage parents to gavage or suction their infants when they visit. These are not the best actions for parents, however, unless the baby will be discharged still needing this type of care. A parent's time is better spent just holding and stroking the infant—being a loving parent, not a technician, to him or her (Figure 45-3).

Two of the biggest dangers to infants in intensive care units are failure of mother-child or parent-child bonding and failure of efforts to give the infant the sensory stimulus required for initial development. When caring for infants in special care settings, implementations such as holding infants, stroking them, looking directly at them so that they have eye-to-eye contact, and singing or talking to them have as much priority as physical interventions. These actions must be as much a part of a nursing care plan as more skill-oriented procedures. Because high-risk newborns are hospitalized for extended periods, sibling visiting, in order to make a new infant real to an older brother or sister, should be allowed also.

A woman, or the father if he will be the primary caretaker, needs to spend enough time with a newborn to be comfortable with him or her before discharge. It is difficult for a first-time parent to learn how to care for a child with

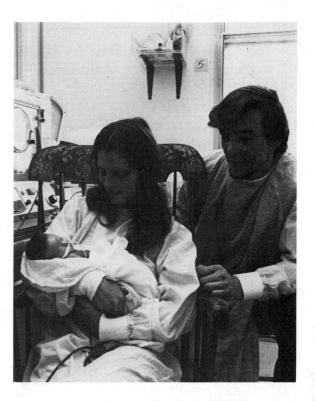

Figure 45-3 *Encourage parents to visit in intensive care nurseries so they can begin parent-child bonding. (Courtesy of the Department of Medical Photography, Children's Hospital, Buffalo, N.Y.)*

enough confidence to feel comfortable about taking the newborn home even when well. When the baby is ill, the situation is compounded. A mother may be able to learn how to feed her hard-to-feed infant in one visit, but she cannot begin to learn in a single visit all her infant's cues that she will need to learn in order to be familiar enough to provide total care. That is the kind of knowledge that comes only with repeated contact.

When people feel self-conscious about their actions, they often do not hold their infant as warmly as they want to. They may feel that talking or singing to an infant will look strange in this setting of machines and technical equipment. Role modeling parental behavior—talking to infants, holding them warmly, counting toes, tickling tummies (all the "motherly" things that new mothers do)—is important in showing parents that such actions are not out of place and they can

Figure 45-2 *Ill or immature neonates are transported to regional care centers in a carrier that provides warmth, oxygen if needed, and easy access for emergency treatment. A. Here the transport carrier is lifted into a transport van by the nurse who will accompany the baby to a regional center. B. A transport carrier is placed aboard a helicopter to transport from a distant site. (Courtesy of the Department of Medical Photography, Children's Hospital, Buffalo, N.Y.)*

Healthy and Unhealthy Parental Reactions to a High-Risk Infant

Healthy Reactions

1. Parents frequently question doctors and nurses about etiology, prognosis, treatment plan, etc.
2. Parents are aware of negative feelings in themselves and can express them.
3. Parents can seek help from friends and relatives.

Unhealthy Reactions

1. Parents make little effort to secure information about their baby's condition.
2. Parents are unable to express feelings of guilt or anger at the baby's early arrival.
3. Parents consistently misinterpret or exaggerate either positive or negative information given to them about the baby's condition and are unable to respond with hope as the condition improves.
4. Parents concentrate conversation and interest on less threatening matters such as welfare of older children.
5. Parents are unable to accept and use help offered them.

Source: Dubois, D. (1975). Indications of an unhealthy relationship between parents and premature infants. *J.O.G.N. Nursing, 4,* 21.

feel comfortable doing them. Although such behaviors are called "motherly," fathers do the same things when they are comfortable with infants. Role modeling when just the father is present is equally as important as with mothers.

Chapter 29 discusses behaviors that mothers usually manifest when they are adjusting well to their newborn and bonding is occurring. These are helpful observations to make with parents of high-risk infants as well. In addition to these behaviors, the box above summarizes behaviors that are indications of healthy and unhealthy relationships between parents and a low-birth-weight baby (Dubois, 1975).

Particularly important in estimating the extent of bonding appears to be the number of times each week that a parent initiates contact with the child, either by a visit or by a phone call if distance interferes with frequent visiting. Nurses in intensive care settings should keep a record of when parents visit or telephone. Infants of parents who make contact less often than twice a week appear to have more difficulty establishing effective parent-child bonding than those whose parents make more frequent contact (Klaus, 1982).

Some parents may be reluctant to telephone a great deal, afraid that they are interrupting important people, that they will be thought of as "nuisances" or overanxious. They need to be told at each contact that their calls are welcome, and even if they must wait a minute sometimes for someone to respond, it is not because no one wants to talk to them but because it takes time to remove a gown or close an Isolette before answering the telephone.

If you are caring for the mother after her infant has been transported to a center, urge her to call the center at least once a day to ask about her child. You may need to dial for her if she has intravenous fluid infusing or is easily intimidated by telephone operators or receptionists who do not fully appreciate the importance of her contact with her newborn. If you are working in a level III center, always initiate contact with the mother after the initial screening and "settling in" procedures for the newly admitted infant. This effort makes a strong impression that you are interested in contact with her and opens the line for communication.

Parents call most readily if they know the name of one person whom they can ask to speak to. The parents should be given the name of their infant's primary nurse and the physician who is their child's doctor. As house staff changes or new associate nurses begin care, parents need to be alerted to the new names and assured that they may now call this new person, lest they lose confidence in the acceptability of their telephoning.

Development of a Sense of Trust

In order that high-risk infants can develop a sense of trust, they must have the same considerations as well newborns: a constant caregiver, active interaction, and sensory stimulation. All high-risk infants need to be assigned a primary nurse and consistent associate nurses so that the number of caregivers they have is as low as possible. These people should spend active time with a child apart from the contacts involving mainly treatments. Sensory stimulation—looking at the child, providing a mobile for the crib or Isolette or some black and white item the infant can see, giving a chance when the infant is out of the Isolette (away from the hum of the motor), to hear a voice or music box, stroking the back of the head or arms or back—should be supplied by everyone who cares for the infant, but the primary care person should accept these actions as a major responsibility. It gains little if an infant is rescued from death at birth by medical intervention but then is never able to relate well to people because nursing intervention to initiate a sense of trust until the mother could take over this function was inadequate.

Return of Infants to Community Facilities

As infants return to wellness again (or achieve it for the first time), at the point that a level I or II nursery could again meet their care needs, ideally they should be transported back to their local communities for care. Such a move almost automatically facilitates bonding by allowing for easier visiting by the parents and more active involvement from the entire family with the infant.

Such a step is not included in some regionalization programs because of problems of infection control (local hospitals are concerned about spread of resident bacteria from the level III center to their site) or lack of continuation of third-party payment. Because a level I nursery loses revenue when an infant is transferred, it is possible that an institution could be reluctant to transport borderline-care infants. If they knew an infant would be returned to them if extended care is unnecessary—or at least as soon as possible—transport decisions could be made without the issue of money being involved. Further health care planning is necessary in order to make regionalization as efficient and supportive a system as it was originally designed to be.

Following High-Risk Infants at Home

It is difficult to predict on discharge from a nursery which infants will do well at home and which ones will have to be returned for care because their families did not understand or could not meet their needs. At each hospital visit it is important to assess the parents' level of knowledge about their child's condition. Do they comprehend that he or she is not only light in weight (2 pounds), but is also immature? The mother who does not understand this connection may think that her infant is unresponsive to her because he does not grasp her finger when she places it in his palm the way her other children did. Knowing that he is too immature to do so will limit her expectations to the responses her child is capable of.

Battle (1975) has devised a number of criteria that can be used to predict whether parents will be able to incorporate a handicapped child into their family. If these factors are absent, a child with a handicap (the one who is going home in a hip spica cast, who will be mentally retarded, who has a cleft palate, for example) is doubly at risk. Not only is the newborn handicapped but also he or she may not be well accepted by the family.

Factors that indicate that a family will probably be able to adjust to caring for a handicapped child are shown in Table 45-3. All families of high-risk infants should be screened for these criteria. You cannot change many of these factors if they are present, but knowledge of their existence serves as an incentive to help the family establish solid support people who can aid in overcoming or minimizing obstacles. These might be people from religious or community groups or a community health nurse.

The High-Risk Infant and Child Abuse

It would seem that if children have been born prematurely or handicapped, the reaction of their parents toward them would be to protect them even more than the average child so that no further harm could come to them. In reality, particularly in reference to low-birth-weight children, the opposite may occur. Low-birth-weight children are at high risk for child abuse.

Table 45-3 Factors That Aid in Acceptance of a Handicapped Child

Factor	Rationale
Support people are available.	Caring for a child is a series of crises during which support people become very important.
A strong marital bond exists between the parents.	A marriage partner can serve as a strong support person.
A good relationship exists between the child's mother and maternal grandmother.	The mother (because she had good care) has a firm sense of trust and the ability to give care to another.
The handicapped child is not a firstborn.	The mother has had practice "mothering."
The family lives close to shopping, schools, and transportation.	The family is not isolated.
The family has a supportive religious faith.	Secondary support systems are important in times of stress.
The parents were told of the child's disability as soon as possible.	Handicapping is easier to accept if parents never thought of the child as totally well.

Source: Battle, C. U. (1975). Chronic physical disease: Behavioral aspects. *Pediatric Clinics of North America, 22,* 525.

Child abuse in this population is probably due to the separation of children from their family at birth, which interferes with bonding. Helfer and Kempe (1968) have identified three factors that must be present before child abuse occurs:

1. *A parent who has the ability to abuse.* All parents grow angry at their children on occasion; only a few are capable of actually hurting a child.
2. *A child who is special in some way.* The child was born prematurely, is more intelligent than the parent, has red hair. . . . The ways that children are "special" are endless.
3. *A triggering event.* The trigger that initiates child abuse can be a major family insult (loss of the father's job, a fire in the house) or a minor incident that serves as the last straw (a plugged toilet, rain on a Sunday picnic).

When following children who are identified as high-risk at birth, it is sound judgment to keep these three criteria in mind: a special person, a special child, a special event. Because one of the circumstances (a special child) is already present, the child is always more vulnerable to abuse than is a nonrisk infant.

Other factors associated with child abuse are lack of support people, alcohol or drug abuse, abuse of the parent as a child, inadequate knowledge of growth and development, and isolation. Serving as a support person or seeing that support people are identified for families with high-risk infants is a means of reducing the possibility that children seen today in a high-risk care setting will be seen tomorrow in the emergency room with burns or scalds.

Helping mothers get to know their children at birth, giving them opportunities to see and touch and care for them as much as possible, provides knowledge of growth and development and aids bonding. With effective bonding, child abuse does not occur under any circumstances.

Suggested Readings

Altemeier, W. A., III, et al. (1982). Antecedents of child abuse. *Journal of Pediatrics, 100,* 823.

American Academy of Pediatrics. (1977). *Standards and recommendations for hospital care of newborn infants* (6th ed.). Evanston, Ill.: The Academy.

Battle, C. U. (1975). Chronic physical disease: Behavioral aspects. *Pediatric Clinics of North America, 22,* 525.

Blackburn, S. (1982). The neonatal ICU—a high-risk environment. *American Journal of Nursing, 82,* 1708.

Blackburn, S. (1983). Fostering behavioral development of high-risk infants. *J.O.G.N. Nursing, 12,* 76s.

Committee on Fetus and Newborn. (1982). Neonatal nurse clinicians: Guidelines. *Pediatrics, 70,* 1104.

Cranley, M. S. (1983). Perinatal risk. *J.O.G.N. Nursing, 12,* 13s.

Cunningham, M. D. (1982). Neonatal intensive care: Is it cost effective? *Perinatology/Neonatology, 6,* 14.

Cushing, M. (1983). "Do not feed" . . . withholding treatment for severely defective newborns. *American Journal of Nursing, 83,* 602.

Dubois, D. (1975). Indications of an unhealthy relationship between parents and premature infants. *J.O.G.N. Nursing, 4,* 21.

Gribbins, R. E., et al. (1982). Stress and coping in the NICU staff nurse: Practical implications for change. *Critical Care Medicine, 10,* 865.

Hansen, F. H. (1982). Nursing care in the neonatal intensive care unit. *J.O.G.N. Nursing, 11,* 17.

Harper, R. G., et al. (1982). The scope of nursing practice in level III neonatal intensive care units. *Pediatrics, 70,* 875.

Hawkins-Walsh, E. (1980). Diminishing anxiety in parents of sick newborns. *M.C.N., 5,* 30.

Helfer, R. E., & Kempe, C. H. (1968). *The battered child.* Chicago: University of Chicago Press.

Holaday, B. (1981). Changing views of infant care. *Pediatric Nursing, 7,* 21.

Klaus, M., & Kennell, J. (1982). *Mother-infant bonding.* St. Louis: Mosby.

Leib, S. A., et al. (1980). Effects of early intervention and stimulation on the preterm infant. *Pediatrics, 66,* 83.

Lubchenco, L. (1976). *The high-risk infant.* Philadelphia: Saunders.

Maloney, J. P. (1982). Job stress and its consequences on a group of intensive care and nonintensive care nurses. *Advances in Nursing Science, 4,* 31.

Marshall, R. E., & Kasman, C. (1980). Burnout in the neonatal intensive care unit. *Pediatrics, 65,* 1161.

McGovern, M. (1984, January 25). Caring for special babies: Separation of the baby from the parents. *Nursing Times, 80,* 28.

Michie, M. M. (1979). Prevention of handicap: The quality of neonatal care in special and intensive care baby units. *Midwives Chronicle, 92,* 13.

Noga, K. M. (1982). High risk infants: The need for nursing follow-up *J.O.G.N. Nursing, 11,* 112.

Reedy, N., et al. (1984). Maternal-fetal transport: A nurse team. *J.O.G.N. Nursing, 13,* 91.

Richards, M. P. M. (1980). Is neonatal special care overused? *Birth and Family Journal, 7,* 225.

Schraeder, B. D. (1980). Attachment and parenting despite lengthy intensive care. *M.C.N., 5,* 37.

Shearer, M. H. (1980). The economics of intensive care for the full-term newborn. *Birth and Family Journal, 7,* 234.

Sniderman, S. (1980). Modifying practices to promote family-centered care in the neonatal intensive care nursery. *Birth and Family Journal, 7,* 255.

Schwartz, D. (1981). Intensive care nurseries: Making them more human. *Children Today, 10,* 42.

Siegel, R. (1982). A family centered program of neonatal intensive care. *Health and Social Work, 7,* 50.

Spikes, J., et al. (1979). Nursing care plans for the special care nursery. *Supervisory Nurse, 10,* 23.

Stewart, M. (1982). Neonatal nurse specialists: Caregivers to the family. *Perinatology/Neonatology, 6,* 79.

Strong, C. (1983). Defective infants and the impact on families: Ethical and legal considerations. *Law of Medicine and Health Care, 11,* 168.

Tappero, E. (1983). Examination of the role of the neonatal nurse clinician: A nurse's view. *Perinatal Press, 7,* 67.

Trotter, C. W., et al. (1982). Prenatal factors and the developmental outcome of preterm infants. *J.O.G.N. Nursing, 11,* 83.

Wikler, L., et al. (1981). Chronic sorrow revisited: Parent vs. professional depiction of the adjustment of parents of mentally retarded children. *American Journal of Orthopsychiatry, 51,* 63.

46

The Newborn with a Congenital Anomaly

OBJECTIVES

Following mastery of the contents of this chapter, you should be able to

1. Describe common congenital anomalies.
2. Assess a newborn who is born with a congenital anomaly.
3. Analyze the potential or actual health problems that can occur as a result of a congenital anomaly and set realistic goals for nursing care.
4. Plan nursing care related to meeting the established goals of care.
5. Complete common nursing implementations in the care of children with congenital anomalies.
6. Evaluate the effectiveness of goal achievement in reference to infants with congenital anomalies.
7. Analyze the impact of a child with a congenital anomaly on the family.
8. Synthesize knowledge of congenital anomalies with nursing process to achieve quality maternal-newborn nursing care.

BUT SOUVENIRS

Daughters may die—but why?
For even daughters can't live with half a heart.

Three days isn't much of a life
But long enough to remember
Thin blue lips
Uneven gasps in incubators
Wracking breaths that caused pain to those who
    watched
Long enough to remember
I never held her, felt her softness
Counted her toes
Knew the color of her eyes,
Long enough to remember
Death paled hands not quite covered
By the gown she was to go home in;
Moist earthy smells, one small casket, and the tears.

I hold in my hand but souvenirs of an occasion:
    A sheet of paper filled with statistics
    A certificate with smudged footprints
    A tiny bracelet engraved "Girl Smith."

You say that you're sorry, that you know how I feel,
But you can't know because I don't feel—not yet.

By Carrol Nessiage Wilkes. (1972). *American Journal of Nursing, 72,* 1596. Reprinted by permission.

FEW THINGS, other than hemorrhage in the mother during delivery, can change the expectant, usually joyous tone of a birthing room faster than the birth of a baby with a congenital anomaly. Physicians or nurse-midwives, who are used to saying "perfect boy" or "beautiful girl" and holding up the infant for the mother's first glance, are suddenly without words and without anywhere to put their hands. They must lift a baby to allow secretions to drain from the mouth; yet at that time, both the mother and father will then know of the defect. You are in the same predicament. Your usual response, "She's beautiful" or "He looks like you," hangs unsaid in the air.

The baby is handed silently away from the table. The feeling of being mortal, with feet of clay, despite the best prenatal care in the world—of impotence to prevent the multitude of congenital anomalies that can occur—fills the room. Health care personnel can become so absorbed in their disappointment and loss at such a happening that they forget the needs of the person or persons in the room who feel this loss the most: the parents of the child.

Informing the Parents

Most physicians and nurse-midwives believe that bearing the news of congenital anomalies to parents is their responsibility. However, because the physician or nurse-midwife must deliver the placenta and suture the perineum if an episiotomy was used for delivery, 10 minutes may pass before this person is ready to make a second inspection of the baby, assess the true extent of the anomaly from the physical symptoms present, and tell the parents about the defect and the baby's prognosis. This delay does one of two things to the parents: It leaves them believing for 10 minutes either that they delivered a perfect child among people who do not share their enthusiasm or that they have just given birth to a child so deformed that all the professional persons in the room find it too horrible to even talk about.

Because parents are very aware of the feeling tone in a birthing room, the second response is by far their more likely one. In terms of parent-child interaction, this response is not healthy. Parents begin anticipatory grieving for a deformed child. Even when they are told later that the defect is not extensive, is easily correctable, and that, as soon as the correction is made, the child will be perfect, the anticipatory grief reaction may be hard to stop. They may continue to cut themselves off emotionally from the child.

Nurses should be familiar enough with the most frequently encountered congenital anomalies to be able to make truthful statements about them and so explain to parents what the problem is. This transfer does not represent a "passing of the buck" by physicians; rather the responsibility then falls to the person who at that moment in the delivery process is free to take it on. If a physician does not feel comfortable in allowing a nurse to take on this care (concerned that it is "diagnosing"), you must be ready to serve as a back-up informant, to answer the questions the parents will have when they are again able to think clearly after having been told that their child has been born less than perfect. (Remember the criterion that most pregnant women set: "I don't care if it's a boy or a girl as long as the baby is healthy.")

It is probably best to explain to parents what the defect is, and what the prognosis for the defect is, before you show the baby to them because parents may find it hard to look at an infant with a cleft lip or palate or exposed abdominal contents and also listen to what you are saying. Their minds are so jammed with the visual image their eyes are sending them, so unlike the child of their imagination, that they cannot hear.

"Your baby's upper lip isn't completely formed. That's called a cleft lip. Your doctor will call one of the plastic surgeons here at the hospital to look at your baby. This is a small problem and can be repaired so well surgically that you'll barely be able to tell your baby was born this way. I'll bring the baby over so you can see her. Remember when you look at her that this can be repaired. She seems perfect in every other way." This is the kind of statement that defines and limits the problem for the parents and gives them direction as to where and how they should proceed in thinking about it and in beginning to seek help for their child.

Parental Self-Esteem

Parents may continue to have difficulty caring for a child with a congenital anomaly because they suffer a loss of self-esteem at the child's birth. Something in the combination of their genes or the prenatal environment they provided has been inadequate. They often feel like "emperors without clothes"—starkly revealed and discredited. Pregnant women may avoid them (a superstitious fear that their disaster could somehow be contracted). They need to hear positive comments about themselves and be given support until they can realize that by caring for the child they are accomplishing more—not less—than other couples.

Parents of children with congenital anomalies are very aware of what people think of their children. They watch closely the way you handle the baby, to see if you are giving as much attention to him or her as to the other babies. It is important for the baby with an anomaly, and for the parents' acceptance of the baby, that you rock the baby as long after feeding as you do any other baby you feed and talk just as you do to the others, and so on. If you, a professional person, find their child distasteful, how will they dare show the child to their family and friends? If you are able to look past the anomaly at the whole child, they begin to feel that way, too. You are setting the stage for later parent-child interaction, whether good or bad, every time you handle an infant born with a congenital anomaly.

Parental Grieving

Parents can be expected to move through stages of grief following the birth of a child with a congenital anomaly because they have, in a sense, lost the "perfect" child they envisioned.

Denial

A mother who delivers an infant under general anesthesia may evidence denial by insisting that children in the nursery must have been interchanged, that because she had no pregnancy symptoms, this child cannot be her child. Even women who see their child in the birthing room immediately after birth say, "This can't be real; it's part of a bad dream; how do I wake from this?" Parents may avoid visiting a child if he or she is transported to another hospital for care; they may hold and feed the infant but ask for the newborn to be returned immediately to the nursery afterward. This "out of sight, out of mind" mechanism helps to protect them from the realization of what has happened (denial).

Other parents hold and visit an infant but only interact from a physical standpoint. They may ask many questions about the child's condition and become very intellectually involved while locking up their emotions. It is very difficult for parents to make decisions at this time because decisions force them to examine the situation, which is too painful. You often have to repeat explanations to be certain that they are "heard." This closure has implications for informed consent. Remember that the purpose of denial is to shield a person from the harsh reality of a situation until he or she has amassed coping strength to deal with it. Supply information as needed, role model good child care but do not try to force a reality orientation too quickly. Allow this first reaction to grief to run its normal course.

Anger

Anger follows rapidly after denial because it is *not* fair that after a perfect pregnancy, the outcome should not also be perfect. Most adults are unable to manifest this anger toward the child. They may manifest it against health care personnel or against each other. It may be difficult to offer care during this time because it is difficult to interact with a person who is directing anger toward you when you have done nothing to cause the anger.

Bargaining

Bargaining may take the form of such statements as "If this can only be fixed, I'll donate my Christmas bonus to the hospital; I'll go back to school and be more responsible. . . ." Be prepared to offer support when you recognize a bargaining stage of grief. When this response proves ineffective in righting the wrong, a person reaches a very low point in grief.

Depression

Depression is the person's first real awareness that the situation is real (and sometimes permanent). During this time the person may begin to ask realistic questions, such as how much risk will be involved in the anticipated surgery or does a mother need to hire professional help to take the child home. Other parents may be so depressed during this time that they do not have energy enough to concentrate on the child.

Acceptance

Many congenital anomalies can be repaired today: At the end of the required surgery, the parents indeed have the perfect child they envisioned in utero. If this result cannot be achieved, the parents may be able to change their goals for the child (they once wanted a son who could take over the family business; now they can modify the goal to a son who will have a positive self-image) so they can accept the child with the limitations he or she will have.

Even if acceptance is achieved, parents can expect to have periods of renewed grieving (often termed *chronic sorrow*) at important points in the child's life (the first birthday, the day he or she would have started grade school or turned "sweet sixteen," etc.). They need anticipatory guidance to be prepared for these difficult times. As a health care provider, you may need to offer additional support at these times.

Anomalies of the Gastrointestinal System

A number of the most common congenital anomalies involve the gastrointestinal system. This tract forms first as a solid tube, then recanalizes. If recanalization does not occur, a blockage or obstruction will be present in the system. Other defects of the tract, such as cleft lip and cleft palate, are the results of midline closure failure extremely early in intrauterine life.

Cleft Lip and Palate

The fusion of the maxillary and median nasal processes normally occurs between the fifth and eighth weeks of intrauterine life. In infants with cleft lip, the fusion fails in varying degrees, with the defect ranging from a small notch in the upper lip to a total separation of the lip and facial structure up into the floor of the nose. Upper teeth and gingiva may be absent. The nose is generally flattened because the incomplete fusion of the upper lip has allowed it to expand in a horizontal dimension. The deviation may be unilateral or bilateral. Cleft lip is more prevalent among males than females. It occurs at a rate of about 1 in every 1,000 live births.

The palatal process closes at about the ninth to twelfth week of intrauterine life. A palate cleft is usually on the midline and may involve just the anterior hard palate, or the posterior soft palate, or both (Figure 46-1). It may be a separate anomaly, but as a rule it occurs in conjunction with a cleft lip. It tends to occur more frequently in females than males, and apparently it is the result of polygenic inheritance or environmental influences.

Parents of a child with a cleft lip or palate should be referred for genetic counseling so that

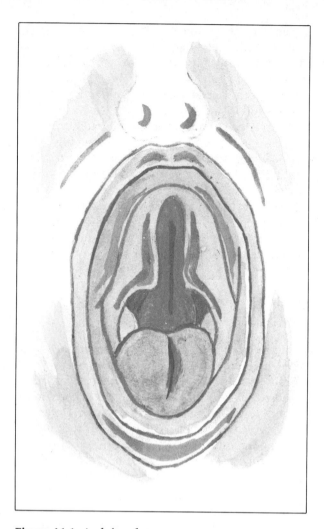

Figure 46-1 *A cleft palate.*

they understand that the phenomenon has a greater-than-normal chance of occurring in their other children.

Assessment

While cleft lip is readily apparent on inspection at birth, cleft palate is not, and it must be assessed for specifically as part of the first physical examination. A good light is necessary, while depressing the tongue with a tongue blade to reveal the total palate and the extent of the defect. As cleft palate is a component of many syndromes, a child with a cleft palate must be assessed for other congenital anomalies.

Analysis

The major nursing diagnoses in reference to cleft lip and palate are interference with nutrition or difficulty establishing parent-child bonding. Goals established must be realistic in terms of the extent of the defect, the timing of anticipated surgery, and stage of grief or readiness for decision

making and planning that the parents have reached.

Implementations

A cleft lip is repaired very shortly after birth, sometimes at the time of the initial hospital stay, sometimes at 1 month of age. Because the deviation of the lip interferes with nutrition, the infant may be a better surgical risk at birth than after a month of poor nourishment. Early repair has an added positive psychological effect in that it corrects the infant's appearance, which potentially encourages bonding.

Today, the results of surgical repair of cleft lip are excellent. It is helpful to parents to see photographs of babies with good repairs (Figure 46-2) so they can be assured that their child's outcome can also be good.

Palate repair is postponed until the child is 12 to 18 months of age, when the anatomic change in the palate contour that occurs during the first year of life has taken place. Repairs made before this change (the palate arch increases) are often ineffective and may have to be rescheduled.

Before the defect is repaired, feeding the infant with a cleft lip or palate is a problem. He or she must take in an adequate amount of food and yet be prevented from aspirating. The best method appears to be to support the baby in an upright position while feeding gently from a small container such as a medicine glass. Contrary to what you might think, newborns do well drinking from glasses in this manner, and it seems safer than using medicine droppers, syringes, or commercial feeders that force formula into the infant's mouth by pressure on a rubber bulb (similar to an Asepto syringe). A hurried nurse or mother can easily cause an infant to aspirate if using one of these methods. Specially designed cleft-lip nipples are available. These do not always work well if the defect is extensive. It may be possible for an infant with a cleft lip to breast-feed as the bulk of the breast tends to form a seal against the injured upper lip. The infant with cleft palate may be able to breast-feed if a breast shield with a cleft nipple is used.

The parents of the infant being discharged prior to surgery (up to a month for the infant with cleft lip and up to 1½ years for the child with cleft palate) must receive detailed instructions on the care and feeding of their baby. Whatever method used for feeding, the infant needs to be held and bubbled well after feeding because of the tendency to swallow a great deal of air due to the inability to grasp a glass or syringe edge securely. Because the infant breathes through the mouth (if the cleft extends to the nares), the mucous membrane there tends to become dry, and the lips may

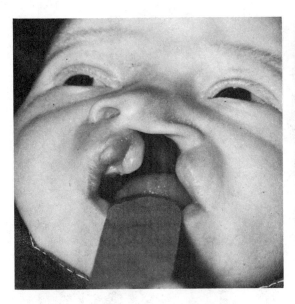 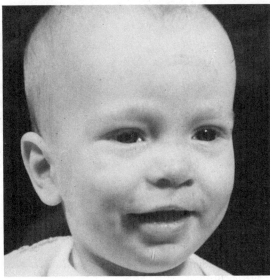

Figure 46-2 *Cleft lip. A. A 2-week-old infant with unilateral cleft lip. B. Same child at 14 months, showing the surgical repair. From Crowley, L. V. (1974).* An introduction to clinical embryology. *Chicago: Year Book Medical Publishers.*

become dry too. The newborn may need small sips of fluid between feedings to keep the mucous membrane of the mouth moist and prevent cracks and fissures that could lead to infection.

Mothers have difficulty learning to feed their infants when they are born with cleft lips. Statements such as "You have to learn this. You'll have to do it at home," although true, are ineffective and sound almost punitive. A positive approach is better: "I think you're doing very well. Try it by yourself now with me sitting right beside you. It takes all babies a few days to be able to eat well. I think she's doing better all the time."

Parents of infants with cleft palate should be encouraged to talk and sing to their babies and to encourage speech sounds, however guttural and harsh, at normal developmental times.

Parents taking a child home to wait for surgery may need a community health nurse referral. Provide a number to call, either the hospital's, a clinic's, or pediatrician's, to ask any questions that arise in the baby's care.

Postoperative Interventions (Cleft lip repair)

Because edema always occurs locally at an incision site and this site is close to the airway, a child must be observed closely in the immediate postoperative period for respiratory distress. Because the infant breathed through the mouth before surgery and now has to breathe through the nose, the change may add to respiratory difficulty. This is not generally a problem, however, because newborns are normally strictly nose breathers.

An infant generally remains on NPO status for 3 to 4 hours following surgery. He or she is then gradually introduced to fluid (clear water or glucose water) in small amounts by a glass or syringe; if this is tolerated, a gradual return is made to regular formula. No tension must be placed on the suture line in order that sutures do not pull apart and leave a large scar; therefore, breastfeeding (any feeding that allows the infant to suck) is contraindicated during this immediate postoperative period.

The best cleft lip repair can end in disaster if crusts are allowed to form on the suture line or the suture line becomes infected. Following every feeding and as many other times a day as serum forms, the suture line must be cleaned. The procedure requires a sterile solution and sterile, cotton-tipped applicators. The solution will depend on the individual surgeon's preference (sterile water, sterile saline, or half-strength hydrogen peroxide in sterile water). It is applied to the suture line by a cotton applicator. Do not rub; dab gently. Rubbing loosens sutures; dabbing cleans. If hydrogen peroxide is used, it will foam as it reacts with the protein particles at the suture line. Next, the suture line is rinsed with sterile water if a cleaning solution, such as half-strength hydrogen peroxide, was used. Again, dab, do not rub. The suture line is then dried by a dry cotton applicator. Remember that the infant has sutures on the inside of the lip as well as those that show; these need the same meticulous care.

Tension on the suture line must be avoided or

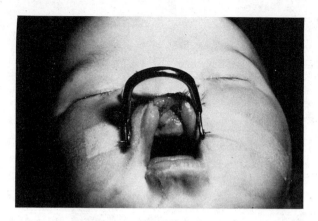

Figure 46-3 A Logan bar in place to protect the surgical incision for a cleft lip repair. Source: Fochtman, D., and Raffensberger, S. G. (1976). Principles of nursing care for the pediatric surgery patient [2nd ed]. Boston: Little, Brown.

it will separate enough to cause a wide, obvious scar. The suture line is held in close approximation by a Logan bar (a wire bow taped to both cheeks) (Figure 46-3) or a Band-Aid simulating a bar. The Logan bar or Band-Aid must be checked after each feeding or cleaning of the suture line to be certain that it is secure and protecting the suture line. An infant should not be allowed to cry because it increases tension on the sutures. This means you have to anticipate the infant's needs. Have formula ready and be ready to feed when the child wishes; do not start to get it ready *after* the newborn is awake and crying. Feedings must be on demand, not by a set hospital schedule. The infant needs to be rocked, jiggled, carried, held, or whatever measure is necessary to feel secure and comfortable. He or she needs to be bubbled well after a feeding because of the tendency to swallow more air than the average infant due to the nonsucking method of feeding employed.

In order that an infant does not irritate the suture line by rubbing at it, the newborn needs to wear a jacket restraint (Figure 46-4). This type of restraint allows the child to exercise but prevents the arm from bending at the elbow in order to bring the hands to the face. If such a jacket is not available, pinning the baby's long shirt sleeves to the diaper on each side is a suitable restraint method. Be certain that an infant does not lie on the abdomen, which makes it easy to rub his or her face against the bedclothes. The baby can lie on either side or sit upright in a comfortable infant chair.

The parents need to interact with the child during the postoperative period. They can be cautioned that the incision does not look as well in the immediate postoperative period as it will

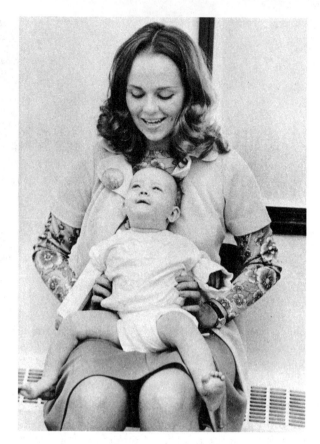

Figure 46-4 An infant arm restraint to protect the infant from bringing his or her hands up to the face.

eventually. After a child's sutures have been removed, the infant may be fed by an ordinary bottle or breast-fed. The breast-feeding mother needs to be cautioned that the infant has never sucked before and so will need time to learn just as a newborn does. An equally difficult time may be had with learning to suck from a bottle.

Notice whether or not parents look at their baby's face while feeding. Help them to understand that any negative feelings of pain or sadness that their baby was born this way, or guilt or responsibility for the baby's defect, are normal for the situation. This support does not instantly make them feel better about the child, but the knowledge that what they are experiencing is normal will help them to begin to deal with such emotions.

Evaluation

Some infants with a cleft lip have a deviated nasal septum, which they may need repaired in later years for good air exchange. Some have a flattened, slightly distorted nose contour, which they may choose to have corrected for cosmetic appearance later in life. Parents may need continued support to view a child as the whole, perfect child which he or she is after repair. If some scar remains, the child may need to be gently taught that what is inside people is more important than what shows on the surface in order to strengthen self-esteem.

Tracheoesophageal Atresia and Fistula

Between the fourth and eighth weeks of intrauterine life, the laryngotracheal groove develops into the larynx, trachea, and beginning lung tissue, and the esophageal lumen is formed. A number of anomalies may be found in infants if the trachea and esophagus do not develop normally. Types of esophageal atresias and fistulas are

1. Esophagus ends in a blind pouch; there is a tracheoesophageal fistula (opening) between the distal part of the esophagus and the trachea.
2. Esophagus ends in a blind pouch. There is no connection into the trachea.
3. A fistula is present between an otherwise normal esophagus and trachea.
4. Esophagus ends in a blind pouch. A fistula connects the blind pouch of the proximal esophagus to the trachea.
5. There is a blind end portion of the esophagus. Fistulas are present between both widely spaced segments of the esophagus and the trachea.

The three most common forms of tracheoesophageal atresia (complete closure) and tracheoesophageal fistula (TEF) are illustrated in Figure 46-5. This defect is always serious because tracheoesophageal atresia interferes with feeding and if a fistula exists, when the infant is fed, milk fills the blind esophagus and overflows into the trachea, causing aspiration. The incidence of tracheoesophageal fistula is about 1 in 3,000 live births.

Assessment

Tracheoesophageal fistula must be ruled out in any infant born to a woman with hydramnios. A normal fetus swallows amniotic fluid during intrauterine life. The infant with a tracheoesophageal fistula cannot swallow, and the amount of amniotic fluid may thus become abnormally large. Many infants are born preterm because of the accompanying hydramnios and thus have the accompanying problem of immaturity. They need to be examined carefully for other congenital anomalies—such as urologic, heart, or intestinal disorders—that could have occurred from the

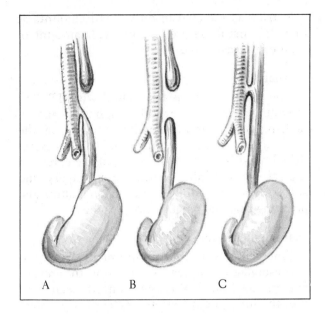

Figure 46-5 *Esophageal atresia and tracheoesophageal fistula. A. The most frequent type of esophageal atresia. The esophagus ends in a blind pouch. The trachea communicates via a fistula with the lower esophagus and stomach (about 90 percent of infants with the defect have this type). B. Both upper and lower segments end in blind pouches (7 to 8 percent of infants have this type). C. Both upper and lower segments communicate with the trachea (2 to 3 percent of infants have this type).*

teratogenic effect at the same week in gestation that caused the TEF.

Tracheoesophageal fistula can be diagnosed with certainty if a catheter cannot be passed through the infant's esophagus to the stomach (be certain that catheters used this way are firm; a soft one will curl in a blind-end esophagus and appear to have passed). If a radiopaque catheter is used, it can be seen coiled in the blind end of the esophagus on X-ray. An X-ray of the abdomen may reveal a stomach distended with air from air passing from the trachea into the esophagus and stomach. A barium swallow will reveal the blind-end esophagus.

Infants who have so much mucus in their mouths that they appear to be blowing bubbles should be suspected of having tracheoesophageal fistula. This possibility may not be considered in some infants who do this bubbling until they are fed for the first time. Then the infant coughs, turns cyanotic, and has obvious difficulty in breathing. For this reason formula-fed infants should first be fed with sterile water. A feeding of either glucose water or formula aspirated into the lungs is more dangerous to the infant because of the glucose or fat content than is sterile water. A breast-fed infant may be fed at the breast because colostrum is secreted in only small amounts at first. If a fistula is present, no great amount of fluid can be aspirated.

Analysis

The major concerns for a child with TEF are providing nutrition, preventing aspiration, and establishing parent-child bonding in light of the early surgery that can be anticipated. Goals established must be realistic in terms of the extent of the defect, the timing of anticipated surgery, and stage of grief or readiness for decision making and planning that the parents have reached.

Implementations

Emergency surgery for an infant with tracheoesophageal fistula is essential to prevent pneumonia from leakage of stomach secretions into the lungs, dehydration, or electrolyte imbalance from lack of oral intake. Prior to surgery, an infant should be kept in an upright position and on the right side to prevent gastric juice from entering the lungs from the fistula. As the baby cannot swallow mucus, he needs frequent oropharyngeal suction to prevent aspiration of collected mucus. A catheter may be passed into the blind-end esophagus and attached to low suction to keep this segment of the esophagus from filling with fluid and causing aspiration. Irrigation of the catheter may be necessary to keep it patent, as mucus tends to dry and plug it. A gastrostomy may be performed (under local anesthesia), and the tube allowed to drain by gravity to keep the stomach empty of secretions and prevent reflux into the lungs. Upper right lobe pneumonia is one of the major complications of this disorder, and antibiotic prophylaxis may be begun as a preventive measure. If surgery will be delayed, an infant may have a cervical esophagostomy (the distal end of the blind esophagus is brought to the surface so that mucus can drain). Use absorbent gauze around the opening to absorb moisture and prevent excoriation of the skin. Apply a protective ointment such as A&D or zinc oxide liberally to protect skin.

An intravenous infusion will be begun to supply fluid and calories because the infant cannot be given oral fluid. He should be kept in an Isolette with high humidity to maintain body heat and liquefy bronchial secretions; close observation must be maintained for respiratory distress. The baby should be kept from crying to prevent air from entering the stomach from the trachea, distending the stomach, and causing vomiting into the lungs. A pacifier may be helpful.

Tracheoesophageal fistula is a perplexing disorder for parents as the infant appears healthy; no obvious deformity is present. The surgical repair is complex, however, so in many instances a child must be transferred to a major center. Parents need a great deal of support, first to realize that their child is that ill, and then to organize their resources to cope with a newborn undergoing major surgery.

Surgery consists of closing the fistula and anastomosing the esophageal segments. It may be necessary to complete the surgery in different stages and to use a portion of the colon to complete the anastomosis if the esophageal segments are far apart from each other.

Postoperative Interventions

Following surgery, because the chest cavity was entered for the repair, the infant will have one or two chest tubes in place. The posterior tube drains collecting fluid; the anterior tube allows air to leave the chest space and the lung to reexpand. A gastrostomy tube in place prevents the stomach from becoming distended and provides a method of feeding without using the esophagus. The infant must be observed closely for respiratory distress in the first few days following surgery. It will be necessary to suction frequently because mucus tends to accumulate in the pharynx from surgery trauma. Suctioning must be done only shallowly, however, so there is no danger that your suction catheter touches the suture line in the esophagus.

The child must be turned frequently to discourage fluid from accumulating in the lungs. This turning and handling generally makes him cry, and he should cry to help expand lung tissue (an older child or adult can be told to take deep breaths; a newborn cannot). An infant laryngoscope and endotracheal tube should be available at the bedside in case extreme edema develops and the infant's airway is obstructed.

A newborn is generally cared for in an Isolette so that body warmth is maintained. He may need oxygen and high humidity to keep respiratory secretions moist. It is best if the chest drainage bottles are attached to the Isolette so they move with the Isolette and will not tip over or be broken (if they should break, room air will enter the chest, collapsing the lungs). Chest bottles should never be raised to the level of the child, or the drainage fluid will flow back into the chest (collapsing the lungs).

The tubing must be observed after the infant is turned and repositioned to see that it is not kinked or twisted. It should be "milked" periodically to remove clots and keep it patent. Be careful that the tubes are not caught or tugged at and that they do not become disconnected when the

Isolette top is raised. They should not be disconnected at any time (to prevent air from entering the chest). Two large hemostats should be taped to the top of the Isolette so that if, in turning the infant or for any other reason, the tubes should become disconnected, they can be clamped close to the infant's chest to prevent air from entering.

An infant is given intravenous fluid for a period of time after surgery until the possibility of vomiting from the anesthetic is decreased. The infant is then begun on feedings through the gastrostomy tube. For feedings, the end of the tube should be raised about 12 inches. The glucose water or formula ordered for a feeding should be introduced into the tube slowly and allowed to run by gravity, never by pressure, to prevent it from entering the esophagus and putting pressure on the suture line. Following the feeding, the end of the tube should be elevated, covered by sterile gauze and kept in that position, perhaps by suspending it from an IV pole. It should not be clamped.

In this way air introduced during the feeding will bubble from the tube, not through the esophagus past the fresh suture line. This arrangement also assures you that if the infant vomits the feeding, the vomitus will be projected into the gastrostomy tube, not past the fresh sutures. Most newborns enjoy sucking a pacifier during gastrostomy feedings for sucking pleasure. If a mother wishes to breast-feed, she can manually express breast milk into a sterile container and bring it to the hospital for the infant's feedings.

An infant may be given sips of clear fluid by mouth as early as the day after surgery, although some infants are kept on NPO status for 7 to 10 days until the suture line is healed. Early introduction of fluid may help to ensure patency of the esophagus since it helps to decrease adhesions from the anastomosis. An infant is introduced to a full oral fluid diet as soon as he begins to tolerate it and the suture line is healed. When the child is taking oral feedings satisfactorily, the gastrostomy tube is removed. In some infants, the esophageal atresia and fistula are so extensive that a number of operations are necessary for repair. If a child is to return home to await a second-stage operation, the mother must be shown how to do gastrostomy feedings. If the gastrostomy tube is only a temporary measure for surgery, she does not need to learn the procedure. Her time is better spent in holding the child (in the Isolette, if necessary), gently stroking or talking to her newborn, and getting to know him better.

In most infants, some stenosis at the anastomosis site occurs and esophageal dilatation at periodic intervals to keep the repaired esophagus fully patent may be necessary. A string is passed from the mouth to the stomach via the esophagus and exits by the gastrostomy site in the stomach. For dilatation, a metal or plastic bougie, or dilator, is attached to the string and pulled through the esophagus. The string remains in place until the child has reached a point where dilatation is no longer necessary.

Evaluation

The prognosis of a newborn with TEF will depend on the extent of the repair necessary, the condition of the child at the time of surgery, and whether or not other congenital anomalies are present. Surgery may need to be scheduled in stages if the distance between the two ends of the esophagus is great. A segment of the intestine may be used to anastomose the esophageal segments.

If surgery can be performed on the child before pneumonia occurs and the defect is amenable to surgical correction, the prognosis is good. However, the mortality rate may be as high as 40 percent. This high a rate is associated with esophageal atresia or tracheoesophageal fistula in the presence of other congenital defects or low birth weight.

Pneumonia is the most frequent complication of a tracheoesophageal repair. Leaks occurring at anastomosis sites are a common complication, most frequently at the seventh to tenth postoperative day when sutures dissolve. Fluid and air leak out into the chest cavity, and pneumothorax occurs.

Omphalocele

An omphalocele is a protrusion of abdominal contents through the abdominal wall at the point of the junction of the umbilical cord and abdomen. The herniated organs are usually intestine, but they may include stomach and liver. They are usually covered and contained by a thin transparent layer of peritoneum. The deviation is evident at birth and reflects an arrest of development of the abdominal cavity at the seventh to tenth week of intrauterine life. At about the sixth to the eighth week of intrauterine life, the abdominal contents are extruded from the abdomen into the base of the umbilical cord. Omphalocele occurs when there is failure of the abdominal contents to return to the abdomen (Figure 46-6). The incidence of omphalocele is as rare as 1 in 10,000 live births. A child may have accompanying defects that also were caused by the teratogen insult which prevented normal intestinal growth.

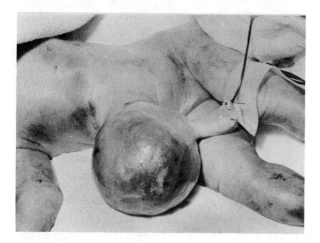

Figure 46-6 *This large omphalocele seen at birth contains intestine and liver. (Courtesy of the Department of Medical Photography, Children's Hospital, Buffalo, N.Y.)*

Assessment

The presence of an omphalocele is obvious on inspection at birth. Record its general appearance and its size in centimeters.

Analysis

The major nursing diagnosis involved with omphalocele is either maintenance of body temperature (a great deal of intestinal surface is exposed), nutrition (the infant cannot be fed, as food in the intestine will make it difficult to return to the abdomen), or interference with bonding (due to the long hospitalization involved). Goals established must be realistic in terms of the extent of the defect, the timing of anticipated surgery, and stage of grief or readiness for decision making and planning that the parents have reached. Omphalocele is a shock to parents: It is an anomaly that is obviously severe and that they probably never knew even existed.

Implementations

It is important that the lining of peritoneum covering the defect not be ruptured or allowed to dry out and crack; otherwise, infection and malrotation of the uncontained intestine will complicate the surgical repair and lead to peritonitis. In order to protect the sac, the omphalocele is usually covered by sterile, saline-soaked gauze until surgery. It is important that the saline used is body temperature. Applying cold saline will lead to a decreased body temperature as so much intestinal surface is involved.

The success of the surgical repair depends on the size of the omphalocele. The viscera may be only partially replaced during surgery; if the entire contents were returned to the abdomen

(which is usually small because it did not need to grow to accommodate abdominal contents), respiratory distress could result from the pressure of the visceral bulk. If replacement is partial, a synthetic material (Silastic) is used to cover the bowel not replaced for about another month, when a second surgical procedure is required to complete the repair. A nasogastric tube will be inserted to prevent intestinal distention and rupture of the sac. The child will be maintained on total parenteral nutrition until the bowel is fully repaired.

Evaluation

Following the final surgical repair, a child with an omphalocele will be the perfect child the parents once envisioned—with the exception of a rather large abdominal scar. If this becomes a problem for the child in later life, plastic surgery can reduce the scar's appearance.

Gastroschisis

Gastroschisis is a condition similar to omphalocele except that the abdominal wall defect is a distance from the umbilicus and abdominal organs are not contained by peritoneal membrane but spill from the abdomen freely. Malrotation of the intestine invariably occurs with gastroschisis so that the repair is more complicated and requires additional surgery stages. An infant's prognosis is guarded until the full surgery repair is complete.

Intestinal Obstruction

If recanalization at one point in the intestine does not occur in utero, an atresia (complete closure) or stenosis (narrowing) of the bowel can occur. The most common site is the duodenal bowel portion.

Obstruction may also occur because of a twisting (rotation) of the mesentery of the bowel as the bowel re-enters the abdomen after being contained in the base of the umbilical cord early in intrauterine life. The same result may be due to severe twisting of the mesentery due to the looseness of the intestine in the abdomen of the neonate (this continues to be a problem for the first sixth months of life). Obstruction can occur due to thicker-than-usual meconium formation (meconium plug or meconium ileus, discussed on page 1083).

Assessment

Intestinal obstruction may be anticipated if a mother had hydramnios during pregnancy (amniotic fluid could not be swallowed effectively) or

Table 46-1 Differentiation Between Regurgitation and Vomiting

Characteristic	Regurgitation	Vomiting
Timing	Occurs with burping at end of feeding.	Timing unrelated to feeding. If following feeding, unassociated with act of burping.
Forcefulness	"Runs out" of mouth with little force.	Is forceful; often projected a foot away from the infant. *Projectile vomiting* is vomiting that is projected as much as 4 feet. This is most often related to increased intracranial pressure in newborns; in infants 4 to 6 weeks of age, pyloric stenosis may be a cause.
Description	Smells barely sour; only slightly curdled; clear water or milk.	Smells very sour and appears curdled; yellow, green, or black in color. Perhaps with fresh blood or old blood stain from swallowed maternal blood.
Distress	Nonpainful; child does not appear to be in distress and may even smile as if the sensation is enjoyable.	Child may cry just prior to vomiting as if abdominal pain is present (and following vomiting as if the force of the action is frightening).
Duration	A quick-one-time-per-feeding occurrence.	Will continue until the stomach is empty and then continue with dry retching even in newborns.
Amount	1 or 2 teaspoons.	As much as a cup in newborns.

more than 30 ml of stomach contents can be aspirated by a nasogastric catheter and syringe at birth. If it is not revealed by these two findings, symptoms of intestinal obstruction in the neonate are the same as at any other time in life. The infant passes no meconium or may pass one stool and then halt (meconium that formed below the obstruction). The abdomen becomes distended. As the effect of the obstruction progresses, the child will vomit.

Obstructions are rare above the ampulla of Vater or the junction of the bile duct with the duodenum, so vomitus will be bile-stained (greenish). Because meconium is black, vomitus may be very dark in color. Bowel sounds increase with obstruction due to the increased peristaltic action as the intestine attempts to pass stool through the point of obstruction. Waves of peristalsis may be apparent across the abdomen. An infant may evidence pain as crying (hard, forceful, indignant crying) and pull his legs up against the abdomen. The child's respiratory rate will increase as the diaphragm is pushed up against the lungs and lung capacity decreases. An abdominal flat plate X-ray will show no gas below the level of obstruction to the intestines. A barium swallow X-ray or barium enema may be used to reveal the position of the obstruction.

Analysis

The most frequent nursing diagnosis concerned with intestinal obstruction is mainte-

nance of nutrition: Once the obstruction is suspected, a child must be kept NPO to not compound the problem and to prevent vomiting and aspiration. Vomiting in neonates is always serious because they lose fluid very rapidly, causing dehydration. They also lose chloride from the hydrochloric acid of the stomach contents. Loss of chloride leads to alkalosis. The body attempts to compensate for the loss of chloride by excreting potassium and so an infant quickly also becomes hypokalemic. Goals should include maintaining hydration, electrolyte balance, and parent-child bonding in light of the early surgery anticipated.

Implementations

A bowel obstruction is a surgical emergency before dehydration, electrolyte imbalance, or aspiration of vomitus occurs. Keep a newborn who vomits NPO until you can contact a physician. Remember that many neonates regurgitate or spit up feedings with burping. This rapid rejection of milk smells barely sour and occurs with burping. Table 46-1 lists the factors that help to differentiate regurgitation from true vomiting in a newborn.

If bowel obstruction is established, the infant's physician may order an orogastric or nasogastric tube inserted for suction or left open to prevent further gastrointestinal distention from swallowed air. Steps for passing an orogastric or nasogastric tube are listed in Procedure 46-1. Al-

Procedure 46-1

**Inserting a Nasogastric Tube
in a Newborn**

Purpose: Provide an access route for relieving air from the stomach or administering feedings.

Plan

1. Wash your hands; identify infant.

2. Assess infant's condition: Analyze appropriateness of the procedure; plan modifications as necessary.

3. Begin implementation by assembling equipment: Wrap to mummy infant; a hemostat or adhesive tape; nonallergic tape; nasogastric tube or small feeding tube 5 to 10F; syringe; cup of sterile water.

4. Use the tube to measure the distance from the bridge of the infant's nose to an earlobe to a midpoint between the umbilicus and xyphoid process. Place hemostat or tape at this point. Wrap infant in a mummy restraint as necessary to contain infant hands during the procedure.

5. Wet tip of tube for lubrication; gently pass it into one nares and with continuing gentle pressure on into the infant's stomach (to the marked point on the catheter).

6. Observe carefully for any respiratory distress that might indicate tube has passed into trachea. Attach syringe and gently aspirate for stomach secretions or insert about 1 ml of air by syringe and listen over stomach for air passage or dip distal end in water cup and assess for bubbling.

7. Place a piece of nonallergic tape on infant's face under nose. Tape tube to this securely. Assess tube does not pull or rub on nares.

8. Close tubing, prepare for gavage feeding or leave it open to air depending on tube's purpose. Reposition infant comfortably.

9. Evaluate infant's condition and effectiveness of procedure. Assess whether further restraint will be necessary to prevent infant from pulling at tube and removing it.

10. Chart placement of tube and infant's response to procedure.

Principle

1. Prevent spread of microorganisms. Assure patient safety.

2. The size of a nasogastric tube varies as to the size of the infant. Use the smallest size practical.

3. Assembling equipment prevents undue exposure or tiring of infant.

4. Marking the tube prevents it from passing too far or not far enough. Restraining is a safety measure.

5. Never use an oil lubricant, which would irritate lungs if it should accidentally pass into them. Use sterile water instead.

6. Do not use dipping method if infant is being ventilated as this may cause aspiration of water in cup.

7. Use nonallergic tape to prevent skin irritation. Securing tube prevents dislodgement.

8. To make the infant comfortable and not exposed to chilling.

9. Evaluation is the final step of nursing process.

10. Document nursing care and patient status.

ways use low suction pressure with decompression tubes in neonates. Greater pressure can cause actual destruction of the stomach lining.

An infant will be begun on intravenous therapy to restore fluid and scheduled for surgery immediately. Repair of the defect (with the exception of meconium plug syndrome) is done through an abdominal incision. The area of stenosis or atresia is removed and the bowel anastomosed. If the repair is anatomically difficult or the infant has other anomalies that interfere with health, a temporary colostomy may be constructed, the infant is discharged, and then returned for surgery at 3 to 6 months of age.

Evaluation

Following final surgery, an infant will be well once more. Abdominal surgery at this age is major surgery, however, so the infant's prognosis is guarded until it is certain that recovery is made from surgery.

Meconium Plug Syndrome

A meconium plug is an extremely hard portion of meconium that completely obstructs the intestinal lumen, causing bowel obstruction. Why it occurs is unknown but it probably reflects normal variations of meconium consistency. Meconium plug formation usually occurs in the lower end of the bowel, where meconium is formed early in intrauterine life and has the best chance to become dry and inspissated.

Because the obstruction is low in the intestinal tract, signs of obstruction such as abdominal distention and vomiting do not occur for at least 24 hours; an infant will be identified first as having no meconium passage in the first 24 hours of life. A gentle rectal examination may reveal the presence of hardened stool, although the plug may be too far removed to be palpated. An X-ray may reveal proximal, air-filled loops of bowel up to the point of obstruction. A barium enema may not only reveal the level of obstruction but be therapeutic in loosening the plug. The administration of saline enemas (never use tap water in newborns, which leads to water intoxication) may cause enough peristalsis to cause expulsion of the plug. Instillation of acetylcysteine proteolytic enzyme rectally may dissolve the plug.

Once the thickened portion of meconium has been passed, these infants should have no further difficulty and, in fact, over the next several hours may pass a great amount of stool. They must be observed for further passage of meconium (at least once daily) over the next 3 days, however, to be certain that further plugs do not exist further up

in the bowel. If an infant is going to be discharged before this time, the mother needs to be instructed on the importance of this observation and the necessity of telephoning her pediatrician should the child have no further stooling at home.

Occasionally a neonate passes a plug of very hardened meconium in the first 1 or 2 days of life—meconium hard enough to cause an obstruction, only no obstruction occurred because of the small size of the particle. Be certain to record and report such a finding because the infant needs the same close observation for continued stooling, as does an infant who actually had an obstruction, to be certain that another larger and truly obstructing plug is not present.

When a meconium plug is discovered, assess the family history for cystic fibrosis, a recessively inherited disorder (which may present as meconium ileus), or aganglionic megacolon (which also may present with absence of meconium), a polygenic inherited disorder. "There's a possibility your child has cystic fibrosis. Is there any of that in your family?" is not a tactful way to broach the subject. Try, "Most babies pass a stool by 24 hours of age. Whenever a baby doesn't, we ask parents if they know of any bowel or stomach disorders in the family. Do you know of anyone who has a disease called Hirschsprung's disease? Megacolon? Cystic fibrosis? Chronic constipation? Lazy bowel?" Hypothyroidism is another disorder that may present with constipation or very hardened stool. Assess an infant for signs of hypothyroidism (large, protruding tongue, lethargy, subnormal body temperature). In some states hypothyroid screening is done along with the PKU screen. Be certain that this blood is obtained in any newborn with a meconium plug.

Meconium Ileus

Meconium ileus is a specific phenomenon that occurs in an infant with cystic fibrosis. With cystic fibrosis, the enzyme that moistens and makes all body fluids free-flowing is absent. All body fluids are therefore thick and tenacious. Cystic fibrosis is most often thought of as a lung disorder because the most severe manifestation of tenacious secretions is in the lung; tenacious lung fluid leads to stasis and infection and alveolar obstruction, reducing air exchange. Intestinal and pancreatic secretions are affected also, however, and the syndrome may be indicated at birth by hardened, obstructive meconium at the ileus level from lack of trypsin secretion from the pancreas (meconium ileus). The usual symptoms of bowel obstruction will follow: no meconium passage, abdominal distention, and vomiting. The obstruction is too high for enemas to be effective; the bowel must be incised and the hardened meconium surgically removed. An infant must be further assessed for cystic fibrosis in the following months.

Biliary Atresia

Obstruction of the bile duct in children generally occurs from congenital atresia, stenosis, or absence of the duct. It can occur from a plugging of biliary secretions, but this is rare. When the bile duct is obstructed, bile cannot enter the intestinal tract. It accumulates in the liver. Bile pigments (direct or conjugated bilirubin) enter the bloodstream. An infant begins to appear jaundiced. This jaundice takes about 2 weeks to develop, and, therefore, differs clinically from physiologic jaundice, which typically occurs on the third day of life or the jaundice of blood incompatibility, which occurs during the first 24 hours of life. Laboratory findings will also distinguish this type of jaundice. Physiologic jaundice and blood incompatibility jaundice occur from a rise in indirect or unconjugated bilirubin, whereas the jaundice of bile duct obstruction is direct bilirubin jaundice.

In the newborn period the most obvious clue that bile duct obstruction is present is the absence of bile salts in the intestine. This causes meconium to be light-colored (acholic) rather than the usual dark black. Once a newborn's stools change to yellow, this color clue may be difficult to establish: Some infants have very light yellow stools that are difficult to distinguish from those that are acholic. Mothers whose infants are born at home should be advised to note the color of newborn stools. If the infant is not seen by a health care provider for 2 or 3 days, the absence of normal meconium will be missed.

Bile duct obstruction is a serious disorder that can cause pressure on the liver and eventually liver destruction. Surgery to relieve the problem is often ineffective; liver transplant may be necessary. Being aware of the color of normal newborn stools and in particular the color of first stools aids in detecting the condition.

Diaphragmatic Hernia

A diaphragmatic hernia is protrusion of an abdominal organ (usually the stomach or intestine) through a defect in the diaphragm into the chest cavity. This condition usually occurs on the left side, and the heart is displaced to the right of the chest; the lung on the left side is collapsed. Its incidence is about 1 in 3,000 live births with no difference in incidence between males and fe-

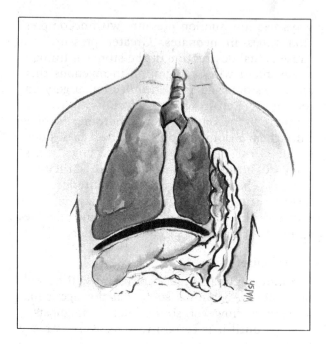

Figure 46-7 *A diaphragmatic hernia. Intestine has invaded the chest cavity, reducing heart and lung function.*

males. Such a defect occurs because early in intrauterine life the chest and abdominal cavity are one; at about the eighth week of growth, the diaphragm forms to divide them. If it does not form completely, intestine will herniate through the diaphragm opening into the chest cavity (Figure 46-7).

Assessment

A newborn with an extensive diaphragmatic hernia will have respiratory difficulty from the time of birth because at least one lung is unable to expand satisfactorily (and may not have formed fully). He will have cyanosis and intracostal or subcostal retractions. The abdomen generally appears sunken because it is not as filled as a normal newborn abdomen. Breath sounds will be absent on the affected side of the chest if the lung is collapsed, and bowel sounds may be heard in the chest cavity by auscultation. A flat plate X-ray of the chest shows the gas-filled bowel in the chest cavity.

Analysis

The major concerns for an infant with a diaphragmatic hernia are maintenance of respirations and nutrition (lung surface is compromised, and becomes compromised even further if oral feeding is started). Be certain that goals established are realistic in terms of the extent of the defect, the timing of anticipated surgery, and stage of grief or readiness for decision making and planning that the parents have reached.

Implementations

Infants with diaphragmatic hernia breathe better with their head elevated, which allows the herniated intestine to fall back as far as possible into the abdomen and provides a maximum of respiratory space. Turning an infant so the compressed lung is down is also a position that allows the good lung to expand most completely and offer optimal aeration. A nasogastric tube or a gastrostomy tube to suction pressure for decompression is usually inserted to prevent distention of the herniated intestine, which would cause further respiratory difficulty. Be certain that the decompression strength is low or the lining of the stomach can be injured. An infant is kept NPO because filling of the intestine with food or active peristaltic motion will further impair lung function. If fed, an infant may vomit due to the twisting and obstruction of the herniated bowel.

Treatment is immediate surgical repair of the diaphragm and replacement of the herniated intestine. Such a repair usually requires a thoracic incision and the placement of chest tubes. If the defect in the diaphragm is large, a Teflon patch may be used in reconstruction. The repair is complicated if there is not room in the abdomen for the intestine to be returned. In these infants, the abdominal incision is not closed but left open to allow the intestine to protrude abdominally. It is covered by a Silastic covering and left to be finally closed at a later date.

Over the following week, the compressed lung (if it is normal) will gradually expand and begin to function. If it is hypoplastic (not functional) from the pressure of the intestine in utero, it will not expand and will be removed at the time of surgery.

Following surgery, infants are maintained in a semi-Fowler's position by an infant chair in order to keep pressure of the replaced intestine off the repaired diaphragm. They may have positive pressure ventilation to increase lung expansion, although this pressure is kept to a minimum to prevent tearing undeveloped or not previously opened lung tissue. They are kept in a warmed, humidified environment to encourage lung fluid drainage, and they should be suctioned as necessary. In order to prevent pressure on the diaphragm by a full bowel, they may be maintained on intravenous or total parenteral nutrition for 1 or 2 weeks. When oral feedings are begun, be certain to burp an infant well following a feeding to reduce the amount of swallowed air and limit bowel expansion.

Evaluation

Unfortunately, the mortality rate of children with diaphragmatic hernia is 25 to 50 percent, with death often due to associated anomalies of the heart, lung, and intestine.

Umbilical Hernia

An umbilical hernia is a protrusion of a portion of the intestine through the umbilical ring, the muscle, and fascia surrounding the umbilical cord. This condition produces a bulging protrusion under the skin at the umbilicus. Rarely noticeable at birth while the cord is still present, the abnormality can be recognized at health care visits during the first year. Umbilical hernias occur most frequently in black children, more often in girls than in boys.

The structure is generally 1 to 2 cm (½ to 1 inch) in diameter but may be as big as an orange when the child cries or strains. The size of the protruding mass is not as important as the size of the fascial ring through which the intestine protrudes. If this fascial ring is under 2 cm, closure will usually occur spontaneously and no repair of the defect will be necessary. If the defect is over 2 cm, surgery for repair will generally be indicated, which is done close to school age.

Inguinal Hernia

Inguinal hernia is protrusion of a section of the bowel into the inguinal ring. It occurs usually in males because, as the testes descend from the abdominal cavity into the scrotum late in fetal life, a fold of parietal peritoneum also descends, forming a tube from the abdomen to the scrotum. In most infants, this tube closes completely. If it fails to close, descent of the intestine into it (hernia) may occur when there is an increase in intraabdominal pressure (Figure 46-8). In girls, the round ligament extends from the uterus into the inguinal canal to its attachment on the abdominal wall. Weakness of the muscle surrounding the round ligament may result in an inguinal hernia.

The hernia appears as a lump in the groin, about 60 percent of the time on the right side. In some instances, the hernia is apparent only on crying (when abdominal pressure increases), and not when the child is less active. Inguinal hernias are painless. Pain at the site implies that the bowel has become incarcerated in the sac, an emergency situation because of the immediate danger of bowel obstruction or compromise to the blood supply of the trapped bowel.

Treatment of inguinal hernia is surgery. The bowel is returned to the abdominal cavity and

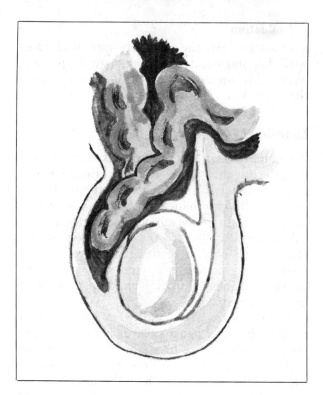

Figure 46-8 *An inguinal hernia. Bowel has protruded through the inguinal ring into the scrotum.*

retained there by the inguinal ring being sealed. Formerly, surgery for inguinal hernia was delayed until a child was 3 or 4 years of age. Today, to prevent the complication of strangulation, which is a surgical emergency, if inguinal hernia is recognized in the newborn surgical correction may be done before hospital discharge or at 1 or 2 months of age.

Volvulus

A volvulus is a twisting of the intestine. The twist leads to obstruction of the passage of feces and compromise of the blood supply to the loop of intestine involved. In fetal life, a portion of the intestine first protrudes into the base of the umbilical cord at about 6 weeks of age. At about 10 weeks, it returns to the abdominal cavity. As the intestine returns to the abdominal cavity, it rotates to its permanent position. After the rotation, the mesentery becomes fixed in this position. In an instance of volvulus, the action is incomplete, so that the mesentery does not attach to a normal position. The bowel is left free to move and twist.

The symptoms are those of intestinal obstruction: intense crying and pain, pulling up of the legs, abdominal distention, and vomiting. Diag-

nosis is made on the history and on abdominal examination, which reveals the abdominal mass. A barium X-ray also will demonstrate the obstruction. Treatment is surgery to relieve the volvulus and reattach the bowel so that it is no longer so free-moving. This action must be taken promptly before necrosis of the intestine occurs from a lack of blood supply to the involved loop of bowel. Preoperative and postoperative care will be the same as for infants with atresia or bowel obstruction.

Aganglionic Megacolon (Hirschsprung's Disease)

Aganglionic megacolon is absence of ganglionic innervation to the muscle of a section of the bowel. In most instances, the lower portion of the sigmoid colon just above the anus is involved. Because no peristalsis is present in the involved segment, it is difficult for formed stool to pass beyond that point. Because newborn stools are normally soft, symptoms of aganglionic megacolon generally do not become apparent in the neonatal period, but only after 6 to 12 months of age. Occasionally an infant will be born with such an extensive section of bowel involved that even meconium cannot pass. The defect is suggested if an infant fails to pass meconium by 24 hours of age, with increasing abdominal distention. On palpation, the rectum is empty of stool. A barium enema will reveal the inactive bowel portion, although this method must be used cautiously as a child cannot expel this substance afterward any more effectively than stool. The definitive diagnosis is by a biopsy of the affected segment that shows the lack of innervation.

Repair of aganglionic megacolon involves dissection and removal of the affected section with anastomosis of the intestine. As this is technically difficult surgery to perform in a small abdomen, the condition is generally treated in the newborn by establishing a temporary colostomy, and the bowel is repaired at 12 to 18 months of age. If a colostomy is not accomplished, daily bowel movements may be achieved by daily enemas. It is important in infants that fluid used for enemas be normal saline (0.9% NaCl), not tap water. Tap water is hypotonic; if it is instilled in the bowel, it moves very rapidly across the intestine into interstitial and intravascular fluid compartments in order to equalize osmotic pressure (by the laws of osmosis, fluid moves from an area of less to greater concentration). This movement has led to death of infants from cardiac congestion or cerebral edema (water intoxication).

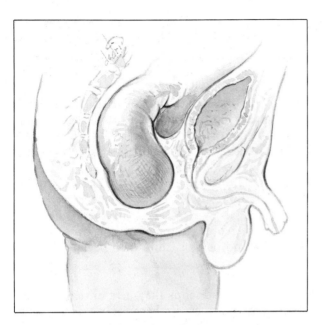

Figure 46-9 *Imperforate anus. The lower bowel ends in a blind pouch. (Courtesy of the Department of Medical Illustration, State University of New York at Buffalo.)*

Imperforate Anus

Imperforate anus (Figure 46-9) is stricture of the anus. In an extreme instance, the intestine ends in a blind pouch a distance from the anus; in less severe involvement, a membrane simply obstructs the rectum. In utero by the seventh week of life, the upper bowel elongates to pouch and combine with a pouch invaginating from the perineum. These two sections of bowel meet, the membranes between them are absorbed, and the bowel is then patent to the outside. If this motion of meeting does not occur or the membrane between the two surfaces does not dissolve, imperforate anus results. It can be a simple problem in a newborn whose bowel needs only the persistent membrane surgically excised. Complications arise when the sections of the bowel are many inches apart and no anus exists. An accompanying fistula to the bladder in males and the vagina in females may be present.

The problem occurs at an incidence of about 1 in 5,000 live births, and more often in males than in females. Imperforate anus may occur as an additional complication of spinal cord defects because the external anal canal and the spinal cord both arise from the same germ tissue layer.

Assessment

Inspection of the perineum may arouse immediate suspicion if no anal formation is seen;

however, it may be very unhelpful if the anus is normal and the defect exists far enough inside that it cannot be discovered on simple inspection. Occasionally a membrane filled with black meconium can be seen protruding from the anus. You may find it impossible to insert a rectal thermometer or rubber catheter into the rectum of a newborn. No stool will be passed, and abdominal distention will become evident. An X-ray or sonogram will reveal the defect if an infant is held in a head-down position to allow swallowed air to rise to the end of the blind pouch of the bowel. This procedure is helpful in estimating the distance the intestine is separated from the perineum. If nerve innervation to the rectum is not intact, a "wink" reflex (touching the skin near the rectum should make it contract) will not be present.

When all newborns stayed in the hospital 4 to 7 days after birth, imperforate anus was always discovered. When an infant failed to pass stools after the first 24 hours, the reason was investigated. Today, when newborns are discharged from health care facilities at 1 day of age or even a few hours after birth, it is normal that the child has not passed a stool in that time. Because imperforate anus is one of the more common congenital anomalies, no infant should be discharged from a health care facility until he or she has passed a stool as proof that the rectum is patent or follow-up must include assessment of stooling. The urine of all infants with imperforate anus should be collected and examined for the presence of meconium to determine whether the child has a rectal-urinary fistula. Placing a urine collector bag over the vagina in females may reveal meconium or the presence of a rectal-vaginal fistula.

Analysis

The most frequent nursing diagnosis in relation to imperforate anus is interference with nutrition: Once the defect is suspected a child should be kept NPO until a surgical consultation is completed. Goals should include maintaining hydration in light of no oral feedings and maintaining parent-child bonding despite early hydrating procedures such as intravenous therapy or total parenteral nutrition and early surgery.

Implementations

The degree of difficulty in repairing an imperforate anus depends on the extent of the problem. If the rectum ends close to the perineum (below or at the level of the levator ani muscle) and the anal sphincter is formed, repair is not difficult.

The task becomes complicated if the end of the rectum is a distance from the perineum (above the levator ani muscle) or the anal sphincter exists only in an underdeveloped or incomplete form. All repairs are complicated if a fistula to the bladder or urethra is present. If the repair will be extensive, a surgeon may create a temporary colostomy, anticipating final repair when the infant is somewhat older (6–12 months of age). A successful repair does not require an internal rectal sphincter, as long as the subrectal muscle is judged to be intact.

Preoperatively, a child must not be fed orally; an intravenous fluid line will be begun to maintain fluid and electrolyte imbalance. A nasogastric tube to low suction pressure for decompression will be inserted to relieve vomiting and prevent the intestine from putting pressure on other abdominal organs or the diaphragm.

Postoperative Interventions

A newborn will return from surgery with a nasogastric tube in place. If a rectal repair was completed, remember that there is a fresh suture line at the rectum. Take axillary temperatures instead of rectal ones. Mark the crib well so that anyone taking temperatures cannot forget and take a rectal temperature by mistake. The infant should have no enemas or any other intrusive rectal procedures. He may be given a stool softener daily to keep the stool from becoming hard and tearing the healing suture line. The suture line must be cleaned well following bowel movements to keep the possibility of infection to a minimum. Irrigations of the suture line following bowel movements with normal saline are an effective means to help keep it clean. It is a help if a diaper is placed under, not on the child, so that bowel movements can be cleansed away as soon as they occur.

Do not place the infant on his abdomen: In this position, newborns tend to pull their knees under them, causing tension in the perineal area. Keep these babies on their side instead. Following removal of the nasogastric tube, small oral feedings, first of glucose water, then of half-strength formula, then of regular formula or breast-feedings are begun.

A child may need rectal dilatation done once or twice a day for a few months following surgery to ensure proper patency of the rectal sphincter. This technique (inserting a lubricated cot-covered finger into the rectum) must be demonstrated to the mother, and she must be able to perform it before the child is discharged in her care. Be certain that she understands the importance of the procedure. The best surgical repair may be unsuc-

cessful if constriction occurs because she does not follow this procedure. If an infant is to be discharged with a prescription for a daily stool softener, be certain that the parent understands why this is important.

Some infants, scheduled for repair in a second-stage operation, are not permitted high-residue foods in order to lessen the bulk of stools. Although this is rarely a problem with infants because their diet naturally is low-residue, do not just assume that a parent knows what low residue means; help her make a list of acceptable beginning foods (allow rice cereal, strained fruits, and vegetables; avoid unrefined rice and grains or vegetables with fibers or fruits with peels).

Evaluation

An imperforate anus may be a difficult anomaly for parents to accept because it affects a body area that they may not feel comfortable discussing. If it involves a temporary (or permanent) colostomy, learning to care for the infant may be difficult. Parents need a great deal of support to accept the child. If a final surgical repair is successful, they can be assured the child will have normal bowel function thereafter (they do not need to be concerned about "lazy bowel" or "irritable bowel"). If a final repair could not be surgically achieved, they have the even harder task of caring for a child with a permanent ostomy. They can be assured that children who always have ostomies accept these well as they grow older because they have never known any other method of defecation.

Care of the Infant with an Ostomy

An ostomy is the construction of an opening of the bowel on the abdominal skin surface. Ostomies in newborns relieve the obstruction of bowel caused by such conditions as ileal atresia, volvulus, and imperforate anus or of bowel illness such as necrotizing enterocolitis or aganglionic megacolon. If the ostomy is made in the ileum (an ileostomy), the stoma (located on the right side of the abdomen) will drain liquid stool, which is extremely irritating to the skin because of the digestive enzymes.

If the ostomy is made in the sigmoid portion of the bowel (a colostomy), the stoma will be on the left lower abdomen and will drain normal newborn stool. An ileostomy requires the use of an ostomy appliance in order to control acid stool and prevent excoriation of the abdominal skin; with a colostomy, parents may choose (with your support and advice) whether it will be better to use an appliance or not. Without an appliance, stool will be discharged on the abdomen 3 or 4 times a day (no different from a normal newborn stool pattern).

Appliance Method

Using an appliance with a newborn has two basic problems: It may be difficult to locate an appliance small enough to contain liquid drainage without leaking and skin may become extremely irritated under the appliance. Clear plastic colostomy bags are often chosen because they do not have a ring or other hard device. They can be cut to adapt readily to the size of the stoma and the contour and size of an infant's abdomen. If even the smallest size of a pediatric stoma appliance is too large, an infant appliance can be constructed using two circles of Stomahesive and a male condom (Harrell-Bean, 1983).

When applying a new appliance, be certain that the skin underneath is clean and dry. Place a gauze square on the stoma opening to absorb any leakage before application. Do not worry about using soap on the stoma or skin (it is potentially drying to newborn skin, but it also cleans better than clear water and reduces friction of your washcloth). Rinse the area well and pat dry to reduce skin irritation.

A commercial skin sealant is helpful to harden the skin surrounding the stoma. Apply according to the brand directions; fan to dry. If a spray is used, shield the infant's face to prevent inhalation of the solution. Apply the chosen stomal collecting appliance. Tuck inside the diaper.

Check the appliance for collecting stool at least every 4 hours. Do not remove it if it is full, but drain collected stool from the bottom of the appliance into a basin or paper cup for disposal. To reduce odor, flush the appliance bag with a warm water and soap solution using an Asepto syringe; rinse with clear water. Change the appliance no more frequently than the point at which leakage occurs (perhaps as long as 1 week) to reduce skin irritation. To remove an appliance that was placed with a sealant, be certain to use the designated solvent to loosen the appliance to prevent pulling or harming underlying skin. A solvent must then be washed away with soap and water or it will become an irritant itself. Soaking in a bathtub will loosen an adhesive-type appliance. As most infants enjoy baths, a long, soaking one is an excellent way to loosen an appliance.

Teach parents to prevent skin excoriation; this is easier than treating it once it has occurred. They should remember to carry a change of appliance while away from home in case it unexpectedly loosens and leaks. Stress that the appliance itself does not need to be changed every day and too frequent changing will excoriate skin. Urge parents when their child is admitted to a health care facility to teach nurses the specific way they maintain skin integrity so it can be maintained in this same excellent condition.

Nonappliance Method

To care for a colostomy without using an appliance, wash and dry the stoma and surrounding skin area well, apply Karaya powder or Karaya powder mixed with a zinc oxide or A&D ointment. Apply ample absorbent gauze (fluffed) and an absorbent pad. Secure in place with nonadhesive tape or a binder (preferred). Check the dressing at diaper changes or about every four hours. Remove and replace when soiled, washing the skin well and applying new powder or ointment as necessary. Without an appliance, stool is kept from touching the skin only by the protection of the ointment and frequent changing of the dressing. Turning a child's position after every feeding from side to side keeps stool from always flowing to one side and may be helpful. Leaving the abdominal skin exposed to air for at least an hour a day is helpful.

If skin excoriation occurs, it may be aided by applying Stomahesive to the affected area, which encourages rapid healing; keeping the skin immediately surrounding the stoma always covered by a ring of Stomahesive may prevent excoriation. Remember that an extremely reddened skin appearance with a sharp border may be a fungal infection (*Monilia*), which is apt to occur in any area of moist skin. Report this problem to the child's physician as an antifungal prescription (nystatin) is then necessary in addition to exposure to air and maintaining the skin in a dry, healing condition.

The mother of an infant who has an ostomy needs to care for the baby in the hospital to become used to the ostomy and its care. Be sure to demonstrate care slowly and be prepared to demonstrate it again and again. This is a frightening, seemingly impossible task for a new mother to undertake. Fortunately, newborn stools do not have the odor of adult stools. Therefore, mothers seem to be much better able to care for infant ostomies than for adult ostomies. In actuality, a mother is doing very little that is different from what the average mother does—all mothers must change their infant's diapers frequently and give diaper-area care. Stress that the stoma has no nerves so the mother can touch it in washing without hurting the child (it looks raw and painful). Stress that compression against the stoma will not hurt it so that the mother feels comfortable laying the infant on his abdomen or holding the baby closely against her body for comfort.

Anomalies of the Nervous System

Anomalies of the nervous system are always potentially serious because there is a danger that the child will be left with enough neurologic disorders to affect total functioning.

Spina Bifida

Although the term *spina bifida* (Latin for "divided spine") is most often used as a collective term for spinal cord involvement, there are well-defined degrees of spina bifida involvement. All these disorders occur because of lack of fusion of the posterior surface of the embryo in early intrauterine life. The incidence is 1 to 3 per 1,000 live births. They may occur as a polygenic inheritance pattern. Women who have had one child born with such a defect have an increased chance of having a second child with such a defect (as great as 1 in 20). For this reason, women who have had one child born with a spinal cord defect are advised to have a maternal serum assay or an amniocentesis done to determine if such a defect exists in a second pregnancy. This is revealed by the presence of alpha-fetoprotein (AFP) in the serum or amniotic fluid escaping from an open cord lesion. These assessments are done at the fifteenth week of pregnancy, when AFP reaches its peak concentration.

Types of Spina Bifida

Spina Bifida Occulta. Spina bifida occulta is a developmental anomaly in which posterior spinal vertebrae fail to close. This anomaly usually involves one or two vertebrae at the sacral or lumbar area, although it may occur at any place along the spinal column. The spot is evident as a depression in the skin. Often there is a tuft of hair growing at the place of the depression (Figure 46-10B).

Meningocele. A meningocele is a pouching of the meninges and cerebrospinal fluid through a defect in the posterior surface of the spinal vertebrae. The meningocele may be covered by a layer of skin, or it may be denuded, with just the fibrous dura mater exposed (Figure 46-10C).

Myelomeningocele. A myelomeningocele is a pouching of the spinal cord, the meninges, and cerebrospinal fluid through a defect in the posterior spinal vertebrae (Figure 46-10D). Often the spinal cord ends at the level of the myelomeningocele, and so there will be no motor or sensory function below this point. As this is lower motor neuron damage, the child will have flaccidity of lower extremities and loss of bowel and bladder control. The infant's legs are lax; the baby does not move them, and urine and stools continually dribble because of lack of sphincter control. It is generally difficult to tell from the gross appearance of the myelomeningocele whether or not it is the simpler meningocele (Figure 46-11).

Figure 46-10 *Degrees of spinal cord defects. A. Normal spinal column. B. Spina bifida occulta. C. Meningocele. D. Myelomeningocele.*

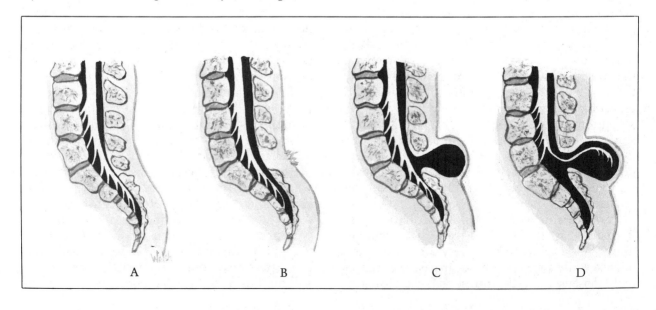

A   B   C   D

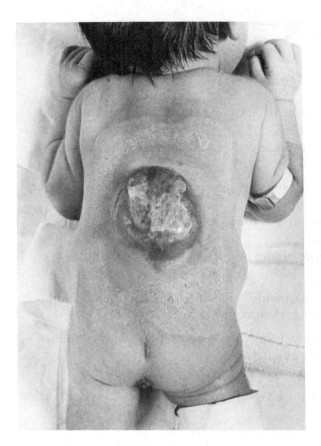

Figure 46-11 *A myelomeningocele protrudes as an obvious deformity of the spine and cord. Note how the area is covered only by a thin membrane, making it prone to trauma and infection. (Courtesy of the Department of Medical Photography, Children's Hospital, Buffalo, N.Y.)*

Encephalocele. An encephalocele is a myelomeningocele occurring at the back of the neck or head. The sac contains brain tissue, as well as spinal cord, meninges, and fluid.

Assessment

All levels of spina bifida but spina bifida occulta are readily visible at birth. They may be discovered during intrauterine life by sonography, fetoscopy, or amniocentesis (discovery of alpha-fetoprotein in amniotic fluid). Observe and record whether an infant has spontaneous movement of lower extremities and the nature and pattern of voiding and stooling. A normal infant appears to be "always wet" from voiding, but actually voids in amounts of about 30 ml and then is dry for 2 or 3 hours before voiding again. An infant without sphincter control voids continually. This pattern is the same for stooling. Observing these features aids in differentiation between meningocele and myelomeningocele. Differentiation may be further established by sonogram of the lesion.

Analysis

With myelomeningocele, there is no correction possible other than palliative repair of the protruding meningeal sac. The child will continue to have paralysis of lower extremities and loss of bowel and bladder function. Nursing diagnoses established with spina bifida defects are concerned with protection of the sac from breakage, prevention of infection, and establishment of maternal-child bonding. Important considerations to use in planning care goals are summarized in the Nursing Care Highlight on page 1092.

Implementations

A spina bifida occulta needs no surgical correction. The parents should be made aware of its existence, however, so that they are not surprised when someone points it out to them later on in the child's life.

Surgical correction of meningocele, myelomeningocele, or encephalocele is scheduled as soon as feasible, before rupture of the sac with loss of cerebral spinal fluid or infection of the fluid (meningitis) can result. An infant must be positioned so as to put no pressure on the sac prior to surgery. Pressure on the outpouching sac increases cerebrospinal fluid pressure. Extreme pressure can result in compressed and nonfunctioning brain tissue. An infant should also be observed closely for signs of increased intracranial pressure: vomiting, lethargy, failure to eat, or a bulging fontanelle. (See the Nursing Care Highlight on page 1092.)

Postoperative Interventions

Following surgery, the nurse must take the same careful precautions against allowing urine or feces to touch the incision area. Continue to observe a child for signs of increased intracranial pressure; vital signs; neurologic signs such as pupillary changes, increase in head circumference, or bulging fontanelles; and behavior changes such as irritability or lethargy.

These children often develop hydrocephalus following surgery, probably because of interference with arachnoid absorption of cerebral spinal fluid (a portion of the arachnoid membrane was removed). It will also be vital for the nurse to help the parents understand and deal with the long-term effects of the disorder.

Evaluation

Eventual prognosis will depend on the extent of the defect. The loss of meninges may limit the rate of absorption of cerebrospinal fluid; it may build up in amount, and hydrocephalus may de-

====== *Nursing Care Highlight* ======

The Child with Myelomeningocele

Preoperative Goals	*Implementations*
Aid diagnosis	Assess for leg motion and voiding and stool patterns to aid diagnosis.
	Measure head circumference daily to detect increasing intracranial pressure.
Protect sac	Prevent pressure on the protruding sac from handling or feeding or trauma.
	Position on abdomen or side to relieve pressure on sac and keep stools from sac.
	Cover sac with sterile saline compresses to prevent drying.
	Construct plastic "bridge" to keep stool from sac.
Protect from hypothermia	Prevent infant from becoming chilled by using Isolette or warm blankets; avoid radiant warmer to prevent drying sac.
Maintain nutrition	Hold to feed if possible, being careful not to press on sac; mother may breast-feed with caution.
	Weigh diapers; measure specific gravity of voidings.
Maintain skin integrity	Clean diaper area skin well q4h; apply A&D ointment to keep urine from skin.
Encourage bonding	Encourage parents to care for child.
	Encourage parents to express grief reaction.

Postoperative Goals	*Implementations*
Prevent hypothermia	Keep from becoming chilled by Isolette.
Assess for complications	Measure head circumference daily to detect increasing intracranial pressure.
	Observe for signs of increased intracranial pressure: lethargy, increased temperature, decreased pulse rate, vomiting, tense fontanelles, pupillary unresponsiveness, high-pitched cry.
Prevent infection	Position on side or abdomen to keep stool and urine from incision line.
	Provide a plastic "bridge" to keep feces from incision line.
	Provide good skin care to prevent excoriation from acid urine.
Encourage bonding	Encourage parents to continue care of infant.
	Encourage to make active contact if infant is transferred for care.
Investigate urine management	If appropriate, begin Credé method of bladder evacuation to maintain continence.
Establish continuing care	Make referral to community health agency as appropriate.
	Be certain parents have a primary caregiver for follow-up care.

velop following repair. If a myelomeningocele is present, a surgeon will close the skin over the area of defect, but the motor and sensory loss below this point cannot be restored.

Parents need a great deal of support to care for a child with a myelomeningocele, because it means their child has a multiple handicap. A number of parents are currently choosing to allow a child born with myelomeningocele to die rather than have palliative surgery to close the defect. This poses an ethical problem in maternal-newborn nursing: Whose rights should be honored—the parents' or the child's?

Hydrocephalus

Hydrocephalus occurs at an incidence of 1 in every 2,000 live births. An increase in the amount of cerebrospinal fluid in the ventricles of the brain (Figure 46-12), the condition may occur because of any one of three reasons: overproduction of fluid by the choroid plexus (rare), lack of arachnoid membrane absorption space, such as could happen with a hemorrhage into this space from the trauma of birth (rare), or a stricture along the path of flow of the fluid, forcing quantities to build up in the ventricles (the most common etiology). An obstruction of this nature usually occurs along the narrow aqueduct of Sylvius from a congenital stricture or hemorrhage; later in life, a tumor growth can cause obstruction at this point.

Assessment

With hydrocephalus, an infant's head is often not enlarged at birth, or is only slightly enlarged.

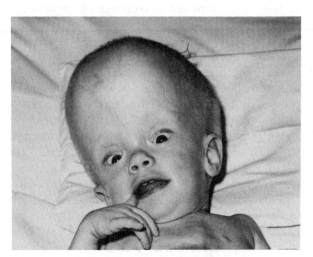

Figure 46-12 *An infant with hydrocephalus. From Marlow, D. (1973). Textbook of pediatric nursing. Philadelphia: Saunders.*

The suture lines, particularly the sagittal suture line, are separated, however, and the fontanelles will feel tense or bulging and may be much longer or wider than normal. Diagnosis is confirmed by CAT scan, sonography, or transillumination that demonstrates the enlarged, fluid-filled ventricles. Head enlargement becomes most apparent during the first 6 weeks of life. All infants who have a documented or suspected intraventricular hemorrhage or meningeal infection should be observed for the possibility of hydrocephalus. As most children who develop hydrocephalus in utero assume a breech delivery position (putting the largest bulk of the body into the uterine fundus) all breech-delivered babies need careful assessment of head circumference during the first 4 weeks of life.

In some infants the fluid increases in amount so rapidly that within the few days of a hospital stay a bulging anterior fontanelle and widely separated sutures appear. An infant's forehead may bulge (termed *bossing*); white sclera is evident above the cornea of the eye (*sundown eyes*) from stretching and pulling up of the upper eyelids. An infant's cry may become high-pitched and shrill. The newborn may be irritable and restless, or he may be lethargic.

Analysis

The most frequent nursing diagnoses established with infants with hydrocephalus are concerned with nutrition and parent-child bonding. Nutrition is affected because with increased intracranial pressure, irritability, lethargy, or vomiting occurs. Bonding is affected because this is a potentially extremely serious defect: If not corrected, the intracranial pressure will eventually destroy brain tissue and leave the child severely mentally retarded and without motor nerve control. Important care measures to help in establishing goals are shown in the Nursing Care Highlight on page 1094.

Implementations

An infant's head circumference should be measured daily. Marking the forehead and the most prominent process of the occiput with a ball-point pen at the points where the tape should pass helps to make measurements accurate even when different people are doing the measuring. The Nursing Care Highlight on page 1094 summarizes other important implementations.

Surgical repair is a shunting procedure, in which, to permit drainage of cerebral spinal fluid, a thin silicone catheter is placed between the ventricle above the obstruction and the base of the brain (the foramen magnum), or threaded under

=== *Nursing Care Highlight* ===

The Child with Hydrocephalus

Preoperative Goals	Implementations
Aid in diagnosis	Measure head circumference daily to detect increasing size.
	Measure size of fontanelles daily.
	Assess for signs of increasing intracranial pressure: increasing temperature, decreasing pulse, lethargy, irritability, vomiting.
Avoid trauma to head	Handle head with open palm in case skull is thin. Support head well when lifting infant to avoid cervical strain.
Maintain nutrition	Hold to feed if possible. Use rocking chair for arm support.
	Mother may breast-feed.
Encourage bonding	Encourage parents to care for infant to aid bonding.
	Allow parents to voice concern or grief over child's condition.
	Educate parents about condition.
	Teach parents about role and flow of CSF, expected surgery, and outcome.

Postoperative Goals	Implementations
Maintain correct intracranial pressure	Position infant as per surgeon's orders (usually flat with shunted side down).
	Pump shunt as ordered to increase CSF flow.
Prevent infection	Assess incision site for redness or inflammation. Keep incision line dry from oral mucus or perspiration.
Maintain nutrition	Begin feedings as ordered cautiously to prevent vomiting (increases intracranial pressure).
Encourage bonding	Encourage parents to care for infant to aid bonding.
	Help parents to maintain contact if infant is transferred for care.
Establish continued care	Ascertain that parents have follow-up care for continued health care of the child for shunt revision.
	Make referral to community health agency as appropriate.

the subcutaneous tissue into the vena cava, a ureter, or the peritoneum (Figure 46-13). Shunts contain a valve and reservoir area to allow sampling of CSF and flushing of the tubing by compressing the pump. The pump rests under the skin behind an ear.

Postoperative Interventions

Following a shunting procedure, the infant's surgeon will write specific orders for positioning (either with the infant's bed flat so that the head remains level with the body and drainage is not encouraged, or with the head elevated to encourage drainage). When bathing and turning the child, make sure you maintain this position. If the head is raised, CSF may flow too rapidly

through the shunt and decompression may occur too rapidly.

Often an infant is not turned to lie on the side opposite the shunt to prevent rapid decompression. If the inserted shunt has a valve, definite orders will be written about how often it must be pressed and fluid forced through the catheter.

Because the head is so heavy, an infant cannot move it freely. If cerebral enlargement occurred the skin of the head is stretched thin, and skin decubitus ulcers tend to occur on the pressure points of the child's head. Wash the head daily. Change position every 2 hours so that no portion of the head rests against the mattress for long periods. A foam rubber or sheepskin pad may help to relieve pressure points. See the Nursing Care

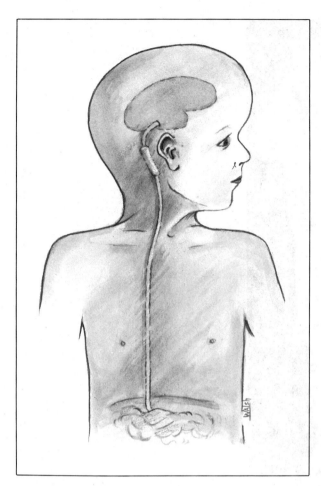

Figure 46-13 *A ventriculoperitoneal shunt to drain cerebral spinal fluid in hydrocephalus.*

Highlight on page 1094 for a summary of postoperative implementations.

Evaluation

Prognosis depends on the location of the stricture that is causing the increased fluid, the success of the shunting procedure, and the amount and site of damage to brain tissue that occurred from compression prior to surgery. An infant may have to be transported to a major center for this repair so bonding may be difficult because of the separation. Following shunting procedures the head may remain larger than normal, but intelligence may be normal. Help a parent to accept a child as well despite the slightly unusual appearance. As a baby grows older, the head will not continue to grow and with overall increased body proportion, the appearance will become less and less obvious.

Following surgery, a mother must be informed of signs of increased intracranial pressure to watch for and must maintain health supervision visits. The shunt can become obstructed and will need its length changed as the child grows.

Arnold-Chiari Deformity

An Arnold-Chiari deformity is caused by overgrowth of the neural tube in the sixteenth to twentieth week of fetal life. The specific anomaly is a projection of the cerebellum, medulla oblongata, and fourth ventricle into the cervical canal. This condition causes the upper cervical spinal cord to jackknife backward. A lumbosacral myelomeningocele is present in about 50 percent of children with the anomaly. Hydrocephalus from aqueduct stenosis also may be present.

Infants with an Arnold-Chiari deformity obviously have the difficulties of a child with both hydrocephalus and myelomeningocele. The ultimate prognosis will depend on the extent of the defect and the surgical procedures possible.

Anomalies of the Genitourinary Tract

The upper urinary tract arises from a different germ layer (the endoderm) than the lower urinary tract (the ectoderm), thus anomalies are usually found in either upper or lower parts of the tract, rarely in both. Although an infant may have accompanying reproductive tract abnormalities, these may not be evident at birth but only become evident with puberty when secondary sex changes do not occur.

Exstrophy of the Bladder

Exstrophy of the bladder is a midline closure defect that occurs during the embryonic period of pregnancy. It occurs more frequently in males than females.

Assessment

In exstrophy of the bladder (Figure 46-14) no anterior wall of the bladder and no anterior skin covering of the lower anterior abdomen forms. The bladder lies open and exposed on the abdomen; it is bright red in color, unable to contain urine, with urine continually draining from it. In males, the penis is often unformed. Pelvic bone defects, particularly nonclosure of the pubic arch, and urethral defects may also be present.

Analysis

Prevention of infection is a major concern in an infant with exstrophy of the bladder; infection of the open bladder may lead to ascending urinary tract or kidney infection. Establishing bonding is a second concern because of the child's obvious defect. Important measures of care are shown in

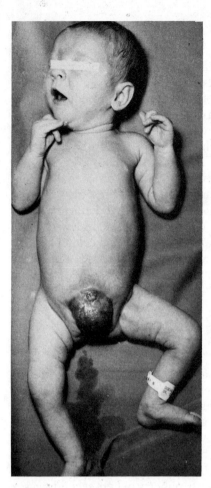 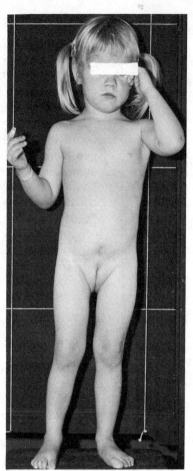

Figure 46-14 *Exstrophy of the bladder. A. Characteristic appearance of exstrophy in a 6-month-old infant. B. Same child at 2 years of age, following surgical reconstruction. From Crowley, L. V. (1974).* An introduction to clinical embryology. *Chicago: Year Book Publishers. Copyright 1974 by Year Book Medical Publishers.*

The Nursing Care Highlight on page 1097 to help you plan care.

Surgical repair is seldom wholly successful. It might be possible to construct a reservoir for urine from the abdominal bladder tissue, but almost impossible to create a system that recognizes when it is filling and empties appropriately. For this reason, in most instances, the bladder is surgically removed and an ileal conduit is constructed (in which the ureters are attached to a separated portion of the small intestine, and urine is voided into a collecting bag attached to the abdomen) or threaded into the wall of the intestine so urine is evacuated with stool (a sigmoid implant).

Patent Urachus

A patent urachus is a fistula between the bladder and the base of the umbilical cord. It forms be-

cause, at an early point in intrauterine life, the bladder is connected to the cord base. A patent urachus is usually detected when urine is seen draining from the base of the cord. Any drainage from an umbilical cord should be tested by Nitrazine paper; urine will show an acid reaction, but other body fluids are invariably alkaline. Surgical repair of a patent urachus is done in the newborn period before infection of the bladder or cord results.

Hypospadias and Epispadias

In hypospadias, the opening of the male urethra is on the ventral or undersurface of the penis. Epispadias is the abnormal placement of the urethra on the upper or dorsal surface of the penis. The meatus may be near the glans, midway back, or at the base of the penis. This usually causes no difficulties in infancy. The defect needs to be cor-

Nursing Care Highlight

The Child with Bladder Exstrophy

Preoperative Goals	*Implementations*
Prevent infection	Cover open bladder with sterile petrolatum gauze.
	Place in infant chair to keep feces away from anterior abdomen.
	Encourage oral intake to dilute urine.
	Cleanse skin frequently to prevent excoriation.
Prevent hypothermia	Keep infant warm (draining urine soaks sheets, which become chilled) by Isolette or radiant warmer.
Encourage bonding	Encourage parents to care for child to aid bonding.
	Allow parents to voice feelings about child to work through grief.
	Help parents to maintain contact if infant is transferred for care.
	Compare care with normal newborn care: All newborns are incontinent of urine.
Educate parents	Teach about child's condition and anticipated surgery and outcome.
Postoperative Goals	*Implementations*
Prevent infection	Protect incision line from feces to prevent infection by using infant chair.
	If sigmoid implant was created, provide good skin care as urine in stool is excoriating to skin.
Aid bonding	Encourage parents to care for ileal conduit if this was created.
	Help to make realistic plans for care of child at home.
Confirm continuing care	Make a referral to community health agency if appropriate.
	Confirm that parents have arrangements for follow-up health care.

rected before the child enters school, however, so that he looks and voids as all the other boys do. It is also important to correct it before reproductive age, so that with coitus the deposition of sperm is near the cervix and not in the distal vagina, which would cause a fertility problem. Infants with hypospadias or epispadias should not be circumcised as the plastic surgeon may want to use the foreskin in the plastic repair. Be certain a mother understands retracting and cleaning the foreskin so that penile infection is prevented prior to surgery.

Imperforate Hymen

Imperforate hymen (Figure 46-15) is a rare disorder and, because the external genitals of female infants are edematous at birth, often difficult to detect. As the genital area may not be included in every health assessment of a child during her growing years, detecting this condition in the newborn period is particularly important. It is

Figure 46-15 *Imperforate hymen in newborn infant. From Crowley, L. V. (1974). An introduction to clinical embryology. Chicago: Year Book Medical Publishers. Copyright 1974 by Year Book Medical Publishers.*

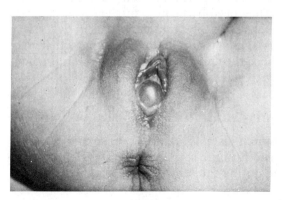

corrected by a simple surgical incision before puberty and menarche.

Ambiguous Genitalia

A few infants have such ambiguous genitalia at birth that it is difficult to tell whether they are male or female. If a mother took an androgen-like hormone during pregnancy, a chromosomally female infant may be born with infant genitalia appearing more male than female. This is a rare occurrence today but happened in the past when a type of synthetic progesterone given during pregnancy acted in an androgen-like manner.

Ambiguous genitalia may occur in a child with adrenogenital syndrome. With this syndrome, the adrenal gland produces androgen instead of adequate cortisone, thus masculinizing female infants.

The true sex of a child can be established by a simple chromosomal test, a Barr body determination. A scraping of cells from the buccal membrane of an infant is taken, stained, and examined under a microscope. If the child has two X chromosomes (female), a black mark (the second X chromosome) will show at the side of the cell nucleus. A more thorough chromosome examination, or karyotype, may also be done. Intravenous pyelography (IVP) establishes whether a child has a full urinary tract, as the urinary tract arises from the same germ tissue as genital tissue. Laparotomy may be necessary to establish whether gonads are present in a child.

Once a child's true sex is known, the extent of necessary reconstructive surgery is determined. This may involve correction of a hypospadias or cryptorchidism, removal of labial adhesions, or surgical removal of an enlarged clitoris. When removal of an enlarged clitoris is involved, the parents must consider what the absence of this organ will mean to the child in terms of later sexual enjoyment.

It is important that the sex of a child be established as soon as possible so that the parents can begin to adjust to claiming and rearing a boy or a girl. They need frequent assurance at health care checkups that the child is normal in every way but this one (assuming that is true) so that they can raise the child to realize his or her full potential with self-esteem intact.

Cryptorchidism

Cryptorchidism is failure of the male testes to descend into the scrotal sac. Testes normally descend during the seventh to ninth months of intrauterine life. They may descend up to 6 weeks after birth; rarely do they descend after that point. Undescended right testes are more common than left. In about 20 percent of boys with undescended testes, both testes are undescended.

An undescended testis may be at the inguinal ring (true undescended testis) or may be an ectopic testis (still in the abdomen). Because testes arise from the same germ tissue as does kidney, children with ectopic testes need to be evaluated for kidney function as well. A buccal smear (Barr body determination) may be used to determine true sex if both testes are undescended.

The cause of undescended testes is often unknown. Fibrous bands at the inguinal ring or inadequate length of spermatic vessels may prevent descent. Testes apparently descend because of stimulation by testosterone; it is possible that lack of testosterone prevents descent.

Assessment

All male infants should be assessed for testes descent in the newborn period. In some children, because of poor examining technique the testes only appear to be undescended. Initiation of a cremasteric reflex (stroking the internal thigh) causes testes to retract, as does cold, stress, or palpation. Testes may often be felt in the scrotal sac when a child is held upright, but not when he is supine; after a warm bath, but not in a chilly examining room.

Implementations

Treatment for cryptorchidism is surgery at preschool age. Children may be given a course of chorionic gonadotropin hormone in the hope of stimulating testes descent, but chances of success with this therapy are limited. It is important that cryptorchidism not be ignored because undescended testes are infertile and may become cancerous if left in the abdomen after puberty.

Anomalies of the Heart and Circulatory System

As many as 1 in 140 live-born infants is born with a congenital heart defect. The mortality of such infants is so high that a third die in the first month of life. Congenital heart disorders occur apparently as a combination of polygenic inheritance patterns and environmental or gene-directed influences. Atrial septal defect, for example, appears to be inherited; many infants with chromosomal abnormalities such as Down's syn-

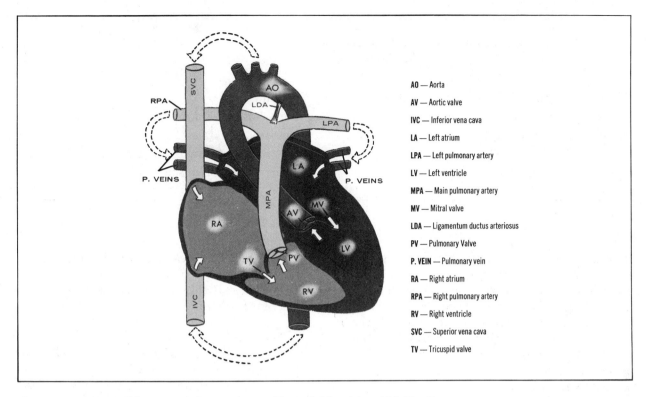

Figure 46-16 *Normal heart circulation. (From Clinical Education Aid, No. 7, Ross Laboratories, Columbus, Ohio, 1970.)*

AO — Aorta

AV — Aortic valve

IVC — Inferior vena cava

LA — Left atrium

LPA — Left pulmonary artery

LV — Left ventricle

MPA — Main pulmonary artery

MV — Mitral valve

LDA — Ligamentum ductus arteriosus

PV — Pulmonary Valve

P. VEIN — Pulmonary vein

RA — Right atrium

RPA — Right pulmonary artery

RV — Right ventricle

SVC — Superior vena cava

TV — Tricuspid valve

drome (trisomy 21) also have heart defects. Infants who contracted viral infections in intrauterine life such as rubella also have a high incidence of heart defects.

The heart is an organ that is prone to defects because it forms first as a single tube (fourth week), then the tube is divided into a left and right section (fifth week), the arteries and veins leading to it are formed (sixth week), and then the valves form (seventh and eighth weeks). Interferences can affect the heart formation at any of these steps, causing inadequate septum, valve, or pulmonary artery or aorta formation. Normal fetal circulation is shown in Figure 14-5. The normal changes that occur in this circulation at birth are discussed in Chapter 31. Normal heart circulation is reviewed in Figure 46-16.

Congenital heart defects are categorized as two types: acyanotic and cyanotic. Acyanotic types are more frequent and milder in occurrence.

Assessment

A number of common symptoms occur in children with congenital heart disorders. These are shown in the box on page 1100. Cyanosis is difficult to assess in a newborn because most newborns have some cyanosis (acrocyanosis). Generalized cyanosis, however, is never normal.

The cyanosis of heart disease can usually be separated from that caused by a lung disorder in that in a child with choanal atresia or a lung disorder, cyanosis usually decreases if the infant cries, since opening the mouth helps to aerate the lungs. The infant with a heart defect usually becomes more cyanotic on exertion and crying because the heart cannot meet the increased metabolic demand caused by the activity of crying. Administering oxygen to a child with a respiratory disorder generally decreases cyanosis; it has little or at least less effect on a child with a heart disorder.

Many of the symptoms of cardiac anomalies are not present in the first days of life because still-functioning fetal circulatory structures, such as the ductus arteriosus and foramen ovale, compensate. A heart murmur in a newborn may be missed because the heart rate is so rapid (120–160 beats per minute) that murmurs are hard to hear; also minimum blood is passing through the pulmonary artery because the lungs still offer a great deal of resistance. With the pressure high in the right ventricle, little blood will pass through a septal opening into the right ventricle.

Clear-cut symptoms that depend on activity to become apparent may not become noticeable during a 3- to 4-day hospital stay, especially if the

Symptoms of Congestive Heart Disease

Tachypnea (respiratory rate over 50 at rest)

Tachycardia (heart rate over 160)

Feeding difficulty (fatigues too easily to finish breast- or bottle-feeding)

Liver palpable over 3 cm

Coughing

Absence of femoral pulses

Cyanosis

Poor capillary filling of extremities

Murmur heard on auscultation

child is relatively inactive from effects of general anesthesia at birth. For this reason, all newborns need close observation for cyanosis, general activity, and auscultation of heart sounds. White room walls help to make cyanosis more noticeable than colored ones; a quiet room is often necessary to hear heart murmurs. The fatigue that occurs from inadequate oxygenation may manifest itself first in a newborn as a feeding problem (too fatigued to breast-feed or bottle-feed well). Rapid respiratory rate also interferes with feeding as the infant has to stop sucking to breathe.

Normal cardiac assessment of newborns is discussed in Chapter 32. The diagnosis of cardiac defects is made on the basis of the signs and symptoms present in the newborn, including cyanosis, abnormal heart sounds, absence of femoral pulses, tachycardia, increased respiratory rate, and feeding difficulty. When listening to newborn hearts, try to wait until the infant as well as other babies in the nursery are not crying. Respect the difficulty involved in auscultation of a newborn heart and quiet babies while an examiner is listening to heart sounds by providing a pacifier; pick up other babies to quiet them; keep conversations low.

A chest X-ray examination or echocardiogram is usually ordered to determine the size of the heart and the state of the pulmonary vasculature. Blood gases will be obtained. Arterial saturation of under 92 percent oxygen is compatible with cyanotic heart disease. An electrocardiogram may be ordered to detect abnormal cardiac electrical activity. The infant may be scheduled for cardiac catheterization. However, cardiac catheterization has a higher risk in newborns than in older children, and if an infant is not in acute distress, the actual diagnosis may be delayed until later in life. Both the American Heart Association and the Academy of Pediatrics recommend that these complex studies be done only in centers performing at least 200 cardiac catheterizations on in-

fants and children yearly and at least 100 heart operations yearly. An infant with a recognized heart defect may thus be transported to a regional center for further studies.

Analysis

Common nursing diagnoses concerned with congenital heart disease are "Interference with nutrition related to the accompanying fatigue and rapid respiratory rate" and "Interference with bonding related to the seriousness of the illness." The Nursing Care Highlight on page 1101 lists goals of care to aid in care planning. When making plans, parents invariably ask at what time of life congenital heart defects will be repaired. With recent advances in heart surgery, heart defects are being repaired at ages earlier than ever before—in some instances, in the first few days of life. All surgical repairs are made individually, on the basis of the extent of the defect and the symptoms in the infant. A major reason for early heart surgery is to prevent subacute bacterial endocarditis from stasis of blood flow at the defect.

Acyanotic Heart Disease

Acyanotic heart defects are heart or circulatory anomalies that involve an obstacle to the flow of blood such as a stenosis or a shunt that moves blood from the arterial to the venous system (oxygenated to unoxygenated blood, or left-to-right shunts). These types of defects do not produce cyanosis but rather create an ineffective pumping action as blood is recirculated through the heart over and over rather than being pumped out to be distributed to the rest of the body. Because the contraction of the left atrium and ventricle is stronger than that of the right side of the heart (contraction must be strong enough to propel blood to the systemic circulation while right heart side contraction only propels it to the lungs), if a defect occurs in the septum wall, blood

—— *Nursing Care Highlight* ——

The Child with Congenital Heart Disease

Goals	Implementations
Conserve energy	Space procedures to provide periods of rest. Provide frequent small feedings rather than large feedings. Breast-feeding may be too fatiguing for the infant.
	Limit tiring procedures such as a full bath.
Prevent infection	Use good hand washing technique with care. Screen health care personnel and visitors for upper respiratory infections.
Prevent hypothermia	Chilling increases metabolic rate, which increases body cell needs. Prevent chilling.
Assess for complications	Assess for signs of congestive heart failure: dyspnea, tachycardia, nasal flaring, retractions, increased liver size, cyanosis, diaphoresis.
	Daily weight; measure intake and output, specific gravity of urine.
Prepare for home care	Review medication schedule with parents.
	Discuss time management (feeding is time-consuming; a knowledgeable person must be with child at all times).
	Review emergency procedures such as knee-chest, resuscitation.
Confirm continuing care	Be certain the parents have arranged for follow-up care as the child will need continued health supervision.

will shunt left to right or create an acyanotic shunt.

Ventricular Septal Defect

The commonest of all congenital cardiac defects, accounting for 22 percent of all instances of congenital heart disease, ventricular septal defects (VSD) are openings in the septum between the two lower chambers of the heart, the right and left ventricles (Figure 46-17A). They occur more frequently in males than in females.

Ventricular septal defects are one of the chief causes of congestive heart failure in a newborn baby. Congestive heart failure results because, with each ventricular beat, blood is forced from the left ventricle across into the right ventricle, overburdening the right side of the heart. Since more than the normal amount of blood is then forced into the pulmonary artery, lung congestion may result as well.

Symptoms of VSD may not be apparent in the newborn because the relatively high pulmonary resistance due to still-unopened alveoli increases pressure in the right ventricle and allows only a small amount of flow across the septal defect. The characteristic murmur heard in older children and adults with VSDs (a grade 3 or 4 rough or

harsh holosystolic murmur, loudest at the fourth left interspace) may be absent. X-ray will not yet show any increase in the size of the right ventricle.

As many as 50 percent of VSDs close spontaneously in the first month of life, especially those that occur in the membranous portion rather than the muscle portion of the septum. The remainder will continue to remain patent and, as the child becomes more active and pulmonary artery tension lowers as alveoli open completely, become important and noticeable. A murmur will become apparent on auscultation, the right ventricle will begin to hypertrophy, and increased pulmonary blood flow will be apparent on X-ray. An electrocardiogram will reveal right ventricular hypertrophy. A cardiac catheterization will reveal the increased oxygen saturation in the right ventricle as well as the increased pressure extending into the pulmonary artery.

If symptoms of congestive heart failure develop early in life and the infant has other associated anomalies or illnesses that make him at risk for a full surgery procedure, pulmonary artery banding, or application of a Teflon band to the pulmonary artery to narrow it and increase the resistance to blood flow even more, may be attempted. This

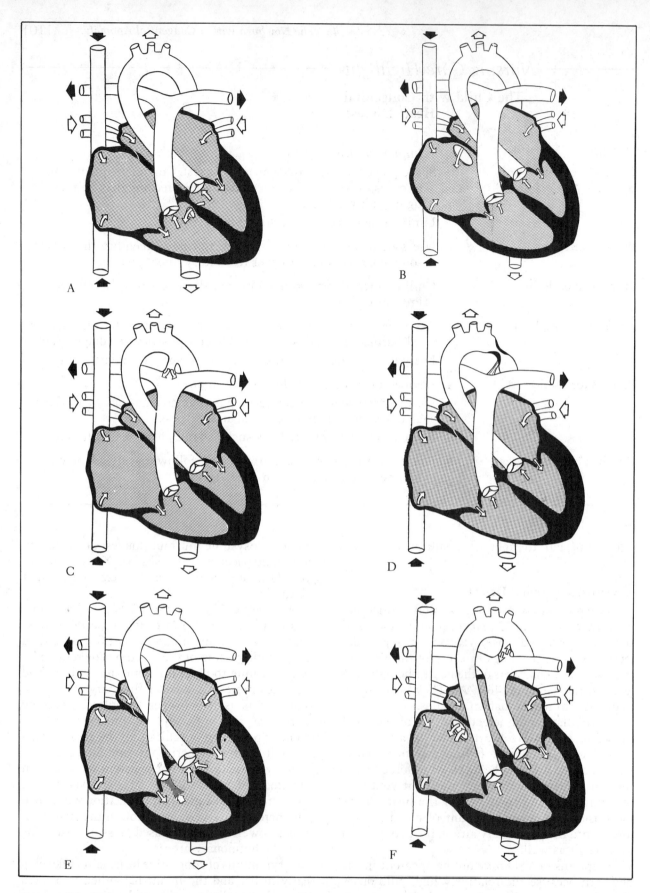

Figure 46-17 *Common congenital heart defects. A. Ventricular septal defect. B. Atrial septal defect. C. Patent ductus arteriosus. D. Coarctation of the aorta. E. Tetralogy of Fallot. F. Complete transposition of great vessels. (From Clinical Education Aid, No. 7, Ross Laboratories, Columbus, Ohio, 1970.)*

forces a buildup in right ventricular pressure and further reduces the amount of blood shunted. When the infant is older, a permanent correction of the defect can be achieved.

An infant who is otherwise well at birth may have permanent surgery performed immediately. This involves simple suturing of the defect if it is only small or application of a Teflon patch to the septal wall (similar to sewing a patch on the knee of jeans). Following the full correction, a child will have follow-up health supervision visits done over the next year but will be a perfectly well child after that time.

Atrial Septal Defect

An atrial septal defect (ASD)—an opening in the septum between the upper chambers of the heart (Figure 46-17B), the right and left atria—is more common in females than males. A defect in the atrial septum may be caused by failure of the foramen ovale to close because of a defective valve flap or may be a more extensive defect of the wall itself (an ostium secundal defect). With atrial defects, the blood shunts from the left to the right atrium or an ineffective pump condition is created. The increased pressure on the right side of the heart from pulmonary resistance allows little blood to cross the defect. The main murmur caused is often barely noticeable in the newborn. As the pulmonary resistance falls, more blood shunts and a murmur (a systolic ejection one) develops. Right heart hypertrophy may occur.

The defect is repaired in early life to prevent subacute bacterial endocarditis due to the relative stasis of blood flow. Repair is by suturing the defect or suturing a Teflon patch in place on the septum.

Endocardial Cushion Defect

The term *endocardial cushion* refers to embryonic growth centers or pads in the heart septum that merge to form the tricuspid and mitral valves and the midportion of the atrial and ventricular septum. An endocardial cushion defect is apt to be major because it potentially involves so many important structures. Such defects may occur as an isolated phenomenon in an otherwise healthy child, but they tend to be most common in children with Down's syndrome (trisomy 21). About 1 in 9 children with Down's syndrome has this type of congenital cardiac defect.

Not only does blood shunt through the imperfect septum but through the valves from the atria to the ventricles (both reflux and regurgitation may occur). A newborn with an endocardial cushion defect has much the same symptoms as does a child with a large VSD. Although the murmurs and chest X-ray films of the two conditions are similar, they are distinguished by electrocardiogram. Repair may not be as successful with endocushion defects because of the valvular involvement.

Patent Ductus Arteriosus

A ductus arteriosus is a prenatal shunt between the pulmonary artery and the aorta. In some infants it fails to close at birth (patent ductus arteriosus) (Figure 46-17C). The flow of blood during intrauterine life is from the pulmonary artery to the aorta because the shunt is used to transport blood away from the nonfunctioning lungs. Because the pressure in the aorta after birth is greater than the pressure in the pulmonary artery after birth, the flow of blood after birth is from the aorta (carries oxygenated blood) to the pulmonary artery (carries unoxygenated blood)—that is, from the arterial to the venous system or an acyanotic or left-to-right shunt. The ductus arteriosus tends to remain open in infants with hypoxia or respiratory difficulty because of increased pulmonary artery pressure. It tends to occur more often in females than males; because many premature infants have respiratory difficulty, it occurs at a higher-than-usual incidence in early-born infants.

In patent ductus arteriosus, a murmur will be heard at the upper left sternal border or under the left clavicle. In older children, it is a continuous (systolic and diastolic) machinery-type murmur. In newborns, the murmur may not be so characteristic, perhaps a short grade 2 or grade 3 harsh systolic murmur. A child's pulse pressure will be wider than normal due to the low diastolic pressure because of the shunt runoff. If the shunt is large, congestive heart failure may develop by the end of the first week as the increased amount of blood pours back into the pulmonary artery, preventing emptying of the right ventricle.

Although surgery for any cardiac problem is severe, a patent ductus arteriosus can be repaired with less risk than can other defects because the repair is actually outside the heart. Repair is made at about 1 year of life or whenever significant symptoms appear; it involves ligation of the unnecessary ductus.

Coarctation of the Aorta

Coarctation of the aorta is a narrowing or stenosis of the aorta. It occurs because as the aorta first forms in utero it is sharply bent; incomplete lumenation can occur at this point (a space just proximal to the ductus arteriosus). One of the commonest malformations causing congestive heart failure during the newborn period (Figure 46-17D), it is suspected if a newborn does not have strong and bilaterally equal femoral pulses. Checking for the presence of both femoral pulses is a procedure that all maternal-newborn nurses should include as part of an initial newborn health status examination.

If the coarctation is slight, absence of the femoral pulses may be the only symptom. If the condition is severe, symptoms of congestive heart failure will be evident, namely, rapid breathing and tachycardia, together with feeding difficulties from the rapid breathing. This combination results from the increased pressure in the left side of the heart. A systolic murmur may be present. X-ray will reveal the enlarged left heart and the indented band of the aorta. Cardiac catheterization will be done to locate the constriction, and surgical correction may be undertaken at this point. If a child is asymptomatic, surgery may be delayed until the child is 4 to 5 years of age.

Pulmonary Stenosis

Pulmonary stenosis is a narrowing of the pulmonary artery or the pulmonary valve that prevents blood from leaving the right ventricle with ease. If the stenosis is sufficiently extensive, back pressure on the right side of the heart can lead to congestive heart failure. The murmur accompanying pulmonary stenosis is usually striking: a grade 4 or 5 rough ejection crescendo-decrescendo systolic murmur loudest at the upper left sternal border. Often a thrill is heard in the same location and in the suprasternal notch.

If the stenosis is severe, the increased pressure on the right side of the heart may reopen the foramen ovale (the fetal opening between the atria), and blood will flow from the right to the left chambers of the heart, perhaps producing a mild cyanosis. Infants with severe stenosis will have a repair (removal of the strictured portion of the artery or repair of the valve) in early infancy; others, with lesser degrees of stenosis, may wait until they are 4 to 5 years old.

Cyanotic Heart Disease

Cyanotic heart disease occurs when blood is being forced or shunted from the venous system to the arterial system; that is, unoxygenated blood is being forced into oxygenated blood (right-to-left shunt).

Tetralogy of Fallot

Tetralogy of Fallot involves four associated defects: pulmonary stenosis, a VSD, an overriding aorta, and right ventricular hypertrophy (Figure 46-17E). Because of the constriction of the pulmonary artery, very little blood enters it. Blood is forced instead across the VSD into the left ventricle. Because the aorta overrides or is abnormally positioned near the septum, blood (still unoxygenated) passes directly into the aorta and out to the body. The right ventricular hypertrophy occurs gradually as extra blood accumulates in the right ventricle because of obstruction in the pulmonary artery.

Although this is an extremely serious form of heart disease, passive newborns may not exhibit a high degree of cyanosis during a brief hospital stay. They shortly will begin to show a poor feeding pattern as they fatigue easily from the effort. Their growth rate will fall from both the poor nutritional intake and poor oxygenation to body cells. With exercise, cyanosis becomes very severe as a child is unable to provide enough oxygen to body cells. When this symptom occurs, the best measure is to trap a quantity of blood in the lower extremities, leaving the infant with less blood, but a supply that he can then manage to oxygenate adequately. Do this by turning an infant prone and pulling the knees underneath him (a knee-chest position). As children grow older, they learn to do this themselves by squatting.

If cyanosis and hypoxic episodes begin to occur frequently, a temporary (palliative) surgical repair may be done, in which a shunt is created between the aorta and the pulmonary artery (a patent ductus arteriosus), allowing blood to leave the aorta and enter the pulmonary artery, be oxygenated in the lungs, and return to the left side of the heart, the aorta, and out to the body (a Potts-Smith-Gibson or Blalock-Taussig procedure). If cyanosis is severe, an infant will have a full surgical repair done as initial surgery.

Transposition of the Great Vessels

With transposition of the great vessels, the aorta arises from the right ventricle, not from the left ventricle, and the pulmonary artery arises from the left ventricle, not from the right ventricle (Figure 46-17F). Blood enters the heart by the vena cava, passes to the right atrium, the right ventricle, and out the aorta to the body, completely bypassing oxygenation. On the left side of the heart, blood enters the left atrium and left ventricle and leaves by way of the pulmonary artery, arising abnormally from the left ventricle. Blood is oxygenated in the lungs, but returns to the left atrium and flows to the left ventricle and pulmonary artery again. This is a closed circulatory system that cannot oxygenate body tissues. Such a defect in its absolute form is incompatible with life. Fortunately, in most infants the ductus arteriosus and foramen ovale remain open and provide a circulatory "mix." A newborn may be administered a prostaglandin with vasodilatation properties to halt closure of the ductus arteriosus and maintain this pathway for blood. Transposition of the great vessels tends to occur in infants who are large for gestation age so these infants should be assessed carefully for cyanosis.

A well-functioning communication between the two blood circulating pathways must be created. This need is usually achieved by passing into the right atrium by cardiac catheterization a polyethylene catheter with an uninflated balloon attached to its end. The catheter is pushed through the leaves of the foramen ovale. The balloon is then inflated and pulled through the foramen ovale, creating an atrial septal defect. This introduction allows blood from the blind circulatory pathways to mix, and, although a child may remain very cyanotic, oxygen will be supplied to the body tissues. Correction of the defect is completed as soon as possible to avoid brain damage from inadequate oxygenation. As this involves total heart reconstruction, it may not be successful.

Hypoplastic Left Heart Syndrome

Hypoplastic left heart syndrome is a cardiac defect that any nurse caring for infants during the newborn time period should be aware of: Although rare, it is a common cause of heart failure in the first week of life. In this syndrome the left ventricle is nonfunctional, and there may be mitral or aortic valve atresia. The right ventricle hypertrophies because it must carry the entire heart load. Cyanosis becomes mild to moderate as the heart fails. The infant rarely lives to be over 2 weeks old; no repair is currently available. Heart transplant is difficult (though possible) in newborns because of the small chest area.

Congestive Heart Failure

Congestive heart failure can develop rapidly in a newborn with a heart anomaly. Tachypnea is often the first symptom. Respirations of more than 50 per minute in the mature infant and 60 in the low-birth-weight infant when the baby is at rest are above normal. In most newborn nurseries, an infant's temperature is taken every 4 hours for the first 24 hours, but respirations are not counted, so the presence of tachypnea may be missed. In these instances feeding difficulty in the infant, such as struggling to free the mouth from the nipple in order to breathe more efficiently, may be the first symptom noted.

Tachycardia follows quickly after tachypnea. Healthy newborns rarely have a heart rate of over

150 beats per minute when at rest. The infant with an insufficient heart output must maintain a more rapid rate to circulate blood.

All maternal-newborn nurses should be skilled enough in physical assessment to be able to palpate and percuss the edge of an infant liver. A normal newborn liver is often palpable 2 cm under the right intercostal margin. A liver palpable more than 3 cm should create suspicion of heart failure if it accompanies other symptoms; the liver enlarges because of back pressure on the portal system. By palpating the chest to determine the point of maximum intensity of the heart beat (the heart apex), or percussing the left side of the chest to reveal the left edge of the heart, one can detect an unusually enlarged heart.

Edema is a late symptom of congestive heart failure in a newborn. If edema is present, it is usually facial. An infant looks puffy, especially about the eyes.

Digoxin and oxygen administration are the mainstays of therapy for the newborn in heart failure. Infants receiving digoxin should be placed on a cardiac monitor to detect cardiac rhythms suggestive of digoxin intoxication (ventricular premature beats or tachycardia). Lasix (furosemide) may be administered to halt sodium retention by the kidney and allow for diuresis. Be conscientious in digoxin administration to ensure that the dose is accurate. As a rule, a dose is omitted if a newborn's heart rate (apical rate) is under 100 beats per minute. Many infants with congenital heart disease are discharged from the hospital with prescriptions for digoxin to be administered at home. The box on page 1106 lists instructions for parents so that they can be certain that they are administering this important drug safely.

Cardiac Catheterization

Cardiac catheterization is the passage of a catheter through a vein (usually the femoral) through the vena cava into the right atrium. The catheter can be further probed into the right ventricle and pulmonary artery or across the foramen ovale into the left side of the heart. Blood samples for oxygen saturation can be withdrawn. Pressures of the blood in different heart chambers can be recorded. If angiogram dye is flushed into the catheter, its path through the heart can be tracked by fluoroscopy and preserved by Polaroid film.

Prior to cardiac catheterization, be certain that no blood is drawn from the anticipated venous entrance site so that a hematoma or infection is not present at the site. Newborns are usually given a sedative so that they rest quietly during

Instructions for Home Administration of Digoxin

1. Always use the same measuring device for doses as different spoons or medicine droppers contain different amounts.
2. Do not change the dose without specific instructions from the primary care physician.
3. Always assess an apical pulse before administration; do not administer under 100 beats per minute (or as specifically instructed).
4. If a single dose is forgotten, give the next dose on time as prescribed.
5. If more than one dose is forgotten, telephone primary care provider for further instructions.
6. Give digoxin 1 hour before or 2 hours after feedings to avoid a dose lost with vomiting.
7. If a dose is vomited within 15 minutes after administration, repeat the dose. If more than 15 minutes has passed since administration, do not repeat.
8. Notify physician if a child vomits more than once a day as vomiting is a sign of digoxin toxicity.
9. Notify nurse if administration of medicine is difficult or timing of dose becomes inconvenient to day's life style.

Source

Modified from Jackson, P. (1979). Digoxin therapy at home: Keeping the child safe. *M.C.N., 4,* 105.

---

the procedure (which can sometimes take up to 2 hours). They can be offered glucose water during the procedure if restless from hunger.

Following cardiac catheterization, apical pulse as well as the pulse in the extremity distal to the catheter insertion site should be recorded every 15 minutes (a complication of cardiac catheterization is venous thrombus formation, occluding the vein and return circulation from the extremity). The catheter insertion site should also be assessed every 15 minutes for bleeding. The femoral vein is a major vein in newborns and if bleeding should occur, an infant can sustain a large blood loss quickly.

Cardiac Surgery

Cardiac surgery carries a risk at any age. It is particularly hazardous in the first few days of life because of the long exposure time required, which causes hypothermia and stress to a circulatory system that is barely adjusted to extrauterine life. An infant who requires surgery during the newborn period, however, is so compromised that the risk of no surgery being performed is greater than the risk of extensive surgery.

Following surgery, before an infant is removed from the operating room, a chest X-ray is taken and the baby is weighed. This is the X-ray and body weight against which future estimates of lung expansion and weight will be checked.

Taking accurate vital signs (about every 15 minutes) for the first 24 hours is a prime nursing responsibility in the immediate postoperative pe-

riod. An infant will have cardiac monitor leads attached to record heart rate and rhythm. Assisted ventilation may be necessary. Blood pressure will probably be electronically monitored by means of an intraarterial catheter, heart and respiratory rate by chest leads. Both a Swan-Ganz catheter into the pulmonary artery and a central venous pressure (CVP) catheter into the right atrium may be inserted to detect heart efficiency. Techniques of CVP reading are discussed in Chapter 39.

An infant needs to be placed in a warmed Isolette or under a radiant heat warmer so he does not become any further chilled and does not need to expend energy maintaining body heat. Be certain that a baby is not exposed to chilling unnecessarily for procedures such as blood drawing or intubation.

The dressing of the surgical incision (often midsternal) and the points of insertion of chest tubes (thoracotomy tubes) must be checked frequently for drainage. Because the chest cavity was entered, thoracotomy tubes must be inserted immediately following surgery to remove air and fluid from the chest to allow the lungs to inflate again. If two tubes are used, the anterior one will drain air, and the posterior one will drain fluid. Chest tubes are connected to underwater-seal drainage bottles (Figure 46-18). Air is kept from entering the chest because the distal end of the tube is immersed in sterile, distilled water about 1 inch (2.5 cm). If two bottles are used, a short tubing connects the first bottle to a second. The second bottle may be connected to a low suction

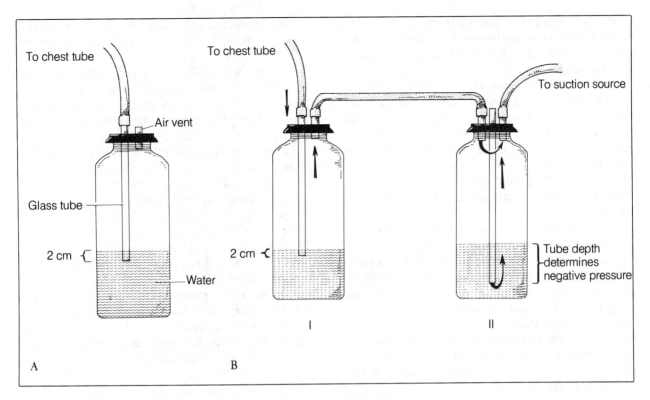

Figure 46-18 *Water-seal drainage. A. One-bottle water-seal drainage. B. Two-bottle water-seal drainage. Bottle I is the water-seal; bottle II is the suction control bottle. From Morrison, M. L. [Ed.],* Respiratory intensive care nursing. *Boston: Little, Brown, 1979.*

source. The amount of suction is controlled by the length of standpipe in the second bottle, which is immersed in water.

The bottles and tubing must be inspected closely when a child is first returned from surgery. The small amount of water that rises in the tubing should fluctuate as the infant inhales, exhales, or coughs. Note carefully whether such fluctuation is present. Absence of such movement in the tube implies that the tube is blocked. This problem might be caused by clot formation within the tube or a kink in the tube. On the third or fourth postoperative day, the fluctuation will cease, indicating that the lungs are fully expanded; then it is time for the tubes to be removed.

Clots may be removed from the tubes by "milking" them gently. If done hourly, this action prevents clot formation. Every time an infant is turned, check the position of the chest tubes to see that they have not become caught under the infant or kinked, causing an obstruction.

Mark the fluid level on the bottles when a child first returns from surgery. Record the amount of drainage from the tubes hourly. Drainage fluid is often blood-tinged but should not contain fresh blood; if it does, this may be an indication that hemorrhage from the heart incision is occurring.

If a tube should accidentally be pulled out of the chest, an infant will immediately develop symptoms of tachycardia, sudden dyspnea, and cyanosis from the resulting pneumothorax. If a connection has come loose and air is leaking slowly, the symptoms may be less dramatic (restlessness and tachypnea) from the gradually decreasing lung space. If a tube is leaking, place a clamp close to the infant's chest wall to seal the tube and prevent any further air from entering the chest. If the tube was pulled out, the chest incision must be closed immediately. This is best done by covering it with petrolatum gauze, which is impervious to air. If such gauze is not immediately available, placing your hand over the puncture wound and holding it there snugly in place until help arrives is the best emergency procedure. An infant may need emergency oxygen administration to counteract the decreased amount of air-exchange space available as a result of partial lung collapse.

Be extremely careful of the rate of flow of intravenous or total parenteral nutrition fluid given during the immediate postoperative period as a newly operated-on heart cannot stand the assault of overload from fluid given too rapidly. It is best if such fluid is administered by means of a mechanical pump so that accidental overloading cannot occur.

An infant's diapers are weighed following surgery so that urine output can be carefully recorded. Individual voidings are tested for specific gravity and pH. For assessment of cardiac and respiratory function, a child will have blood gases determined along with hemoglobin, hematocrit, clotting time, and electrolytes (particularly sodium and potassium) during the postoperative course.

Infants tend to have hypervolemia following cardiac surgery because of increased production of aldosterone by the adrenal gland and an increase in antidiuretic hormone secretion by the pituitary gland, as a response to the shock of such extreme surgery. If a heart-lung machine was used during surgery, some fluid may have been shifted from the intravascular system to the interstitial system during surgery; after surgery, this fluid returns by osmosis to the vessels, which is manifested by hypervolemia.

Infants cannot cough and deep breathe in order to keep respiratory secretions from pooling. Postural drainage must be begun in order to do this action for them by clapping (striking the chest with a cupped palm) or vibrating (placing the hand on the chest and vibrating it). Because an adult hand covers almost all of a newborn chest, clapping with a nipple or an infant resuscitation mask may be more effective. This is discussed in Chapter 47 because it is also used with other newborn illnesses.

The Newborn with a Pacemaker

Occasionally it is discovered during labor that a fetus has a persistent bradycardia (slow heart rate). Following delivery, the slow rate does not improve as the infant has a congenital heart block from ineffective sinoatrial node function (difficulty initiating a sufficient heart rate) or ineffective atrioventricular node function (difficulty transferring the heart impulse to the ventricles). An infant usually has accompanying dyspnea, lethargy, and perhaps cyanosis as a persistent bradycardia is not sufficient to supply his high metabolic needs.

These children are fitted with pacemakers in the first few hours of life. Initially an external pacemaker will be used; following full diagnosis, an internal pacemaker may be implanted. Infants are fitted with *demand pacemakers*, which are activated only when the heart does not beat on its own. It is reassuring to parents to know that the pacemaker is not going to compete with the heart's natural beat but will only act to supplement it.

Parents of a child with a pacemaker must be taught how to take the child's pulse accurately. It should be taken apically and for a full minute. They will need to do this at home daily and report any alterations to their physician.

Parents often worry that a child's pacemaker batteries will suddenly stop operating and therefore stay awake at night or worry on vacations. They can be assured that pacemaker batteries last a long time (5 to 10 years) and, when batteries do grow old, they lose power slowly, not abruptly. There is ample time for the battery weakness to be recognized and the pacemaker replaced before a child's heart fails.

Occasionally, pacemaker leads in the right ventricle may lie in such close proximity to the diaphragm in an infant that they stimulate the diaphragm to contract with each ventricular contraction. This association causes constant hiccoughing. If prolonged hiccoughing occurs, an infant should be seen by the physician. The leads may need a positional adjustment.

Pacemaker function is affected by electromagnets and microwaves. The parents must learn to screen the child's environment for possible problem areas (a microwave oven or a toy that uses an electric current).

Home Care of the Newborn with Heart Disease

The day a child with a heart defect is taken home from the hospital is difficult for most parents. They have many questions to which they need full answers before they can feel confident enough to take their baby home. They should have ample opportunity to handle and feed the baby in the hospital, so that they can feel secure in managing at home.

Parents generally ask, "Can we let the baby cry?" If a baby has tetralogy of Fallot or other heart defects in which cyanotic spells tend to develop, or if there is a severe aortic stenosis, the baby should not be allowed to cry for long periods of time. Crying for a few minutes while a bottle is prepared or a fresh diaper is folded will not harm the baby with a less severe heart defect.

"What do we feed him?" Babies with heart defects are usually fed normal newborn and infant diets. Only rarely is salt restricted. If it is the infant can be placed on a low sodium formula such as Similac PM 60/40 or SMA S-26. If salt is not restricted, breast-feeding is advantageous in that milk is always prepared so the infant does not have to wait for formula to be prepared; breast-feeding takes more energy, however, so an infant who tires readily may thrive better on formula.

"What are the chances any other children we have will be born with this kind of defect?" This is a question for a genetic counselor. Although congenital heart disease is not inherited, certain forms tend to be familial. Patent ductus arteriosus and atrial septal defect are two such forms.

Anomalies of the Respiratory Tract

Respiratory tract deviations can be immediately life-threatening. They demand prompt assessment so that interventions can be started quickly.

Choanal Atresia

Choanal atresia, or blockage of the posterior nares, may be unilateral or bilateral. It may be caused by a simple membrane or a hard bony process. Bilateral choanal atresia causes acute respiratory difficulty in newborns because they are invariably nose breathers. They may be a month old before they can coordinate opening the mouth to breathe if necessary.

Assessment

An infant may appear to breathe well in the immediate moments after birth while he is crying (with mouth open). The baby may become cyanotic and begin retracting after stopping crying and closing the mouth. He may become cyanotic during a feeding when forced to breathe through the nose. You may hear snoring noises as air is sucked through a partial obstruction. As nasal mucus cannot drain backward, an infant may have a clear nasal discharge. The diagnosis is confirmed by inability to pass a catheter through the infant's posterior nares.

If a mother received reserpine in the two days before delivery (used to lower blood pressure), her infant may be born with symptoms similar to choanal atresia: stuffy and distended mucous membrane, nasal discharge, retractions, and cyanosis. The baby may need an oral airway inserted to carry him through the first 5 days, until the effect of the drug is no longer apparent. Cysts and tumors of the nose, mouth, or pharynx may cause similar airway symptoms.

Analysis

The primary concern of an infant with a respiratory disorder is maintenance of respiratory function. Because these are frightening conditions, encouraging bonding is also a frequent nursing diagnosis. Be certain that goals are realistic in light of a child's condition and the parents' stage of grief and coping.

Implementations

An oral airway must be inserted and taped in place, if the atresia is bilateral and complete (a nipple with a cutoff tip may serve this purpose), until surgery to relieve the obstruction can be performed. The infant may need to be fed by gavage or orogastric tube (or kept NPO with intravenous therapy for immediate surgery).

Evaluation

Following surgery, the respiratory obstruction will be relieved with no further difficulty.

Pierre Robin Syndrome

Pierre Robin syndrome is a combination of micrognathia (abnormal smallness of the jaws), glossoptosis (a dropping backward of the tongue), and cleft palate. Apparently in utero, before the ninth week of development, hypoplasia of the mandible forces the developing tongue to press up against the palate, resulting in incomplete closure of the palate. Etiology is unknown except that some interference with fetal formation occurred early in pregnancy. It may be inherited by a polygenic pattern with variable levels of expression from mild to severe. Accompanying defects such as cardiac defects, central nervous system involvement, and glaucoma may be also present. Respiratory obstruction occurs because the prominent tongue obstructs the airway as it is pulled even further backward on inspiration.

Assessment

Respiratory distress is usually obvious at birth and resuscitation is difficult because of the occluded airway.

Analysis

Nursing diagnosis is usually relevant to the airway obstruction and interference with bonding due to a multiply handicapped infant.

Implementations

The respiratory difficulty may be temporarily relieved by placing the infant on the stomach, so that the tongue falls forward. Insertion of an airway to keep the tongue forward may be necessary. Some surgeons provide temporary airway relief by placing a suture in the anterior tongue and pulling it forward, free of the airway, by traction. The presence of a cleft palate and the abnormal tongue position creates secondary feeding problems because an infant may be unable to suck effectively. He may need to be fed by gavage, or a gastrostomy tube may be inserted for feedings.

Evaluation

The prognosis for an infant depends on the degree of involvement. As an infant's mandible grows in the coming months, the respiratory problem decreases as the tongue is able to fall into a normal position. The cleft palate can be repaired at 15 to 18 months of age. By early school age, assuming that no other anomalies are present, the mandible, tongue size, and respiratory function are essentially normal.

Congenital Stridor

Laryngeal stridor is marked by a characteristic "crowing" sound on inspiration. The cause of the stridor may be congenital laryngeal webs, cysts, or stenosis or laryngeal malacia (an immature or soft trachea).

Assessment

Listen to the sounds that infants make as they breathe (not always easy to do in a noisy nursery) to discover this problem. The exact diagnosis and plan for repair is determined by direct laryngoscopy.

Analysis

The usual nursing diagnosis established for an infant with congenital stridor is maintenance of respiratory function. Bonding is also important as this condition is very frightening for parents to cope with in a newborn (they are inexperienced and they are going to be asked to care for a child at home with signs of respiratory obstruction).

Implementations

Placing an infant prone often relieves stridor by allowing the soft wall of the trachea to fall forward and widen the trachea lumen. Suction the oropharynx as necessary to keep it clear of mucus. Congenital stridor will increase if an infant develops an upper respiratory infection. Screen health care givers and visitors to be certain they are free of infection. Unless the stridor is caused by a cyst or webbing that will be surgically removed, an infant is discharged after the mother has grown comfortable in care. Caution the parents that they must call their primary caregiver at the earliest sign of upper respiratory infection in the infant: associated inflammation could cause serious tracheal obstruction.

Evaluation

At the point that the trachea matures (about 6 months) and becomes sturdier, the problem fades.

Anomalies of Bone or Muscle

Orthopedic anomalies are usually detected on routine newborn physical assessment. It is important that they be identified at this time in order to be corrected before they interfere with locomotion or development.

Subluxated or Dislocated Hip (Hip Dysplasia)

Subluxated or dislocated hip is commonly referred to as *congenital hip*. It is a flattening of the acetabulum of the pelvis, which prevents the head of the femur from remaining in the acetabulum and rotating adequately. The acetabulum may be soft because ossification may be incomplete. In *subluxated* hip, the femur "rides up" because of the flat acetabulum; in *dislocated* hip, the femur rides so far up that it actually leaves the acetabulum (Figure 46-19). Why the defect occurs is unknown, but it may be from a polygenic inheritance pattern; it may occur from a uterine position that causes less-than-usual pressure of the femur head on the acetabulum.

The defect is found in females six times more frequently than in males, possibly because the hips are normally more flaring in females and possibly because the hormone relaxin causes the pelvic ligaments to be more relaxed, preventing effective pressing of the femur into the acetabulum. It is usually, but not always, unilateral involvement.

Assessment

Subluxated or dislocated hip is noticed on physical assessment, when the affected hip does not abduct. With a baby lying on his back, the leg will flex onto the abdomen but will then not abduct to lie almost flat against the mattress, as will the normal newborn leg (Figure 46-19D). An audible sound (a click) may be present as the femur slides to the top of the acetabulum. Other less important signs that may be present are unequal creases on the posterior thighs and abnormal heights of knees when the infant is laid supine and the knees and hips are flexed.

An X-ray may be ordered to document the extent of the acetabulum involvement as a baseline for correction. It is important that hip dysplasia

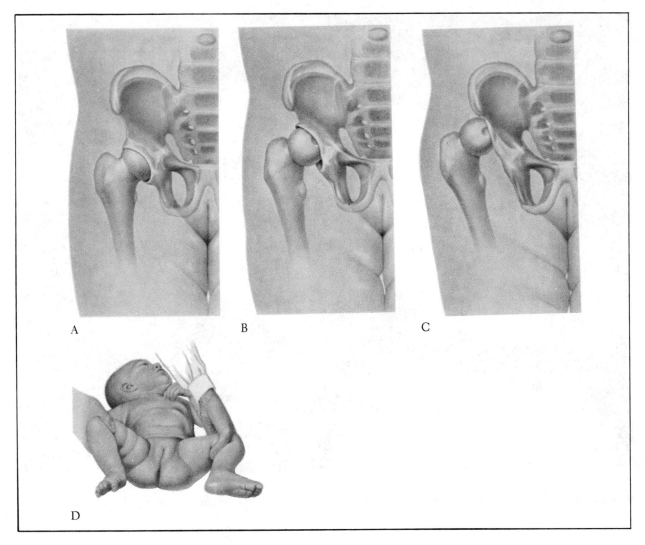

Figure 46-19 *Congenital hip anomalies. A. Normal hip. B. Subluxated hip. C. Dislocated hip. D. Limitation of abduction on affected side. (From Clinical Education Aid, No. 15, Ross Laboratories, Columbus, Ohio, 1965.)*

be detected in the newborn period because the longer it goes undetected, the more difficult it is to correct. If it is not detected by the time a child begins to ambulate, the child will walk with a "pull-toy" or rolling gait. Correction at that point may require surgery or an extremely long period of casting.

Detection of hip dysplasia is difficult in an infant who delivered from a footling breech presentation as the knees are stiff and do not flex readily.

Analysis

Nursing diagnoses related to congenital hip disorders are concerned with maintenance of correction of the defect and bonding. If splints or casts are used in the initial correction, an infant is difficult to carry or hold.

Implementations

Correction of subluxated and dislocated hip involves positioning the hip into a flexed abducted (externally rotated) position in order to press the femur head against the acetabulum and deepen its contour by the pressure. Either splints or casts may be used. Often splint correction is begun during a newborn's initial hospital stay. The easiest form of splint (to hold the legs in a frog-leg position) is use of not one, but two or three, diapers on an infant. The extra bulk of cloth between the child's legs effectively separates and spreads them. Another form of splint is made of plastic and buckles onto a child as a huge confining diaper (a Frejka splint) (Figure 46-20).

If the hip is dislocated or the subluxation is severe, an infant may be placed immediately in a "frog leg" cast or a cast to maintain the externally

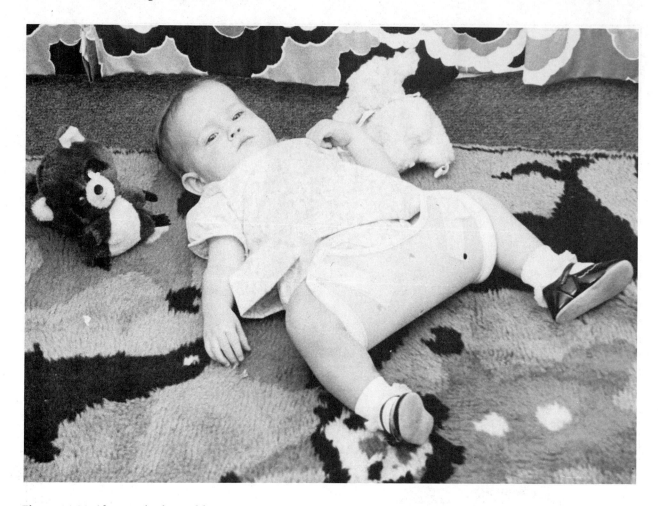

Figure 46-20 *Therapy for hip subluxation. A plastic (Frejka) splint for correction.*

rotated hip position. These casts (Figure 46-21) are very heavy and so wide that dressing an infant or containing him in an infant car seat or bassinette is difficult. A newborn is unable to report that a cast is causing circulatory constriction: Hourly assessment must be done for the first 24 hours the cast is in place and daily thereafter. The checks involved are listed in the box on page 1113. A mother must be taught to do them accurately before she takes the infant home to prevent circulatory compression from a rapidly growing limb outgrowing a cast.

Mothers should handle their infants enough before they are discharged from the hospital to be familiar with the equipment they will need to use. If only bulky diapers are called for, be certain a mother understands that, although this may not seem like an important measure (as might a more complicated splint or cast), it is important that she continue to use the extra diapers. Mothers are taught that swaddling babies tightly is comforting for the baby; be certain this mother understands that bringing the child's legs together with a tight swaddling blanket will not be good therapy. Some Native American mothers still use a swaddling board for their children. Be sure a mother does not straighten the legs to swaddle a child with a board.

Evaluation

Be sure that the parents have an appointment for follow-up care before discharge. A child will need further evaluation and cast and splint changes during the first year.

The Talipes Deformities

Talipes is a Latin word formed from the words *talus* and *pes*, meaning "foot" and "ankle." The talipes deformities are ankle-foot deformities, popularly called *clubfoot* (Figure 46-22). That term implies permanent crippling to many people and should not be used when discussing talipes deformities with parents. With good orthopedic correction techniques available today, correction should leave a child with no permanent deformity

Circulation and Neurologic Assessments for a Child in a Cast

Blanch a toe nail distal to the cast. It should blanch white and immediately fill within 5 seconds.

Assess for warmth of toes. Toes should be warm to touch.

Assess for normal color. Color should be normal skin tone.

Assess that cast is not indented and pressing on casted part.

Assess cast for areas of bleeding or drainage.

Assess for crying or restlessness that could denote pain.

---

of the foot. About 1 in every 1,000 live-born children has a talipes deformity; it occurs more often in males than in females. Probably inherited as a polygenic pattern, it usually occurs only as a unilateral problem.

Some newborns have a pseudotalipes deformity from intrauterine position. In these infants the foot can be brought into a good position by manipulation, in contrast to true defects, in which the foot cannot be properly aligned without surgical intervention. If you discover a pseudo situation on a newborn examination, be certain to demonstrate to the mother that the foot can easily be brought into line or is not deformed. Otherwise the first time she fits booties or shoes on the

infant, she will notice its difference and worry that the foot is misshapen. Such intrauterine varus positions need no therapy.

Assessment

The earlier a true deformity is recognized, the better is the correction. Make a habit of straightening all newborn feet to the midline as part of initial assessment to detect this defect.

Analysis

The usual nursing diagnoses associated with a talipes deformity concern maintenance of the correction and bonding. Parents are asked to care for a child in a cast, which is difficult for new parents. Goals of care are shown in the Nursing Care Highlight on page 1114.

Implementations

Most infants will have casts to above their knees applied during the newborn period for correction. The cast must be left exposed to the air

Figure 46-21 *Therapy for hip subluxation. A hip spica cast for correction.*

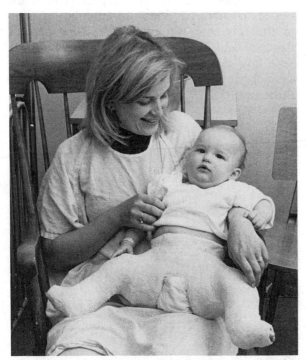

Figure 46-22 *Talipes equinovarus deformity. (From Clinical Education Aid, No. 15, Ross Laboratories, Columbus, Ohio, 1965.)*

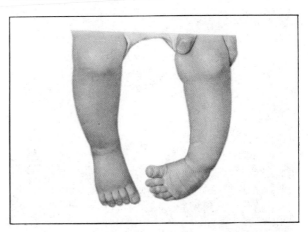

═══ *Nursing Care Highlight* ═══

The Child with a Talipes Defect

Goal	*Implementations*
Maintain circulation	Handle cast with open hand until dry to avoid indenting it.
	Perform hourly circulation and neurologic checks of foot of leg with cast for the first 24 hours.
	Assess for unexplained crying or restlessness that could be signs of pain.
	Smooth edges of cast with adhesive tape to prevent skin irritation.
Prevent hypothermia	Keep all of child but cast covered until cast dries as a wet cast can lower body temperature appreciably.
	Do not use a blower or other measure to dry cast that can cause it to dry unevenly.
Aid bonding	Encourage parents to care for child.
	Teach parents care of child at home.
	Teach possible long-term nature of disorder as child may need ankle exercises or special shoes for the next year.
Maintain cast integrity	Use plastic-covered, disposable diapers or rubber pants to keep urine from cast.
	No tub baths with cast in place.
Confirm continuing care	Make referral to community health agency as appropriate.
	Confirm that parents have appointments for continuing care as cast will need to be changed frequently (as often as every 2 weeks) because a newborn grows so rapidly.

until thoroughly dry; it must be handled gently, so that your hands do not make impressions that can result in pressure points and impaired circulation. A newborn must be changed frequently, so that a wet diaper does not touch the cast and cause it to become urine- or meconium-soaked (a mother should put plastic pants on the infant or use disposable, plastic-lined diapers). Check the toes of an infant frequently for circulation (press on the toes and watch whether they become blanched and then immediately pinken again). Note any restlessness or crying that might be signs of pain resulting from poor circulation due to the cast.

Figure 46-23 *Polydactyly. (Reproduced with permission of Mead Johnson & Company, Evansville, Ind.)*

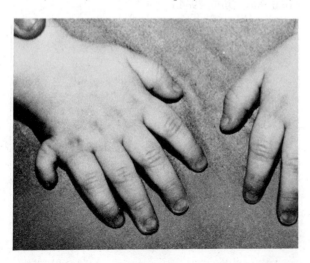

Figure 46-24 *Syndactyly, or webbing of the fingers, together with supernumerary digit. (Reproduced with permission of Mead Johnson & Company, Evansville, Ind.)*

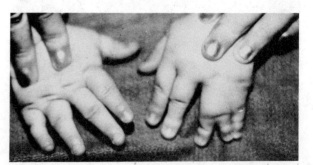

Evaluation

Be certain a mother handles the infant enough in the hospital to be comfortable being on her own. Be sure she understands that she must keep the cast dry. Be sure she has an appointment for follow-up care before discharge.

Polydactyly

Polydactyly is a developmental anomaly in which extra digits are present (Figure 46-23). Most of the additional digits do not include bone and so are removed simply by ligating them in the early months of life.

Syndactyly

Syndactyly is the presence of a webbing or joining of toes or fingers (Figure 46-24). The defect is usually corrected by surgical separation. Unless the bone is also fused, separate fingers usually can be constructed.

Utilizing Nursing Process

An infant born with a congenital anomaly is immediately at threat because of the compromise of function in some way. In order that nursing care will be adequate to meet his special needs, nursing process must be used as the basis for care.

Assessment

All infants need careful assessment at birth in order that congenital anomalies can be identified. A gross inspection should be done immediately after birth; as soon as the parents have had a chance to see and visit with the infant, the baby needs a detailed assessment. Techniques such as passing a catheter through the nares into the stomach and aspirating stomach contents, then passing the tube rectally rules out many anomalies. Measuring head circumference, counting respiratory rate, externally rotating hips, and observing an infant's feeding pattern are other important assessments to detect congenital anomalies.

Analysis

A nursing diagnosis is never a medical diagnosis so the congenital anomaly itself is never the nursing diagnosis. "Fear related to birth of a child with an anomaly," "Grief related to a child born with a diaphragmatic hernia"; or a "well" diagnosis of "Good adaptation to birth of a child with a congenital anomaly" are diagnoses frequently used. Be certain when setting goals related to an infant or the parents that they are realistic to the condition and the parents' ability to cope with the circumstance.

Unfortunately, not all outcomes will be perfect; some children will die or be left permanently impaired. Remember that a current philosophy of care of newborns is to maintain a positive outlook or present an explanation of, "Of course some infants have poor surgery outcomes, but we have every reason to believe that John's outcome will be good," not, "No one can readily predict surgery outcome until it happens." This approach prevents parents form beginning anticipatory grief for a child's death, or "turning off" bonding. Bonding that is interrupted in this way at birth may be difficult to "turn on" later if the infant does live.

Planning

A need of parents of a child with a congenital anomaly is to learn about the child's condition. A great deal of planning, therefore, needs to be done about the best means of fulfilling this need. Chapter 21 discusses teaching-learning principles. Because parents of a child born with a congenital anomaly are under great stress, they need content reduced to a level they can understand fully; they often need information "layered," or offered to them one step at a time so they can hear and accept it. Do not be afraid to draw illustrations of body parts or show parents photos of anatomy or surgical outcomes to help them understand their child's condition and what surgery can accomplish.

Implementations

Nursing care of neonates with congenital anomalies is important because preventing complications following surgical repair and educating parents to give care or understand a child's problem better can make the difference in the child being a productive citizen in the future. Important considerations include always doing procedures without chilling or tiring an infant. Remember that parents observe very carefully health care providers' actions toward their child. Your role modeling of parenting helps them to more quickly begin this role.

Allow parents to do those procedures that a child will need to have continued at home. If the procedure is a temporary one, such as a gavage feeding, the parents' time with the child is probably better spent in holding and comforting than in

Important Considerations for Neonatal Surgery

Consideration	Nursing Responsibility
Infant must be kept in a balanced fluid and electrolyte state.	Regulate any intravenous fluid infused exactly. Report any vomiting or diarrhea. Record intake and output hourly.
Blood loss must be kept to a minimum.	Account for and record the amount of blood withdrawn for testing. Check dressings frequently postoperatively for drainage.
Blood loss must be replaced milliliter for milliliter.	Conscientiously monitor blood transfusions. Warm any blood administered to room temperature to prevent chilling.
Infant must be kept from cold exposure.	Do not expose the infant unnecessarily during procedures. Cover head and extremities. Transport to surgery in a warmed Isolette. Advocate the use of radiant heat warmers during surgery. Following surgery, place infant in an Isolette for warmth.
A minimum of preoperative and operative analgesia and anesthesia must be used.	Calculate fractional dosages accurately. Sooth by rocking, holding.
Good lung aeration must be established postoperatively.	Provide postural drainage and percussion postsurgery as infant cannot cough. Reposition every 1–2 hours.
Parent's anxiety must be reduced as much as possible.	Prepare for child's appearance after surgery (tubes, IVs, etc.). Help to make contact with appropriate parents' group for support. Encourage questions; give explanations of procedures.

doing the procedure (learning to be a parent, not a technician). Advocate for breast-feeding unless it is strictly contraindicated by a child's condition. Expressing milk daily to bring to an infant is a very real contribution that parents can make toward their child's care and a method of increasing their interaction and chances for successful bonding with the child. Many children with a congenital anomaly have a surgical correction. Considerations for the newborn undergoing surgery are shown in the box above.

Evaluation

Evaluation of the goals of a child with a congenital anomaly are ongoing because some goals are long-range and cannot be evaluated until the child reaches adulthood. Be certain that psychosocial goals are evaluated as well as physical ones. Children who had full surgical repairs but who do not feel good about themselves, or have parents who do not feel good about them, have not achieved high-level wellness.

Nursing Care Planning

Bobby McFadden is a 1-day-old infant born with a cleft lip and cleft palate.

Problem Area. Nutrition.

Assessment

Unilateral cleft present in left upper lip extending through into floor of nose. Gingiva absent. Sucking reflex present but ineffective. Rooting reflex present. Midline cleft palate extending through soft and hard palate present. Uvula intact and midline.

Analysis

Potential for inadequate nutrition related to congenital cleft lip and palate.

Locus of Decision Making. Shared, parent and nurse.

Goal. Patient to ingest adequate amounts of breast milk daily to fulfill RDA requirements.

Criteria. Patient will not lose more than 10% of birth weight; skin turgor remains adequate.

Nursing Orders

1. Mother to express breast milk by pump q4h.
2. Teach mother to feed 1–2 oz mother's breast milk by sterile medicine glass q4h.
3. Teach mother to hold baby in arms; position baby in upright position for feeding to prevent aspiration through cleft palate.
4. Teach to bubble well following feeding as infant swallows excess air.
5. Cleanse cleft lip following feeding with clear water and cotton applicator. Cleanse cleft palate by a final swallow of clear water following breast milk feeding.
6. Use no pacifier (M.D. order).
7. Weigh daily; assess skin turgor q8h. Weigh diapers and measure output and specific gravity for each voiding.

Problem Area. Bonding.

Assessment

Mother originally asked for rooming-in; now has changed mind due to "fatigue." Tried feeding infant once but stated, "He doesn't like me to feed him. You do it." Father states, "He's too little for me to handle."

Analysis

Potential for inadequate bonding related to congenital anomaly in child.

Goal. Parent-child bonding to be evident by 1 week.

Criteria. Mother to hold infant for feedings; to look at him and speak to him. Father to demonstrate support of family unit.

Nursing Orders

1. Role model accepting care of infant.
2. Encourage parents to express feelings about child's condition.
3. Educate parents about surgery plans and prognosis.
4. Encourage parents to hold and feed infant by remaining close by for support.
5. Support child's positive attributes (pretty hair, long fingers, etc.)

On the third day of life, Bobby has surgery completed to repair the cleft lip. A nursing care plan made the first hour following surgery is shown below.

Problem Area. Nutrition.

Assessment

Twelve microsutures present in a Z-shaped incision; area nonreddened; dry; no crusting present. Logan bow in place.

Analysis

Potential for inadequate nutrition related to inability to suck.

Goal. Patient will ingest adequate nutrition during period of surgery healing.

Criteria. Patient to ingest a minimum 45 ml of breast milk or supplemental formula q4h.

Nursing Orders

1. Mother to continue to express breast milk q4h; remind to use sterile container.
2. Sucking contraindicated as force of motion would disrupt recent suture placement. Offer infant 2 oz of breast milk or 2 oz iron-fortified formula q4h by sterile glass.
3. Encourage mother to hold infant to feed; remind her to hold child upright to prevent aspiration through cleft palate.
4. Burp well following each ounce of feeding as he swallows excess air.
5. Weigh diapers and measure specific gravity of urine with each voiding.
6. Daily weight and chart.
7. Assess for skin turgor, mucous membrane moisture q8h.
8. Record intake and output.

Problem Area. Cosmetic results of surgical repair.

Assessment

Suture line is free of tension with Logan bar in place. All sutures intact. No erythema or crusting present.

Analysis

Potential for poor cosmetic appearance related to possibility of tension or infection of sutures.

Goal. Patient to have maximum healing and correction of cleft lip.

Criteria. Patient to have well-healed, nonscarred suture line by 2 weeks.

Nursing Orders

1. Logan bar to remain in place at all times. Check and secure appropriately following each feeding.
2. Following feeding, do suture line care: Swab line with cotton-tipped applicators dipped in ½ strength H_2O_2 and distilled H_2O. Rinse with cotton-tipped applicator and sterile distilled H_2O. Dry with dry cotton-tipped applicator.
3. No dressing on suture line. Leave exposed to air.
4. Assess qh for crusting and use suture line care to remove.
5. Keep infant restraint jacket in place.
6. Remove jacket q4h for passive ROM exercises of upper extremities. Ask for assistance to contain hands while jacket is removed.
7. Position on side or supine, never on abdomen to prevent rubbing suture line on mattress.
8. No pacifier to prevent sucking.
9. Keep from crying by anticipating needs.

Problem Area. Safety.

Assessment

Upper lip noticeably swollen. Respiratory rate 30 per minute. Some difficulty controlling oral mucus.

Analysis

Potential for aspiration related to edema from surgical repair.

Goal. Patient will develop no respiratory complication in postoperative period.

Criteria. Infant will not experience aspiration following surgical repair.

Nursing Orders

1. Observe for airway obstruction by assessing rate of respirations and general appearance.
2. Observe for bleeding at surgery site.
3. Maintain upright in infant chair or on side (never prone) until oral mucus is diminished.

Questions for Review

Multiple Choice

1. Baby Boy Ontkean is born with tracheoesophageal fistula. Which finding during pregnancy would have caused you to suspect this might be present?
   a. a difficult second stage of labor
   b. hydramnios
   c. bleeding at 32 weeks of pregnancy
   d. oligohydramnios

2. Tracheoesophageal fistula should be assessed for in all newborn infants. Which procedure below would be safest in order to detect this anomaly with a first feeding?
   a. offer a dilute commercial formula
   b. give 1 ounce of glucose water orally
   c. prevent the infant from using a pacifier after feeding
   d. allow the infant to breast-feed

3. Baby Boy Ontkean will be transported to a center for care. Before transport, which position would you maintain him in?
   a. on his right side
   b. prone
   c. semi-Fowler's
   d. on his left side

4. Baby Girl Dee's physician asks you to observe her carefully for signs of congenital heart disease. Which of the following is a common symptom?
   a. a voracious appetite
   b. yellow, sallow complexion
   c. bradycardia
   d. tachypnea

5. Baby Girl Dee is diagnosed as having transposition of the great vessels. Your best advice to give the parents regarding this condition is
   a. "This is a minor form of heart disease, easily repaired."
   b. "This is a defect for which there is no therapy."
   c. "The child may have a temporary palliative procedure done."
   d. "The child will not be cyanotic with this."

6. If Baby Girl Dee becomes extremely cyanotic and dyspneic, which position would be best to place her in?
   a. semi-Fowler's to cause descent of the diaphragm
   b. on her left side
   c. prone with her knees brought under her
   d. on her right side

7. Baby Riviera has a meconium ileus causing a bowel obstruction. Symptoms you would expect to see him begin to develop are
   a. regurgitation of all feedings.
   b. frequent, small, ribbon-like stools.
   c. a sunken abdomen from the empty intestine.
   d. no passage of meconium.

8. Baby Riviera's mother asks you why her physician wants to do a sweat test on her infant. Your most factual answer would be
   a. "All babies born with meconium ileus develop cystic fibrosis."
   b. "Cystic fibrosis will develop if bowel necrosis occurs."
   c. "Cystic fibrosis is caused by meconium ileus."

d. "Meconium ileus is a symptom of cystic fibrosis."

9. Baby Kristos is born with a myelomeningocele. The best position for her prior to surgery is
   a. semi-Fowler's in an infant chair.
   b. on her left side with head elevated.
   c. prone.
   d. on her right side.

10. An assessment you would expect to see ordered for Baby Kristos is
    a. level of consciousness q4h.
    b. paracervical reflex daily.
    c. measurement of urine output q8h.
    d. daily head circumference.

Discussion

1. Bobby Adams is a newborn who is going to have to have surgery. What are the specific risks of surgery in a child this age?

2. Helen is a newborn with a minor congenital anomaly of one hand. Her parents appear to be experiencing an intense grief reaction because of this. What measures could you take to help the parents at this difficult time in life?

3. Joel is an infant with myelomeningocele who will have an early ventriculoperitoneal shunt placed. What preoperative and postoperative nursing care would you plan for him?

Suggested Readings

Campbell, D. L. (1982). Congenital abdominal wall defects: Gastroschisis and omphalocele. *Neonatal Network, 1,* 18.

Carey, B. E. (1982). Prostaglandin E-1 treatment for neonatal heart defects. *Dimensions of Critical Care Nursing, 1,* 275.

Clarkson, J. D. (1982). Self-catheterization training of a child with myelomeningocele. *American Journal of Occupational Therapy, 36,* 95.

Cohen, S., et al. (1982). Newborn respiratory paralysis for severe respiratory distress: A nursing protocol. *Dimensions of Critical Care Nursing, 1,* 340.

Colten, J. M. (1984). A comprehensive nursing approach to the neonate with myelomeningocele. *Neonatal Network, 2,* 7.

Drane, J. F. (1984). The defective child: Ethical guidelines for painful dilemmas. *J.O.G.N. Nursing, 13,* 42.

Epstein, M. F. (1982). Neonatal and pediatric respiratory care: An update on research. *Respiratory Care, 27,* 295.

Foster, S. D. (1981). Tolazoline therapy in the hypoxic neonate. *M.C.N., 6,* 425.

Gottesfeld, I. B. (1979). The family of the child with congenital heart disease. *M.C.N., 4,* 101.

Harrell-Bean, H. A., et al. (1983). Neonatal ostomies. *J.O.G.N. Nursing, 12,* 69.

Hazle, N. (1981). An infant who survived gastroschisis. *M.C.N., 6,* 35.

Hibbard, B. M. (1982). Screening for neural tube defects. *Midwife Health Visitor and Community Nurse, 18,* 460.

Ho, E. (1983). Neural tube defects. *Nursing Mirror, 2,* 156.

Holland, S. H. (1983). Up to date home care of a baby in a hip spica cast. *Pediatric Nursing, 9,* 114.

Jackson, P. L. (1983). Peritoneal shunting for hydrocephalus. *Critical Care Update, 10,* 33.

Jeffries, J. S., et al. (1982). Behavioral management of fecal incontinence in a child with myelomeningocele. *Pediatric Nursing, 8,* 267.

Korones, S. B. (1981). *High-Risk Newborn Infants* (3rd Ed.). St. Louis: Mosby.

MacKenzie, J. (1983). Congenital and developmental problems. *Nursing (Oxford), 2,* 463.

Neal, W. A., & Morgan, M. F. (1981). Care of the critically ill neonate with heart disease. *Critical Care Quarterly, 4,* 47.

Norris, S., et al. (1982). Nursing procedures and alterations in transcutaneous oxygen tension in premature infants. *Nursing Research, 31,* 330.

Pearce, J. M. (1983). The use of ultrasound in the diagnosis of congenital anomalies. *Midwife Health Visitor and Community Nurse, 19,* 82.

Pinyerd, B. J. (1983). Siblings of children with myelomeningocele: Examining their perceptions. *Maternal Child Nursing Journal, 12,* 61.

Pressman, S. D. (1981). Myelomeningocele: A multidisciplinary problem. *Journal of Neurosurgical Nursing, 13,* 323.

Shaw, L. M. (1982). A teaching plan for cerebrospinal shunting . . . for hydrocephalus. *Association of Operating Room Nurses Journal, 35,* 893.

Slota, M. (1982). Pediatric cardiac catheterization: Complications and interventions. *Critical Care Nurse, 2,* 22.

Smith, K. M. (1979). Recognizing cardiac failure in neonates. *M.C.N., 4,* 98.

Vogel, M. (1979). When a pregnant woman is diabetic: Care of the newborn. *American Journal of Nursing, 79,* 458.

Wallis, M. (1982). Emergency surgery for the newborn. *Nursing Mirror, 155,* 22.

Weinberg, J. S. (1982). Human sexuality and spinal cord injury. *Nursing Clinics of North America, 17,* 407.

Williams, R. (1982). Congenital diaphragmatic hernia: A review. *Heart Lung, 11,* 532.

47

The Newborn Who Is Ill at Birth

OBJECTIVES

Following mastery of the contents of this chapter you should be able to

1. Describe common illnesses that occur in newborns.
2. Assess a newborn who is ill in the neonatal period.
3. List nursing diagnoses concerned with illness in newborns.
4. Establish plans for care, respecting priorities in order to be able to help a newborn stabilize body systems.
5. Describe implementations for the care of ill newborns.
6. Evaluate outcome criteria established for ill newborns.
7. Analyze measures to prevent illness in newborns and help newborns to recover from illness to a state of high-level wellness.
8. Synthesize knowledge of illness in newborns with nursing process to achieve quality maternal-newborn nursing care.

ALL HIGH-RISK INFANTS need skilled health care personnel in attendance during birth and the first few days of life, not only to save a life, but also to protect well-being and thereby prevent neurologic disorders and mental retardation. All women should be screened during pregnancy and again at a pregnancy's end for the factors that lead to high-risk infants (see Chapter 45).

Being able to predict that an infant will be high-risk makes it possible to arrange beforehand for adequate health care personnel to be present at the delivery. This ability is extremely important, because a high-risk infant may have difficulty establishing respirations and may need resuscitation at birth. All newborns should be closely observed at birth for initiation of normal respirations, and they should be carefully assessed all during the neonatal period until it is confirmed that they have no difficulty and are doing well. Not all instances of high risk can be predicted. It is not unusual to discover that an infant of a "perfect" pregnancy is born needing special care or develops a problem over the next few day's time that necessitates special interventions.

Priorities in First Days of Life

All infants have eight needs that take precedence over all others in the first few days of life: initiation and maintenance of respirations, establishment of extrauterine circulation, control of body temperature, intake of adequate nourishment, establishment of waste elimination, prevention of infection, establishment of an infant-parent relationship, and adequate stimulation for mental development. These are also the eight priority needs of high-risk infants, but with such infants the means to meet them may have to be modified for their particular problems. They may require special equipment or care measures.

Initiation and Maintenance of Respirations

The ultimate prognosis of an infant depends a great deal on how the first moments of life are managed. Most deaths in the first 48 hours after delivery are the result of an inability to establish or maintain adequate respirations. An infant who has difficulty accomplishing effective respiratory action in the first hours of life and yet survives may pay the penalty of residual brain damage. Extremely thorough care is necessary to make interventions during this time maximally effective: Little victory can be had in a race that ultimately ends in cerebral palsy, recurrent convulsions, or mental retardation.

Most infants are born with some degree of respiratory acidosis, but the spontaneous onset of respirations rapidly corrects it. If respiratory activity does not begin immediately, respiratory acidosis will increase. The blood pH and buffer base will fall, and newborn defense mechanisms are inadequate to reverse the process. Therefore, an effort to establish respirations must be begun in the first 2 minutes after birth; by 2 minutes, the development of severe acidosis is well under way.

Any infant who sustains some degree of asphyxia in utero such as could have occurred from cord compression, maternal anesthesia, placenta previa, or premature separation of the placenta will already be in serious threat from acidosis at birth and have difficulty before 2 minutes.

Resuscitation

Factors that make infants high-risk for requiring resuscitation are shown in Table 47-1. Resuscitation comprises three organized steps: establishment and maintenance of an airway, expansion of the lungs, and initiation and maintenance of effective ventilation that reduces the

Table 47-1 Factors that Make Infants High-Risk for Respiratory Difficulty in the First Few Days of Life

Low birth weight
Mothers with a history of diabetes
Premature rupture of membranes
Mothers with a history of reserpine use
Mothers who used barbiturates or narcotics close to
  delivery
Meconium staining
Irregularities detected by fetal heart monitor during
  labor
Cord prolapse
Lowered Apgar score (under 7)
Postmaturity
Small size for gestation age
Breech birth
Multiple birth
Chest, heart, or respiratory tract anomalies

PCO$_2$ and increases the PO$_2$. If respiratory depression becomes severe, the heart will fail and resuscitation must then also include cardiac massage.

In order that resuscitation can be undertaken effectively, every birthing and delivery room should have available the equipment listed in Table 47-2. In addition to this necessary equipment, adequate personnel separate from that needed to care for a mother must be available,

Table 47-2 Necessary Resuscitation Equipment at Birth

An oxygen supply and a source of suction separate
  from those needed for the mother
A warm blanket to dry the infant
A radiant heat table with thermocontrol on which
  procedures can be performed without cooling the infant (more efficient than an Isolette because the infant is more accessible)
A suction bulb and suction catheters (8F or 10F, attached to a DeLee mucus trap)
An infant laryngoscope with premature- and infant-
  sized blades
An infant endotracheal tube and pharyngeal airway
An infant and preterm bag and mask or resuscitator
Emergency drugs such as naloxone, sodium bicarbon-
  ate, calcium gluconate, epinephrine diluted
  1 : 10,000, glucose, salt-poor albumin, and isopro-
  terenol
A heart rate and respiratory monitor and leads
Equipment for intravenous administration of fluids
  and medicine for a neonate; plasmanate
Equipment for umbilical vein catheterization
A good light source

along with someone to perform blood gas analysis. It is important that this equipment be checked on a routine basis on each nursing shift and again immediately before any delivery. Check not only that equipment is present but is functioning by testing suction pressure and the light in the laryngoscope. Check that extra batteries and bulbs are available.

The First Breath

An infant takes a first breath because of a combination of a buildup of PCO$_2$ that stimulates the respiratory center and the shock of a change in temperature from the birth passageway (99°F, or 37.2°C) to outside air (68–72°F, or 20–22.2°C). The squeezing of chest muscles during vaginal delivery also causes a "recoil" action on chest muscles that causes inspiration.

The first breath requires a great deal of muscle strength as the infant must overcome the force of closed alveoli (or nearly closed, because they contain lung fluid). The required pressure is about 44 cm H$_2$O. Following this first breath, subsequent breaths require only 10 to 15 cm H$_2$O. If the first breath is successful, fetal cardiac shunts begin to close as the expansion of the lungs decreases the pulmonary vascular resistance. Increased pressure on the left side of the heart (systemic circulation pressure is increased with clamping of the cord) causes the closure of the foramen ovale; lower pressure in the pulmonary artery causes the ductus arteriosus to collapse.

If breathing is not effective, circulatory shunts (particularly the ductus arteriosus) fail to close. Because left side heart pressure is stronger than right side, blood circulates through a patent ductus arteriosus left to right or from the aorta to the pulmonary artery, creating ineffective pump action in the heart. Struggling to breathe and circulate blood, an infant uses available serum glucose quickly and so may become hypoglycemic, compounding the problem still further.

For all these reasons, resuscitation becomes an important implementation for an infant who fails to take a first breath or has difficulty maintaining adequate respiratory movements on his or her own.

Establishment of an Airway

Establishment of an airway is the first step in any resuscitation effort. Immediately after birth, all infants should be dried briskly but gently with a warm sterile blanket and placed on a radiant heat table on their side with their head slightly lowered (15 to 30 degrees Trendelenburg) to allow mucus to drain from the nose and throat. The 1-minute Apgar score serves as a useful guide to whether resuscitation will be necessary and if so, its extent.

The Infant with an Apgar Score of 7 to 10. An infant with a score of 7 to 10 rarely needs resuscitation. A score this high is possible only if respiratory and cardiac functions have been established. The most care needed is bulb syringe suction to establish a clear airway and prevent aspiration of mucus and amniotic fluid with the first breath (Figure 47-1).

BULB SYRINGE SUCTION. A bulb syringe is adequate for removing secretions from the mouth and nose of the average infant unless mucus is meconium-stained; meconium is too sticky to be pulled easily through a bulb syringe.

To suction, depress the bulb first, then insert it into an infant's mouth. Gradually release the compressed bulb to suction mucus. Always be sure to compress the syringe *before* inserting it; otherwise the compression of the syringe will push mucus further back into the infant's pharynx rather than remove it.

Newborns are nose breathers. Always suction the nose following removal of secretions from the mouth to ensure a clear airway, but always suction the mouth first. Stimulating the nose may cause an infant to breathe in the secretions in the mouth and posterior pharynx.

Suctioning by a bulb syringe is gentle, so there is little danger of causing trauma to tissue. Its disadvantage is in achieving only local mouth and

Figure 47-1 *A bulb syringe used for suctioning an infant's nose and mouth following birth.*

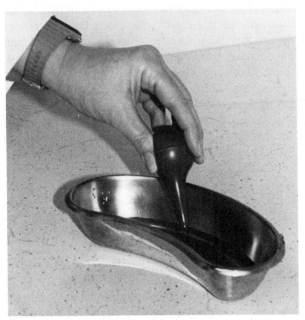

nose suction, not lower airway suction. It is often performed first after delivery of the head as well as after an infant is laid on a radiant warmer.

The Infant with an Apgar Score of 3 to 6. An infant with a score of 3 to 6 is moderately depressed. Such a baby generally has heart action but has not yet breathed; generalized cyanosis is present; and muscle tone and reflex irritability are poor.

Alert the physician or nurse-midwife to the low Apgar score; suction the infant's nose and mouth and rub the back (skin stimulation may initiate respirations). Be certain an infant is dry, including the hair and head. Evaporation of amniotic fluid will cause the body temperature to drop dramatically. The newborn's attempts to raise this again will increase his need for oxygen (which the baby cannot supply).

SUCTION. To clear the airway, secretions should be aspirated from the nose and mouth after delivery of the head, and again before any mechanical resuscitation measures are initiated— not only to allow air to enter the infant's lungs but to prevent aspiration of mucus or amniotic fluid at the first breath. Aspiration of the nose, mouth, and pharynx may alone initiate respirations.

NEGATIVE MOUTH SUCTION. For deeper suction than is possible by a bulb syringe, place an infant on his back, slide a folded towel or pad under the shoulders to raise them a small amount, and slightly extend the head. Slide a catheter (8F to 12F) over the infant's tongue to the back of the throat. Suck on the distal end of the catheter as if drinking fluid through a straw. Using a mucus trap such as a DeLee trap between the infant and yourself prevents mucus from being sucked into your mouth. It also allows for easy inspection of the fluid removed. There is little danger that suction will lead to tissue damage if you only use mouth suction.

MECHANICAL SUCTION. When introducing a suction catheter with a mechanical suction source, be certain that the power is off during insertion and turned on only during withdrawal (Figure 47-2). The catheter will not pass well with the suction source on as it tends to cling to the walls of the pharynx and can cause tissue damage from prolonged tissue tension. Do not suction for longer than 10 seconds at a time (count seconds as you suction) to avoid removing excessive air from an infant's lungs. Use a gentle touch. Bradycardia

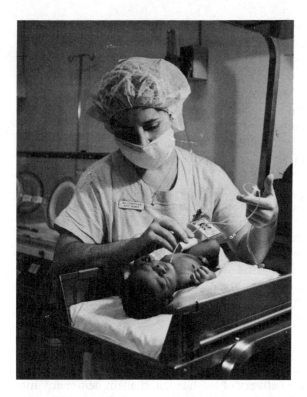

Figure 47-2 *Suctioning a newborn with mechanical suction controlled by a finger valve. Suction is applied as the catheter is withdrawn. If the catheter is rotated as it is withdrawn, the risk of traumatizing membrane is reduced. From Roberts, J. E. (1973). Suctioning the newborn.* American Journal of Nursing, 73, 63.

or cardiac arrhythmias can occur because of vagus stimulation from vigorous suctioning.

Be certain to keep the infant under a radiant heat source to prevent chilling during establishment of a clear airway. If you do not have an overhead radiant source for some reason, keep the baby wrapped as much as possible to conserve body heat.

The Infant with an Apgar Score of 0 to 2.

An infant with an Apgar score as low as 0 to 2 is severely depressed. Generally no respirations and no heartbeat (or a very slow one) can be found; the infant appears blue and limp.

These infants require immediate laryngoscopy so that their airway can be opened and deep-suctioned, an endotracheal tube can be inserted, and oxygen can be administered by a pressure source.

In the first few seconds of life, a severely depressed infant may take several weak gasps of air, then almost immediately stop. This period of halted respirations is termed *primary apnea*. Following a minute of two of apnea, the infant again tries to initiate respirations with a few strong

gasps. He cannot maintain this effort longer than 4 or 5 minutes, however; his respiratory effort will become weaker and weaker until he stops the gasping effort altogether. He then enters a period of *secondary apnea* (Klaus, 1979).

During the period of the first gasps or primary apnea, resuscitation attempts are generally successful. If an infant is allowed to enter the secondary apnea period, however, resuscitation measures are very difficult and may not be effective. It is important, therefore, that the person caring for the baby (often a nurse) recognizes the degree of the infant's distress and initiates or secures someone to initiate resuscitation measures before the last gasp occurs.

Be certain that an infant is kept warm so the newborn does not have to increase his metabolic rate. Cover the cord with a sterile, wet saline compress: With this degree of respiratory distress, the umbilical vein will probably be used as an intravenous route for medication. If the cord dries appreciably under the radiant heat, entering the cord becomes difficult because its veins sclerose.

LARYNGOSCOPE INSERTION. Someone (obstetrician, pediatrician, neonatologist, anesthesiologist, or nurse with extended skills) who is adept at passing infant endotracheal tubes should be present at the delivery of all identified high-risk infants. Laryngoscope insertion is easy in theory; in practice, the wide variation in the sizes of infants' posterior pharynx and trachea combined with the emergency conditions always present can make it very difficult.

A tube of the Cole type that widens 2 cm from the tip is preferred, since it prevents overinsertion. The size of the tube used varies from an 8F to a 12F, depending on the size of the infant. Because premature infants are prone to hemorrhage due to capillary fragility, extra gentleness must be used in passing an endotracheal tube with these high-risk infants.

For intubation, an infant should be placed on his back on a flat surface; a folded towel or pad is slipped under the shoulders to raise them slightly and hyperextend the neck (Figure 47-3). Open the mouth by pressing down on the lower jaw and slide the laryngoscope blade gently along the side of the tongue on the right side of the mouth. At the rear of the mouth, the blade is brought to the midline and the tongue pushed to the side so that it is depressed and does not obscure the view of the pharynx.

With the laryngoscope at the entrance to the pharynx, the epiglottis is generally easily visualized. It is a slit-like opening. Elevating the tip of the laryngoscope blade brings the vocal cords into

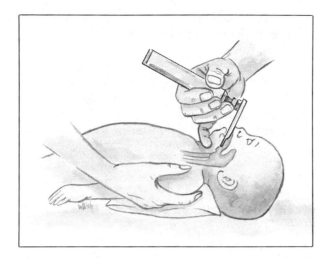

Figure 47-3 *Intubation. The head should be slightly hyperextended by a towel under the shoulders. The blade of the laryngoscope is inserted to reveal the vocal cords. An endotracheal tube for ventilation would then be passed into the trachea, past the laryngoscope.*

view. Any mucus or meconium present on the vocal cords is suctioned away with a catheter. An endotracheal tube is inserted through the laryngoscope down into the trachea about an inch beyond the vocal cords. The laryngoscope is removed; deeper suction may be done through the endotracheal tube.

If a laryngoscope does not pass readily, the difficulty is generally that the infant's neck is hyperextended too far. Reducing the neck extension generally allows the tube to pass freely. Once an endotracheal tube is in place, it is important that it is not dislodged. Even a small degree of slipping will allow it to enter one bronchi or the other and therefore reach either the left or right lung but not both.

Manually hold it securely in place. Secure a piece of eyetape to the space between the infant's upper lip and nose. Applying tincture of benzoin under the tape allows better adhesion and toughens skin to permit removal of the tape later without injuring delicate facial skin. Secure the tube immediately by adhesive tape to this protective eye tape. Mark with a magic marker the point of insertion on the tube so that any slippage is readily apparent.

Expansion of the Lungs

Once a clear airway has been established, an infant next needs the lungs expanded.

The Infant with an Apgar Score of 7 to 10.
The infant with a high Apgar score inflates his lungs adequately with the first breath. The sound of a baby crying is proof that lung expansion is good: Vocal sounds are produced by a free flow of air over the vocal cords.

The Infant with an Apgar Score of 3 to 6.
Following suction this infant may need oxygen by mask to initiate lung expansion. An infant mask should cover both the mouth and the nose to be effective. It should not cover the eyes, as it can cause eye injury by mechanical injury or drying of the cornea. If no respirations are present or the infant's heart rate is below 100, administer oxygen by face mask and pressure bag at a rate of about 40 compressions a minute. Oxygen up to 100 percent concentration can be used. To prevent cooling, oxygen should be administered both warmed (between 32–34°C, or 89.6–93.2°F) and humidified (between 60–80 percent) (Klaus, 1979).

Remember that the pressure needed to open lung alveoli for the first time is about 40 cm of water pressure. After that, pressures of 10 to 15 cm H_2O are generally adequate to reinflate alveoli. The pressure from bags of the MIE type (used by anesthesiologists) is controlled by the pressure of your hand; other types of bags such as the AMBU can be set with a "blowoff" valve so the pressure in the apparatus does not exceed a certain limit.

It is important that no pressure above what is necessary is used: The force may rupture lung alveoli. To be certain that oxygen is reaching the lungs, the chest should be auscultated simultaneously with the oxygen administration. In many infants this degree of resuscitation will initiate responsive respirations and a strong heartbeat. Color, muscle response, and reflexes will improve.

If an infant's amniotic fluid is meconium-stained, do not administer air or oxygen under pressure or you will push meconium down into the infant's airway and compromise respirations even further. Give oxygen by mask without pressure and wait for a laryngoscope to be passed and the trachea to be deep-suctioned before oxygen under pressure is given.

The Infant with an Apgar Score of 0 to 2.
This infant will need to have oxygen administered by an endotracheal tube following laryngoscope insertion. Whether oxygen is administered by mask or by endotracheal tube, initial lung pressure will need to be higher than continuing pressure in order to cause initial lung expansion. Pressure of oxygen over 44 cm H_2O should be used with extreme caution; an effort to open atelectatic areas by increased pressure may

rupture lung areas already fully expanded. On the other hand, if adequate insufflation is not achieved, an infant stands little chance of survival.

Listen with a stethoscope to both lungs as oxygen is administered to be certain that both sides are being aerated. If air can be heard on only one side, the endotracheal tube is probably at the bifurcation of the trachea and blocking one of the main stem bronchi. Drawing it back half a centimeter will usually free it and allow oxygen flow to both lungs.

When oxygen is given under pressure to a newborn, not only the lungs but also the stomach quickly fills with oxygen. Inserting an oral-gastric tube and leaving the distal end open will deflate the stomach and decrease the possibility that vomiting and aspiration of stomach contents will occur. You can pass this tube moments after an endotracheal tube is in place.

DRUG THERAPY. Stimulants have very little place in resuscitation unless an infant's respiratory depression appears to be related to the administration of a narcotic such as morphine, meperidine (Demerol), or anileridine (Leritine). In these instances, a narcotic antagonist such as naloxone (Narcan) injected into an umbilical vessel will relieve the depression.

MOUTH-TO-MOUTH RESUSCITATION. When you find yourself the only person at a birth to establish respirations and you are untrained in the use of an endotracheal tube or other resuscitation methods, mouth-to-mouth resuscitation is the wisest step.

Aspirate the mouth and pharynx of an infant with a bulb syringe to clear secretions. A clean piece of gauze may be placed over an infant's mouth (although it is questionable that this technique prevents spread of microorganisms). Place your mouth over the infant's mouth and nose and begin mouth breathing at a rate of about 40 breaths per minute. Use only the air in your mouth administered with short, sharp puffs. This small amount of air presents little danger of rupturing either the pulmonary alveoli or the stomach, which fills with air during resuscitation. Allow time for a child to exhale between each of your exhalations (by elastic recoil of the lungs). Note rising of the chest to determine the effectiveness of the mouth-to-mouth breathing. The chest wall should rise and fall if the lungs are being filled.

Slapping the soles of an infant's feet to initiate respirations may be tried. Procedures such as spanking, slapping the baby's back, tubbing, or squeezing the thorax do more harm than good and should not be attempted.

Maintenance of Effective Ventilation

In order to allow an infant to adjust to and maintain cardiovascular changes during the newborn period, effective ventilation (continued respirations) must be maintained. A healthy infant accomplishes this task on his own. The ill infant may need support.

The Infant with an Apgar Score of 7 to 10. This infant continues to breathe alone and therefore needs only careful watching for the first 24 hours of life with special emphasis on respiratory rate and assessment that the airway is free of mucus.

The Infant with a Low Apgar Score. All infants who have trouble breathing at birth should be carefully observed in the next few days to be certain that the problem does not continue.

Respiratory difficulty occurring after an initial establishment of respirations generally begins subtly. Picking up the first presenting signs is a nursing responsibility. Make a habit of counting a newborn's respiratory rate before you disturb the infant to begin to undress him. An increasing respiratory rate is often the first sign of obstruction or respiratory compromise. If the respiratory rate is increased, undress the baby's chest and look for retractions. Retractions are an inward sucking of the anterior chest wall on inspiration. They reflect the difficulty the infant is having in drawing in air (tugging so hard to inflate the lungs that the anterior chest muscles are pulled in, too). Retractions can be subcostal (below the last rib), intercostal (between ribs), or supracostal (above the ribs).

An infant who is retracting generally has an increased heart rate. If intervention to aid breathing is not begun at this point, cyanosis and an ever faster heart rate will occur. Cyanosis is first localized around the mouth (circumoral), then becomes facial, then total body. An infant will begin to have apneic episodes (pauses or cessation of breathing for over 15 seconds), irregular respirations, and flaring of the nares. Sounds of airway obstruction such as expiratory grunting or inspiratory stridor may be heard.

Auscultating the chest in most newborns reveals rhonchi (the loud harsh sound of mucus in the throat). If respiratory distress is present, the sound of rales (air being pulled through fluid in alveoli, a sound simulating the crinkle of cellophane) may be heard; diminished or absent breath sounds of atelectasis may be noted.

Infants who are having difficulty with breathing should have the weight of clothing removed from the chest. They generally appear to be in less distress if they are positioned on their backs with the head of the mattress elevated about 15 degrees to allow abdominal contents to fall away from the diaphragm and afford optimal breathing space.

Keeping the infant warm is important. The infant can then use his energy for respiratory effort, not for maintaining temperature. If secretions are accumulating in the respiratory tract, they should be suctioned. Bagging an infant for a minute prior to suction will improve the PO_2 level and prevent it from dropping to dangerous levels during suctioning. An infant may need glucose in order to prevent hypoglycemia resulting from activity and extreme respiratory effort. At the same time, infants with respiratory distress cannot suck well to obtain glucose because of their rapid breathing. Intravenous fluid may be necessary. Oxygen may have to be administered or ventilation begun. The cause of the respiratory distress must be determined and appropriate interventions such as oxygen administration, postural drainage, and apnea monitoring to correct the difficulty undertaken.

Oxygen Administration. Low levels of oxygen may be administered to infants in Isolettes by flooding the Isolette with a certain concentration of oxygen (Figure 47-4). This method is ineffective for supplying high levels of oxygen because when the portholes are opened to give the baby care a proportion of the concentration always escapes.

An oxygen hood (a plastic box with inlet connections that fits across the infant's head) allows for high concentrations of oxygen to be given yet provides easy access to the infant for other procedures (Figure 47-5). Using a hood inside an Isolette prevents large fluctuations of oxygen level when the Isolette is opened for care. Oxygen hoods tend to become very warm; the temperature of the hood needs to be checked every 30 to 60 minutes. The hood should be placed so that the stream of oxygen does not blow directly on an

Figure 47-4 *An Isolette used as a means of administering oxygen. (Courtesy of the Department of Medical Photography, Children's Hospital, Buffalo, N.Y.)*

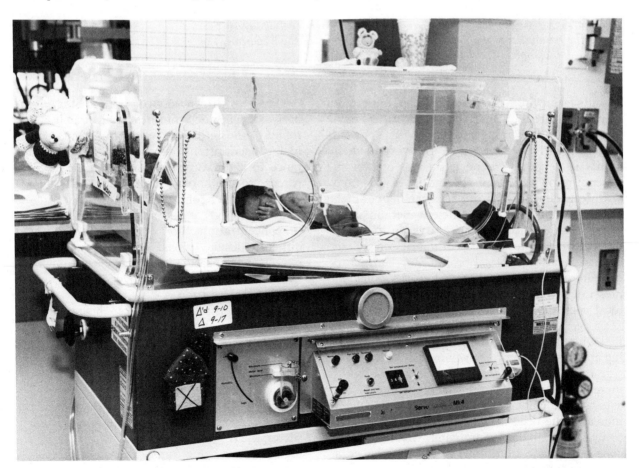

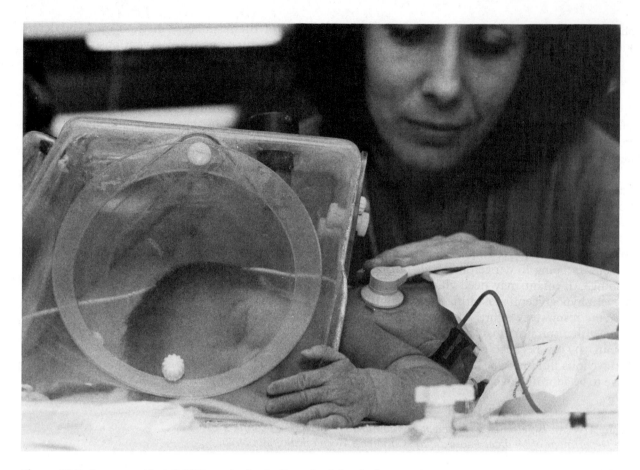

Figure 47-5 *An oxygen hood. This method supplies a high level of oxygen yet leaves the remainder of the infant's body free. (Courtesy of the Department of Medical Photography, Children's Hospital, Buffalo, N.Y.)*

infant's face, which can chill the baby. Important responsibilities for care of the infant with an oxygen hood are shown in Table 47-3.

Masks with free-flowing oxygen vary in their ability to deliver high concentrations of oxygen, depending on the fit of the mask. Masks used with resuscitation pressure bags can deliver high concentrations. The most efficient method of delivering high concentrations of oxygen to a neonate is with a pressure bag or ventilator and an endotracheal tube. Nasal prongs may be used to deliver oxygen to newborns, but the constant pressure of the prongs in the nares tends to cause local necrosis.

Oxygen must always be warmed and humidified when given to newborns. Cold oxygen blowing across the face of a newborn affects temperature receptors in the face and causes the baby to increase his metabolism (local cold is interpreted as systemic cold). This increase in metabolism increases the need for oxygen. Dry oxygen leads to drying of mucous membrane. Cracks in mucous membrane from extreme drying can be a source of infection.

OXYGEN CONCENTRATION. At one time, on the basis of occurrences of retrolental fibroplasia (atrophy of the retina) in immature infants due to high concentrations of oxygen, there was a reluctance to give oxygen in concentrations over 40 percent to newborns. An infant who needs oxygen in a greater concentration, however, in order to maintain PO₂ at normal limits, may receive it in concentrations up to 100 percent without difficulty (Klaus, 1979). Problems occur when the oxygen concentration is given in excess of what is needed or when high levels (over 60%) are needed for an extended time.

The concentration of oxygen being administered must be checked by an oxygen analyzer to be certain that it is as high as desired but not higher. Oxygen analyzers must be calibrated daily against a 100 percent concentration to make sure they are registering correctly.

Despite the concentration of oxygen in the hood or Isolette or being administered by a ventilator, the true test of how much oxygen is reaching alveoli or being transported across alveoli is the level of the arterial PO₂. Oxygen must not be

Table 47-3 Nursing Responsibilities and Interventions for Use of Oxygen Hood

Responsibility	Interventions
Maintain prescribed FIO$_2$ (Freely inspired oxygen concentration)	Know how to operate and calibrate oxygen analyzer Place sensor near infant's nose Analyze and document FIO$_2$ hourly Avoid fluctuations in oxygen concentration
Maintain patent airway and optimal position	When supine, slightly hyperextend neck with roll under neck and shoulders; place in prone position if umbilical artery catheter not in place Gently suction nasal passages and oropharynx as needed; aspirate stomach every 4 hours Do not restrict air exchange with nasogastric tube or phototherapy eye pads
Prevent drying of mucous membranes	Humidify (sterile water) all inspired gases Give oral care with glycerin swabs as needed
Prevent cold stress	Warm all inspired gases to infant's neutral thermal range Keep thermometer in hood at all times Maintain constant temperature in hood Note and document hood temperature with vital signs
Prevent CO$_2$ buildup in hood	Provide at least a 2 liter flow of gas through hood
Monitor clinical response to oxygen therapy	An arterial blood gas should be obtained at least every 4 hours, and 10 to 20 minutes after each change in FIO$_2$ Notify physician if PaO$_2$ > 80 or < 50 mm Hg; PCO$_2$ > 50 mm Hg; pH < 7.30 Monitor hourly: skin color, breath sounds, quality of respirations, and vital signs Alert physician to changes in clinical status

Source: Nugent, J. (1983). Acute respiratory care of the newborn. *J.O.G.N. Nursing, 12,* 31s.

given to newborns except in emergencies unless blood gas analysis is available.

In an emergency, if an infant is cyanotic, it is safe to administer oxygen to the point of decreasing cyanosis. Raise the oxygen level to the point at which cyanosis disappears; lower it at 10 percent intervals until cyanosis appears again. Raise it at 5 percent intervals until cyanosis disappears again. Administer it at that level. At the end of 15 minutes, repeat the process to test that the same level of oxygen is still needed. Arrangements must be made for transport to a center where blood gas analysis is available rather than relying on this assessment for any length of time.

BLOOD GASES. The normal PO$_2$ in a newborn is 50 to 80 mm Hg. Cyanosis does not become apparent until the PO$_2$ is 40 to 50 mm Hg (Klaus, 1979). With respiratory distress, when an infant is unable to ventilate the lungs, the PO$_2$ level will fall and the PCO$_2$ level will rise. Many newborns are unable to pull in enough oxygen, however, due to not-yet-inflated alveoli; thus, the PO$_2$ level falls but carbon dioxide is still eliminated from the lungs due to lung recoil. Thus the marked increase in PCO$_2$ occurring in adults will not be found in newborns.

As an immediate response to hypoxia (low PO$_2$ levels), blood vessels to nonessential organs become constricted to save oxygen for essential organs. In a newborn, a low level of circulating oxygen can cause reopening of the ductus arteriosus through a simulation of uterine conditions. An infant begins shunting blood, creating an ineffective circulatory pattern or adding to the already compromised breathing efforts.

As the hypoxia increases, oxygenation of body cells fails and anaerobic metabolism begins. This complication involves formation of lactic acid as an end product rather than of the carbon dioxide and water normally produced and leads to a metabolic acidosis. Free fatty acids in the bloodstream compete with indirect bilirubin for binding sites on albumin molecules and increase the amount of indirect bilirubin in the bloodstream. High levels of indirect bilirubin can cause brain damage due to kernicterus. Anaerobic metabolism uses larger-than-usual amounts of glucose. If an infant is not receiving a glucose supplement, he quickly depletes glycogen stores and becomes hypoglycemic.

Table 47-4 Blood Gases

Determination	Normal Value	Assessment
Oxygen saturation	96–98%	The proportion of hemoglobin that is filled and carrying oxygen. If oxygen cannot reach the bloodstream to unite with hemoglobin, saturation level will be low.
PO_2	60–80 mm Hg	The partial pressure of oxygen in arterial blood. Values under normal denote hypoxia; values above normal are dangerous to the neonate in that they can cause lung and eye damage.
PCO_2	35–45 mm Hg	The partial pressure of carbon dioxide in the arterial blood. Levels under normal denote respiratory alkalosis; levels above normal denote respiratory acidosis.
pH	7.35–7.45	The acidity of the blood or the proportion of hydrogen ions present. A level under 7.25 is clinical acidosis; infants cannot live for a long period with extreme acidosis. Acidosis can be caused by poor excretion of carbon dioxide leading to excess carbonic acid in the blood (respiratory acidosis) or the excess production of nonvolatile acids from metabolism (metabolic acidosis). Alkalosis can occur from vomiting or removal of stomach contents before gavage feedings.
Base excess	+2 or −2	The amount of bicarbonate in arterial blood. Bicarbonate buffers or counteracts acids. Low base excess levels suggest that an infant has used reserve buffering potential and is in acute danger of acidosis.

To counteract metabolic acidosis (caused by the formation of lactic acid), infants attempt to use their buffering system or increase the amount of bicarbonate in the bloodstream. Over a very short time, newborns exhaust their ability to do this. To counteract the respiratory acidosis occurring (the accumulation of PCO_2), an infant must be ventilated.

Babies who are being ventilated need frequent blood gas measurements for both PO_2 and PCO_2 levels plus pH, base excess, and oxygen saturation levels. If ventilation is too rapid, too much carbon dioxide is removed and the PCO_2 level will be low; the PO_2 may be increased too much and oxygen toxicity can occur. Remember that it is not true that in relieving distress, if a little oxygen is good for an infant, a lot will be even better. Normal blood gas values are shown in Table 47-4.

Blood gas measurements must be made from arterial blood. In many instances in newborns, the blood is obtained from the umbilical artery by catheterization. If a syringe with a dilute heparin solution is attached to the catheter to keep the tubing patent, blood can be withdrawn from the site at frequent intervals without reinsertion of a catheter. Sterile technique must be used when irrigating umbilical vessels or withdrawing blood samples from this site; the umbilical artery enters a major infant vessel (the aorta), and septicemia will easily result if pathogens are introduced at this point. Brachial, radial, or temporal arteries may be used for blood gas determinations. A heelprick may be used. This method is accurate for PCO_2 and pH values; it is questionable for PO_2 values. The heel should be warmed prior to the prick by application of a warm, moist pack, which dilates heel capillaries and brings arterial blood into them.

In a baby with a patent ductus arteriosus, blood drawn from an artery proximal to the shunt, such as the right radial artery, offers better evaluation of the oxygen reaching the brain and eyes than does blood drawn from the umbilical artery. This is an important determination because the eye is one organ that excessive oxygen levels can destroy.

Blood gas determinations should be taken about 15 to 30 minutes after any change in amount of oxygen being administered or rate or depth of ventilator settings so that the true condition of the infant following the adjustment can be determined. Blood gas specimens should be placed in ice for transport to the laboratory for analysis. If blood remains at room temperature, the pH level will fall, the PCO_2 will rise, and the accuracy of the sample will be lost.

A new method of obtaining oxygen levels is by use of transcutaneous electrodes. The PO_2 level obtained by this method correlates well with that obtained by drawing arterial blood, and this method has the added advantages of being noninvasive and of removing no blood from the infant. One problem with ill neonates is that so much blood is drawn for frequent laboratory determinations that they develop a blood loss anemia to add to their already disease-stressed state.

TRANSCUTANEOUS OXYGEN MONITORING. For transcutaneous oxygen monitoring ($TcPO_2$), an electrode heated to 44°C is attached to the infant's chest, abdomen, or back (or any surface area large enough to allow an airtight seal). The purpose of the heat is to cause vasodilation underneath the electrode, which brings peripheral arterial blood to the surface under the electrode and allows it to be read for oxygen content. Occasionally the heat of the electrode may cause a skin blister, but this side effect can be prevented if the electrode site is changed every 2 hours.

In addition to efforts to prevent skin complications, an electrode must be removed, recalibrated, and reapplied every 3 to 6 hours in order for accuracy to be maintained. Such electrodes always leave a temporary erythematous area on the skin under the site of attachment. Do not interpret this mark as an injury but rather as evidence that the seal of the electrode was tight and accurate.

$TcPO_2$ correlates well with intraarterial PO_2 unless an infant is extremely acidotic, anemic, or has hypothermia. It has the advantage of being noninvasive and prevents blood loss from frequent sampling. When an arterial blood gas is drawn, note the $TcPO_2$ reading and record it so that the accuracy of the reading can be documented (or inaccuracy determined).

Having a continuous readout of PO_2 values allows you to modify your care appropriately. If an oxygen level begins to fall while you are handling a baby, for example, you would immediately stop care until the infant's PO_2 again returns to normal. Transcutaneous electrodes can be helpful in identifying whether a patent ductus arteriosus exists. If one electrode is placed in a preductal site (the baby's upper right chest) and one on a postductal site (below the chest nipple line), a comparison of the two values will reveal different levels of oxygen (the preductal electrode reading will be higher) if a patent ductus arteriosus is present. An interesting finding that transcutaneous monitoring of oxygen has revealed is that infants seem to oxygenate their bodies better and more efficiently when they are gently stroked or "mothered." Use transcutaneous monitors to show parents how their infant improves with mothering actions in order to encourage bonding.

CONTINUOUS POSITIVE AIRWAY PRESSURE. Continuous positive airway pressure (CPAP) is a method of ventilatory assistance initiated by endotracheal tube, nasopharyngeal tube, face mask, hood chamber, or nasal prongs that causes an infant to continuously breathe out against pressure. It increases residual capacity and oxygenation, while decreasing CO_2 levels and the work of breathing by ensuring that lung alveoli do not collapse on expiration—a common problem with a newborn illness such as respiratory distress syndrome. Once alveoli collapse, an opening pressure three times that normally required must be used with each breath to continue respirations (each breath is like a first breath). CPAP, then, reduces the effort a child must make to breathe and allows for easy entry of oxygen to alveoli. If nasal prongs are used, the nares must be inspected frequently for areas of pressure that could lead to tissue breakdown.

CPAP is usually begun if an infant has a PO_2 under 50 mm Hg while breathing 60 percent oxygen. It is begun with a low pressure of 4 to 6 cm H_2O and then increased by 2-cm increments until adequate oxygenation is achieved. An infant is usually not removed suddenly from CPAP but gradually weaned by 2-cm decrements in pressure. Cardiac output can be stressed during therapy due to the increased pressure in thoracic veins and reduced venous return to the heart. Nursing responsibilities with CPAP are shown in Table 47-5.

MECHANICAL VENTILATION. Mechanical ventilation is used if CPAP fails and an infant's PO_2 falls below 50 mm Hg in 100 percent oxygen at a pressure of 10 to 12 cm H_2O. Other indications are a pH below 7.25 or PCO_2 above 60 mm Hg in 60 percent oxygen. When an infant is placed on a ventilator, be certain that high and low pressure alarms, high and low oxygen alarms, apnea, heart rate, blood pressure, and power disconnect controls are set for safety.

Oxygen equipment of this level is often held in place by a head cradle that both immobilizes an infant and cushions the infant's head while it supports the tubing for a ventilator off the infant's face. Lambswool padding prevents decubiti on the back of an infant's head and cushions the sound level at the ears. Explain to parents why a cradle which makes the equipment seem bigger than the infant is being used. Table 47-6 summarizes nursing responsibilities with an infant on a ventilator.

POSITIVE END-EXPIRATORY PRESSURE. Positive end-expiratory pressure (PEEP) can be added to ventilatory assistance to accomplish the same

Table 47-5 Nursing Responsibilities and Intervention for Use of Constant Positive Airway Pressure

Responsibility	Intervention
Maintain prescribed constant positive airway pressure	Check manometer readings frequently Document distending pressure on flow sheet Adjust pressure when infant is quiet Be alert for leaks or loose connections Maintain nasal prongs securely and properly angled in nares
Maintain prescribed FIO_2	Monitor in-line oxygen concentrations hourly Document FIO_2 on flow sheet
Maintain adequate humidity	Constant positive airway pressure tubing should be fogged evenly with humidity Avoid excessive humidity, which causes pooling and increases danger of near-drowning
Maintain adequate temperature of inspired gases	Maintain in-line thermometer in system close to infant In-line temperature should be 1 to 2 degrees below body temperature Check and document temperature with vital signs
Prevent airway obstruction	Suction endotracheal tube, nares, and oral pharynx as needed Clean nasal prongs every 2 hours
Be alert for signs of pneumothorax	Auscultate and document quality of breath sounds hourly Pneumothorax is evidenced by decreased breath sounds and chest movement, shift in point of maximal impulse, bradycardia, cyanosis, and decreased pulse pressure Action: ventilate with 100% oxygen, alert physician, call for stat chest X-ray, prepare for needle aspiration and/or chest tube placement
Prevent abdominal distention	Insert orogastric tube, leave open to atmospheric pressure Periodically use syringe to decompress stomach
Prevent skin breakdown	Secure prongs or endotracheal tube to prevent excessive movement or displacement Keep skin dry and clean Support constant positive airway pressure tubing to prevent excessive pressure points Turn infant every 2 hours Use of water bed may be indicated
Maintain good oral hygiene	Assess nares and mouth frequently for irritation; apply antibiotic ointment if indicated Apply glycerine to prevent cracking or drying of mouth
Monitor clinical response to constant positive airway pressure	Obtain arterial blood gas at least every 4 hours and 10 to 20 min past change in pressure or FIO_2 Be alert for hypercapnea ($PCO_2 > 50$ mm Hg), hypoxia ($PO_2 < 50$ mm Hg), and acidosis (pH < 7.30) Monitor temperature, pulse, respiration, and blood pressure every 1 to 2 hours Observe closely: skin color, quality of respirations, and peripheral perfusion

Source: Nugent, J. (1983). Acute respiratory care of the newborn. *J.O.G.N. Nursing, 12,* 31s.

Table 47-6 Nursing Responsibilities and Interventions for Use of Ventilator

Responsibility	Intervention
Maintain patent airway Alert to extubation	Clinically evidenced by audible crying, distinct ventilator sounds auscultated in stomach, decreased breath sounds, and sudden deterioration in color and heart rate Action: remove tube, ventilate with bag and mask, place orogastric tube to decompress stomach, set up for reintubation
Provide CPT* regimen	Follow prescribed technique for percussion, vibration, and suctioning; frequency dictated by individual assessment

Table 47-6 (continued)

Responsibility	Intervention
Maintain prescribed ventilator parameters (PIP,† PEEP,‡ FIO₂**, rate, I:E ratio§)	Have working knowledge of ventilator Check and record ventilator parameters hourly Properly humidify inspired gases Keep in-line temperature of gases 97°F (36°C)
Assess infant's response to mechanical ventilation	
Arterial blood gases	Obtain blood gas 10 to 20 min postparameter change Subsequent gases should be obtained at least every 4 hours Use blood gas data to assess ventilation (PCO_2), oxygenation (PO_2), acid-base balance (pH, HCO_3), and response to therapy Follow serially to detect deterioration, i.e., acidosis, hypoxia, hypercapnea
Clinical	Auscultate breath sounds hourly to assess: quality of ventilation, adequate placement of endotracheal tube or occurrence of pneumothorax Assess vital signs: temperature, pulse, respirations, and blood pressure hourly Observe closely for deterioration in color, heart rate, blood pressure, activity, and tone Document findings on flow sheet
Detect malfunctioning equipment	
Preventive measures	Check ventilator parameters frequently Maintain alarms ON at all times Check all connections hourly to make sure they are snug Respond promptly to sounding of alarm
Occurrence of malfunction	Evidenced by sounding of alarm, sudden change in ventilator parameters, and sudden deterioration of infant Action: remove infant from ventilator, ventilate with bag, and get assistance in locating problem
Safe administration of muscle relaxants	Know dosage, side effects, antidotes Maintain all alarm systems ON Close observation is imperative Assess respiratory paralysis after each administration of drug; note duration of effect and any changes in cardiorespiratory systems Maintain good alignment of body parts Credé bladder every 2 hours as needed Assess need for continuation of neuromuscular block prior to each dose
Prevent decubiti formation	Evidenced by inflammation or skin breakdown Keep skin clean, dry and free from pressure points Turn infant every 1 to 2 hours Use water bed if pressure points occur Secure endotracheal tube to prevent excessive movement
Maintain good oral hygiene	Assess nares and mouth frequently for irritation; apply antibiotic ointment if indicated. Apply glycerine to prevent cracking or drying of mouth.
Prevent gastrointestinal insufflation	Insert orogastric tube Aspirate with a syringe to decompress stomach every 2 hours

* CPT—Chest physiotherapy.
** FIO₂—Freely inspired oxygen concentration.
† PIP—Peak inspiratory pressure.
‡ PEEP—Positive end-expiratory pressure.
§ I:E ratio—Inspiration/expiration ratio.

Source: Nugent, J. (1983). Acute respiratory care of the newborn. *J.O.G.N Nursing, 12,* 31s.

Table 47-7 Common Positions for Postural Drainage

Lung Area	Patient Position	Area To Be Clapped and Vibrated
Upper lobes		
Apical segment	Sit upright, leaning forward slightly	Upper back and shoulders above shoulder blades
Right posterior segment	Sims' position on left side, bed flat	Area surrounding right scapula
Left posterior segment	Bed flat, Sims' position on right side	Area surrounding left scapula
Anterior portion	Bed flat, supine position	Upper anterior chest below clavicle
Lingula (middle segment of left lung)	Raise foot of bed 15–30 degrees. Position infant turned partially to back and partially to right side.	Left lateral chest at nipple line
Middle lobe of right lung	Raise foot of bed 15–30 degrees. Position infant turned partially to back and partially to the left side.	Right lateral chest at nipple line
Lower lobes		
Superior segments	Bed flat; supine position	Area over lower third of anterior rib cage
Posterior segments	Raise foot of bed 30 degrees; prone position	Lower third of posterior rib cage
Anterior segments	Raise foot of bed 30 degrees; supine position	Lower anterior ribs
Left lateral segment	Raise foot of bed 30 degrees; right side position	Lower third of left lateral rib cage
Right lateral segment	Raise foot of bed 30 degrees; left side position	Lower third of right lateral rib cage

goals as with CPAP. It adds pressure at the end of the expiratory phase rather than continuously to prevent alveoli from collapsing, allowing better oxygen entry with the next inspiration and less breathing effort.

Postural Drainage. Postural drainage is the use of gravity to drain secretions from bronchi. Even newborns have a cough reflex, but, since they do not use it effectively, most infants with respiratory difficulty need some outside intervention such as postural drainage to help them clear their respiratory tract of secretions and raise sputum.

Changing infants from side to side every 1 or 2 hours aids in preventing stasis of fluid. Tilting them so that the chest is lower than the abdomen aids in the drainage of secretions. There is a risk in placing infants who are prone to intracranial hemorrhage in this position as it increases blood pressure in the head and may lead to bleeding.

Specific positions for draining lung lobes are shown in Table 47-7.

CUPPING AND VIBRATING. Cupping is manual percussion of lung areas to loosen secretions (Figure 47-6). It is done with the hand held in a "cupped," or dome-shaped, position or with a cupping device such as a nipple or resuscitation mask (which better localizes the action). When the chest is struck with the hand in this position, it produces a hollow, echoing sound. Vibration is simply what it implies: placing the hand on the skin surface and vibrating it. The combination of these two measures, done for 30 to 60 seconds over a lung area, loosens secretions. Suctioning an infant after the procedure will remove loosened secretions.

Although cupping and vibrating sounds forceful, it is not painful. Parents need to understand this concept or they will be reluctant to have the

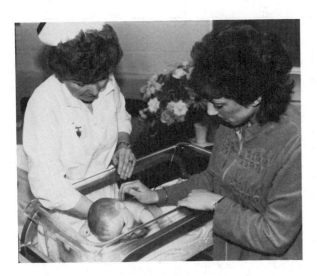

Figure 47-6 *Using a teaching doll, a new mother is shown a clapping technique of postural drainage she will need to use with her newborn infant.*

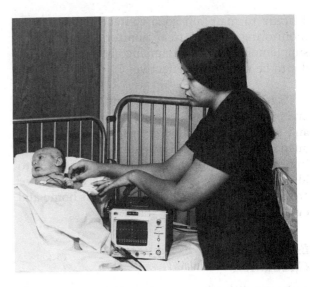

Figure 47-7 *Placement of respiratory monitor leads to detect sudden cessation of respirations. (Courtesy of the Department of Medical Photography, Children's Hospital, Buffalo, N.Y.)*

technique used with their child. Demonstrating it on a parent is the easiest way to show that it is not painful.

Postural drainage and cupping may be tasks assumed by respiratory therapists or by nurses. Such techniques for drainage should not be used after feedings as they may lead to regurgitation and aspiration.

Ventilation Assessment. In addition to direct observation of respiratory rate, a number of mechanical devices may be used to assess ventilation.

APNEA MATTRESS MONITORS. Apnea is a halt in respirations of at least 20 seconds. An apnea mattress is a pressure-sensitive pad that, when placed under an infant, registers any halt in the infant's respirations by means of a connection to a display box. The device can be set to respond by an alarm to breath delays of 10, 15, or 20 seconds.

Apnea mattresses have many advantages for the neonate because they involve no attachment of monitor leads to cause possible skin irritation. A disadvantage is that a mattress may continue to record breathing as adequate because chest movement is present even though air exchange is ineffective. It will be ineffective if a child squirms and moves his chest away from the pad.

All monitoring devices need to be supplemented with careful nursing observations in order to be maximally effective.

THORACIC IMPEDANCE MONITORS. Thoracic impedance monitors are based on the principle that a small electric current passing through the

thorax flows easily through blood and interstitial fluid but is impeded or slowed by air. Two chest leads placed symmetrically on the chest must be used in order to complete the electrical current. Leads function best if they are placed approximately 2 cm below the axilla on the right and left midaxillary line (Figure 47-7). They must be applied with a conductive gel to ensure close contact.

With the majority of impedance systems, the chest leads return to a monitor, which both counts and digitally displays the number of respirations per minute. An alarm that sounds if a lapse in respirations occurs is also included. A graph which displays the depth and pattern of respiration may be included.

A disadvantage of impedance monitors is that the leads used may misinterpret a strong ventricular heart contraction as respiratory activity and thereby fail to alarm even with apnea present. This occurs because with apnea, bradycardia will result. Cardiac stroke volume must increase to maintain cardiac output. The large difference between empty and filled ventricles is so extreme that it may be interpreted by the monitor leads as a respiratory movement. This error in interpretation will prevent the alarm from sounding until bradycardia becomes so extreme that the space between heartbeats is longer than the 10- to 15-second apnea alarm space.

A monitor will alarm if one or both leads become loose or are accidentally placed on the abdomen, not the chest. Leads should be removed, wiped dry, and replaced with new gel about every

4 hours to maintain good contact and continue monitoring. All electrical monitoring needs to be supplemented by close nursing observation in order to be maximally effective.

PNEUMOGRAM. A pneumogram is a continuous monitor readout showing the respiratory rate and rhythm, amplitude of inspiration, and frequency and duration of any apnea using thoracic impedance monitoring. A pneumogram is used to identify infants who are susceptible to apnea or are candidates for apnea monitoring at home and evaluation of therapy for apnea.

Establishment of Extrauterine Circulation

Although difficulty in the establishment of respirations is the usual critical problem at an infant's birth, lack of cardiac function may be present concurrently—or, if respiratory function is not quickly restored, develop. If there is no cardiac function at birth, or if cardiac arrest subsequently occurs because of the lack of respirations, closed chest massage should be started. This technique is accomplished by placing the index and middle finger of the right hand on an infant's chest over the middle third of the sternum or holding the infant with your fingers on the back and pressing your thumbs against the sternum (Figure 47-8). Depress the sternum about 1 or 2 cm, at a rate of 100 to 120 times per minute.

If pressure and rate of massage are adequate, you will be able to palpate a femoral pulse. If heart sounds are not resumed after a minute of massage, an intracardiac injection of epinephrine may be ordered. Intravenous glucose and sodium bicarbonate (2–3 mEq per kilogram of body weight diluted 1 : 1) will be necessary to maintain blood glucose levels and reduce acidosis. Lung ventilation at a rate of 40 times per minute should be carried out concurrently with the cardiac massage in the proportion of three heart contractions, then one ventilation, three heart contractions, etc.

Infants who had difficulty initiating cardiac function need to be transferred to a transitional or high-risk nursery for continuous surveillance of their cardiac function.

Blood Pressure Monitoring

Because blood pressure is such a strong indicator of cardiac health, continuous monitoring of the blood pressure of a newborn is often used to monitor the effect of medication, stress, and intravenous fluid and to monitor circulating blood

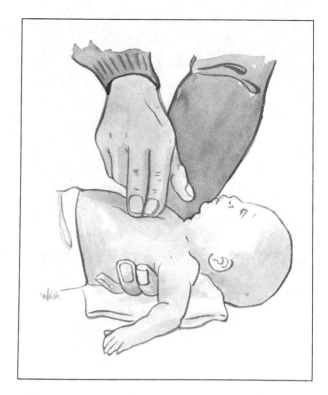

Figure 47-8 External cardiac massage in a newborn. The sternum is depressed with the pressure of only two fingers.

volume and cardiac output. Blood pressure may be monitored by either noninvasive or invasive techniques. Noninvasive techniques are auscultation, palpation, flush, and Doppler methods.

Auscultation methods are notoriously inaccurate in newborns because of inability to fit the infant with the proper size cuff (no more than one-third of the upper arm or leg), inability to fit the diaphragm of a stethoscope snugly enough into the antecubital space to hear Korotkoff sounds clearly, and inaccuracy of the results if an infant cries during the procedure due to the extent of the manipulation.

Palpation is also very inaccurate. To palpate blood pressure, locate the radial pulse; inflate the blood pressure cuff on the upper arm until the pulse disappears to your touch. Gradually lower the pressure in the cuff until the pulse is again discernible to your touch. This is the child's systolic pressure. An advantage of palpating blood pressure is that the size of the cuff is less important than with auscultation. A disadvantage is that the systolic pressure obtained by this method is not as accurate as by auscultation or intraarterial monitoring.

Flush Method. A flush method of blood pressure recording can be used when you do not have a blood pressure cuff small enough to obtain an auscultated one accurately on an infant. This technique is discussed in Chapter 31.

Doppler Method. Ultrasound blood pressure monitoring is based on the principle that ultrasound "bounces off" different tissue with different densities at different rates. When a blood pressure cuff with an ultrasound attachment is placed on an infant's arm, inflated, and the pressure gradually decreased, a pulsing sound will be heard at the point of systolic pressure; the sound muffles at the diastolic level, while simultaneously a monitor displays a digital readout of the systolic, diastolic, and mean blood pressure. This system of blood pressure reading is convenient with infants with illness: You do not have to restrain the infant in order to hold a stethoscope in place against the arm.

Intraarterial Technique. New intraarterial techniques offer very accurate methods of determining systemic blood pressure; if used continuously they can detect changes in blood pressure at the first possible point and therefore, hopefully, allow measures to restore the pressure to be instituted most quickly. The catheter inserted facilitates arterial blood sampling for blood gases or electrolytes. Intraarterial blood pressure is not without risk; in order to be done safely, skilled and knowledgeable nursing care personnel must be present.

The normal systolic and mean blood pressures of infants are shown in Table 47-8. The reading most frequently used with small infants is the mean pressure because it is less influenced by a child's respiratory cycle or size of the catheter. Figure 47-9 depicts an intraarterial wave pattern. The wave length surges upward rapidly during heart systole (compression of the ventricles) or correlates with the QRS pattern of an ECG. After peaking, the wave sweeps downward again to form a *dicrotic notch*, which represents closure of

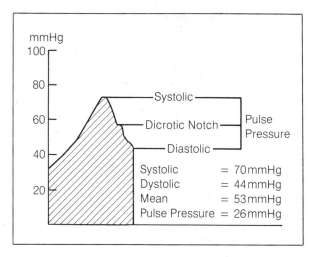

Figure 47-9 *Arterial pressure wave form. From Nugent, J. (1982). Intra-arterial blood pressure monitoring in the neonate.* J.O.G.N Nursing, 11, *281.*

the aortic valve. It then continues downward to a low point before it rises again with a new systole. The highest point of the wave is the systolic blood pressure. The lowest point is the diastolic pressure. Pulse pressure (the difference between systolic and diastolic pressure) can be determined from these levels. Mean pressure refers to the average pressure during the cardiac cycle.

It is important to note when reading wave forms that the upstroke is rapid and sharp and that a clear dicrotic notch is noticeable. To simplify interpretation, the systolic, diastolic, and mean pressures may be shown as a digital readout on the monitor as well as the wave form.

For intraarterial blood pressure monitoring, a catheter is threaded into either an umbilical artery or peripheral artery (radial, brachial, posterior tibial, or dorsalis pedis). The radial artery is the most commonly used peripheral site because the site is relatively easy to locate and the nearby ulnar artery provides good collateral circulation to the hand while the monitoring catheter is in place. The disadvantage of a peripheral site is that the catheter is in a very narrow vessel. Thus only a very slow infusion rate of fluid to maintain catheter patency can be used and the solution must be strictly isotonic in order to avoid vasospasm and thrombus formation. The site should not be used for medication administration for the same reason. Finger pricks should not be performed in the hand or foot distal to the insertion because blood supply to the foot or hand may be limited.

Because of these problems, the umbilical artery is the site of choice in newborns. An umbilical artery catheter is threaded into the aorta until it

Table 47-8 Blood Pressures of Newborns

Birthweight (gm)	Systolic	Diastolic	Mean
1,000–2,000	49–52	26–31	35–40
2,000–3,000	57–64	32–38	41–45
Over 3,000	65–70	39–43	50–54

Source: Kitterman, J. A., et al. (1969). Aortic blood pressure in normal newborn infants during the first 12 hours of life. *Pediatrics, 44,* 959.

rests just below the origin of the renal arteries (about L3–4) or above the level of the diaphragm (T10). Because placement at these points places the tip of the catheter in an area of high blood flow, any solution administered through the catheter will be quickly diluted and thus be less irritating to the vessel. This position avoids blocking the renal or inferior or superior mesenteric arteries and possibly having the blood supply to the kidneys or major abdominal organs disrupted. Following placement, the catheter location is determined by X-ray. Make a habit, when inspecting an X-ray of an infant with an umbilical artery catheter in place, always to confirm tip placement (the lower rib is T12; count down to L3–4 or up to T10).

With an umbilical artery catheter in place, heel pricks for blood samples should not be performed as the blood flow to lower extremities may be altered. The color of the lower extremities should be assessed immediately following catheter insertion to be certain that vasospasm of the aorta and constriction of blood flow to the lower extremities has not occurred (legs appear pale or cyanotic). Following the catheter insertion, the catheter is connected to tubing filled with a sterile intravenous solution; this connects via a stopcock to a transducer that reads the systolic, diastolic, and mean blood pressure and transmits it to a monitor screen in the wave form pattern.

Be certain to check the color, pulse, and warmth of the extremity distal to the catheter insertion every hour. Be certain the transducer is calibrated at 0 before the catheter is inserted, after a change in the system, and every nursing shift. Transducers should be kept on the mattress of an infant's Isolette or radiant warmer to keep the transducer at right atrial heart level. Change lines daily to prevent infection. While changing the proximal stopcock, be certain to clamp the catheter securely or hemorrhage could occur. Tape connections to hold them securely. All bubbles must be removed from the system to prevent damping the wave form.

It is easy for an umbilical artery catheter to clot because internal pressure is high enough that the intravenous fluid infusing by gravity may not enter readily to maintain patency. Connecting a continuous intravenous infusion to a pump such as an IVAC can be used to allow fluid to be continually infused. Adding heparin to the fluid also helps to prevent thrombus formation.

Blood Sampling

Blood samples are obtained in neonates to establish both blood gas and blood composition determinations. Such samples are often obtained by capillary prick (heel prick). A capillary hematocrit or hemoglobin may be higher than those obtained for either venous or arterial sites because red blood cells pool in newborn capillaries due to reduced peripheral blood flow. In order to mobilize red blood cells, the heel can be warmed prior to the sampling. Always mark on a laboratory slip the site of the sample (heel, umbilical artery, catheter, etc.) and whether a peripheral site was warmed or not prior to the puncture so that a difference in two samples is not over- or underinterpreted. Heel punctures should not be used if an umbilical artery catheter is in place, as blood flow to the infant's extremities may be decreased due to the catheter.

Fluid and Electrolytes

Fluid is often necessary for an infant who is ill in the newborn period to prevent hypoglycemia from breathing effort and dehydration from insensible water loss. Fluid commonly used is Ringer's lactate or 5 percent dextrose in water; electrolytes (particularly sodium and potassium) are added as necessary after initial hydration is achieved.

High fluid intake may lead to patent ductus arteriosus as well as congestive heart failure. Thus careful control of volume is necessary. If a radiant warmer is used, more fluid may be required because of increased insensible water loss. An infant under 1,250 grams may be unable to tolerate increased insensible loss or tolerate the fluid load required to replace it.

Urine output and urine specific gravity need monitoring; if output under 2 milliliters per kilogram per hour or a specific gravity over 1.010 to 1.015 occurs, an infant needs more fluid (Schreiner, 1981). Elevated specific gravity may also be caused by inappropriate antidiuretic hormone secretion or kidney failure due to the primary illness.

If an infant has hypotension without hypovolemia, a vasopressor such as dopamine may be used to increase blood pressure. With hypovolemia there will be tachypnea, pallor, tachycardia, decreased arterial blood pressure, decreased central venous pressure, and decreased tissue perfusion of peripheral tissue, with progressive metabolic acidosis. The hematocrit may be normal for some time following acute blood loss as blood cells present are in proportion to plasma. Plasma expanders (whole blood or a protein solution) may be administered to increase blood volume. Control the rate carefully with such infusions to prevent congestive heart failure, patent ductus arteriosus, or intracranial hemorrhage from fluid pressure overload.

Temperature Regulation

Any high-risk infant may have difficulty maintaining a normal temperature. In addition to stress from an illness or immaturity, he is often exposed because of such procedures as resuscitation, blood drawing, and intravenous regulation.

Special efforts to prevent chilling must be taken in the birthing or delivery room. Wet infants must not be allowed to be exposed while resuscitation or physical assessment is carried out. Such infants may arrive at a special care nursery cyanotic and so cold that their temperature is unrecordable. To avoid this situation, an infant should be wiped dry and wrapped in a warm blanket or placed immediately in a warmed Isolette or under a prewarmed radiant heat warmer.

Controlling environmental air by placing an infant in an Isolette or under a radiant heat source is done to keep a baby's metabolic rate, and therefore oxygen consumption, at its lowest. Below a neutral environmental temperature, the infant must increase his metabolic rate to keep his temperature from falling. Increased oxygen is required. Body cells become hypoxic. In order to save oxygen for essential body functions, vasoconstriction of blood vessels occurs. If the process continues too long, pulmonary vessels are affected and pulmonary perfusion will be decreased. The infant's PO_2 level will fall and PCO_2 increase. The infant begins to become acidotic. The decreased PO_2 level may open fetal right-to-left shunts again. In order to supply glucose to maintain increased metabolism, the infant begins anaerobic glycolysis, which pours acid into the bloodstream.

Because he is cold, the infant has become acidotic and cyanotic. With acidosis, the risk of kernicterus (invasion of brain cells with unconjugated bilirubin) rises as more bilirubin-binding sites are lost and more free bilirubin passes out of the bloodstream into brain cells.

The temperature necessary to keep an infant in the neutral zone of lowest metabolic rate is highest in the first 2 days of life. Axillary temperatures (see Figure 34-11) are preferred to rectal temperatures to prevent excessive stooling (which could lead to loss of body fluids and electrolytes). The axillary temperature should be maintained at 97.8°F (36.5°C). Some Isolettes have servocontrol mechanism units that monitor infants' temperatures and automatically change the temperature of the Isolette as needed.

Radiant heat sources have servocontrol probes so that an infant's temperature can be continually monitored. Abdominal skin temperature measured by a probe this way should be 97°F (35.1°C). Tape the probe or disk in place on an infant's abdomen between the umbilicus and the xyphoid process. Be sure that it is not over the rib cage or the thinness of subcutaneous tissue at that point will not allow it to record an accurate reading.

Incubator temperature for infants under 1,500 gm (3 pounds, 4 ounces) should be about 93°F to 95°F (34.3°C to 35°C) for the first days. Babies over 2,500 gm (5 pounds, 8 ounces) usually need an incubator temperature of 89.6°F to 93°F (32°C to 34.3°C) for their first days. Infants between 1,500 gm and 2,500 gm require a temperature of 91°F to 93°F (32.9°C to 34.3°C) (Klaus, 1979).

An infant in an incubator should be undressed except for a diaper so that the flow of air will contact the body surface. Portholes must remain closed to keep the temperature steady and as a safety measure (small infants can fit through a porthole and fall).

The temperature of Isolettes varies with the amount of time portholes are open and the temperature of the area where the Isolette is placed. Direct sunlight or a warm radiator can increase the temperature. Isolette temperature must be checked at frequent intervals to be certain the temperature level designated is being maintained. Use of an additional plexiglass shield inside the Isolette prevents heat loss when portholes are opened for care.

Once an infant's temperature is stabilized, incubator temperature should not be changed at will. Otherwise, a change in the infant's temperature, which might be the first indication of disease, may be misinterpreted as a change in the temperature of the incubator.

Infants who are cold need to be warmed, but warming too rapidly can cause periods of apnea and severe acidosis as the infant's metabolism rate increases. Proper warming can be done by setting an incubator temperature 2°F (1.2°C) above the infant's temperature. Wait for the infant's temperature to increase those two degrees, then reset two more degrees, and so forth until the infant's temperature reaches normal.

Weaning an infant from an incubator is done the same way: Dress the infant as if he were going to be in a bassinet, then set the incubator slightly lower step by step until Isolette temperature is room temperature. If the infant cannot maintain temperature as the incubator temperature level is brought down, he is not yet ready for room temperature air and the weaning process needs to be slowed or stopped until the baby is more mature or better ready to self-regulate temperature. Be certain that during procedures, an infant is not placed directly on cool X-ray plates, scales, or an unheated radiant warmer. In the event of power failure, wrapping infants with plastic bubble wraps or tin foil is a method to maintain body heat.

Nutrition and Elimination

Because a high-risk infant may tire easily or have a congenital anomaly that interferes with sucking, obtaining nourishment by bottle- or breast-feeding may not be possible. A mother who wants to breast-feed must have a realistic appraisal of her child's needs. If a child is almost mature enough to suck, or will have only a brief extended hospital stay for other reasons, she can manually express breast milk to initiate and continue her milk supply until the infant is mature enough or otherwise ready for breast-feeding. Expressed breast milk may be used as the infant's feeding. If the hospital stay will be lengthy, however, she might be well advised to bottle-feed the baby. This decision will rest with the mother, and the depth of her interest in breast-feeding will affect it.

All babies who cannot be fed by bottle or breast need oral stimulation and should be supplied with a pacifier at feeding times. Exceptions are infants too immature to have a sucking reflex and infants who must not swallow air, such as those with a tracheoesophageal fistula awaiting surgery.

Gavage-Feeding

Gavage-feeding (Figure 47-10) is a means of supplying adequate nutrition to an infant who is unable to suck or tires too easily to suck. To prepare for single gavage feedings, the space from the bridge of an infant's nose to a point halfway between the umbilicus and the xyphoid process is measured against a Number 8 or 10 gavage tube. Mark the tube at this point by a small Kelly clamp or piece of tape. It is important that the tube be measured this way to ensure that it enters the stomach after it is passed. A tube passed too far will curl and end up in the esophagus; a tube passed not far enough will also be in the esophagus. Both situations could cause the feedings to be aspirated into the lungs.

Swaddle a baby to be certain the arms will be out of the way and lay him supine. The head should be slightly hyperextended. The tip of the catheter may be lubricated by sterile water. An oil lubricant should never be used. Although the tube is going to be passed into the stomach, it is occasionally passed into the trachea accidentally. Oil left in the trachea could lead to lipoid pneumonia, a complication that an infant already bur-

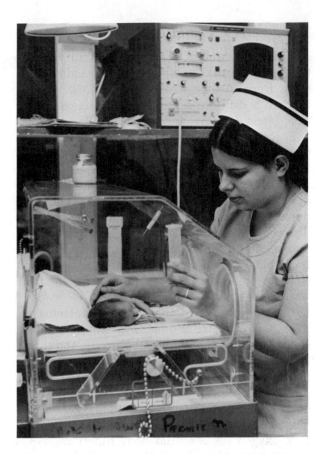

Figure 47-10 *A gavage feeding. Formula enters the gavage tube by the force of gravity only. (Courtesy of the Department of Medical Photography, Children's Hospital, Buffalo, N.Y.)*

dened with a deviation from the normal may not be able to survive.

Whether gavage catheters should be passed through the nares or the mouth is controversial. Because newborns are nose breathers, it seems reasonable that passing the catheter through the mouth will lead to less infant distress than passing it through the nose.

The catheter is passed with gentle pressure to the point of the Kelly clamp or tape. If the catheter is inadvertently passed into the trachea rather than the esophagus, the infant usually has some dyspnea, and the catheter should be withdrawn and replaced. The catheter must be checked for position (that it is not in the trachea) before any feeding is given. This check can be made in one of three ways. The time-honored method is to remove the clamp from the tube and dip the distal end of the tube into a glass of sterile water. Because of possible air in the stomach, one bubble, or possibly two bubbles, may rise from the catheter if the proximal end is in the stomach. If bubbles appear in the water with each expiration, however, the catheter is in the trachea, not in the esophagus. This method should not be used if an infant is being ventilated. The active inspiratory pressure of a ventilator might draw the water from the glass into the lungs, causing aspiration.

An alternative way to test placement is to inject 0.5 to 1.0 ml of air into the tube while you listen over the epigastric area (over the stomach) for the sound of air. In very small babies this is often a difficult task as your stethoscope tip tends to hear lung sounds as well.

A third way to test that the catheter is in the stomach is to attach a syringe to the tube and aspirate stomach contents. There is an advantage of detecting placement by this route in that it allows you to measure the amount of fluid in an infant's stomach prior to feeding. If it is excessive—over 1 to 2 ml—the infant may not be digesting all the food being given to him. If the present feeding schedule is maintained, the baby may begin to vomit from overfeeding. Vomiting always carries with it the danger of aspiration. As a rule, you want to return aspirated stomach contents to the infant's stomach prior to feeding. Constantly removing stomach secretions this way and discarding them can cause an alkalosis.

Once you are assured the catheter is in the stomach, a syringe or a special feeding funnel is attached to the tube. The specific kind and amount of formula ordered is then poured into the syringe or funnel and allowed to flow by gravity drainage into the infant's stomach. The tube should not be elevated more than 12 inches above the infant's abdomen, so that the gravity flow is not too fast. Feedings should never be hurried by using the plunger of the syringe or a bulb attachment for more pressure. These methods lead to stomach overflow and aspiration.

In order to avoid overfeeding, the amount of stomach contents aspirated at the beginning of the feeding is sometimes ordered to be subtracted from the total amount of feeding given; that is, if the feeding ordered was 20 ml, but you drew back and replaced 1 ml, give only 19 ml. Some physicians like a quantity of sterile water added at the end of the feeding to flush the last of the milk into the stomach; others calculate the amount of formula so as to account for the additional amount remaining in the tubing: If you flushed the tubing amount in, you would be giving too much. Ask about the specific technique used in the nursery where you give care.

When the total feeding has passed through the tubing, the tube is reclamped securely and then gently but rapidly withdrawn. Clamping the tube before it is withdrawn is important, because it prevents any milk remaining in the tube from flowing out as the tube is removed and, again, reduces the risk of aspiration.

A baby should be bubbled following gavage-feeding as he would be after a bottle- or breast-feeding. This extra handling not only prevents regurgitation of formula along with bubbles after an infant is laid down but serves to give an infant close contact similar to that a bottle- or breast-fed infant experiences. The infant should be unswaddled and placed on the side or stomach following a feeding.

Polyethylene feeding tubes may be passed through a nostril and left in place for 2 or 3 days at a time for permanent gastric feedings. The advantages of permanent feeding tubes is that they do not have to be replaced every 3 or 4 hours. A disadvantage is the possible nasal irritation or breaks in the nasal membrane, which can result and lead to infection.

Because infants are obligate nose breathers, some infants do poorly with nasally placed catheters. Measuring the tube for placement is done in the same way as for oral insertion except that the catheter is measured from the bridge of the nose to the earlobe, then to the point halfway between the xyphoid process and the umbilicus (Figure 47-11).

After any feeding, procedures such as cupping and vibrating should be postponed for at least an hour. The infant's stomach then has time to di-

Figure 47-11 *A nasogastric tube is measured from the bridge of the nose to the earlobe to a point halfway between the umbilicus and the xyphoid process.*

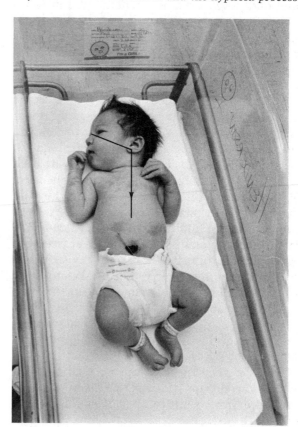

gest the feeding, and vomiting is not likely to occur.

Infants are usually weaned gradually from gavage-feedings to bottle- or breast-feedings, with the number of bottle- or breast-feedings increased each day until the infant is able to take all the feedings by conventional methods.

Nasal-Jejunal Feeding

Infants may be fed by having a long feeding tube threaded through the nares into the stomach, past the pyloric sphincter, and on into the jejunum. It takes a number of hours for a tube to pass this far. That the tube has passed the pyloric valve can be determined by aspirating and analyzing contents from the tube. Stomach secretions are acid; intestinal secretions are alkaline. Placement may also be confirmed by X-ray film as the tubing is opaque on X-ray.

Feedings through a nasal-jejunal tube are usually given by slow, continuous feedings although small feedings every 2 hours may be given. There are many questions as to the wisdom of using nasal-jejunal feedings. An association can be made between the method and the development of necrotizing enterocolitis in low-birth-weight infants. Intestinal perforation has occurred in some infants.

Intravenous Fluid

Infants who cannot ingest adequate amounts of fluid orally will have intravenous fluid lines inserted. Because it is often difficult (and poor absorption from small muscles may make it ineffective) to inject medication intramuscularly in newborns, intravenous lines are used as a major route for medication as well as fluid therapy.

The sites of intravenous infusion in newborns vary considerably. Antecubital veins are seldom used in infants as an infant does not understand the necessity of keeping the elbow straight and so the site infiltrates easily. Small veins in the back of the hand are easily accessible and may be used. Scalp veins are often chosen because they are larger and, if an infant's head is restrained from moving, do not infiltrate easily (Figure 47-12). Parents are generally apprehensive at seeing a scalp vein insertion. It is not a site they are familiar with. They may worry that fluid is infusing into their child's brain. Parents need an explanation of any tube inserted into their baby before they see the baby so they can understand the purpose of the device and view it as a helping, not a harmful, apparatus.

Small 27-gauge needles can be used to begin intravenous therapy in newborns. Infants must be restrained firmly while intravenous fluid lines are

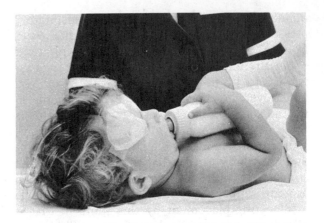

Figure 47-12 *A scalp vein used for intravenous administration. The inverted medicine cup over the insertion site protects the site if the infant turns.*

inserted. The prick of the needle is painful, and even an ill newborn struggles forcefully against painful procedures. The needle and tubing should be taped firmly in place as even the thrashing of arms when an infant cries can dislodge tubing.

At the same time, the insertion site should not be covered so completely with tape that you cannot judge readily whether infiltration is occurring there. The use of a paper or plastic cup to cover a site is questionable when the actual protection it offers is contrasted to the degree it obscures the site.

If the fluid line is begun in a hand, the wrist and arm need to be restrained by an arm board, which is then pinned to the child's mattress by tape "wings" attached to the board (Figure 47-13). If a scalp vein is used, placing firm blanket rolls or sandbags on both sides of the infant's head prevents him from turning too forcefully.

Extremities with intravenous fluid lines in them should be freed every 1 to 4 hours and passively exercised to prevent lack of circulation in the body part (being extremely careful not to dislodge and infiltrate the fluid line).

All intravenous fluid in newborns should be administered by means of a Minidrip and a safety reservoir (a buret) containing no more than 1 hour's worth of parenteral fluid. Thus even if the clamp to the child should be faulty, no more fluid than 1 hour's supply can flow into the child. Fluid should be administered by means of an infusion pump to safeguard against overhydration. If no infusion pump is available, the drip rate must be counted as frequently as every 15 minutes to ensure that the fluid is not being infused too rapidly.

The infusion site should be checked at least hourly to ensure that it is not infiltrated. Check for tissue swelling and coolness. If a scalp vein is

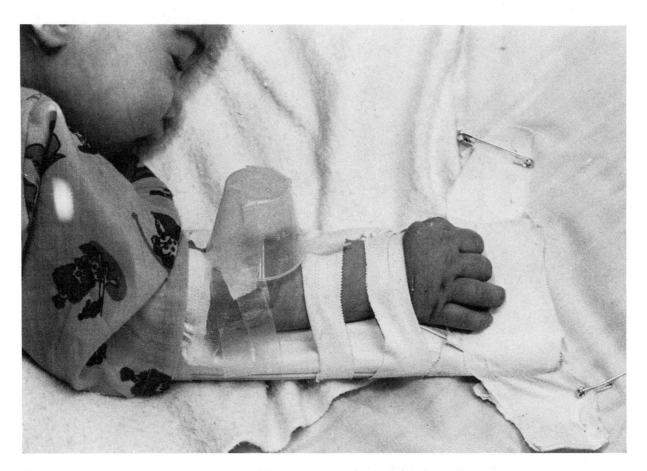

Figure 47-13 *An intravenous site is guarded by an arm board. Wings on the ends can be pinned to the bed surface to prevent motion.*

used, look posteriorly to the site; when a scalp vein infusion infiltrates, swelling most often occurs there because fluid collects by gravity in that area.

At the same time check for signs of dehydration (sunken fontanelles, poor tissue turgor, dry mucous membranes) and signs of overhydration (rales on chest auscultation, cardiac arrhythmias). Infants receiving intravenous fluid should be weighed every 24 hours (more often if fluid balance is tenuous) as an excessive increase in weight indicates that the infant is becoming overhydrated.

All infants with intravenous fluid should have their output determined as well as their input. All voidings should be measured (by weighing diapers rather than using urine collectors, to prevent skin breakdown). The specific gravity of each specimen should be determined (use a syringe to collect urine from the diaper).

Fluid administration sets should be changed every 24 to 48 hours to ensure that bacteria will not begin to grow in the sugar-rich solution. Intravenous fluid in neonates should never be stopped abruptly but tapered as the infant begins to ingest

adequate oral fluid. Sudden stopping of intravenous fluid may lead to hypoglycemia from the sudden loss of glucose in the solution.

Restraints and Intravenous Fluid. To restrain a newborn for a procedure such as beginning intravenous fluid, generally no equipment other than your hands is necessary. If the newborn is exceptionally strong, he may be "mummied" by means of a newborn blanket. The infant is laid on the blanket and the right side of the blanket is brought over the infant's arm and tucked under the body; the left side of the blanket is brought across the trunk and tucked under on the right side (Figure 47-14). By this method, the arms are restrained by the weight of the body. It is a secure feeling for the infant and not uncomfortable.

During intravenous therapy, infants should be restrained only the minimum amount necessary. If the intravenous line is into a scalp vein, for example, an infant may have to have the arms restrained so he cannot raise them to his head; the legs need no restraint. Restraints should not be in place when someone is with the newborn; they should be removed every hour so that the

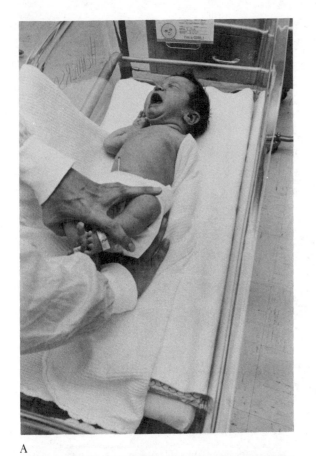

A

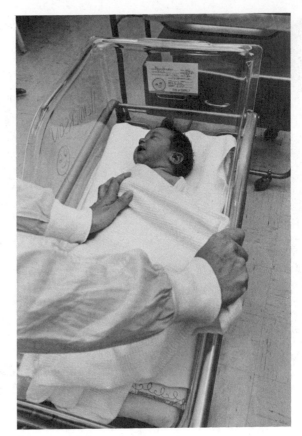

B

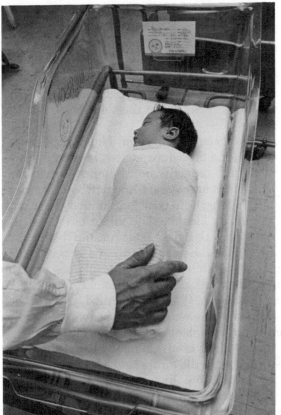

C

Figure 47-14 *A mummy restraint. A. A sheet or blanket is placed under the infant and brought over one arm. B. The sheet or blanket is brought from the opposite side. C. When it is tucked under the baby, the baby is sharply restrained yet secure in the wrapping. (Courtesy of the Department of Medical Photography, Children's Hospital, Buffalo, N.Y.)*

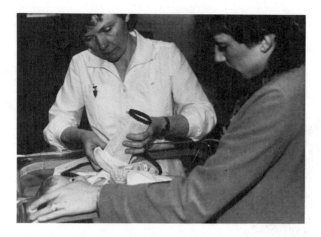

Figure 47-15 *An arm restraint can be used to effectively immobilize arms. Here a new mother learns the art of placing one on an infant.*

baby can exercise the part and the skin condition can be examined. Since eye coordination in newborns may be encouraged by hand movements (movement of the hand gives the newborn something to focus on) "spread-eagling" for long periods may delay newborn development.

If an arm or leg is going to be restrained, a commercial jacket or arm restraint or a "clove-hitch" restraint with soft muslin should be the only type used. Infant jackets are infant shirts with tongue blades slipped into special pockets in the sleeves. The rigid sleeves prevent the child from bending the elbow. The axillary region must be checked frequently to see that the top of a tongue blade is not pressing into the important nerves and blood vessels that cross there. "No-No" sleeves are commercial plastic arm restraints (Figure 47-15).

A clove hitch restraint is made as shown in Figure 47-16. This type of restraint cannot grow tight on an arm or leg and so will not compromise circulation.

Total Parenteral Nutrition

An infant who is unable to take oral feedings even by gavage for prolonged periods of time needs intravenous supplementation to prevent starvation. Traditional intravenous feedings contain electrolytes and sugars but do not contain protein and fat, substances that are essential for the maintenance and growth of body tissue. In total parenteral nutrition, all a baby's nutritional needs can be met by intravenous therapy: The method consists of intravenous administration of a solution containing glucose, vitamins, electrolytes, minerals, and protein. Transfusion of lipids in a second solution supplies an infant with essential fatty acids.

The solution is usually administered by a catheter inserted through the right external jugu-

Figure 47-16 *A clove-hitch restraint. A soft strip of cloth (A) is formed into a figure eight with both ends of cloth folded on top of the figure eight (B). Bring the loops together (C) and pull the two ends to adjust the loop to the size of the child's wrist or ankle (D).*

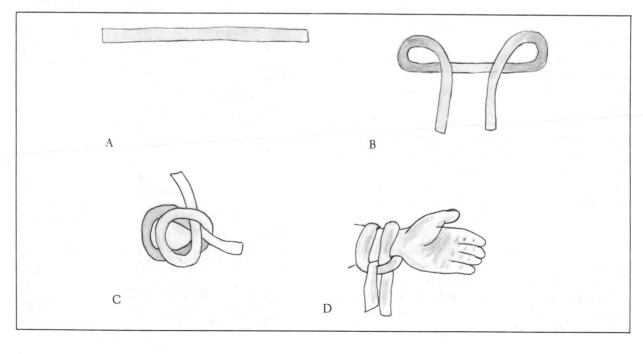

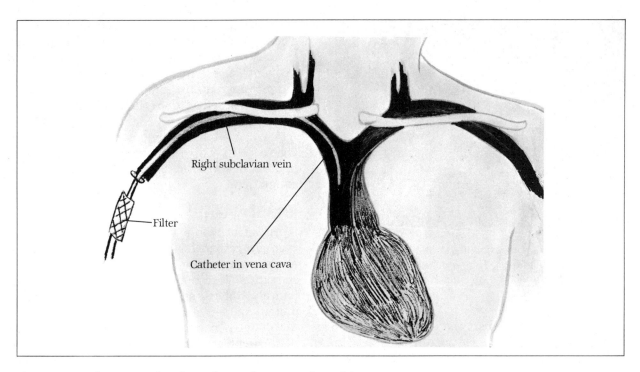

Figure 47-17 *Placement of catheter for total parenteral nutrition.*

lar vein or subclavian to the superior vena cava (Figure 47-17). A major vein of this nature is chosen to avoid inflammation reactions and resulting venous thrombosis. The distal end of the catheter (the end not in the vena cava) may be passed under the skin (subcutaneously) to the parietal head area, where it exits through a stab wound and is connected to the solution tubing. Displacing the catheter entrance this way protects against infection; there is less likelihood of contamination by nasal or oral secretions; and the catheter cannot be displaced by thrashing newborn hands. Placement of the catheter must be done under sterile conditions; in many hospitals it is done in the operating room to ensure sterility.

The solution is administered to an infant by means of a constant infusion pump, so that the rate can be governed. The amount of fluid may be as low as 60 ml per kilogram of body weight per day, or it may be as high as 120 ml per kilogram, depending on the child's needs and whether or not he can take limited oral feedings (Figure 47-18).

Infection is a major danger of total parenteral nutrition; the solution used is a perfect medium for the growth of microorganisms, particularly *Candida* organisms. The dressing covering the insertion site and the intravenous tubing must be changed daily to avoid infection; the tubing

Figure 47-18 *An infant receiving total parenteral nutrition. (Courtesy of the Department of Medical Photography, Children's Hospital, Buffalo, N.Y.)*

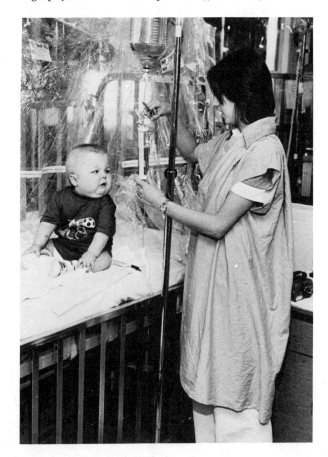

should not be used for drawing blood or for the addition of medications, since such use may introduce infection. Good technique is necessary in changing bottles of solution so that the tubing is not contaminated during changes.

A second major problem of total parenteral nutrition is dehydration. The solution contains about twice the amount of glucose normally administered to infants. This amount ensures that the amino acids of the solution will not be used for energy but for the synthesis of protein. Dehydration may occur as the body tries to dilute the amount of glucose recognized by the kidneys as excessive and begins excreting it (the same phenomenon that leads to high urine output in persons with diabetes). The urine of an infant undergoing total parenteral nutrition needs to be assessed for glucose by a test such as Clinitest at least every 4 hours. If two or more consecutive samples reveal a 3+ or 4+ glucose level, either the rate of the infusion or the amount of glucose in the solution will be decreased. Urine is also tested for specific gravity and protein and measured for volume. Dextrostix determinations for blood glucose are taken about every 4 hours.

After the first few days of total parenteral nutrition, a rebound effect (the baby's body produces increased insulin) may cause hypoglycemia. A urine sample that is suddenly negative for sugar after a series that has been highly positive is therefore not necessarily an encouraging sign but may be a warning that a lethally low sugar level is present.

Total parenteral nutrition is used with infants who have undergone gastrointestinal tract surgery and in the extremely small or ill infant who is not able to suck or has such a small stomach capacity that gavage-feeding is not highly successful. It is helpful for an infant with a respiratory disorder whose respiratory rate is so rapid that sucking and swallowing are difficult.

Total parenteral nutrition may be done by peripheral vein. Glucose concentrations must be less when given by this route or the solution will be so irritating to the vein that phlebitis will occur. Sites must be watched conscientiously because if infiltration occurs tissue sloughing can be extensive.

Infants receiving total parenteral nutrition need sucking stimulation. Offering a pacifier every 2 to 4 hours at the time of normal infant feedings provides this need. If a sucking reflex is not stimulated at birth, it fades. When the infant is ready for oral feedings, he may have difficulty learning to suck effectively unless this reflex is encouraged.

Signs of Dehydration

Infants born under general anesthesia who are too lethargic to suck well in the first few hours of life or infants born with a congenital anomaly that prevents sucking or swallowing (cleft lip or tracheoesophageal fistula) are in danger of becoming dehydrated in the first day of life. They should be observed closely for signs of this problem: a sunken fontanelle, dry mucous membranes, decreased skin turgor, decreased urination, and an increasing specific gravity level of urine. To assess fontanelles, always raise a child to a sitting position. In some infants the fontanelle appears tense and bulging in a supine position and only reveals the extent of the true tension when the head is elevated. To assess skin turgor, raise a portion of skin on an infant's abdomen or thigh between your finger and thumb as if you were going to pinch the baby. In a well-hydrated infant, after you remove your hand, the skin returns to its previous contour. In a dehydrated infant, the skin remains raised in a ridge.

Maintaining Adequate Output

Ill neonates need close observation for adequate urine output, which reflects their kidney function. Kidney function depends on adequate blood flow and fluid intake and is therefore an indirect measure of these rates.

A single urine specimen should be collected by application of a plastic urine collector (Figure 47-19). Be certain the infant's skin is dry and no powder or ointment is present so that the collector adheres well. It is difficult to measure continuous urine output by plastic urine collectors in neonates as their skin is so delicate and application of tape or the constant moisture of a collector causes excoriation and skin breakdown. Measuring urine output may be done by weighing diapers. Weigh the diaper before it is placed on the infant; weigh it again after it has been wet. The difference in weight in grams reflects the milliliters of urine in the diaper.

In order that blood pressure can be maintained to ensure kidney function, the amount of blood withdrawn for analysis must be carefully calculated. A newborn's total blood volume is 80 ml per kilogram of body weight. Thus a 6-pound neonate (3 kg) only has a total of 240 ml of blood. If 5 ml is removed every hour for analysis of blood gases, within 24 hours, half of the child's blood volume would be removed.

Evaluation

The box on page 1148 summarizes criteria that indicate an infant is receiving adequate nutrition.

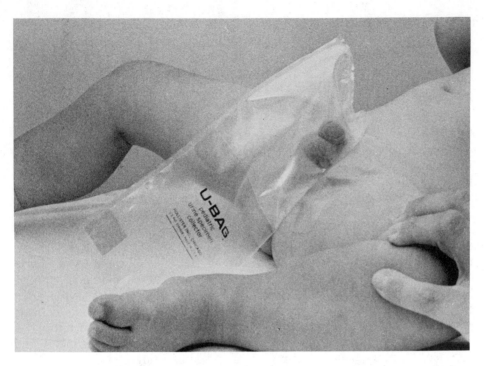

Figure 47-19 *An infant urine collector in place.*

Stimulation and Parent Bonding

It is easy to assume that ill newborns need to conserve strength for healing and therefore should be kept as quiet and motionless as possible. In order to develop normally, however, even very ill infants need stimulation. Such activity apparently aids in myelination of nerve tissue and promotes psychosocial development.

As with well newborns, stimulation for ill newborns should include activities that appeal to the infant's senses. In addition, vestibular stimulation such as that provided by a rocking chair or water bed may be used to help reduce apnea.

Visual Stimulation

Infants respond best to a human face and to black and white designs that resemble a human face or are in a geometric pattern. Encourage the infant's parents to bring in a large black and white photo to place where the infant can view it (as close as 20 cm for immature infants). Hang a mobile where it can be easily seen. Be certain to turn your head when speaking to an infant so your face is in line with his (*en face*). Infants grow tired of the same visual stimulation after 3 or 4 days. Have new stimuli prepared to use at that point.

Auditory Stimulation

Infants respond best to the sounds of a human voice or to soft music. Ask parents to tape record their voices and play these for the infant for 2 or 3 minutes at a time. Turn on music boxes or tape recorded music during care. Speak and sing to the infant and encourage the parents to do this when they visit (Figure 47-20).

Assessment for Adequate Feeding

1. No more than 15 percent weight loss in first 3 days of life
2. Continued weight gain after this point
3. Urine output maintained at 1–3 ml/kg/hr
4. Specific gravity of urine maintained at 1.003 to 1.030
5. No hypoglycemia (Dextrostix over 45 mg/100 ml)
6. No hyperglycemia (Dextrostix under 130 mg/100 ml)
7. No glycosuria by dipstick

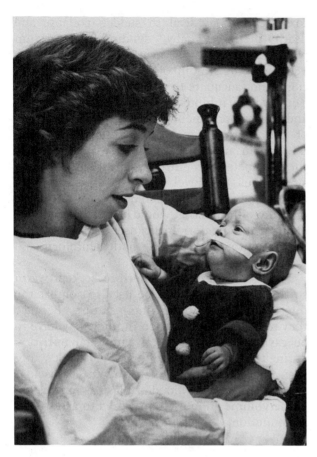

Figure 47-20 *A nurse speaks to and rocks an ill neonate for stimulation. Note the infant's attentiveness. (Courtesy of the Department of Medical Photography, Children's Hospital, Buffalo, N.Y.)*

Olfactory Stimulation

Ask parents to provide sachets of the mother's favorite perfume or the father's shaving lotion. Allow the infant to smell breast milk provided for him by his mother for gavage feedings. Avoid obnoxious odors, particularly in an Isolette, where it takes a long time for the odor to dissipate.

Tactile Stimulation

Stroke the infant's head and back following feedings; provide sheepskin or deep pile velvet for the infant to lie on for additional touch sensations.

Gustatory Stimulation

Provide a pacifier for the infant during gavage feedings. Do not discourage thumb sucking.

Vestibular Stimulation

Place the infant on an oscillating water bed or hammock or rock him in a rocking chair for 10-minute periods. Rocking of this nature may en-

courage memory development and help regulate respiratory function (Chaze, 1984).

Prevention of Infection

The last thing that a high-risk infant needs during the first few days of life is to contract an infection. In some instances, such as premature rupture of the membranes, it is the development of infection (pneumonia or skin lesions, for example) that places the infant in the high-risk category.

Infections may have prenatal, perinatal, or postnatal causes. The most common viruses to affect infants in utero are the cytomegalovirus and the rubella virus. An infant with either of these infections may be born with congenital anomalies. Infants who contract rubella in utero may be born infectious to other babies and must be isolated from the regular nursery at birth. Thus, it is important to ask a woman on admission to the labor service whether she knows of any diseases or rashes she had during pregnancy. In that way congenital anomalies can be anticipated, and at the same time other newborns and health care personnel can be protected from exposure to the rubella virus.

The most prevalent perinatal infections are those contracted from the vagina during delivery: group B streptococcal septicemia, and thrush from *Candida* infection.

Postnatal infection is invariably spread to an infant from health care personnel. Persons caring for infants must observe strict nursery technique to keep the possibility of infection to a minimum. Health care personnel with infections have a moral obligation not to work in newborn nurseries.

Assessment

It is often said that newborns do not manifest symptoms when they contract an infection. A more accurate statement would be that they do not manifest *the same symptoms as adults*. The first noticeable sign may be inactivity or poor feeding. Fever may not be present; many newborns evidence hypothermia with infection. An infant may become jaundiced from inability of the liver to perform under stress, and cyanosis may develop from failure of circulation due to decreased blood pressure. The white blood count is not always helpful in establishing the presence of infection in newborns because it is normally elevated from the trauma of birth.

Following these nonspecific symptoms, specific symptoms will appear: diarrhea and vomiting if the infection is gastrointestinal; skin lesions if the infection begins with surface contact; bulging fontanelle and nuchal rigidity if the infection is in the central nervous system; shock if it becomes a septicemia.

The body's natural resistance to infection depends on the ability of the white blood cells, the reticuloendothelial system, and the immune system to function effectively. In a newborn, none of these defense systems is fully developed. Thus, even a slight infection, if allowed to go untreated, may spread rapidly throughout the newborn's body, becoming a severe and generalized infection that can result in death. Even the smallest skin lesion or slightest suspicion that an infant is acting ill therefore warrants reporting.

Sepsis Workup. When it is suspected that a newborn has an infection, a sepsis workup is ordered. Each hospital has a policy concerning the parts of this workup, but common procedures you will need to assist with or carry out are cultures of body fluids (cerebrospinal fluid obtained by a lumbar puncture, urine obtained by suprapubic catheterization, gastric secretions obtained by nasogastric tube aspiration); body cultures from the umbilical cord, external auditory canal, nose, throat, and rectal areas; and blood cultures. Additional blood will be drawn for white blood count and differential, hematocrit and hemoglobin, platelet count, sedimentation rate, serum immunoglobulin, and possibly serologic tests.

Analysis

Nursing diagnoses established with the newborn with an infection usually concern nutrition because of associated nausea and vomiting or bonding because isolation to prevent spread of the infection may be necessary.

Implementations

Newborns with infections are removed from a central nursery to an isolation nursery to protect other infants. If there is not enough nursing personnel available to staff a separate nursery and make frequent observations of an ill child, the child may be isolated from the other infants in the central nursery by being placed in a closed Isolette. Nursing personnel caring for an ill infant in a central nursery must be extremely meticulous in their technique or the infection will spread throughout the nursery.

As with adults, specific antibiotics based on sensitivity studies are used to treat newborn infections. A number of antibiotics are toxic to newborns and are avoided in newborn care. Chloramphenicol is poorly excreted by newborns; toxic levels of the drug develop rapidly. These toxic levels may lead to sudden collapse and death (the "gray baby" syndrome). Potassium penicillin G can cause heart block in newborns because of the buildup of potassium if renal function is not adequate to excrete excess potassium. Tetracycline inhibits the growth of long bones and causes permanent yellowish-brown staining of the tooth enamel. The sulfonamides and novobiocin are dangerous to newborns because they compete with bilirubin for albumin-binding sites. Thus the level of indirect bilirubin increases and kernicterus and death occur at levels of serum bilirubin that would normally be considered safe. Cephaloridine causes nephrotoxicity. Nitrofurantoins may cause both neurologic and kidney impairment.

Infants with infections need to be kept warm so that their energy will be used to combat the infection, not maintain temperature. Because they may suck poorly when ill, they may have to be gavaged or fed by total parenteral nutrition during the course of the infection. If shock symptoms should occur, an infant may need vascular support with whole blood or plasma transfusion. Urine volume should be measured to assess kidney function.

Infections in Newborns

Congenital Syphilis

If a woman has syphilis during the last half of pregnancy, the organism of syphilis, *Treponema pallidum*, may cross the placenta and cause congenital syphilis. Severely infected infants are stillborn; others, less infected, are born with congenital anomalies. Moist areas of an infant (the cord and nasal secretions) contain the organism and are generally infectious at birth.

Adult syphilis is described in Chapter 36. The infected newborn does not develop a chancre, the typical, painless ulcer lesion of adult first-stage syphilis, but about a week after birth a copper-colored rash, most prominent over the face, soles of the feet, and palms of the hands, may appear. This is an unusual rash as most rashes do not cover the soles of the feet or the palms of the hands. The infant's nose may show a severe rhinitis (snuffles). X-ray study of the long bones may reveal changes of epiphyseal lines at about 1 to 3 months of age.

Assessment

All women during pregnancy have tests for syphilis (VDRL or FTA-ABS) done at their first prenatal visit, and again at delivery. An FTA-ABS test (fluorescent treponemal antibody absorption) is a specific test for IgM antibodies against syphilis and may be helpful also for diagnosis in the newborn. Be certain that blood is drawn for syphilis screening on all pregnant women; this "routine" is easy to forget if the mother is ill or something unusual is happening to her during pregnancy or labor.

Analysis

The nursing diagnosis concerning congenital syphilis usually deals with nutrition: The infant is ill and so may not suck well. It may also concern prevention of complications from spread of the disease or with any defect present, along with parent-child bonding because the parents may feel guilty that their child has been born infected or with congenital anomalies.

Implementations

An infant born of a woman who has a positive serologic test is isolated at birth and given a course of penicillin. Isolation is maintained until culture reports are returned as negative or penicillin has been administered for 24 hours. It is important that health care personnel who are pregnant not care for the infant until the course of penicillin is complete so that they do not contract the disorder. The infant needs careful assessment in order to be certain that nutritional intake is adequate and respiratory/cardiac conversion to extrauterine life proceeds normally. Make certain a mother has the opportunity to visit the isolation nursery and touch and hold the infant in order that bonding can proceed. Even though the mother has had syphilis she still needs to use isolation technique (hand washing and gowning) for infant care. No immunity exists for syphilis so that she could contract it again. If a mother was not treated during pregnancy, both she and her sexual partner need treatment with penicillin postpartally.

Evaluation

The child needs long-term follow-up because other manifestations of the disease will develop as he grows older. As the permanent teeth erupt at 5 or 6 years, they may be pegged or notched (Hutchinson's teeth). All teeth tend to be of poor quality and decay easily. If the disease remains untreated, interstitial keratitis (inflammatory reaction of the cornea with vascular infiltration) may result when a child is between 6 and 14 years of age. This scarring may cause blindness. If not treated at birth, the disease will progress, and may become tertiary or lead to neurologic manifestations.

Gonococcal Conjunctivitis

If a woman has gonorrhea at the time of delivery, an infant delivered vaginally may contract gonorrhea of the conjunctiva or *ophthalmia neonatorum*.

Assessment

This infection is generally bilateral. The eye conjunctivae become fiery red, there is thick pus present, and the eyelids are edematous, all on the first to the fourth day of life. Gonococcal conjunctivitis should be considered as a possibility when a conjunctivitis occurs in any child under 30 days of age. Occasionally silver nitrate drops cause a severe chemical conjunctivitis; this reaction fades by 24 hours, however; gonococcal conjunctivitis does not.

Analysis

This is an extremely serious form of conjunctivitis because, if it is left untreated, the infection extends to corneal ulceration and destruction, which results in opacity of the cornea and blindness. Nursing diagnoses are usually concerned with the potential for blindness and difficulty with bonding.

Implementations

The prophylactic instillation of 1% silver nitrate or erythromycin, penicillin, or tetracycline ointment into the eyes of newborns prevents gonococcal conjunctivitis.

If the disease does occur, the newborn must be isolated; this condition is extremely contagious. The baby is treated with large doses of penicillin given both locally by instillation and systemically. The eyes are washed with saline irrigations to clear the copious discharge of pus. When irrigating eyes, use a sterile medicine dropper or sterile bulb syringe. The solution should be at room temperature and sterile. Direct the stream of the irrigation fluid laterally so that it does not enter and contaminate the other eye. If some fluid should splash into your own eye, you must have penicillin administered or you may contract the disease.

Evaluation

Parents of an infant with the infection should be given a realistic report of the seriousness of this disease. However, parents can be assured that with early diagnosis and treatment the prognosis for normal eyesight in the child is good. The mother needs treatment for gonorrhea herself before fallopian tube sterility or pelvic inflammatory disease results. Any recent sexual contacts of the mother should be treated so that the spread of the disease can be halted.

Candidiasis

Candida albicans is the fungus responsible for candidal infections. *Candida* organisms grow in the vagina of many adult women (monilial vaginitis). Pregnant women are particularly susceptible to candidal infections because of the change in vaginal pH during pregnancy. If infection is present at the time of birth, an infant may develop an infection of the mucous membrane of the mouth (thrush) if he is born vaginally.

Assessment

Thrush is characterized by white plaques on an erythematous base on the buccal membrane and the surface of the tongue. It resembles milk curds left from a recent milk feeding. Thrush plaques do not scrape away, however, whereas milk curds do. The child's mouth is painful, and he does not eat well because of the inflammation and local pain. Since thrush usually appears on the fourth to seventh day of life, it may not be seen in newborn nurseries as much as by community health nurses or nurses in ambulatory health care facilities.

Candida albicans also causes a severe, bright red, sharply circumscribed diaper-area rash. Satellite lesions may appear. The rash is marked by its intense color and by the fact that it does not improve with the usual diaper-rash remedies, such as the use of talcum, frequent changing of diapers, exposure to air, or an ointment such as A&D. It tends to occur in infants who have been treated with an antibiotic; suppression of normal skin flora may allow for overgrowth of fungal organisms.

Analysis

The nursing diagnosis concerned with candidal infections usually deals with potential for insufficient nutrition (the child's mouth is tender, which prevents good sucking) although it may involve instead the discomfort related to a diaper-area rash.

Implementations

Nystatin is an antifungal drug that is effective against both the oral and diaper-rash form of illness. For thrush, it is supplied as a liquid. It should be dropped into an infant's mouth about four times a day following feedings so that the drug remains in contact with the oral mucosa for a period of time rather than being washed away immediately by a feeding. A mother who is breast-feeding should apply topical nystatin to her nipples prior to each feeding or manually express milk for about 2 days to avoid contracting a mastitis (breast infection) from the infant. For diaper rash, a nystatin ointment is prescribed to use with diaper changes.

Evaluation

If a newborn infant develops a candidal infection, the mother is usually treated also with nystatin vaginal suppositories to eradicate the cause of infection. The woman's sexual partner may need treatment also, or the infant will have the infection again in another few weeks after it has been spread from the man back to the mother and from the mother back to the infant. Be certain that a mother understands the importance of using the liquid or ointment and how to administer it correctly.

Group B Hemolytic Streptococcal Infection

The major cause of infection in newborn infants today is the group B hemolytic streptococcal organism. Between 50 and 300 infants in every 1,000 live births display a positive culture for this organism. The organism is contracted at the time of delivery from secretions in the birth canal. It may be spread from baby to baby if good hand washing technique is not used in handling newborns.

Colonization by group B hemolytic streptococci may result in early-onset or late-onset illness. With the early-onset form, symptoms of pneumonia become apparent in the first few hours of life. An infant will have tachypnea and apnea and symptoms of shock such as decreased urine output, extreme paleness, or hypotonia. He may develop an expiratory grunt. The grunting sound is made by air being forced past contracted vocal cords. This is a compensatory mechanism of newborns to maintain pressure in the alveoli on expiration and prevent alveolar collapse. Pneumonia may develop so rapidly that as many as 90 percent of infants who contract the infection die within 24 hours of birth.

With the late-onset type, instead of pneumonia being the infection focus, meningitis tends to occur. About a week after the infant returns home, he gradually becomes lethargic and develops a fever and upper respiratory symptoms. The fontanelles will bulge from increased intracranial pressure. Mortality from the late-onset type is not as high as from the early-onset form (15% compared to 90%), but neurologic consequences may occur in up to 50 percent of infants who survive.

Gentamicin, ampicillin, and penicillin are all effective against group B hemolytic streptococcal infections. It is difficult for parents to understand how their infant could suddenly become this ill. They may need a great deal of support to care for an infant if he does survive the infection but is left neurologically handicapped.

Congenital Rubella

In urban areas of the United States, about 15 to 20 percent of women of childbearing age are susceptible to rubella. The greatest risk to the embryo from the rubella virus is during the second to sixth week of intrauterine life. The frequency of malformations is about 50 percent if the virus invasion is during these early weeks.

The classic symptoms of the rubella syndrome are thrombocytopenia; cardiac, sight, and hearing defects; and motor and mental retardation. The thrombocytopenia is manifested by purpura: red-purple macula with a blueberry muffin–like appearance. The cardiac defects that are most common are patent ductus arteriosus, pulmonary stenosis, and atrial and ventricular septal defects. Deafness with the rubella syndrome is generally neural, uncorrectable, and bilateral. Serious eye defects seen are cataract and congenital glaucoma. The retina of the eye is often covered by discrete, patchy black pigmentation that, while it does not interfere with sight, is so often present that it is an aid in diagnosis. The diagnosis is confirmed by identifying IgM antibodies against rubella in the child's serum. IgM antibodies do not cross the placenta, so they could not have come from the mother; they must have been produced by the fetus in response to invasion by the rubella antigen.

Live rubella virus may be cultured from nasopharyngeal secretions of affected infants at birth. At 1 year of age, about 10 percent of these infants are still shedding live virus. These infants must be isolated during the days they spend in the hospital at birth as this virus is airborne-spread. Treatment is symptomatic, depending on the defects present. The prognosis will also depend on the number and extent of the defects.

Herpesvirus II Infection

A herpesvirus II infection can be contracted by a fetus across the placenta. More often, however, it is contracted at birth from the mother who has active herpetic vulvovaginitis at the time of birth.

Assessment

If the infection was acquired during pregnancy, an infant may be born with vesicles covering the skin. If an infant acquires the infection at birth, about the fourth to seventh day of life he shows a loss of appetite, perhaps a low-grade fever, and lethargy. Stomatitis or a few vesicles on the skin appear. Herpes vesicles are always clustered, pinpoint in size, and surrounded by a reddened base. Following the appearance of the vesicles, the infant becomes extremely ill. He will develop dyspnea, jaundice, purpura, convulsions, and shock. Cultures are obtained from representative vesicles as well as other common culture points in newborns. Serum is analyzed for IgM antibodies.

Analysis

A nursing diagnosis concerning a herpes infection usually involves the problems of sustaining life functions and encouraging the parents to grieve for a newborn who is so seriously ill.

Implementations

There is some evidence that adenine arabinoside (Ara-A), a drug that inhibits viral DNA synthesis, may be effective in combating this overwhelming infection. At the moment, however, prevention is the newborn's best protection. Women with herpetic vulvar lesions should be delivered by cesarean birth. Infants with an infection should be isolated from other infants. Women with herpes lesions on their face (herpes simplex or cold sores) should not feed or hold their newborns until lesions are crusted and no longer contagious. Health care personnel who have herpes simplex infections must not care for newborn infants. Although herpes simplex lesions are probably caused by herpesvirus type I, this limitation in contact does not seem excessive in light of the severity of the disease if they should be herpes type II lesions. A woman who is isolated from her newborn at birth needs to view the infant from the nursery window. She should be kept informed of how well the baby is eating and of anything special (how her newborn likes to be wrapped firmly, how he follows a finger eagerly) so that maternal bonding will not be seriously impaired.

Evaluation

Death may occur within hours or days in infants who develop the disease. Children who survive generalized herpesvirus infections in the newborn period may have permanent central nervous system sequelae.

Cytomegalic Inclusion Disease

The cytomegalovirus was originally named the *salivary gland virus* because it was first isolated from salivary glands. It is similar to the herpes simplex virus.

Cytomegalic inclusion disease may be transmitted across the placenta to the fetus. The infant who has severe involvement from this virus invasion may have gross central nervous system damage, such as microcephaly, blindness, deafness, and mental retardation. He may show signs of jaundice, lethargy, convulsions, splenomegaly, and hepatomegaly. Management is supportive, depending on the problems present.

Pneumonia

Pneumonia may occur in the first few days of life in an infant whose membranes were ruptured more than 24 hours before delivery, or in the infant who aspirates vaginal secretions or meconium-stained amniotic fluid. The infant may have manifested delayed respirations at birth, with subsequent development of dyspnea, tachypnea, retractions, and cyanosis. The mature infant may have an accompanying fever; a less mature baby may evidence hypothermia as a response to infection. A chest X-ray film will reveal densities suggestive of pneumonia.

An infant needs warmth, oxygen administration, and possibly assisted ventilation and an antibiotic. Pneumonia is always a serious finding in a neonate, as it is a severe infection and is difficult for a newborn to combat with limited reserves.

Prolonged Rupture of the Membranes

If membranes rupture more than 24 hours prior to delivery, a very great chance is created that organisms have invaded the open uterus and the infant will be born with bacterial contamination. Pneumonia or skin infections may result. Blood and surface cultures should be obtained from the infant at birth. If any sign of infection (lethargy or shock) is found, blood, cerebrospinal fluid, urine, gastric aspiration, throat, ear canals, umbilicus, axilla, and rectum all need to be examined by culture.

The infant will be treated with an antibiotic appropriate for the organism identified.

Metabolic Illness

A number of metabolic illnesses can occur in newborns.

Hypoglycemia

Hypoglycemia is low blood serum glucose. If hypoglycemia is going to occur it usually occurs in the first few hours or days of life. The ability to regulate glucose is an important skill of a newborn's metabolism. Maintaining an adequate level of blood glucose is crucial because the brain can neither make nor store glucose; it must have a ready supply available from the circulation for cell metabolism. Hypoglycemia, therefore, results in brain cell destruction. The circulating glucose level depends on glucose input (from oral feedings), glucose released by the liver (glucogenesis, or production of glucose, and the amount of glucose uptake by body tissues. Infants who have respiratory distress and cannot suck well may not be able to take in an adequate amount of glucose. An immature infant does not have adequate liver stores to use for glucogenesis. An infant who is cold or hypoxic uses glucose rapidly for metabolism and thus quickly depletes liver stores.

During fetal life, glucose is supplied to the fetus by placental transfer. This occurs at a constant, rapid rate, although the levels of fetal glucose never exceed those of the mother.

The average level of glucose in cord blood varies from 60 to 80 mg per 100 ml of blood. An infant can be considered hypoglycemic if the glucose level falls below 30 mg per 100 ml in the first 72 hours of life and below 40 mg per 100 ml thereafter (Klaus, 1979).

Blood glucose values are usually lower in low-birth-weight infants than in mature infants. A premature infant is therefore ordinarily not considered hypoglycemic until the glucose level is under 20 mg per 100 ml. Factors that make babies particularly prone to hypoglycemia are shown in Table 47-9.

Assessment

Hypoglycemia may be asymptomatic, or the infant may be jittery, limp, apathetic, tachypneic, or cyanotic, may refuse to nurse, or may have convulsions. Few of these signs are specific for hypoglycemia. Cyanosis and tachypnea occur in respiratory distress, jitteriness in hypocalcemia, and convulsions in central nervous system injury. Refusal to eat and apathy are seen in an infant with an infection or possibly with heart disease. The symptoms therefore require an investigation into the cause, and the investigation will reveal the hypoglycemia.

Blood glucose values fall rapidly in the first hours after birth. Infants should have at least one test for glucose blood level in the early hours of life before they are fed. Glucose levels can be

Table 47-9 Factors that Make Infants Prone to Hypoglycemia

Factors	Result
Born of poorly controlled diabetic mother	The fetus produces a high level of insulin because of maternal hyperglycemia; after birth, the high insulin level lowers the level of circulating glucose in the infant.
Born of mother with pregnancy-induced hypertension	Poor placental perfusion limits the amount of glucose the fetus has stored.
Hemolytic disease	The liver stores little glucose due to its level of intrauterine stress.
Difficulty establishing respirations	The infant uses glucose during the period of respiratory stress.
Twinning	Twin transfusion has occurred or the smaller twin receives less glucose than the other.
Immaturity	The infant has inadequate glucose stores.
Small for gestation age	The infant has inadequate glucose stores.
Postmaturity	Glucose stores are exhausted during the additional time in utero.
Intrauterine or extrauterine stress	The infant uses glucose stores during the period of stress.
Failure to suck well	Infant is unable to take in adequate glucose.

monitored by heel pricks. The technique for Dextrostix determination is shown in Procedure 47-1. A reading of under 45 mg per 100 ml on a Dextrostix should be reported, and interventions to increase the glucose level must be begun.

Analysis

Nursing diagnoses concerned with hypoglycemia often reflect the difficulty with glucose metabolism or the parents' fear regarding the illness of their infant.

Implementations

To correct blood glucose levels, early oral feeding or intravenous administration of a dextrose solution will be required. Administration of glucogon or epinephrine to convert glycogen into glucose is usually ineffective in newborns because their glycogen stores are generally inadequate. If the glucose level is only slightly lowered, giving a baby oral glucose water will cause a rapid rise. A rapid rise in glucose level will bring a compensatory increase in insulin production, however, which in another hour will again reduce the glucose level. Offering an infant formula rather than glucose water prevents this sequence of events. Since formula is absorbed slower, it does not cause such a rebound effect.

If an infant has difficulty sucking, feeding may be given by gavage. If the glucose level must be raised immediately, an intravenous line is necessary. If a bolus of glucose is given by intravenous push, it will quickly relieve the hypoglycemia. A rebound effect of insulin production will also quickly lower the glucose level again, however. After the initial corrective measure, therefore, a slow infusion of glucose must be maintained to keep this effect from happening; the glucose is gradually tapered off. The infant must have continued assessment for blood glucose levels for at least 24 hours to determine whether the level has stabilized and is not still fluctuating.

Infants who are delivered under general anesthesia and who do not suck well in the early hours of life require particular observation. Breast-fed infants who do not take readily to breast-feeding may need a supplemental feeding after breast-feeding to maintain a glucose level. Most mothers who are breast-feeding do not want their infants to have supplemental feedings in order that the infant will suck vigorously at feedings and fully empty the breasts; but then, neither do they want a retarded child with brain damage due to decreased glucose levels. Explaining the reason for the supplemental feeding will eliminate misunderstanding and any feeling that the hospital personnel are trying to undermine breast-feeding (you are trying to undermine mental retardation).

Evaluation

Monitoring glucose levels of high-risk infants can be a time-consuming task in a high-risk or transitional nursery. Because maintaining adequate circulating glucose levels protects against brain damage, however, the time spent in testing and regulating intravenous infusions is time very well spent.

The Infant of a Diabetic Mother

The infant of a diabetic woman whose disease is poorly controlled during pregnancy is typically longer and weighs more than other babies (Figure

Procedure 47-1

Blood Glucose Determination by Dextrostix

Purpose: To assess blood glucose level by a rapid dipstick technique.

Procedure	*Rationale*
1. Wash hands; don protective gown.	1. Protect infant from microorganisms.
2. Assess infant for lesions of heel; analyze appropriateness of procedure; plan variations based on special circumstances.	2. Skin puncture is contraindicated if lesions exist over the puncture point.
3. Implement procedure by assembling necessary equipment: Dextrostix container with test strips, sterile blood lancet, alcohol swab, dry cotton ball, Band-Aid.	3. Assembling supplies prevents unnecessary exposure of infant. Use blood lancets in preference to scalpel blades to avoid penetrating too deeply and injuring periosteum of bone.
4. Expose only one foot of infant and locate acceptable puncture site (lateral sides of heel). (Figure 47-21)	4. Prevent cold exposure; using lateral surfaces, not center of heel avoids puncture of plantar artery or tibial nerve.
5. Grasp foot firmly to steady it; wipe selected site vigorously with alcohol swab; puncture with lancet with a quick firm thrust.	5. Infant will move foot when hurt; a firm grasp prevents puncture at the wrong site.
6. Wipe first drop of blood away with sterile dry cotton ball; allow a second drop to fall on to end of Dextrostix.	6. First drop of blood is diluted with alcohol and tissue fluid. Do not squeeze foot as this will add tissue juice and distort results.
7. Time carefully for 1 minute, then rinse excess blood from Dextrostix. Compare color change immediately against color chart on side of bottle.	7. Timing is crucial as color change will continue and result will be read inaccurately.
8. Apply pressure to puncture site to halt bleeding; apply Band-Aid.	8. Bleeding could continue unnoticed under blanket if it is not halted before infant is re-wrapped.
9. Record result on infant chart. Report finding over 175 mg/100 ml or under 45 mg/100 ml.	9. Values under 45 mg/100 ml suggest hypoglycemia. Values over 175 mg/100 ml suggest hyperglycemia.
10. Evaluate procedure for safety, efficiency, and cost effectiveness. Plan health teaching for parents about necessity for puncture and importance of observing site for bleeding if infant will be with them for the next hour.	10. Health teaching is an integrated part of all nursing care.

Postprocedure Precaution: Assess puncture site q15min for next hour to be certain that complete hemostasis has been achieved.

47-22), and has a greater chance of having a congenital anomaly than do other infants. Most such babies have a cushingoid (fat and puffy) appearance. They tend to be lethargic or limp in the first days of life. The large size results from overstimulation of pituitary growth hormone during pregnancy and extra fat deposits due to high levels of glucose during pregnancy. The infant's large size is deceptive. Such babies are often immature, born at 36 to 38 weeks' of gestation. The lungs may be very immature. A term frequently used for these infants, which implies the amount of care they need, is *fragile giant.*

Infants of diabetic women tend to have polycythemia. They will have their cord clamped early at delivery to prevent an overload of red blood cells from passing into them from the placenta. An infant of a diabetic mother loses a greater proportion of weight in the first few days of life than does the average baby, because of the

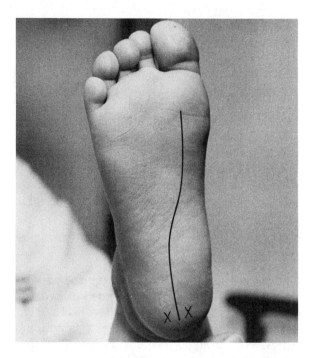

Figure 47-21 *Sites for a heel prick for a blood sample. Avoid the exact center of the heel to avoid the medial plantar artery.*

loss of extra fluid accumulation. The baby needs to be observed closely to be certain that this large weight loss actually represents a loss of extra fluid and that dehydration is not occurring. Because congenital anomalies occur more often in infants of diabetic mothers than in other infants, such infants should have a careful newborn

Figure 47-22 *Infant of a diabetic mother. Note the large size and the chubbiness. Although exceptionally large, the child is immature, a fragile giant. (Courtesy of the Department of Medical Photography, Children's Hospital, Buffalo, N.Y.)*

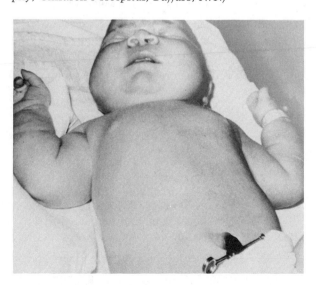

anomaly appraisal. Respiratory distress syndrome (hyaline membrane disease) occurs frequently in these infants because lecithin pathways do not mature as rapidly in them. High insulin secretion during pregnancy by the fetus to counteract the hyperglycemia may interfere with cortisol release; this blocks the formation of lecithin or prevents lung maturity.

Immediately after birth, an infant tends to be hyperglycemic because the mother was probably slightly hyperglycemic during the pregnancy, allowing excessive glucose to diffuse across the placenta. The fetal pancreas responded to the high glucose level by islet cell hypertrophy, resulting in matching high levels of insulin. Following delivery, the glucose level in the infant begins to fall because the mother's circulation is no longer supplying the infant. The overproduction of insulin causes the development of severe hypoglycemia, which makes the first 6 hours of life an infant's most hazardous. The problem remains a real possibility for the first 24 hours.

Assessment

The clinical signs of hypoglycemia are tremors, lethargy, poor sucking, apnea, hypotonia, hypothermia, and convulsions from lack of glucose to body cells. An infant should have a Dextrostix determination done at birth, which is repeated every 30 minutes until the glucose level has stabilized. Although most infants with hypoglycemia show definite signs, a few may appear asymptomatic and yet have severe hypoglycemia. Rely on the Dextrostix determination in infants of diabetic mothers, not on your intuition.

Hyperbilirubinemia also tends to occur in these infants, probably because they are unable to clear bilirubin from their system at this immature age. An infant therefore needs bilirubin levels monitored, so that treatment may be initiated if the level rises above safe limits.

It is difficult to think of babies of diabetic mothers as immature because they are so large. They *are* immature, however, so they may have more difficulty with mucus than more mature babies.

If a mother had class D diabetes, the infant tends to be small for gestation age because of poor placental perfusion. The problems of hypoglycemia, hypocalcemia, and hyperbilirubinemia remain the same.

Analysis

Nursing diagnoses concerned with infants of diabetic mothers usually involve the potential for hypoglycemia or difficulty with bonding. Bonding is apt to be a problem because the infant may have to be transferred to a special center for care.

Implementation

Early oral or intravenous feeding of a glucose solution is almost always necessary to prevent severe hypoglycemia. In addition to blood sugar determinations, an infant should have a calcium level obtained, since hypocalcemia often accompanies hypoglycemia in these infants. Parathyroid glands, which regulate the calcium level, appear to hypertrophy in utero, also, and so a similar rebound effect occurs. The baby may need supplemental calcium administration as well.

An infant must have follow-up care after discharge from the hospital because of the risk of becoming diabetic at a later date. Diabetes will develop in about 2 percent of these infants by the time they are 20 years of age.

Evaluation

The mother needs frequent assurance that the infant is well, assuming that the baby has made the transition from intrauterine life to extrauterine life without trauma. Only when she thinks of the child as well can she begin deep maternal-child interaction.

Hypocalcemia

Hypocalcemia is a lowered blood calcium level. Phosphorus and calcium levels are maintained in indirect proportion to each other in the bloodstream. That is, if phosphorus levels rise, calcium levels decrease; if calcium levels rise, phosphorus levels decrease. Hypocalcemia may be due, therefore, to changes in either calcium or phosphorus metabolism.

Hypocalcemia tends to occur in infants who had birth anoxia (phosphorus is released with anoxia), immature infants (the parathyroid gland, which controls calcium metabolism is immature), and infants of diabetic mothers (parathyroid glands are hypertrophied). It may be caused by the imbalance between phosphorus and calcium in milk (such an imbalance does not exist in breast milk and is modified in commercial formulas). If tetany is going to be caused by cow's milk, it occurs at about the seventh day of life. A community health nurse making a follow-up visit after a home birth might recognize the problem initially.

Latent Tetany

The chief sign of hypocalcemia is neuromuscular irritability, often referred to as *latent tetany*. This occurs when the serum calcium level is less than 7.5 mg per 100 ml of blood. The newborn is jittery when handled or cries for extended periods.

Manifest Tetany

If the serum calcium level falls well under 7 mg per 100 ml of blood, manifest tetany may result. Muscular twitching and carpopedal spasms are the usual signs of this kind of tetany. A *carpal* (hand) spasm involves abduction of the hand and flexion of the wrist with the thumb positioned across the palm. In *pedal* (foot) spasm, the foot is extended, the toes flex, and the sole of the foot cups. Generalized seizures may occur. There may be spasm of the larynx, during which an infant emits a high-pitched crowing sound on inspiration because of the constricted airway. If the spasm is prolonged, respirations may cease.

Assessment

There are four ways to produce the clinical manifestations of tetany for diagnosis of hypocalcemia; these are all useful tests (see Table 47-10) to determine or suggest whether newborn jitteriness is from hypocalcemia, a central nervous system problem, or some other cause.

The presence of hypocalcemia is confirmed by a low serum calcium level on laboratory testing.

Table 47-10 Assessment for Hypocalcemia

Sign	Description
Chvostek's	When the skin anterior to the external ear (just over the sixth cranial nerve) is tapped, the facial muscles surrounding the eye, nose, and mouth contract unilaterally.
Trousseau's	When the upper arm is constricted by a tourniquet for 2 to 3 minutes and the area becomes blanched, carpal spasm is elicited (the hand abducts, the wrist flexes, and the thumb is positioned across the cupped palm).
Peroneal	When the fibular side of the leg over the peroneal nerve is tapped, the foot abducts and dorsiflexes.
Erb's	Although this test is a dramatic one to see demonstrated, it requires a mild galvanic current and so cannot be used routinely as a test in a newborn nursery. A newborn with tetany has greater muscular irritability than a person with a normal calcium level. When mild current is applied to the infant, usually over the peroneal nerve just below the head of the fibula, the foot on that side will abduct and dorsiflex.

Analysis

Nursing diagnoses concerned with the newborn with hypocalcemia usually involve the potential for difficulty with respiratory function due to laryngeal spasm.

Implementations

Treatment for hypocalcemia is aimed toward increasing the serum calcium level in the blood to the point above the level that leads to latent tetany. Calcium may be administered orally as 10 percent calcium chloride if the infant can and will suck. It can be given intravenously as a 10 percent solution of calcium gluconate if the tetany has progressed to a point at which the child does not have enough muscular coordination to take oral fluid safely. Calcium gluconate should not be given intramuscularly or subcutaneously, since necrosis may occur at the injection site. If the newborn is having generalized seizures, he may require sodium phenobarbital in addition to the calcium gluconate to halt the seizures. Emergency equipment for intubation to relieve laryngospasm should be available.

Following the immediate therapy to increase the low serum blood levels, the infant will be placed on oral calcium therapy until it can be demonstrated that the calcium level has been regulated. Since vitamin D is necessary for the absorption of calcium and phosphorus from the gastrointestinal tract, an infant may be given a vitamin D supplement also.

Evaluation

The infant needs continued careful observation until it is confirmed that calcium metabolism is stabilized.

Disorders of the Hemopoietic System

Disorders of the hemopoietic system are always potentially serious disorders in newborns because of the importance of cardiovascular function for life. Diagnosis of these disorders depends on nursing observation because they generally begin with subtle signs and symptoms.

Hemorrhagic Disease of the Newborn

Hemorrhagic disease of the newborn is excessive bleeding in the newborn period due to low vitamin K levels. With the routine administration of AquaMEPHYTON to all newborns at birth, this entity is almost never seen today.

Vitamin K deficiency leads to deficiency of blood clotting factors II, VII, IX, and X. Hemorrhagic disease of the newborn typically begins on the second to fifth day of life. It involves massive hemorrhages in many parts of the body, including the meninges, ventricles of the brain, pulmonary alveoli, and liver. This tragic development could be easily prevented by a prophylactic measure at birth. When difficulty occurs at birth (the infant needs resuscitation or the mother hemorrhages), personnel are often so geared to giving emergency care that routine measures can be forgotten. An infant born at home may not receive vitamin K at birth. Be certain to check that all newborns receive this prophylactic treatment against hemorrhage.

Polycythemia

Polycythemia (an increased number of red blood cells) must be interpreted in the light of normal newborn values or many newborns would be considered to have polycythemia. In a newborn, a normal hemoglobin level is 14 to 21 gm per 100 ml; a normal hematocrit is 50 to 53 percent. Polycythemia in a term newborn is therefore defined as a hemoglobin over 22 gm per 100 ml or a hematocrit over 65 percent (Avery, 1981).

This problem may occur from maternal-fetal transfusion, twin-to-twin transfusion (the recipient twin), delayed cord clamping (which allows more than the usual amount of blood to infuse into a child), and placental insufficiency (which may reduce the amount of plasma in relation to red blood cells).

The increased viscosity of blood caused by the high percentage of red blood cells makes it more difficult for a child to pump blood through the circulating system; this inability can lead to respiratory distress (if unable to circulate blood well through the lungs) and congestive heart failure. Infants appear unusually ruddy in complexion. They are prone to thrombus formation. As the extra red blood cells are destroyed, they become prone to hyperbilirubinemia.

If an infant has an elevated hematocrit but no clinical signs other than a ruddy complexion, he may be merely observed closely and screened frequently for indirect bilirubin level. Assess the fluid intake carefully so that the baby does not become dehydrated, which will further increase the viscosity of the blood. Prevent extensive crying, which can result in increased insensible fluid loss from the lungs. If placed under bilirubin lights, the infant may need glucose water offered every 2 hours in addition to breast- or formula-feeding in order to be certain that hydration is maintained.

It is possible for the infant's blood supply to be

diluted by exchange transfusion of plasma. Just transfusing plasma without removing red cells would overload the circulation and complicate, not relieve, the blood picture.

Hyperbilirubinemia

When hyperbilirubinemia occurs in a newborn, it is usually the result of immature liver function, hemolytic disease of the newborn (erythroblastosis), infection, or bruising. Factors that make infants prone to hyperbilirubinemia are listed in Table 47-11.

Physiologic Jaundice

It is common for infants to have immature liver function at birth—so common that jaundice from this cause occurring after the third day of

Table 47-11 Factors that Make Infants Prone to Hyperbilirubinemia

Factor	Result
Premature birth	Liver is immature.
Blood group incompatibilities	Liver is unable to process the bilirubin released from the excessive breakdown of red blood cells.
Sepsis	Under stress the liver is unable to process indirect bilirubin.
Gastrointestinal obstruction	Bilirubin is reabsorbed from the bowel.
Increased red blood cell volume (polycythemia)	The liver is unable to process the bilirubin released from excessive breakdown of red blood cells.
Extensive ecchymosis	As ecchymotic blood is absorbed and destroyed, excessive bilirubin is released.
Cephalhematoma	As the blood from the cephalhematoma is absorbed and destroyed, excessive bilirubin is released.
Intrauterine infections	Under stress, the liver is unable to process indirect bilirubin.
Breast-feeding	The breakdown product of progesterone (pregnanediol) interferes with the process of bilirubin degradation.
Congenital hypothyroidism or galactosemia	Under stress and altered metabolism, the liver is unable to process indirect bilirubin.

life is normal in newborns. This type of jaundice occurs because fetal red blood cells are broken down rapidly after birth as the excess red blood cells needed during intrauterine life to transport oxygen are no longer needed. As red blood cells are destroyed, heme and globin, a protein, are released. Globin is reused by the body, and heme is further broken down into iron and protoporphyrin. Iron is reused by the body. Protoporphyrin breaks down into indirect bilirubin. Indirect bilirubin is fat-soluble and therefore cannot be excreted by the kidneys. It is transported bound to serum albumin to the liver, where it must be converted to direct bilirubin (which is water-soluble and incorporated into bile for excretion) by the liver enzyme glucuronyl transferase.

When liver function is immature, glucuronyl transferase cannot convert all the indirect bilirubin to direct bilirubin. Indirect bilirubin thus begins to accumulate in the infant's bloodstream, causing jaundice. If levels of indirect bilirubin rise above 20 mg per 100 ml, a lethal condition, kernicterus, may develop (the indirect bilirubin level in brain tissue rises and destroys brain cells). Symptoms such as poor feeding, lethargy, and loss of the Moro reflex are the beginning signs of kernicterus. Also present may be opisthotonos and a high-pitched cry. Many babies in whom the symptoms of kernicterus develop die. The rest may be left mentally retarded or with neuromotor retardation. The exact level at which kernicterus will occur cannot be predicted in individual infants. Those who are acidotic or immature or have decreased serum albumin may have damage at much lower levels of indirect bilirubin than infants without these factors present.

In jaundice due to immature liver function (physiologic jaundice), indirect bilirubin rarely rises above 12 mg per 100 ml in a mature infant. It seldom becomes apparent before the third day of life or lasts past the first week of life.

Infants who are small for gestation age or are of low birth weight tend to have higher indirect bilirubin levels than do mature infants. Their bilirubin levels need to be monitored closely; although they have physiologic jaundice, levels can rise to toxic amounts in these infants.

Hemolytic Disease of the Newborn

The term *hemolytic* is Latin for "destruction" (lysis) of red blood cells. Traditionally, hemolytic disease of the newborn (HDN) is thought of as occurring from an Rh incompatibility. Because prevention of Rh antibody formation has been available for over 20 years, the disorder is now most often caused by an ABO incompatibility. In both these instances, a mother builds antibodies against the fetal red blood cells, leading to cell hemolysis (destruction). The destruction of red blood cells causes severe anemia and severe hyperbilirubinemia.

Rh Incompatibility. Theoretically no direct connection exists between the fetal and maternal circulation so no fetal blood cells enter the maternal circulation. In actuality, occasional placental villi break and a drop or two of fetal blood does enter maternal circulation. If a mother is Rh negative and the fetal blood is Rh positive (contains the D antigen) sensitization occurs—or the mother begins to form IgG D antibodies against it. Very few antibodies form this way, however. Most form in the mother's bloodstream in the first 72 hours following birth because of the exchange of fetal-maternal blood as placental villi loosen and the placenta is delivered.

With a second pregnancy, this interaction will cause a high level of antibody D in the mother's bloodstream acting to destroy the fetal red blood cells at the beginning of the pregnancy. By the end of a second pregnancy, the fetus may be severely compromised by the action of these antibodies crossing the placenta to destroy red blood cells. Some fetuses will need to receive intrauterine transfusions to combat red cell destruction. They may be delivered early because of the destructive maternal environment.

Hemolytic disease of the newborn can be predicted by finding a rising anti-Rh titer or rising level of antibodies (indirect Coombs' test) in the mother during pregnancy. It can be confirmed by detecting antibodies on the infant's erythrocytes in cord blood (positive direct Coombs' test) at birth. The mother in this situation will always have Rh-negative blood (dd), and the baby will be Rh positive (DD or Dd).

An infant may not appear pale at birth despite the red cell destruction that has gone on in utero, because the acceleration of red cell production during the last few months in utero may have compensated for the destruction to some degree. He does not appear jaundiced as the maternal circulation has evacuated the rising bilirubin level. Enlargement of the liver and spleen from an attempt to produce new blood cells may be present. If the number of red cells present has fallen drastically, blood in the vascular circulation will have become hypotonic to interstitial fluid; fluid will have shifted from the lower isotonic to higher isotonic pressure by the law of osmosis, causing extreme edema and congestive heart failure from the severe anemia present.

Hydrops fetalis is an old term for the appearance of a severely involved infant at birth, referring to the edema (hydrops) and the lethal state. Despite the fall in the level of red blood cells in normal newborns after birth, the hemoglobin of newborns actually increases during the first day of life. This increase is due in part to transfusion of placental blood and in part to a shift of fluid from the intravascular to the extravascular spaces. By age 7 to 10 days, the hemoglobin level returns to that observed in the cord blood. These infants will show a decrease in hemoglobin during the first week of life to a level less than that of cord blood, indicative of blood loss or hemolysis. Progressive jaundice, usually occurring within the first 24 hours of life, will reveal that a hemolytic process is at work. Progressive hypoglycemia occurs with Rh hemolytic disease because of liver stress in at least 20 percent of infants, compounding their initial problem.

ABO Incompatibility. Hemolysis of a newborn may occur in the first pregnancy if an ABO incompatibility is present. In most of these instances, the maternal blood type is O and the fetal blood type is A; it may occur when a fetus has type B or AB blood. An infant with B blood often has the most serious reaction.

Hemolysis can become a problem with a *first* pregnancy in which there is an ABO incompatibility because the production of antibodies to A and B cell types are naturally occurring antibodies or are present from birth in individuals whose red cells lack these antigens. Unlike the antibodies formed against the Rh D factor, these antibodies are the large IgM class and so do not cross the placenta well. The infant with an ABO incompatibility therefore is not born anemic, as is the Rh-sensitized child. Hemolysis of the blood begins with birth, however, when blood and antibodies are exchanged as maternal and fetal blood mixes, with loosening of the placenta. This leads to early jaundice in the newborn as red blood cells are lysed.

Interestingly, low-birth-weight infants do not seem to be affected by ABO incompatibility. This immunity may be because the receptor sites for anti-A or anti-B antibodies do not appear on red cells until late in fetal life. Even in the mature newborn, the direct Coombs' test may only be weakly positive because of the few anti-A or anti-B sites present. The reticulocyte count (immature or newly formed red blood cells) is usually elevated and reveals the infant's attempt to replace destroyed cells.

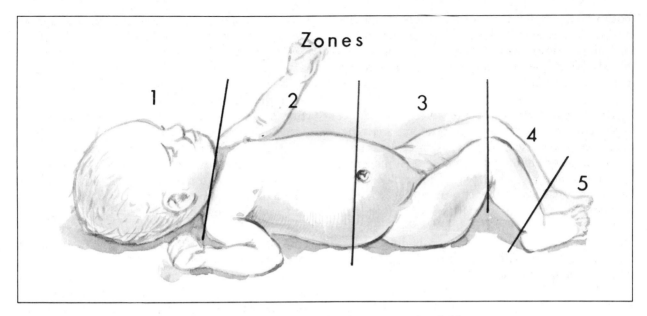

Figure 47-23 *Jaundice may be estimated to some degree by the zone on the child that it has reached. The indirect bilirubin level of zone 1 is 4 to 8 mg per 100 ml; of zone 2, 5 to 12 mg per 100 ml; of zone 3, 8 to 16 mg per 100 ml; of zone 4, 11 to 18 mg per 100 ml; of zone 5, 15 mg per 100 ml. (Based on data from Kramer, L. D. (1969). Advancement of dermal icterus in the jaundiced newborn. American Journal of Diseases of Children, 118, 454.)*

Assessment

Jaundice becomes clinically apparent at about 7 mg of bilirubin per 100 ml of blood. At first, jaundice is seen only on the face. As it increases in severity, it affects the child's body also. The degree of bilirubin present may be estimated to some degree by observing how much of the infant's body is jaundiced (Figure 47-23).

Infants with extensive bruising (large babies, breech babies, immature babies) must be watched carefully for indirect bilirubin levels. Assess whether any tissue bruising is present. Bruising at birth leads to hemorrhage of blood into the subcutaneous tissue or skin. This blood is removed as bruising heals by breakdown of blood components. As the red blood cells are hemolyzed, indirect bilirubin is released. Cephalhematoma, or a collection of blood under the periosteum of the skull bone, can lead to the same phenomenon.

Assess for intestinal function. Indirect bilirubin is converted to direct bilirubin in the liver, becomes bile, and is excreted with stool. It is what gives stool its typical dark color. If intestinal obstruction is present and stool is not being evacuated, intestinal flora may break down bile back into its basic components and release indirect bilirubin into the bloodstream. Early feeding of newborns, then, promotes intestinal movement and excretion of meconium and prevents indirect bilirubin buildup from this source.

Analysis

Nursing diagnoses for infants with jaundice generally concern the potentials for injury from kernicterus, dehydration or interference with bonding related to phototherapy.

Planning

Suspension of breast feeding, phototherapy, and exchange transfusion may all be necessary to reduce indirect bilirubin levels in an infant affected by ABO or Rh incompatibility.

Suspension of Breast-Feeding. Pregnanediol, the breakdown product of progesterone, is excreted in breast milk until the high levels of progesterone that were present during pregnancy are excreted. Pregnanediol interferes with the conjugation of indirect bilirubin. Breast-fed babies, therefore, may evidence more jaundice than bottle-fed babies. Temporary suspension of breast-feeding for 24 hours may be necessary to reduce an accumulating indirect bilirubin level in some infants. If a mother manually expresses breast milk while feeding is halted, her milk supply will be maintained; this therapy is not a permanent contraindication to breast-feeding.

Phototherapy. An infant's liver processes little bilirubin in utero because the mother's circulation does this action for him. With birth, ex-

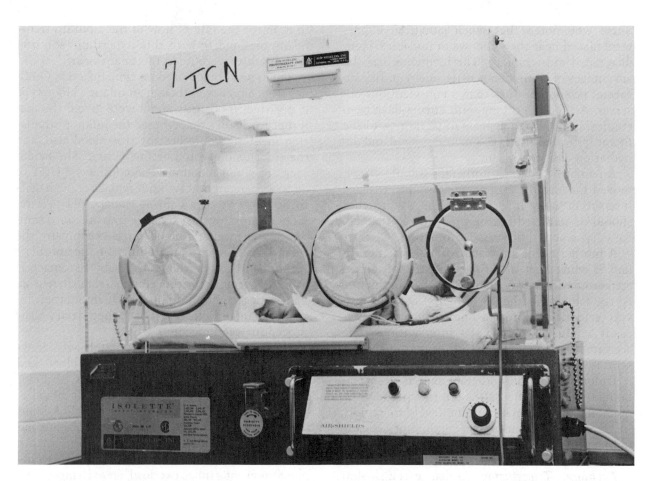

Figure 47-24 *A newborn receiving phototherapy. The infant is undressed except for the diaper. Notice how snugly the eyes are covered to protect them from the light source. (Courtesy of the Department of Medical Photography, Children's Hospital, Buffalo, N.Y.)*

posure to light apparently triggers the liver to assume this function. In many infants, liver immaturity causes its efficiency to be in doubt for the first few days of life; additional light appears to speed the conversion potential of the liver and reduce indirect bilirubin levels. Phototherapy is the light technique that is most often used today. In phototherapy, an infant is continuously exposed to three to six fluorescent light tubes with a total strength of 200 to 500 foot-candles. Although lights may be placed above an open bassinet they are usually placed over an Isolette; the infant is undressed except for the diaper, so that as much skin surface as possible is exposed to the light (Figure 47-24). The Plexiglass top of the Isolette should always be in place when the lights are on because it protects the infant from ultraviolet lights and burning.

Continuous exposure to a bright light may be harmful to a newborn's retina, and thus the eyes must be covered for the entire time the infant is under bilirubin lights. The infant's eyes are closed and then covered with eye dressings or cotton balls, which are then secured firmly in place by an additional dressing. The infant must be checked frequently to be certain the dressings have not slipped and are not causing corneal irritation.

The stools of an infant under bilirubin lights are often bright green from the excessive bilirubin that is excreted as a result of the therapy. They are also frequently loose and may be irritating to the skin; therefore good skin care is necessary with diaper changes. Urine may be dark colored from urobilinogen formation. An infant may lose considerable fluid through insensible water loss because of the temperature of the lights above him. Skin turgor should be assessed along with intake and output to ensure that dehydration is not occurring. Maintaining the infant's temperature between 96.8°F and 98.6°F (36°C and 37°C) prevents a baby from overheating under the bright lights. Increase the fluid intake by offering glucose water every 2 hours.

Phototherapy is a relatively new technique, only available since the early 1960s. It was first discovered to be effective due to the reports of a nurse who noted that when jaundiced infants were placed near the windows in nurseries, jaundice faded most rapidly. The technique has the advantages of being inexpensive and requiring no special personnel other than a conscientious observer. Although no long-term effects have been studied as yet, there appears to be no risk to the infant, provided the eyes remain covered and dehydration does not occur.

An infant under phototherapy should be removed for feeding so that he continues to have interaction with his mother. The eye patches should be removed during this time so that the baby has a period of visual stimulation.

A mother needs an explanation of why her infant is being kept under special lights. Isolettes are automatically associated with very ill infants. At the same time, the use of lights does not seem very scientific (almost a home remedy). She is easily confused by the two interventions, one seemingly serious and the other seemingly not serious at all.

Unfortunately, phototherapy may take several hours to have an effect. It is not the first method of choice, therefore, if bilirubin levels are rapidly rising. In that instance, the method of clearing indirect bilirubin levels is exchange transfusion.

Exchange Transfusion. Exchange transfusion may be used for any condition that leads to hyperbilirubinemia or polycythemia. When used as therapy for blood incompatibility, it removes about 85 percent of sensitized red cells. It reduces the serum concentration of indirect bilirubin and often prevents congestive heart failure in infants. Because indirect bilirubin levels rise at relatively predictable levels, exchange transfusion would be performed if the bilirubin concentration exceeds 5 mg per 100 ml at birth, 10 mg per 100 ml at 8 hours, 12 mg per 100 ml at 16 hours, and 15 mg per 100 ml at 24 hours of age or if serum bilirubin is rising more than 0.5 mg per hour in Rh incompatibility, 1.0 mg per hour in an ABO incompatibility (Klaus, 1979). These criteria prevent indirect serum bilirubin level reaching kernicterus levels: 20 mg per 100 ml of blood in mature infants; 8 to 12 mg per 100 ml in immature infants.

The infant must be kept warm during exchange transfusion so he does not expend energy on metabolism. The blood being given must be maintained at room temperature, or shock can result. Warm blood this way only by using a commercial blood warming unit, not by hot towels or a radiant heat warmer to avoid destroying red cells. Albumin may be administered 1 to 2 hours prior to the procedure to increase the number of bilirubin-binding sites available and increase the efficiency of the transfusion. Be extremely careful

to monitor the rate of flow of the albumin transfusion as rapid flow of this hypertonic solution will quickly overburden the infant heart.

The type of blood used for transfusion is O Rh-negative blood even though an infant's blood type is positive; if positive blood were given, the maternal antibodies that entered the infant's circulation in utero would destroy this blood also, and the transfusion would be ineffective. The hematocrit of donor blood used should have a HCT of 45 to 55 percent or it will not replace enough cells to be effective. If a baby is transported to a regional center for the exchange transfusion, a sample of the mother's blood must accompany the infant, so that cross-matching on the mother's serum can be done there. The baby's stomach is aspirated prior to the procedure so that there is no danger of aspiration due to the manipulation involved. The umbilical vein is catheterized for the procedure (see Procedure 47-2).

Exchange transfusion is alternately withdrawing minute amounts of the infant's blood and then replacing it with equal amounts of donor blood. About 2 to 4 ml of the infant's blood is withdrawn and discarded and 2 to 4 ml of donor blood is infused, and so forth for the procedure (an aliquot may be as large as 20 ml in a term infant). Because the blood must be exchanged at this slow rate to prevent cardiac overload, an exchange transfusion takes 1 to 2 hours. An automatic pump is being devised that can take over this exhausting ritual. A hematocrit, bilirubin, electrolytes (especially calcium), glucose determination, and blood culture are determined at the end of the procedure by using the last aliquot of blood withdrawn.

A baby must be carefully monitored during an exchange transfusion; heart rate, respirations, and venous pressure all must be observed. The amount of blood given is usually calculated as follows: 85 ml × weight (in kilograms) × 2. The average blood volume of a newborn is 86 ml per kilogram, but an amount equal to twice the blood volume is used because this quantity will ensure an exchange of erythrocytes that is 85 to 90 percent effective. Because stored blood for transfusion contains acid-citrate-dextrose (ACD) (which can lower blood calcium levels and cause acidosis) added to it as an anticoagulant, calcium gluconate should be given through the exchange catheter after each 100 ml of blood to counteract its effect. If citrate-phosphate-dextrose (CPD) is used as a preservative, the reaction is less severe than with ACD, but the problems of decreased calcium and acidosis are still present. Because a load of glucose is given during the transfusion by administration of the calcium gluconate, the infant may become hyperglycemic during the transfusion; this will be followed by insulin

Procedure 47-2

Assisting with Umbilical Vessel Catheterization

Purpose: Assist with provision of a vessel site for fluid administration or a port for blood drawing.

Plan	*Principle*
1. Wash your hands; identify patient.	1. Prevent spread of microorganisms; assure patient safety.
2. Assess patient status; analyze appropriateness of procedure; plan any modifications necessary.	2. Nursing care is always individualized to meet patient needs.
3. Implement care by assembling supplies: sterile pack containing forceps, scissors, needle holder, hemostat, syringe, umbilical tape or suture material, 3-way stopcock, drape; umbilical catheter 3.5–5F; tincture of benzoin; intravenous fluid and tubing (flushed to remove all air); infusion pump; heparinized solution for flushing catheter.	3. Organizing equipment prevents undue exposure of the infant.
4. Place infant in a supine position on a prewarmed radiant heat warmer. Apply servocontrol lead to abdomen. Attach cardiac monitor leads and check function of monitor. Restrain infant arms and legs as necessary. Provide a good light source.	4. Maintaining the infant's temperature during the procedure is a major nursing responsibility.
5. Assist primary caregiver to scrub hands and don mask, cap, sterile gown and gloves.	5. Prevent spread of microorganisms.
6. Assist as needed while the umbilical cord is scrubbed with bacteriocidal solution and a drape is placed over umbilical area. A purse-string suture is placed around the cord or sterile umbilical tape is secured around the cord. The umbilical cord is then cut 1 cm from the abdomen. The vessels are identified, dilated with a forceps; the umbilical catheter is threaded into the chosen vessel.	6. Be certain to keep infant still as a sudden movement could cause the umbilical cord to be torn.
7. Attach IV tubing to catheter by a 3-way stopcock; adjust to designated flow rate or assist with filling of catheter with flush solution.	7. Prevent blood clotting in catheter which could lead to embolus.
8. Apply tincture of benzoin to abdomen; tape catheter in place.	8. Avoid dislodgement of catheter.
9. Assist with X-ray as necessary.	9. An X-ray is taken to demonstrate position of catheter.
10. Assess pulse, respiratory rate, and color and temperature of lower extremities.	10. Cyanosis, mottling, or cool temperature suggests that the catheter blocks lower extremity circulation, necessitating position adjustment or removal.
11. Evaluate effectiveness of procedure; plan health teaching such as advantage of umbilical site to parents.	11. Health teaching is an independent action always included in nursing care.
12. Record procedure, and condition of infant.	12. Document nursing care and patient status.

overproduction and hypoglycemia following the transfusion. If heparinized blood is used, the heparin content may interfere with clotting following the transfusion, and, as it has a relatively low glucose concentration, it may also lead to hypoglycemia. Administering protamine sulfate following the exchange aids in the metabolism of heparin and restoration of clotting ability.

Following the transfusion, an infant must be observed closely for umbilical bleeding and changes from normal in vital signs (take vital signs every 15 minutes for 1 hour, then every 30 minutes for 3 hours). Do a Dextrostix reading every hour postexchange for 2 hours. In addition, the infant needs bilirubin levels monitored for 2 or 3 days following transfusion, to make certain that the level of bilirubin is not rising again and another transfusion is necessary.

Necrotizing endocolitis may occur following exchange transfusion. Thus an infant needs to be monitored for signs of this problem (see page 1203). Assess the umbilical vein for signs of infection (warmth and redness).

Blood Transfusion. Infants who have had hemolytic disease of the newborn tend to have a progressive drop in the hemoglobin concentration during the first 6 months of life as the bone marrow fails to increase its production of erythrocytes in response to some continuing hemolysis. The infant may need a transfusion of blood in order to correct this late anemia.

A newborn can be transfused by a peripheral vein but thrombophlebitis may occur at the site due to the stretching and irritation from such a viscous fluid as blood infusing. Blood is often, therefore, infused by the umbilical vein or artery. The umbilical vein is easier technically to catheterize than an umbilical artery so is often used for transfusion of blood or blood expansion products such as plasma.

Blood Loss Anemia

Blood loss anemia may occur for a number of reasons: fetal-maternal transfusion (placental blood going in to the mother's circulation), twin transfusion (blood is shunted away from one twin to the other), traumatic blood loss from a tear in the cord or spleen, or internal bleeding such as hemorrhage into the ventricles.

Fetal Maternal Transfusion

As mentioned in the discussion on blood incompatibility, some fetal blood enters the maternal circulation in at least 50 percent of all pregnancies as the placenta loosens. If the exchanged amount is over 40 ml (7% of the infant's circula-

tion), it can result in symptomatic anemia. This complication can also occur if an amniocentesis is traumatic (a placenta is punctured); it may be more frequent with oxytocin infusion used to induce labor because of the force of the uterine contractions. That fetal red cells are present in the maternal blood can be demonstrated by a laboratory test for their different composition.

Twin-to-Twin Transfusion

Twin-to-twin transfusion can occur if twins are identical (share the same placenta) and abnormal arteriovenous shunts occur that direct more blood to one twin than the other. The process may occur in as many as one-third of all identical twin pregnancies but only enough blood is exchanged to be clinically important in 15 percent of such pregnancies. The result of this shift of blood will lead to anemia in the donor twin and polycythemia in the receiving twin. The anemic twin may also be small for gestational age because of the lack in nutrients or oxygen for growth; and this same small-for-gestational-age twin will be prone to hypoglycemia from lack of glucose stores. He or she will appear pale next to the polycythemic twin, who is prone to hyperbilirubinemia as the excessive red blood cell level is broken down.

All identical twins should have hemoglobin determinations done at birth and the results compared. A difference of over 5.0 gm per 100 ml is enough to suggest that a transfusion has occurred. Each twin needs therapy as indicated by the extent of the distribution. The donor twin may need a transfusion to establish a functioning blood level; the recipient twin may need an exchange transfusion to reduce the polycythemia and viscosity of his blood.

Birth Trauma

A torn umbilical cord, a placenta previa, or lacerated placenta at cesarean birth may be sources of blood loss at birth. Normal cord blood has a hemoglobin level of 17 to 18 gm per 100 ml. A level below 13.5 gm per 100 ml indicates anemia.

An infant with blood loss anemia appears pale. Respirations may be grunting and distressed because of poor lung perfusion. Although an infant seems to be in respiratory distress, little cyanosis is seen (cyanosis is caused by unoxygenated hemoglobin; if little hemoglobin is present—under 5 gm/100 ml—cyanosis will not be evident) and oxygen administration does not improve color.

The cord blood may not reflect the degree of blood loss if bleeding is continuing. Blood must be drawn from the infant for a true picture. For all forms of anemia, blood transfusion may be necessary. Replacement of iron stores by an oral iron preparation over the next few months may be indicated.

Postbirth Hemorrhage

Newborn infants rarely hemorrhage externally; they can hemorrhage internally, however, from the pressure and trauma of birth. If the hemorrhage is extensive, signs and symptoms may occur immediately. As a rule, however, bleeding is slow but steady and so symptoms do not become evident until 24 to 72 hours after birth. In a preterm infant, hemorrhage into the ventricles or subarachnoid space may occur following hypoxic episodes. These will produce neurologic symptoms that are severe. They will cause jaundice as the pooled blood is broken down and reabsorbed.

Iatrogenic Blood Loss

Iatrogenic means related to health care procedures. Iatrogenic anemia can occur, especially in preterm infants, if sample after sample of blood is removed for laboratory analysis with no concern toward replacing it. Anemia begins to develop at the point that 10 to 15 percent of an infant's blood is removed over 24 to 48 hours. Keeping an accurate record of the amount and time of each blood sample withdrawn allows transfusion to replace removed blood as necessary. A newborn has a blood supply of 85 ml per kilogram of body weight. Thus a 7-pound infant has a total blood volume of about 300 ml, and 30 ml, then, represents 10 percent of the blood volume. In a 4-pound preterm infant, 10 ml represents this critical level.

Respiratory Illness

Respiratory illness in a newborn is always potentially serious because of the importance of respiratory function.

Transient Tachypnea of the Newborn (Respiratory Distress, Type II or TTN)

At birth, a newborn may have a rapid rate of respiration, up to 80 breaths per minute when crying; within an hour this rapid rate slows to between 30 and 50. In some infants, respiratory rate remains at a high level, between 80 and 120 per minute. The infant does not appear to be in a great deal of distress aside from the tiring effort of breathing so fast. Mild retractions can be noted but no marked cyanosis. Mild hypoxia and hypercapnia may be present. Feeding is difficult for the child, who cannot suck and breathe this rapidly at the same time. A chest X-ray reveals some fluid in the central lung but aeration is adequate.

Transient tachypnea appears to result from slow absorption of lung fluid. This delay limits the amount of alveolar surface available to the infant for oxygen exchange, and he must increase the respiratory rate and depth to better use the surface available. Transient tachypnea of the newborn occurs more often in infants who are born by cesarean birth and in preterm infants. These infants are probably more prone to development of respiratory distress because the thoracic cavity is not compressed by the force of vaginal birth and so less lung fluid is expelled than normally.

An infant needs close observation to see that the increased effort is not too tiring. Another concern is that the signs are not simply slow absorption of lung fluid but rather the beginning signs of a more serious disorder (a rapid rate of respirations is often the first sign of respiratory obstruction in infants). Transient tachypnea of the newborn peaks in intensity at about 36 hours of life, then begins to fade until by 72 hours it disappears as the lung fluid is absorbed and respiratory activity becomes effective.

Meconium Aspiration Syndrome

An infant who has hypoxia in utero has a vagal reflex relaxation of the rectal sphincter with release of meconium into the amniotic fluid. Babies born breech may expel meconium into the amniotic fluid. The appearance of meconium-stained fluid is green to greenish black.

At the time of the initial distress or with the first breath, if the infant inhales any of the fluid, he aspirates meconium. Meconium may cause severe respiratory distress in two ways: It can bring about inflammation of bronchioles because it is a foreign substance, or it may block small bronchioles by mechanical plugging. Hypoxemia, CO_2 retention, and intra- and extrapulmonary shunting occur. A secondary infection of injured tissue may lead to pneumonia. Meconium staining occurs in approximately 10 percent of all pregnancies, and in about 10 percent of pregnancies with meconium staining, the fetus aspirates fluid with meconium (Bancalari 1978).

Assessment

Infants with meconium-stained amniotic fluid may have difficulty establishing respirations at birth (those who were not breech-born have had a hypoxic episode in utero to cause the meconium to be in the amniotic fluid). The Apgar score is apt to be low. Almost immediately, tachypnea, retractions, and cyanosis occur. Oxygen under pressure (bag and mask) should not be administered until the infant has been intubated and suctioned so that the pressure of the oxygen does not drive small plugs of meconium farther down into the lungs, worsening the irritation and obstruction.

Following the initiation of respirations, an infant's respiration rate may remain elevated (tachypnea); coarse bronchial sounds may be heard on auscultation. The baby may continue to have retractions; the inflammation of bronchi tends to trap air in alveoli—the way an asthmatic traps alveolar air. The chest may become enlarged in its anteroposterior diameter (barrel chest) due to this air trapping. Blood gases will reveal the poor exchange of air. A chest X-ray film will show bilateral coarse infiltrates in the lung with spaces of hyperaeration (a peculiar honeycomb effect). The diaphragm will be pushed downward.

Analysis

Nursing diagnoses concerned with infants with meconium aspiration generally include their threat to oxygenation and bonding because the infant will need to be transferred to a level III center for care.

Implementations

An infant may require continued oxygen administration and assisted ventilation. Unfortunately, lung tissue is fairly noncompliant following meconium aspiration and so high inspiratory pressure may be necessary. This technique can cause pneumothorax or pneumomediastinum. Infants who are trapping air in alveoli must be observed closely for signs of this because alveoli can expand only so far and then will rupture, sending air into the pleural space. Because of the high pulmonary resistance, the ductus arteriosus may remain open, causing blood to shunt from the aorta into the pulmonary artery, compromising cardiac efficiency. An infant needs to be observed closely for signs of congestive heart failure (increased heart rate, exhaustion) that indicate this is happening. He must be kept in a thermal neutral environment to prevent the metabolic rate from rising and increasing the need for oxygen while the baby already has difficulty supplying cells due to this unfortunate birth trauma.

Postural drainage with clapping and vibration may be helpful to encourage removal of flecks of remaining meconium from the lungs. An infant may be treated with an antibiotic to forestall development of pneumonia as a secondary problem. Provided that an infant did not suffer a hypoxic incident in utero or during therapy that left him with neurologic impairment, the infant can be expected to recover completely in a number of days.

Pneumothorax

A pneumothorax is collection of air in the pleural space. This condition may occur at birth from overinflation and rupture of alveoli with the first breath, but it usually occurs as a result of ventilatory assistance. Air in the pleural space prevents the lung from expanding, making it difficult for the infant to inspire (negative pressure is lost); and atelectasis occurs (Figure 47-25).

An infant quickly develops extremely distressed respirations. The chest may appear asymmetrical; the trachea may be displaced away from the affected side. Cyanosis develops rapidly. The infant's abdomen may become distended from pressure on the diaphragm.

The heart will be displaced toward the unaffected side. A chest X-ray film will reveal the air-filled chest space. Transillumination is an easy, noninvasive procedure to use to detect pneumothorax. A bright light held behind an infant's chest will cause it to glow from the air-filled space taking the place of the collapsed lung.

The infant needs immediate oxygen, but it must be administered by hood or mask, not by pressure, or the problem may be compounded. The air in the pleural space must be withdrawn in order to allow the affected lung to reexpand. This can be done by needle aspiration. Chest tubes may be inserted to continue removal of air.

A pneumothorax is a shocking happening to the child's system, reducing respiratory capacity by 50 percent in a second's time. If treatment measures can be instituted promptly, an infant's prognosis from this sudden, possibly devastating occurrence is good.

Pneumomediastinum

Pneumomediastinum is collection of air in the mediastinal space. This condition leads not only to lung collapse but compression on the heart as well. Both respiratory and cardiac function is severely compromised. Air is removed in the same ways as with pneumothorax.

The Infant of a Drug-Dependent Mother

Infants of drug-dependent women tend to be small for gestation age. It is often difficult during pregnancy to predict a delivery date for many of these infants because of their small size and the woman's uncertainty about the date of her last menstrual period (women with drug dependence have irregular menses). Urine estriol levels are usually low in drug-addicted women and so are not a good guide to use to determine a due date;

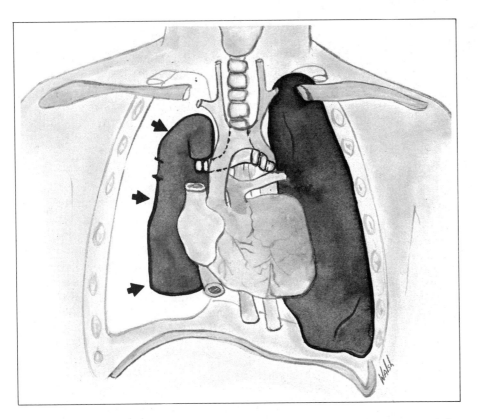

Figure 47-25 *Pneumothorax. Air has entered the pleural space and collapsed the right lung.*

they give false information as to placental status. The best guide to assess maturity seems to be the lecithin/sphingomyelin ratio of amniotic fluid (see Chapter 15).

Assessment

An infant born of a woman who is addicted to a narcotic such as morphine, heroin, or methadone will show withdrawal symptoms shortly after birth. Some women will tell you or the physician on admission to a hospital labor unit that they are addicted to such drugs to warn the health care personnel that their infant will have withdrawal symptoms. Other women, afraid of exposing their habit, will not reveal this information. Be suspicious of addiction in a woman who appears to obtain little relief from normal amounts of analgesics (remembering that there is a great deal of difference in people's pain thresholds), or who is overly anxious to be discharged shortly after delivery. Look for reddened streaks over veins or blackened needle puncture marks on the skin of a woman over the brachial or popliteal veins. Women who use cocaine have no nasal hair and possibly have inflamed nasal membranes.

Babies of drug-dependent women are usually irritable, with disturbed sleep patterns. They move so constantly that they cause abrasions on their elbows, knees, or nose. They may have tremors and may sneeze frequently. They may have a shrill, high-pitched cry like that of a brain-damaged infant. Hyperreflexia and clonus (neuromuscular irritability) may be present, and convulsions may occur. Many such infants have tachypnea (rapid respirations) so severe that hyperventilation and alkalosis develop. An infant may have frantic sucking activity. Vomiting and diarrhea may begin, leading to large fluid losses and secondary dehydration. These symptoms usually occur in the first 24 hours of life, although they may appear as late as at 7 days of age in heroin addiction, 2 weeks of age in methadone addiction, and 2 months of age in phenobarbital addiction.

Methadone-addicted infants tend to have an increased incidence of seizures as compared with heroin-addicted infants. One of the most frequent findings in methadone-addicted infants at 2 to 3 months of age is an excessive amount of fluid intake (40 to 50 ounces per day).

Narcotic metabolites or quinine (heroin is often mixed with quinine) may be obtained from an infant's urine in the first hour after birth. These products are quickly cleared from the body, however, and by the time symptoms become severe, detection of narcotic substances may no longer be possible. A neonatal drug withdrawal scoring system is shown in Table 47-12. Assessment using

Table 47-12 Items Used to Score Neonatal
Abstinence in the Nursery Newborn

Signs and Symptoms	Score
High-pitched cry	2
Continuous high-pitched cry	3
Sleeps less than 1 hour after feeding	3
Sleeps less than 2 hours after feeding	2
Sleeps less than 3 hours after feeding	1
Hyperactive Moro reflex	2
Markedly hyperactive Moro reflex	3
Mild tremors when disturbed	1
Marked tremors when disturbed	2
Mild tremors when undisturbed	3
Marked tremors when undisturbed	4
Increased muscle tone	2
Generalized convulsion	5
Frantic sucking of fists	1
Poor feeding	2
Regurgitation	2
Projectile vomiting	3
Loose stools	2
Watery stools	3
Dehydration	2
Frequent yawning	1
Sneezing	1
Nasal stuffiness	1
Sweating	1
Mottling	1
Fever less than 101°F	1
Fever greater than 101°F	2
Respiratory rate over 60 per minute	1
Respiratory rate over 60 per minute with retractions	2
Excoriation of nose	1
Excoriation of knees	1
Excoriation of toes	1

Source: Kron, R. E., et al. (1977). Behavior of infants born to drug-dependent mothers. Effects of prenatal and postnatal drugs. In Rementería, J. L. (Ed.), *Drug abuse in pregnancy and neonatal effects.* St. Louis: Mosby.

the scale is made hourly for the first 24 hours, every 2 hours for the next 24 hours, and every 4 hours thereafter. If an infant receives a score under 7 by this scale, he probably does not need drug withdrawal therapy. Such assessment can be done as an independent nursing action.

Analysis

Nursing diagnoses with infants of drug-dependent mothers usually concern nutrition or potential for injury related to an unsafe home environment.

Implementation

Infants of drug-dependent mothers usually seem most comfortable when firmly swaddled

(Figure 47-26). They should be kept in an environment free from excessive stimuli (a small isolation nursery, not a large, noisy one). Some quiet best if the room is darkened. Many infants of heroin-addicted women suck vigorously and continuously and seem to find comfort and quiet if given a pacifier. Infants of methadone-addicted women may have extremely poor sucking ability and may have difficulty getting enough fluid intake unless gavaged.

Specific therapy for an infant is individualized according to the nature and severity of the symptoms. The infant must have his electrolyte and fluid balance maintained. If he has vomiting or diarrhea, intravenous administration of fluid may be indicated. The drugs used to counteract withdrawal symptoms include paregoric, phenobarbital, codeine, methadone, chlorpromazine (Thorazine), and diazepam (Valium). An infant should not be breast-fed by an addicted mother to prevent additional drug being passed to him in breast milk.

Evaluation

Infants of heroin-addicted women are rarely jaundiced, probably because their liver matures faster in utero in response to its need to metabolize the heroin it is receiving. This does not apply to those women who were treated with methadone to relieve heroin addiction; their infants tend to have a higher-than-normal incidence of jaundice. Infants of heroin-addicted women also are likely to have a low incidence of respiratory distress syndrome despite their small size, again implying that they mature faster than usual in utero.

Once an infant is identified as having been exposed to drugs in utero, the mother needs treatment for withdrawal symptoms and follow-up care as much as does the infant. Whether an environment that allowed for this much drug abuse will be safe for an infant must be evaluated before the baby is discharged into the parent's care.

The Infant of an Alcohol-Dependent Mother (Fetal Alcohol Syndrome)

Alcohol crosses the placenta in the same concentration that it is present in the maternal bloodstream. When a woman ingests more than 3 ounces (two drinks) of 100 percent alcohol per day, her child may be born severely affected as a direct result of the alcohol or its oxidation product acetaldehyde on fetal growing cells. As the exact minimum amount of alcohol that could cause defects is not known, any amount of al-

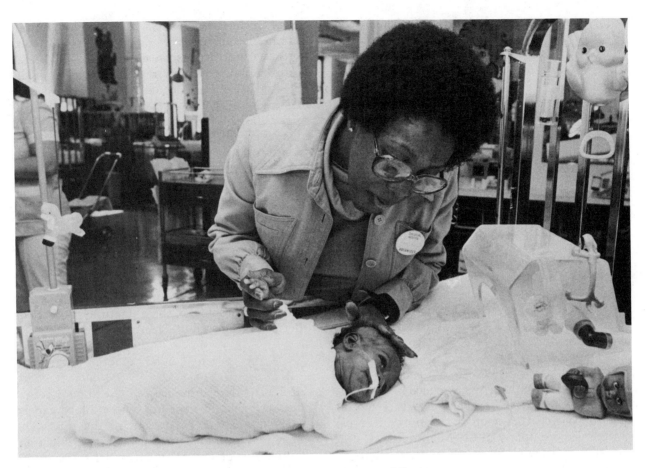

Figure 47-26 *Infants born of drug-addicted mothers enjoy tight swaddling at birth, as shown here. (Courtesy of the Department of Medical Photography, Children's Hospital, Buffalo, N.Y.)*

cohol ingested during pregnancy could have an effect on fetal growth and development.

Assessment

A mother with a high alcohol intake during pregnancy should be discovered by history taking. Frequent consequences in infants are prenatal and postnatal growth retardation, mental retardation, microcephaly, and joint and cardiac anomalies. Perinatal growth retardation is unusual in that these infants are short in length in comparison with weight. Usually with intrauterine growth retardation, weight is decreased in comparison with length. A baby may have difficulty feeding in the newborn period because of poor sucking. He may be irritable, tending to be always awake or always asleep, depending on the alcohol level of the mother close to delivery.

Analysis

Nursing diagnoses established with an infant are usually concerned with nutrition because the infant sucks poorly and with specific interventions related to congenital defects. Bonding may be a problem because the mother may feel guilty about the problem (and guilt makes it hard to deal with problems) and the child is irritable and hard to satisfy.

Implementations

Being a mother is a new role for a woman, a new beginning with perhaps greater status than she had before. It may be a time when a mother is willing to initiate help for herself through a group such as Alcoholics Anonymous. Investigate to see if this is a possibility and help her make a contact. On the other hand, do not assume that every mother of an infant with fetal alcohol syndrome is alcohol dependent. The syndrome can occur if alcohol is ingested on only *one* day of susceptible growth during the pregnancy.

Evaluation

An infant needs long-term follow-up so the full extent of involvement can be determined during growth and proper educational programs can be planned. Double-check that the mother understands what care is needed at home. Many women who are alcoholic have few support people and have no one to turn to if they have a problem with newborn care. Evaluate whether a home is safe before discharging a baby from the hospital.

Birth Injury

Birth is a stress to an infant and during the process a number of neuromuscular injuries can occur.

Erb-Duchenne Paralysis

Erb-Duchenne paralysis is caused by birth injury and is seen much less often with modern techniques. In this type of paralysis, the arm is adducted close to the chest and internally rotated. It is held straight at the elbow with the forearm pronated. Erb-Duchenne paralysis is caused by stretching, hemorrhage, or tearing of the anterior fifth and sixth cervical nerve roots, such as might occur if the fetal head is overextended laterally to effect delivery of wide fetal shoulders. It is important to observe the symmetrical movement of newborns, particularly in the Moro reflex, to detect the presence of this birth injury. Diaphragmatic paralysis may occur in conjunction with this from the same cause. All infants with Erb-Duchenne paralysis need to be observed closely for tachypnea or other symptoms of respiratory distress to detect that diaphragmatic paralysis is not also present.

Therapy for Erb-Duchenne paralysis is to hold the arm in an abducted, externally rotated, and supinated position to rest the paralyzed muscle. Usually a cotton restraint is tied around a newborn's wrist, and the infant's arm is raised over the head and tied to the head of the bassinet. Unless the damage to the nerve root was extensive (avulsion), the paralysis is temporary, and arm function will return.

If the root of the nerve was actually torn, this will be a permanent deformity. The child will need long-term follow-up to be certain that his potential is realized despite the handicap. The parents may need some help accepting the unexpected injury in an otherwise healthy child.

Diaphragmatic Paralysis

Injury to the phrenic nerve at birth may result in paralysis of the diaphragm and resulting respiratory distress. Phrenic nerve injury usually occurs in connection with injury to the brachial plexus (the network supplying the arm). Infants who had a difficult breech birth or those who delivered ver-

tex with shoulder dystocia are most likely to suffer phrenic nerve injury, since a lateral hyperextension of the head is usually the cause. An X-ray examination will show a slight elevation of the diaphragm on the affected side. Atelectasis may be present. If the injury is mild, the child's condition usually improves over the first week of life; if it is severe, surgery may be necessary to lower the position of the diaphragm to reduce interference with lung expansion.

Intracranial Hemorrhage

The pressure of delivery on the fetal head may cause tentorial membrane tears (the membrane separating the cerebellum and parietal brain portions), resulting in hemorrhage from torn blood vessels into the cerebellum or brain stem. This is primarily a problem of the immature infant and is therefore discussed in Chapter 48.

Seizures

In older children, the cause of seizures is often unknown, but in neonates, the etiology can be established about 75 percent of the time. The cause may be anoxia, perinatal injury, infection, kernicterus, or a metabolic disorder.

Anoxia may result from placenta previa or premature separation of the placenta. Perinatal injury involves some form of trauma to the newborn head: an unusually tight maternal cervix or ineffective use of forceps, causing trauma. Subdural hematomas caused from the pressure of the birth canal do not as a rule lead to convulsions; the skull suture lines are so expandable at birth that pressure such as a blood accumulation is not acute. The metabolic disorders that lead to seizures are hypoglycemia, hypocalcemia, and lack of pyridoxine (vitamin B_6).

Occasionally, neonates will have an infection of the central nervous system that is manifested by convulsions. Newborns whose membranes were ruptured for 24 hours or more before delivery are more prone to infection than infants whose membranes ruptured closer to delivery. Seizures that occur after the third day of life are much more likely to be caused by infection than by trauma.

Kernicterus, in which high bilirubin levels in the blood destroy brain cells, resulting from either physiologic jaundice or jaundice caused by blood incompatibility, may lead to seizures.

Assessment

Seizures in the newborn period may be difficult to recognize because they may consist only of some twitching of the head, arms, or eyes or slight cyanosis or apnea. The infant may be limp and flaccid afterward. Electroencephalograms in the newborn may be normal despite extensive disease. Thus, an abnormal electroencephalogram this early in life usually denotes a particularly severe involvement and a poor prognosis. Lumbar puncture in newborns may not give meaningful results, because about 20 percent of all newborns have abnormal cerebrospinal fluid at birth. Protein is increased and a few red blood cells may be present from rupture of subarachnoid capillaries during passage through the birth canal.

Analysis

The nursing problems identified in relation to convulsions are usually prevention of aspiration during a seizure and provision of adequate nutrition. Aspiration is a problem because the infant cannot swallow saliva during a convulsion. Nutrition is a problem for the infant who is having frequent seizures, who is thus unable to suck effectively; trying to feed the baby while he is convulsing may lead to aspiration.

Implementations

During a convulsion, turn an infant to the side to prevent aspiration of oral secretions and allow the tongue to fall away from the back of the throat. Do not restrain the infant or attempt to place a padded tongue blade in the mouth as these actions do more harm than good. Neonates metabolize drugs more rapidly than do older infants, children, or adults, and so the dosage of anticonvulsant medication used during the newborn period to prevent further convulsions is high. The dosage of phenobarbital, for instance, is about 1.5 mg per kilogram per day for adults; in newborns, the dosage may be 8 to 12 mg per kilogram per day. An infant will need intravenous fluid to keep from becoming dehydrated until the seizures are controlled and it is safe for the baby to suck orally again.

Evaluation

Infants who develop recurrent seizures in the newborn period need long-term follow-up as their dosage of medication will change as they grow older. They also need follow-up to be certain that their parents are treating them as normal children and allowing them normal childhood experiences, not sheltering them needlessly (though still respecting safe limits, such as never allowing them to swim alone). The child may be multiply handicapped because the insult that caused the seizure activity may also have caused additional neurologic destruction.

Utilizing Nursing Process

An infant who is ill at birth or becomes ill in the newborn period is under serious threat because he has difficulty in just regulating the new body processes; having to regulate them in the face of illness may be far more than the newborn is able to accomplish. In order that the infant can survive this period, nursing care planning should be implemented with use of the nursing process.

Assessment
Assessment of a newborn with an illness begins with a history of the infant's pregnancy. Important aspects to inquire about are the level of nutrition, gestation length, and the events of labor and delivery. Be certain that every newborn receives a thorough physical examination immediately after birth and again at about 24 hours of age. Be alert whenever you are caring for newborns to observe them for circulatory and respiratory function and intake and output; be certain that they have achieved an adaptation to extrauterine life without difficulty or illness.

Analysis
Nursing diagnoses used with ill newborns must consider not only the pathophysiology of the disease process, such as "Potential for electrolyte disturbance related to calcium imbalance," but the difficulty with parent-child bonding that may occur due to separation of the infant or anticipatory grief. Be certain that goals are realistic in light of a newborn's limited physiologic capabilities.

Planning
Be certain in planning care of ill newborns that you include the parents in planning so that they feel comfortable with the plans and are able to participate in the infant's care.

Implementation
Implementation of care for ill newborns must include good handwashing and strict precautions with aseptic techniques so that an infant does not contract a serious infection in addition to the initial illness. Be certain that it includes a balanced program of rest and stimulation and continuity of care so that an infant can continue to develop as well as recover from the illness. Many interventions of care involve the use of monitors for respiratory or cardiac function. Be certain that their use is explained to the parents and they are encouraged to actively participate in care despite all the equipment that may surround their baby.

Evaluation

Evaluation of goals for the ill newborn should include not only whether an infant is recovering from an illness but whether he has any residual effects from the illness and if the family is prepared to accept the baby as a full member of the family (even in light of a continuing handicap).

Nursing Care Planning

John Baco is an infant admitted to your Careful Watch Nursery following birth.

Problem Area. Potential for disturbance in glucose metabolism.

Assessment

Vigorously crying large male infant. Infant 38 weeks' gestation age, mother a gestational diabetic. No FHR abnormalities during labor; vaginal delivery. Mother given continuous insulin infusion during labor. Blood sugars were always between 90 and 105. Weight: 9 lbs, 6 oz (over 90th %). Dextrostix at birth: 90 mg. Dextrostix now at 1 hour of age: 45–90 mg.

Analysis

Potential for hypoglycemia related to hyperglycemic intrauterine environment.

Locus of Decision Making. Parents and nurse.

Goal. Infant stabilizes glucose metabolism.

Criteria. Infant maintains blood glucose over 45 mg/100 ml.

Nursing Orders

1. Infant to be fed at 1 hour of life with 2 oz Similac (M.D. order).
2. Admit to Isolette for warmth.
3. Dextrostix q½h for first 4 hours.
4. Observe for jitteriness, clonus, or lethargy q30min for first 4 hours.

Problem Area. Potential for respiratory or jaundice development related to immaturity.

Assessment

No jaundice at present. Lungs are clear to auscultation (mild rhonchi present). No retractions; respiratory rate at 40/min.

Analysis

Potential for respiratory or jaundice development related to immaturity.

Locus of Decision Making. Shared, parents and nurse.

Goal. Infant will develop no respiratory or jaundice complications during neonatal period.

Criteria:

1. Infant's bilirubin level will remain under 12 mg/100 ml.
2. Infant will develop no pulmonary problems such as respiratory distress syndrome.
3. Infant's temperature will stabilize with Isolette protection.

Nursing Orders

1. Admit to Isolette for warmth.
2. Do gestational assessment at 1 hour to evaluate true gestation age.
3. Observe for jaundice using daylight q4h.
4. Prick heel for bilirubin level at 4 and 8 hours (M.D. order).

Questions for Review

Multiple Choice

1. All infants need to be observed for hypoglycemia in the newborn period. Based on the following facts obtained from pregnancy history, which infant below would be most likely to develop hypoglycemia?

   a. Jane, whose labor began with ruptured membranes
   b. Bobby, who had difficulty establishing respirations at birth
   c. Tom, who has marked acrocyanosis of his hands and feet

   d. Susan, whose mother craved chocolate during pregnancy

2. A usual sign of an infant with hypoglycemia is

   a. prolonged jaundice.
   b. limpness or jitteriness.
   c. spasm of the sixth cranial nerve.
   d. excessive hunger.

3. Hypoglycemia in a mature infant is defined as a blood glucose level below which number?

   a. 100 mg/100 ml whole blood
   b. 80 mg/100 ml whole blood

c. 40 mg/100 ml whole blood

d. 30 mg/100 ml whole blood

4. Baby Green does not breathe spontaneously at birth. You administer oxygen by bag and mask. If oxygen is entering the lungs, you should notice that

   a. the abdomen rises while the chest falls with bag compressions.

   b. the infant's pupils dilate after 3 minutes.

   c. the infant's neck veins become prominent and palpable.

   d. the chest rises with each bag compression.

5. To administer oxygen by bag and mask to a newborn, you would position the baby

   a. in Trendelenburg's position.

   b. on the back with the neck slightly flexed.

   c. on the back with the head slightly extended.

   d. position is unimportant as long as the tongue is pulled forward.

6. If Baby Green needs cardiac massage, you would initiate this at what rate?

   a. 40 beats/minute

   b. 80 beats/minute

   c. 120 beats/minute

   d. 180 beats/minute

7. Before feeding Baby Green by gavage, which method would be best to use to test whether his indwelling catheter is in place?

   a. Assess if the tube is curled in his mouth.

   b. Aspirate stomach contents from the catheter.

   c. Inject sterile water into the tube and listen for bowel sounds.

   d. Check that the tape holding the tube to his nose is secure.

8. Baby Bargnesi is the infant of an Rh-sensitized mother. At birth, the problems that he must be assessed for most are

   a. polycythemia and hypercalcemia.

   b. small for gestation age and hypocalcemia.

   c. congenital anomalies and hypoglycemia.

   d. anemia and hyperbilirubinemia.

9. A positive direct Coombs' test means that

   a. the infant's red blood cells are free of maternal antibodies.

   b. the infant's red blood cells have maternal antigens attached to them.

   c. the infant's red blood cells have maternal antibodies attached to them.

   d. the infant's red blood cells are microcytic from destruction.

10. Baby Bargnesi is placed under phototherapy lights. Under lights, it would be most important to observe him for

    a. shock from hypovolemia.

    b. dehydration due to loose stools.

    c. hypobilirubinemia due to excess hemolysis.

    d. intestinal obstruction due to constipation.

Discussion

1. Nasogastric feedings are often used with newborns with respiratory distress. What precautions would you take pre-and post-feeding to prevent aspiration with this type of feeding?

2. Oxygen must be administered to newborns with precautions. What is a safe method of administering oxygen to a cyanotic newborn?

3. Caring for an infant under phototherapy lights is a primary nursing responsibility. What are important aspects of care for an infant during such therapy?

Suggested Readings

Allen, D. A., et al. (1982). The predictive validity of neonatal intensive care nurses' judgments of parent-child relationships: A nine month followup. *Journal of Pediatric Psychology, 7*, 125.

Anderson, R. A. (1982). The possible role of paternal alcohol consumption in the etiology of the fetal alcohol syndrome. In Abel, E. L. (Ed.) *Fetal alcohol syndrome*, Boca Raton, Florida, CRC Press.

Avery, G. B. (Ed.) (1981). *Neonatology*, 2nd ed. Philadelphia, Lippincott.

Bacon, K. K., et al. (1981). Care of the neonate after cesarean section. *Association of Operating Room Nurses Journal, 34*, 860.

Bancalari, E., & Berlin, J. (1978). Meconium aspiration and other asphyxial disorders. *Clinical Perinatology, 5*, 317.

Battle, C. U. (1975). Chronic physical disease: Behavioral aspects. *Pediatric Clinics of North America, 22*, 525.

Beckham, R. W., et al. (1982). Sound levels inside in-cubators and oxygen hoods used with nebulizers and humidifiers. *Respiratory Care, 27*, 33.

Braune, K. W., & Lacey, L. (1983). Common hematologic problems of the immediate newborn period. *J.O.G.N. Nursing, 12*, 19s.

Budd, R. A. (1982). The Logan Bow method for securing endotracheal tubes in neonates. *Critical Care Nurse, 2*, 27.

Carey, B. E. (1982). Converting micrograms/kilograms/minutes to microdrops. *Dimensions of Critical Care Nursing, 1*, 338.

Carey, B. E. (1983). Intraventricular hemorrhage in the preterm infant. *J.O.G.N. Nursing, 12*, 60s.

Chaze, B. A., et al. (1984). Sensory stimulation in the NICU. *American Journal of Nursing, 84*, 68.

Cloutier, J., & Measel, C. P. (1982). Home care for the infant with congenital heart disease. *American Journal of Nursing, 82*, 100.

Clyman, R. I., et al. (1979). What pediatricians say to mothers of sick newborns. *Pediatrics, 63*, 719.

Dingle, R. E., et al. (1980). Continuous transcutaneous O_2 monitoring in the neonate. *American Journal of Nursing, 80,* 890.

Duncan, J. A., & Webb, L. Z. (1983). Teaching families home apnea monitoring. *Pediatric Nursing, 9,* 171.

Generra, S. (1980). Necrotizing enterocolitis: Detecting it and treating it. *Nursing 80, 8,* 52.

Glasper, A., et al. (1984). Observation of the sick infant. *Nursing (Oxford), 2,* 655.

Griggs, C. C. (1982). What is the prune-belly syndrome? *M.C.N., 7,* 253.

Haddock, N. (1980). Blood pressure monitoring in neonates. *M.C.N., 5,* 131.

Halliday, H. L., et al. (1981). Transient tachypnoea of the newborn: Two distinct clinical entities? *Archives of Diseases of Children, 56,* 322.

Hubner, L., et al. (1982). Aeromedical physiology: Implications for neonatal nurses. *Neonatal Network, 1,* 10.

Jay, S. (1982). The effects of gentle touch on mechanically ventilated very-short-gestation infants. *Maternal Child Nursing Journal, 11,* 199.

Johnson, M. (1981). Nursing responsibilities for neonatal fluid therapy. *Journal of National Intravenous Therapy, 4,* 330.

Klaus, M., & Fanaroff, A. (1979). *Care of the high-risk neonate.* Philadelphia: Saunders.

Korones, S. B. (1981). *High-risk infants—the basis for intensive nursing care* (2nd ed.). St. Louis: Mosby.

Kraus, A. N. (1983). Recent advances in hyaline membrane disease. *Pediatric Annals, 12,* 24.

LaRossa, M. M., et al. (1982). Foster grandmothers in the premature nursery. *American Journal of Nursing, 82,* 1834.

Lemons, P. M. (1981). Prenatal addiction: A dual tragedy. *Critical Care Quarterly, 4,* 79.

Long, J. G., et al. (1980). Excessive handling as a cause of hypoxemia. *Pediatrics, 65,* 203.

Martin, R. J., et al. (1979). Effect of supine and prone positions on arterial oxygen tension in the preterm infant. *Pediatrics, 63,* 528.

McFadden, R. (1981). Decreasing respiratory compromise during infant suctioning. *American Journal of Nursing, 81,* 2158.

Nugent, J. (1982). Intra-arterial blood pressure monitoring in the neonate. *J.O.G.N. Nursing, 11,* 281.

Nugent, J. (1983). Acute respiratory care of the newborn. *J.O.G.N. Nursing, 12,* 31s.

Robarge, J. P., et al. (1982). Increased child abuse in families with twins. *Research in Nursing Health, 5,* 199.

Ruegsegger, D. R. (1982). Radiation exposure levels in an intensive care nursery. *Pediatric Nursing, 8,* 244.

Samson, L. F. (1982). Use of a preemie needle . . . a 27 gauge IV needle designed for use with small infants. *Critical Care Nurse, 2,* 6.

Schreiner, R. L., & Kisling, J. A. (1981). Treatment of the newborn in respiratory distress. *Critical Care Quarterly, 4,* 19.

Schreiner, R. L. (Ed.). (1981). *Care of the newborn.* New York: Raven Press.

Seaman, C. K. (1981). Monitoring the critically ill neonate. *Critical Care Quarterly, 4,* 9.

Shogan, M. (1984). Intensively caring . . . neonatal nursing. *Critical Care Nurse, 4,* 32.

Strodtbeck, F. (1981). Critical care concepts related to neonatal septicemia and septic shock. *Critical Care Quarterly, 4,* 71.

Sullivan, R., et al. (1979). Determining a newborn's gestational age. *M.C.N., 4,* 38.

Thompson, S. W. (1983). How to use the Heimlich maneuver on choking infants and children. *Pediatric Nursing, 9,* 13.

Webb, L. Z., & Duncan, J. A. (1983). Selecting the right home apnea monitor. *Pediatric Nursing, 9,* 179.

48

The Infant with Altered Gestational Age or Birth Weight

OBJECTIVES

Following mastery of the contents of this chapter, you should be able to

1. Define the terms *small-for-gestational, average-for-gestational,* and *large-for-gestational* age, and *preterm* and *postmaturity.*
2. Assess the unusual-for-gestational-age or -birth-weight infant.
3. State a nursing diagnosis regarding an infant with unusual age for gestational or birth weight.
4. Plan nursing interventions for an infant with an unusual gestational age or birth weight.
5. Implement nursing care for an infant with an unusual gestational age or birth weight, recognizing the special needs of the neonate with an alteration in growth or birth weight in such areas as respiratory function, cardiovascular adjustment, temperature regulation, nutrition, bonding, and stimulation.
6. Evaluate goal criteria to ensure that established goals for care have been met.
7. Analyze the special crisis imposed on families when alterations of growth in utero or length of pregnancy occur.
8. Synthesize knowledge of the infant with altered gestational age or birth weight with nursing process to achieve quality maternal-newborn nursing care.

APPROXIMATELY 7 PERCENT of all pregnancies for white infants and 14 percent of pregnancies for black infants end before term, and about 10 percent continue after term. All newborns should have their birth weight plotted on a growth chart such as the Colorado (Lubchenco) Intrauterine Growth Chart (Figure 31-1), so that their birth weight may be compared with their gestational age. These charts have been recently updated to reflect current intrauterine weights (slightly heavier than in past years because mothers eat more calories during pregnancy) and new mortality rates due to improved neonatal care. If this process of recording birth weight is routinely carried out, infants may be placed in one of three categories: low birth weight (an infant who would have been normal weight if carried to term); small for the length of the pregnancy (intrauterine growth retardation), and large for gestational age.

These are important differentiations. A low-birth-weight infant appears to have been growing normally in utero. The stay in utero was unfortunately prematurely terminated. In the second category of infants, growth appears to have been impaired, and a pathologic process in the fetus or placenta is suggested. In the third category the accelerated growth is not necessarily optimal for newborn health.

Infants Who Are Small for Gestational Age

An infant is small-for-gestational-age (small for dates) if the birth weight is below the tenth percentile on an intrauterine growth curve. The infant may be born before term (before 38 weeks' gestation); he or she may be a full-term infant (38 to 42 weeks of gestation) or a post-term infant (past 42 weeks) who weighs less than 2,500 gm (5½ pounds). About a third of all newborns weighing less than 2,500 gm are small-for-gestational-age infants. Such infants (preterm, term, or post-term) are a separate group of infants from those merely born with a low birth weight.

Causes of the Problem

Infants fall into the small for gestational age category because they have suffered intrauterine growth retardation (IUGR). Causes are largely placental: Either nutrients did not reach the placenta, or the placenta could not transfer them adequately to the fetus. A mother's nutrition during pregnancy plays a major role in fetal growth. Adolescents who have poor nutritional habits have a high incidence of small-for-gestational-age babies.

Damage to the placenta, such as partial placental separation with bleeding, might be a cause. The area of placenta that separated becomes infarcted and fibrosed, reducing placental surface for exchange. The placenta may have a developmental defect that prevents it from functioning properly. A mother with advanced diabetes mellitus who has vascular involvement may have an IUGR infant. Pregnancy-induced hypertension, which leads to vascular spasm and decreased blood flow to the placenta, may also be associated with small-for-gestational-age infants. Women over 35 and those with systemic diseases, such as hypertension, chronic renal or cardiovascular disease and those who smoke heavily or use narcotics tend to have them as well.

In some pregnancies the placental supply of nutrients is adequate, but the infant is unable to use them. Infants with intrauterine infections such as rubella or toxoplasmosis have this problem. Babies with chromosomal abnormalities may be small for their gestational age as well as suffering from a chromosomal difficulty. One of twins may be IUGR because the majority of nutrients passed to the other twin.

Assessing These Infants

Assessment of the small-for-gestational-age infant begins with a pregnancy history. Ask specifically about the presence of accompanying disease such as diabetes, symptoms of hypertension of pregnancy, and the mother's nutrition during pregnancy.

A small-for-date infant may be detected in utero as the recorded fundal height during pregnancy becomes progressively less than the expected fundal height. If a woman is unsure of the date of her last menstrual period, this discrepancy will be hard to substantiate. Serial sonograms will show the small increase in weight and growth. The adequacy of placental function may be assessed by collecting 24-hour urines for estriol determination. Low estriol levels (below 12 mg) indicate poor fetal or placental function. A nonstress test may be done to further estimate placental function. If poor placental function is apparent from such determinations, the infant will probably do poorly during labor; periods of hypoxia would lead to neurologic damage. Cesarean birth would then be the delivery method of choice in such circumstances.

Physical Examination

Early in intrauterine life, fetal growth consists primarily of an increase in the number of body cells (hyperplastic growth). Late in intrauterine life, growth is achieved primarily by an increase in cell size (hypertrophic growth). During either period of growth, if the nutritional supplies to the fetus become inadequate, the brain, heart, and lungs are little affected. In contrast, the liver, adrenals, and spleen are very susceptible to the amount of nutrients present and fail to grow in size or function.

An infant who suffered nutritional deprivation early in pregnancy is generally below average in weight, length, and head circumference. An infant who suffered deprivation late in pregnancy may only have a reduction in weight. Regardless of the time of deprivation, infants have an overall wasted appearance. They may have a small liver, which causes a great deal of difficulty in regulating glucose and protein levels. They have dull, listless hair and a lack of lanugo. Infants generally appear to have a large head because the rest of the body is small. Skull sutures may be widely separated from lack of normal bone growth. They may have poor skin turgor because of lack of body fluid or subcutaneous fat. The abdomen may be sunken. The cord often appears dry and may be yellow-stained.

Because an infant's age is more advanced than the weight implies, he may have quite well developed neurologic responses, hair texture, sole creases, and ear cartilage. The skull is firmer than that of the average infant of the same weight, and the baby may seem unusually alert and active for weight achieved.

The small-for-gestational-age infant needs careful assessment for congenital anomalies: The poor nutrition available in the intrauterine environment makes him very susceptible to prenatal injury (or a congenital anomaly may have interfered with nutritional use of available substances) (Figure 48-1).

Establishment of Respirations

A pediatrician should be present at the birth of a small-for-gestational-age infant because many of these infants need resuscitation at birth. They need close observation for both respiratory rate and character in the first few hours of life because their chest muscles may be underdeveloped and so not able to maintain the rapid respiratory rate of newborns. They may develop meconium aspiration syndrome due to anoxia during labor.

Cardiovascular Competence

Blood studies at birth on small-for-gestational-age infants show a high hematocrit level (less plasma in proportion to red blood cells than is normal) and an increase in the total number of red blood cells present (polycythemia). The increase in red blood cells is probably due to the state of anoxia

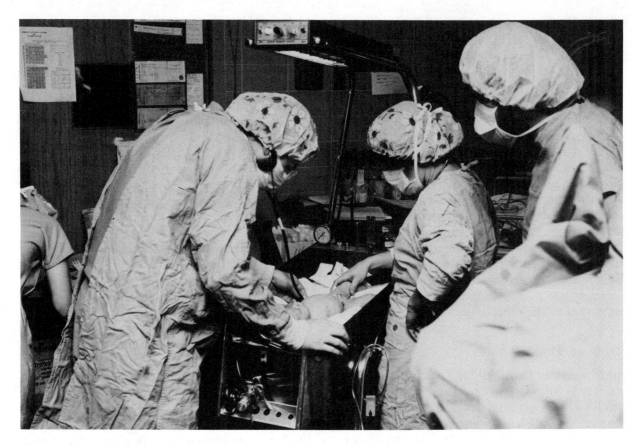

Figure 48-1 *An infant being examined at birth. Note the radiant heat warmer.*

during intrauterine life. The infant produced an unusual number of red blood cells while attempting to supply oxygen to body cells. This phenomenon also occurs in infants with cyanotic heart disease.

The high hematocrit may reflect not only an increase in red blood cells but a lack of plasma due to lack of fluid in utero. The polycythemia present results in increased blood viscosity, which puts extra work on the heart because of the resulting difficulty in circulating blood effectively. Persistent acrocyanosis (blueness of the hands and feet) may be a telltale sign. If the polycythemia is extreme, blocked vessels and thrombus formation can result. If the hematocrit is over 65 percent, an exchange transfusion to dilute the concentration of blood may be necessary.

Nutritional Needs

Since small-for-gestational-age infants have decreased glycogen stores one of the most common problems in neonatal life is hypoglycemia. They may need intravenous glucose to sustain blood sugar until they are able to suck vigorously enough to take sufficient oral feedings.

Temperature Regulation

Temperature control in these infants is poor because of the lack of subcutaneous fat. They need their environment carefully controlled so that it is always in a neutral zone.

Bonding

Although these infants may gain weight and appear to thrive in the first few days of life, their mental development is often impaired because of lack of oxygen and nourishment in utero. Babies who were growing normally in utero but whose gestation was interrupted prematurely (true prematures) usually gain in weight and height so rapidly that by the end of the first year of life the majority are nearing the fiftieth percentile on growth charts. Small-for-date infants may always be below normal on standard growth charts. This inability to reach normal levels of growth and development may interfere with bonding as a child does not meet the parents' expectations, and it can interfere with the child's development of self-esteem if he is never able to meet self-expectations.

Stimulation

A small-for-gestational-age infant needs stimulation during the infant period in order to reach normal growth and development milestones. Because the child is small for his age, parents need to be cautioned to supply toys that are suitable for this chronological age, not size.

Infants Who Are Large for Gestational Age

An infant is large for gestational age if birth weight is above the ninetieth percentile on an intrauterine growth chart. These babies' appearance is deceptive at birth because they are term babies by weight, but a gestational examination will reveal immaturity. It is important that large-for-gestational-age infants be identified immediately at birth: They are at great risk if treated as term newborns and not as having achieved a less-than-optimal gestational age.

A large-for-gestational-age baby is born most frequently to a mother who has poorly controlled diabetes due to overproduction of growth hormone in utero. Some women who will become diabetic late in life have these infants—as if, although clinical symptoms of diabetes are not yet present, some of the pathology of the disease that will lead to clinical symptoms later on may already be present. A woman with multiple parity may have a large baby (babies tend to grow larger with succeeding pregnancies). For an unknown reason, infants with transposition of the great vessels tend to be large for gestational age. One rare condition, Beckwith's syndrome, manifested by overgrowth and congenital anomalies such as omphalocele, results in large-for-gestational-age infants.

A fetus's unusual size for age can be suspected during pregnancy when the size of the mother's uterus appears to be more stretched than it should be. Because a fetus assumes such a flexed position, however, a 10-pound fetus does not occupy a great deal more space than a 7-pound fetus. If a fetus is growing more rapidly in utero than is normal, a nonstress test may be done to assess the placenta's ability to sustain the fetus during labor. An infant's lung maturity may be assessed by amniocentesis. This condition may first be recognized during labor when descent fails to occur because the infant's size is out of proportion to the mother's pelvis. It can be revealed by X-ray pelvimetry at term. A sonogram determination may show the biparietal diameter to be above average for intrauterine age.

Cesarean birth may be necessary for delivery because of cephalopelvic disproportion (the biparietal diameter is closer to 10 cm than the usual 9 cm). A baby may have extensive bruising or a birth injury such as a broken clavicle or Erb-Duchenne paralysis from trauma to the cervical nerves if delivered vaginally. Because the head is large it may be submitted to unusual pressure, and the possible increased intracranial pressure at birth could lead to permanent neurologic damage, such as seizures or an intracranial bleed.

All infants should have a gestational age exam done in the first few hours of life. The immature reflexes or low rating score of this type of infant shows that, although they are large, they are immature and so must be cared for with the extra precautions in effect for immature infants. Specific factors to examine for at an initial or continuing assessment of a large-for-gestational-age infant are shown in the box on page 1182.

Establishment of Respirations

Many large-for-gestational-age infants have difficulty establishing respirations at birth because of birth trauma or because they were delivered by cesarean birth. Increased intracranial pressure from delivery of the larger-than-usual head may lead to edema and pressure on the respiratory center that decreases respiratory function. A diaphragmatic paralysis may occur due to cervical nerve trauma as the head is bent laterally to allow for delivery of the large shoulders. This accommodation prevents active lung motion on the affected side. Observe large-for-gestational-age infants well not only for the rate of respirations but the type and symmetry of chest movements. If diaphragmatic paralysis has occurred, paralysis of the arm on that side may be present too. This problem is revealed by rigid extension and pronation of the arm or lack of response in the arm on a Moro reflex.

Circulatory Competence

Circulatory shunts can be expected to close in large-for-gestational-age infants as in other infants. Such infants need to be observed carefully at birth, however, for heart rate and the presence of cyanosis. Transposition of the great vessels, a very serious heart anomaly, tends to occur most often (for unknown reasons) in large-sized infants. They may have polycythemia, which developed in an attempt to fully oxygenate all tissue. They must be observed closely after birth for hyperbilirubinemia from absorption of blood due to bruising and polycythemia.

Important Assessments for Large-for-Gestational-Age Infants

Assessment	*Rationale*
Skin color for ecchymosis, jaundice, and erythema.	Bruising occurs with vaginal delivery. Jaundice may occur from breakdown of ecchymotic collections of blood. Polycythemia causes ruddiness of skin.
Motion of extremities on spontaneous movement and in response to a Moro reflex to detect clavicle fracture (crepitus or swelling may then be palpated at the fracture site) and palsy due to edema of the cervical nerve plexus.	Clavicle or cervical nerve injuries may occur due to problem of delivery of wider-than-normal shoulders.
Asymmetry of the anterior chest or unilateral lack of movement to detect diaphragmatic paralysis from edema of the phrenic nerve.	The cervical nerve may be stretched by delivery of wide shoulders.
Eyes for evidence of unresponsive or dilated pupils, vomiting, bulging fontanelles, and a high-pitched cry suggestive of increased intracranial pressure.	Compression of third, fourth, and sixth cranial nerves by increased pressure limits eye response. Other signs of increased intracranial pressure may occur.
Activities such as jitteriness, lethargy, uncoordinated eye movements that suggest seizure activity.	Seizures may be caused by increased intracranial pressure; seizures in newborns often produce only vague symptoms.

Nutritional Needs

Large-for-gestational-age infants need to be assessed carefully for hypoglycemia in the early hours of life because they use up nutritional stores readily in order to sustain greater-than-normal weight. If born to a diabetic mother, an infant lived with an increased blood glucose level during pregnancy, resulting in elevated levels of insulin during fetal life. After birth, the increased levels of insulin will continue for the first few hours of life and cause a rebound hypoglycemia.

As a rule, a large-for-gestational-age infant needs to be fed early (by four hours after birth) in order to prevent hypoglycemia. He may need supplemental glucose water following breast-feeding to supply enough fluid and glucose for size.

It is easy to overestimate a large-for-gestational-age infant's ability to feed at birth (it seems breast-feeding would be easy because the baby is already the size of a 2-month-old; instead the infant sucks too ineffectively to obtain an adequate supply of milk).

Temperature Regulation

The necessity for temperature regulation may be underestimated in the large-for-gestational-age infant, who appears larger and more competent than he actually is. As a rule of thumb, protect *all* infants from chilling in the first few days of life so the immature infant who is term size will not be missed.

Bonding

Parents may overestimate an infant's needs in the newborn period because of the excessive size. Their newborn seems so large and healthy they may be confused about why he needs careful-watch care. They may read more into a child's condition than is present (he must be sick in some way that they are not being told about), and so bonding does not happen as instinctively as it might. If a woman received a cervical or perineal tear or had to have a cesarean birth she needs some time to talk about the experience or the excess pain she has so she can understand the infant is not at "fault." She cannot bond well to an infant whom she holds something against.

Stimulation

A large-for-gestational-age infant needs just as much stimulation as do other infants. Rocking, talking, stroking the back, providing a mobile are as necessary for this child as for other gestational age infants. Be certain that parents begin to think of the newborn as needing this nourishing type of care and not as already grown beyond this need.

Infants Who Are Low-Birth-Weight

By traditional definition, a low-birth-weight infant is a live-born infant weighing less than 2,500 gm (5 pounds, 8 ounces) at birth. A live birth was defined by the World Health Assembly in 1950 as follows:

> . . . the complete expulsion or extraction from its mother of a product of conception . . . which, after such separation, breathes or shows any other evidence of life such as beating of the heart, pulsation of the umbilical cord or definite movement of the voluntary muscles, whether or not the umbilical cord has been cut or the placenta is attached.

Incidence of Low-Birth-Weight Infants

The incidence of low-birth-weight infants in nonwhites is twice that in whites (14% vs 7%). Countries from the Eastern world use different standards to define low birth weight as babies born in these countries are typically lighter in weight than in Western countries. Burma and Thailand, for example, use 2,250 gm, India uses 2,150 gm, and Malaya uses 2,000 gm as their definition of low birth weight. Because black infants normally tend to be lighter in weight than Caucasian infants, it has been suggested that black infants be evaluated on the standard of 2,350 gm.

Another way to differentiate low-birth-weight infants is not by their weight but by their length or weeks of gestation. By these criteria, other infants traditionally put in the low-birth-weight group are live-born infants measuring 47 cm (18.5 inches) or less in length, or live-born infants of less than 37 weeks of gestation.

Increasingly, the maturity of an infant is being evaluated on the basis of physical findings such as sole creases, skull firmness, ear cartilage, and neurologic findings that reveal gestational age.

It is important that low-birth-weight babies be separated from small-for-gestational-age babies (which also may be low birth weight) at birth, as the two groups result from different situations and therefore the babies have different problems adjusting to extrauterine life.

Low-birth-weight infants appear to have been doing well in utero; for an unexplained reason, the trigger that initiates labor was activated too early and so, even though they are immature, they are born. With small-for-gestational-age ba-

bies, something was going wrong in utero with the placenta or its ability to transfer nutrients to the child and therefore the pregnancy was ended. The latter infants are ill from the effects of intrauterine malnutrition; the former are well, merely very immature and small. Characteristics of small-for-gestational-age and low-birth-weight infants are compared in Table 48-1.

Infants who are born before 20 weeks' gestation are generally categorized as products of abortions, not as low-birth-weight children. Their chances of survival are very slight. Infants who are born before 30 weeks of gestation (a weight of about 500 to 1,500 gm; 1 pound, 3 ounces to 3 pounds, 5 ounces) are extremely immature. They need level III care from the moment of birth to give them their best chance of survival without neurologic aftereffects due to their being so critically close to the age of viability. A lack of lung surfactant makes them extremely vulnerable to respiratory distress syndrome.

An infant born between 31 and 36 weeks of gestation (a birth weight between 1,500 and 2,500 gm; 3 pounds, 5 ounces and 5 pounds, 8 ounces) is moderately immature. The chance for survival is good.

An infant of 37 to 38 weeks' age (a birth weight close to 2,500 gm; 5 pounds, 8 ounces) is only slightly immature. If immaturity is recognized by a gestational age assessment and the specific problems of prematurity such as respiratory distress syndrome, hypoglycemia, and intracranial hemorrhage are watched for, chances of survival are very good.

Causes of Low Birth Weight

Because deaths of low-birth-weight infants account for 80 to 90 percent of mortality in the first year of life, discovering and correcting the causes of premature birth—and thus bringing more pregnancies to term—would dramatically reduce infant mortality rates.

The exact cause of early birth, however, is rarely known. There is a high correlation between low socioeconomic level and early termination of pregnancy. In women from the middle and upper socioeconomic groups, only 4 to 8 percent of pregnancies are terminated early; in women from low socioeconomic levels, 10 to 20 percent end before term. The major influencing factor in these instances appears to be inadequate nutrition before pregnancy in both parents, and during pregnancy in the woman, as a result of either insufficient purchasing power or ignorance of what constitutes good nutrition. Other contributing factors are the higher incidence of pregnancy-induced hypertension and chronic disease in women with

Table 48-1 Differences Between Small-for-Gestational-Age Infants and Low-Birth-Weight Infants

Characteristic	Small-for-Gestational Age Infant	Low-Birth-Weight Infant
Gestation age	28–42 weeks	Under 37 weeks
Birth weight	Under tenth percentile	Normal for age
Congenital malformations	A strong possibility	A possibility
Pulmonary problems	Meconium aspiration Pulmonary hemorrhage Pneumothorax	Respiratory distress syndrome
Hyperbilirubinemia	A possibility	A very strong possibility
Hypoglycemia	A very strong possibility	A possibility
Intracranial hemorrhage	A strong possibility	A possibility
Apnea episodes	A possibility	A very strong possibility
Feeding problems	Most likely to be due to accompanying problem such as hypoglycemia	Small stomach capacity; sucking reflex not mature
Weight gain in nursery	Rapid	Slow
Future retarded growth	May always be under tenth percentile	Not likely to be retarded in growth

poor nutrition. Additional factors that seem to be related to early termination of pregnancy are shown in the box on page 1185.

It is unfortunate when a fetus is born prematurely because labor was induced. Tests of fetal immaturity by amniocentesis limit the number of instances when this happens today. The decline of labor by induction or elective cesarean birth has limited prematurity from these iatrogenic causes. Labor, however, may still be induced in a woman with severe preeclampsia, Rh incompatibility, or diabetes to remove the fetus from an environment that is more detrimental than extrauterine existence.

Assessment of the Low-Birth-Weight Infant

Assessment of a low-birth-weight infant begins with a detailed pregnancy history in an attempt to determine possible causes for the early birth (not only to aid in care of the child but to prevent another occurrence of low birth weight in a future pregnancy for that mother).

Pertinent information includes the age of the mother, date of the last menstrual period (LMP), contraceptive method used previous to pregnancy, if any, reproductive health, nutrition (special reference to early months when organs were forming and perhaps nausea and vomiting in the mother were present as well as a recent 24-hour recall history), rest, activity, work patterns, socioeconomic pattern, history of past pregnancies, interval since last pregnancy, complications such as vaginal spotting, ingestion of medication or alcohol or cigarette smoking, trauma, X-ray, infection, and psychological stress during the pregnancy, and events that followed first signal of early labor, including any complications.

In many instances, the pregnancy history of a low-birth-weight infant is normal up to the point that labor began (the mark of a low-birth-weight infant is good growth in utero; unfortunately, delivery occurred before maturity was reached). Women are usually very concerned and worried when discussing their pregnancy, examining the factors themselves for a possible cause of this happening. They may be very fearful that you *will* discover a suggested cause, that this *is* somehow their fault and they will have to live with the guilt for the rest of their lives.

Be careful with your interviewing technique that you do not convey disapproval of an action such as cigarette smoking or working a 12-hour workshift during pregnancy. The average woman who does these things during pregnancy does not do them maliciously; she is probably not aware that they could be detrimental to the fetus (she

Factors Associated with Low Birth Weight

Low socioeconomic level

Poor nutritional status

Lack of prenatal care

Multiple pregnancy

Prior previous early birth (perhaps a low gestational capacity)

Race (nonwhites have a higher incidence of prematurity than whites, which is perhaps a reflection of their general lower socioeconomic status rather than of race)

Cigarette smoking

The age of the mother (the highest incidence is in mothers under 20)

Order of birth (early termination is highest in first pregnancies and in those beyond the fourth)

Closely spaced pregnancies

Abnormalities of the reproductive system such as intrauterine septum

Infections (especially urinary tract infection)

Obstetric complications such as premature rupture of membranes or premature separation of the placenta

Multiple gestation

Early induction of labor

Elective cesarean birth

---

did not "hear" prenatal teaching or did not believe bad luck could happen to her) or perhaps was forced to do these things due to her economic situation. Now that the infant is born, she needs good self-esteem and all of her resources in order to sustain herself through this crisis. Being overburdened by guilt will not help her adjustment and may be very detrimental to bonding with this new, very small infant. Answer her direct inquiries about cause by a statement such as, "In the final analysis, no one knows what causes prematurity."

In many instances, premature labor could have been halted if a woman had only recognized that what she was feeling was not the normal Braxton-Hicks contractions of pregnancy, but true labor. If this was a woman's first labor, however, the feeling of contractions is so unique that it is easy for her to misjudge what is happening (she imagined labor contractions would be agonizingly painful and so discounted a sensation of pure contraction as anything important). Some women have watched so many women on television sitcoms announce, "I'm in labor" or "this is it" very certainly (and then proceed to deliver within the half-hour show) that they simply do not realize labor usually begins with subtle signs and not with a dramatic announcement. Even if she is a multipara, because each labor with each pregnancy tends to be different, a woman may miss the early signs until labor is too far advanced to be reversed. Again, assure women that labor is such a unique sensation that it is understandable they did not realize what was happening to them until

cervical dilatation had occurred and labor could not be reversed.

Physical Examination

A low-birth-weight infant appears small and underdeveloped to gross inspection (Figure 48-2). The head is disproportionately large (3 cm or more greater than chest size). Skin is generally unusually ruddy because of little subcutaneous fat, veins are easily noticeable, and a high degree of acrocyanosis may be present. The infant has

Figure 48-2 *An immature infant. Notice the frog-leg or lax position from immature muscle contraction. (Courtesy of the Department of Medical Photography, Children's Hospital, Buffalo, N.Y.)*

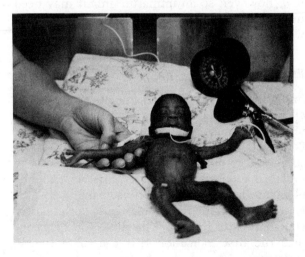

little vernix caseosa, a substance formed late in pregnancy. Lanugo is usually extensive, covering the back, forearms, forehead, and sides of the face. Both anterior and posterior fontanelles are small.

The eyes of most immature infants appear small. A pupillary reaction is present, although it is difficult to elicit. Ophthalmoscopic examination is extremely difficult and often unrewarding, since the vitreous humor may be hazy. The premature infant has varying degrees of myopia (nearsightedness) because of lack of depth to the eye globe.

The cartilage of the ear is immature and allows the pinna to fall forward. The ears appear large in relation to the head. The level of ears should be carefully inspected to rule out chromosomal abnormalities.

Examination of the pharynx is difficult because of its small size and the necessity for gentleness to prevent bruising. The gag reflex may be immature.

Neurologic function in the immature child is difficult to evaluate. The observations of spontaneous movement and provoked movement may yield as important findings as the reflex tests. If tested, reflexes such as sucking and swallowing may be absent; deep tendon reflexes such as the Achilles are markedly diminished. During an examination, an immature infant moves far less than a mature infant and rarely cries. If he does cry, the sound is often weak and high-pitched. Assessment charts, such as those by Kempe shown in Figure 48-3, are helpful in determining what neurologic activity should be apparent in a low-birth-weight baby.

Laboratory Findings

Laboratory values of immature infants compared to term infants are shown in Appendix G. Average values are similar; the range of values is narrow, however, so an immature infant may need intervention to correct levels before a term infant would.

Planning Care

Immature infants have the same priority needs of all newborn infants; but because of immaturity, techniques must be adapted to meet their needs. Because an immature infant has few body resources, both physiologic and psychological stress must be reduced as much as possible and implementations must be initiated rapidly to prevent depletion of resources. Close observation and analysis of findings will allow you to recognize the first indication that the infant needs assistance.

Initiation and Maintenance of Respirations

It is helpful in the delivery of an immature infant if a mother is given oxygen by mask during the delivery to allow the infant to be born with optimal oxygen saturation. Keeping analgesia and anesthesia to a minimum also gives an infant the best chance of initiating respirations effectively. Immature infants have great difficulty initiating respirations at birth because the pulmonary capillary bed continues to mature and proliferate throughout intrauterine life. When a pregnancy is terminated early, pulmonary ventilation may not have achieved its normal efficiency. Lung surfactant may be inadequate, leading to alveolar collapse with each expiration and requiring the infant to use maximum strength to reinflate the alveoli each time. Since infants turn to a vertex presentation late in pregnancy, an immature infant may present breech, resulting in an aspiration of vaginal secretions or meconium that compounds his or her respiratory problem in yet another way.

A pediatrician or neonatologist should be present at all preterm deliveries to supervise resuscitation procedures. Alerting this person that a premature birth is imminent is often a nursing responsibility.

Most infants are born with a temporary respiratory acidosis. Once respirations are established, the temporary condition quickly clears, however. Because an immature infant is unable to initiate effective respirations as quickly, he is prone to irreversible acidosis. The newborn must establish adequate ventilation or be resuscitated within 2 minutes after birth to prevent this development. An infant must be kept warm during resuscitation procedures so that the metabolic rate is not raised to maintain temperature. All procedures must be carried out with great gentleness; an immature infant's tissues are more sensitive to trauma than are those of the term infant. They can be easily damaged or bruised by a roughly applied oxygen mask. Reabsorption of blood from bruising can lead to hyperbilirubinemia and yet another problem.

Giving 100 percent oxygen to immature infants during resuscitation or to maintain respirations poses the dangers of pulmonary edema and retrolental fibroplasia (blindness of prematurity). The development of both these conditions depends on saturation of the blood with oxygen (a PO_2 above 100 mm Hg), however; as long as an infant is cyanotic, the blood saturation level of oxygen is not likely to be high.

The Committee on the Fetus and Newborn of the American Academy of Pediatrics (1978) rec-

Nursing Care Highlight

Oxygen Administration and Low-Birth-Weight Infants

When a newborn infant needs extra oxygen, it must be administered with great care because there is a causal relationship between a higher-than-normal (60 to 100 mm Hg) oxygen tension in arterial blood and retrolental fibroplasia (retinopathy of prematurity). When the normal oxygen tension is exceeded, there is an increased risk of retrolental fibroplasia. The upper limit of arterial oxygen tension and its duration that are safe for these infants is not known. It is probable that even concentrations of 40 percent oxygen in inspired air (formerly considered safe) could be dangerous for some infants.

An inspired oxygen concentration of 40 percent may be insufficient for infants with cardiorespiratory disease to raise the oxygen tension of arterial blood to a normal level. In such instances, an inspired oxygen concentration of 60 percent, 80 percent, or higher may be necessary. However, it is difficult to judge by clinical signs the concentration of inspired oxygen necessary to maintain effective oxygenation of tissues in these infants. An infant may have peripheral cyanosis and yet may have a normal, or even an elevated, arterial oxygen tension. Therefore, arterial blood gas measurements are extremely important for regulation of the concentration of inspired oxygen when an oxygen-enriched environment is considered necessary.

---

ommends the precautions in the administration of oxygen to high-risk and low-birth-weight infants shown in the Nursing Care Highlight above.

The immature infant may continue to need oxygen administration beyond that given for resuscitation measures because he often has difficulty maintaining respirations. The soft cartilage of the ribs of the immature infant tends to create respiratory problems because the ribs may collapse on expiration. The accessory muscles of respiration may be undeveloped, so that, unlike the mature infant, the immature infant has no backup muscles to use when fatigued from trying to maintain respirations. Many preterm infants tend to have higher PO_2 levels when placed prone than when supine (Martin, 1979).

Many immature babies, particularly those under 32 weeks of age, have a very irregular respiratory pattern (a few quick breaths, a period of 5 to 10 seconds without respiratory effort, a few quick breaths again, and so on). There is no bradycardia or cyanosis with this irregular pattern (sometimes termed *periodic respirations*); the pattern seems to be a result of immaturity and uncoordinated respiratory efforts.

Apnea

Many immature infants may have periods of true apnea as a result of fatigue or the immaturity of their respiratory mechanisms. With true apnea, the pause in respirations is more than 20 seconds and bradycardia (heart rate under 100 beats per minute) occurs. Babies with secondary stresses such as hyperbilirubinemia, hypoglycemia, or hypothermia tend to have a high incidence of apneic occurrences. If you gently shake an infant or flick the sole of the foot, often the baby begins to breathe again, almost as if he needs to be "reminded" to maintain this function. If an infant does not respond to these simple measures, resuscitation by bagging and oxygen administration is necessary. Immature infants must have extremely close observation to detect these apneic episodes. Apnea monitors that record respiratory movements are invaluable tools to detect failing respirations and sound a warning that an infant needs attention. An infant with frequent or difficult-to-correct episodes will be placed on a ventilator to provide respiratory coordination until he becomes more mature.

To prevent episodes of apnea, maintain thermal neutrality and use gentle handling to avoid excessive fatigue. Always suction gently to minimize nasopharyngeal irritation, which can cause bradycardia due to vagal stimulation. Using indwelling nasogastric tubes rather than intermittent ones can also reduce the amount of vagal stimulation. Following feeding, observe an infant carefully as the stomach puts pressure on the diaphragm. Careful burping helps to reduce this effect. Never take rectal temperatures: Resulting vagal stimulation can change the heart rate (bradycardia), which could lead to apnea.

Infants with apnea may be administered theophylline. The mechanism by which theophylline reduces the incidence of apnea episodes is unclear, but the drug appears to increase an in-

Examination First Hours

WEEKS GESTATION (20–48)

PHYSICAL FINDINGS		Findings (by gestational week)
Vernix		Appears (20) · Covers body, thick layer (23+) · On back, scalp, in creases (38–40) · Scant, in creases (40–41) · No vernix (42+)
Breast tissue and areola		Areola and nipple barely visible, no palpable breast tissue (24+) · Areola raised (34–35) · 1–2 mm nodule (36) · 3–5 mm (38–39) · 5–6 mm (40) · 7–10 mm (40–41) · ?12 mm (44–45)
Ear	Form	Flat, shapeless (22) · Beginning incurving superior (34–35) · Incurving upper 2/3 pinnae (36) · Well-defined incurving to lobe (38+)
	Cartilage	Pinna soft, stays folded (23) · Cartilage scant, returns slowly from folding (32–33) · Thin cartilage, springs back from folding (36–37) · Pinna firm, remains erect from head (42)
Sole creases		Smooth soles without creases (24) · 1–2 anterior creases (32–33) · 2–3 anterior creases (34–35) · Creases anterior 2/3 sole (36) · Creases involving heel (38) · Deeper creases over entire sole (42)
Skin	Thickness & appearance	Thin, translucent skin, plethoric, venules over abdomen, edema (25–30) · Smooth, thicker, no edema (32–33) · Pink (36–37) · Few vessels (40) · Some desquamation pale pink (40–41) · Thick, pale, desquamation over entire body (42+)
	Nail plates	Appear (20–21) · Nails to finger tips (33) · Nails extend well beyond finger tips (44)
Hair		Appears on head (22) · Eye brows and lashes (24) · Silky, single strands, lays flat (36–37) · ?Receding hairline or loss of baby hair, short, fine underneath (44)
Lanugo		Appears (21) · Covers entire body (22) · Vanishes from face (34) · Present on shoulders (38) · No lanugo (42)
Genitalia	Testes	Testes palpable in inguinal canal (28+) · In upper scrotum (36–37) · In lower scrotum (40–41)
	Scrotum	Few rugae (29) · Rugae, anterior portion (36) · Rugae cover (40) · Pendulous (42)
	Labia & clitoris	Prominent clitoris, labia majora small, widely separated (30–31) · Labia majora larger, nearly cover clitoris (36) · Labia minora and clitoris covered (42)
Skull firmness		Bones are soft (23) · Soft to 1" from anterior fontanelle (30) · Spongy at edges of fontanelle, center firm (35) · Bones hard, sutures easily displaced (38–39) · Bones hard, cannot be displaced (42)
Posture	Resting	Hypotonic, lateral decubitus (22) · Hypotonic (27) · Beginning flexion, thigh (30) · Stronger hip flexion (32) · Frog-like (34) · Flexion, all limbs (36) · Hypertonic (38–39) · Very hypertonic (42)
	Recoil - leg	No recoil (20) · Partial recoil (33) · Begin flexion, no recoil (34) · Prompt recoil (38)
	Arm	No recoil (20) · Prompt recoil, may be inhibited (36) · Prompt recoil after 30" inhibition (42)

Week scale: 20 21 22 23 24 25 26 27 28 29 30 31 32 33 34 35 36 37 38 39 40 41 42 43 44 45 46 47 48

Confirmatory Neurologic Examination To Be Done After 24 Hours

Weeks Gestation: 20 21 22 23 24 25 26 27 28 29 30 31 32 33 34 35 36 37 38 39 40 41 42 43 44 45 46 47 48

Tone — Physical Findings

Finding	Progression across weeks
Heel to ear	No resistance (≈20–24) → Some resistance (≈30) → Impossible (≈35)
Scarf sign	No resistance (≈20) → Elbow passes midline (≈30–33) → Elbow at midline (≈37) → Elbow does not reach midline (≈44)
Neck flexors (head lag)	Absent (≈20) → Head in plane of body (≈38) → Holds head (≈43)
Neck extensors	Head begins to right itself from flexed position (≈34) → Good righting cannot hold it (≈37) → Holds head few seconds (≈39) → Keeps head in line with trunk > 40° (≈41) → Turns head from side to side (≈45)
Body extensors	Straightening of legs (≈34) → Straightening of trunk (≈37) → Straightening of head and trunk together (≈41)
Vertical positions	When held under arms, body slips through hands (≈30) → Arms hold baby, legs extended? (≈33) → Legs flexed, good support with arms (≈38)
Horizontal positions	Hypotonic, arms and legs straight (≈30) → Arms and legs flexed (≈37) → Head and back even, flexed extremities (≈40) → Head above back (≈44)

Flexion angles

Finding	Progression across weeks
Popliteal	No resistance (≈20) → 150° (≈30) → 110° (≈33) → 100° (≈35) → 90° (≈39) → 80° (≈41)
Ankle	90° (≈30) → 45° (≈33) → 20° (≈37) → 0 (≈41)
Wrist (square window)	90° (≈30) → 60° (≈33) → 45° (≈37) → 30° (≈39) → 0 (≈41)

Reflexes

Finding	Progression across weeks
Sucking	Weak, not synchronized with swallowing (≈27) → Stronger, synchronized (≈33) → Perfect (≈35) → Perfect, hand to mouth (≈39) → Perfect (≈43)
Rooting	Long latency period slow, imperfect (≈28) → Hand to mouth (≈31) → Brisk, complete, durable (≈35) → Complete (≈44)
Grasp	Finger grasp is good, strength is poor (≈29) → Stronger (≈33) → Can lift baby off bed, involves arms (≈39) → Hands open (≈46)
Moro	Barely apparent (≈25) → Weak, not elicited every time (≈30) → Stronger (≈33) → Complete with arm extension, open fingers, cry (≈35) → Arm adduction added (≈40) → ?Begins to lose Moro (≈46)
Crossed extension	Flexion and extension in a random, purposeless pattern (≈30) → Extension, no adduction (≈33) → Still incomplete (≈36) → Extension, adduction, fanning of toes (≈39) → Complete (≈44)
Automatic walk	Minimal (≈31) → Begins tiptoeing, good support on sole (≈33) → Fast tiptoeing (≈37) → Heel-toe progression, whole sole of foot (≈40) → A pre-term who has reached 40 weeks walks on toes (≈44) → ?Begins to lose automatic walk (≈47)
Pupillary reflex	Absent (≈20) → Appears (≈30)
Glabellar tap	Absent (≈20) → Appears (≈33)
Tonic neck reflex	Absent (≈20) → Appears (≈29)
Neck-righting	Absent (≈20) → Appears (≈35); Present after 37 weeks

Figure 48-3 *Clinical estimation of gestational age. An approximation based on published data. (From Kempe, C. H., Silver, H. K., & O'Brien, D. O. (1974). Current pediatric diagnosis and treatment (3rd ed.). Los Altos, Calif.: Lange.)*

fant's sensitivity to carbon dioxide, ensuring better respiratory function.

Those infants who had had an apneic episode severe enough to require resuscitation are high risk for the development of sudden infant death syndrome (SIDS). The mortality rate for such infants from this may be as high as 10 percent (Kelly, 1982). In order to prevent this from happening, such infants may be discharged with home apnea monitoring until 1 year of age.

Sudden Infant Death Syndrome. SIDS occurs in 2 out of 1,000 live births. It is the most frequent cause of death of infants between 1 month and 1 year of age (Merritt, 1984). Although the cause of SIDS is unknown, it tends to occur at a higher than usual rate in the infants of adolescent mothers, infants of closely spaced pregnancies, and underweight male infants. Also prone to SIDS are infants with bronchopulmonary dysplasia, preterm infants, Native American infants, Alaskan native infants, economically disadvantaged black infants, twins, and siblings of a child with SIDS.

Although the cause of SIDS is unknown, a number of theories about its cause have been advanced. In addition to prolonged but unexplained apnea, a viral respiratory or botulism infection may occur. Familial distorted breathing patterns may be involved.

The affected infant is typically well nourished but has a slight head cold; he or she has been put to bed at night or is in bed for a nap. The infant is found dead a few hours later. Infants who die this way do not appear to make any sound as they die, which indicates that they die with laryngospasm present. Although many infants are found with blood-flecked sputum or vomitus in their mouths or on the bedclothes, this seems to occur as the result of death, not as its cause. An autopsy often reveals petechiae in the lungs and mild inflammation and congestion in the respiratory tract, but these symptoms are not severe enough to cause sudden death. It is clear that children do not suffocate from bedclothes or choke from overfeeding or underfeeding or from crying.

At the time of the death, parents need to talk about the things that they fear may have caused the death. (They heard the child crying but did not go to him right away; if only they had. . . . They fed her in a hurry because they were leaving to catch an early show; if only they had been more patient. . . .) They can be assured that the child did not die because of any of these things they did or did not do. Children with SIDS do not die crying; the time they heard crying was not the time the infant died.

Parents have a difficult time accepting the death of a child when it happens so suddenly. In discussing the child, they often use both the past and present tense, as if they are not yet aware of the death. Many parents experience a period of physical symptoms such as nausea, stomach pain, or vertigo. These are somatic symptoms that occur with acute grief.

Parents may move from the home or apartment where the death occurred, unable to live there any longer. They may separate if one parent believes that the other could or should have prevented the child's death. Parents should be counseled by a nurse or some other well-prepared person at the time of the infant's death; they usually need to talk to the same person a week or a month or many months later to resolve grief further. The National Foundation of Sudden Infant Death has chapters in most large cities. It is helpful for parents to join this organization so they can understand that the feelings they are experiencing are not unique but happen to everyone at such times of crisis. This realization keeps many parents from believing that they are becoming insane.

The National Foundation suggests that mandatory autopsies be performed on all children who die from SIDS, in the hope that a cause for the phenomenon can be identified. It is helpful to parents if autopsy reports are given to them as soon as they are available (if toxicology tests are included in the autopsy, results are not available for weeks). Reading a report that the child died an unexplained death helps reassure them that this was not their fault. They need this assurance so that they are not afraid to plan for other children. When another child is born, the parents can be expected to become extremely frightened at any sign of illness in the child. They need support to see them through the first few months of the second child's life. Some parents need support to view a second child as an individual child and not as a replacement for the one who died. Older children in the family need assurance that SIDS is a disease of infants and that the strange phenomenon that invaded their home and killed a brother or sister will not also kill them. If they wished the infant dead (all children wish siblings were dead on some days), they need to be assured that their wishes are not as powerful as this, and that they did not cause the baby's death.

Some infants have been discovered cyanotic and limp in their beds but have survived after mouth-to-mouth resuscitation by parents. These children are categorized as "near-miss" SIDS.

For some premature infants who show a tendency toward periods of apnea, those children who have had "near-miss" episodes, and the sib-

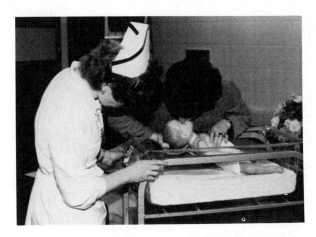

Figure 48-4 *All mothers of high-risk infants should learn mouth-to-mouth resuscitation before their baby is discharged from the hospital. Here a mother practices on a teaching doll.*

ling of a child who died from SIDS, a monitoring device that rings when a period of apnea occurs may prevent SIDS. If a mother is going to use an apnea monitor at home, explore with her questions such as: Can she hear it in all parts of the house? Usually the alarm is not loud enough to be heard in the basement from an upstairs bedroom. She will have to plan on not using the basement area when the infant is sleeping upstairs. This means that many women are not able to wash clothes until someone else is at home. Can she hear the alarm over the sound of the family room television? Another child's radio? The vacuum cleaner, a hair dryer, or shower water? Does she know how to reposition leads? Is she comfortable enough with the apparatus to see past it to the child? All parents of high-risk infants should be taught mouth-to-mouth resuscitation before their infant is discharged from the hospital. Be certain these parents know the technique well (Figure 48-4).

The impact of caring for the child on an apnea monitor usually becomes the mother's chief responsibility. Parents describe the impact of the monitor on the marriage as ranging from worsening of the relationship (about 14 percent) to improving the relationship (about 26 percent) (Cain, 1980). Arranging for a babysitter (or trusting care of the child to a babysitter) is often described as a major problem.

Most parents with a baby on an apnea monitor at home appreciate a community nurse referral so that they have a second opinion about the baby's condition as well as a listening ear to discuss the strain of having always to be alert for a sound that means their infant has stopped breathing.

They appreciate having someone review with them periodically what steps they should take if the alarm should sound (jiggle the baby; begin mouth-to-mouth resuscitation; call the emergency squad). They are parents under a tremendous strain, accentuated because when other parents sleep, they do not; a part of them is always listening for an alarm to ring.

Sudden infant death syndrome is a baffling disease. Parents of an infant born prematurely live with the fear of it until their child reaches a year of age.

Pneumothorax

Pneumothorax is leakage of air from lung alveoli into the pleural space surrounding the lung. Because this also occurs in term infants, it is discussed in Chapter 47.

Temperature Regulation

An immature baby has a great deal of difficulty maintaining body heat because of the relatively large surface area per pound of body weight and therefore rapid cooling from evaporation can occur, especially because these babies do not flex their body well but remain in an extended position due to immaturity.

The infant has little subcutaneous fat for insulation, and the poor muscular development does not allow active movement to produce body heat. He or she has a limited amount of brown fat, the special tissue in newborns that maintains body heat. Unable to shiver, which is a useful mechanism to increase body temperature, the baby is also unable to sweat to reduce body temperature because of immature central nervous system and hypothalamic control. He is thus dependent on the environmental temperature provided. The best course is a radiant heat warmer in a delivery room because delivery rooms are typically kept at a temperature of 62° to 68°F (16.6° to 20°C). A 1,500 gm infant exposed to this low a temperature loses 1 degree centigrade of body heat every 3 minutes if not protected.

Unless there are obvious abnormalities noted when a child is born, physical assessment of the infant—even weighing—should be delayed until the newborn is placed in the warmth of an Isolette or under a radiant warmer with a servocontrol.

In order to conserve energy, the infant's axillary temperature should be maintained at 97.8°F (36.5°C). He must have radiant heat for any procedure that has to be performed outside the Isolette. If a baby is going to be transported to a department within the hospital, such as the X-ray de-

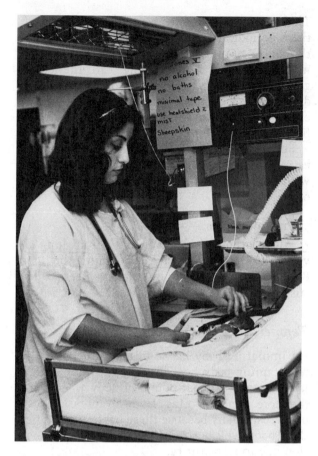

Figure 48-5 *Caring for an infant on a radiant heat warmer allows easier access to the child in the event of an emergency. (Courtesy of the Department of Medical Photography, Children's Hospital, Buffalo, N.Y.)*

partment or to a regional center for specialized care, he must be provided warmth during transport. Remember that infants lose heat by radiation. Even though an Isolette is warm, therefore, if it is placed near a cold window or air conditioner, an infant will lose heat to the distant source. Keep this fact in mind if transporting infants on cold days. An ambulance must be pulled in close to the hospital door; it, as well as the Isolette, must be prewarmed. An additional heat shield may be placed over an infant inside an Isolette to help conserve heat. A radiant heat source may be placed above the Isolette to further ensure heat in the Isolette. When using a radiant heat source, be certain the servocontrol to the infant is taped securely to the abdomen and covered with a piece of gauze to protect it from direct heat. If the probe should fall off, the radiant heat source will increase in intensity and possibly overheat the newborn; if the infant is turned on the abdomen so the probe is underneath, it may overheat and the radiant heat source will decrease, allowing hypothermia. Infants in radiant heat warmers have a higher insensible heat loss than those in Isolettes. Keep careful records of intake and output so that the infant receives enough fluid intake.

A preterm baby is typically left undressed except for a diaper in the Isolette or lying on a radiant warmer so that the chest and respiratory activity can be carefully observed (see Figure 48-5). Be certain whenever a baby is removed from an Isolette or warmer that he is wrapped warmly. Covering an infant's head covers a large surface area and helps a great deal to conserve heat in a small baby.

Nutritional Needs

Nutritional problems arise with an immature infant because his body continues to, or attempts to continue to, maintain the rapid rate of intrauterine growth after birth. The newborn therefore requires a larger amount of nutrients in the diet than the mature infant to prevent hypocalcemia or azotemia (low protein level in blood). Delayed feeding may also add to hyperbilirubinemia, a problem he is already high-risk to develop because of the extremely high hematocrit.

Nutritional problems occur because, as much as the small infant needs calories and protein, he has difficulty swallowing and sucking due to immature reflexes and small stomach capacity, and a distended stomach may cause respiratory distress. Increased activity, necessitated by ineffective sucking, may increase the metabolic rate and oxygen requirements and require even more calories (120 to 150 kcal/kg/day). The immature cardiac sphincter (between the stomach and esophagus) allows regurgitation to occur readily.

The lack of a cough reflex may lead the immature newborn to aspirate regurgitated formula. Digestion and absorption of nutrients in the stomach and intestine may be immature.

The immature infant is apparently unable to manufacture all nonessential amino acids from essential amino acids. The amino acids histidine, tyrosine, cystine, and taurine must be supplied in formula for these infants. Such infants are also unable to digest formula that has a higher casein than whey content. Thus premature formulas are designed with this distribution (as is human breast milk). A high insensible water loss follows from the large body surface. Since the baby is unable to concentrate urine well, he excretes a high proportion of fluid from the body. All these factors make it important that the immature baby receive 160 to 200 ml of fluid per kilogram of body weight daily. In order that he has enough calcium for rapidly growing skeletal growth, both calcium and vitamin D supplements are recommended (Ziegler, 1983).

Immature babies need intravenous fluid begun within hours after birth to begin to fulfill this fluid requirement and provide glucose to prevent hypoglycemia. Intravenous fluid should be given by a continuous infusion pump to ensure a constant infusion rate. A volume control meter must be used to prevent accidental overload if a tube clamp should slip and allow fluid rate to change. Intravenous sites must be checked conscientiously as the lack of subcutaneous tissue makes infiltration very damaging to tissue. Specially designed 27-gauge needles are available to enter small-lumened veins. Many immature infants have no peripheral veins of a size necessary for even this small a needle and so receive intravenous fluid by an umbilical vein or artery catheter.

The baby's weight, specific gravity and amount of urine, and serum electrolytes all must be monitored to ensure that fluid intake is adequate. Too little fluid and calories leads to dehydration and starvation, acidosis, and weight loss. Overhydration leads to weight gain, pulmonary edema, and heart failure.

An immature infant should void (and pass meconium) by 24 hours after birth. Urine output should be measured by weighed diapers to limit the number of urine collectors necessary (the constant changing of collectors leads to skin irritation and breakdown). The range of urine output for the first few days of life in low-birth-weight babies is high in comparison with that of the term baby—40 to 100 ml per kilogram per 24 hours, compared to 10 to 20 ml per kilogram. The specific gravity is low, rarely over 1.012 (normal term babies may concentrate urine up to 1.030). Doing Dextrostix tests every 4 to 6 hours helps to determine hypo- or hyperglycemia (level should be over 20 mg/ml). Be certain to keep a record of all blood drawn so that a child does not become hypovolemic. Hematest stools to determine that they do not contain blood (gastrointestinal bleeding with the introduction of milk).

Hyperglycemia caused by the glucose infusion may lead to spillage of glucose in the urine and an accompanying diuresis. If the glucose being supplied is too low and body cells are using protein for metabolism, ketone bodies will appear in urine; therefore, urine specimens are tested for glucose and ketones as well as for amount and specific gravity.

Feeding Patterns

Calorie requirements for an immature infant are higher than for the term infant in order to provide calories for rapid growth: 120 to 150 calories per kilogram body weight per day compared to 100 to 110 calories per kilogram weight per day. Protein requirements are 3 to 4 grams per

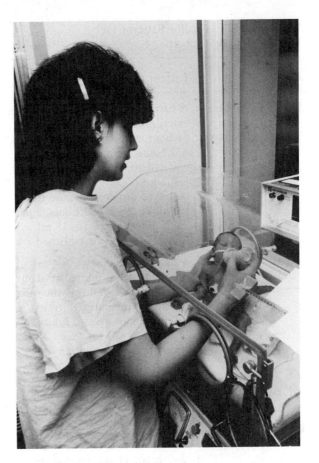

Figure 48-6 *Feeding a low-birth-weight infant. Notice the small bottle used. (Courtesy of the Department of Medical Photography, Children's Hospital, Buffalo, N.Y.)*

kilogram weight compared to 2.0 to 2.5 grams per kilogram weight in a term newborn. An immature infant's small stomach capacity precludes large feedings, so frequency is necessary. An infant under 1,200 gm is fed as often as every 2 hours; over 1,200 gm, about every 3 hours (Figure 48-6). Feeding patterns for various weight infants are shown in Table 48-2. Common formulas used with immature infants are shown in Table 48-3.

Formulas used may have a higher calorie count than those for term infants to enable more calories to be given in small amounts. Thus, the caloric concentration of formula for immature babies may be 24 or 27 calories per ounce in comparison to 20 calories per ounce for a term baby.

Minerals such as calcium and phosphorus and electrolytes such as sodium, potassium, and chloride may have to be supplemented, depending on blood studies. An immature infant needs supplementary A, C, D, and E vitamins. Vitamin K should be administered at birth, as with a term baby, except that the amount is more often 0.5 ml instead of 1 ml. Vitamin E seems to be important in preventing hemolytic anemia in immature in-

Table 48-2 Oral Feeding Patterns for
Low-Birth-Weight Infants

Infant	Pattern
Under 1,000 gms	A first oral feeding of 1–2 ml of sterile water is offered at about 1 hour of age: During the next 72 hours, premature formula is offered about every hour. The amount is increased 1 ml every other feeding to a maximum of 5 ml. Following 72 hours, a pattern of feeding of 10–15 ml every 2 hours is established.
Between 1,001 and 1,500 gms	A first oral feeding of 3–4 ml sterile water is offered at about 2 hours of age. During the next 72 hours, premature formula is offered about every 2 hours. The amount is increased 1 ml every other feeding to a maximum of 10 ml. Following 72 hours, a pattern of feeding of 20–28 ml every 2–3 hours is established.
Between 1,501 and 2,000 gms	A first oral feeding of 4–5 ml sterile water is offered at about 2–3 hours of age. During the next 72 hours, premature formula is offered about every 2–3 hours. The amount is increased 2 ml every other feeding to a maximum of 15 ml. Following 72 hours, a pattern of feeding of 28–37 ml every 3 hours is established.
Over 2,000 gms	A first oral feeding of 10 ml sterile water is offered at about 3 hours of age. During the next 72 hours, premature formula is offered about every 3 hours. The amount is increased 5 ml every other feeding to a maximum of 20 ml. Following 72 hours, a pattern of feeding of 37–50 ml every 3–4 hours is established.

Source: Avery, G. B. (Ed.) (1981). Neonatology, 2nd. ed. Philadelphia, Lippincott.

fants. Iron supplements interfere with the absorption of vitamin E and so are not added to formula until an infant has gained an average birth weight.

The lack of an iron supplement is confusing to parents because they have always been told that iron helps to build strong blood. Now they are told that in their particularly vulnerable infant, iron is not being given because it will interfere with blood cell integrity. They need an explanation of the particular blood problem that must be prevented. Iron supplements will be started on discharge from the hospital or at least by 3 months of age. Again, parents should have an explanation of what is happening. By the time of discharge, their infant has reached term maturity, and iron deficiency anemia due to low iron stores then becomes the chief problem.

With the early administration of intravenous fluid to prevent hypoglycemia and supply fluid, gastrointestinal feedings may be safely delayed until the infant has stabilized respiratory effort from birth. Feedings should be begun, however, by gavage or bottle as soon as he is able to tolerate them. If a baby is going to be bottle-fed, the feeding pattern should be started with sterile water. If the infant should aspirate this first feeding, the insult of sterile water on lung tissue is less than that of either glucose water or formula.

Because of the small stomach capacity of preterm infants, feedings are very small in amount—as little as 1 or 2 ml in the smallest infants. The amount is gradually increased as the infant gains weight and stomach capacity enlarges. Increases in amount must be very small (1 or 5 ml) to prevent regurgitation.

There is accumulating evidence that, although the immature infant needs the increased caloric distribution of commercial formulas, the best milk for immature babies, as well as for term babies, is breast milk. The immunologic properties of breast milk play a major role in preventing neonatal necrotizing enterocolitis, a destructive intestinal disorder that occurs in low-birth-weight babies.

A mother who wants to breast-feed can manually express breast milk for her infant's gavage feedings. Women in the community who have excess breast milk or who have discontinued breast-feeding and want to express breast milk and supply it to special care nurseries are urged to do so to maintain a milk bank for immature babies. In most programs of this nature, the expressed breast milk is frozen for safe transport and storage. Whether freezing destroys the antibodies or factors that make breast milk preferable for sensitive digestive tracts is being investigated. The sodium content of breast milk in a mother whose infant has been born prematurely is higher than that of milk at term. It is best if an infant receives his own mother's breast milk rather than pooled breast milk in order to receive this high level of sodium (necessary for fluid retention in an immature infant). Low-birth-weight infants may be fed

Table 48-3 Formulas Commonly Used with Immature Infants

| Formula | Caloric Content | Carbohydrate | | Protein | | Fat | | Osmolality |
		g/dL	Type	g/dL	Whey/ Casein Ratio	g/dL	Type	mosm/kg H₂O
Enfamil 24 Premature Formula	24 kcal/30 ml	9.1	60% polycose 40% lactose	2.4	60/40	4.1	40% MCT 40% corn	300
Similac Special Care Infant Formula	24 kcal/30 ml	8.6	50% lactose 50% polycose	2.2	60/40	4.4	50% MCT	290
Similac PM 60/40	20 kcal/30 ml	6.9	lactose	1.6	60/40	3.8	60% coconut	260
SMA 24	24 kcal/30 ml	4.2	lactose	1.8	60/40	4.2	oleo, soy, coconut	364

Source: From Avery, G. B. (Ed.)(1981). *Neonatology.* 2nd ed. Philadelphia, Lippincott, p. 1026.

by total parenteral nutrition until they are mature enough for other means. With adequate nutrients, an immature infant gains about 20 to 30 grams a day and increases in length 1 cm a week.

Gavage-Feeding

Immature infants of low birth weight are begun on gavage feedings by permanently placed nasogastric tubes. (See Procedure 48-1.) As they mature, bottle-feeding is gradually introduced. A mother who wants to breast-feed and has preserved her milk supply during the time the infant could not suck may visit daily and, as the infant grows strong enough, begin breast-feedings.

Infants are 32 weeks of gestation before their gag reflex is intact. They are 34 weeks of gestation before they can consistently coordinate sucking and swallowing.

As long as an infant is being gavage-fed, stomach secretions are usually aspirated, measured, and replaced prior to the feeding. An infant who has a stomach content of over 2 ml just prior to a feeding is receiving more formula than he can digest in the time allowed. Feedings should not be increased but possibly even cut back to ensure better digestion and decrease the possibility of regurgitation and aspiration. Inability to digest this way is also a symptom of necrotizing enterocolitis.

Immature infants must be observed closely after an oral or gavage feeding to be certain that the filled stomach is not causing them respiratory distress. As soon as a sucking reflex is present, offering a pacifier will strengthen this reflex and better prepare an infant for bottle-feeding as well as provide oral satisfaction.

Prevention of Infection

As noted, the skin of immature babies is easily traumatized and therefore offers less resistance to infection than the skin and mucous membrane of mature babies. Immature infants have difficulty producing phagocytes to localize infection, and they have a deficiency of IgM antibodies because of insufficient production.

Linen and equipment used with an immature infant must be sterile to reduce the chances of infection. Staff members must be free of infection, and hand washing and gowning regulations must be enforced.

Bonding

The periods of reactivity normally observed in newborns at 1 hour and 4 hours of life (see Chapter 31) are delayed in an immature infant. In some infants, no period of increased activity or tachycardia may appear until 12 to 18 hours of age. If the purpose of a period of reactivity is to stimulate respiratory function, this places the immature infant in even greater threat of respiratory failure. A second consequence of periods of reactivity is the interaction between parents and child that occurs during this time. With delayed periods of reactivity, this stimulation for parent-

---

Procedure 48-1

Gavage Feeding

Purpose: Offer nutrition to infant who cannot suck effectively—or has another contraindication to bottle or breast feeding—through a previously placed nasogastric tube.

Plan	*Principle*
1. Wash your hands; identify the infant.	1. Prevent spread of microorganisms. Promote patient safety.
2. Assess the infant's condition; analyze appropriateness of procedure; plan modifications as necessary.	2. Do not feed if respiratory distress or symptoms such as vomiting are present.
3. Begin implementation by assembling equipment: breast milk or formula in designated amount; sterile water for rinse (if designated); wrap for swaddling infant; syringe and stethoscope; measuring tape.	3. Assembling equipment prevents undue exposure or tiring of infant.
4. Measure abdominal circumference to detect distention if infant is high risk for development of necrotizing enterocolitis. Swaddle infant in mummy restraint to contain infant hands. Turn infant to right side; elevate infant's chest and head slightly. Provide pacifier for oral stimulation (if appropriate).	4. Infants at high risk for necrotizing enterocolitis are those who have suffered anoxia. Elevating chest will prevent aspiration. Gustatory stimulation aids normal development.
5. Assess that gavage tube is in stomach by aspirating stomach contents. Measure contents removed and return to tube.	5. Assessing placement prevents aspiration. Returning stomach contents prevents alkalosis.
6. Attach feeding syringe or funnel and add formula or milk. Elevate no more than 12 inches over infant's stomach and allow fluid to flow by gravity.	6. Allowing feeding to infuse by gravity prevents stomach overflow and aspiration.
7. Observe color of infant during feeding. Discontinue feeding if apnea, cyanosis, or coughing should occur.	7. Respiratory distress can occur from stomach overflow or pressure on diaphragm.
8. Finish feeding with water rinse if ordered. At completion of feeding, reclamp tubing; sit infant upright and gently rub back to allow any air bubbles in stomach to rise.	8. If air remains in stomach, it will cause discomfort and possibly aspiration.
9. Remove restraint; reposition infant comfortably on side with head and chest still slightly elevated. Assess for need for additional hand restraints.	9. Keep chest elevated for 20 minutes to prevent aspiration.
10. Evaluate patient status and effectiveness of procedure. Plan health teaching for parents regarding procedure such as need for feeding method.	10. Health teaching is an independent measure always incorporated in nursing care.
11. Chart type, and amount of feeding and patient response.	11. Document nursing care and patient status.

child contact is also decreased. Because the infant is often transported for care, separation from the infant may lead to decreased bonding.

Common Illnesses of Immature Infants

In the neonatal period, immature infants are particularly susceptible to the following: anemia (since it is in the last few weeks of intrauterine life that iron is stored in the liver); failure to thrive due to feeding difficulty; failure of cardiac shunts to close due to increased lung resistance; dehydration due to feeding difficulty and inefficient concentration of urine; infection, principally of the respiratory tract and skin; hypoglycemia (since glycogen deposits are not yet stored); and hypothermia (as little subcutaneous fat has been deposited). These conditions are discussed in Chapter 47 since they also occur in term infants. In addition, immature infants may develop a number of additional conditions: hemorrhage, persistent fetal circulation, respiratory distress syndrome, retrolental fibroplasia, necrotizing enterocolitis, and kernicterus.

Hemorrhage

Because immature infants are born with exceedingly low levels of vitamin K, they have a greater tendency to hemorrhage than do mature infants. Hemorrhage from vitamin K deficiency responds within a few hours to the administration of vitamin K or to the infusion of fresh whole blood. It can be prevented by the routine prophylactic administration of vitamin K to all infants immediately after birth (a procedure that can be easily missed in the stress of a preterm infant's birth).

A second form of bleeding that occurs chiefly among preterm infants is the result of a combination of (a) increased capillary fragility, (b) prolonged bleeding time, and (c) a decreased amount of blood factor V. It is clinically difficult to distinguish this form of hemorrhagic disease from vitamin K deficiency. It is found most often in infants who have had hypoxia or infection. Vitamin K deficiency bleeding tends to occur in the gastrointestinal tract, the nose, and around the eyes; in this second form of bleeding, the lungs and the central nervous system are the most common sites of hemorrhage. The increased capillary fragility is apparently a manifestation of immaturity. Extremely gentle handling minimizes

the occurrence of bleeding episodes, although such bleeding may occur during delivery, particularly in the form of intracranial hemorrhage, and may severely damage or be lethal to the immature infant.

Intracranial Hemorrhage

One of the greatest hazards to the immature infant at birth is intracranial hemorrhage. This is also a possibility any time an infant has a period of hypoxia during neonatal life.

If the tentorial membrane is torn because of birth trauma, the bleed will be into the basic structures below, or the pons, cerebellum, and medulla oblongata. As the regulatory mechanisms for heart and respiratory function are located in these parts, a bleed here is obviously life-threatening.

The fact that an intracranial bleed has occurred is evidenced by signs of respiratory distress and cyanosis; hypotension may occur, and seizures may occur. The infant may have a high, shrill cry. He may show signs of cardiovascular shock. The reflexes, particularly the Moro reflex, are no longer present. Other neurologic signs such as jitteriness, hypothermia, or hypotonia may occur. If the bleed is into the subarachnoid space, the cerebrospinal fluid will be blood-tinged on lumbar puncture. Subdural bleeding (equally serious because it causes compression of brain tissue) will not stain cerebrospinal fluid.

A fall in the infant's hematocrit level may reveal that a bleed has occurred. A computerized tomography (CT) scan or a sonogram will reveal the extent of the bleed. The infant should be placed in a position with the head elevated to minimize intracranial pressure. The infant needs oxygen and assisted ventilation as a rule, to overcome the shock to the system. The ability to suck may be poor, so the baby needs intravenous fluid to maintain water and caloric balance. Hyperbilirubinemia may occur as the trapped blood is reabsorbed.

The infant has been severely compromised by an intracranial bleed. It is difficult for parents to understand what has happened since they know little about brain anatomy. They need day-to-day reports of progress and the accumulating evidence (the infant cannot sustain respiratory function without assisted ventilation; the vital signs are becoming less and less steady) to help them understand the seriousness of their child's condition. Some infants do survive an intracranial bleed during this time but are left with permanently impaired neurologic and mental incapabilities.

Persistent Fetal Circulation/Persistent Pulmonary Hypertension Syndrome

In utero, the resistance in the pulmonary artery is high because lung alveoli are not open. At birth, pulmonary vascular resistance decreases not only in response to the opening of alveoli but to an increased oxygen tension in blood vessels. In an infant whose PO_2 levels remain compromised, pulmonary resistance remains high in the pulmonary artery. This prevents closure of the ductus arteriosus and perhaps the foramen ovale. Blood pressure in the pulmonary artery is so high that blood continues to shunt as it did in fetal life from the venous to the arterial circulation (a right-to-left shunt or cyanotic heart disease).

That a right-to-left shunt is operating is suspected when an infant needs more than 80 percent concentration of oxygen to maintain a normal PO_2. A patent ductus shunt is suggested by a lower PO_2 level in arterial blood sampled from lower extremity arteries (postductal blood) than in temporal or right radial arteries (preductal blood or blood that arises from the aorta proximal to the shunt). If blood is being shunted by the foramen ovale, this assessment will not demonstrate a difference (all blood is postductal).

Echocardiography can be used to identify a shunt. For this examination, a bolus of saline is injected into the inferior vena cava. This pocket of a lower concentration of fluid can be followed by echocardiography as it follows the shunt across into the arterial circulation.

Administering indomethacin, a prostaglandin inhibitor, causes closure of the patent ductus arteriosus. Indomethacin has the side effects of decreased renal function, decreased platelet count, and gastric irritation. All infants who receive it need urine output carefully recorded and observation for bleeding, especially at blood puncture sites. Be certain the infant is not overhydrated to limit hypervolemia, which may contribute to poor ductus closure. Pulmonary vasculature may be vasodilated by the administration of isoproterenol or tolazoline. Both these drugs have side effects that may make them unacceptable. Isoproterenol causes tachycardia; an infant with an already increased heart rate due to respiratory distress may not be able to tolerate the additional insult. Tolazoline causes systemic vasodilatation as well as pulmonary vasodilatation. This may lead to such hypotension that it cannot be used; an antihypertensive such as dopamine hydrochloride may need to be administered concurrently to maintain systemic blood pressure.

Administering these agents through an intravenous line directly into a pulmonary artery catheter may cause only local effects. Another choice is scalp vein administration because blood from the superior vena cava entering the heart tends to go directly to the right ventricle and pulmonary artery, rather than crossing the foramen ovale. While such drugs are infusing, systemic blood pressure and blood gases must be continually monitored.

Alkalinization, or maintaining the infant's blood pH well above an acidotic level (pH 7.5 or above), also appears to be helpful in patent ductus arteriosus closure. In addition, in the presence of an alkaline pH, tolazoline and isoproterenol are more effective and pulmonary vessel vasodilatation more efficient.

Respiratory Distress Syndrome

Respiratory distress syndrome (RDS) (formerly termed *hyaline membrane disease*) most commonly occurs in immature infants; in infants of diabetic mothers or mothers who have had vaginal bleeding during pregnancy, such as occurs with placenta previa or premature separation of the placenta; and in infants born by cesarean birth. The pathologic feature of RDS is a hyaline-like (fibrous) membrane, composed of products formed from an exudate of the infant's blood that lines the terminal bronchioles, alveolar ducts, and alveoli. This membrane prevents exchange of oxygen and carbon dioxide at the alveolar-blood interface. The cause of RDS is a low level of phosphotidyl glycerol and the lecithin component of surfactant, the phospholipid that indicates lung maturity at birth and maintains surface tension in the alveoli on expiration to keep them from collapsing on expiration.

Very high pressure is required to fill the lungs with air for the first time and overcome the pressure of lung fluid. It takes a pressure between 40 to 70 cm H_2O to inspire a first breath, but only 6 to 8 H_2O to maintain quiet, continued breathing in the immature infant. When alveoli collapse with each expiration, however, it continues to take forceful inspiration to inflate them.

As areas of hypoinflation occur, pulmonary blood resistance in the lung is increased. This high tension in the pulmonary artery may cause blood to shunt through the foramen ovale and the ductus arteriosus as it did during fetal life (persistent fetal circulation), when passage of blood through the lungs could not be accomplished. With poor lung cell blood perfusion, the production of surfactant decreases even further. Infants with persistent fetal circulation are most prone to become ventilator-dependent and to develop pulmonary dysplasia.

The poor oxygen exchange leads to systemic tissue hypoxia. Tissue hypoxia causes the release of lactic acid. This, combined with an increasing carbon dioxide level resulting from the formation of the hyaline membrane on the alveolar surfaces, leads to severe acidosis. Acidosis causes vasoconstriction. Decreased pulmonary perfusion from vasoconstriction limits surfactant production still further.

With decreased surfactant production, the ability to stop alveoli from collapsing with each expiration is even further impaired. This vicious cycle continues until oxygen–carbon dioxide exchange in the alveoli is no longer adequate to sustain life.

Assessment

Most infants who will later develop RDS have difficulty initiating respirations; after resuscitation at birth, they appear to have a period of hours or a day when they are free of symptoms. However, during this time, subtle signs such as low body temperature, nasal flaring, sternal and subcostal retractions, and tachypnea (over 70 respirations per minute) may be present. Within several hours, expiratory grunting becomes apparent. Expiratory grunting indicates a prolonged expiratory time. The sound denotes closure of the glottis. Glottis closure increases the pressure in alveoli on expiration, helps to keep alveoli from collapsing, and makes oxygen exchange more complete. Thus, expiratory grunting is a compensatory mechanism.

Even with this attempt at better oxygen exchange, however, as the disease progresses, most infants become cyanotic in room air. On auscultation, there may be fine rales and diminished breath sounds because of poor air entry. As distress increases, the infant shows seesaw respirations (on inspiration, the anterior chest wall retracts and the abdomen protrudes; on expiration, the sternum rises). An infant's heart begins to fail, the urine output decreases, and there may be edema of the extremities. The child's temperature falls. Color becomes a pale gray; periods of apnea occur, and bradycardia becomes apparent.

Diagnosis of RDS is made on clinical signs of grunting, cyanosis in room air, tachypnea, nasal flaring, and retractions and shock. A chest X-ray will reveal a diffuse pattern of radiopaque areas of ground glass (haziness). Blood gas studies (blood is taken from an umbilical vessel catheter) will reveal respiratory acidosis. The infant obviously is gravely ill. Echocardiography is used to identify whether a patent arteriosus is present.

A Group B hemolytic streptococcal infection may mimic RDS. This infection is so severe in newborns that with the insult to the lungs, sur-

Table 48-4 Respiratory Therapy Score: Scoring System Using Five Clinical and Laboratory Measurements Available in Community Hospitals

Measurement	Score		
	0	1	2
Birth weight (gm)	Over 2,000	1,500–2,000	Under 1,500
Clinical score	3 or under	4–5	6 and over
FiO₂[a]	49 or under	50–65	65 and over
PCO₂[b]	Under 40	40–45	Over 45
pH[b]	7.35 or over	7.34–7.30	7.30 and lower
Totals	—	—	—
TOTAL SCORE	_____		

[a]Inspired oxygen concentration necessary to maintain the infant's skin color pink.
[b]Venous blood sample.

Source: Peckham, G. J., et al. (1979). A clinical score for predicting the level of respiratory care in infants with respiratory distress syndrome. Clinical Pediatrics, 18, 716.

factant production may stop. Cultures of blood, CSF, and skin are taken and antibiotic therapy (penicillin or ampicillin) and an aminoglycoside (gentamicin or kanamycin) may be begun until accurate reports are available.

When newborns of low birth weight are born in community hospitals, one of the most serious decisions that must be made is whether the infant needs to be transferred to a regional center for respiratory therapy for RDS. Using a scoring system such as the one shown in Table 48-4 helps decide if the newborn will need more respiratory therapy than a small hospital can provide. To use the scoring system, points are given for birth weight, a clinical score, the percentage of oxygen needed to keep the infant's skin color pink, and venous blood CO₂ and pH. The clinical score is obtained by using Table 48-5.

Infants who score from 0 to 3 (Table 48-4) probably can be managed with oxygen by hood. Infants scoring 4 or 5 usually need CPAP therapy. Infants who score over 6 are likely to need mechanical ventilation. Whether to transfer an infant is a physician's responsibility, but the preceding scoring system can guide you in evaluating the infant.

Analysis

The most frequent nursing diagnoses established with an infant with RDS are ineffective oxygen-carbon dioxide exchange and a potential interference with bonding. It is difficult for parents to maintain bonds with a child if he is transferred to a special care nursery. Goals for care are

Table 48-5 Clinical Respiratory Distress Scoring System

	Score		
Measurement	0	1	2
Respiratory rate (per minute)	60	60–80	Over 80 or apneic episodes
Cyanosis	None	In air	In 40% oxygen
Retractions	None	Mild	Moderate to severe
Grunting	None	Audible with stethoscope	Audible without stethoscope
Air entry (crying)*	Clear	Delayed or decreased	Barely audible

* Air entry represents the quality of inspiratory breath sounds as heard in the midaxillary line.

Source: Downes, J., et al. (1970). Respiratory distress syndrome of newborn infants. New clinical scoring system with acid-base and blood-gas correlates. *Clinical Pediatrics, 9,* 325.

summarized in the Nursing Care Highlight on page 1201.

Implementations

An infant with RDS needs care in a unit specially designed to meet the needs of such infants. He must be kept warm, because cooling increases acidosis in all infants, and may increase it in these infants to lethal levels. In this way also the metabolic rate does not have to increase to maintain an adequate temperature, which reduces the oxygen need as well. The newborn may need correction of acidosis by intravenous sodium bicarbonate administration. The infant will need intravenous fluid and glucose or gavage-feeding for hydration and nourishment because respiratory effort makes him too exhausted to suck.

Administration of oxygen is generally necessary to maintain correct PO_2 and pH levels. Continous positive airway pressure (CPAP) or assisted ventilation with positive end expiratory pressure (PEEP) will exert pressure on the alveoli at the end of expiration and keep alveoli from collapsing. This management greatly improves the oxygen exchange. Complications are pneumothorax and impairment of cardiac output from lung pressure. A possible risk of increased intracranial and venous pressure and hemorrhage exists. Limiting fluid intake may decrease pulmonary artery pressure. The administration of indomethacin will cause closure of a patent ductus arteriosus and make ventilation more efficient. Indomethacin has the side effects of decreased renal function, decreased platelet count, and gastric irritation. All infants who receive it need urine

output carefully recorded and observation for bleeding, especially at blood puncture sites.

Yet another method of increasing pulmonary blood flow and oxygenation is by the use of muscle relaxants. Pancuronium (Pavulon) is administered intravenously to a point of abolishing spontaneous respiratory action. This allows mechanical ventilation to be accomplished at lower pressures because there is no normal muscle resistance to overcome. Pneumothorax is then less likely, while PO_2 increases. Obviously an infant who has no spontaneous respiratory function needs critical observation and frequent arterial blood gases: He or she is totally dependent on caregivers at that point. The effects of pancuronium decrease as the life of the drug expires; its effect can be interrupted by the administration of atropine or Prostigmin.

When pancuronium is being administered, both atropine and Prostigmin should be immediately available. The infant's nursing care plan should be specially marked that pancuronium therapy is being used so that, in the event of a power failure, manual ventilatory assistance can be immediately begun.

Normally, inspiration is shorter than expiration or an inspiratory/expiratory ratio (I:E) is 1:2. It is difficult to deliver enough oxygen to stiff, noncompliant lungs in this usual ratio without forcing the air into the lungs at such a high pressure and rapid rate that pneumothorax becomes a constant fear. New infant ventilators are devised with a reversed I:E ratio (2:1). Use of these allows a greater amount of air to be administered at lower pressures. Their use has reduced the problem of pneumothorax and appears to relieve the problem of bronchopulmonary dysplasia as well. High-frequency oscillatory ventilation (HFOV) and "jet" ventilation are other new methods of introducing oxygen to infants with noncompliant lungs. As the name implies, these systems maintain a high airway pressure and then intermittently "jet" or oscillate at a very rapid rate (up to 600 times a minute) an additional amount of air to inflate alveoli.

Parental Needs. Parents of a child with RDS should be able to visit the special nursing unit to which the child is admitted as often as they choose, wash and gown, and actually touch the child. This opportunity makes the child's birth more real to them, and, should the baby not survive the illness, it will make the death more real. Only when both birth and death seem real can parents begin to work through their feelings and accept these events. Parents may have to work

Nursing Care Highlight

The Infant with Respiratory Distress Syndrome

Goal of Care	*Implementations*
Aid in diagnosis	Identify high-risk population: immature infant; infant with respiratory insult at birth.
	Assess respiratory rate and evidence of retraction or grunting; periods of apnea.
	Auscultate for sound of patent ductus arteriosus.
	Obtain cultures for *Streptococcus* B differentiation.
Provide respiratory support	Assist with ventilatory support such as CPAP or PEEP.
	Provide ventilatory assistance with reversed I:E ratio as ordered.
	Observe for pneumothorax and ventilatory dependence.
	Administer pancuronium to maintain muscle relaxation.
Maintain circulation	Administer indomethacin or other agent to aid closure of ductus arteriosus.
	Maintain thermal neutrality to prevent vasoconstriction.
	Aid in maintaining alkaline blood serum.
Provide nutrition	Gavage-feed or sustain by total parenteral alimentation to prevent need to expend energy for sucking.
Aid bonding	Encourage parents to visit and care for infant.
	Keep parents informed of infant's progress.

through a great many feelings concerning their child's birth. If the baby is premature, a mother may need assurance that nothing she did (ate too much dinner the day of labor and so crowded out the baby; forgot to take her iron pill for 2 days) caused the premature birth and therefore this illness. If she had to have a cesarean birth, she may feel inadequate as a woman and may need assurance that being able to give vaginal birth is not a measure of a woman's worth. If the parents are young and have not planned well to provide for medical expenses, they may be extremely concerned about the hospital bill and may wonder whether the child will receive good care once the cashier learns that they have no hospital insurance.

All mothers handle newborn babies tentatively until they have "claimed" them or have become better acquainted. The mother of a child who has been very ill at birth may take months before she can handle the baby comfortably and confidently. The parents need to spend time in the intensive care nursery as the baby improves, so that they can begin the process of claiming. They need to

have access to health care personnel after discharge, to help them in caring for the child with confidence at home.

If an infant dies, the parents often wish to see the body. They may never have seen their newborn without a great deal of surrounding equipment and may need this time to reassure themselves that in every other way except lung function, he was a perfect baby. This realization gives them confidence to plan for other children and to continue their lives.

Evaluation

Despite current therapy, about 20 to 30 percent of children who develop RDS will not survive. In infants with moderate disease, a peak is reached in about 3 days; after that time, the condition will gradually improve.

The ultimate therapy for infants with RDS will be the administration of surfactant to lung surfaces to replace that which is not being produced, just as insulin is administered to people with diabetes. Both animal and synthetic surfactant is now available on an experimental basis. The results garnered from the animal form are encouraging, although not as dramatic as first expected. Findings suggest that animal surfactant is not totally identical to human surfactant and that chemical analysis must have missed some factor in it. The synthetic form, although apparently identical, still must lack some vital component also. Methods of administering surfactant so that it reaches closed alveoli are yet another problem. The side effects or long-term effects of the direct administration are not yet known.

Preventing Respiratory Distress Syndrome

RDS rarely occurs in mature infants. Dating a pregnancy by sonogram determination and L/S ratio of amniotic fluid are important means of assessing whether an infant delivered by cesarean birth or induced is mature enough that RDS is not apt to occur. (If the level of lecithin in surfactant exceeds that of sphingomyelin by 2:0, the lungs are mature and RDS is not likely to occur.) Preventing labor by the use of tocolytic agents such as ritodrine helps to prevent immature infants from being born.

It may be possible to prevent RDS in infants by administering glucocorticosteroids (betamethasome is a common type) to the mother 24 hours prior to delivery. Steroids appear to act to quicken the formation of lecithin production pathways. Unfortunately, there is often no warning that premature birth is imminent until hours before delivery. Even if this becomes a feasible means of preventing the syndrome, some labors and deliveries will progress too rapidly to be prevented by this measure.

Retrolental Fibroplasia

Although retrolental fibroplasia (RFP) is rarely seen today, it is a possibility that must be kept in mind by all health care personnel caring for infants of interrupted pregnancies.

Retrolental fibroplasia is an acquired ocular disease that leads to partial or total blindness in children due to vasoconstriction of immature retinal blood vessels. It was first recognized as an eye disorder in 1942, occurring in 5 to 25 percent of surviving infants whose birth weights were under 1,800 gm (4 pounds) and replacing gonococcal ophthalmia neonatorium as the leading cause of blindness in children. It was 10 years before it was established that a high concentration of oxygen is the causative agent. High concentrations of oxygen cause the vasoconstriction of retinal blood vessels and a secondary proliferation of endothelial cells in the layer of nerve fibers in the periphery of the retina in the immature infant, often resulting in detachment of the retina and blindness.

An infant who is receiving oxygen must have blood PO_2 levels monitored. If PO_2 levels are kept within normal limits, there is no danger. With PO_2 levels over 100 mg Hg, the danger of retrolental fibroplasia is great. The recommendations of the American Academy of Pediatrics for oxygen administration (see page 1187) are designed to protect infants from receiving concentrations of oxygen that will damage retinal tissue (Figure 48-7).

Vitamin E may reduce the incidence of RFP as it modifies tissue response to the effect of oxygen. Monitoring PO_2 by transcutaneous monitoring is the best method to be certain that an infant's oxygen level is continually well controlled.

A person experienced in recognizing retrolental fibroplasia should examine the eyes of all infants born at less than 36 weeks' gestation or weighing less than 2,000 gm who have received oxygen therapy. Examination should be made at discharge from the nursery and again at 3 to 6 months of age.

Figure 48-7 *Excessive oxygen administration is the cause of retrolental fibroplasia in the immature infant. The amount of oxygen given to any newborn must be monitored carefully by health care personnel. (Courtesy of the Department of Medical Photography, Children's Hospital, Buffalo, N.Y.)*

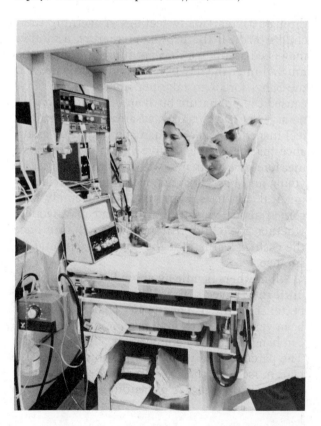

Kernicterus

Kernicterus, which results from high concentrations of indirect bilirubin in the blood due to excessive breakdown of red blood cells, occurs in about 5 percent of mature infants and in 10 to 40 percent of immature infants. Because many immature infants are acidotic, their brain cells may be more susceptible to the effect of indirect bilirubin than are those of the more mature infant, and they may have less serum albumin to bind indirect bilirubin and therefore inactivate its effect. Hence kernicterus may occur at lower levels of indirect bilirubin in these infants than in mature infants. Thus, it is as important or more important to monitor indirect bilurubin levels in immature infants if jaundice occurs, so that phototherapy or exchange transfusion can be begun before an infant becomes toxic. This point may be as low as 8 to 12 mg per 100 ml in immature infants.

Necrotizing Enterocolitis

Necrotizing enterocolitis (NEC) is a condition that develops in about 5 percent of all infants in intensive care nurseries. The bowel develops necrotic patches, interfering with digestion and possibly leading to a paralytic ileus. Perforation and peritonitis may follow.

The necrosis appears to result from ischemia or poor perfusion of blood vessels in sections of bowel. The ischemic process may occur when, owing to shock or hypoxia, there is vasoconstriction of blood vessels to nonessential organs such as the bowel. The entire bowel may be involved, or it may be a localized phenomenon. The incidence of NEC is highest in very immature infants and those who have suffered anoxia or shock; it may occur following an exchange transfusion. Infants with infections may develop it as a further complication of their already stressed state.

There is a low incidence of the condition in infants who are fed breast milk. Intestinal organisms grow more profusely with cow's milk than breast milk. The combination of decreased bowel perfusion and a response to the foreign protein in cow's milk probably starts the necrotic process.

Assessment

Signs that the condition is beginning usually appear in the first week of life. The abdomen becomes distended and tense. The infant does not empty the stomach by the next feeding time because of poor intestinal action, so if you aspirate for fluid before a gavage feeding you will find a return of undigested milk over 2 ml. Stool may be positive for occult blood. Periods of apnea may begin, or worsen in amount if they were already present. Signs of blood loss due to intestinal bleeding such as lowered blood pressure and inability to stabilize temperature may be present.

Abdominal X-ray films reveal a characteristic picture of air invading the intestinal wall; if perforation has occurred, there will be free air in the abdominal cavity. The abdomen's increase in size can be ascertained by measuring the abdominal circumference every 4 to 8 hours. The measurement is made just above the umbilicus.

Implementations

Gavage or bottle feedings must be discontinued and the infant maintained on intravenous or total parenteral nutrition solutions to rest the gastrointestinal tract. A course of an antibiotic may be given to limit secondary infection. The abdomen must be handled gently to lessen the possibility of bowel perforation. The infant may need a temporary colostomy performed to relieve obstruction. If the area of necrosis appears to be localized, surgery to remove that portion of the bowel may be successful. If a large portion of the bowel is removed, the infant may be prone to "short-bowel" syndrome or have a problem with digestion of nutrients in the future.

Evaluation

NEC is a grave insult to an infant already stressed by immaturity. The prognosis is guarded until it can be demonstrated that he can again take oral feedings without bowel complication.

Hypoglycemia

Glycogen stores are laid down in the late months of pregnancy. Thus an immature infant is apt to have few glycogen stores. If establishing respirations at birth is difficult, a baby uses a great deal of any glucose available in the effort. If chilled the infant's use of glucose is even more rapid.

An immature infant should have frequent blood sugar levels taken in the first hours of life by Dextrostix determinations (on nursery admission and then every 4 hours times 6) until stable, and while IV fluid is infusing and at the completion of IV fluid. A level below 30 mg is considered hypoglycemia in a term infant; under 20 mg is hypoglycemia in an immature infant.

Assess urine for glycosuria to detect if a level is being spilled. Clinical signs of hypoglycemia are more difficult to detect in an immature infant than the term infant because lethargy, poor feeding, and hypotonia may already be present; immature CNS control may mimic the jittery motion of immaturity.

The administration of intravenous glucose or constant parenteral nutrition may be necessary to maintain a functioning glucose level until further maturity is reached.

The Immature Infant and Parent-Child Interaction

At one time, immature infants were handled as little as possible by hospital staff in order to conserve their energy and not interfere with respiration. Parents were strictly isolated from the nursery to prevent the introduction of infection. Parents isolated themselves because they felt intimidated by the equipment and complicated procedures they saw being used with their children.

When a child reached a magic weight of 4½ or 5½ pounds, the parents were called and told that their child was ready to be discharged. The more enlightened nursery personnel offered to allow a mother to feed her infant once under their supervision before the day of discharge. In other nurseries, a mother was simply handed the smallest infant she had ever seen and told to take him home and "mother" this stranger.

Premature infants could be detected during their preschool years for the unusually flat sides of their heads caused by lying continually in one position during their first month of life and for behavior problems. A "premature personality," was defined as that of a spoiled, undisciplined, hard-to-manage child.

Today, it is recognized that, although both conserving the immature infant's strength and gentle handling are extremely important, the immature infant needs to be handled, rocked, and touched as much as the mature infant if he is to begin to develop a sense of trust and relate satisfactorily to people. Parents need to begin interaction in as near normally a way as possible in order that parent bonding can occur. (See the Nursing Research Highlight on page 1205.)

Responses to the Infant's Problems

A number of reactions of parents of the immature infant can be anticipated.

Guilt

When "rethinking" a pregnancy, almost every parent can identify some factor that was not perfect (the mother slipped on ice a week before delivery; forgot to take a prenatal vitamin supplement one day; worked an hour overtime). It is important that parents be allowed to voice these occurrences that they believe caused the early birth. As long as the parents feel responsible for the early birth, they have a difficult time interacting with the child (they are worried the child will not like them because they "caused" this problem).

Lack of Reality

A mother organizes her life around a pregnancy due date (she will work until 2 weeks before then, then take a leave of absence; she will vacation well in advance; she must buy a crib by then, and so forth). When birth occurs a month before expected, she has difficulty believing that it has occurred. Following delivery and a nap, she wakes and turns to her back and immediately worries because she does not feel fetal movements; she sits up thinking "something is wrong" and takes a long moment to realize that the child is no longer inside her. This feeling of unreality is heightened if the infant is hospitalized in a distant health care facility.

Fear

Parents were told at their first prenatal visit that the reason that they must take certain precautions during pregnancy and come for prenatal care is because a fetus is immeasurably safer in utero than extrauterinely until maturity. Now that the child has been born prematurely, the worst has happened. They cannot help but be afraid that the child will die. This level of fear blocks off interaction with the child (fear that they will hurt him further by touching and handling).

Grief

Anticipatory grief, or mourning the loss of the child while he is still alive, is apt to occur as a psychological preparation for the child's actual death. Anticipatory grief proceeds through the usual stages: denial, anger, bargaining, depression and finally acceptance.

Denial. All parents know that birth anomalies and low-birth-weight infants are born. At the same time, all parents are surprised to discover that it has happened to *them.* Using denial allows them to be protected from the realization that it has happened to them. A typical parent's comment during this time would be: "I can't believe this has happened." They may not listen to what you are saying about a high-risk parent's support group because they do not identify themselves as parents of a high-risk infant.

Nursing Research Highlight

Preterm and Low-Birth-Weight Infants

Preterm Infants—Are They Developmentally Delayed?

A retrospective analysis was conducted to determine the developmental outcome of 101 sick preterm infants cared for at a teaching hospital's neonatal intensive care unit. Developmental testing was performed on all infants at a post-conceptual age of 12 months and compared with significant perinatal factors such as birth weight, gestational age, neonatal mortality index, respiratory distress syndrome severity, and high-risk pregnancy factors. Mental or neurologic delays were noted in 18 percent of all infants studied. These data suggested an improved prognosis for the low-birth-weight and preterm infant as compared to data reports from the 1970s.

Reference

Trotter, C. W., Chang, P. N., & Thompson, T. (1982). Perinatal factors and the developmental outcome of preterm infants. _J.O.G.N. Nursing, 11_(2), 83.

Discharge Planning Tool—Effective?

When high-risk infants are ready for discharge, families need to be prepared to care for them at home. There are many questions that should be addressed regarding families' readiness and needs. Could a structured discharge planning program be developed to meet each family's special needs while standardizing and documenting the nursing role in this planning? Two researchers (Cagan & Meier, 1983) developed a tool and implemented a pilot study to determine the usefulness of such a tool. Once this was determined a follow-up study was then done.

Consistent use of the discharge planning tool resulted in parents' increased feeling of preparedness for discharge of their high-risk infants. Clinically a discharge planning tool can enhance and support the characteristics of the discharge planning process and would provide an effective means of communication between the hospital and community. It can be concluded from this study that parents are willing and need to be involved in the discharge planning process. The project also validates the need for discharge planning to be organized and have consistent follow-through by health professionals.

Reference

Cagan, J., & Meier P. (1983). Evaluation of a discharge planning tool for use with families of high-risk infants. _J.O.G.N. Nursing, 12_(4), 275.

Tactile and Kinesthetic Stimulation—Effective?

The premature neonate is prone to many problems including feeding difficulties, unstable temperature regulation, and respiratory problems. In a study conducted by Rausch (1981), 40 infants, divided equally in a treatment and a control group, were assessed to determine the effect of compensatory tactile and kinesthetic stimulation on their clinical course. The study focused specifically on caloric intake, stooling, and weight. The treatment and control group were cared for according to the nursery routine but the treatment group were given the tactile/kinesthetic treatment regimen for 15 minutes each day of admission to the study.

Results from the study indicate that tactile and kinesthetic stimulation treatment improves the clinical course of premature infants. This study suggests that nurses or other caregivers could positively affect the clinical course of prematurely born infants.

Reference

Rausch, P. B. (1981). Effects of tactile and kinesthetic stimulation on premature infants. _J.O.G.N. Nursing, 10_(1), 34.

Anger. Anger is a typical second reaction. The parent's comments change from "This couldn't have happened" to "It's not fair this happened." Some parents may feel a strong need to point out to you how unfair it is this happened (they did everything they were supposed to do during the pregnancy; they pay their income tax; they go to church, and so forth). It is often difficult to give care to their child during this time, because the underlying message to their anger is: "Make it fair again. Tell us this really didn't happen to us."

Bargaining. Bargaining is an attempt to "buy off" the situation or substitute a better deal for the present one. A typical parent comment during this time might be: "If he only lives, I'll go to school and be a better person." "I can accept him being small; just so he's not mentally retarded." Bargaining is a difficult stage to watch parents pass through because you may realize that their "bargain" will not be honored: Their baby *is* likely to be retarded or probably will not live. Remember that when a parent's bargaining does fail, he is at a very low point in grief.

Depression. Depression or sadness occurs as a parent finally faces the reality of the situation: The newborn is very small and very apt to die. If the baby does survive, he may be limited in capabilities. A parent may cry easily during this time. Problem-solving ability is severely lessened. This stage may not be reached until the child dies or is discharged from the hospital with a handicap. As long as the newborn was hospitalized, hope that things could be changed was kept alive.

Acceptance. Acceptance is the final stage of grief and represents a change from "This is happening to me" to "It's all right this is happening to me." A parent may not reach this stage until months after the child's birth. If the child will have a permanent handicap, the parent may never reach this stage but continue to have chronic grief for the remainder of the child's life.

In order to limit an anticipatory grief reaction, it is important for a parent to be given explanations of what is happening to the child as soon as they occur, as well as to see and touch the child as soon as possible after birth. This makes the child real and limits the grief reaction in that parents do not grieve for imagined problems but only for a real situation.

If the infant cannot be removed from an Isolette or radiant heat warmer, he should be handled and stroked in the Isolette or warmer prior to and following feeding (Figure 48-8). As soon as the mother can be out of bed, she needs to visit the nursery and observe her baby (in 4 to 8 hours if the baby is housed in the same hospital). If she wishes to do so, she should be encouraged to touch the baby inside the Isolette. Touching is important in terms of initiating claiming of her

Figure 48-8 *Mothers should be encouraged to visit with immature infants to establish bonding. (Courtesy of the Department of Medical Photography, Children's Hospital, Buffalo, N.Y.)*

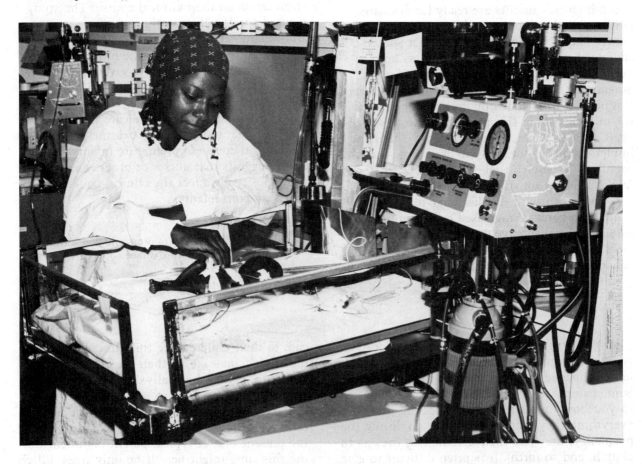

infant and making the birth of her infant real. She was not psychologically ready for birth, and it is much harder for her to believe she has had a child than it is for the mother who has delivered at term. A mother can be encouraged to express breast milk if the infant is too young to nurse. As soon as the infant is taking bottle- or breast-feedings, the mother should be encouraged to visit the hospital and give the feedings. Feeding the child or actively expressing milk is direct participation in her newborn's care and welfare.

If a baby is transferred to a regional center for care, the mother should have an opportunity to see him or her before the transfer. Having a Polaroid photo to keep is helpful and makes the birth more real to her. After she is discharged, she needs to go to the hospital to visit the infant in the nursery. She needs to be encouraged to telephone the nursery as often as she wants to ask about the baby. Notes taped to the Isolette or warmer about the baby's health, written as if they are from the baby, are helpful (do not mail these with ill infants as a parent may find them an intense hurt if one arrives after the baby has died).

Parents visiting in a high-risk nursery should have a great deal of attention and support from nursing personnel. Remember that, although incubators and ventilators and monitoring equipment are commonplace to you, they are frightening to parents. They may want to touch their infant very much but be so afraid that they might touch a button or monitor that they stand by a wall with their arms folded.

Parents need to be able to telephone the nursery and ask about the child's condition on days they cannot visit. They should be able to feel by the day of discharge that they are taking home "their" baby, a baby they know well and are ready to love.

Making parents and the baby's siblings welcome in a high-risk nursery is a major role for the nurse of high-risk infants (Figure 48-9). Because immature infants are hospitalized for long periods of time, the parents will be baffled by being told information by a parade of different health care professionals, or even a different person every time they visit. Primary nursing is the system that allows them to have one constant person to relate to. It can improve care because that single person has a clear picture of what has been tried in the past or the total health picture of the child.

Sensory Stimulation

Immature infants need rest in order to reserve energy for growth and to combat hypoglycemia or

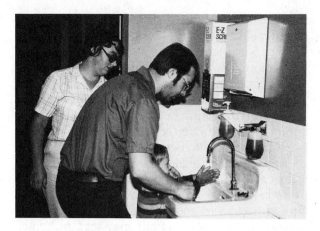

Figure 48-9 *Parents and siblings should be able to visit in high-risk nurseries with their new family member. Here a family washes preparatory to gowning. (Courtesy of the Department of Medical Photography, Children's Hospital, Buffalo, N.Y.)*

infection or stabilize temperature. Procedures should be organized, therefore, so that rest time is available. If this is not specifically planned, the infant can constantly be awakened for procedure after procedure and never rest.

At the same time, an infant needs planned periods of sensory stimulation. Like all newborns, immature infants respond best to stimulation that appeals to their senses—sight, sound, and touch.

The view from inside an Isolette may be distorted by the Plexiglas dome. It is most natural for people to view an infant in an Isolette from the side. Thus the infant's face is rarely in the same line of vision as the adult's (an *en face* position). You need to provide some time during each nursing shift for looking directly at the infant in the straightforward position so that he has the stimulation of a human face. If you put your head at the level of the infant's and look to each side, you may discover that there is nothing to see except a gray intravenous pole or a light green ventilator or a white wall. Even very immature infants should have a mobile or a black or white object in their view. As the infant's position is changed from side to stomach to opposite side, the object should be moved in line with the vision.

Infants in closed Isolettes may be able to hear nothing but the sound of the Isolette motor. They may see people looking at them, nodding at them—they may see their mouths move—but they cannot benefit from the sound of their voices because it is obscured by the continuous hum of the motor. Some talk time—words spoken softly but clearly to the ear—should be provided each nursing shift.

Even an infant who cannot be removed from the Isolette should not suffer from lack of touch. Gently stroking the infant's back or smoothing the back of the head is not a tiring motion. There should be time during every nursing shift for this interaction, particularly if clinical interventions with the infant include hurting procedures such as suctioning or blood drawing. As soon as the baby can be out of his Isolette or removed from a warmer, he or she needs special time, aside from procedures, to be rocked and held. Prolonged or rough handling of an infant may lead to hypoxemia. Transcutaneous oxygen determinations allow you to recognize the point where handling is comforting and the point where it is tiring.

As soon as the parents can visit, their visit should include touching and talking to their newborn. This type of intervention not only is beneficial to the infant but enhances parent-child bonding.

A number of studies have shown that infants with increased stimulation through an auditory or tactile stimulus gain weight more rapidly, have decreased stooling (which helps prevent dehydration) and fewer apneic spells. (Chaze, 1984). Special times of stimulation during the day should be included in the child's care plan as certainly as plans for nutrition and sleep.

Health Maintenance

Before discharge from a health care facility, parents of a low-birth-weight infant need to learn any special method of care necessary with adequate time to practice it before discharge. Most parents have a tendency to overprotect low-birth-weight infants (allowing no visitors, not taking the infant outside, waking constantly at night to check on him or her). Discussing that this is often a problem is helpful before discharge. It does not necessarily alleviate the problem, but it does make the parents feel "normal" in light of their concern.

Health maintenance of the low-birth-weight infant after discharge from the hospital follows the usual pattern of well-child care, with the exception of basic immunizations, which are delayed until the child reaches what would have been 2, 4, and 6 months of life if he had been born at term. This timing is necessary because the immunologic system must be mature enough to form antibodies before immunizations will be successful. In many communities a level III health facility maintains its own well-baby conferences for infants who were hospitalized there;

this arrangement accomplishes long-term follow-up studies on the effect of oxygen or drug therapy. Many parents enjoy bringing their infant back to the level III facility for health care rather than establishing a new network of health care. They have confidence in a health care facility that allowed their child to live. This choice also increases their self-esteem as they hear nursing and medical staff's delight in the growth of all their efforts.

Infants can be followed by any health care provider, however, and if the level III center is a distance away a transfer of care is often wiser. Remember when plotting height and weight of low-birth-weight infants to account for their early birth on the growth chart by double charting, i.e. plotting the child's weight and height according to chronological age (a pattern that probably places a baby in the early months below the tenth percentile); and then in another color, plotting the height and weight according to the "set back" age, or the age the child would be if he or she had been born at term. A low-birth-weight baby typically gains "catch-up" weight in the first 6 months of life, reaching by 1 year of age over the tenth percentile on a growth chart without accounting for a set-back age.

Evaluate growth and development of an infant by the same manner. A low-birth-weight infant can be expected to meet first-year milestones not by chronological age but by a set-back age. Ask at health promotion visits if parents are beginning to feel more comfortable with a child. Ask if they are able to allow the child to stay with a babysitter or another family member, if the shock of having such a fragile infant has begun to diminish, and if the infant is beginning to be incorporated normally into their family life.

The Postmature Infant

A pregnancy is normally 38 to 42 weeks in length. An infant is postmature (post-term) if he or she remains in utero longer than 42 weeks. An infant who stays in utero past the time to be born is at risk because a placenta appears to be a timed structure; it lasts effectively for 40 weeks, then seems to lose function. The post-term infant who remains in utero with a failing placenta may develop a *postmature syndrome.*

Postmature infants have many of the characteristics of the small-for-gestational-age infant: dry, cracked, almost leather-like skin from lack of fluid; and absence of vernix. They may be light in weight from a recent weight loss. Fingernails are grown well beyond the end of the fingertips. They may demonstrate an alertness much more like a 2-week-old baby than a newborn. They may be meconium-stained; the amount of amniotic fluid at delivery may be less than normal.

When a pregnancy becomes post-term, a sonogram may be obtained to measure the biparietal diameter of the fetus. Estriol levels may be assessed and a nonstress test done to establish whether the placenta is still functioning adequately. An amniocentesis will show whether the infant's lungs are mature by the production of surfactant. Many postmature infants are delivered by cesarean birth if a nonstress test reveals a placenta that will be extremely compromised during labor because of its failing ability to provide nutrients and oxygen to the fetus.

At birth, these babies are likely to have difficulty establishing respirations. They may have meconium aspiration. In the first hours of life, hypoglycemia may develop as they do not have adequate stores of glycogen. They have used available stores to support themselves in the last weeks of intrauterine life. Because of low levels of subcutaneous fat, which was also used during the predelivery weeks, temperature regulation may be difficult. These babies must be protected from chilling at birth or in transport to a special care center. Polycythemia may have resulted due to decreased oxygenation in the preterm weeks. The hematocrit may be elevated because of the polycythemia and dehydration, which lowers the circulating plasma level.

Bonding

Any woman is anxious when she does not deliver on her due date. She becomes extremely anxious when her pregnancy is more than 42 weeks long. She may be angry when she is told that the baby appears to be postmature (she said over and over that she knew her dates were right, but no one listened to her). It may seem to her that the longer a baby stays in utero the stronger and healthier he should be. Why then, is the baby being transferred for special care? She may feel guilty in that she did not provide well for the infant in the last few weeks of pregnancy, that she has let her newborn down.

A mother needs to spend time with her newborn to assure herself that, although delivery was not triggered, everything else about the baby appears to be normal; that with appropriate interventions to control the hypoglycemia or meconium aspiration she will have a well baby. All postmature infants need continued follow-up of developmental abilities until at least 4 or 5 years of age. The lack of nutrients and oxygen in utero may have left them with neurologic symptoms that will not become apparent until such children attempt fine motor tasks.

Utilizing Nursing Process

Nursing care of newborns with an abnormal weight for gestational age must speak to all the major areas of newborn care: establishing respiratory and cardiovascular function, maintaining temperature, nutrition, prevention of infection, and the formation of parent-child bonding and infant stimulation.

Assessment

All infants need assessment at birth for gross congenital anomalies and true gestational age; both these determinations can be done by the nurse who first inspects the infant at birth. Be certain that these assessments are made with the infant under a radiant heat warmer (that was prewarmed) to safeguard the infant who appears to be a term newborn but is actually a large-for-gestational-age preterm infant.

Continuing assessment of low-birth-weight infants involves the use of instrumentation such as cardiac, apnea, and blood pressure monitors. When working with monitors, be sensitive to a small increment or decrement that is consistently occurring. A heart rate that, increases one beat per minute every 20 minutes does not seem to be changing significantly; but over a 24 hour period, this type of increase can lead to tachycardia. No matter how many monitors are in use, they never replace the role of common sense observation. Evaluate carefully any comments from fellow nurses that an infant "isn't himself" or "is acting different." These comments, although not scientific, are the same observations that a mother who knows her baby well reports at health visits. A nurse who knows an infant well from having cared for him for a consistent length of time "senses" changes before a monitor or other equipment begins to put a quantitative measurement on the factor.

Analysis

In order to use nursing diagnosis with infants of unusual gestational age, you must be aware of the normal values of this population. Nursing diagnoses generally center on the six main areas of care although a problem in any area can be identified. The North American Association on Nursing Diagnosis has accepted no diagnoses specific to the unusual gestational age infant. Common diagnoses used are "Fear related to birth of preterm infant," "Potential for altered oxygen/carbon dioxide exchange related to immaturity," or "Potential for lack of stimulation related to Isolette care." Be certain that goals established are consistent with the infant's potential. A goal that implies complete recovery from a major illness may not be realistic.

Planning

Planning for an infant who is ill at birth must be done carefully so that all aspects of care can be accomplished yet the infant's energy conserved. Be certain in establishing plans that the parents are included. Coming into a nursery to bathe or hold an infant may be the mechanism that makes the child real to parents.

Implementation

The mark of implementation for an infant who is ill at birth is consistency in caregivers (a primary nursing pattern) and performance in such a manner as to conserve energy and prevent chilling.

Evaluation

Infants who are ill at birth need long-term followup so that any consequence of their illness such as minimal neurologic injury can be evaluated and special schooling or counseling be arranged as needed during the preschool and school years.

Nursing Care Planning

Baby Harrington is a 32 week gestation, lowbirth-weight infant (2 pounds, 6 oz) you care for. Below is a nursing care plan you might design for him.

Problem Area. Establishment of respirations.

Assessment

No spontaneous respiratory effort at birth; resuscitated by Ambu respirator and placed on Baby Bird Ventilator for transport to level III nursery. PO_2 40 mm Hg on arrival at Central Nursery.

Analysis

Inability to maintain adequate ventilation related to lung immaturity.

Locus of Decision Making. Shared: parents and nurse.

Goal. Patient will maintain adequate respiratory function with mechanical intervention.

Criteria. Infant's PO_2 will be maintained between 60–100 mm Hg.

Nursing Orders

1. Position infant with head and chest elevated to allow for maximum lung space.
2. Maintain body temperature in neutral thermal environment to prevent need for excess oxygen.
3. Observe q15min for respiratory rate, sternal retractions.
4. Auscultate q30min for rales, respiratory grunting.
5. Suction nares as necessary to maintain airway patency.

6. Withdraw blood for umbilical catheter for PO_2 q1h.
7. Maintain ventilation at prescribed values.

Problem Area. Maintenance of body temperature.

Assessment

Axillary temperature 97.6°F with infant in servocontrol Isolette.

Goal. Patient to maintain temperature at neutral thermal temperature.

Criteria. Patient's temperature to be maintained at 97.6°F with servocontrol.

Nursing Orders

1. Place in servocontrol Isolette; attach temperature probe to abdomen.
2. Use radiant heat warmer for all procedures outside Isolette.
3. If chilling should occur, warm slowly to limit apnea.
4. Change diapers frequently to keep dry to prevent chilling from evaporation.
5. Position Isolette away from air conditioner or window to limit radiation cooling.
6. Assess and record body temperature q30min.
7. Cover infant's head with cap and wrap warmly when removed from Isolette for feeding.

Problem Area. Nutrition

Assessment

Taking 20 ml of breast milk q3h by gavage-feeding. No residual aspirated from stomach before feedings. Weight gain: 25 gm for last 24 hours.

Analysis

Potential for inadequate nutrition related to immaturity.

Goal. Infant to ingest adequate breast milk for calorie and protein needs.

Criteria. Infant to continue weight gain consistent with preterm rate.

Nursing Orders

1. Calculate amount of breast milk by 120 cal/kg/day; divide by 8 feedings (per M.D. order).
2. Maintain intravenous fluid of 5% dextrose/water at 5 ml/hr.
3. Gavage feed q3h; feed with "preemie" nipple q other feeding.
4. Aspirate stomach contents before feeding; return amount of aspirate before feeding. Reduce feeding amount by aspirate amount.
5. Burp well following nipple- or gavage-feeding.
6. Weigh all diapers and S.G. urine.
7. Weigh daily.
8. Dextrostix q4h.
9. Record blood loss for blood samples.
10. Assess for skin turgor, mucous membrane moisture q4h.
11. Assess BP q1h intraarterially.

Problem Area. Prevention of infection.

Assessment

Abraided areas present on elbows and knees from irritation of sheets during transport. Axillary temperature 97.6°F by servocontrol probes. No apnea.

Analysis

Potential for infection related to broken skin and immaturity.

Goal. Patient to remain free of infection.

Criteria. Patient to have negative blood and urine cultures.

Nursing Orders

1. Encourage mother to continue to supply breast milk for antibody protection.
2. Apply A&D ointment to dry skin 4× daily to prevent skin cracking.
3. Use sterile gavage technique; provide sterile bottles for mother to collect breast milk.
4. Use sterile linen.
5. Enforce hand washing before care; use cover gown when holding infant.
6. Remind parents to wash hands and wear cover gown.
7. Daily bath with clear water only to prevent skin drying.
8. Reposition frequently to prevent any further debraided areas.

Problem Area. Bonding.

Assessment

Mother has not seen infant because she is still hospitalized at community hospital. Father has visited twice but touched infant only once. He states: "He's not going to make this." Said not to name him because he doesn't want to "waste" name on a baby who will die.

Analysis

Potential for inadequate bonding due to separation of child and anticipatory grief.

Goal. Family to develop normal parent-child attachment.

Criteria. Both parents to visit and hold infant and express interest in child by day 7.

Nursing Orders

1. Inform both parents of ability to visit any time.
2. Give Polaroid snapshot of infant to father to take to mother.
3. Urge mother to telephone daily about child's progress. Stress importance of her breast milk for child.
4. Encourage father to touch and hold infant at visits.
5. Role model "parenting" at parent visits.

Problem Area. Stimulation.

Assessment

Infant focuses on smiling face; "attunes" to spoken words.

Analysis

Potential for inadequate stimulation related to necessary equipment for care.

Goal. Patient to receive necessary stimulation for normal growth and development.

Criteria. Infant to meet expected growth and development milestones at periodic health assessments.

Nursing Orders

1. Maintain "en face" position by turning head to speak to infant in Isolette.
2. Speak to infant whenever he is out of Isolette away from sound of motor.
3. Secure mobile for over Isolette; stroke back and head a minimum of 4× daily.

Questions for Review

Multiple Choice

1. Amy is a preterm baby of 32 weeks who will be started on formula. In planning care for her, you can anticipate that the formula used will most likely be
   a. diluted with glucose water.
   b. a 20 cal/oz formula.
   c. a 24 cal/oz formula.
   d. an iron-supplemented formula.

2. Amy has an umbilical vessel catheter inserted so that blood can be drawn readily. Which implementation below would be most important during this procedure?
   a. Prevent her from crying.
   b. Be certain she is kept warm.
   c. Assess her cranial vascular tension.
   d. Evaluate her urinary output.

3. At an amniocentesis just prior to birth, Amy's lecithin/sphingomyelin ratio was determined to be 1:1. Based on this, she is prone to which type of respiratory problem following birth that you must plan for?
   a. wheezing from excess fluid accumulation
   b. bronchial constriction from room air
   c. alveolar collapse on expiration
   d. inspiratory constricture from air contaminants

4. Amy develops respiratory distress syndrome. Circulatory impairment is apt to occur because, with increased lung tension,
   a. the ductus arteriosus remains open.
   b. the foramen ovale closes prematurely.
   c. the aorta or aortic valve strictures.
   d. the pulmonary artery remains open.

5. Amy is transferred to an intensive care nursery at a distant hospital. When her mother visits her, which would be the most important action you would urge Amy's mother to do?
   a. Call Amy by her name.
   b. Touch and hold Amy.
   c. Stand so Amy can see her.
   d. Bring a piece of clothing for Amy.

6. Amy needs ventilatory assistance and is placed on a volume control ventilator. In light of her lung pathology, which additional ventilatory measure would you anticipate you would need to plan for:
   a. administration of chilled oxygen to reduce lung spasm
   b. increased inspiratory pressure; decreased expiratory pressure
   c. administration of dry oxygen to avoid overhumidification
   d. positive end expiratory pressure to increase oxygenation

7. With the administration of oxygen, Amy's PO_2 level is carefully monitored. It is important to keep this level under which value to prevent retrolental fibroplasia?
   a. 40 mm Hg
   b. 50 mm Hg
   c. 100 mm Hg
   d. 180 mm Hg

8. Following a respiratory insult, Amy develops necrotizing enterocolitis. An important assessment for revealing this happening is
   a. formula remaining in stomach before a gavage-feeding.
   b. mottled appearance to her extremities.
   c. a decreasing abdominal circumfrence.
   d. excess fat in stools.

9. Amy will be hospitalized for an extended time. Which environment would you devise as the one most suitable for her?
   a. Keep her environment free of color to reduce eye strain.
   b. Provide a mobile she can see no matter how she is turned.
   c. Place her Isolette near the window so she can see outside.
   d. Bring her open bassinet near the desk area so she sees people.

Discussion

1. Mrs. Harris visits the nursery daily where her low-birth-weight infant is cared for but states she doesn't want to come in to the nursery and touch him for fear of hurting him. What measures could you initiate to encourage better bonding between Mrs. Harris and her infant?
2. Maintaining body heat in an immature infant is always important. What precautions would you take with Baby Harris to maintain his body temperature?
3. Immature infants may be small for gestational age, average for gestational age, or large for gestational age. What specific problems would you need to plan for at the births of these three types of infants?

Suggested Readings

Ariagno, R. L. (1984). Evaluation and management of infantile apnea. *Pediatric Annals, 13*, 210.

Avery, G. B. (Ed.) (1981). *Neonatology*, 2nd ed. Philadelphia, Lippincott.

Blackburn, S. (1983). Fostering behavioral development of high-risk infants. *J.O.G.N. Nursing, 12*, 765.

Bragdon, D. B. (1983). A basis for the nursing management of feeding the premature infant. *J.O.G.N. Nursing, 12*, 515.

Brooten, D. (1983). Issues for research on alternative patterns of care for low-birth-weight infants. *Image, 15*, 80.

Cain, L. P., et al. (1980). Parents' perceptions of the psychological and social impact of home monitoring. *Pediatrics, 66,* 37.

Chaze, B. A., et al. (1984). Sensory stimulatiton in the NICU. *American Journal of Nursing, 84,* 68.

Collinge, J. M., et al. (1982). Demand vs scheduled feedings for premature infants. *J.O.G.N. Nursing, 11,* 362.

Committee on the Fetus and Newborn. (1978). *Standards and recommendations for hospital care of newborn infants.* Evanston, Ill., American Academy of Pediatrics.

Duxbury, M. L., et al. (1984). Caregiver disruptions and sleep of high-risk infants. *Heart Lung, 13,* 141.

Griffith, R. A., et al. (1981). Care of the low-birth-weight infant. *Perinatology/Neonatology, 5,* 19.

Jacobson, H. N. (1983). Prevention of prematurity. *Perinatology/Neonatology, 7,* 17.

Harper, R. G., et al. (1982). The scope of nursing practice in level III neonatal intensive care units. *Pediatrics, 70,* 875.

Kelly, D. H., & Shannon, D. C. (1982). Sudden infant death syndrome and near sudden infant death syndrome: A review of the literature, 1964 to 1982. *Pediatric Annals of North America, 29,* 1241.

Klaus, M., & Kennell, J. (1982). *Mother-Infant Bonding.* St. Louis, Mosby.

Koops, B. L., et al. (1982). Neonatal mortality risk in relation to birth weight and gestational age: An update. *Journal of Pediatrics, 101,* 969.

Kuller, J. M., et al. (1983). Improved skin care for premature infants. *M.C.N., 8,* 200.

LaRossa, M. M., et al. (1982). Foster grandmothers in the premature nursery. *American Journal of Nursing, 82,* 1834.

Lemons, P. M. (1983). Breast-feeding the premature newborn. *Perinatal Press, 7,* 83.

Martin, R. J., et al. (1979). Effect of supine and prone positions on arterial oxygen tension in the preterm infant. *Pediatrics, 63,* 528.

Merritt, T. A., & Valdes-Dapena, M. (1984). SIDS research update. *Pediatric Annals, 13,* 193.

Norris, S. C., et al. (1982). Nursing procedures and alterations in transcutaneous oxygen tension in premature infants. *Nursing Research, 31,* 330.

Norris, S. C. (1983). Apnea of prematurity. *Critical Care Nurse, 3,* 56.

Ogata, E. S. (1983). Metabolic problems of the premature infant. *Perinatology/Neonatology, 7,* 49.

Reich, V., et al. (1982). Sudden infant death syndrome and apnea of prematurity. *Current Reviews in Respiratory Therapy, 5,* 43.

Schwartz, D. (1981). Intensive care nurseries: Making them more human. *Children Today, 10,* 42.

Shields, W. D., et al. (1983). Ultrasound evaluation of neonatal intraventricular hemorrhage. *Perinatology/Neonatology, 7,* 19.

Sinatra, F. R., et al. (1983). Nutritional needs of the premature infant. *Perinatology/Neonatology, 7,* 61.

Smith, J. C. (1984). Psychosocial aspects of infantile apnea and home monitoring. *Pediatric Annals, 13,* 219.

Stewart, M. (1982). Neonatal nurse specialists: Caregivers to the family. *Perinatology/Neonatology, 6,* 79.

Thibeault, D. W., et al. (1983). Drug therapy in neonatal lung disease. *Perinatology/Neonatology, 7,* 39.

Walker, C. H. M. (1982). Neonatal intensive care and stress. *Archives of Diseases of Children, 57,* 85.

Ziegler, E. E., et al. (1983). Nutritional requirements of the premature infant. In R. M. Suskind (ed.), *Symposium on pediatric nutrition.* New York, Raven Press.

Our Antenatal Care Methods," in *Contemporary Ob/Gyn* 22 (1984). Reprinted by permission.

Figure 18–21: From J. M. Belizan et al., "Diagnosis of Intrauterine Growth Retardation by a Simple Clinical Method: Measurement of Uterine Height," in *American Journal of Obstetrics and Gynecology* 131. Reprinted by permission.

Table 19–1, Figure 19–6: From M. Barman, "Advising Pregnant and Postoperative Working Patients," in *Contemporary Ob/Gyn* 23. Reprinted by permission of the author.

Table 23–6, 23–7, 23–15: From E. Friedman, *Labor, Clinical Evaluation and Management*, Second Edition. Reprinted by permission of Appleton-Century-Crofts.

Figure 24–1: The Century Birthing Chair. Reprinted by permission of Century Manufacturing Company.

Figure 27–3, 27–4, 27–5: From J. Hellmuth, (editor), *Exceptional Infant: Studies in Abnormalities*, Volume 2. Reprinted by permission of Brunner/Mazel.

Table 27–1: From B. Bishop, "A Guide to Assessing Parenting Capabilities," in *American Journal of Nursing*. Reprinted by permission.

Table 27–2: From M. Gruis, "Beyond Maternity: Postpartum Concerns of Mothers," in *M.C.N.* Reprinted by permission.

Table 31–1: From A. Moss, "Indirect Methods of Blood Pressure Measurement," in *Pediatric Clinics of North America* 25 (1978). Reprinted by permission.

Figure 31–1: From B. L. Koops, L. J. Morgan and F. C. Battaglia, "Neonatal Mortality Risk in Relation to Birth Weight and Gestational Age: An Update," in *Journal of Pediatrics* 101, 969 (1952). Reprinted by permission.

Table 31–2: Adapted from M. Moore, *The Newborn and the Nurse*. Reprinted by permission of W. B. Saunders Company, a division of CBS Publishing, Inc.

Table 31–3: From M. Desmond et al., "The Clinical Behavior of the Newly Born: The Term Baby," in *Journal of Pediatrics* 62 (1963). Reprinted by permission.

Table 32–2: From R. Usher et al., "Judgment of Fetal Age," in *Pediatric Clinics of North America* 13 (1966). Reprinted by permission.

Figure 32–5, 32–6: From J. Ballard et al., "A Simplified Assessment of Gestational Age," in *Pediatric Research* 11 (1977). Reprinted by permission.

Figure 34–5: From R. J. Meyer et al., "Accidental Injury to the Preschool Child," in *Journal of Pediatrics* 63 (1963). Reprinted by permission.

Table 34–3: From G. Van Leeuwen and L. Glenn, "Screening for Hidden Congenital Anomalies," in *Pediatrics* 41 (1968). Reprinted by permission of American Academy of Pediatrics.

Table 36–1: From the Criteria Committee of the New York State Heart Association, Nomenclature and Criteria Diagnosis of *Diseases of the Heart and Blood Vessels*, Eighth Edition (1979). Reprinted by permission of Little, Brown and Company (Inc.).

Table 36–5: From P. White, "Classification of Obstetric Diabetes," in *American Journal of Obstetrics and Gynecology* 135 (1978). Reprinted by permission.

Table 39–6: From L. D'Angelo and R. Sokol, "Prematurity: Recognizing Patients at Risk," in *Geromata: Care* 2 (1978). Reprinted by permission.

Table 40–2: From J. Spranger et al., "Errors of Morphogenesis: Concepts and Terms," in *Journal of Pediatrics* 100, 160. Reprinted by permission.

Table 42–2: From P. J. Placek, S. Taffel and M. Moien, "Cesarean Section Delivery Rates: United States, 1981," in *American Journal of Public Health* 73, 861 (1983). Reprinted by permission.

Table 42–7: From S. Taffel and P. Placek, "Complications in Cesarean and Non-cesarean Deliveries," in *American Journal of Public Health* 73, 856 (1983). Reprinted by permission.

Table 43–5: From E. Bishop, "Pelvic Scoring for Elective Induction," in *Obstetrics and Gynecology* 24, 266 (1964). Reprinted by permission.

Table 45–2: From American Academy of Pediatrics, *Standards and Recommendations for Hospital Care of Newborn Infants*, Sixth Edition (1977). Copyright 1977 American Academy of Pediatrics. Reprinted by permission.

Table 45–3: From C. U. Battle, "Chronic Physical Disease: Behavioral Aspects," in *Pediatric Clinics of North America* 22, 525 (1975). Reprinted by permission.

Figure 46–18: From M. L. Morrison (Editor), *Respiratory Intensive Care Nursing* (1979). Reprinted by permission of Little, Brown and Company (Inc.).

Table 47–3, 47–5, 47–6: From J. Nugent, "Acute Respiratory Care of the Newborn," in *J.O.G.N. Nursing* 12, 31 (1983).

Table 47–8: From J. A. Kitterman et al., "Aortic Blood Pressure in Normal Newborn Infants During the First 12 Hours of Life," in *Pediatrics*, 44, 959 (1969). Reprinted by permission.

Figure 47–9: From J. Nugent, "Intra-arterial Blood Pressure Monitoring in the Neonate," in *J.O.G.N. Nursing* 11, 281 (1982). Reprinted by permission.

Table 47–12: From R. E. Kron et al., "Behavior of Infants Born to Drug-dependent Mothers," in J. L. Rementeria (Editor) *Drug Abuse in Pregnancy and Neonatal Effects*. Reprinted by permission of C. V. Mosby Company.

Table 48–2, 48–3: From G. B. Avery (Editor), *Neonatology*, Second Edition (1981). Reprinted by permission of J. B. Lippincott.

Table 48–4: From G. J. Peckham et al., "A Clinical Score for Predicting the Level of Respiratory Care in Infants with Respiratory Distress Syndrome," in *Clinical Pediatrics* 18, 716. Reprinted by permission.

Table 48–5: From J. Downes et al., "Respiratory Distress Syndrome of Newborn Infants. New Clinical Scoring System with Acid-base and Blood-gas Correlates," in *Clinical Pediatrics* 9, 325. Reprinted by permission.

Appendix A
Drug Compendium

Drugs included are those that tend to be specific to and encountered in maternal-newborn nursing. Because of this association, these are the drugs most likely to be considered in planning nursing care.

Acetaminophen (Tylenol)

Pharmacology: Inhibits the synthesis of prostaglandins, causing analgesic and antipyretic actions.

Uses: The relief of mild to moderate pain and for reduction of fever.

Side effects: Hypersensitivity is the side effect most seen, but it is not very common. Overdose of acetaminophen may be fatal, because very large doses are extremely hepatotoxic.

Dose: 650 mg (2 tablets) every 4 to 6 hours as needed.

Nursing responsibilities:

1. Monitor body temperature; acetaminophen should reduce body temperature in conditions in which it is elevated.
2. Assess pain; when alleviating pain, ask patient if the drug seems to help, since this assurance is the best indicator of how the drug is working.

Acyclovir (Zovirax Ointment)

Pharmacology: An antiviral agent, effective against herpes simplex virus types I and II.

Use: The treatment of herpes genitalis in limited, nonlife-threatening situations, in immunocompromised patients.

Side effects: Include burning, stinging, pruritus, rash, and vulvitis. All of the effects appear only as often as they did with placebo-treated patients.

Dose: Apply every 3 hours (6 times daily) for 1 week.

Nursing responsibilities:

1. Monitor for local irritation, as this may be caused by the drug, and not placebo (burning, stinging, etc.).
2. Apply ointment with rubber gloves or a finger cot so as to decrease the chance of spreading the infection.
3. Apply thoroughly over all lesions.
4. Exercise caution in pregnant and nursing women; the effects for the child or fetus are unknown.

Americaine (see Anorectal Products)

Source: Compiled by Jayson B. Bulmahn, R.P.H., Pharmacist, DeGraff Hospital, North Tonawanda, New York.

Anorectal Products

Pharmacology:

Corticosteroids are used to reduce and control inflammation.

Products: Anusol-HC, Proctocort, Corticaine.

Side effects: Local effects such as burning, irritation, itching, and dryness. With prolonged use, the steroid may be absorbed through the skin into the circulation; after a period of time, this tendency could lead to adrenal suppression.

Local anesthetics relieve the symptoms of pain, itching, and irritation.

Products: Anusol, Proctodon, Nupercainal, Rectal Medicone, Americaine.

Side effects: Sensitization to the drug, which causes urticaria, edema, lesions, or contact dermatitis. Local irritation such as burning and swelling are also possible. Systemic absorption of the drug can lead to CNS toxicity. The effects seen are the same as from lidocaine toxicity: stimulation, nervousness, dizziness, blurred vision, tremors, and convulsions. These effects are very rare and only seen with frequent, excessive, long-term use.

Vasoconstrictors decrease the swelling and congestion by constricting the blood vessels.

Products: Epinephricaine Rectal, Pazo Hemorrhoidal.

Side effects: Rare.

Astringents "pull" water from the hemorrhoid, thus decreasing the swelling.

Products: Tucks.

Side effects: Rare.

Nursing responsibilities:

1. Assess effectiveness of treatment. If the patient feels better, is more comfortable, etc., the treatment selected is working and should be continued. If, however, no relief is obtained, another product should be suggested, preferably from another category (if a local anesthetic was ineffective, a steroid or astringent might provide relief).
2. Side effects are usually local and of minor importance. If the patient is sensitive to, or is irritated by, one product, another one may be more acceptable.

Acetylsalicylic Acid (Aspirin [ASA])

Pharmacology: Inhibits the synthesis of prostaglandins, causing analgesic, anti-inflammatory, and antipyretic actions.

Uses: Relief of low to moderate pain. Reduction of fever. Reduces inflammation (as in rheumatoid arthritis).

Side effects: Aspirin causes gastric ulceration, which causes blood loss and may lead to anemia. An increase in platelet aggregation time; prolongation of labor and gestation. Long-term large doses may lead to renal damage.

Interactions: **Anticoagulants.** Due to the platelet effects of aspirin, an increased bleeding time results from this combination. The GI lesion that may result would create a place for bleeding to take place. **Oral Hypoglycemics.** ASA causes a further decrease in blood sugar. **Other anti-inflammatory drugs** run an increased risk of GI ulceration.

Dose: 650 mg (2 tablets) every 4 to 6 hours as needed.

Nursing responsibilities:

1. Assess CBC. The hemoglobin and hematocrit may be decreased, indicating anemia.
2. Body temperature. ASA should reduce the body temperature in conditions in which it is elevated.
3. Pain. When alleviating pain, ask the patient if the drug seems to help, as this is the single best indicator of how the drug is working.
4. Inflammation. By palpating the site of inflammation and asking the patient how it feels, one can get a good idea of how effective the ASA is.
5. Blood sugar. In diabetics, this should be monitored, as it may be decreased enough to warrant changing the dose of an oral hypoglycemic.
6. Any signs of stomach ulceration such as pain and burning should be watched for.
7. ASA should be avoided in pregnancy, especially in the last trimester, as its use causes increased duration of labor and prolonged gestation. ASA is also harmful to the fetus as its antiplatelet effects give an increased risk of bleeding.
8. Patients may be allergic to aspirin and may exhibit asthma-type symptoms as a result.

Betamethasone (Celestone, Soluspan)

Pharmacology: A glucocorticoid capable of accelerating fetal lung maturation by increasing production of surfactant. It is optimal if delivery can be delayed until 24 hours after administration.

Use: Administered to a woman in premature labor to prevent respiratory distress syndrome in her infant. May be effective in fetuses as early as 28 weeks gestation but best results are obtained between 30 and 32 weeks. More effective with female than male infants.

Side effects: Sodium retention, hypertension, GI bleeding.

Dose: 12 mg IM one time daily for 2 days. May need to be repeated after 1 week if delivery has not occurred by then.

Interactions: The concomitant administration of a tocolytic agent may result in pulmonary edema.

Nursing responsibilities:

1. Assess for GI bleeding.
2. Estriol urine levels will be inaccurate as a measure of fetal welfare following administration.
3. Assess respiratory rate and for rales to detect pulmonary edema.

4. Assess for sodium retention (weight gain and edema).
5. Should be administered into a major muscle as local atrophy can occur if a smaller muscle is used.
6. Assess newborn for signs of hypoglycemia (jitteriness, limpness) or by Dextrostix for glucose serum level.
7. Assess newborn for urine output and specific gravity of urine as aldosterone levels may be suppressed up to 2 weeks following delivery.

Breast Care Products (Massé, Mammol, A&D Ointment, Vitamin E Ointment, Lanolin)

Pharmacology: Emollients. These ointments moisten the skin (nipple) by forming an occlusive barrier. This allows the skin to retain its own moisture, thus preventing dryness and cracking. The vitamins A,D, and E have no proven effect on the nipple, even though many people believe otherwise.

Use: Care of the nipples in pregnant and nursing mothers. Start to prepare the nipple for nursing up to 2 months prior to birth.

Side effects: Tenderness, irritation, redness. These effects can be caused by two different mechanisms. One is a sensitization to a preservative. The other is overhydration (similar to soaking a hand in water for a couple of hours).

Dose: When applying, rub in approximately 1 inch of ointment with a gentle and outward motion one to two times daily. Once nursing is started, wash area, dry, and apply. Do this after each feeding.

Nursing responsibilities:

1. If any irritation should occur, discontinue use.
2. Use of these products is intended to prevent cracking of the nipples. If there is no cracking, then therapy is effective.

Bromocriptine Mesylate (Parlodel)

Pharmacology: A nonhormonal, nonestrogenic dopamine receptor agonist that causes an inhibition of prolactin secretion by the pituitary gland.

Uses and dose: Galactorrhea (breast milk secretion) and amenorrhea, which are associated with hyperprolactinemia. Treat with 2½ mg twice to three times daily for up to 6 months. Also used for the prevention of physiologic lactation after birth, abortion, or stillbirth. Start therapy no later than 4 hours after birth with 2½ mg orally two times daily for 14 days. Some patients may require treatment for 21 days.

Side effects: Hypotension. This is significant, and caution should be exercised during the first few days of therapy. Effect is additive with other hypotensive drugs, such as diuretics. Other side effects are nausea, vomiting, headache, dizziness, and drowsiness.

Interactions: The pharmacology of phenothiazines is opposite to that of bromocriptine. Phenothiazines often cause Parkinson-type adverse reactions; it is for this reason that bromocriptine is effective in the treatment of Parkinson's disease.

Nursing responsibilities:

1. Assess blood pressure. Delay initial administration until blood pressure is stable following delivery. Observe for hypotensive effects, and caution the patient of this possibility. Advise such things as getting out of bed slowly.
2. Assess serum prolactin levels. If drawn during treatment, this level should be decreased.
3. Milk production should decrease, and then stop. If the secretion of milk has not stopped in 14 days, notify the physician, in which instance 7 more days of treatment may be necessary.
4. This drug should be taken with food or meals so as to avoid any possible GI upset. Educate the patient to do this.

Chlorotrianisene (Tace)

Pharmacology: Estrogen.
Uses and doses: Postpartum breast engorgement; 12 mg qid for 7 days, or 72 mg bid for 2 days. The first dose should be given within 8 hours of delivery for optimal effects. Vasomotor symptoms associated with menopause (hot flashes)—12–25 mg qd for 30 days, given cyclically. Atrophic vaginitis—12–25 mg qd cyclically for 30 to 60 days. Female hypogonadism—12–25 mg qd for 21 days, then progestins for 5 days, then repeat.
Side effects: Estrogen related. Increased blood pressure, due to sodium and water retention. This water retention often leads to weight gain. Thromboembolic disease such as pulmonary embolism, thrombophlebitis, myocardial infarction, and stroke are all at an increased risk with estrogen treatment. Nausea and vomiting are very common with estrogens. Breakthrough bleeding, dysmenorrhea, gallbladder disease, and neoplastic disease are all increased in patients treated with estrogens.

Nursing responsibilities:

1. Assess blood pressure; will be increased if the patient has any significant fluid retention. Intake and output should be assessed, as well as any physical signs of edema.
2. Due to the increased risk of embolus formation, the patient should be assessed carefully for development of any early signs of formation. These include warm, red, painful legs, positive Homan's Sign, shortness of breath, or any chest pain.
3. Women with diabetes should be aware that estrogens cause a decrease in glucose tolerance, which may require additional insulin.
4. Assess serum calcium. Estrogens generally cause an increase. This, however, is easily monitored.
5. Caution patients of the possibility of photosensitivity. Prolonged exposure to sunlight should be avoided.
6. Assess for jaundice. If during treatment the patient develops jaundice, the estrogen should be

considered as a cause. This may require stopping the drug.
7. Avoid use in nursing mothers. Estrogens are secreted in the milk and may cause harm to the infant.
8. If a change in the menstrual flow develops, notify the doctor, as this is probably due to the estrogen.
9. Have the patient take this drug with food to minimize the nausea and vomiting associated with its use.

Clomiphene Citrate (Clomid)

Pharmacology: Binds to, and thus causes a net decrease in the number of, estrogen receptors. This effect in turn causes the body to "read" a low estrogen level. It responds by increasing the secretion of luteinizing hormone (LH), follicle-stimulating hormone (FSH), and also gonadotropins, leading to ovarian stimulation and ultimately ovulation.
Uses: Treatment of ovarian failure in patients without pituitary, adrenal, or other organ failure. This drug has also been used investigationally for the treatment of male infertility.
Side effects: "Hot flashes"—a vasomotor side effect related to estrogens. Abdominal discomfort, nausea, vomiting, and weight gain are also estrogen-related side effects seen. Other effects include headache, insomnia, dizziness, polyuria, depression, skin rashes, and blurred vision. There is an increased risk of birth defects with clomiphene-treated mothers; therefore, if pregnancy is suspected, the drug should be discontinued immediately. Multiple gestation may occur.
Dose: 50 mg daily for 5 days beginning on the fifth day of the menstrual cycle. This may be increased to 100 mg daily for 5 days. If there is still no response, dosage may be increased to 100 mg daily for 5 days again.

Nursing responsibilities:

1. The patient should be aware of the possibility of birth defects and multiple gestation.
2. This drug should not be given to patients with liver disease, as it may cause liver damage.
3. This drug should never be given during pregnancy. If the patient suspects that she is pregnant, she should stop treatment immediately.
4. Caution the patient of possible visual disturbances, which may cause a problem driving or when doing anything in which keen eyesight is necessary. If visual problems occur, the physician should be notified, as treatment by an ophthalmologist may be necessary.
5. Any uterine bleeding should be reported to the physician, as this is sufficient cause not to use clomiphene in a patient.

Clotrimazole (Gyne-Lotrimin)

Pharmacology: Antifungal with fungicidal activity against *Candida.*
Use: Treatment of vaginal moniliasis.
Side effects: Mild burning due to local irritation or

sensitivity to the drug, which gives itching, rash, and redness.

Dose: One applicatorful, or one vaginal tablet at bedtime daily for 7 to 14 days.

Nursing responsibilities:

1. Assess for sensitivity (itching, rash, and redness). The patient should notify her physician, as she may wish to use another drug. There are good alternatives.
2. Have the patient use a sanitary napkin to avoid staining of clothing.
3. This medication should be inserted high into the vagina with the applicator provided.
4. Coitus during treatment should be avoided (or the male should use a condom), to prevent reinfection.
5. Treatment should be uninterrupted and for the full course (do not discontinue treatment for the menstrual period).

Ergonovine Maleate, Methylergonovine Maleate (Ergotrate, Methergine)

Pharmacology: Ergot alkaloid that is a potent uterine stimulant causing uterine contractions.
Use: Prevention and treatment of postpartum and postabortal hemorrhage due to uterine atony.
Side effects: Nausea and vomiting; hypertension. Allergic reactions to these drugs are also reported. Another is ergotism, a condition caused by too much drug in the body. See the nursing responsibilities section below for explanation.
Dose: 0.2 mg IM after delivery of the placenta. Then 0.2 mg orally every 6 to 12 hours for 1 to 2 days after delivery.

Nursing responsibilities:

1. Assess blood pressure. As a guide, do not administer if blood pressure is over 140/90.
2. Assess the amount of uterine bleeding and fundal consistency. When bleeding stops, the drug is no longer needed.
3. Assess for ergotism. Signs include vomiting, diarrhea, headache, and dizziness. Less frequently, thirst, tingling, itching, cold skin, rapid, weak pulse, and confusion. Marked vasoconstriction may also result, leading to coldness, paleness, and numbness in the feet and hands. There is the possibility that pain and ultimately gangrene will ensue. Ergotism may also present with tachycardia, bradycardia, hypotension, or hypertension. Watch carefully for the above signs and symptoms; should any of these appear, notify the physician immediately.

Estrogens (Premarin, diethylstilbestrol [DES])

Pharmacology: The estrogens have many pharmacologic effects. For this reason, the pharmacology of the estrogens is included under the uses and side effect categories.
Uses: To decrease the vasomotor symptoms associated with menopause. The symptoms are due to the decrease in estrogen production in the body. Hence, these exogenous estrogens replace what the body is no longer producing. To decrease symptoms of female hypogonadism, female castration, and primary ovarian failure. The goal here, too, is to replace the estrogens that the body is not producing. Postpartum breast engorgement can be treated with estrogens; however, the necessity is questionable. To prevent osteoporosis due to estrogen deficiency. Estrogens do help prevent this from happening, and may or may not help to reverse it. As postcoital birth control— only an investigational use of the drug.
Side effects: There is an increased risk of breast and uterine cancer in estrogen-treated patients. For this reason the lowest possible dose for the shortest period of time should be used. Gallbladder disease— Postmenopausal women treated with estrogens have twice to three times the incidence of gallbladder disease of those who do not take estrogens. Sodium and water retention leading to elevated blood pressure, weight gain, and edema. Increased risk of thromboembolic disease. Patients being treated for breast cancer may develop hypercalcemia. Nausea and vomiting are common. The patient may take estrogens with food to help stop this effect. Also, after a time, resistance will ensue, and this will no longer be a problem. Estrogens have many effects on the GU tract. Breakthrough bleeding, a change in menstrual flow, amenorrhea, dysmenorrhea, vaginal candidiasis, and a premenstrual-like syndrome. Effects on the breast include tenderness, enlargement, and emission of secretions. The effect of estrogens on the corneal curvature may prevent patients from wearing contact lenses.
Dose: 1 mg DES, 80 mcg mestranol, 5 mg conjugated estrogens (Premarin), 50 mcg estradiol. With vasomotor symptoms, treatment should be cyclic (3 weeks of drug, then 1 week off). This should last 3 to 6 months with therapy being tapered or stopped at this time. Estrogen replacement therapy should also be given cyclically.

Nursing responsibilities:

1. Estrogens should not be given during pregnancy because of the possibility of birth defects. They should only be given to nursing mothers if absolutely necessary.
2. The breasts, cervix, vagina, kidneys, and liver should all be examined for neoplasms during and after estrogen therapy; there is an increased risk with administration.
3. Assess blood pressure and intake and output to detect any sodium or water retention. Edema may also indicate some water retention.
4. Pain in the legs, shortness of breath, symptoms of stroke, and chest pain are all signs of thromboembolic disease. This risk is even greater if the patient smokes.
5. Assess serum calcium; may increase enough to require treatment.
6. Blood sugar should be monitored in women with

diabetes because these patients may experience impaired glucose tolerance.

7. Give these drugs with food to decrease nausea and vomiting.
8. Any abnormal vaginal bleeding should be reported to the physician, as a dosage change may be necessary.
9. If pregnancy is suspected, the physician should be notified and the drug discontinued.
10. Assess for jaundice as this may be indicative of gallbladder or liver disease.

Flagyl (see Metronidazole)

Erythromycin Ophthalmic Ointment (Ilotycin)

Pharmacology: Bacteriostatic ointment.
Use: Prophylactic therapy for ophthalmia neonatorum.
Side effects: Mild edema, inflammation or sensitivity reactions may occur. Ability to focus eyesight may be temporarily effected.
Dose: A one quarter inch ribbon of ointment is applied to each lower conjunctival rim; one application only.

Nursing responsibilities:

1. Do not irrigate eyes after administration to prolong the drug's action.
2. Assess for signs of hypersensitivity or edema or inflammation following application.

Heparin

Pharmacology: Blocks the effects of certain clotting factors, thus increasing the time it takes for blood to clot. Heparin, however, has little or no effect on the bleeding time, which is a function of the platelets. Heparin has no effect on existing clots (does not dissolve clots).
Uses: Following venous thrombosis and pulmonary embolism, it prevents the formation of further clots and decreases the probability of clots breaking off in large pieces, which may then lodge in the heart, etc. Subcutaneous, lower doses are used postoperatively in patients who are at a high risk of deep venous thrombosis or pulmonary embolism. Heparin is also used in cardiovascular surgery to prevent clot formation during the procedure.
Side effects: Hemorrhage, which is caused by too much heparin in the body (overanticoagulation). Hypersensitivity is not uncommon because this drug is derived from bovine and porcine sources. Local irritation is why heparin should never be given IM. This causes hematoma formation and histamine-like reactions.
Dose: SC. 10,000–20,000 Units IV bolus, then 10,000 to 12,000 Units SC q8–12h.
IV Intermittent. 10,000 Units IV bolus, then 5,000 to 10,000 Units IV q4–6h.
IV Continuous. 5,000 Units IV bolus as a loading dose, then 10,000 to 40,000 Units per day.
Low Dose SC Therapy. 5,000 Units SC 2 hours prior to surgery, then 5,000 Units SC 18–12h for 7 days.

Interactions: With antiplatelet drugs such as aspirin, nonsteroidal antiinflammatory agents (Indocin), and diprimadole (Persantine). This interaction causes an increase in bleeding and bleeding time; it can be very severe.

Nursing responsibilities:

1. Assess partial thromboplastin time (PTT). For optimal anticoagulation, this value should be increased to 1½ to 2½ times the normal value. If this value is less than 1½ times normal, the patient is not anticoagulated, whereas if the PTT is over 2½ times normal, the patient runs the risk of hemorrhage.
2. Assess for hemorrhage. Signs include black, tarry stool, hematuria, or any other bleeding that might occur (gumline, etc). While on heparin, women may experience an increased menstrual or lochia flow.
3. Assess CBC. A decrease in hemoglobin/hematocrit may be an indicator of some undetected bleeding.
4. Caution should be exercised in disease states if there is an increased risk of hemorrhage—for example, cardiovascular disease with hypertension; GI disease such as ulcerative colitis or any ulceration of the GI tract. Certain blood diseases such as hemophilia certainly increase the risk of hemorrhage to the patient as do threatened abortion, severe hepatic or renal disease. Any one or a combination of these disease states leads to an increased risk of hemorrhage to anticoagulated patients.
5. Heparin, unlike warfarin, does not cross the placenta and is not secreted in human milk; this makes heparin the drug of choice in treating lactating women.

Magnesium Sulfate ($MgSO_4$)

Pharmacology: A CNS depressant.
Use: Acts to block neuromuscular transmission reducing the possibility of seizures in the woman with hypertension of pregnancy.
Side effects: Flushing of face, sweating. Patients receiving digitalis may develop serious alterations of heart conduction.
Toxic effects: Absence of deep tendon reflexes, decreased respiratory rate, decreased urine output.
Dose: Initial dose is 4 gm administered IV in 250–500 ml intravenous fluid or 10 gm of 50% solution administered IM; initial dose is followed by individually calculated IV rate or 5 gm every 4 hours (50% solution) IM. Should not be administered if deep tendon reflexes are absent, respiratory rate is under 16, or urine output is under 30 ml per hour. 0.5–1 ml of procaine should be added to IM injection to decrease pain of administration.

Nursing responsibilities:

1. Assess maternal blood pressure continuously with IV administration and every 15 minutes with IM administration.

2. Do not administer drug if toxic symptoms are present.
3. Provide calcium gluconate (10 ml of 10% solution) at bedside as antagonist.
4. Divide IM injection in two and inject into large muscle groups because of large size of injection. Massage injection site following administration to increase absorption.
5. Monitor FHR continuously during IV administration.
6. Magnesium sulfate is administered for 24 hours after delivery to prevent postpartal occurrence of seizures.

Methergine (see Ergonovine Maleate)

Metronidazone (Flagyl)

Pharmacology: Antibacterial, antiprotozoal. Good activity against *Trichomonas* and anaerobes, such as bacteroides.
Uses: Treatment of trichomoniasis in males and females and amebiasis such as amebic dysentery. Treatment of serious infections that are caused by anaerobes. The IV form of metronidazole should be used here. Intraabdominal infections such as peritonitis, liver abscess, and intraabdominal abscess are often caused by bacteroides and treated with metronidazole.
Side effects: Seizures. Should a seizure occur, the drug should be discontinued. Peripheral neuropathy, or numbness or paresthesia of the extremities. Animal studies have shown a possibility of tumor induction by metronidazole. This has not been proven in humans, however. GI side effects such as nausea, vomiting, diarrhea, pain, and constipation. A metallic taste in a patient's mouth. *Candida* overgrowth in the mouth or vagina has been reported during therapy. Allergic reactions are also seen, such as urticaria, rash, and flushing.
Dose: Trichomoniasis —2 gm po once, or 250 mg po three times daily for 7 days. The woman as well as all sexual partners should be treated in this manner. Amebiasis: 750 mg po tid for 5 to 10 days. Anaerobic infections: Dosage varies by the severity and location of the infection.
Interactions: With *alcohol*. The effect is similar to alcohol mixed with disulfiram (Antabuse), which is used to discourage alcoholics from using alcohol. Concurrent administration gives nausea, vomiting, flushing, and headache. With *warfarin*. Potentiates the effects of warfarin. This in turn gives an increase in the prothrombin time and puts a patient in danger of hemorrhage.

Nursing responsibilities:

1. Assess for seizures. Any signs of CNS stimulation such as dizziness, vertigo, irritability can be a forewarning of future seizure activity.
2. Any numbness in the extremities should be reported to the physician. This is how peripheral neuropathies will present.

3. Caution the patient about alcohol use. Make sure any medication the patient may be taking does not contain any alcohol.
4. Impress upon the patient with trichomoniasis the importance of treating all sexual partners, so as to avoid any reinfection.
5. This drug should not be used during the first trimester of pregnancy.
6. This drug should also be avoided in nursing mothers due to the possibility of tumor induction.
7. Watch for *Candida* growth in the mouth or vagina (white patches). This condition can easily be treated with other agents.

Miconazole (Monistat 7)

Pharmacology: Antifungal with fungicidal activity against *Candida*.
Use: Moniliasis.
Side effects: Sensitivity to the drug seen as burning, itching, and rash.
Dose: One applicatorful at bedtime for 7 days.

Nursing responsibilities:

1. Assess for sensitivity, shown as burning, itching, and rash. The patient should notify her physician, who may wish to use another drug. There are good alternatives.
2. Have the patient use a sanitary napkin to avoid staining clothing.
3. The medication should be inserted high into the vagina with the applicator provided.
4. Coitus during treatment should be avoided (or the male should use a condom) to prevent reinfection.
5. Treatment should be uninterrupted and for the full course (do not discontinue treatment during the menstrual period).

Motrin (see Nonsteroidal Anti-inflammatory Agents)

Naloxone Hydrochloride (Narcan)

Pharmacology: A narcotic antagonist that acts to reverse CNS depression effects of narcotics by displacing drugs from organ receptor sites.
Use: To reverse respiratory depression in neonates whose mothers received narcotics during labor and delivery. Usually administered through umbilical vein catheter. Effect is apparent in 1–2 minutes; effect lasts 1–2 hours. Dose may be repeated after 1–2 hours to sustain effect.
Dose: 0.01 mg/kg body weight.
Interactions: Naloxone should not be administered with alkaline solutions.

Nursing responsibilities:

1. Assess depth and rate of respirations following administration and at end of 1–2 hours when drug effect diminishes (because a narcotic has an effect for 3–4 hours, respiratory depression may occur again at this time).
2. Naloxone must not be administered to neonates

who have respiratory depression from other non-narcotic related causes or naloxone will produce depression effects of its own.

3. Administer with caution to infants of narcotic-dependent women as severe withdrawal symptoms may occur.

Nonsteroidal Anti-inflammatory Agents (NSAIA)
Ibuprofen (Advil, Nuprin, Motrin), Naproxen Sodium (Anaprox), Fenoprofen (Nalfon), Indomethacin (Indocin)

Pharmacology: Anti-inflammatory, analgesic, antipyretic. These drugs are prostaglandin inhibitors, which is how they are believed to exert their actions.
Use: Reduce uterine inflammation postpartally.
Side effects: GI upset and ulceration, therefore, administer these drugs after meals or with antacids. Signs of gastric irritation include pain, cramps, heartburn, bleeding, nausea, vomiting, and diarrhea. Inhibition of platelet aggregation, which gives an increase in bleeding time. Anemia due to prolonged blood loss via the GI tract. Some edema due to water retention. Vision changes have been reported in some people. CNS effects include dizziness, insomnia, and drowsiness. Renal side effects such as urinary tract infections, hematuria, changes in serum creatinine, and BUN are all possible with the use of the drugs. Allergic reactions such as skin rashes or asthma are sometimes seen.
Doses: Motrin: 300 to 600 mg po q6–8h. Anaprox: 275 mg q8–12h. Nalfon: 300 to 600 mg q6–8h.
Interactions: With anticoagulants (warfarin and heparin). NSAIA cause an increased prothrombin time when given with warfarin, resulting in an increased risk of hemorrhage. Another important factor that may lead to an increased risk of hemorrhage is that many of these NSAIA cause an ulcer in the GI tract, where bleeding can occur.

Nursing responsibilities:

1. Assess for GI bleeding. Signs include black, tarry stools and a decrease in hemoglobin and hematocrit.
2. Assess for GI ulceration. Signs include pain and heartburn.
3. Assess for fluid retention. Watch for an increase in blood pressure, edema, weight gain. Monitor the intake and output, as this may show fluid retention.
4. Any change in vision should be reported to the physician, as this may require treatment by an ophthalmologist.
5. Assess renal function. BUN and serum creatinine should be monitored as there is a small degree of renal toxicity with these agents.
6. Assess for hypersensitivity. Any signs of asthma, such as wheezing or shortness of breath, should be reported to the physician.
7. Teach the patient to take the medicine with food, milk, or antacids; and if GI upset continues, notify her physician.

Nystatin (Mycostatin Vaginal Tablets)

Pharmacology: Antifungal effective against a wide variety of yeasts and yeast-like fungi, including *Candida.*
Use: Moniliasis.
Side effects: Very few side effects have been reported with nystatin use. Rarely irritation or sensitization is seen.
Dose: One tablet (100,000 Units) inserted vaginally daily for 2 weeks.

Nursing responsibilities:

1. Have the patient use a sanitary napkin to avoid staining clothing.
2. The medication should be inserted high into the vagina with the applicator provided.
3. Coitus during treatment should be avoided (or the male should use a condom), so as to prevent reinfection.
4. Treatment should be uninterrupted and for the full course (do not discontinue treatment during the menstrual period).
5. No adverse effects have been seen in infants born to nystatin-treated mothers. This is an argument for the use of nystatin in pregnant women rather than other antifungal agents.

Oxytocin IV (Pitocin, Syntocinon)

Pharmacology: Drug is a pituitary hormone that stimulates uterine contraction.
Uses: Primarily for the induction or improvement of uterine contractions. Oxytocin is not indicated for elective induction of labor in which the patient is free from any medical problems. If, however, the patient, for some medical reason, must be induced, oxytocin may be used. Oxytocin is also used for the control of postpartum bleeding.
Side effects: Oxytocin can lead to water intoxication due to its intrinsic antidiuretic effect. Other side effects include nausea, vomiting, premature ventricular contractions, and fetal bradycardia.
Dose: Based on uterine response. Use a constant infusion pump and a nonhydrating IV solution to deliver the drug; nonhydrating so as to decrease the chance of water intoxication (0.9% NaCl). For control of postpartum bleeding, 10 Units IM after delivery of the placenta is recommended.

Nursing responsibilities:

1. Assess intake and output and electrolytes. You will probably see a decrease in serum electrolytes and hemoglobin/hematocrit values if water intoxication is present. These values should be monitored; and if they start to decrease, necessary action should be taken (notify the physician).
2. Ventricular rhythm should be followed while a woman is receiving oxytocin infusions. Watch for any premature ventricular contractions, as these will require a dosage adjustment.
3. Assess maternal blood pressure, pulse and the duration, frequency, and resting tone of the contrac-

tions before any increase in oxytocin infusion rate.

4. The fetal heart rate should also be monitored. If bradycardia should occur, a dosage adjustment may be necessary.
5. Other signs of water intoxication are signs of edema. These include any increase in blood pressure, shortness of breath, and weight gain.
6. Discontinue administration of oxytocin if sustained uterine contractions, fetal distress, or no relaxation between contractions occurs.

Oxytocin Nasal

Use: Indicated to encourage initial milk let-down.
Dose: One spray into both nostrils 2 to 3 minutes before nursing or pumping of breasts. The patient should be sitting down, holding the bottle upright when using this spray.
Side effects and monitoring: Parameters are the same as for oxytocin IV.

Parlodel (see Bromocriptine)

Prenatal Vitamins

Uses: Vitamin supplementation in pregnant and lactating women, as these women require an increased intake. Folic acid is most important; as much as 50 mcg is lost each day in breast milk alone.
Dose: One tablet daily.
Products: Materna 1.60, Natabec Rx, Natalins Rx, Stuartnatal 1 + 1, Filibon F.A.
Side effects: If taken as directed, side effects are not usually present.

Nursing responsibilities:

1. Stress the importance of compliance.
2. Urge women to not substitute an over-the-counter vitamin preparation as these do not contain folic acid.

Progestins (Progesterone)

Pharmacology: These drugs transform the proliferative endometrium into a secretory endometrium. Progestins also inhibit the secretion of pituitary gonadotropins, thus preventing follicular maturation and ovulation. These agents also have estrogenic, anabolic, and androgenic effects. One agent may exhibit more or less of one property than another.
Uses: Secondary amenorrhea. Functional uterine bleeding. Some progestins are used to treat endometriosis.
Side effects: Estrogen-related effects: water retention leading to edema, increased blood pressure, and weight gain, thrombophlebitis, thromboembolism, cerebrovascular accidents. Other side effects (not estrogen-related) include photosensitivity, hypersensitivity, depression, acne, hirsutism, breakthrough bleeding, and spotting. Vision changes can occur; and if so, the patient should notify her physician, because complete vision loss has been reported. Amenorrhea

is a result of the inhibition of maturation and ovulation. Local reactions at the site of injection are possible.
Dose: Provera, 5–10 mg po qd for 5 to 10 days; withdrawal bleeding will usually occur in 3 to 7 days.

Nursing responsibilities:

1. Should the patient experience any changes in vision, the physician should be notified immediately.
2. Any signs of thrombotic disorders such as pain, redness, or warmth in a leg (phlebitis). Neurologic changes such as numbness in an extremity that might indicate a CVA; shortness of breath or angina that might indicate a pulmonary embolism.
3. This drug is not recommended for use during the first 4 months of pregnancy.
4. Assess blood pressure increases, weight gain, and intake and output to detect any fluid retention.
5. Caution the patient of possible photosensitivity reactions upon exposure to direct sunlight.
6. When a patient is administered this drug for the first time, she must be given a patient package insert. This does not apply to patients being treated for cancer.

Prostaglandins

Pharmacology: Stimulation of the myometrium, causing contractions similar to those during labor at full-term pregnancy. Stimulates the smooth muscle of the GI tract. Contracts vascular smooth muscle, thus causing an increase in blood pressure. Causes an increase in body temperature.
Use: Induced abortion.
Side effects: The attempted abortion may be incomplete, in which instance other measures should be taken to complete the abortion. GI side effects due to smooth muscle stimulation. These include nausea, vomiting, and diarrhea. Pretreatment with antidiarrheal and antiemetic drugs is of some benefit. Along with an increase in body temperature, you will see flushing, chills, and hot flashes. The temperature returns to normal upon discontinuing the drug. It is interesting to note that aspirin inhibits prostaglandins, and it is by this mechanism that fever reduction is achieved. Endometritis, retained fragments of the placenta, and excessive uterine bleeding are all complications of prostaglandin administration that require additional treatment.

Nursing responsibilities:

1. Assess for GI side effects. While pretreatment is of some benefit, additional therapy may be required.
2. Assess body temperature, which will increase. If the body temperature rises excessively, treatment may be required. The temperature should return to normal within 12 to 24 hours after the drug is discontinued.
3. Assess for endometritis. Signs include a fever 3 days after the drug is used; there will be necrosis of the endometrium, lymphocytes will be present, and hemorrhage will be evident. The uterus may also be tender.

4. Assess for any signs of uterine bleeding, which may be severe and require immediate treatment.

Ritodrine (Yotopar)

Pharmacology: Drug is a sympathomimetic. Ritodrine has beta 2 receptor specificity. This means that it stimulates the sympathetic nervous system, with specificity for certain receptors, namely beta 2. Uterine smooth muscle is an example of an area in the body that contains these receptors. When stimulated with ritodrine (or any beta 2 stimulant), the result is an inhibition of uterine contractility.

Uses: The treatment of preterm pregnancy, but only in suitable patients. The initial treatment should be intravenous, followed with oral treatment so as to prevent a relapse of contractions.

Side effects: Are due to the beta 2 stimulation at other sites in the body. Almost always, the heart rate is increased, along with the blood pressure and blood glucose. About half the time, palpitations, tremor, nausea, vomiting, and headache are present. Less frequently, nervousness, emotional upset, anxiety, hyperventilation, dyspnea, chills, drowsiness, and weakness occur.

Interactions: With steroids, this combination can lead to pulmonary edema. If this happens, both drugs should be stopped, and the edema should be treated. With other sympathomimetic drugs, the effect is additive. Overstimulation may result. With beta blockers, the effects of ritodrine are blocked, therefore allowing uterine contractions to go on unaltered.

Dose: Based on the uterine response and on the side effects. The intravenous infusion is begun at 1 mg per minute, and increased at a rate of 0.05 mg per minute every 10 minutes, until a response is achieved. The infusion should be continued for 12 hours after uterine contractions stop. The infusion should be followed with 10 mg orally, the first dose being given before the IV is discontinued, then 10 mg every 2 hours for 24 hours; or 10 mg to 20 mg every 4 to 6 hours based on the side effects. The maximum daily dose should not exceed 120 mg.

Nursing responsibilities:

1. Assess uterine contractions. These should be suppressed completely. If not, the IV rate should be increased until contractions stop. However, if side effects appear, a further increase in dose may not be suggested.
2. Assess beta 2 stimulation in other areas of the body—heart rate, blood pressure, fetal heart rate. If these increase excessively, the dose must be decreased. Other side effects that may warrant a dosage reduction are palpitations, respiratory rate changes, tremor, and increased serum glucose. All of the effects are direct results of beta 2 stimulation.

3. This drug should not be given before 20 weeks of gestation as uterine muscle is not responsive to its action until then.

Silver Nitrate Ophthalmic Solution

Pharmacology: Anti-infective, applied to mucous membranes as a germicide and astringent.

Use: For the prevention of ophthalmia neonatorum.

Side effects: Chemical conjunctivitis. Silver nitrate may also cause cauterization of the cornea with repeated applications, which could lead to blindness. Silver nitrate is caustic and irritating to the skin and mucous membranes.

Dose: After proper cleansing of the eye, two drops in each eye. The lid should then be separated from the eyeball so a lake of solution may lie over the eyeball for a half minute. Make sure the solution has come in contact with all parts of the eye.

Nursing responsibilities:

1. Assess for chemical conjunctivitis. The conjunctiva will be reddened; mucus is pustular.
2. Assess for cauterization of the cornea (irregular, distorted cornea).

Vitamin K (Phytonadione, Aquamephyton)

Pharmacology: Vitamin K is a necessary component in the liver for production of certain coagulating factors (II, VII, IX, and X).

Uses: The prophylaxis and treatment of hemorrhagic disease in newborns. Vitamin K is also used in the treatment of warfarin overdose.

Side effects: Local irritation, such as pain and swelling at the site of injection. Allergic reactions to the drug are not uncommon, especially when the drug is given IV. Deaths have occurred from anaphylactic shock, cardiac and respiratory failure. Due to this possibility, IV vitamin K should only be used in severe illness.

Dose: Prophylaxis—0.2–2 mg IM once in the newborn. For treatment of hemorrhagic disease, 1–2 mg IM or SC daily; the prothrombin time should be normal in 2 to 4 days.

Nursing responsibilities:

1. Assess prothrombin time. This is the single best indicator of vitamin K-dependent clotting factors.
2. Assess for any sign of bleeding—black tarry stool, hematuria, decreased hemoglobin/hematocrit (anemia), bleeding from open wounds, etc. These would be indicators that more vitamin K is necessary, as control of bleeding has not been achieved.
3. IM injections should be given into large muscles: Adults—upper outer quadrant of the buttocks. Infants—anterolateral muscle of the thigh.

Appendix B

Organizations Concerned with Maternal-Child Health

American Academy of Husband-Coached Childbirth
P.O. Box 5224
Sherman Oaks, CA 91413

American Academy of Pediatrics
P.O. Box 1034
Evanston, IL 60204

American College of Home Obstetrics
2821 Rose Street
Franklin Park, IL 60131

American College of Nurse Midwifery
330 W. 58th Street
New York, NY 10019

American College of Obstetrics and Gynecology
1 East Wacker Drive
Chicago, IL 60601

American National Red Cross
17 & D Street, N.W.
Washington, D.C. 20006

American Nurses Association
2420 Pershing Road
Kansas City, MO 64108

American Society for Psychoprophylaxis in Obstetrics, Inc.
1523 L Street, N.W.
Washington, D.C. 20005

Association for Childbirth at Home, International
P.O. Box 1219
Cerritos, CA 90701

Cesarean Association for Research, Education, Support and Satisfaction in Birthing (CARESS)
Burbank, CA 91510

Cesarean/Support, Education and Concern (C/SEC, Inc.)
66 Christopher Road
Waltham, MA 02154

Childbirth Without Pain Education Association
20134 Snowden Avenue
Detroit, MI 48235

Childbirth Without Pain Education League
3940 Eleventh Street
Riverside, CA 92501

Council of Childbirth Education Specialists, Inc.
168 West 86th Street
New York, NY 10024

Home Oriented Maternity Experience (HOME)
511 New York Avenue
Takoma Park, MD 20012

International Childbirth Education Association
Box 20048
Minneapolis, MN 55420

La Leche League International, Inc.
9616 Minneapolis Avenue
Franklin Park, IL 60131

Maternity Center Association
48 West 92nd Street
New York, NY 10028

National Association of Parents and Professionals for Safe Alternatives in Childbirth (NAPSAC)
P.O. Box 1307
Chapel Hill, NC 27514

National Council for Prevention of Child Abuse
Box 2866
Chicago, IL 60690

National Foundation March of Dimes
1707 H Street, N.W.
Washington, D.C. 20006

National League for Nursing
10 Columbus Circle
New York, NY 10019

National Sudden Infant Death Syndrome Foundation
310 South Michigan Avenue
Chicago, IL 60604

Nurses Association, American College of Obstetrics and Gynecology
1 East Wacker Drive
Chicago, IL 60601

Parents Without Partners
80 Fifth Avenue
New York, NY 10011

Planned Parenthood Federation of America
810 Seventh Avenue
New York, NY 10019

Appendix C

Joint Position Statement on the Development of Family-Centered Maternity/Newborn Care in Hospitals

The Interprofessional Task Force on Health Care of Women and Children, June 1978

Definition of Family-Centered Maternity/Newborn Care

Family-centered maternity/newborn care can be defined as the delivery of safe, quality health care while recognizing, focusing on, and adapting to both the physical and psychosocial needs of the client-patient, the family, and the newly born. The emphasis is on the provision of maternity/newborn health care which fosters family unity while maintaining physical safety.

Position Statement

The Task Force organizations, The American College of Obstetricians and Gynecologists, The American College of Nurse-Midwives, The Nurses Association of the American College of Obstetricians and Gynecologists, The American Academy of Pediatrics, and The American Nurses' Association, endorse the philosophy of family-centered maternity/newborn care. The development of this conviction is based upon a recognition that health includes not only physical dimensions, but social, economic, and psychologic dimensions as well. Therefore, health care delivery, to be effective and satisfying for providers and the community alike, does well to acknowledge all these dimensions by adhering to the following philosophy.

That the family is the basic unit of society;

That the family is viewed as a whole unit within which each member is an individual enjoying recognition and entitled to consideration;

That childbearing and childrearing are unique and important functions of the family;

That childbearing is a developmental opportunity and/or a situational crisis, during which the family members benefit from the supporting solidarity of the family unit.

To this end, the family-centered philosophy and delivery of maternal and newborn care is important in assisting families to cope with the childbearing experience and to achieve their own goals within the concept of a high level of wellness, and within the context of the cultural atmosphere of their choosing.

The implementation of family-centered care includes recognition that the provision of maternity/newborn care requires a team effort of the woman and her family, health care providers, and the community. The composition of the team may vary from setting to setting and include obstetricians, pediatricians, family physicians, certified nurse-midwives, nurse practitioners, and other nurses. While physicians are responsible for providing direction for medical management, other team members share appropriately in managing the health care of the family, and each team member must be individually accountable for the performance of his/her facet of care. The team concept includes the cooperative interrelationships of hospitals, health care providers, and the community in an organized system of care so as to provide for the total spectrum of maternity/newborn care within a particular geographic region.

Appendix D

The Pregnant Patient's Bill of Rights

American parents are becoming increasingly aware that health professionals do not always have scientific data to support common American obstetrical practices and that many of these practices are carried out primarily because they are part of medical and hospital tradition. In the last forty years many artificial practices have been introduced which have changed childbirth from a physiological event to a very complicated medical procedure in which all kinds of drugs are used and procedures carried out, sometimes unnecessarily, and many of them potentially damaging for the baby and even for the mother. A growing body of research makes it alarmingly clear that every aspect of traditional American hospital care during labor and delivery must now be questioned as to its possible effect on the future well-being of both the obstetric patient and her unborn child.

One in every 35 children born in the United States today will eventually be diagnosed as retarded; one in every 10 to 17 children has been found to have some form of brain dysfunction or learning disability requiring special treatment. Such statistics are not confined to the lower socioeconomic group but cut across all segments of American society.

New concerns are being raised by childbearing women because no one knows what degree of oxygen depletion, head compression, or traction by forceps the unborn or newborn infant can tolerate before that child sustains permanent brain damage or dysfunction. The recent findings regarding the cancer-related drug diethylstilbestrol have alerted the public to the fact that neither the approval of a drug by the U.S. Food and Drug Administration nor the fact that a drug is prescribed by a physician serves as a guarantee that a drug or medication is safe for the mother or her unborn child. In fact, the American Academy of Pediatrics Committee on Drugs has recently stated that there is no drug, whether prescription or over-the-counter remedy, which has been proven safe for the unborn child.

The Pregnant Patient has the right to participate in decisions involving her well-being and that of her unborn child, unless there is a clear-cut medical emergency that prevents her participation. In addition to the rights set forth in the American Hospital Association's "Patient's Bill of Rights" (which has also been adopted by the New York City Department of Health), the Pregnant Patient, because she represents TWO patients rather than one, should be recognized as having the additional rights listed below.

Source: Reprinted by permission of the Committee on Patient's Rights, Box 1900, New York, N.Y. 10001.

1. *The Pregnant Patient has the right,* prior to the administration of any drug or procedure, to be informed by the health professional caring for her of any potential direct or indirect effects, risks or hazards to herself or her unborn or newborn infant which may result from the use of a drug or procedure prescribed for or administered to her during pregnancy, labor, birth, or lactation.

2. *The Pregnant Patient has the right,* prior to the proposed therapy, to be informed, not only of the benefits, risks, and hazards of the proposed therapy but also of known alternative therapy, such as available childbirth education classes which could help to prepare the Pregnant Patient physically and mentally to cope with the discomfort or stress of pregnancy and the experience of childbirth, thereby reducing or eliminating her need for drugs and obstetric intervention. She should be offered such information early in her pregnancy in order that she may make a reasoned decision.

3. *The Pregnant Patient has the right,* prior to the administration of any drug, to be informed by the health professional who is prescribing or administering the drug to her that any drug which she receives during pregnancy, labor and birth, no matter how or when the drug is taken or administered, may adversely affect her unborn baby, directly or indirectly, and that there is no drug or chemical which has been proven safe for the unborn child.

4. *The Pregnant Patient has the right,* if cesarean section is anticipated, to be informed prior to the administration of any drug, and preferably prior to her hospitalization, that minimizing her and, in turn, her baby's intake of nonessential preoperative medicine will benefit her baby.

5. *The Pregnant Patient has the right,* prior to the administration of a drug or procedure, to be informed if there is NO properly controlled follow-up research which has established the safety of the drug or procedure with regard to its direct and/or indirect effects on the physiological, mental and neurological development of the child exposed, via the mother, to the drug or procedure during pregnancy, labor, birth, or lactation—(this would apply to virtually all drugs and the vast majority of obstetric procedures).

6. *The Pregnant Patient has the right,* prior to the administration of any drug, to be informed of the brand name and generic name of the drug in order that she may advise the health professional of any past adverse reaction to the drug.

7. *The Pregnant Patient has the right,* to determine for herself, without pressure from her attendant, whether she will accept the risks inherent in the proposed therapy or refuse a drug or procedure.

8. *The Pregnant Patient has the right* to know the name and qualifications of the individual administering a medication or procedure to her during labor or birth.

9. *The Pregnant Patient has the right* to be informed, prior to the administration of any procedure, whether that procedure is being administered to her for her or her baby's benefit (medically indicated) or as an elective procedure (for convenience or teaching purposes).

10. *The Pregnant Patient has the right* to be accompanied during the stress of labor and birth by someone she cares for, and to whom she looks for emotional comfort and encouragement.

11. *The Pregnant Patient has the right* after appropriate medical consultation to choose a position for labor and for birth which is the least stressful to her baby and to herself.

12. *The Obstetric Patient has the right* to have her baby cared for at her bedside if her baby is normal, and to feed her baby according to her baby's needs rather than according to the hospital regimen.

13. *The Obstetric Patient has the right* to be informed in writing of the name of the person who actually delivered her baby and the professional qualifications of that person. This information should also be on the birth certificate.

14. *The Obstetric Patient has the right* to be informed if there is any known or indicated aspect of her or her baby's care or condition which may cause her or her baby later difficulty or problems.

15. *The Obstetric Patient has the right* to have her and her baby's hospital medical records complete, accurate, and legible and to have their records, including Nurses' Notes, retained by the hospital until the child reaches at least the age of majority, or alternatively, to have the records offered to her before they are destroyed.

16. *The Obstetric Patient*, both during and after her hospital stay, *has the right* to have access to her complete hospital medical records, including Nurses' Notes, and to receive a copy upon payment of a reasonable fee and without incurring the expense of retaining an attorney.

It is the obstetric patient and her baby, not the health professional, who must sustain any trauma or injury resulting from the use of a drug or obstetric procedure. The observation of the rights listed above will not only permit the obstetric patient to participate in the decisions involving her and her baby's health care, but will help to protect the health professional and the hospital against litigation arising from resentment or misunderstanding on the part of the mother.

Appendix E
Conversion Tables

Conversion of Pounds and Ounces to Grams for Newborn Weights

						Ounces										
	0	1	2	3	4	5	6	7	8	9	10	11	12	13	14	15
Pounds																	Pounds
0	—	28	57	85	113	142	170	198	227	255	283	312	430	369	397	425	0
1	454	482	510	539	567	595	624	652	680	709	737	765	794	822	850	879	1
2	907	936	964	992	1021	1049	1077	1106	1134	1162	1191	1219	1247	1276	1304	1332	2
3	1361	1389	1417	1446	1474	1503	1531	1559	1588	1616	1644	1673	1701	1729	1758	1786	3
4	1814	1843	1871	1899	1928	1956	1984	2013	2041	2070	2098	2126	2155	2183	2211	2240	4
5	2268	2296	2325	2353	2381	2410	2438	2466	2495	2523	2551	2580	2608	2637	2665	2693	5
6	2722	2750	2778	2807	2835	2863	2892	2920	2948	2977	3005	3033	3062	3090	3118	3147	6
7	3175	3203	3232	3260	3289	3317	3345	3374	3402	3430	3459	3487	3515	3544	3572	3600	7
8	3629	3657	3685	3714	3742	3770	3799	3827	3856	3884	3912	3941	3969	3997	4026	4054	8
9	4082	4111	4139	4167	4196	4224	4252	4281	4309	4337	4366	4394	4423	4451	4479	4508	9
10	4536	4564	4593	4621	4649	4678	4706	4734	4763	4791	4819	4848	4876	4904	4933	4961	10
11	4990	5018	5046	5075	5103	5131	5160	5188	5216	5245	5273	5301	5330	5358	5386	5415	11
12	5443	5471	5500	5528	5557	5585	5613	5642	5670	5698	5727	5755	5783	5812	5840	5868	12
13	5897	5925	5953	5982	6010	6038	6067	6095	6123	6152	6180	6209	6237	6265	6294	6322	13
14	6350	6379	6407	6435	6464	6492	6520	6549	6577	6605	6634	6662	6690	6719	6747	6776	14
15	6804	6832	6860	6889	6917	6945	6973	7002	7030	7059	7087	7115	7144	7172	7201	7228	15
	0	1	2	3	4	5	6	7	8	9	10	11	12	13	14	15

Temperature Conversion Chart: Fahrenheit to Celsius

Celsius	Fahrenheit		Celsius	Fahrenheit		Celsuis	Fahrenheit
34.0	93.2		37.0	98.6		40.0	104.0
34.2	93.6		37.2	99.0		40.2	104.4
34.4	93.9		37.4	99.3		40.4	104.7
34.6	94.3		37.6	99.7		40.6	105.2
34.8	94.6		37.8	100.0		40.8	105.4
35.0	95.0		38.0	100.4		41.0	105.9
35.2	95.4		38.2	100.8		41.2	106.1
35.4	95.7		38.4	101.1		41.4	106.5
35.6	96.1		38.6	101.5		41.6	106.8
35.8	96.4		38.8	101.8		41.8	107.2
36.0	96.8		39.0	102.2		42.0	107.6
36.2	97.2		39.2	102.6		42.2	108.0
36.4	97.5		39.4	102.9		42.4	108.3
36.6	97.9		39.6	103.3		42.6	108.7
36.8	98.2		39.8	103.6		42.8	109.0
						43.0	109.4

(°C) × (9/5) + 32 = °F.
(°F − 32) × (5/9) = °C.

Appendix F
Growth Charts

Birth to 36 Months, Height and Weight, Boys and Girls

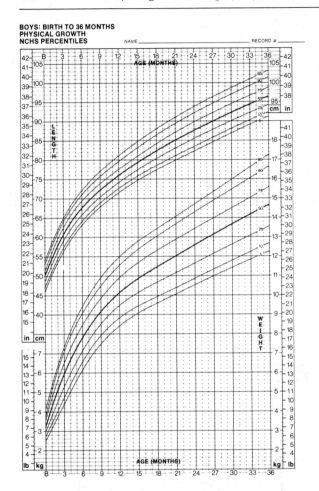

Source: Ross Laboratories, Columbus, Ohio. Adapted from National Center for Health Statistics, NCHS Growth Charts, 1976. Data from the Fels Research Institute, Yellow Springs, Ohio.

1983 Metropolitan Height and Weight Table for
Women

Height		Weight*		
Feet	Inches	Small Frame (lb)	Medium Frame (lb)	Large Frame (lb)
4	10	102–111	109–121	118–131
4	11	103–113	111–123	120–134
5	0	104–115	113–126	122–137
5	1	106–118	115–129	125–140
5	2	108–121	118–132	128–143
5	3	111–124	121–135	131–147
5	4	114–127	124–138	134–151
5	5	117–130	127–141	137–155
5	6	120–133	130–144	140–159
5	7	123–136	133–147	143–163
5	8	126–139	136–150	146–167
5	9	129–142	139–153	149–170
5	10	132–145	142–156	152–173
5	11	135–148	145–159	155–176
6	0	138–151	148–162	158–179

*Weight in pounds according to frame (in indoor clothing weighing 3 pounds, shoes with 1-inch heels).

Source of basic data: 1979 Build Study, Society of Actuaries and Association of Life Insurance Medical Directors of America, 1980.

Birth to 36 Months, Head Circumference, Boys and Girls

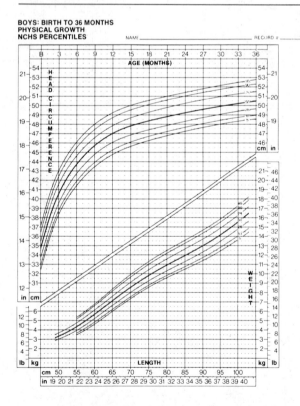
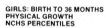
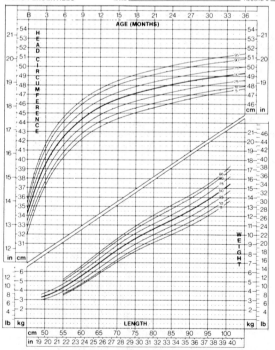

Source: Ross Laboratories, Columbus, Ohio. Adapted from National Center for Health Statistics, NCHS Growth Charts, 1976. Data from the Fels Research Institute, Yellow Springs, Ohio.

Appendix G

Laboratory and Assessment Values

Laboratory Values for Nonpregnant and Pregnant Women

	Nonpregnant	Pregnant
Hematologic Values		
Complete Blood Count (CBC)		
Hemoglobin, g/100 ml	12–16[a]	10–14[a]
Hematocrit, %	37–47	32–42
Red cell volume, ml	1600	1900
Plasma volume, ml	2400	3700
Red blood cell count, million/cu mm	4–5.5	4–5.5
White blood cells, total per cu mm	4500–10,000	5000–15,000
Polymorphonuclear cells, %	54–62	60–85
Lymphocytes, %	38–46	15–40
Erythrocyte sedimentation rate, mm/hr	≤20	30–90
MCHC, g/dl packed RBCs (mean corpuscular hemoglobin concentration	30–36	No change
MCH/(mean corpuscular hemoglobin per picogram [less than a micromicrogram])	29–32	No change
MCV/cu μm (mean corpuscular volume per cubic micrometer)	82–96	No change
Blood Coagulation and Fibrinolytic Activity[b]		
Factors VII, VIII, IX, X		Increase in pregnancy, return to normal in early puerperium; factor VIII increases during and immediately after delivery
Factors XI, XIII		Decrease in pregnancy
Prothrombin time (protime)	60–70 sec	Slight decrease in pregnancy
Partial prothrombin time (PTT)	12–14 sec	Slight decrease in pregnancy and again decrease during second and after third stage of labor (indicates clotting at placental site)
Bleeding time	1–3 min (Duke) 2–4 min (Ivy)	No appreciable change
Coagulation time	6–10 min (Lee/White)	No appreciable change
Platelets	150,000 to 350,000 cu mm	No significant change until 3–5 days after delivery, then marked increase (may predispose women to thrombosis and gradual return to normal)
Fibrinolytic activity		Decreases in pregnancy, then abrupt return to normal (protection against thromboembolism)
Fibrinogen	250 mg/dl	400 mg/dl
Mineral/Vitamin Concentrations		
Serum iron, μg	75–150	65–120
Total iron-binding capacity, μg	250–450	300–500
Iron saturation, %	30–40	15–30
Vitamin B$_{12}$, folic acid, ascorbic acid	Normal	Moderate decrease
Serum proteins		
Total, g/100 ml	6.7–8.3	5.5–7.5
Albumin, g/100 ml	3.5–5.5	3.0–5.0
Globulin, total, g/100 ml	2.3–3.5	3.0–4.0

Laboratory Values for Nonpregnant and Pregnant Women

	Nonpregnant	Pregnant
Mineral/Vitamin Concentrations (Continued)		
Blood sugar		
Fasting, mg/100 ml	70–80	65
2-hour postprandial, mg/100 ml	60–110	Under 140 after a 100 g carbohydrate meal is considered normal

[a]At sea level. Permanent residents of higher levels (e.g., Denver) require higher levels of hemoglobin.
[b]Pregnancy represents a hypercoagulable state.

Source: Benson, R.C. (1977). *Handbook of obstetrics and gynecology* (6th ed.). Los Altos, California: Lange Medical Publications. Reprinted by permission of Lange Medical Publications.

Hematology Values for Preterm and Term Infants

Determination (whole blood unless otherwise indicated)	Age	Normal Value
Hematocrit (vol %)	Premature	45–60%
	Newborn	44–64%
	Neonate	35–49%
Hemoglobin	Premature	15.6–20 gm/100 ml
	Newborn	14–24 gm/100 ml
	Neonate	11–20 gm/100 ml
Hemoglobin, fetal (Hb F)	Premature	55–85%
	Newborn	40–70% of total
	Neonate	20–40% of total
Nucleated red blood cells	Cord	250–500/mm^3
	Day 1	200–300/mm^3
	Day 2	20–30/mm^3
	Thereafter	0
Platelet count	Premature	100–300 000/mm^3
	Newborn	140–300 000/mm^3
	Neonate	150–390 000/mm^3
Red blood cell count (RBC)	Premature	4–6 million/mm^3
	Newborn	4.8–7.1 million/mm^3
	Neonate	4.1–6.4 million/mm^3
Blood indices		
MCH	Newborn	32–34 μμg
MCV	Newborn	98–108 μ^3
MCHC	Newborn	32–33%
Reticulocyte count	Newborn	2.5–6.5% total RBC
	Neonate	0.1–1.5% total RBC
Erythrocyte sedimentation rate (ESR) (uncorrected)	Newborn	0–2 mm/hr
	Neonate	3–13 mm/hr
White blood cell count (WBC)	Premature	10,000–15,000/mm^3
	Newborn, total	9,000–30,000/mm^3
	% neutrophils	≅61%
	% lymphocytes	≅31%
	1 wk, total	5,000–21,000/mm^3
	% neutrophils	≅45%
	% lymphocytes	≅41%
	4 wk, total	5,000–19,500/mm^3
	% neutrophils	≅35%
	% lymphocytes	≅56%

Source: V. C. Vaughan, III, and R. J. McKay, Jr. (Eds.). (1983). *Textbook of pediatrics* (12th ed.). Philadelphia: Saunders. Reprinted by permission of W. B. Saunders.

Blood Chemistry Values for Preterm and Term Infants

Determination	Specimen[a]	Age	Normal Value
Ascorbic acid			0.5–1.5 mg/100 ml
Bilirubin, total			Premature/full term
		Cord	<2 <2 mg/100 ml
		0–1 day	<8 <6 mg/100 ml
		1–2 day	<12 <8 mg/100 ml
		3–5 day	<16 <12 mg/100 ml
		Thereafter	<2 <1 mg/100 ml
Bilirubin, direct			0–1 mg/100 ml
Calcium, total		Premature	6.1–11.6 mg/100 ml
		Newborn	3.7–7.0 mEq/liter
Calcium, ionized			2.1–2.6 mEq/liter
Carbon dioxide (CO_2) content	Venous (arterial 2 mEq/L less)	Cord	14–22 mEq/liter
		Newborn	19–27 mEq/liter
Carbon dioxide, partial pressure (PCO_2)	Whole blood, arterial		35–45 mm Hg
	Whole blood, venous		40–50 mm Hg
Chloride		Premature	100–104 mEq/liter
		Cord	96–104 mEq/liter
		Newborn	93–112 mEq/liter
Cholesterol, total		Cord	45–100 mg/100 ml
		Newborn	45–170 mg/100 ml
Cholesterol, esters		Newborn	42%–71% of total
Creatinine clearance (endogenous)	Serum and urine	Newborn	40–65 ml/minute/1.73 m^2

Electrophoresis, protein (cellulose acetate)

	Total Protein	Albumin	a_1-globulin	a_2-globulin	β-globulin	γ-globulin	Units
Premature	4.3–7.6	3.1–4.2	0.1–0.5	0.3–0.7	0.3–1.2	0.3–1.4	g/100 ml
Newborn	4.6–7.4	3.6–5.4	0.1–0.3	0.3–0.5	0.2–0.6	0.2–1.2	g/100 ml

Determination		Age	Normal Value
Fibrinogen		Newborn	150–300 mg/dl
Galactose		Newborn/infant	0–20 mg/dl
Glucose, fasting (FBS)		Premature	20–60 mg/dl
		Newborn	30–80 mg/dl
Immunoglobulin levels	Serum		

	IgG (mg/dl)	IgM (mg/dl)	IgA (mg/dl)	Total Ig (mg/dl)
Newborn	645–1244	5–30	0–11	660–1439
1–3 months	272–762	16–67	6–56	324–699

Determination	Age	Normal Value
Iodine, total serum organic (PBI)	Newborn	4–14 μg/100 ml
	6 weeks–16 years	5–9 μg/100 ml
Iodine, butanol extractable (BEI)	Newborn	3–13 μg/100 ml
	6 weeks–16 years	4–8 μg/100 ml
Iodine, T_3 (Triosorb)		
Normal		25%–35%
Hyperthyroidism		>35%
Hypothyroidism		<25%
Iodine, T_4-by-column (thyroxine)	Newborn	3–12 μg/100 ml
	Thereafter	3.4–6.2 μg/100 ml

Blood Chemistry Values (continued)

Determination	Specimen[a]	Age	Normal Value
Iodine, T_4/comp. protein binding (throxine)		Newborn	3–12 µg/100 ml
		Thereafter	3–7 µg/100 ml
Iron		Newborn	100–200 µg/100 ml
		4 months–2 years	40–100 µg/100 ml
Iron-binding capacity (IBC)		Newborn	60–175 µ/dl 100 ml
		4 months–2 years	100–400 µg/dl 100 ml
Lead, normal	Whole blood, venous		0–40 µg/dl
Abnormal, nontoxic			40–80 µg/dl
Toxic			>80 µg/dl
Lipids, total		Newborn–2 years	170–450 mg/dl
Magnesium		Newborn	1.4–2.9 mEq/liter
Oxygen, partial pressure (PO_2)	Whole blood, arterial		75–100 mm Hg
	Whole blood, venous		20–50 mm Hg
Oxygen, % saturation	Whole blood, arterial	Newborn	40%–95%
		Thereafter	95%–98%
	Whole blood, venous	Newborn	30%–80%
		Thereafter	35%–85%
pH (37°C)[b]	Whole blood, arterial	Premature (cord)	7.15–7.35
		Premature (48 hours)	7.35–7.50
		Newborn	7.27–7.47
		Thereafter	7.35–7.45
Phenylalanine			0.5–2.0 mg/dl
Phosphorus		Premature	5.4–10.9 mg/100 ml
		Newborn	3.5–8.6 mg/dl
Potassium		Premature (cord	5.0–10.2 mEq/liter
		Premature (48 hours)	3.0–6.0 mEq/liter
		Newborn (cord)	5.6–12.0 mEq/liter
		Newborn	5.0–7.7 mEq/liter
Protein, total		Premature	4.3–7.6 gm/dl
		Newborn	4.6–7.6 gm/dl
Sodium		Premature (cord)	116–140 mEq/liter
		Premature (48 hours)	128–148 mEq/liter
		Newborn (cord)	126–166 mEq/liter
		Newborn	139–162 mEq/liter
Transaminases			
Glutamic oxaloacetic (SGOT) (aspartate, 30°C)s		Newborn/infant	5–70 IU/liter
Glutamic pyruvic (GPT) (alanine, 30°C)		Newborn/infant	5–50 IU/liter
Transferrin			0.2–0.3 gm/dl
Urea nitrogen (BUN)		Premature	16.22 mg/100 ml
		Newborn/infant	5–15 mg/dl

[a] Serum or plasma unless otherwise indicated.
[b] Arterial blood is approximately 0.03 pH units greater than circulating venous blood.

Source: Adapted from V. C. Vaughan, II, and R. J. McKay, Jr. (Eds.). (1983). *Textbook of pediatrics* (12th ed.). Philadelphia: Saunders; and Cloherty, J. P., and Stark, A. R. (Eds.). (1980). *Manual of neonatal care.* Boston: Little, Brown. Used by permission of W. B. Saunders and Little, Brown and Co.

Mean Blood Pressure at Wrist and Ankle in Infants (Flush Technique)

	Blood Pressure at Wrist		Blood Pressure at Ankle	
Age	Mean	Range	Mean	Range
1–7 days	41	22–66	37	20–58
1–3 months	67	48–90	61	38–96
4–6 months	73	42–100	68	40–104
7–9 months	76	52–96	74	50–96

Source: A. J. Moss. (1978). Indirect methods of blood pressure measurement. *Pediatr. Clin. North Am. 25, 3.*
Data from A. J. Moss and F. H. Adams. (1962). *Problems of Blood Pressure in Childhood.* Springfield, Ill.: Thomas.

Average Blood Pressures in American Females

		White Women		Black Women	
	Age	Average (mm Hg)	S.D.	Average (mm Hg)	S.D.
Systolic	Under 20	111.0	13.7	112.7	13.2
	20–29	116.9	13.8	119.1	14.7
	30–39	121.4	16.3	128.1	20.2
	40–49	129.3	19.6	138.3	22.8
Diastolic	Under 20	69.3	9.8	70.0	10.1
	20–29	73.7	7.2	75.4	9.7
	30–39	76.9	10.7	82.0	13.0
	40–49	80.6	11.6	86.9	13.9

S.D. = standard deviation.

Source: Adapted from J. Stamler et al. (1976). Hypertension screening of one million Americans. *J.A.M.A. 235,* 2299. Copyright © 1976, American Medical Association.

Normal Vital Sign Measurements in Newborns

Sign	Value
Pulse rate	100–120
Respiration rate	30–50
Temperature	97.6 axillary
Blood pressure	$80 \pm 16/46 \pm 16$

Appendix H

Health Maintenance Schedule for the First Year of Life

Assessment	Assessment Measures	Frequency
Meeting developmental milestones	History, observation	Every visit
	Formal Denver Developmental Screening Test	At 3 months and 1 year
Meeting growth milestones	Height, weight plotting on standard growth chart	Every visit
	Physical exam	
Determining nutritional problems	History, observation	Every visit
	Height, weight information	
Assessing parent-child relationship	History, observation	Every visit
Visual and hearing defects	Grossly by observation and history	Every visit
Dental assessment	History, physical exam	Every visit after teeth erupt
Anemia	Hematocrit	9th month visit
Immunizations	History and past records	Diphtheria, pertussis, and tetanus: 2nd, 4th, and 6th month visit
		Trivalent oral poliomyelitis at 2nd, 4th, and (optional) 6th month visit
Tuberculosis identification	Skin test	Tine test at 12th month visit
Counseling	Infant care, growth, and development	Every visit

Note: The above procedures vary in different communities and change with new health prevention knowledge. They should serve as a guide for independent nursing function toward ensuring that children receive adequate health maintenance care. The frequency of visits is every 1, 2, or 3 months, depending on the mother's experience in childrearing.

Appendix I

Answers to Chapter Multiple-Choice Questions

I Maternal-Newborn Nursing

1 A Framework for Maternal-Newborn Nursing
1. d   3. d   5. c
2. c   4. d   6. a

2 Trends in Maternal-Newborn Nursing
1. d   3. a   5. c
2. b   4. b   6. b

3 Ethics and Legal Aspects of Maternal-Newborn Nursing
1. b   4. c   7. b   10. d
2. d   5. c   8. a
3. c   6. a   9. c

II Childbearing in Today's World

4 Individual, Family, and Community Dynamics
1. a   5. a   9. b
2. c   6. b   10. a
3. d   7. b   11. b
4. b   8. b   12. d

5 The Culture of Childbearing
1. d   3. a   5. a
2. c   4. d   6. c

6 Genetic Assessment and Counseling
1. d   4. c   7. d
2. a   5. c   8. c
3. b   6. d   9. a

III The Interpartal Period

7 Developmental Readiness for Childbearing
1. b   3. a   5. d   7. a
2. c   4. a   6. a

8 Physiological Readiness for Childbearing
1. d   4. a   7. a   10. c
2. c   5. d   8. b
3. b   6. d   9. c

9 The Physiology of Menstruation
1. a   3. a   5. d
2. d   4. d

10 Sexuality
1. b   3. b   5. d   7. d
2. d   4. b   6. a

11 Reproductive Life Planning
1. b   4. a   7. b   10. a
2. c   5. d   8. c
3. c   6. b   9. b

12 The Couple Who Is Infertile
1. a   4. c   7. a
2. c   5. a   8. a
3. c   6. c

IV The Prepartal Period: Preparing for Parenthood

13 Psychological Aspects of Pregnancy
1. b   4. a   7. c
2. a   5. a
3. b   6. a

14 Growth and Development of the Fetus
1. b   4. c   7. d
2. b   5. a   8. a
3. b   6. d   9. b

15 Fetal Assessment
1. a   4. c   7. d
2. a   5. b   8. b
3. d   6. d

16 Physiologic Changes in Pregnancy
1. a   5. a   8. a
2. c   6. a   9. c
3. c   7. c   10. b
4. a

17 The Diagnosis of Pregnancy
1. a   4. d   6. c
2. b   5. c   7. b
3. d

18 Health Care: The First Prenatal Visit
1. d   5. c   8. c
2. c   6. b   9. c
3. a   7. d   10. a
4. b

19 Health Promotion During Pregnancy
1. b   5. b   8. b
2. b   6. d   9. a
3. b   7. c   10. a
4. c

20 Nutrition During Pregnancy
1. d   5. b   8. a
2. b   6. b   9. b
3. a   7. c   10. d
4. b

21 Preparation for Parenthood
1. d   4. b   7. a
2. c   5. c   8. a
3. a   6. d   9. b

V The Period of Parturition

22 Psychological Aspects of Labor
1. c   3. b   5. b
2. c   4. d

23 The Labor Process
1. c   5. b   8. a
2. a   6. d   9. c
3. c   7. c   10. a
4. a

24 Nursing Care During the Labor Experience
1. a   5. b   8. b
2. a   6. b   9. d
3. c   7. a   10. c
4. d

25 Analgesia and Anesthesia in Labor and Delivery
1. a   3. c   5. c
2. b   4. d

26 Alternative Birth Settings
1. b   3. a   5. b
2. d   4. c   6. d

VI The Postpartal Period: Parenthood

27 Psychological Aspects of the Postpartal Period
1. c   3. d   5. d
2. c   4. b   6. a

28 Physiology of the Postpartal Period
1. c   3. c   5. d
2. d   4. b   6. d

29 The Postpartal Experience: Nursing Implementations
1. c   4. d   7. b   10. b
2. b   5. d   8. c
3. a   6. a   9. c

VII The Newborn

30 Personality Development in the Newborn
1. c   3. b   5. a
2. b   4. b   6. b

31 Physiologic Development in the Newborn
1. b   4. d   7. a   10. d
2. b   5. d   8. d
3. c   6. b   9. d

32 Health Assessment of the Newborn
1. b   4. d   7. c   10. b
2. a   5. d   8. d
3. b   6. a   9. c

33 Nutritional Needs of the Newborn
1. a   4. b   7. b
2. d   5. b   8. c
3. a   6. d   9. b

34 Newborn Care: Nursing Implementations
1. c   4. c   7. d
2. b   5. b   8. b
3. a   6. b

VIII High-Risk Pregnancy

35 Identifying the High-Risk Mother
no questions

36 The Woman with Preexisting Illness
1. c   5. d   9. d
2. a   6. b   10. c
3. c   7. d   11. a
4. c   8. a

37 Pregnancy at Age Extremes
1. b   5. c   8. a
2. b   6. c   9. c
3. a   7. d   10. b
4. d

38 The Handicapped Woman
1. c   4. d   7. d
2. b   5. a   8. a
3. d   6. b   9. b

39 The Woman Who Develops a Complication of Pregnancy
1. d   5. b   9. a   12. b
2. a   6. a   10. c   13. b
3. c   7. d   11. d   14. b
4. c   8. b

40 Teratogens and Fetal Health
1. d   4. d   7. a
2. b   5. d
3. b   6. b

41 Trauma and Pregnancy
1. a   5. c   9. a
2. a   6. b   10. c
3. a   7. c   11. c
4. c   8. c   12. a

42 Cesarean Birth
1. a   3. d   5. c
2. b   4. c   6. b

43 The Woman Who Develops a Complication During Labor or Delivery
1. a   4. c   7. c
2. d   5. b   8. a
3. b   6. b   9. a

44 The Woman Who Develops a Complication During the Puerperium
1. a   4. c   7. d
2. b   5. a   8. d
3. b   6. c   9. b

IX The High-Risk Newborn

45 Identifying the High-Risk Newborn
no questions

46 The Newborn with a Congenital Anomaly
1. b   4. d   7. d   10. d
2. d   5. c   8. d
3. c   6. c   9. c

47 The Newborn Who Is Ill at Birth
1. b   4. d   7. b   10. b
2. b   5. c   8. d
3. c   6. c   9. c

48 The Infant with Altered Gestational Age or Birth Weight
1. c   4. a   7. c
2. b   5. b   8. a
3. c   6. d   9. b

Glossary

Abdominal pregnancy (also called **Abdominal gestation**). A pregnancy occurring in the abdominal cavity exterior to the uterus.

Abdominal hysterectomy. Surgical removal of the uterus through an incision in the anterior abdominal wall.

Abortion. The expulsion of the products of conception before 20 weeks' gestation or before an age of viability.

> *Complete abortion.* All the products of conception are expelled and no therapy is required.

> *Habitual abortion.* An abortion that occurs following two previous consecutive abortions.

> *Incomplete abortion.* An abortion in which not all of the products of conception are expelled. Further therapy is necessary to halt potential hemorrhage.

> *Induced abortion.* Termination of pregnancy by medical intervention.

> *Inevitable abortion.* A situation where irreversible uterine evacuation has begun; the internal cervical os is dilated. At this point the pregnancy will inevitably be lost.

> *Missed abortion.* A fetal death in which the products of conception have not yet been expelled.

> *Threatened abortion.* Unexplained vaginal bleeding but without cramping or cervical os dilatation.

Abruptio placentae. A normally implanted placenta that separates prematurely (between the twentieth week of gestation and birth of the infant).

Acceleration. An increase in a baseline rating such as a fetal heart rate.

Acini cells. Milk-producing cells of the breasts.

Acme. The peak or strongest intensity point of a uterine contraction.

Acrocyanosis. Mottled cyanosis of hands and feet. Normal finding in newborns.

Acromion. An extension of the scapula, forming the highest point of the shoulder.

Acrosome. The head of a sperm; contains the germ cell nucleus and its genetic material.

Adenomyoma. A tumor that grows from smooth muscle tissue; found in the uterus, popularly termed *fibroid tumor.*

Adnexae. Reproductive tract structures other than the uterus such as fallopian tubes, ligaments, and ovaries.

Adolescence. The time span of life during which biologic and psychosocial maturity occurs, generally 13 to 18 years of age.

Afibrinogenemia. Absence of fibrinogen in the blood plasma causing a decrease in blood coagulation ability. Associated with complications of pregnancy.

Afterbirth. Lay term for placenta, as it is delivered after the fetus.

Afterpains. Alternating contracting and relaxation of the uterine muscle following birth to accomplish involution. Most noticeable in women who are multigravida and nursing.

Agalactia. Absence of the secretion of milk.

Albuminuria. Albumin (protein) in urine.

Allele. Alternate forms of a gene found at the same chromosome locus.

Alopecia. Loss of hair.

Ambient. Surrounding; used to describe oxygen concentration.

Amelia. Absence of a limb.

Amenorrhea. Absence of menstrual flow.

Amniocentesis. Withdrawal of amniotic fluid from the uterus by means of introduction of a needle through the abdominal wall.

Amniography. X-ray of the uterus and its contents following introduction of a contrast medium into the amniotic sac.

Amnion. The inner membrane that encases the fetus during intrauterine life and covers the fetal surface of the placenta. Secretes amniotic fluid.

Amnionitis. Infection of amniotic fluid.

Amnioscope. A lighted instrument introduced through the cervical canal to view amniotic fluid.

Amniotic fluid. The fluid that surrounds the developing fetus. Contained within the amnion and chorion.

Amniotic sac. The sac formed by the amnion and chorion membranes; contains the fetus and amniotic fluid.

Amniotomy. Rupture of the amnion and chorion membranes to release amniotic fluid. Abbreviated AROM for artificial rupture of membranes.

Ampulla. The outer one third of the fallopian tube. Division where fertilization generally occurs.

Analgesic. Pharmacologic agent that relieves pain.

Anaphase. The phase of mitosis in which the chromosomes migrate to opposite poles of the cell.

Androgen. A male hormone.

Android. Male-like.

Anencephaly. Absence of brain formation.

Anemia. A decrease in the number or quality of red blood cells.

Anesthesia. Loss of sensation.

Anomaly. A malformation of a body organ or structure.

Anovulation. Absence of ovulation.

Anoxia. Decreased level of oxygen in body cells.

Antenatal (also, *Antepartal*). Occurring prior to birth.

Anthropoid. Used to describe a pelvis with a short anteroposterior diameter.

Antibody. A specific protein developed in response to a specific protein invader in order to destroy it.

Antigen. A protein that initiates an antibody response.

Apnea. Cessation of respirations.

Areola. The pigmented circle of epidermis that surrounds the nipple of the breast.

Arnold-Chiari malformation. A congenital disorder in which cerebellar tissue herniates into the foramen magnum; a cause of hydrocephaly.

Artificial insemination. The artificial introduction of semen into the female vagina to initiate fertilization.

Aschheim-Zondek test. A test for the diagnosis of pregnancy; utilizes urine from a pregnant woman injected into laboratory mice.

Asphyxia. Deprivation of oxygen.

Asphyxia neonatorum. Deficient or absent respiration in a newborn.

Asymptomatic bacteriuria. Urinary tract infection without symptoms.

Asynclitism. A fetal presentation where the head is not parallel to the pelvis.

Atelectasis. Collapse of the lung alveoli.

Atony. Loss of muscle tone.

Atresia. Closure of a normally patent tube.

Attitude. A reference to the relationship of the fetal parts to each other or the degree of flexion of the fetal head.

Augmentation. Assistance.

Auscultation. Assessing through listening, either with an unassisted ear or with an instrument.

Autosome. A paired chromosome.

Axis. An imaginary line drawn through the center of the body.

Azoospermia. Absence of spermatozoa.

Bag of waters. Lay term for fetal membranes containing amniotic fluid.

Ballottement. The sensation of an object rebounding after being pushed by an examining hand. Used for pregnancy diagnosis.

Bandl's ring. A pathologic retraction ring. Danger sign of labor.

Barr body. A dark-staining chromatin mass evident in the cell nucleus of a female body cell. Used to diagnose sex identity.

Bartholin's glands. Two glands located on the perineum bilateral to the vagina. Secretion moistens inner surface of the labia.

Basal body temperature. Body temperature at rest or at its lowest metabolic activity. Measured before rising in the morning.

Basal body temperature method. A method of family planning based on the rhythm method. Ovulation is detected by assessment of a daily basal body temperature, which rises at the time of ovulation from the release of progesterone produced by the corpus luteum.

Battledore placenta. A placenta with the umbilical cord inserted on the periphery rather than the center.

Bicornate uterus. A uterus that has two fundal horns; it may have an accompanying septum.

Bilirubin. A breakdown product from the destruction of red blood cells. It is unconjugated or insoluble and toxic to body cells until it is conjugated and made soluble to water by the liver. Also referred to as indirect (insoluble) and direct (soluble).

Billing's method. The ovulation method of family planning.

Bimanual examination. The assessment of a body part using both hands. Most often used to refer to a two-handed pelvic examination in which the uterus and adnexa are examined by one hand placed abdominally and two fingers of the other placed vaginally.

Biopsy. Surgical removal of a tissue for examination and diagnosis.

Birth rate. The number of live births to 1,000 population during a specified year.

Blastocyst. A hollow sphere of cells that forms in very early fetal development.

Bonding. The attachment that occurs between the parents and infant at birth.

Bradley's method. A method of preparation for childbirth. Also called husband-coached childbirth. Based on the theory that childbirth should be a natural, peaceful, and painless time.

Bradycardia. Slow heart rate.

Braxton Hicks contractions. Painless, erratic uterine contractions that occur toward the end of pregnancy. They ready the cervix for labor but cervical dilatation does not occur with them.

Brazelton assessment. A scale for determining interactional behavior of the neonate.

Breast. A mammary or milk-producing gland.

Breech. Buttocks; used to denote a delivery presentation.

Bregma. The junction of the coronal and sagittal sutures on the fetal skull.

Brim. The inlet of the pelvis.

Broad liagment. Two large folds of peritoneum that are attached bilaterally to the uterus. They extend to the pelvic walls and give uterine support.

Brown fat. Unique fat located between the scapula, around the neck, kidneys, and adrenals and behind the sternum that has a rich nerve and blood supply and generates heat in the neonate.

Bulbourethral glands. Two small structures located bilateral to the male urethra just below the prostate gland. Secretion adds bulk to seminal fluid. Also called Cowper's glands.

Café au lait spots. Light brown marks (the color of coffee with cream) on the skin; more than five such marks suggest the neurologic disorder neurofibromatosis exists.

Caking of milk. Milk accumulation in the lacteriferous ducts of the breast and not coming forward; has the potential to lead to mastitis.

Calendar method. A method of contraception that uses a principle of calculating fertile days by subtracting 11 from the woman's longest period and 18 from her shortest period.

Candida albicans. A fungus that commonly causes infections in the vagina and mouth (moniliasis and thrush).

Caput succedaneum. A localized edematous area on the scalp of a newborn caused by pressure on the presenting part of the head against the cervix during labor.

Carcinoma. A malignant (cancerous) tumor.

Caudal anesthesia. Injection of an anesthetic agent into the extrathecal space of the spinal canal through the nonclosure of the laminae of the last sacral vertebra; causes regional anesthesia.

Caul. A hood. A child born with the membranes still intact is said to be born "under a caul." Hamlet was born this way.

Cautery. A method of destroying tissue by heat; used to treat cervical conditions.

Cauterization. The act of destroying tissue by heat.

Centromere. The narrow junction point of a chromosome at which the two chomatids are joined.

Cephalic. Pertaining to the head; used to denote delivery presentation.

Cephalhematoma. An elevated area on a newborn head caused by the extravasation of blood between the skull bone and its periosteum from the pressure of birth.

Cephalopelvic disproportion (CPD). A delivery condition in which the mother's pelvis is too small or too misshaped to allow the infant's head to pass through. The most common reason for which cesarean birth is performed.

Cervical canal. The opening in the cervix between the internal and external os.

Cervical cap. A mechanical barrier contraceptive device that fits over the cervix and is held in place by suction.

Cervicitis. Infection of the cervix.

Cervix. The lowermost portion of the uterus; the portion that dilates at birth to allow fetus to be expelled.

Cesarean birth. Birth of an infant by surgical incision on the mother's abdomen and uterus.

Chadwick's sign. A change in color of the mucous membrane of the vagina from a pink to a deep violet because of increased vascularity due to pregnancy. A presumptive sign of pregnancy.

Chancre. A painless ulcer that is a primary syphilitic lesion.

Change of life. Lay term for menopause.

Chemical method. A conception method that relies on the introduction of spermacidal agents into the vagina.

Chloasma. Dark brown pigment causing discoloration of the face during pregnancy (the mask of pregnancy).

Choanal atresia. Obstruction of the posterior nares by membrane or bone; always assessed for in newborns.

Chorioamnionitis. Infection and inflammation of fetal membranes and amniotic fluid.

Choriocarcinoma. A malignant tumor that occurs following a hydatidiform mole. One of the most curable forms of malignancy.

Chorion. The outer of the two membranes that form the amniotic sac and contain the amniotic fluid and developing fetus during intrauterine life.

Chorion laeve. The outer surface of the chorion that develops a smooth appearance.

Chorionic somatomammotropin, human (HCS). A hormone produced by the placenta in pregnancy; helps to regulate maternal glucose levels. Formerly termed *human placental lactogen hormone.*

Chorionic villi. Projections of the trophoblast that produce human chorionic gonadotropin and begin osmosis of nutrients to the embryo.

Chromatids. Two coiled threads of DNA joined together by the centromere of a chromosome.

Chromosomal aberration. An abnormality of the structure or number of chromosomes.

Chromosome. A rod-shaped structure composed of DNA and found within the nuclei of cells; carries genetic information.

Cilia. The hairlike processes on the lining of the fallopian tubes that help propel the ovum to the uterus.

Circumcision. The surgical removal of the foreskin of the penis.

Circumoral cyanosis. A bluish appearance around the mouth.

Circumvallate placenta. A placenta with a fibrous ring at the edge.

Cleavage. Rapid mitotic division of the zygote.

Cleft lip and/or palate. Incomplete fusion of the lip or palate during intrauterine life.

Climacteric. Originally male menopause. Now used to denote either a male or female slowing of reproductive ability.

Clitoris. The female organ of sexual arousal.

Coccyx. Five fused bones at the base of the spinal column.

Coitus. Sexual intercourse.

Coitus interruptus. Withdrawal of the penis from the vagina just prior to ejaculation as a form of contraception.

Colostrum. The light yellow fluid secreted as the first milk following delivery.

Colpectomy. Surgical excision of the vagina.

Colporrhapy. Suturing of the vagina.

Colposcope. An instrument used to inspect the vagina and cervix by magnification of tissue.

Colposcopy. An examination using a colposcope.

Colpotomy. Surgical incision of the vagina; generally done in the posterior vaginal fornix to allow for direct visualization of the pelvic organs.

Conception. Impregnation of the female ovum by the male spermatozoon.

Conceptional age. The age of the fetus measured from the time of conception; estimated as 2 weeks less than gestational age as actual conception date is unknown.

Conceptus. The products of conception: the fetus, umbilical cord, fetal membranes, amniotic fluid, and placenta.

Condom. A mechanical barrier device used by the male for contraception.

Condylomata accuminata. A wart-like lesion found on the vulva.

Congenital. A condition present at the time of birth.

Conization. A surgical procedure done to excise a cone-shaped portion of the cervix for pathologic examination.

Conjoined twins. Twins formed from a single ovum that did not completely separate from each other in intrauterine life. May or may not be able to live independently of each other.

Conjugate. The anteroposterior diameter of the pelvic inlet.

Conjunctivitis. Inflammation of the mucous membrane lining the eyelid.

Contraction. Tightening of the uterine muscles during labor to cause effacement and dilatation of the cervix.

Coombs' test. A test for Rh antibodies on the red blood cells. Indirect: Demonstrates antibodies in maternal blood. Direct: Determines maternal Rh antibodies in fetal cord blood.

Copper 7 (Cu 7). An intrauterine contraceptive device wound with copper and in the shape of a seven.

Copulation. Sexual intercourse; coitus.

Corona radiata. The crown-like grouping of cells that surrounds the ovum immediately after ovulation.

Coronal. The suture formed by the junction of the frontal and two parietal bones.

Corpora cavernosa. Two cylindric, spongy structures located in the body of the penis; fill with blood to cause erection.

Corpus luteum. The yellow body formed in the Graafian follicle after ovulation.

Corpus uteri. The body of the uterus.

Cotyledon. A subdivision of the maternal surface of the placenta. Filled with maternal blood to allow for osmosis of nutrients to the fetal placental villi.

Couvade syndrome. Somatic symptoms experienced by the father during pregnancy simulating those of the pregnant mother.

Couvelaire uterus. Board-like rigidity and discoloration of the uterus due to accumulation of blood in the myometrium from hemorrhage into the muscle wall; can occur with premature separation of the placenta.

Cowper's glands. See bulbourethral glands.

CPD. Abbreviation for cephalopelvic disproportion.

Cradle cap. Lay term for seborrheic dermatitis; a salmon-colored crusting of the scalp due to sebaceous gland secretion.

Craniosynostosis. Premature closure of cranial sutures.

Credé's eye prophylaxis. Instillation of 2% silver nitrate into the eyes of the neonate following birth to prevent ophthalmia neonatorum. Currently used to denote any eye prophylaxis treatment at birth.

Credé's placental extraction. A technique of assisted placental delivery in which a hand is placed on the uterine fundus and the fundus gently massaged.

Cri du chat syndrome. A chromosomal disorder caused by partial deletion of the short arm of chromosome number 5; child is mentally retarded and has a cat-like cry.

Crisis. A self-limiting period of disorganization due to stress. May be maturational (predictable) or situational (unexpected).

Crowning. The appearance of the presenting part of the fetus at the vaginal orifice.

Cryosurgery. Controlled freezing of tissue to destroy abnormal cells.

Cryptorchidism. Undescended testes.

Cul-de-sac of Douglas. The pouch formed behind the posterior surface of the cervix by the vaginal wall.

Cunnilingus. Oral-genital sex.

Curettage. Scraping of the endometrial lining of the uterus.

Cutis marmorata. Purplish discoloration of skin on exposure to cold.

Cystocele. Pouching of the bladder into the anterior vaginal wall.

Cyesis. Pregnancy.

Deceleration. A decrease in the baseline reading of a fetal heart rate.

Decidua. The uterine endometrium during pregnancy. Is shed as lochia following birth.

  Decidua basalis. The decidua portion under the implanted blastocyst.

  Decidua capsularis. The portion of endometrium that covers the blastocyst.

  Decidua vera. The portion of the decidua covering the nonimplanted portion of the uterus.

Decrement. A decrease in intensity.

Deletion. Loss of part of a chromosome.

Delivery. The expulsion of a child during the second stage of labor.

Deoxyribonucleic acid (DNA). The basic structural material of genes that allows them to carry genetic information generation to generation.

Dermatoglyphics. The patterns of skin configurations on fingers and toes.

Descent. The maneuver of delivery following internal rotation.

Desquamation. Peeling of the epithelium.

Development. Maturation or an increase in the ability to perform tasks.

Developmental task. An activity for which a specific age group is "ripe." If the opportunity for accomplishing the task is lost, development proceeds with difficulty from that point.

Diagonal conjugate. Distance from the sacral promontory to the lower posterior border of the symphysis pubis.

Diaphragm. A mechanical barrier contraceptive device fitted over the cervix in the woman. Must be used with a spermacidal jelly for optimum effectiveness.

Diaphragmatic hernia. Protrusion of the intestinal contents through a defect in the respiratory diaphragm into the thoracic cavity.

Diastasis recti. A separation of the rectus abdominis muscle.

Diffusion. The transfer of substances from one body area to another.

Dilatation. Opening of the cervix to allow for delivery.

Dilatation and curettage (D&C). Surgical evacuation of uterine contents by scraping the internal walls of the uterus.

Dilatation and evacuation (D&E). Surgical evacuation of uterine contents using mechanical suction.

Diploid. Two sets of chromosomes.

Disparate twins. Twins that are unlike each other.

Disseminated intravascular coagulation (DIC). A

clotting disorder in which serum fibrinogen is used up so no further coagulation can occur.

Dizygotic. Arising from two zygotes.

Döderlein bacillus. A gram-positive bacteria found normally in the vagina.

Dominant trait. A characteristic that will be expressed in a heterozygous union.

Down's syndrome. A mental retardation syndrome caused by the presence of an extra number 21 chromosome (trisomy 21).

Dry labor. A lay term to describe labor when labor begins with rupture of the membranes.

Ductus arteriosus. A blood vessel joining the pulmonary artery and aorta in fetal life; closes at birth.

Ductus venosus. A blood vessel joining the umbilical vein and the inferior vena cava in fetal life; closes at birth.

Duncan presentation. A placenta delivered with the maternal surface evident.

Dyscrasia. An abnormal or incompatible condition; used to describe blood disorders.

Disfunctional uterine bleeding. Abnormal bleeding from the uterus from hormonal influences; innocent except for excessive blood loss.

Dysmenorrhea. Painful menstruation.

Dyspareunia. Pain on sexual intercourse.

Dystocia. Difficult delivery.

Ecchymosis. Extravasation of blood into the subcutaneous tissue; bruising.

Eclampsia. Severe pregnancy-induced hypertension after the point a woman has convulsed.

Ectocervix. The outer surface of the cervix.

Ectoderm. One of the layers of primary germ cell tissue in the embryo.

Ectopic pregnancy. A pregnancy implanted outside the uterine cavity; generally located in a fallopian tube.

EDC. Abbreviation for expected date of confinement.

Effacement. Thinning and shortening of the cervical canal.

Effleurage. Light, circular massage of the abdomen used as a distraction technique in prepared childbirth.

Ejaculation. Emission of semen from the male due to orgasm contraction.

Ejaculatory ducts. The two tubes through which semen is ejected from the seminal vesicles.

Embryo. The intrauterine growth period from the time following implantation until organogenesis is complete (tenth day to 5 to 8 weeks).

Enanthema. A rash on the mucous membrane.

Endocervix. The inner surface of the cervix.

Endoderm. One of the layers of primary germ cells in the embryo.

Endometrial aspiration. Menstrual extraction.

Endometriosis. Abnormal implantation sites of endometrial cells outside uterus.

Endometrium. Inner layer of the uterus that is shed as menstruation.

En face. A position in which one person looks at another with his or her face in the same vertical plane as the other; typical position a mother holds her newborn.

Engagement. Descent of the fetal head to the midlevel of the maternal pelvis or the level of the ischial spines.

Engorgement. Local congestion of the breasts associated with lactation.

Entoderm. One of the layers of primary germ cells in the embryo.

Enzygotic. Development from the same fertilized ovum.

Epididymis. The portion of the male testis where spermatozoa are stored after formation.

Epicanthus. A fold of skin that covers the inner canthus of the eye extending from the edge of the nose to the median end of the eyebrow.

Epidural. The space just below the dura membrane of the spinal cord. Used as a site for anesthesia to give regional anesthesia effect.

Episiotomy. A surgical incision in the perineum to enlarge the vaginal introitus for childbirth.

Epispadias. A urethral opening on the dorsal surface of the penis.

Epstein's pearl. An innocent, round, white epithelial cyst located on the palate of neonates. Caused by excess calcium formation during intrauterine life.

Erb's palsy. Paralysis of the brachial plexus leaving impairment in an arm; a birth injury. Also: brachial palsy.

Ergot. A pharmacologic agent that causes uterine contraction.

Erosion. Chronic irritation or infection of the uterine cervix.

Erythema toxicum neonatorum. Rash of the newborn marked by minute papules on an erythematous base caused from the first exposure to environmental contaminants.

Erythroblastosis fetalis. Severe hemolytic anemia due to Rh incompatibility.

Esophageal atresia. A congenital defect in which the esophagus ends in a blind pouch. Usually associated with a fistula that connects the blind esophagus to the trachea.

Estriol (E_3). A form of estrogen produced by the theca cells of the ovary. Also: the breakdown product of estrogen excreted in the urine. Used as a measure of fetal well-being.

Estradiol (E_2). A form of estrogen produced by the theca cells of the ovary. The main estrogen of premenopausal women.

Estrogen. The female hormone produced by the ovaries and, during pregnancy, the placenta. A combination of estrone, estradiol, and estriol.

Estrone (E_1). A component of estrogen. Produced only in small amounts by ovaries; large amount by liver. The estrogen of postmenopausal women.

Eugenics. The science that deals with the improvement of the human race through the control of genetic factors.

Exanthem. A rash of the skin.

Exchange transfusion. The replacement of 80 percent of a newborn's blood by withdrawing it in small amounts and injecting donor blood in equal amounts; used to reduce dangerously high indirect bilirubin blood levels.

Expected date of confinement (EDC). Calculated date on which birth will occur.

Expiratory grunt. A noise made by expiration against a closed larynx; typical sign of respiratory distress syndrome in newborns.

External rotation. Movement of the fetal head after expulsion from the birth canal to a transverse position to allow the shoulders to assume an anterior-posterior position. Also termed *restitution*.

External os. The junction of the cervical canal with the vagina.

Extrophy of the bladder. A congenital defect in which the bladder is open and exposed on the anterior abdominal wall.

Facies. Pertaining to the face; used to describe typical facial appearances in congenital syndromes.

Failure to thrive. A syndrome of ineffective growth related to poor mother-child attachment.

Fallopian tubes. Oviducts. Bilateral tubular structures that attach to the uterine body and extend to the ovaries. Serve to transport the ovum following ovulation and serve as the place of fertilization.

False labor. Uterine contractions that appear strong but do not cause cervical dilatation.

False pelvis. The area of the pelvis above the linea terminalis.

Familial. Description of a trait that occurs frequently in a family but does not appear to follow rules of Mendelian inheritance.

Fecundation. See Fertilization.

Fern test. Vaginal secretions allowed to dry on a glass slide will present a ferning pattern due to the level of sodium chloride present.

Fertility. The ability to reproduce.

Fertility rate. The number of births per 1,000 women of childbearing age in a given population per year.

Fertilization. The union of the sperm and ovum.

Fetal alcohol syndrome. A fetus with growth retardation; mental deficiencies; and facial, cardiac, and joint anomalies caused by the mother's consumption of alcohol during pregnancy.

Fetal death. Death of a fetus past the age of viability (500 gm or 20 weeks' gestation).

Fetal death rate. Number of fetal deaths per 1,000 live births.

Fetoscope. A head stethoscope for listening to fetal heart sounds.

Fetus. The developing structure from the eighth week postfertilization until birth.

FHR. Abbreviation for fetal heart rate.

Fibroid. An adenomyoma or benign tumor of the uterus.

Fimbria. The finger-like projections that line the fallopian tubes and help propel the ovum toward the uterine body.

Flexion. The degree to which a fetus in utero has the head bent forward on the chest; the more flexion, the smaller the head diameter presents to the birth canal.

Fluorescent treponemal antibody absorption test (FTA-ABS). Laboratory test for the detection of syphilis.

Follicle. A small fluid-filled cavity.

Follicle stimulating hormone (FSH). A gonadotrophic hormone released by the anterior pituitary gland to cause development of the ovarian follicles.

Fontanelles. Spaces of connective tissue at the anterior and posterior ends of the sagittal suture line in neonates. Referred to as *soft spots* by mothers.

Footling. A breech presentation in which one or both feet are the presenting fetal part.

Foramen ovale. An opening between the atria of the heart during intrauterine life.

Forceps. Metal instruments used to aid in delivery.

Foreskin. The prepuce of the penis; tissue removed by circumcision.

Fornix. An arch formed by the junction of the cervix and vagina.

Fourchette. The perineal surface posterior to the labia majora.

Fraternal twins. Two infants from two separate ova; also dizygotic twins.

Frenulum. The attachment of the inferior surface of the tongue to the oral mucous membrane.

Friedman's test. A modification of the Aschheim-Zondek test for pregnancy; performed with female rabbits.

Friedman's curve. A plotted curve of the pattern of normal labor.

FSH. Abbreviation for follicle-stimulating hormone.

Fundal dominance. Contractions during labor begin at the fundus and flow from the fundus to the cervix.

Fundus. The upper part of the uterus located between the insertions of the fallopian tubes.

Funic souffle. A soft blowing sound produced by the umbilical cord, heard on auscultation of fetal heart sounds.

Funis. Umbilical cord.

Furuncle. A pus-filled skin lesion; usually caused by a *Staphylococcus organism*.

Galactagogue. An agent or stimulus whose action is to cause or increase the flow of milk.

Galactorrhea. Excessive flow of milk.

Gamete. A mature sexual cell such as an unfertilized ovum or spermatozoon.

Gametogenesis. Maturation of sperm and ova.

Gastroschisis. A congenital anomaly in which the intestines are outside the abdominal cavity.

Gate theory. A theory of pain control in which a person's perception of pain can be altered by interruption of the sensory input of pain.

Gavage. To feed by means of a tube passed into the stomach; used with immature newborns.

Genitalia. Reproductive organs.

Gene. A segment of DNA material that carries character traits generation to generation.

Genetics. The science that deals with the gene transmission of characteristics generation to generation.

Genotype. The genetic constitution of an individual.

Gestation. Pregnancy.

Gonorrhea. A sexually transmitted disease caused by the *Neisseria gonorrhoeae*.

Gestational age. The number of weeks of fetal development calculated from the first day of the last menstrual cycle.

Glycosuria. The presence of glucose in the urine.

Gonad. A sex gland; an ovary in the female, a testis in the male.

Gonadostat. The unknown control mechanism that stimulates the hypothalamus to begin stimulation for puberty changes.

Gonadotropin. A hormone that stimulates activity of the sex glands.

Goodell's sign. Softening of the cervix; a probable sign of pregnancy.

Graffian follicle. A mature ovarian follicle containing the ovum and surrounding estrogen-enriched fluid.

Granulosa cells. Cells surrounding the oocyte as it matures.

Gravid. Pregnant.

Gravida. The number of pregnancies a woman has had; a pregnant woman.

Growth. An increase in physical size.

Gynecoid pelvis. A pelvis with the contours best for childbirth.

Gynecologic examination. The physical examination of the internal and external organs of reproduction, including breasts of a woman.

Gynecologist. A physician who specializes in the diseases and conditions of women.

Gynecology. The study of conditions and diseases of women.

Habitual abortion. See Abortion, habitual.

Haploid. A single set of chromosomes or half the usual number. In humans, this is 23.

Harlequin sign. A marked distinction in color of the newborn, the upper most surface appearing white, the lower surface appearing red. Caused by initial difficulty establishing peripheral circulation. An innocent finding.

HCG. Abbreviation for human chorionic gonadotropin hormone.

Hegar's sign. Softening of the lower uterine segment. A probable sign of pregnancy.

Hemagglutination-inhibitor test (Pregnosticon R). A pregnancy test based on the presence of HCG in the woman's urine.

Hemangioma. A collection of blood vessels.

Hematocrit. The volume of red blood cells per 100 ml of blood; expressed as volume percent.

Hematoma. A swelling from a collection of blood in the subcutaneous tissue.

Hemoconcentration. An increase in the number of red blood cells compared to plasma volume.

Hemoglobin. The iron-containing portion of red blood cells responsible for the transportation of oxygen to body cells.

Hemorrhagic disease of newborn. Hemorrhage in the newborn caused by inadequate level of vitamin K.

Hemorrhoid. A distended vein near the anus. May be internal (not evident) or external (evident).

Hereditary. Capable of being passed from one generation to the next through genes.

Herpes genitalis. An infection manifested as a lesion of grouped minute vesicles transmitted by the herpes II virus; a sexually transmitted disease.

Heterozygous. Possessing two different genes for a character trait.

Hirschsprung's disease. A congenital disorder in which there is absence of ganglion cells in the submucosal portion of the colon just proximal to the rectum. Leads to constipation and possible abdominal obstruction.

Homan's sign. Pain in the calf of the leg on dorsiflexion of the foot; an indication of a thrombophlebitis of a vein in the calf.

Homologue. A structure similar in origin to another.

Homosexual. An individual whose sexual relations are with those of his or her own sex.

Homozygous. Possessing two like genes for a character trait.

Hormone. A substance produced by one organ to cause an effect in other.

Human chorionic gonadotropin (HCG). A hormone produced by the chorionic villi to ensure continued function of the corpus luteum; used as the basis for pregnancy testing.

Human placental lactogen (HPL). See Chorionic somatomammotropin.

Hyaline membrane disease. See Respiratory distress syndrome (RDS).

Hydatidiform mole. Abnormal growth or proliferation of the trophoblast cells. No fetus forms and clear fluid-filled grape-like vesicles form in place of the placenta.

Hydramnios. An excessive amount of amniotic fluid (generally over 2,000 ml).

Hydrocele. A collection of fluid in the sac surrounding the testis.

Hydrocephalus. An abnormally enlarged head size due to accumulated cerebral spinal fluid distending the cerebral ventricles.

Hydrops fetalis. An older name for erythroblastosis fetalis.

Hymen. A thin fold of mucous membrane that partially covers the vaginal orifice. Obliterated with first sexual intercourse or often by physical exercise or prior pelvic examination.

Hymenal tag. Swollen hymen tissue apparent in females at birth due to maternal hormone influence.

Hyperbilirubinemia. Excessive bilirubin in the blood.

Hypercapnia. Increased carbon dioxide level in the blood.

Hyperemesis gravidarum. Extreme vomiting during pregnancy or vomiting beyond the third month of pregnancy.

Hyperplasia. Increase in the size of cells to increase the size of an organ.

Hypertelorism. Excessive width between the eyes.

Hypertrophy. An increase in size.

Hyperventilation. Rapid shallow breathing that leads to excessive loss of carbon dioxide; symptoms include dizziness, confusion, and numbness of extremities.

Hypofibrinogenemia. A decrease in the level of fibrinogen in the bloodstream.

Hypogalactia. A reduced amount of milk flow.

Hypophysis. The pituitary gland.

Hypoplasia. Decrease in the size of cells to decrease the size of an organ.

Hypospadias. Opening of the urethra on the ventral surface of the penis.

Hypovolemic shock. A decrease in the volume of circulating blood leading to lowered blood pressure and rapid pulse rate.

Hypoxemia. Decreased level of oxygen in circulating blood.

Hypoxia. Decreased level of oxygen in body cells.

Hysterectomy. Surgical removal of the uterus.

Hysterosalpingography. X-ray of the uterus and fallopian tubes after the instillation of a contrast dye through the vagina to outline the structures; a test for patency.

Hysterotomy. A surgical incision into the uterus.

Iatrogen. A stimulus by a health care provider that causes initial or increased problems for a patient.

Iatrogenic. A condition caused by a health care provider or health care environment.

IDM. Abbreviation for infant of diabetic mother.

Ilium. The upper flared portion of the innominate bone.

Imperforate anus. Congenital closure of the anus not allowing meconium to pass.

Imperforate hymen. A hymen that completely covers and obstructs the vaginal opening not allowing for menstrual flow.

Implantation. Nidation; the attachment of the zygote to the uterine endometrium.

Impotence. Inability of the male to achieve or maintain an erection.

Inborn error of metabolism. A hereditary deficiency of an enzyme needed for metabolism.

Incompetent cervix. A defect of the cervix that makes it unable to remain closed through pregnancy; premature delivery occurs at about 20 weeks.

Induction of labor. Using a stimulus to cause labor to begin.

Inertia. A halt in activity; used to describe inactivity of uterine contractions.

Infant. A child from birth to 1 year of age.

Infant mortality rate. The number of infant deaths during the first year of life per 1,000 live births.

Infertility. The state of being unable to reproduce; sterile.

Infundibulopelvic ligament. The outer portion of the broad ligament that extends from the ovarian end of the fallopian tube to the pelvic wall. Also termed the *suspensory ligament.*

Infundibulum. The funnel-shaped portion of the fallopian tube.

Inlet. The upper brim of the pelvic cavity.

Innominate bones. The two large bones on the sides of the pelvis; join in front to form the pubic arch.

Inspection. Assessment by visual observation.

Intensity. The strength of a uterine contraction.

Internal genitalia. The uterus, fallopian tubes, and ovaries in the female; the testes, urethra, and prostate gland in the male.

Internal os. The junction of the cervical canal with the uterine isthmus.

Internal rotation. Turning of widest diameter of the fetal head from the transverse aspect in which it entered the pelvic inlet to the anterioposterior aspect of the pelvic outlet. Follows descent.

Interphase. The stage of cell division during which DNA replication occurs.

Introitus. The external opening of the vagina.

Interstitial. The portion of the fallopian tube adjoining the uterine body.

Intervillous space. An open space in the placenta in which maternal blood collects for exchange of nutrients with the placental villi.

Intrapartum. The period during labor and delivery.

Intrathecal. The space beneath the arachnoid membrane of the spinal cord.

Intrauterine device (IUD). A contraceptive device inserted into the uterine cavity.

Intrauterine growth retardation (IUGR). An infant born with a weight below normal due to an adverse environment.

Introitus. The external opening to the vagina.

In utero. Inside the uterus.

Inversion. To turn inside out.

In vitro fertilization. Fertilization outside the uterine body by extraction of the oocyte by laparoscopy and union with the sperm under laboratory conditions.

Involution. A retrograde process of regaining a previous state.

Ischial spines. The bony prominences on the sides of the ischium at the midlevel of the true pelvis. Serve as landmarks for engagement.

Ischium. The lower portion of the innominate bone at the side of the pelvis.

IUD. Abbreviation for intrauterine device.

IUGR. Abbreviation for intrauterine growth retardation.

Jaundice. A yellow color of the skin or mucous membrane. Caused by an increase in bilirubin.

Karyotype. A display of the number, size, and shape of chromosomes of a representative body cell.

Kegal's exercises. Exercises used to improve the tone of perineal muscles. The perineal muscles are alternately contracted and then relaxed.

Kernicterus. Accumulation of indirect bilirubin in brain cells causing cell destruction.

Klinefelter's syndrome. A chromosomal abnormality caused by the presence of an extra X chromosome in a male (an XXY pattern).

Labia majora. The outermost folds of skin that form the sides of the female vulva.

Labia minora. The inner folds of skin on the sides of the female vulva.

Labor. The mechanism by which the fetus and accompanying structures are expelled from the uterus and vagina; parturition.

Laceration. A tear in tissue of the perineum as a result of childbirth.

Lactation. The production of and secretion of milk from the mammary glands; also the time of milk secretion.

Lactiferous ducts. The tubules that transport secreted milk from the glands to the nipple of the breast.

Lactosuria. Lactose in the urine.

Lamaze method. A method of preparation for childbirth based on conditioned reflexes. Developed by Fernand Lamaze in France; also termed the *psychoprophylactic technique.*

Lambdoidal. The suture between the occipital and two parietal bones.

Lanugo. The fine, downy hair formed on the shoulders and back of the fetus.

Laparoscope. An instrument introduced through a small abdominal surgical incision for visual examination of the abdominal cavity.

Laparoscopy. Examination of the abdominal cavity using a laparoscope.

Laparotomy. A surgical incision into the abdominal cavity.

Large for gestational age (LGA). A fetus or newborn whose growth is excessive in relation to the in-utero time period.

Latex agglutination test (Gravindex or pregnosticon slide test). A pregnancy test.

Lay midwife. A person who gives care during the prenatal, labor and delivery, and postpartal periods but who is not also a nurse.

Leopold's maneuvers. A series of steps of abdominal palpation to determine fetal presentation and position.

Let-down reflex. A reflex initiated by an infant's suckling that releases oxytocin from the posterior pituitary, contracts the myoepithelial cells surrounding milk glands, and brings hindmilk forward to the nipple.

Letting-go phase. Rubin's last stage of postpartal adjustment during which the mother redefines her new role as a mother.

Leukocytosis. An increase in the number of white blood cells.

Leukopenia. A decreased number of white blood cells.

Leukorrhea. A whitish vaginal discharge.

Levator ani muscle. The large muscle that rises from the pelvic surface of the ischial spines and inserts at the midpoint of the perineum, anococcygeal area, and coccyx.

Leydig's cells. The cells of the testes that secrete the male hormone testosterone.

LGA. Abbreviation for large for gestational age.

LH. Abbreviation for luteinizing hormone.

Lie. The relationship between the long axis of the mother and the long axis of the fetus.

Ligation. The action of tying closed.

Lightening. Descent of the fetus into the pelvis at about 2 weeks prior to delivery; also engagement.

Linea nigra. A line of brown pigment that extends from the umbilicus to the pubis during pregnancy.

Linea terminalis. An imaginary line that separates the true from the false pelvis.

Liquor amnii. The fluid contained within the fetal membranes. Also amniotic fluid.

Lithotomy position. An examining or delivery position with the patient lying supine; knees are flexed and heels are elevated in stirrups.

Lochia. The vaginal discharge during the postpartal period that is a sloughing of the uterine decidua.
Lochia alba. A whitish vaginal discharge.
Lochia rubra. A vaginal discharge similar to a menstrual flow.
Lochia serosa. A pinkish or brown vaginal discharge.

LMP. Abbreviation for last menstrual period.

L/S ratio. The ratio of the two component factors of surfactant, lecithin and sphingomyelin, to each other. Relationship is used to establish fetal lung maturity.

Lunar month. A 28-day month derived from the phase of the moon. Length of pregnancy is estimated in lunar rather than calendar months.

Luteal phase. The second half of a menstrual cycle.

Luteinizing hormone (LH). A gonadotrophic hormone secreted by the anterior pituitary gland that stimulates ovulation in the female, and the cells of the testes to secrete testosterone in the male.

Mammary glands. The breasts.

Mask of pregnancy. See Chloasma.

Mastalgia. Pain or tenderness of the breast.

Mastectomy. Surgical removal of the breast.

Mastitis. Inflammation of breast tissue.

Masturbation. Self-stimulation of genitals.

Maturation. Coming of age or adulthood.

Maternal attachment. The unique bonding that occurs between a mother and child.

Maternal mortality. The death of a woman during pregnancy, childbirth, or the postpartal period as a direct result of gestation.

Maternal mortality rate. The number of maternal deaths per 100,000 live births.

Meatus. The external opening of the urethra.

Meconium. The first stool of the newborn, dark green or black in color.

Meiosis. A process whereby a cell divides and reduces its chromosome number by half; reduction cell division.

Menarche. The first menstrual period.

Meningomyelocele. A midline neural tube defect in which the spinal cord and meninges herniate through a defect in the vertebrae.

Menopause. The time at which menstruation ceases; change of life.

Menorrhagia. An excessively profuse menstrual flow.

Menses. The periodic monthly flow of blood from the uterus.

Menstruation. The cyclic discharge of vaginal bleeding due to hormonal influences.

Menstrual cycle. The time interval from the beginning of one menstrual flow to the next.

Menstrual aspiration. The removal of the endometrial lining of the uterus by suction following a missed menstrual flow.

Menstrual phase. The phase of a menstrual cycle during which the endometrium sloughs and the vaginal flow occurs.

Mentum. The chin.

Mesoderm. One of the layers of primary germ cell tissue in the embryo.

Mesonephric duct (wolffian duct). The undifferentiated embryonic structure that matures to become the male vas deferens.

Metrorrhagia. Vaginal bleeding between normal menstrual cycles.

Microcephaly. A head circumference smaller than normal.

Midwife. A person who assists a woman at the time of birth.

Migration. The passage of the ovum from the ovary to the uterus.

Milia. Minute, white papules commonly found on the nose and cheeks of neonates; unopened sebaceous glands.

Miscarriage. Lay term for abortion.

Mitosis. A type of cell division in which the new cell contains the same number of chromosomes as the original cell. Daughter cell division.

Molding. Shaping of the fetal head to accommodate the shape of the birth canal.

Mongolian spot. A slate gray area of pigment on the skin of the neonate.

Moniliasis. An infection caused by the *Candida albicans* organism. Termed thrush when it occurs in the mouth.

Monosomy. A chromosome pattern in which only one chromosome of a pair is present.

Monzygotic. Derived from one zygote.

Mons veneris. The pubic or area of pubic hair.

Montgomery's tubercles. The small nodular glands on the areolae surrounding the nipples.

Morbidity. Illness.

Morning sickness. The nausea and vomiting that normally occur during the first 3 months of pregnancy.

Moro reflex. A neurologic reflex in newborns manifested by sudden abduction and then adduction of arms and legs.

Mortality. The incidence of deaths in relation to a specific population.

Morula. The developing blastomere structure as it multiplies rapidly and forms a bumpy surface.

Mottling. Discoloration of the skin in response to chilling or poor oxygen perfusion.

Mucous plug. A collection of thickened mucus that blocks the cervical canal during pregnancy; also operculum.

Müllerian duct. The undifferentiated embryonic structure that matures to form the female reproductive organs.

Multigravida. A woman who is having or has had more than one pregnancy.

Multiple pregnancy. A pregnancy with one or more fetus in utero.

Multipara. A woman who has delivered more than one child who was live at birth.

Mutation. The occurrence of the formation of an individual with a diffrent genetic structure than could be predicted.

Myometrium. The muscle layer of the uterus.

Nägele's rule. A method of calculating the expected date for the birth of a child. Add 7 days and subtract 3 months from the date of the last menstrual period.

Natal. Referring to birth.

Natural childbirth. Childbirth for which the parents are prepared with knowledge of the birth process and techniques to aid in the control of pain during labor.

Navel. The umbilicus.

Neonatal. Pertaining to the newborn or the first 28 days of life.

Neonatal mortality rate. The number of deaths of infants in the first 28 days of life per 1,000 live births.

Neonate. An infant during the first 28 days of life.

Neurofibromatosis. A neurologic disorder marked by tumors that form along nerve pathways; the child characteristically has more than five café au lait spots present on the skin at birth.

Nevus. A mole; a sharply circumscribed pigmented area on the skin at birth.
Nevus cavernosus. A network of large venous channels in the deep subcutaneous tissue.
Nevus flammeus. A port-wine birthmark.
Nevus vasculosus. A strawberry-color birthmark; a red, raised network of subcutaneous venous connections.

Nidation. Implantation or attachment of the fertilized ovum to the endometrium.

Nondisjunction. Failure of two paired chromosomes to separate during cell division; leads to the trisomy disorders.

Nuclear family. A family consisting of only parents and children; lacks extended family members.

Nulligravida. A woman who has never been pregnant.

Nullipara. A woman who has never given birth.

Nurse-midwife. An R.N. with extended knowledge in care of the family during the prenatal, natal, and postnatal periods. Abbreviated as C.N.M. for certified nurse midwife.

Nystagmus. Involuntary oscillation of the eyeball; seen normally when a person looks laterally.

Obstetrics. The branch of medicine concerned with the care of women during pregnancy, childbirth, and the postpartal period.

Occiput. The posterior part of the skull.

Occipitobregmatic. An anterioposterior diameter of the fetal head from the junction of the coronal and sagittal sutures to the occiput.

OCT. Abbreviation for oxytocin challenge test.

The first movement of the fetus per-
◾e mother.

A lay term for a urine-based pregnancy

◾iation for Respiratory Distress Syn-

◾ trait that will not be expressed unless
◾gous genes for the trait are present.
◾turn to a position of flexion after being

◾erniation of the rectum into the poste-
◾ wall.
◾xamination.   Examination of the poste-
◾ the vagina by palpation of the wall
◾ rectum.
◾voluntary movement.
◾ormone secreted by the corpus luteum
◾ relaxation of the body joints to aid in

◾or.   Factor secreted by cells of the hy-
◾ that stimulates or inhibits pituitary en-
◾vity.
◾isk.   A woman is in jeopardy of having
◾iculty producing a well infant or main-
◾own health during pregnancy or child-

◾.   Urine remaining in the bladder after

◾tress syndrome (RDS).   A lung disorder
◾ infants caused by lack of surfactant se-
◾lveoli; alveoli collapse on expiration,
◾iration difficult each time.
◾See external rotation.
◾ Artificial respiration and cardiac mas-
◾re vital functions.
◾nta.   A placenta that fails to deliver.
◾raw up.
◾A uterus that is bent backward just
◾rvix.
◾oplasia.   The formation of fibrotic tis-
◾e lens of the eye causing blindness; oc-
◾ature infants from hyperoxemia.
◾A uterus that is tipped abnormally

◾protein component found on the red
◾ 85 percent of the population. Those
◾actor are Rh-negative.
◾d harsh sounds heard on auscultation
◾ in the upper airways; clears with

◾d.   A method of contraception based
◾ation of fertile periods each month.
◾d (RNA).   A basic component of ge-
◾l that serves as a messenger for the
◾netic information.
◾used to describe the softening of the
◾ior to labor.
◾er.   A technique used to control deliv-
◾d by lifting it upward and forward.
◾ postpartal care philosophy in which
◾ays in the mother's room rather than a

---

ir of the perineum.
sion into the perineum.
een the vagina and the

nbrane covering the in-
l walls and coating the

erted into the vagina to
apse.
ple spot caused by capil-

of an individual in rela-

mino acid.
essively inherited men-
o inability to metabolize

e of the foreskin of the

vein.
itis of the femoral vein.
tion of arms or legs.
crease plasma bilirubin

ent jaundice resulting
n of red blood cells in

uch beneath the skin at

the ear.
of oxytocin. Often re-

lketonuria.
lar structure that serves
en the mother and fetus
term is *afterbirth*.
adherence of the pla-
aking placental delivery

that is implanted in the
hat it touches or covers
ix.
with a short or flat an-

nce due to an excessive
of red blood cells.
st cavity causing a lung

fetus to change fetal lie

number of red blood
l.
n hand or foot.
ion of milk.
s.
f urine output.
arbitrary portion of the
of the mother's pelvis.
finding that definitely
ent.
rn that has remained
onal age in utero.

Postnatal. Occurring after birth.

Postpartal. Occurring after birth.

Precipitate delivery. Unusually rapid progression of labor and delivery; also used to denote a birth where no physician was in attendance.

Preeclampsia. The former name for pregnancy induced hypertension.

Pregnancy. The state of having a fetus in utero.

Pregnancy Induced Hypertension (PIH). A complication of pregnancy manifested by hypertension, edema, and albuminuria.

Premature infant. An infant who weighs 2,500 gm or less at birth or is less than 38 weeks' gestation age.

Prenatal. Prior to birth.

Prepuce. The skin that covers the glans of the penis in the male and the clitoris in the female.

Presentation. The lie of the fetus.

Presenting part. Designation of that part of the fetus which is presenting to the internal cervical os.

Presumptive signs of pregnancy. Findings that suggest but do not confirm that a pregnancy is present.

Preterm infant. An infant born before 38 weeks' gestation.

Primigravida. A woman who is having her first pregnancy.

Primipara. A woman who has given birth to one live-born child.

Primordial. Original or elemental in nature.

Probable signs of pregnancy. Findings that suggest but do not confirm that a pregnancy is present.

Prodromal. Expectant period, or the period during which a disease is infectious before clinical symptoms appear.

Progesterone. A hormone secreted by the corpus luteum. Prepares and maintains the endometrium for the growth of the fertilized ovum. Produced by the placenta during pregnancy.

Prolactin. A hormone produced by the anterior pituitary gland that stimulates milk production in the mammary glands.

Prolapsed cord. An umbilical cord that precedes the fetus in delivery.

Prophylactic. A preventive measure; also a male contraceptive device.

Proteinuria. Protein in the urine.

Pseudocyesis. A psychological condition in which a woman believes she is pregnant when she is not.

Psychoprophylaxis. A method of prepared childbirth; also the Lamaze method.

Puberty. The stage of development at which the reproductive organs mature.

Pudendal block. Injection of an anesthetic agent into the perineum to achieve anesthesia of the pudendal nerve.

Pudendum. The external genital parts.

Puerperal sepsis. Infection of the reproductive organs following childbirth due to organisms introduced at the time of childbirth.

Puerperium. The first 6 weeks following childbirth.

Pyelonephritis. Urinary tract infection extending to the pelvis of the kidney.

Quickening.
ceived by t

Rabbit test.
test.

RDS. Abbre
drome.

Recessive.
two homoz

Recoil. To
extended.

Rectocele.
rior vagina

Rectovaginal
rior wall
through the

Reflex. An i

Relaxin. A
that causes
childbirth.

Releasing fac
pothalamu
docrine acti

Reproductive
unusual dif
taining her
birth.

Residual urin
voiding.

Respiratory di
of immatur
cretion by
making ins

Restitution.

Resuscitation
sage to rest

Retained plac

Retract. To

Retroflexion.
above the c

Retrolental fib
sue behind
curs in imm

Retroversion.
backwards.

Rh factor. A
blood cell
without the

Rhonchi. Lo
from mucu
coughing.

Rhythm meth
on the calcu

Ribonucleic a
netic mater
transfer of g

Ripe. A term
cervix just p

Ritgen maneu
ery of the h

Rooming-in.
the neonate

separate nursery in order to encourage maternal-infant bonding.

Rooting reflex. A newborn reflex; infant turns head to the side where his or her cheek is touched.

Rotation. Turning. Delivery involves both internal and external maneuvers.

Round ligaments. Ligaments located on each side of the uterus that terminate in the upper portion of the labia majora and serve to anteriorly stabilize the uterus.

Rubella titer. The percentage of antibodies against rubella present in blood serum. A low titer suggests the woman would be susceptible to a rubella infection.

Rubin's test. A test to determine the patency of the fallopian tubes accomplished by introduction of carbon dioxide into the uterus through the vagina.

Rugae. Folds of tissue found on the scrotum and in the vagina that allow for expansion of tissue.

Sacroiliac. The joint between the sacrum and the ilium.

Sacrum. Five fused bones that form part of the posterior surface of the pelvic ring.

Saddle block. Low spinal anesthesia that anesthesizes those body surfaces that would touch a saddle.

Sagittal suture. The junction of the two parietal bones of the skull.

Salpingo-oophorectomy. The surgical removal of the fallopian tube and its accompanying ovary.

Scanzoni's maneuver. Rotation of the fetal head from a posterior to an anterior position using forceps.

Scaphoid. Slightly indented; used to describe abdominal contour in adults.

Scarf sign. A test of immaturity in newborns; accomplished by assessing position of elbow when arm is drawn across chest.

Schultze's placenta. A placenta that delivers with the fetal surface presenting.

Scrotum. The pouch that holds the male testes.

Seborrhea dermatitis. Cradle cap; greasy, salmon-colored scales that form on an infant's scalp.

Secondary sex characteristics. Those characteristics that accompany maturation of the reproductive tract such as pubic and axillary hair, voice changes, and breast changes.

Secondary areola. An increased area of pigment that forms surrounding the areola during pregnancy.

Secretory phase. The second phase of a menstrual cycle that begins with ovulation and ends with menstruation.

Second stage of labor. The phase of labor from complete dilatation of the cervix to expulsion of the fetus.

Secundines. Placental and fetal membranes.

Semen. The fluid that contains and transports sperm.

Seminal vesicle. A pouch adjoining the vas deferens that secretes part of the seminal fluid.

Seminiferous tubules. The coiled tubules of the testes that secrete testosterone and serve as storage for sperm.

Septa. A partition.

Sex chromatin. A Barr body.

Sex chromosomes. The X and Y chromosomes that are responsible for sex determination.

Sex-linked trait. A characteristic transmitted by genes on the X chromosome.

Sexual identification. The sexual gender that a person perceives him- or herself and feels satisfaction in being.

Show. A lay term for release of the cervical mucous plug at the beginning of labor.

Simian line. A single palmar crease associated with Down's syndrome.

Singleton. A pregnancy with a single fetus.

Skene's glands. Two glands located laterally to the female urethra; they secrete a clear mucus fluid.

Small for gestational age (SGA). A fetus whose weight is below the tenth percentile for weeks in utero.

Smegma. Cheese-like secretion produced under the prepuce of the clitoris and penis.

Souffle. A soft, blowing sound heard on auscultation caused by blood passing through vessels.

Spermatogenesis. The formation and maturation of spermatozoa.

Spermatozoa. The male gamate cell produced by the testes. Abbreviated as *sperm*.

Sphincter. A muscle that is capable of constricting or closing a passage.

Spina bifida occulta. A spinal defect where a posterior vertebral surface is absent. A term often used wrongly to denote herniation of spinal cord contents into the defect.

Square window. The angle formed at the wrist when a newborn's palm is flexed toward the forearm.

Station. The relationship of the presenting part of the fetus to the ischial spines.

Sterility. Inability to conceive or produce children.

Stillbirth. The birth of a dead infant.

Strabismus. Deviation of gaze due to neural or muscular involvement.

Striae gravidarum. Red marks that appear on the abdomen during pregnancy due to stretching of abdominal skin.

Subinvolution. Failure of the uterus to return to its nonpregnant size following childbirth.

Sucking reflex. Involuntary sucking in a newborn when an object touches his or her lips.

Supernumerary nipples. Additional nipples formed along mammary lines.

Surfactant. A lipoprotein secreted by the alveoli cells to reduce surface tension on expiration.

Suture. A fibrous connection between bones.

Symphysis pubis. The anterior joint of the pelvic ring.

Syndactyly. Webbing or joining of fingers or toes.

Syphilis. A sexually transmitted disease caused by the *Treponema pallidum* organism.

Tachycardia. Rapid heart rate.

Tachypnea. Rapid respirations.

Taking-hold phase. The second phase of postpartal adjustment in which the mother begins to take an active role in child care.

Taking-in phase. The first phase of postpartal adjustment in which the mother is chiefly interested in her own care.

Talipes equinovarus. Congenital deformity of the foot.

Teratogen. An agent capable of causing abnormality in a fetus.

Term infant. An infant born at 38 to 42 weeks of gestational age.

Testis. A male gonad.

Testosterone. A steroid hormone secreted by the Leydig cells of the male testes.

Theca cells. Cells of the ovarian follicle that secrete estrogen.

Thermal neutral environment. An environment that provides for optimum newborn temperature regulation without excessive expenditure of energy.

Thrombophlebitis. Inflammation of a vein with accompanying thrombus formation.

Tonic neck reflex. A newborn reflex; in an infant lying supine, when he turns the head to the right, right arm and leg extend, left arm and leg contract. When head turns left, the opposite happens.

Toxemia. Older term for hypertension of pregnancy.

Tracheoesophageal fistula. A congenital defect in which there is an abnormal connection between the trachea and esophagus.

Transient tachypnea of the newborn (TTN). Increased respiratory rate in newborns probably due to poor absorption of lung fluid.

Transition. The period of time just prior to the second stage of labor.

Translocation. Abnormal placement of chromosomal material.

Trichomoniasis. A vaginal infection from *Trichomonas vaginalis.*

Trimester A 3-month period.

Trisomy. A chromosomal defect in which there are three rather than two matched chromosomes.

Trophoblast. The outer layer of cells of the blastocyst that will become the placenta.

Ultrasonography. A study made by high frequency sound waves.

Umbilical cord. The structure composed of two veins and one artery that connects the placenta to the fetus.

Umbilicus. The point at which the umbilical cord enters the fetal abdomen.

Urethritis. Inflammation of the urethra.

Uterine prolapse. Malposition of the uterus into the vagina.

Uterine souffle. A soft, blowing sound heard on auscultation that is produced by the flow of blood through the uterine vessels; rate is the same as the maternal pulse.

Uterus. The hollow muscular organ in which a fetus grows.

Vacuum curettage. See dilatation and evacuation.

Vacuum extraction. Delivery of a fetus by suction applied to the presenting part.

Vagina. The distensible structure that connects the uterine cervix with the perineum. Serves as the birth canal.

Varicose veins. Permanently distended veins of the legs or vulva.

Vas deferens. The tubular structure that carries spermatozoa from the semininferous tubules to the urethra.

Vasectomy. A surgical ligating of the vas deferens that results in male sterility.

Venereal disease. A sexually transmitted disease.

Venereal disease research laboratory test (VDRL). A laboratory test for the detection of syphilis.

Vernix caseosa. The cheese-like covering of the fetus to protect it from water maceration.

Version. To turn a fetus into a more favorable position for delivery.

Vertex. The crown of the head.

Vestibule. The portion of the female vulva between the labia minora in which the urinary meatus and vagina are located.

Viable. Capable of living outside the uterus.

Vulva. Female external genitalia.

Vulvectomy. Surgical excision of the vulva.

Wharton's jelly. The gelatinous substance that gives bulk to the umbilical cord.

White's classification. A system for classifying women with diabetes who are pregnant according to the severity of their illness.

Witch's milk. The thin, white discharge from breasts of newborns due to maternal hormone stimulation.

Wolffian duct. The duct that differentiates to become the male organs of reproduction; the mesonephric duct.

Womb. A lay term for uterus.

Zona pellucida. A layer of fluid that surrounds the ovum at ovulation.

Zygote. A fertilized ovum.

Index